CONNECT CORE CONCEPTS IN HEALTH

SEVENTEENTH EDITION

Claire E. Insel
*California Institute of
Human Nutrition*

Walton T. Roth
Stanford University

Paul M. Insel
Stanford University

Mc
Graw
Hill

CONNECT CORE CONCEPTS IN HEALTH, SEVENTEENTH EDITION

1 2 3 4 5 6 7 8 9 LWI 24 23 22 21

ISBN   978-1-264-14911-7 (bound edition)
MHID 1-264-14911-5 (bound edition)
ISBN   978-1-264-14465-5 (loose-leaf edition)
MHID 1-264-14465-2 (loose-leaf edition)

Portfolio Manager: *Erika Lo*
Product Development Manager: *Dawn Groundwater*
Product Developer: *Kirstan Price*
Senior Marketing Manager: *Meredith Leo DiGiano*
Content Project Managers: *Mary E. Powers (Core), Vanessa McClune (Assessment)*
Buyer: *Laura Fuller*
Designer: *David W. Hash*
Content Licensing Specialist: *Jacob Sullivan*
Cover Image: *FatCamera/Getty Images*
Compositor: *Aptara®, Inc.*

Library of Congress Cataloging-in-Publication Data

Names: Insel, Claire, author. | Roth, Walton T., author. | Insel, Paul M., author.
Title: Connect core concepts in health : big / Claire E. Insel, California Institute of Human Nutrition, Walton T. Roth, Stanford University, Paul M. Insel, Stanford University.
Description: Seventeenth edition. | Dubuque : McGraw Hill Education, [2022] | Includes index.
Identifiers: LCCN 2020038734 (print) | LCCN 2020038735 (ebook) | ISBN 9781264149117 (hardcover) | ISBN 9781264144655 (spiral bound) | ISBN 9781264149124 (ebook) | ISBN 9781264149148 (ebook other)
Subjects: LCSH: Health.
Classification: LCC RA776 .C83 2022 (print) | LCC RA776 (ebook) | DDC 613–dc23
LC record available at https://lccn.loc.gov/2020038734
LC ebook record available at https://lccn.loc.gov/2020038735

BRIEF CONTENTS

CONTENTS

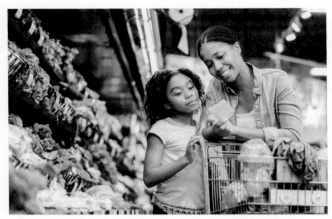

SDI Productions/E+/Getty Images

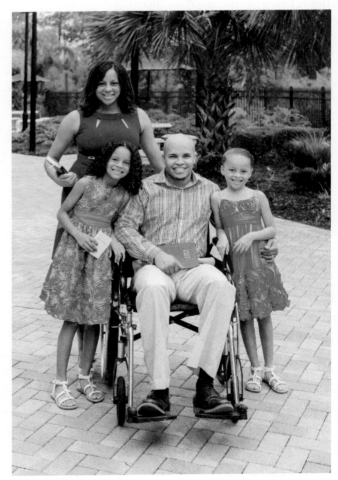

Lokibaho/Getty Images

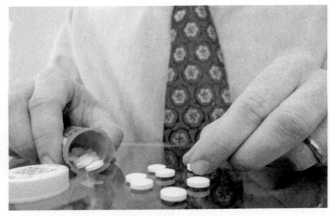
RBFried/iStock/Getty Images

PART THREE

SUBSTANCE USE DISORDERS: MAKING RESPONSIBLE DECISIONS

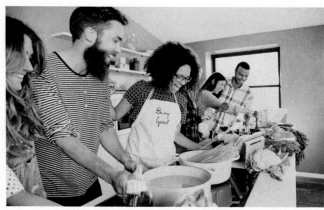
Flamingo Images/Shutterstock

PART FOUR

GETTING FIT

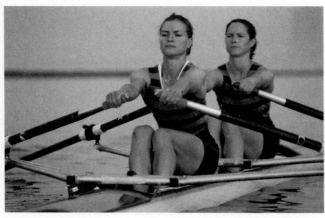

Dann Tardif/Getty Images

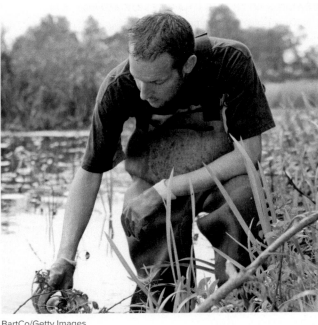
BartCo/Getty Images

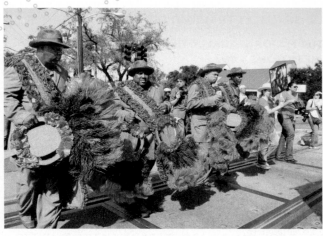

Ninette Maumus/Alamy Stock Photo

PROVEN, SCIENCE-BASED CONTENT

Now in its seventeenth edition, *Connect Core Concepts in Health* remains the leading health textbook in U.S. higher education. In 2020, *Connect Core Concepts in Health* won the Textbook and Academic Authors McGuffey Award for Excellence and Longevity. The book's unique psychological approach to mind-body health encourages students to take proactive self-assessments. Students can stay current on the latest studies while learning how to negotiate cross-cultural ideas of what it means to be healthy and how to live in our diverse, consumer-oriented society. McGraw Hill Education's digital and teaching learning tools also integrate *Connect Core Concepts in Health's* authoritative, science-based content.

Assess Yourself helps students analyze their own health and health-related behavior.

Take Charge challenges students to take meaningful action toward personal improvement.

Critical Consumer helps students navigate the numerous and diverse health-related products available on the market.

Diversity Matters introduces the many ways that cultural and gendered ideas of health come to influence our health strengths, risks, and behaviors.

Wellness on Campus focuses on health issues, challenges, and opportunities that students are likely to encounter on a regular basis.

Behavior Change Strategy offers specific behavior management/modification plans related to the chapter topic.

Ask Yourself: Questions for Critical Thinking and Reflection encourages critical reflection on students' own health-related behaviors.

Quick Stats updated for the seventeenth edition, focuses attention on particularly striking statistics related to the chapter content.

Tips for Today and the Future ends each chapter with a quick, bulleted list of concrete actions readers can take now and in the near future.

CONNECT IS PROVEN EFFECTIVE

McGraw Hill Connect

***McGraw Hill Education Connect*®** is a digital teaching and learning environment that improves performance over a variety of critical outcomes; it is easy to use and proven effective. Connect® empowers students by continually adapting to deliver precisely what they need, when they need it, and how they need it, so your class time is more engaging and effective. Connect for *Core Concepts in Health* offers a wealth of interactive online content, including health labs and self-assessments, video activities on timely health topics, and practice quizzes with immediate feedback.

PERSONALIZED LEARNING

McGraw Hill SMARTBOOK

Available within Connect, ***SmartBook 2.0*®** makes study time as productive and efficient as possible by identifying and closing knowledge gaps. SmartBook 2.0 identifies what an individual student knows and doesn't know based on the student's confidence level, responses to questions, and other factors. SmartBook 2.0 builds an optimal, personalized learning path for each student, so students spend less time on concepts they already understand and more time on those they don't. As a student engages with SmartBook 2.0, the reading experience continuously adapts by highlighting the most impactful content that person needs to learn at that moment. This ensures that every minute spent with SmartBook 2.0 is returned to the student as the most value-added minute possible. The result? More confidence, better grades, and greater success.

SmartBook 2.0 is now optimized for phones and tablets. Its interactive features are also accessible for students with disabilities Just like our new ebook and ReadAnywhere app, SmartBook 2.0 is available both online and offline.

Using Food Labels
1 — 2

WELLNESS WORKSHEET

Informed Food Choices

Be sure to complete all portions of the lab. There are two parts, appearing on two separate screens. Once you complete all content in a particular part, you will be able to navigate to the next screen using the navigation map at the top or bottom of the activity.

USING FOOD LABELS

Choose three food items to evaluate. You might want to select three similar items, such as regular, low-fat, and fat-free salad dressing, or three very different items. Record the information from their food labels in the table below.

To receive an initial score of complete, fill out all fields in the table. Enter a zero (0) in a field if a food does not contain a particular nutrient. Enter only whole numbers and decimals in the log. For example, enter a half gram of dietary fiber as 0.5, not 1/2.

Food Items			
Serving size			

Physical Responses to Stressors

Imagine a close call: As you step off the curb, a car careens toward you. With just a fraction of a second to spare, you leap safely out of harm's way. In that split second of danger and in the moments following it, you experience a predictable series of physical reactions. Your body goes from a relaxed state to one prepared for physical action to cope with a threat to your life.

Two systems in your body are responsible for your physical response to stressors: the nervous system and the endocrine system. Through rapid chemical reactions affecting almost every part of your body, you are primed to act quickly and appropriately in time of danger.

The Nervous System The **nervous system** consists of the brain, spinal cord, and nerves. Part of the nervous system is under voluntary control, as when you tell your arm to reach for a chocolate. The part that is *not* under conscious supervision—for example, the part that controls the digestion of the chocolate—is the **autonomic nervous system**. In addition to digestion, it controls your heart rate, breathing, blood pressure, and hundreds of other involuntary functions. The autonomic nervous system consists of two divisions:

- The **parasympathetic division** is in control when you are relaxed. It aids in digesting food, storing energy, and promoting growth.
- The **sympathetic division** is activated when your body is stimulated, for example, by exercise, and when there is an emergency, such as severe pain, anger, or fear.

- Perspiration increases to cool the skin.
- The brain releases **endorphins**—chemicals that inhibit or block sensations of pain—in case you injured.

As a group, these nearly instantaneous physio changes are called the **fight-or-flight reaction.** changes give you the heightened reflexes and streng

stress response The physical and emotional reactions to a stressor.

stress The general physical and emotional state that the stressor produces.

nervous system The brain, spinal cord, and nerves.

autonomic nervous system The part of the nervous system that controls certain basic body processes; consists the sympathetic and parasympathetic divisions.

parasympathetic division The part of the autonomic nervous system that moderates the excitatory effect of the sympathetic division, slowing metabolism and restoring en supplies.

sympathetic division Division of the autonomic nervous system that reacts to danger or other challenges by accele body processes.

endocrine system The system of glands, tissues, and that secrete hormones into the bloodstream to influence metabolism and other body processes.

hormone A chemical messenger produced in the body transported in the bloodstream to target cells or organs for specific regulation of their activities.

DIETARY ANALYSIS TOOL

NutritionCalc Plus is a suite of powerful dietary self-assessment tools that help students track their food intake and activity and analyze their diet and health goals. Students and instructors can trust the reliability of the ESHA database while interacting with a robust selection of reports. This tool is provided at no additional charge inside Connect Personal Health.

APPLICATION-BASED ACTIVITIES

New to this edition, Application-Based Activities help your students to assess their own health and behavior. Twelve new self-assessments and five new Portfolio Health Profiles include privacy controls to protect student data.

WRITING ASSIGNMENT

McGraw Hill's new Writing Assignment tool delivers a learning experience that improves students' written communication skills and conceptual understanding with every assignment. Assign, monitor, and provide feedback on writing more efficiently and grade assignments within McGraw Hill Connect®. Writing Assignment gives students an all-in-one place interface, so you can provide feedback more efficiently.

Features include:
- Saved and reusable comments (text and audio)
- Ability to link to resources in comments
- Rubric building and scoring
- Ability to assign draft and final deadline milestones
- Tablet ready and tools for all learners

CHAPTER-BY-CHAPTER CHANGES

The seventeenth edition focuses current events, health trends, and content changes informed by the COVID-19 pandemic.

Chapter 1: Taking Charge of Your Health
- A new figure illustrating how lifestyle choices correlate to overall health.
- Expanded discussion of how healthy habits relate to quality of life and reduced risk of death.
- New Diversity Matters feature about health inequality and the COVID-19 pandemic.
- Updated data about the leading causes of death among college-age Americans.
- Updated data about the top 10 health issues affecting college students' academic performance.
- Hot-off-the-press *Healthy People 2030* targets.

Chapter 2: Stress: The Constant Challenge
- Inclusion of the freeze response to describe physiological reactions to stress.
- Expanded discussion of the social stressors that impact girls and women more than men.
- Updated research about how social media can affect stress in young people.

Chapter 3: Psychological Health
- Updated language surrounding social anxiety disorder.
- New questions for reflection about digital technology, fear of missing out, and mental health.
- New discussion of the correlation between education about psychological symptoms and the number of college students who report seeking help for mental illness.

Chapter 4: Sleep
- New discussion of circadian rhythm variation among individuals.
- Revised content about circadian rhythm disruptions and their impact.
- Revised discussion of how the homeostatic sleep drive and the circadian system work together to regulate sleep.
- Revised explanation about how sleep quality and duration change across the life span.

Chapter 5: Intimate Relationships and Communication
- Expanded discussion of gender roles, culture, and their effects on individuals.
- New content about nonsexual intimate relationships, including peer relationships.
- Expanded discussion of premarital sex, sex education, and the average age of Americans' first sexual experiences.
- New content about how to recognize unhealthy relationships and how these standards have changed over time.
- Revised discussion of how social media and digital tools affect relationships, including a discussion of online bullying, stalking, and violations of privacy.
- New discussion of cultural norms for finding and choosing romantic partners, including the role of online dating.
- Updated examination of marriage, cohabitation, and the factors that influence these trends, including an expanded discussion of trends surrounding the decision to remain single.
- Revised discussion of how spousal and parent roles have changed over time. This includes an updated exploration of single parenthood and blended families.

Chapter 6: Sex and Your Body
- Updated discussion of intersex conditions, how doctors assign genders, and how intersex individuals make key choices about their sex and gender.
- Expanded explanations of consent have been added throughout the chapter to highlight this important topic.

Chapter 7: Contraception
- Revised Wellness on Campus feature about contraception use and pregnancy among college students.
- New figure with updated data about contraceptive effectiveness.
- Updated content about how attitudes about gender differences can influence contraception choices, including discussing options with a partner, sharing the costs of contraception, and policies to support contraceptive health care.
- Revised Diversity Matters box about barriers to contraceptive use.

Chapter 8: Abortion

- Updated discussion of the long-term mental health impact of having an abortion as opposed to being turned away.
- New figure illustrating access to abortion facilities in all 50 states.
- New coverage of policies that affect abortion in the United States, including refusal laws and state legislation that challenges *Roe v. Wade*.

Chapter 9: Pregnancy and Childbirth

- Discussion of fetal programming has been removed.
- Expanded discussion of first-trimester screening tests.

Chapter 10: Drug Use and Addiction

- Updated data on drug use among high school seniors, including vaping marijuana (newly added), smoking marijuana, and prescription painkillers. This includes new data about high school drug use and race/ethnicity.
- Revised content about gender differences in drug use, overdose deaths, and substance use disorder.
- Expanded discussion of how addiction works on a physiological level, including drug effects on neurotransmitters, receptors, and neurons.
- Revised discussion of the opioid epidemic, including updated data and the role of synthetic opioids.
- Revised discussion of use and abuse of stimulant ADHD medications.
- New content about the United Nations' findings about addiction as a public health issue. This includes the costs of treatment and drug-related incarceration and recommendations for addressing addiction.

Chapter 11: Alcohol: The Most Popular Drug

- Revised discussion of gender differences in alcohol use and alcohol's effects.
- Updated discussion of driving under the influence, including updated data and discussion questions.

Chapter 12: Tobacco Use

- Expanded discussion of e-cigarettes, including updated data, a new discussion of vaping THC and CBD products, and new recommendations from the Centers for Disease Control.
- New figure illustrating tobacco and e-cigarette use among high school and college students.
- Updated discussion of federal regulation of e-cigarettes and vaping products and devices.

Chapter 13: Nutrition Basics

- Updated material on the forthcoming *2020–2025 Dietary Guidelines for Americans*.

- Revised discussion of the risks and regulation of trans fats.
- New practical advice for how students can afford to eat healthier on a budget.
- Expanded discussion of plant-based products and meat alternatives, including those that mimic meat.

Chapter 14: Exercise for Health and Fitness

- Revised explanation of the physical activity pyramid to enhance clarity.
- Updated material based on the recently released second edition of the U.S. Department of Health and Human Services's *Physical Activity Guidelines for Americans*.

Chapter 15: Weight Management

- New section explaining the various models to describe individual differences in weight and the underlying factors that determine a person's weight, including genetics, body composition, hormones, culture, behavior, and the microbiome.
- Revised Wellness on Campus feature providing practical ways to change behavior for healthy weight management.
- New discussion of intermittent fasting as a weight loss strategy.
- Expanded discussion of how to assess safe and effective weight loss programs.
- Updated explanation of avoidant restrictive food intake disorder (ARFID), a new DSM-5 diagnosis (previously referred to as "selective eating disorder.")

Chapter 16: Cardiovascular Health

- New Take Charge box about using online health tools for cardiovascular health.
- Simplified atherosclerosis figure and technical language throughout the chapter.

Chapter 17: Cancer

- New explanation of CAR-T cell immunotherapy.
- Current numbers of cancer cases and deaths for groups of different genders, ages, and ethnicities.

Chapter 18: Immunity and Infection

- Updated discussion of 2019 measles outbreak, including the role of reduced vaccination rates and the long-term effects of measles.
- New section on the COVID-19 pandemic, including the virus's symptoms, epidemiology, and similarity to other coronaviruses. It also includes sections on the response of the global public health sector.
- New section on the prevention of COVID-19 and similar viruses, and the reasons behind COVID-19's quick spread and difficult treatment. This includes specific behaviors students can take in public and at

home to reduce their risk of infection and treat symptoms.

- Updated discussion of the risks of antibacterial soaps in generating drug-resistant bacteria.

Chapter 19: Sexually Transmitted Infections

- Extensive data updates about long-term trends in sexually transmitted infections.
- New Diversity Matters box about global disparities in cases of HIV/AIDS.
- Revised Wellness on Campus feature about the risks of a range of sexual behaviors, trends in STI contraction, and how to prevent infection.
- Updated discussions of treatment and diagnoses of HIV cases globally and in the United States.
- Revised feature about STI screening and prevention on college campuses, including strategies for protection.

Chapter 20: Environmental Health

- Updated discussion of the impact of climate change, including recent wildfires in California, Australia, and the Amazon rainforest.

Chapter 21: Conventional and Complementary Medicine

- New table showing common alternative mind-body therapies used in the United States.
- Updated statistics about the increased popularity of yoga and meditation in the United States.

Chapter 22: Personal Safety

- Updated content about preventing distracted driving and the digital tools available to support safe driving.

- Updated explanation of harassment, including strategies for better understanding what type of behavior and communication is appropriate.

Chapter 23: Aging: An Ongoing Process

- Revised discussion of data about gerontology and the study of aging.
- Revised content about the social effects of aging, including the impact of retirement, the death of a spouse, and divorce.
- Revised section about elderly people being vulnerable to crime.
- Reorganized and updated sections about hearing loss, arthritis, falls, sexual functioning, and cognitive changes.
- Revised discussion of the gender gap in life expectancy and differences in aging between men and women.
- Revised discussion of living and care options.

Chapter 24: Dying and Death

- Revised discussion of advance directives and specific tools for planning them.
- Updated discussion of organ donation, including how to register and what process is used for donating organs.
- Updated discussion of physician-assisted death, including legislation affecting death-with-dignity laws.

YOUR COURSE, YOUR WAY

McGraw Hill Education Create® is a self-service website that allows you to create customized course materials using McGraw Hill Education's comprehensive, cross-disciplinary content and digital products. You can even access third-party content such as readings, articles, cases, videos, and more.

- Select and arrange content to fit your course scope and sequence.
- Upload your own course materials.
- Select the best format for your students—print or eBook.
- Select and personalize your cover.
- Edit and update your materials as often as you'd like.

Experience how McGraw Hill Education's Create empowers you to teach your students your way: http://create.mheducation.com.

Remote Proctoring & Browser-Locking Capabilities

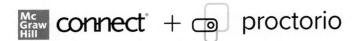

New remote proctoring and browser-locking capabilities, hosted by Proctorio within Connect, provide control of the assessment environment by enabling security options and verifying the identity of the student.

Seamlessly integrated within Connect, these services allow instructors to control students' assessment experience by restricting browser activity, recording students' activity, and verifying students are doing their own work.

Instant and detailed reporting gives instructors an at-a-glance view of potential academic integrity concerns, thereby avoiding personal bias and supporting evidence-based claims.

Campus

McGraw Hill Education Campus® is a groundbreaking service that puts world-class digital learning resources just a click away for all faculty and students. All faculty—whether or not they use a McGraw Hill title—can instantly browse, search, and access the entire library of McGraw Hill instructional resources and services, including eBooks, test banks, PowerPoint slides, animations, and learning objects—from any Learning Management System (LMS), at no additional cost to an institution. Users also have single sign-on access to McGraw Hill digital platforms, including Connect, Create, and Tegrity, a fully automated lecture caption solution.

INSTRUCTOR RESOURCES

Core Concepts in Health offers an array of instructor resources for the personal health course:

Instructor's manual. The instructor's manual provides a wide variety of tools and resources for presenting the course, including learning objectives and ideas for lectures and discussions.

Test bank. By increasing the rigor of the test bank development process, McGraw Hill has raised the bar for student assessment. Each question has been tagged for level of difficulty, Bloom's taxonomy, and topic coverage. Organized by chapter, the questions are designed to test factual, conceptual, and higher-order thinking.

Test Builder. New to this edition and available within Connect, Test Builder is a cloud-based tool that enables instructors to format tests that can be printed and administered within a Learning Management System. Test Builder offers a modern, streamlined interface for easy content configuration that matches course needs, without requiring a download.

Test Builder enables instructors to:

- Access all test bank content from a particular title
- Easily pinpoint the most relevant content through robust filtering options
- Manipulate the order of questions or scramble questions and/or answers
- Pin questions to a specific location within a test
- Determine your preferred treatment of algorithmic questions
- Choose the layout and spacing
- Add instructions and configure default settings

PowerPoint. The PowerPoint presentations highlight the key points of the chapter and include supporting visuals. All slides are WCAG compliant.

ACKNOWLEDGMENTS

We are grateful for the contributors and reviewers who provided feedback and suggestions for enhancing this seventeenth edition:

ACADEMIC CONTRIBUTORS

Anna Altshuler, MD, MPH
California Pacific Medical Center
Abortion

Melissa Bernstein, PhD, RD, LD, FAND
College of Health Professions and Chicago Medical School
Rosalind Franklin University of Medicine and Science
Nutrition Basics
Weight Management

Thomas D. Fahey, EdD
California State University—Chico
Exercise for Health and Fitness

Tanya Gupta, MD
Stanford University
Cancer

Nancy Kemp, MD, MA
Board Certified in Hospice and Palliative Medicine
Aging: An Ongoing Process
Dying and Death

Christine Labuski, PhD
Virginia Tech
Sex and Your Body

Candice McNeil, MD, MPH
Wake Forest University School of Medicine
Sexually Transmitted Infections

Carol Chapnick Mukhopadhyay, PhD
San Jose State University
Intimate Relationships and Communication

Michael Joshua Ostacher, MD, MPH, MMSc
Stanford University School of Medicine
Psychological Health

David Ouyang, MD
Stanford University School of Medicine
Cardiovascular Health

Johanna Rochester, PhD
ICF
Environmental Health
Personal Safety

Heidi Roth, MD
University of North Carolina—Chapel Hill
Sleep

Pir Rothenberg, PhD
California Institute of Human Nutrition
Contraception
Drug Use and Addiction

Marcia Seyler, MPhil
California Institute of Human Nutrition
Immunity and Infection

Jeroen Vanderhoeven, MD
Swedish Medical Center
Pregnancy and Childbirth

Estefânia de Vasconcellos Guimarães, PhD
Stress

ACADEMIC ADVISORS AND REVIEWERS

Phoebe Ajibade, North Carolina A&T State University
Jeremy Barnes, Southeast Missouri State University
Dipavali Bhaya, Bucks County Community College
Amanda Brace, Towson University
Bruce Ferguson, Taft College
Kathy Lyn Finley, Indiana University, Bloomington
Dave Opon, Joliet Junior College
Natascha Romeo, Wake Forest University
Karla Rues, Ozarks Technical Community College
Sharon Woodard, Wake Forest University

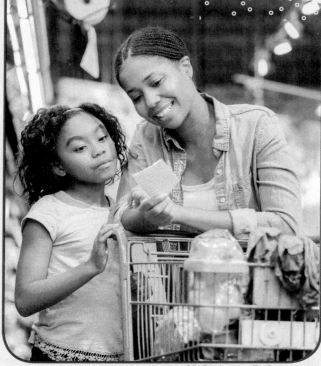
SDI Productions/E+/Getty Images

Taking Charge of Your Health

CHAPTER **1**

CHAPTER OBJECTIVES

- Define wellness as a health goal
- Explain two major efforts to promote national health
- Describe factors that influence wellness
- Explain methods for achieving wellness through lifestyle management
- List ways to promote lifelong wellness for yourself and your environment

TEST YOUR KNOWLEDGE

1. **Which of the following lifestyle factors influence wellness?**
   a. Managing your finances
   b. Cultivating a support group
   c. Exercising regularly

2. **The terms *health* and *wellness* mean the same thing.**
   True or False?

3. **What is the leading cause of death for college-age students?**
   a. Alcohol misuse
   b. Motor vehicle accidents
   c. Cancer

4. **A person's genetic makeup determines whether he or she will develop certain diseases (such as breast cancer), regardless of that person's health habits.**
   True or False?

ANSWERS

1. **ALL THREE.** All of these practices affect your sense of well-being.

2. **FALSE.** The term *health* refers to the overall condition of the body or mind and to the presence or absence of illness or injury. The term *wellness* refers to optimal health and vitality, encompassing the dimensions of well-being.

3. **B.** Motor vehicle accidents are the leading cause of death for people aged 15–24 years.

4. **FALSE.** In many cases, behavior can counter the effects of heredity or environment. For example, diabetes may run in families, but this disease is also associated with controllable factors, such as being overweight and inactive.

When was the last time you felt truly healthy? Not just free from illness, but energized, hungry, and flexible, like all your muscles just got a good stretching or workout? Many of us do not feel this way. We're overweight; we smoke; we eat a lot of sugar; we don't sleep well. We are surrounded by people who might be contagious, or we might be contagious.

The good news? There is always something we could be improving. This book can help you learn about the many aspects of life that work together to get you feeling on top of your game. Let's set some goals and make some changes!

WELLNESS AS A HEALTH GOAL

Generations of people have viewed good health simply as the absence of disease, and that view largely prevails today. The word **health** typically refers to the overall condition of a person's body or mind and to the presence or absence of illness or injury. **Wellness** expands this idea of good health to include living a rich, meaningful, and energetic life. Beyond the simple presence or absence of disease, wellness can refer to optimal health and vitality—to living life to its fullest. Although we use the words *health* and *wellness* interchangeably, they differ in two important ways:

• *Health*—or some aspects of it—can be determined or influenced by factors beyond your control, such as your genes, age, and family history. Consider, for example, a 50-year-old man with a family history of early heart disease. This factor increases his risk of having a heart attack at an earlier age than might be expected.

• *Wellness* is determined largely by the decisions you make about how you live. That same 50-year-old man can reduce his risk of an early heart attack by eating sensibly, exercising, and having regular screening tests. Even if he develops heart disease, he may still live a long, rich, meaningful life. To achieve wellness he should choose not only to care for himself physically but also to maintain a positive outlook, enjoy his relationships with others, challenge himself intellectually, and nurture other aspects of his life.

Wellness, therefore, involves conscious decisions that affect **risk factors** that contribute to disease or injury. We cannot control risk factors such as age and family history, but we can control lifestyle behaviors.

Dimensions of Wellness

The process of achieving wellness is continual and dynamic, involving change and growth. The encouraging aspect of

health The overall condition of body or mind and the presence or absence of illness or injury.

TERMS

wellness Optimal health and vitality, encompassing all the dimensions of well-being.

risk factor A condition that increases your chances of disease or injury.

wellness is that you can actively pursue it. Here are nine dimensions of wellness:

• Physical
• Emotional
• Intellectual
• Interpersonal
• Cultural

• Spiritual
• Environmental
• Financial
• Occupational

These dimensions are interrelated and may affect each other, as the following sections explain. Figure 1.1 lists specific qualities and behaviors associated with each dimension.

Physical Wellness Your physical wellness includes not just your body's overall condition and the absence of disease but also your fitness level and your ability to care for yourself. The higher your fitness level, the higher your level of physical wellness. Similarly, as you develop the ability to take care of your own physical needs, you ensure greater physical wellness. The decisions you make now, and the habits you develop over your lifetime, will determine the length and quality of your life.

Emotional Wellness Trust, self-confidence, optimism, satisfying relationships, and self-esteem are some of the qualities of emotional wellness. Emotional wellness is dynamic and involves the ups and downs of living. It fluctuates with your intellectual, physical, spiritual, cultural, and interpersonal health. Maintaining emotional wellness requires exploring thoughts and feelings. *Self-acceptance* is your personal satisfaction with yourself—it might exclude society's expectations—whereas *self-esteem* relates to the way you think others perceive you; *self-confidence* can be a part of both acceptance and esteem. Achieving emotional wellness means finding solutions to emotional problems, with professional help if necessary.

Intellectual Wellness Those who enjoy intellectual wellness constantly challenge their minds. An active mind is essential to wellness because it detects problems, finds solutions, and directs behavior. People with active minds often discover new things about themselves.

Interpersonal Wellness Satisfying and supportive relationships are important to physical and emotional wellness. Learning good communication skills, developing the capacity for intimacy, and cultivating a supportive network are all important to interpersonal (or social) wellness. Social wellness requires participating in and contributing to your community and to society.

Cultural Wellness Cultural wellness refers to the way you interact with others who are different from you in terms of ethnicity, religion, gender, sexual orientation, age, and customs. It involves creating relationships with others and suspending judgment of other's behavior until you have "walked in their shoes." It also includes accepting and valuing the different cultural ways people interact in the world. The extent to which you maintain and value cultural identities is one measure of cultural wellness.

PHYSICAL WELLNESS	EMOTIONAL WELLNESS	INTELLECTUAL WELLNESS
• Eating well • Exercising • Avoiding harmful habits • Practicing safer sex • Recognizing symptoms of disease • Getting regular checkups • Avoiding injuries	• Optimism • Trust • Self-esteem • Self-acceptance • Self-confidence • Ability to understand and accept one's feelings • Ability to share feelings with others	• Openness to new ideas • Capacity to question • Ability to think critically • Motivation to master new skills • Sense of humor • Creativity • Curiosity • Lifelong learning

INTERPERSONAL WELLNESS	CULTURAL WELLNESS	SPIRITUAL WELLNESS
• Communication skills • Capacity for intimacy • Ability to establish and maintain satisfying relationships • Ability to cultivate a support system of friends and family	• Creating relationships with those who are different from you • Maintaining and valuing your own cultural identity • Avoiding stereotyping based on race, ethnicity, gender, religion, or sexual orientation	• Capacity for love • Compassion • Forgiveness • Altruism • Joy and fulfillment • Caring for others • Sense of meaning and purpose • Sense of belonging to something greater than oneself

ENVIRONMENTAL WELLNESS	FINANCIAL WELLNESS	OCCUPATIONAL WELLNESS
• Having abundant, clean natural resources • Maintaining sustainable development • Recycling whenever possible • Reducing pollution and waste	• Having a basic understanding of how money works • Living within one's means • Avoiding debt, especially for unnecessary items • Saving for the future and for emergencies	• Enjoying what you do • Feeling valued by your manager • Building satisfying relationships with coworkers • Taking advantage of opportunities to learn and be challenged

FIGURE 1.1 **Qualities and behaviors associated with the dimensions of wellness.** Carefully review each dimension and consider your personal wellness strengths and weaknesses.

Spiritual Wellness To enjoy spiritual wellness is to possess a set of guiding beliefs, principles, or values that give meaning and purpose to your life, especially in difficult times. The spiritually well person focuses on the positive aspects of life and finds spirituality to be an antidote for negative feelings such as cynicism, anger, and pessimism. Organized religions help many people develop spiritual health. Religion, however, is not the only source or form of spiritual wellness. Many people find meaning and purpose in their lives through their loved ones or on their own—through nature, art, meditation, or good works.

Environmental Wellness Your environmental wellness is defined by the livability of your surroundings. Personal health depends on the health of the planet—from the safety of the food supply to the degree of violence in society. To improve your environmental wellness, you can learn about and protect yourself against hazards in your surroundings and work to make your world a cleaner and safer place.

Financial Wellness Financial wellness refers to your ability to live within your means and manage your money in a way that gives you peace of mind. It includes balancing your income and expenses, staying out of debt, saving for the future, and understanding your emotions about money. See the "Financial Wellness" box.

Occupational Wellness Occupational wellness refers to the level of happiness and fulfillment you gain through your work. Although high salaries and prestigious titles are gratify-

ing, they alone may not bring about occupational wellness. An occupationally well person enjoys his or her work, feels a connection with others in the workplace, and takes advantage of the opportunities to learn and be challenged. Another important aspect of occupational wellness is recognition from managers and colleagues. An ideal job draws on your interests and passions, as well as your vocational skills, and allows you to feel that you are making a contribution in your everyday work.

The Long and the Short of Life Expectancy

Can we control how long we will live, or is our life span determined by our genes? Studies suggest that our genes can determine up to 25% of the variability in life span. Some genes influence lifestyle factors, such as alcohol consumption and addiction. A new study found correlations among genes, behavior, and how long we might expect to live.

Researchers at the University of Edinburgh looked at the genomes of over 600,000 people in Europe, Australia, and North America and at their parents' life spans. They found that the strongest correlations between genes and mortality are susceptibility to coronary artery disease and modifiable behaviors such as cigarette smoking. Also correlated to a shorter life span are obesity, susceptibility to lung cancer, and insulin resistance. Greater longevity can happen for people who give up smoking, maintain their high-density lipoprotein cholesterol levels, attain more education, and cope well with stress.

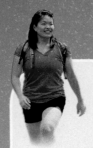

TAKE CHARGE
Financial Wellness

Many students feel less prepared to manage their money than to handle almost any other aspect of college life. Compared to a 2016 study on students' financial behaviors, an identical 2019 study reveals that fewer students reported paying bills on time, saving money, and avoiding spending money they don't have. Compared to college graduates and those who did not complete college, students were least likely to know their credit score; they also scored lower on tests about financial literacy and money management skills. *Financial wellness* means having a healthy relationship with money. Here are strategies for establishing that relationship:

Follow a Budget

A budget is a way of tracking where your money goes and making sure you're spending it on the things that are most important to you. To start one, list your monthly income and expenditures. If you aren't sure where you spend your money, track your expenses for a few weeks or a month. Then organize them into categories, such as housing, food, transportation, entertainment, services, personal care, clothes, books and school supplies, health care, credit card and loan payments, and miscellaneous. Knowing where your money goes is the first step in gaining control of it.

Now total your income and expenditures and examine your spending patterns. Use this information to set guidelines and goals for yourself. If your expenses exceed your income, identify ways to make some cuts.

Be Wary of Credit Cards

Students have easy access to credit but little training in finances. A little more than half of students use a credit card, with an average monthly balance of $1,183. Many pay credit card bills late, pay only the minimum amount, and have large total outstanding credit balances.

Shifting away from credit and toward debit cards is a good strategy for staying out of debt. More students now use mobile payment services like PayPal and Venmo, and the majority link their debit cards to it. Familiarity with financial terminology helps as well. Basic financial literacy with regard to credit cards involves understanding terms like *APR* (annual percentage rate—the interest you're charged on your balance), *credit limit* (the maximum amount you can borrow), *minimum monthly payment* (the smallest payment your creditor will accept each month), *grace period* (the number of days you have to pay your bill before interest or penalties are charged), and *over-the-limit* and *late fees* (the amounts you'll be charged if you go over your credit limit or your payment is late).

Manage Your Debt

One-fifth of students with a debt are behind on their payments. When it comes to student loans, having a direct, personal plan for repayment can save time and money, reduce stress, and help you prepare for the future. However, only about 10% of students surveyed feel they have all the information needed to pay off their loans. Work with your lender and make sure you know how to access your balance, when to start repayment, how to make payments, what your repayment plan options are, and what to do if you have trouble making payments. Information on managing federal student loans is available from https://studentaid.ed.gov/sa/.

If you have credit card debt, stop using your cards and start paying them off. If you can't pay the whole balance, try to pay more than the minimum payment each month. It can take a very long time to pay off a loan by making only the minimum payments. For example, paying off a credit card balance of $2000 at 10% interest with monthly payments of $20 would take 203 months—nearly 17 years. Check out an online credit card calculator like http://money.cnn.com/calculator/pf/debt-free/. If you carry a balance and incur finance charges, you are paying back much more than your initial loan.

Start Saving

If you start saving early, the same miracle of compound interest that locks you into years of credit card debt can work to your benefit (for an online compound interest calculator, visit http://www.interestcalc.org). Experts recommend "paying yourself first" every month—that is, putting some money into savings before you pay your bills. If you work for a company with a 401(k) retirement plan, contribute as much as you can every pay period.

Become Financially Literate

Most Americans have not received any basic financial training. For this reason, the U.S. government has established the Financial Literacy and Education Commission (http://MyMoney.gov) to help Americans learn how to save, invest, and manage money better. Developing lifelong financial skills should begin in early adulthood, as money-management experience appears to have a more direct effect on financial knowledge than does education. For example, when tested on their basic financial literacy, students who had checking accounts had higher scores than those who did not.

SOURCES: Smith, C., and G. A. Barboza. 2013. The role of trans-generational financial knowledge and self-reported financial literacy on borrowing practices and debt accumulation of college students. Social Science Research Network (http://ssrn.com/abstract=2342168); EverFi. 2016. *Money Matters on Campus: Examining Financial Attitudes and Behaviors of Two-Year and Four-Year College Students* (www.moneymattersoncampus.org); Sallie Mae and Ipsos Public Affairs. 2019. *Majoring in Money 2019.* (https://www.salliemae.com/assets/about/who_we_are/Majoring-In-Money-Report-2019.pdf).

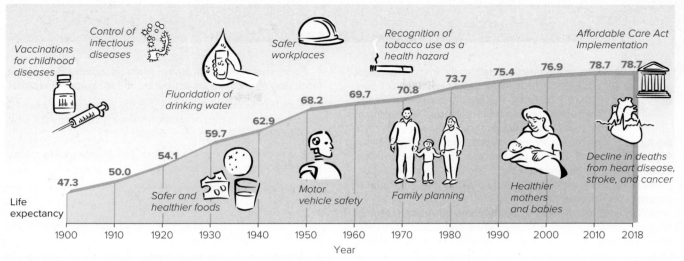

FIGURE 1.2 Public health, life expectancy, and quality of life. Public health achievements during the 20th century are credited with adding more than 25 years to life expectancy for Americans, greatly improving quality of life, and dramatically reducing deaths from infectious diseases. Public health improvements continue into the 21st century, including greater roadway safety and a steep decline in childhood lead poisoning. Between 2014 and 2017, U.S. life expectancy declined, likely due to the opioid and obesity epidemics. Life expectancy rose 0.1 year in 2018.

SOURCES: Centers for Disease Control and Prevention. 2011. Ten great public health achievements—United States, 2001–2010. *MMWR* 60(19): 619–623; Centers for Disease Control and Prevention. 1999. Ten great public health achievements—United States, 1900–1999. *MMWR* 48(50): 1141; Xu, J. Q., et al. 2020. Mortality in the United States, 2018. NCHS Data Brief, no 355. Hyattsville, MD: National Center for Health Statistic (https://www.cdc.gov/nchs/products/databriefs/db355.htm).

Why does education help us live longer? Consider smoking to understand the effect of education on life span. People with more education smoke less, so they have a lowered risk for lung cancer. For example, smoking a pack of cigarettes per day over 20 years reduces **life expectancy** by seven years. Each year spent in higher education correlates to an additional year of life.

Other factors, such as obesity and drug use, also strongly correlate to life span (Figure 1.2). The effect of obesity can be measured by cases of coronary artery disease. Except for smoking, no other modifiable risk factor contributes to a shorter life span than obesity. (See box "Life Expectancy and the Obesity Epidemic.")

In the United States, opioid use disorders stand out as a contributor to years of life lost. In 2018, there were over 67,000 drug-related deaths, two-thirds of which involved opioids.

In the early 20th century, **morbidity** and **mortality rates** (rates of illness and death, respectively) from common **infectious diseases** (e.g., pneumonia, tuberculosis, and diarrhea) were much higher than Americans experience today. By 1980, life expectancy had nearly doubled, due largely to the development of vaccines and antibiotics to fight infections and to public health measures such as water

purification and sewage treatment to improve living conditions. After over two decades of Americans' living increasingly longer, life expectancy declined between 2014 and 2017. This decline is generally attributed to drug overdose, suicide, and obesity. By 2018, suicide rates had continued to rise, but death rates from overdoses, cancer, accidents, and other diseases were lower, resulting in an increase in life expectancy. Regardless of the general rise in life expectancy, many would agree that it's the quality of our lives during those years that matters most. The major difference between life span (how long we live) and **health span** (how long we stay healthy) is freedom from chronic or disabling disease (Figure 1.3).

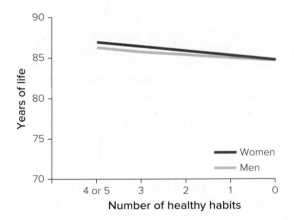

FIGURE 1.3 How long people at age 50 can expect to live if they don't develop cancer, CVD, or type 2 diabetes. Note that life expectancy increases with more healthy habits: not smoking, getting exercise, eating well, drinking alcohol in moderation, and maintaining a normal body weight.

SOURCE: Yanping, L., et al. 2020. Healthy lifestyle and life expectancy free of cancer, cardiovascular disease, and type 2 diabetes. *British Medical Journal* 368 (2020): l6669.

TERMS

life expectancy   The period of time a member of a given population is expected to live.

morbidity rate   The relative incidence of disease among a population.

mortality rate   The number of deaths in a population in a given period; usually expressed as a ratio, such as 75 deaths per 1000 members of the population.

infectious disease   A disease that can spread from person to person, caused by microorganisms such as bacteria and viruses.

health span   How long we stay healthy and free from chronic or disabling disease.

TAKE CHARGE
Life Expectancy and the Obesity Epidemic

Life expectancy consistently increased each decade in the United States since 1900 (see Figure 1.3). But the upward trend has reversed, and some researchers point to the significant increase in obesity among Americans as a potential cause. According to estimates released in 2020, about 42% of adults and 19% of children are obese. The problem isn't confined to the United States: The 2018 European Congress on Obesity estimates that by 2045, 22% of the global population will be obese.

Along with increases in obesity come increased rates of diabetes, chronic liver disease, heart disease, stroke, and other chronic diseases that are leading causes of death. Of course, medical interventions for these conditions have improved over time, lessening the impact of obesity to date. Still, medical treatments may be reaching their limits in preventing early deaths related to obesity. Moreover, people are becoming obese at earlier ages, exposing them to the adverse effects of excess body fat over a longer period of time. The magnitude of the obesity problem has brought predictions that an overall decline in life expectancy will take place in the United States by the mid-21st century.

What can be done? For an individual, body composition is influenced by a complex interplay of personal factors, including heredity, metabolic rate, hormones, age, and dietary and activity habits. But many outside forces—social, cultural, and economic—shape our behavior, and some experts recommend viewing obesity as a public health problem that requires an urgent and coordinated public health response. A response in health care technology such as gastric bypass surgery, medications, and early screening for obesity-related diseases has helped in the past, but if obesity trends persist, especially among children, average life spans may begin to decrease.

What actions might be taken? Suggestions from health promotion advocates include the following:

- Change food pricing to promote healthful options; for example, tax sugary beverages and offer incentives to farmers and food manufacturers to produce and market affordable healthy choices and smaller portion sizes.

- Limit advertising of unhealthy foods targeting children.

- Require daily physical education classes in schools.

- Fund strategies to promote physical activity by creating more walkable communities, parks, and recreational facilities.

- Train health professionals to provide nutrition and exercise counseling, and mandate health insurance coverage for treatment of obesity as a chronic condition.

- Promote the expansion of work site programs for improving diet and physical activity habits.

- Encourage increased public investment in obesity-related research.

In addition to indirectly supporting these actions, you can directly do the following:

- Analyze your own food choices, and make appropriate changes. Nutrition is discussed in detail in Chapter 13, but you can start by shifting away from consuming foods high in sugar and refined grains.

- Be more physically active. Take the stairs rather than the elevator, ride a bike instead of driving a car, and reduce your overall sedentary time.

- Educate yourself about current recommendations and areas of debate in nutrition.

- Speak out, vote, and become an advocate for healthy changes in your community.

See Chapters 13–15 for more on nutrition, exercise, and weight management.

SOURCES: Hales, C. M., et al. 2020. Prevalence of obesity and severe obesity among adults: United States, 2017–2018. NCHS Data Brief, No 360. Hyattsville, MD: National Center for Health Statistics (https://www.cdc.gov/nchs/data/databriefs/db360-h.pdf); Ludwig, D. S. 2016. Lifespan weighed down by diet. *JAMA* (published online April 4, 2016, DOI:10.1001/jama.2016.3829); Olshansky, S. J., et al. 2005. A potential decline in life expectancy in the United States in the 21st century. *New England Journal of Medicine* 352(11): 1138–1145; National Center for Health Statistics. 2016. *Health, United States, 2015: With Special Feature on Racial and Ethnic Health Disparities*. Hyattsville, MD: National Center for Health Statistics; International Food Policy Research Institute. 2016. *Global Nutrition Report 2016: From Promise to Impact: Ending Malnutrition by 2030*. Washington, DC: International Food Policy Research Institute; U.S. Department of Agriculture. 2015. *Scientific Report of the 2015 Dietary Guidelines Advisory Committee* (http://www.health.gov/dietaryguidelines/2015-scientific-report); Fottrell, Q. 2018. Almost a quarter of the world's population will be obese by 2045. MarketWatch.com, May 26.

Most Americans contend with some level of physical and cognitive impairment during the last 15% of our lives. Another important factor to quality of life is our level of happiness. An analysis of responses to the Health and Retirement Study yielded data from 11,964 older adults and found that happiness and cognitive impairment are not closely linked; we can expect to live substantially more years happy than cognitively impaired.

People also have some control over whether they develop **chronic diseases.** Table 1.1 and Figure 1.4 both show **lifestyle choices** that most affect the length and the quality of our lives. The numbers in Figure 1.4 give an idea that both

chronic disease A disease that develops and continues over a long period, such as heart disease, cancer, or diabetes.

lifestyle choice A conscious behavior that can increase or decrease a person's risk of disease or injury; such behaviors include smoking, exercising, and eating a healthful diet.

TERMS

Table 1.1 — Leading Causes of Death in the United States, 2018

RANK	CAUSE OF DEATH	NUMBER OF DEATHS	PERCENTAGE OF TOTAL DEATHS	LIFESTYLE FACTORS				
1	Heart disease	655,381	23.1	D	I	S	A	O
2	Malignant neoplasms (cancer)	599,274	21.1	D	I	S	A	O
3	Unintentional injuries (accidents)	167,127	5.9		I	S	A	
4	Chronic lower respiratory diseases	159,486	5.6			S		O
5	Cerebrovascular diseases (stroke)	147,810	5.2	D	I	S	A	O
6	Alzheimer's disease	122,019	4.3					
7	Diabetes mellitus	84,946	3.0	D	I	S		O
8	Influenza and pneumonia	59,120	2.1	D	I	S	A	
9	Kidney disease	51,386	1.8			S		O
10	Intentional self-harm (suicide)	48,344	1.7				A	
11	Chronic liver disease and cirrhosis	42,838	1.5				A	O
12	Septicemia (systemic blood infection)	40,718	1.4				A	
13	Hypertension (high blood pressure)	35,835	1.3	D	I	S	A	O
14	Parkinson's disease	33,829	1.2					
15	Lung inflammation due to solids and liquids	19,239	0.7				A	
	All other causes	571,853	20.1					
	All causes	2,839,205	100.0					

Key
D Diet plays a part.
I Inactive lifestyle plays a part.
S Smoking plays a part.
A Excessive alcohol use plays a part.
O Obesity is a contributing factor.

NOTE: The 2020 cause-of-death data will reflect the impact of the SARS-CoV-2 pandemic.

SOURCE: Xu, J., et al. 2020. Mortality in the United States, 2018. National Center for Health Statistics Data Brief No. 355 (https://www.cdc.gov/nchs/products/databriefs/db355.htm).

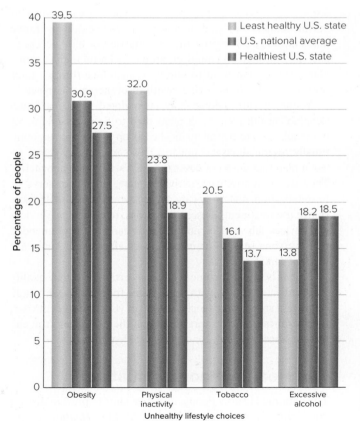

lifestyle choices and external circumstances—such as where we live and how easily we can access health care—influence our general health. Two of the most important contributors to health are obesity and smoking. Notice that obesity results from more than just physical inactivity—diet control is vital. The need to make good choices is especially true for teens and young adults. For Americans aged 15–24, for example, the leading cause of death is unintentional injuries (accidents), with the greatest number of deaths linked to car crashes, followed by drug overdose deaths (Table 1.2).

Sudden, large-scale outbreaks of infectious disease, such as the coronavirus that began in 2019, have the widespread feel of natural disasters but can be greatly affected by individual and joint, worldwide efforts to curb the tide.

FIGURE 1.4 **Key behaviors to avoid for a longer, healthier life.** America's Health Ranking reports assess the nation's health state by state, based on factors including behaviors, public policies, access to health care, poverty, education and environmental conditions. The poorer, less educated areas of the country also fare the worst.

SOURCE: United Health Foundation. 2020. *America's Health Rankings Annual Report, 2019.* (https://assets.americashealthrankings.org/app/uploads/ahr_2019annualreport.pdf).

Table 1.2	Leading Causes of Death among Americans Aged 15–24, 2018		
RANK	CAUSE OF DEATH	NUMBER OF DEATHS	PERCENTAGE OF TOTAL DEATHS
1	Unintentional injuries (accidents):	12,044	47.9
	Motor vehicle	6,308	25.1
	Unintentional poisoning (drug overdose)	4,245	17.0
	All other unintentional injuries	1,491	6.0
2	Suicide	6,211	25.0
3	Homicide	4,607	18.0
4	Cancer	1,371	5.5
5	Heart disease	905	3.5
	All causes	25,138	100.0

SOURCE: Centers for Disease Control and Prevention. 2020. Fatal Injury Data: Leading Causes of Death 1981–2018 (https://www.cdc.gov/injury/wisqars/index.html).

Ask Yourself

QUESTIONS FOR CRITICAL THINKING AND REFLECTION

How often do you feel exuberant? Vital? Joyful? What makes you feel that way? Conversely, how often do you feel downhearted, de-energized, or depressed? What makes you feel that way? Have you ever thought about how you might increase experiences of vitality and decrease experiences of discouragement?

PROMOTING NATIONAL HEALTH

Wellness is a personal concern, but the U.S. government has financial and humanitarian interests in it, too. A healthy population is the nation's source of vitality, creativity, and wealth. Poor health drains the nation's resources and raises health care costs for all. The primary **health promotion** strategies at the government and community levels are public health policies and agencies that identify and discourage unhealthy and high-risk behaviors and that encourage and provide incentives for positive health behaviors. At the federal level in the United States, the National Institutes of Health (NIH) and the Centers for Disease Control and Prevention (CDC) are charged with promoting the public's health. These and other agencies translate research results into interventions and communicate research findings to health care providers and the public. There are also health promotion agencies and programs at the state, community, workplace, and college levels. Take advantage of health promotion resources at all levels that are available to you.

Health Insurance Options

The Affordable Care Act (ACA), also called "Obamacare," was signed into law on March 23, 2010. It has remained in

health promotion The process of enabling people to increase control over their health and its determinants, and thereby improve their health.

effect under President Trump, but certain provisions have been altered. Health insurance costs will likely increase as a result.

Finding a Plan Under the ACA, health insurance marketplaces, also called health exchanges, facilitate the purchase of health insurance at the state level. The health exchanges provide a selection of government-regulated health care plans that students and others may choose from. Those who are below income requirements are eligible for federal help with the premiums. Many employers and universities also offer health insurance to their employees and students. Small businesses and members of certain associations may also be able to purchase insurance through membership in a professional group.

Benefits to College Students The ACA continues to permit students to stay on their parents' health insurance plans until age 26—even if they are married or have access to coverage through an employer. Students not on their parents' plans who do not want to purchase insurance through their schools can do so through a health insurance marketplace.

Young, healthy people may be tempted to buy a "catastrophic" health plan. Such plans tend to have low premiums but require you to pay all medical costs up to a certain amount, usually several thousand dollars. This can be risky if you select a plan that does not cover the ACA's 10 essential benefits. They are: preventive care, outpatient care, emergency services, hospitalization, maternity care, lab tests, mental health and substance use treatment, prescription drugs, rehabilitative services and devices, lab services, and pediatric care. It's recommended that everyone select a plan that covers all of these important types of care.

Students whose income is below a certain level may qualify for Medicaid. Check with your state. Individuals with non-immigrant status, which includes worker visas and student visas, qualify for insurance coverage through the exchanges. You can browse plans and apply for coverage at HealthCare.gov.

The Healthy People Initiative

The national Healthy People initiative aims to prevent disease and improve Americans' quality of life. *Healthy People*

Table 1.3	Healthy People 2030 Targets		
		BASELINE (% IN 2016–2018)	TARGET (% BY 2030)
Increase proportion of people with health insurance		89.0	92.1
Reduce proportion of adults with hypertension		29.5 (2013–2018)	27.7
Reduce proportion of obese adults		38.6 (2013–2016)	36.0
Reduce proportion of adults who engaged in binge drinking in past 30 days		26.6	25.4
Increase proportion of adults who meet federal guidelines for exercise		24.0	28.4
Reduce current use of any tobacco products by adults		20.1	16.2

SOURCE: U.S. Department of Health and Human Services. *Healthy People 2030* data search (https://health.gov/healthypeople).

reports, published each decade since 1980, set national health goals based on 10-year agendas. *Healthy People 2030* proposes the eventual achievement of the following broad national health objectives:

- Eliminate preventable disease, disability, injury, and premature death.
- Achieve health equity, eliminate disparities, and improve health literacy.
- Create social, economic, and physical environments that promote good health for all.
- Promote healthy development and healthy behaviors across every stage of life.
- Engage leadership and the public to design effective health policies.

This continues a trend set by *Healthy People 2020*. Both emphasize the importance of health determinants—factors that affect the health of individuals, demographic groups, or entire populations. Health determinants are social (including factors such as ethnicity, education level, or economic status) and environmental (including natural and human-made environments). Thus one goal is to improve living conditions in ways that reduce the impact of negative health determinants.

Examples of individual health-promotion goals from *Healthy People 2030* appear in Table 1.3.

Health Issues for Diverse Populations

We all need to exercise, eat well, manage stress, and cultivate positive relationships. We also need to protect ourselves from disease and injuries. But some of our differences—both as individuals and as members of groups—have important implications for wellness. These differences can be biological (determined genetically) or cultural (acquired as patterns of behavior through daily interactions with family, community, and society); many health conditions are a function of biology and culture combined.

Eliminating health disparities is a major focus of *Healthy People*. But not all health differences between groups are considered **health disparities,** which are those differences linked with social, economic, and/or environmental disadvantage. They affect groups who have systematically experienced greater obstacles to health based on characteristics that are historically linked to exclusion or discrimination. For example, the fact that women have a higher rate of breast cancer than men is a health *difference* but is not considered a disparity. In contrast, the higher death rates from breast cancer for black women compared with non-Hispanic white women is considered a health disparity.

You share patterns of influences with certain others, and information about those groups can help you identify areas that may be of concern to you and your family.

Sex and Gender   *Sex* refers to the biological and physiological characteristics that define men, women, and intersex people. In contrast, *gender* encompasses how people identify themselves and also the roles, behaviors, activities, and attributes that a given society considers appropriate for them. Examples of gender-related characteristics that affect wellness include the higher rates of smoking and drinking found among men and the lower earnings found among women (compared with men doing similar work). Although men are more biologically likely than women to suffer from certain diseases (a sex issue), men are less likely to visit their physicians for regular exams (a gender issue). Men have higher rates of death from injuries, suicide, and homicide, whereas women are at greater risk for Alzheimer's disease and depression. On average, men and women also differ in body composition and certain aspects of physical performance.

Race and Ethnicity   Among America's racial and ethnic groups, striking disparities exist in health status, access to and quality of health care, and life expectancy. However, measuring the relationships between ethnic or racial backgrounds and health issues is complicated for several reasons. First, separating the effects of race and ethnicity from socioeconomic status is difficult. In some studies, controlling for social conditions reduces health disparities. For example, a study from the Exploring Health Disparities in Integrated

health disparity   A health difference linked to social, economic, or environmental disadvantage that adversely affects a group of people.

TERMS

Communities project found that in a racially integrated community where blacks and whites had the same earnings, disparities were eliminated or reduced in the areas of hypertension, female obesity, and diabetes.

In other studies, even when patients shared equal status in terms of education and income, insurance coverage, and clinical need, disparities in care persisted. For example, compared with non-Hispanic whites, blacks and Hispanics are less likely to get appropriate medication for heart conditions or to have coronary artery bypass surgery; they are also less likely to receive kidney transplants or dialysis.

Second, the classification of race (a social construct) itself is complex. How are participants in medical studies classified? Sometimes participants choose their own identities; sometimes the physician/researcher assigns identities; sometimes both parties are involved in the classification; and sometimes participants and researchers may disagree.

Despite these limitations, it is still useful to identify and track health risks among population groups. Some diseases are concentrated in certain gene pools, the result of each ethnic group's relatively distinct history. Sickle-cell disease, for example, is most common among people of African ancestry. Tay-Sachs disease tends to afflict people of Eastern European Jewish heritage and French Canadian heritage. Cystic fibrosis is more common among Northern Europeans.

In addition to biological differences, many cultural differences occur along ethnic lines. Ethnic groups vary in their traditional diets; the fabric of their family and interpersonal relationships; their attitudes toward tobacco, alcohol, and other drugs; and their health beliefs and practices. All these factors have implications for wellness.

In tracking health status, the federal government collects data on what it defines as five race groups (African American/black, American Indian or Alaska Native, Asian American, Native Hawaiian or Other Pacific Islander, and European American/white) as well as two categories of ethnicity (Hispanic or Latino; not Hispanic or Latino); Hispanics may identify as being of any race group.

• *African Americans* have the same leading causes of death as the general population, but they have a higher infant mortality rate and lower rates of suicide and osteoporosis. Health issues of special concern for African Americans include high blood pressure, stroke, diabetes, asthma, and obesity. African American men are at significantly higher risk of prostate cancer than men in other groups.

• *American Indians and Alaska Natives* typically embrace a tribal identity, such as Sioux, Navaho, or Hopi. American Indians and Alaska Natives have lower death rates from heart disease, stroke, and cancer than the general population, but they have higher rates of early death from causes linked to smoking and alcohol use, including injuries and cirrhosis. Diabetes is a special concern for many groups.

• *Asian Americans* include people who trace their ancestry to countries in the Far East, Southeast Asia, or the Indian subcontinent. Asian Americans have lower rates of coronary heart disease and obesity. However, health differences exist among these groups. For example, Southeast Asian American men have higher rates of smoking and lung cancer, and Vietnamese American women have higher rates of cervical cancer.

• *Native Hawaiian and Other Pacific Islander Americans* trace their ancestry to the original peoples of Hawaii, Guam, Samoa, and other Pacific Islands. Pacific Islander Americans have a higher overall death rate than the general population and higher rates of diabetes and asthma. Smoking and obesity are special concerns for this group.

• *Latinos* are a diverse group, with roots in Mexico, Puerto Rico, Cuba, and South and Central America. Many Latinos are of mixed Spanish and American Indian descent or of mixed Spanish, Indian, and African American descent. Latinos on average have lower rates of heart disease, cancer, and suicide than the general population; areas of concern include gallbladder disease, obesity, diabetes, and lack of health insurance.

Poverty and low educational attainment are key factors underlying ethnic health disparities, but they do not fully account for the differences. Access to appropriate health care can be a challenge. Nonwhite racial and ethnic groups, regardless of income, are more likely to live in areas that are medically underserved, with fewer sources of high-quality or specialist care (see the box "Health Inequality and COVID-19"). Language and cultural barriers, along with racism and discrimination, can also prevent people from receiving appropriate health services.

Income and Education Income and education are closely related. Groups with the highest poverty rates and the least education have the worst health status. They have higher rates of infant mortality, traumatic injury, violent death, and many diseases, including heart disease, diabetes, tuberculosis, HIV infection, and some cancers. They are also more likely to eat poorly, be overweight, smoke, drink, and use drugs. And to complicate and magnify all these factors, they are also exposed to more day-to-day stressors and have less access to health care services. Researchers estimate that about 250,000 deaths per year can be attributed to low educational attainment, 175,000 to individual and community poverty, and 120,000 to income inequality.

Disability People with disabilities have activity limitations or need assistance due to a physical or mental impairment. About one in four people in the United States has some level of disability, and the rate is rising, especially among younger segments of the population. People with disabilities are more likely to have obesity, heart disease, diabetes, and to smoke. Many also lack access to health care services.

Geographic Location About one in four Americans currently lives in a rural area—a place with fewer than 10,000 residents. People living in rural areas are less likely to be physically active, use seat belts, or obtain screening tests for preventive health care. They have less access to timely emergency services and much higher rates of some diseases

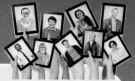

Pandemics illuminate social disparity. People most vulnerable to disease are typically the ones with fewer resources—less wealth, less access to health care, and less control over where they live. In the United States, groups hardest hit by COVID-19 have been elderly people and people of nonwhite ethnicity.

The novel virus began in late 2019 in the city of Wuhan, China, and spread the world over. Younger people had fewer symptoms and recovered from the disease more easily, although evidence of longer-term and unexpected symptoms continues to unfold. By contrast, the severity of this infection increases with age in people 50 and older; at least 20% of national deaths occurred in nursing homes. Age-related differences are not fully understood, but they may be attributable to children's flexible immune systems. As we age, our immune responses narrow to fight off specific pathogens we've already encountered; young children are still primed to deal with new viruses and have more weapons in their arsenal.

By April 2020, a racial breakdown of COVID-19 cases and deaths showed that in addition to older people, nonwhite ethnic groups were disproportionately affected—especially African Americans, Latinos, Asian Americans, and American Indian or Alaska Natives (AIANs).

When race was reported, 34% of cases involved African Americans, although they make up only 13% of the total population. They also died at higher rates and were far more likely to be hospitalized. In many parts of the country, black people accounted for over half of all coronavirus deaths.

In New Mexico and Arizona, AIAN people made up a larger share of confirmed infections and deaths. During the worst of the outbreak in New York City, more Latinos per capita were hit than any other ethnic group. Although infections and deaths for Asian Americans did not stand out as starkly disproportionate as those for African Americans, Asian Americans accounted for half of all COVID-19 deaths in San Francisco in May 2020.

One explanation for the disproportionate numbers is the presence of underlying medical conditions. Heart disease and diabetes occur at higher rates among black, Latino, and AIAN populations, and these are also risk factors for COVID-19 infection. However, social inequities detrimentally affect even nonwhite individuals without preexisting medical conditions.

Members of less affluent communities have fewer resources to protect themselves from infection, to find and receive testing, and to be treated. Lack of resources like stable housing, access to health care, and family members who can take time off work to help a sick relative all compromise people's ability to cope with infectious disease. Outbreaks of the coronavirus have been twice as likely in nursing homes where a significant number of residents are black or Latino. The workers in these homes are also disproportionately nonwhite. For example, African Americans make up 12% of the workforce but 30% of nurses.

Poorer communities have fewer options for staying home from work. If you can't work from home, or afford to take a break from work, you are at greater risk of infection from the virus. The U.S. Bureau of Labor Statistics reported that over 80% of black workers and about 85% of Latino workers have to leave home to work. About two-thirds of Latino adults said they could not get paid leave for more than two weeks.

Pandemics and other crises remind us about the importance of education and science-based research, to keep our society healthy. They remind us to identify and continue working to solve the social disparities that let some groups fall through the cracks.

SOURCES: Artiga, S., et al. 2020. Growing data underscore that communities of color are being harder hit by COVID-19. *Kaiser Family Foundation*, 21 April (https://www.kff.org/coronavirus-policy-watch/growing-data-underscore-communities-color-harder-hit-covid-19/); Landon, E. 2020. COVID-19: What we know so far about the 2019 novel coronavirus. At the Forefront: The University of Chicago Medicine, 8 May (https://www.uchicagomedicine.org/forefront/prevention-and-screening-articles/wuhan-coronavirus); Palomino, J. 2020. Why has coronavirus taken such a toll on SF's Asian American community? Experts perplexed over high death rate. *San Francisco Chronicle*, 20 May (https://www.sfchronicle.com/health/article/Why-has-coronavirus-taken-such-a-toll-on-SF-s-15282096.php); Wadman, M., et al. 2020. How does coronavirus kill? Clinicians trace a ferocious rampage through the body, from brain to toes. *Science* (https://www.sciencemag.org/news/2020/04/how-does-coronavirus-kill-clinicians-trace-ferocious-rampage-through-body-brain-toes); Zhang, S. 2020. Why the coronavirus hits kids and adults so differently. *The Atlantic*, 15 May (https://www.theatlantic.com/science/archive/2020/05/covid-19-kids/611728/).

and injury-related deaths than people living in urban areas. They are also more likely to lack health insurance. Children living in dangerous neighborhoods—rural or urban—are less likely to play outside and are four times more likely to be overweight than children living in safer areas.

Sexual Orientation and Gender Identity Lesbian, gay, bisexual, and transgender (LGBT) health was added as a new topic area in *Healthy People 2020*. Questions about sexual orientation and gender identity have

> **QUICK STATS**
>
> More than
> ## 34 million
> American adults have diabetes, and 21% of them don't know it.
> —Centers for Disease Control and Prevention, 2020

not been included in many health surveys, making it difficult to estimate the number of LGBT people and to identify their special health needs. However, research suggests that LGBT individuals may face health disparities due to discrimination and denial of their civil and human rights. LGBT youth have high rates of tobacco, alcohol, and other drug use as well as an elevated risk of suicide; they are more likely to be homeless and are less likely to have health insurance and access to appropriate health care providers and services.

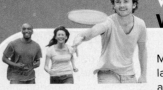

WELLNESS ON CAMPUS
Wellness Matters for College Students

Most college students, in their late teens and early twenties, appear to be healthy. But appearances can be deceiving. Each year, thousands of students lose productive academic time to physical and emotional health problems—some of which can continue to plague them for life.

The following table shows the top 10 health issues affecting students' academic performance, according to the spring 2019 American College Health Association–National College Health Assessment II.

HEALTH ISSUE	STUDENTS AFFECTED (%)
Stress	34.2
Anxiety	27.8
Sleep difficulties	22.4
Depression	20.2
Cold/flu/sore throat	14.8
Concern for a friend/family member	11.7
Relationship difficulties	9.5
Death of a friend/family member	6.2
Attention deficit/hyperactivity disorder	6.0
Sinus or ear infection, strep throat, bronchitis	4.5

Each of these issues is related to one or more of the dimensions of wellness, and most can be influenced by choices students make daily. Although some troubles—such as the death of a friend or family member—cannot be controlled, students can moderate their physical and emotional impact by choosing healthy behaviors. For example, there are many ways to manage stress, the top health issue affecting students (see Chapter 2). By reducing unhealthy choices (such as using alcohol to relax) and by increasing healthy choices (such as using time management and relaxation techniques), students can reduce the impact of stress on their lives.

The survey also estimated that, based on students' reporting of their height and weight, nearly 23% of college students are overweight and 14.9% are obese. Although heredity plays a role in determining your weight, lifestyle is also a factor in weight management.

In many studies over the past few decades, a large percentage of students have reported behaviors such as the following:

- Overeating
- Frequently eating high-fat foods
- Using alcohol and binge drinking

Clearly, eating behaviors are often a matter of choice. Although students may not see (or feel) the effects of their dietary habits today, the long-term health risks are significant. Overweight and obese persons run a higher-than-normal risk of developing diabetes, heart disease, and cancer later in life. We now know with certainty that improving one's eating habits, even a little, can lead to weight loss and improved overall health.

Other Choices, Other Problems

Students commonly make other unhealthy choices. Here are some examples from the 2019 National College Health Assessment II:

- Only 43.4% of students reported that they used a condom during vaginal intercourse in the past 30 days.
- About 16% of students had seven or more drinks the last time they partied.
- About 6% of students had smoked cigarettes at least once during the past month; 13% used an e-cigarette; and 22% used marijuana.

What choices do you make in these situations? Remember: It's never too late to change. The sooner you trade an unhealthy behavior for a healthy one, the longer you'll be around to enjoy the benefits.

SOURCE: American College Health Association. 2019. *American College Health Association–National College Health Assessment IIc: Reference Group Executive Summary Spring 2019.* Hanover, MD: American College Health Association. (https://www.acha.org /documents/ncha/NCHA-II_SPRING_2019_US_REFERENCE_GROUP _EXECUTIVE_SUMMARY.pdf).

FACTORS THAT INFLUENCE WELLNESS

Optimal health and wellness come mostly from a healthy lifestyle—patterns of behavior that promote and support your health and promote wellness now and as you get older. In the pages that follow, you'll find current information and suggestions you can use to build a healthier lifestyle; also, see the "Wellness Matters for College Students" box.

Our behavior, family health history, environment, and access to health care are all important influences on wellness. These factors, which vary for both individuals and groups, can interact in ways that produce either health or disease.

Health Habits

Research continually reveals new connections between our habits and health. For example, heart disease is associated with smoking, stress, a hostile attitude, a poor diet, and being sedentary. Poor health habits take hold before many Americans reach adulthood.

Other habits, however, are beneficial. Regular exercise can help prevent heart disease, high blood pressure, diabetes, osteoporosis, and depression. Exercise can also reduce the risk of colon cancer, stroke, and back injury. A balanced and varied diet helps prevent many chronic diseases. As we learn more about how our actions affect our bodies and minds, we can make informed choices for a healthier life.

Heredity/Family History

Your **genome** consists of the complete set of genetic material in your cells—about 25,000 genes, half from each of your parents. **Genes** control the production of proteins that serve both as the structural material for your body and as the regulators of all your body's chemical reactions and metabolic processes. The human genome varies only slightly from person to person, and many of these differences do not affect health. However, some differences have important implications for health, and knowing your family's health history can help you determine which conditions may be of special concern for you.

Errors in our genes are responsible for about 3500 clearly hereditary conditions, including sickle-cell disease and cystic fibrosis. Altered genes also play a part in heart disease, cancer, stroke, diabetes, and many other common conditions. However, in these more common and complex disorders, genetic alterations serve only to increase an individual's risk, and the disease itself results from the interaction of many genes with other factors. An example of the power of behavior and environment can be seen in the more than 60% increase in the incidence of diabetes that has occurred among Americans since 1990. This huge increase is not due to any sudden change in our genes; it is the result of increasing rates of obesity caused by poor dietary choices and lack of physical activity.

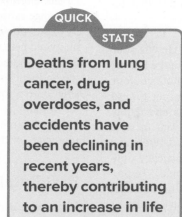

QUICK STATS

Deaths from lung cancer, drug overdoses, and accidents have been declining in recent years, thereby contributing to an increase in life expectancy.

—National Center for Health Statistics, 2020

Environment

Your environment includes substances and conditions in your home, workplace, and community. Are you frequently exposed to environmental tobacco smoke or the radiation in sunlight? Do you live in an area with high rates of crime and violence? Do you have access to nature?

Today environmental influences on wellness also include conditions in other countries and around the globe, particularly weather and climate changes occurring as a result of global warming. The burning of fossil fuels causes not only climate change but also outdoor air pollution, which damages our hearts and lungs; a growing collection of studies is discovering how air pollution also damages our brains. Indoor air pollution caused by toxic gases (e.g., carbon monoxide and radon), household cleaning products, formaldehyde, and mold can also lead to serious health problems for people who are exposed. Industrial waste, including lead and cancer-causing chemicals, can leach into our water and compromise our health.

Access to Health Care

Adequate health care helps improve both quality and quantity of life through preventive care and the treatment of disease. For example, vaccinations prevent many dangerous infections, and screening tests help identify key risk factors and diseases in their early treatable stages. As described

earlier, inadequate access to health care is tied to factors such as low income, lack of health insurance, and geographic location. Cost is one of many issues surrounding the development of advanced health-related technologies.

Personal Health Behaviors

In many cases, behavior can tip the balance toward good health, even when heredity or environment is a negative factor. For example, breast cancer can run in families, but it also may be associated with being overweight and inactive. A woman with a family history of breast cancer is less likely to develop the disease if she controls her weight, exercises regularly, and has regular mammograms to help detect the disease in its early, most treatable stage.

Similarly, a young man with a family history of obesity can maintain a normal weight by balancing calorie intake against activities that burn calories. If your life is highly stressful, you can lessen the chances of heart disease and stroke by managing and coping with stress (see Chapter 2). If you live in an area with severe air pollution, you can reduce the risk of lung disease by not smoking. You can also take an active role in improving your environment. Behaviors like these can make a difference in how great an impact heredity and environment will have on your health.

REACHING WELLNESS THROUGH LIFESTYLE MANAGEMENT

As you consider the behaviors that contribute to wellness, you may be doing a mental comparison with your own behaviors. If you are like most young adults, you probably have some healthy habits and some habits that place your health at risk. For example, you may be physically active and have a healthful diet but spend excessive hours on your cell phone or on social media. You may be careful to wear your seat belt in your car but skip meals. Moving in the direction of wellness means cultivating healthy behaviors and working to overcome unhealthy ones. This approach to lifestyle management is called **behavior change.**

As you may already know, changing an unhealthy habit (such as giving up cigarettes) can be harder than it sounds. When you embark on a behavior change plan, it may seem

TERMS

genome The complete set of genetic material in an individual's cells.

gene The basic unit of heredity, containing chemical instructions for producing a specific protein.

behavior change A lifestyle management process that involves cultivating healthy behaviors and working to overcome unhealthy ones.

like too much work at first. But as you make progress, you will gain confidence in your ability to take charge of your life. You will also experience the benefits of wellness—more energy, greater vitality, deeper feelings of appreciation and curiosity, and a higher quality of life.

Getting Serious about Your Health

Before you can start changing a wellness-related behavior, you have to know that the behavior is problematic and that you *can* change it. To make good decisions, you need information about relevant topics and issues, including what resources are available to help you change.

Examine Your Current Health Habits How is your current lifestyle affecting your health today and in the future? Think about which of your current habits enhance your health and which detract from it. Begin your journey toward wellness with self-assessment: Talk with friends and family members about what they have noticed about your lifestyle and your health, and take the quiz in the box titled "Wellness: Evaluate Your Lifestyle." Challenge any unrealistically optimistic attitudes or ideas you may hold—for example, "To protect my health, I don't need to worry about quitting smoking until I'm 40 years old" or "Being overweight won't put *me* at risk for diabetes." Health risks are very real and can become significant while you're young; health habits are important throughout life.

Many people consider changing a behavior when friends or family members express concern, when a landmark event occurs (such as turning 30), or when new information—like receiving high cholesterol results—raises their awareness of risk. If you find yourself reevaluating some of your behaviors as you read this text, take advantage of the opportunity to make a change in a structured way.

Choose a Target Behavior Changing any behavior can be demanding. Start small by choosing one behavior you want to change—called a **target behavior**—and working on it until you succeed. Your chances of success will be greater if your first goal is simple, such as resisting the urge to snack between classes. As you change one behavior, make your next goal a little more significant, and build on your success.

Learn about Your Target Behavior Once you've chosen a target behavior, you need to learn its risks and benefits—both now and in the future. Ask these questions:

• How is your target behavior affecting your level of wellness today?

• Which diseases or conditions does this behavior place you at risk for?

• What effect would changing your behavior have on your health?

As a starting point, use this text and the resources listed in the "For More Information" section at the end of each chapter. See the "Evaluating Sources of Health Information" box for additional guidelines.

Find Help Have you identified a particularly challenging target behavior or condition—something like overuse of alcohol, binge eating, or depression—that interferes with your ability to function or places you at a serious health risk? If so, you may need help to change a behavior or address a disorder that is deeply rooted or too serious for self-management. Don't let the problem's seriousness stop you; many resources are available to help you solve it. On campus, the student health center or campus counseling center can provide assistance. To locate community resources, consult the yellow pages, your physician, or the internet.

Building Motivation to Change

Knowledge is necessary for behavior change, but it isn't usually enough to make people act. Millions of people have sedentary lifestyles, for example, even though they know it's bad for their health. This is particularly true of young adults, who feel healthy despite their unhealthy behaviors. To succeed at behavior change, you need strong motivation. The sections that follow address some considerations.

Examine the Pros and Cons of Change Health behaviors have short-term and long-term benefits and costs. Consider the benefits and costs of an inactive lifestyle:

• *Short-term.* Such a lifestyle allows you more time to watch TV, use social media, do your homework, and hang out with friends, but it leaves you less physically fit and less able to participate in recreational activities.

• *Long-term.* It increases the risk of heart disease, cancer, stroke, and premature death.

To successfully change your behavior, you must believe that the benefits of change outweigh the costs.

Carefully examine the pros and cons of continuing your current behavior and of changing to a healthier one. Focus on the effects that are most meaningful to you, including those that are tied to your personal identity and values. For example, engaging in regular physical activity and getting adequate sleep can support an image of yourself as an active person who is a good role model for others. To complete your analysis, ask friends and family members about the effects of your behavior on them.

target behavior An isolated behavior selected as the object for a behavior change program.

TERMS

The short-term benefits of behavior change can be an important motivating force. Although some people are motivated by long-term goals, such as avoiding a disease that may hit them in 30 years, most are more likely to be moved to action by shorter-term, more personal goals. Feeling better, doing better in school, improving at a sport, reducing stress, and increasing self-esteem are common short-term benefits of health behavior change.

Many wellness behaviors are associated with immediate improvements in quality of life. For example, surveys of Americans have found that nonsmokers feel healthy and full of energy more days each month than do smokers, and they report fewer days of sadness and troubled sleep; the same is true when physically active people are compared with sedentary people. Over time, these types of differences add up to a substantially higher quality of life for people who engage in healthy behaviors.

Boost Self-Efficacy   A big factor in your eventual success is whether you feel confident in your ability to change. **Self-efficacy** refers to your belief in your ability to successfully take action and perform a specific task. Strategies for boosting self-efficacy include developing an internal locus of control, using visualization and self-talk, and getting encouragement from supportive people.

LOCUS OF CONTROL   Who do you believe is controlling your life? Is it your parents, friends, or school? Is it "fate"? Or is it you? **Locus of control** refers to the extent to which a person believes he or she has control over the events in his or her life. People who believe they are in control of their lives are said to have an *internal locus of control.* Those who believe that factors beyond their control determine the course of their lives are said to have an *external locus of control.*

For lifestyle management, an internal locus of control is an advantage because it reinforces motivation and commitment. An external locus of control can sabotage efforts to change behavior. For example, if you believe that you are destined to die of breast cancer because your mother died from the disease, you may view regular screening mammograms as a waste of time. In contrast, if you believe that you can take action to reduce your risk of breast cancer despite hereditary factors, you will be motivated to follow guidelines for early detection of the disease.

If you find yourself attributing too much influence to outside forces, gather more information about your wellness-related behaviors. List all the ways that making lifestyle changes will improve your health. If you believe you'll succeed, and if you recognize that you are in charge of your life, you're on your way to wellness.

VISUALIZATION AND SELF-TALK   One of the best ways to boost your confidence and self-efficacy is to visualize yourself successfully engaging in a new, healthier behavior. Imagine yourself going for an afternoon run three days a week or no longer smoking cigarettes. Also visualize yourself enjoying all the short-term and long-term benefits that your lifestyle change will bring.

You can also use *self-talk,* the internal dialogue you carry on with yourself, to increase your confidence in your ability to change. Counter any self-defeating patterns of thought with more positive or realistic thoughts: "I am a strong, capable person, and I can maintain my commitment to change."

ROLE MODELS AND SUPPORTIVE PEOPLE   Social support can make a big difference in your level of motivation and your chances of success. Perhaps you know people who have reached the goal you are striving for. They could be role models or mentors for you, providing information and support for your efforts. Gain strength from their experiences, and tell yourself, "If they can do it, so can I." Find a partner who wants to make the same changes you do and who can take an active role in your behavior change program. For example, an exercise partner can provide companionship and encouragement when you might be tempted to skip your workout.

Identify and Overcome Barriers to Change   Don't let past failures at behavior change discourage you. They can be a great source of information you can use to boost your chances of future success. Make a list of the problems and challenges you faced in any previous behavior change attempts. To this, add the short-term costs of behavior change that you identified in your analysis of the pros and cons of change. Once you've listed these key barriers to change, develop a practical plan for overcoming each one. For example, if you are not getting enough sleep when you're with certain friends, decide in advance how you will turn down their next late-night invitation.

Enhancing Your Readiness to Change

The transtheoretical, or "stages of change," model has been shown to be an effective approach to lifestyle self-management. According to this model, you move through distinct stages of action as you achieve your target behavior. First, determine your target behavior, the final stage where your goals are accomplished; then determine what stage you are in now so that you can choose appropriate strategies to progress through the cycle of change. This will help you enhance your readiness and intention to change. Read the following sections to determine what stage you are in. Let's use exercise as an example of changing sedentary behavior to active, engaging behavior.

self-efficacy   The belief in your ability to take action and perform a specific task.

TERMS

locus of control   The extent to which a person believes he or she has control over the events in his or her life.

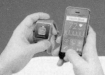

ASSESS YOURSELF
Wellness: Evaluate Your Lifestyle

All of us want optimal health, but many of us do not know how to achieve it. Taking this quiz, adapted from one created by the U.S. Public Health Service, is a good place to start. The behaviors covered in the quiz are recommended for most Americans. (Some of them may not apply to people with certain diseases or disabilities or to pregnant women, who may require special advice from their physician.) After you take the quiz, add up your score for each section.

Tobacco Use

If you never use tobacco, enter a score of 10 for this section and go to the next section.

	ALMOST ALWAYS	SOME TIMES	NEVER
1. I avoid smoking tobacco.	4	1	0
2. I avoid using a pipe or cigars.	2	1	0
3. I avoid spit tobacco.	2	1	0
4. I limit my exposure to environmental tobacco smoke.	2	1	0

Tobacco Score: _____

Alcohol and Other Drugs

1. I avoid alcohol or I drink no more than one drink (women) or two drinks (men) a day.	4	1	0
2. I avoid using alcohol or other drugs as a way of handling stressful situations or problems in my life.	2	1	0
3. I am careful not to drink alcohol when taking medications, such as for colds or allergies, or when pregnant.	2	1	0
4. I read and follow the label directions when using prescribed and over-the-counter drugs.	2	1	0

Alcohol and other drugs score: _____

Nutrition

1. I eat a variety of foods each day, including seven or more servings of fruits and vegetables.	3	1	0
2. I limit the amount of saturated and trans fat in my diet.	3	1	0
3. I avoid skipping meals.	2	1	0
4. I limit the amount of salt and added sugar I eat.	2	1	0

Nutrition score: _____

Exercise/Fitness

1. I engage in moderate-intensity exercise for 150 minutes per week.	4	1	0
2. I maintain a healthy weight, avoiding overweight and underweight.	2	1	0
3. I exercise to develop muscular strength and endurance at least twice a week.	2	1	0
4. I spend some of my leisure time participating in physical activities such as gardening, bowling, golf, or baseball.	2	1	0

Exercise/fitness score: _____

Emotional Health

1. I enjoy being a student, and I have a job or do other work that I like.	2	1	0
2. I find it easy to relax and express my feelings freely.	2	1	0
3. I manage stress well.	2	1	0
4. I get along well with other people.	2	1	0
5. I participate in group activities (such as church and community organizations) or hobbies that I enjoy.	2	1	0

Emotional health score: _____

Support

	ALMOST ALWAYS	SOME TIMES	NEVER
1. I volunteer one or more times each year.	2	1	0
2. I enjoy helping other people.	2	1	0
3. I feel free to ask others for help.	2	1	0
4. I have close friends with whom I can talk about personal matters.	2	1	0
5. I acknowledge the success and achievements of others.	2	1	0

Support score: _____

Safety

1. I wear a seat belt while riding in a car.	2	1	0
2. I avoid driving while under the influence of alcohol or other drugs.	2	1	0
3. I obey traffic rules and speed limits when driving.	2	1	0
4. I read and follow instructions on the labels of potentially harmful products or substances, such as household cleaners, poisons, and electrical appliances.	2	1	0
5. I avoid using a cell phone while driving.	2	1	0

Safety score: _____

Disease Prevention

1. I know the warning signs of cancer, diabetes, heart attack, and stroke.	2	1	0
2. I avoid overexposure to the sun and use sunscreen.	2	1	0
3. I get recommended medical screening tests (such as blood pressure checks and Pap tests), immunizations, and booster shots.	2	1	0
4. I do not share needles to inject drugs.	2	1	0
5. I am not sexually active, or I have sex with only one mutually faithful, uninfected partner, or I always engage in safer sex (using condoms).	2	1	0

Disease prevention score: _____

What Your Scores Mean

Scores of 9 and 10 Excellent! Your answers show that you are aware of the importance of this area to your health. More important, you are putting your knowledge to work for you by practicing good health habits. As long as you continue to do so, this area should not pose a serious health risk.

Scores of 6 to 8 Your health practices in this area are good, but there is room for improvement.

Scores of 3 to 5 Your health risks are showing.

Scores of 0 to 2 You may be taking serious and unnecessary risks with your health.

CRITICAL CONSUMER
Evaluating Sources of Health Information

Surveys indicate that college students are smart about evaluating health information. They trust the health information they receive from health professionals and educators and are skeptical about popular information sources, such as magazine articles and websites.

How good are you at evaluating health information? Here are some tips.

General Strategies

Whenever you encounter health-related information, take the following steps to make sure it is credible:

• **Go to the original source.** Media reports often simplify the results of medical research. Find out for yourself what a study really reported, and determine whether it was based on good science. What type of study was it? Was it published in a recognized medical journal? Was it an animal study, or did it involve people? Did the study include a large number of people? What did the authors of the study actually report?

• **Watch for misleading language.** Reports that tout "breakthroughs" or "dramatic proof" are probably hype. A study may state that a behavior "contributes to" or is "associated with" an outcome; this does not prove a cause-and-effect relationship.

• **Distinguish between research reports and public health advice.** Do not change your behavior based on the results of a single report or study. If an agency such as the National Cancer Institute urges a behavior change, however, follow its advice. Large, publicly funded organizations issue such advice based on many studies, not a single report.

• **Remember that anecdotes are not facts.** A friend may tell you he lost weight on some new diet, but individual success stories do not mean the plan is truly safe or effective. Check with your physician before making any serious lifestyle changes.

• **Be skeptical.** If a report seems too good to be true, it probably is. Be wary of information contained in advertisements.

An ad's goal is to sell a product, even if there is no need for it.

• **Make choices that are right for you.** Friends and family members can be a great source of ideas and inspiration, but you need to make health-related choices that work best for you.

Internet Resources

Online sources pose special challenges; when reviewing a health-related website, ask these questions:

• **What is the source of the information?** Websites maintained by government agencies, professional associations, or established academic or medical institutions are likely to present trustworthy information. Many other groups and individuals post accurate information, but it is important to look at the qualifications of the people who are behind the site. (Check the home page or click the "About Us" link.)

• **How often is the site updated?** Look for sites that are updated frequently. Check the "last modified" date of any web page.

• **Is the site promotional?** Be wary of information from sites that sell specific products, use testimonials as evidence, appear to have a social or political agenda, or ask for money.

• **What do other sources say about a topic?** Be cautious of claims or information that appear at only one site or come from a chat room, bulletin board, newsgroup, or blog.

• **Does the site conform to any set of guidelines or criteria for quality and accuracy?** Look for sites that identify themselves as conforming to some code or set of principles, such as those established by the Health on the Net Foundation or the American Medical Association. These codes include criteria such as use of information from respected sources and disclosure of the site's sponsors.

Precontemplation At this stage, you think you have no problem and don't intend to change your behavior. Your friends have commented that you should exercise more, but you are resistant. You have tried to exercise in the past and now think your situation is hopeless. You are unaware of risks associated with being sedentary, and you also blame external factors like other people for your condition. You believe that there are more important reasons *not* to change than there are reasons to change.

To move forward in this stage, try raising your awareness. *Research* the importance of exercise, for example. Look up articles, websites, and other resources that address the issue. How does exercise affect the body and mind? *Look also at the mechanisms you use to resist change,* such as denial or

rationalization. Find ways to counteract these mechanisms of resistance.

Seek social support. Friends and family members can help you identify target behaviors (e.g., fitting exercise into your time schedule or encouraging you while you work out). *Other resources* might include exercise classes or stress management workshops offered by your school.

Contemplation You now know you have a problem and within six months intend to do something about it, such as join a gym or take an exercise class. You realize that getting more exercise will help decrease your stress level. You acknowledge the benefits of behavior change but are also aware that the barriers to change may be difficult to overcome. You consider possible courses of action but don't know how to proceed.

To take charge, start by *keeping a journal*. Record what you have done so far and include your plan of action. *Do a cost-benefit analysis:* Identify the costs (e.g., it will cost money to take an exercise class) and benefits (e.g., I will probably stick to my goal if someone else is guiding me through the exercise). *Identify barriers to change* (e.g., I hate getting sweaty when I have no opportunity to shower). Knowing these obstacles can help you overcome them. Next, *engage your emotions.* Watch movies or read books about people with your target behavior. Imagine what your life will be like if you don't change.

Other ways to move forward in the contemplation stage include *creating a new self-image* and thinking before you act. *Imagine what you'll be like* after changing your unhealthy behavior. Try to think of yourself in those new terms right now. *Learn why you engage in the unhealthy behavior.* Determine what "sets you off" and train yourself not to act reflexively.

Preparation   You plan to take action within a month, or you may already have begun to make small changes in your behavior, like taking the stairs instead of the elevator. You may have discovered a place to go jogging but have not yet gone regularly or consistently.

Work on creating a plan. Include a start date, goals, rewards, and specific steps you will take to change your behavior. *Make change a priority.* Create and sign a contract with yourself.

Practice visualization and self-talk. Say, "I see myself jogging three times a week and going to yoga on Fridays." "I know I can do it because I've met challenging goals before." *Take small steps.* Successfully practicing your new behavior for a short time—even a single day—can boost your confidence and motivation.

Action   You outwardly modify your behavior and your environment. Maybe you start riding your bike to school or work. You put your stationary bicycle in front of the TV, and you leave your yoga mat out on your bedroom floor. The action stage requires the greatest commitment of time and energy, and people in this stage are at risk of relapsing into old, unhealthy patterns of behavior. *Monitor your progress.* Keep up with your journal entries. *Make changes* that will discourage the unwanted behavior—for example, park your car farther from your house or closer to the stairs. *Find alternatives* to your old behavior. Make a list of things you can do to replace the behavior.

Reward yourself. Rewards should be identified in your change plan. *Praise yourself* and focus on your success. *Involve your friends.* Tell them you want to change, and ask for their help. Don't get discouraged. Real change is difficult.

Maintenance   You have maintained your new, healthier lifestyle for at least six months by working out and riding your bike. Lapses have occurred, but you have been successful in quickly reestablishing the desired behavior. The maintenance stage can last months or years.

Keep going. Continue using the positive strategies that worked in earlier stages. And *be prepared for lapses.* If you find yourself skipping exercise class, don't give up on the whole project. Try inviting a friend to join you and then keep the date. *Be a role model.* Once you successfully change your behavior, you may be able to help someone do the same thing.

Termination   For some behaviors, you may reach the sixth and final stage of termination. At this stage, you have exited the cycle of change and are no longer tempted to lapse back into your old behavior. You have a new self-image and total control with regard to your target behavior.

Dealing with Relapse

People seldom progress through the stages of change in a straightforward, linear way. Rather, they tend to move to a certain stage and then slip back to a previous stage before resuming their forward progress. Research suggests that most people make several attempts before they successfully change a behavior, and four out of five people experience some degree of backsliding. For this reason, the stages of change are best conceptualized as a spiral in which people cycle back through previous stages but are farther along in the process each time they renew their commitment (Figure 1.5).

If you experience a lapse (a single slip) or a relapse (a return to old habits), don't give up. Relapse can be demoralizing, but it is not the same as failure; failure means stopping before you reach your goal and never changing your target behavior. During the early stages of the change process, it's a

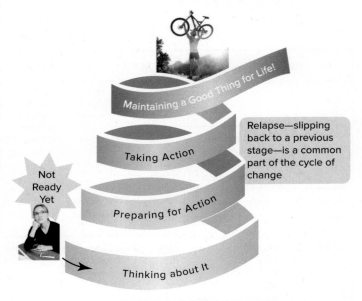

Relapse—slipping back to a previous stage—is a common part of the cycle of change

FIGURE 1.5   The stages of change: A spiral model.

SOURCE: Adapted from Centers for Disease Control and Prevention. n.d. *PEP Guide: Personal Empowerment Plan for Improving Eating and Increasing Physical Activity.* Dallas, TX: The Cooper Institute. Bottom left: Glow Images; Top right: UpperCut Images/Alamy Stock Photo

good idea to plan for relapse so that you can avoid guilt and self-blame and get back on track quickly. Follow these steps:

1. *Forgive yourself.* A single setback isn't the end of the world, but abandoning your efforts to change could have negative effects on your life.

2. *Give yourself credit for the progress you have already made.* You can use that success as motivation to continue. Don't compare yourself with others.

3. *Move on.* You can learn from a relapse and use that knowledge to deal with potential future setbacks.

If relapses keep occurring or you can't seem to control them, you may need to return to a previous stage of the behavior change process. If this is necessary, reevaluate your goals and strategy. A different or less stressful approach may help you avoid setbacks when you try again.

Developing Skills for Change: Creating a Personalized Plan

Once you are committed to making a change, put together a plan of action. Your key to success is a well-thought-out plan that sets goals, anticipates problems, and includes rewards.

1. Monitor Your Behavior and Gather Data Keep a record of your target behavior and the circumstances surrounding it. Record this information for at least a week or two. Keep your notes in a health journal or notebook or on your computer (see the sample journal entries in Figure 1.6). Record each occurrence of your behavior, noting the following:

- What the activity was
- When and where it happened
- What you were doing
- How you felt at that time

Tracking your activities will help, for example, if your goal is to start an exercise program, and you want to determine how to make time for workouts.

2. Analyze the Data and Identify Patterns After you have collected data on the behavior, analyze the data to identify patterns. When are you most likely to overeat? To skip a meal? What events trigger your appetite? Perhaps you are especially hungry at midmorning or when you put off eating dinner until 9:00. Perhaps you overindulge in food and drink when you go to a particular restaurant or when you're with certain friends. Note the connections between your feelings and such external cues as time of day, location, situation, and the actions of others around you.

3. Be "SMART" about Setting Goals If your goals are too challenging, you will have trouble making steady progress and will be more likely to give up altogether. If, for example, you are in poor physical condition, it will not make sense to set a goal of being ready to run a marathon within two months. If you set goals you can live with, it will be easier to stick with your behavior change plan and be successful.

Experts suggest that your goals meet the "SMART" criteria; that is, your behavior change goals should be

- *Specific.* Avoid vague goals like "eat more fruits and vegetables." Instead state your objectives in specific terms, such as "eat two cups of fruit and three cups of vegetables every day."

- *Measurable.* Your progress will be easier to track if your goals are quantifiable, so give your goal a number. You

Date	November 5			Day	M	TU	W	TH	F	SA	SU			
Time of day	M/ S	Food eaten	Cals.	H		Where did you eat?	What else were you doing?	How did someone else influence you?	What made you want to eat what you did?	Emotions and feelings?	Thoughts and concerns?
7:30	M	1 C Crispix cereal 1/2 C skim milk coffee, black 1 C orange juice	110 40 — 120	3		home	looking at news headlines on my phone	alone	I always eat cereal in the morning	a little keyed up & worried	thinking about quiz in class today
10:30	S	1 apple	90	1		hall outside classroom	studying	alone	felt tired & wanted to wake up	tired	worried about next class
12:30	M	1 C chili 1 roll 1 pat butter 1 orange 2 oatmeal cookies 1 soda	290 120 35 60 120 150	2		campus food court	talking	eating w/ friends; we decided to eat at the food court	wanted to be part of group	excited and happy	interested in hearing everyone's plans for the weekend
	M/S = Meal or snack			H = Hunger rating (0–3)							

FIGURE 1.6 Sample health journal entries.

might measure your goal in terms of time ("walk briskly for 20 minutes a day"), distance ("run two miles, three days per week"), or some other amount ("drink eight glasses of water every day").

• *Attainable.* Set goals that are within your physical limits. For example, if you are a poor swimmer, you might not be able to meet a short-term fitness goal by swimming laps. Walking or biking might be better options.

• *Realistic.* Manage your expectations when you set goals. For example, a long-time smoker may not be able to quit cold turkey. A more realistic approach might be to use nicotine replacement patches or gum for several weeks while getting help from a support group.

• *Time frame–specific.* Give yourself a reasonable amount of time to reach your goal, state the time frame in your behavior change plan, and set your agenda to meet the goal within the given time frame.

Using these criteria, sedentary people who want to improve their health and build fitness might set a goal of being able to run three miles in 30 minutes, to be achieved within a time frame of six months. To work toward that goal, they might set a number of smaller, intermediate goals that are easier to achieve. For example, their list of goals might look like this:

WEEK	FREQUENCY (DAYS/WEEK)	ACTIVITY	DURATION (MINUTES)
1	3	Walk < 1 mile	10–15
2	3	Walk 1 mile	15–20
3	4	Walk 1–2 miles	20–25
4	4	Walk 2–3 miles	25–30
5–7	3–4	Walk/run 1 mile	15–20
⋮			
21–24	4–5	Run 2–3 miles	25–30

Of course you may not be able to meet these goals, but you never know until you try. As you work toward meeting your long-term goal, you may need to adjust your short-term goals. For example, you may find that you can start running sooner than you thought, or you may be able to run farther than you originally estimated. In such cases, you may want to make your goals more challenging. In contrast, if your goals are too difficult, you may want to make them easier in order to stay motivated.

For some goals and situations, it may make more sense to focus on something other than your outcome goal. If you are in an early stage of change, for example, your goal may be to learn more about the risks associated with your target behavior or to complete a cost-benefit analysis. If your goal involves a long-term lifestyle change, such as reaching a healthy weight, focus on developing healthy habits rather than targeting a specific weight loss. Your goal in this case might be exercising for 30 minutes every day, reducing portion sizes, or eliminating late-night snacks.

4. Devise a Plan of Action Develop a strategy that will support your efforts to change. Your plan of action should include the following steps:

• *Get what you need.* Identify resources that can help you. For example, you can join a community walking club or sign up for a smoking cessation program. You may also need to buy some new running shoes or nicotine replacement patches. Get the items you need right away; waiting can delay your progress.

• *Modify your environment.* If you have cues in your environment that trigger your target behavior, control them. For example, if you typically have alcohol at home, getting rid of it can help prevent you from indulging. If you usually study with a group of friends in an environment that allows smoking, move to a nonsmoking area. If you always buy a snack at a certain vending machine, change your route so that you don't pass by it.

• *Control related habits.* You may have habits that contribute to your target behavior. Modifying these habits can help change the behavior. For example, if you usually plop down on the sofa while watching TV, try putting an exercise bike in front of the set so that you can burn calories while watching your favorite programs.

• *Reward yourself.* Giving yourself instant, real rewards for good behavior will reinforce your efforts. Plan your rewards; decide in advance what each one will be and how you will earn it. Tie rewards to achieving specific goals or subgoals. For example, you might treat yourself to a movie after a week of avoiding snacks. Make a list of items or events to use as rewards. They should be special to you and preferably unrelated to food or alcohol.

• *Involve the people around you.* Tell family and friends about your plan and ask them to help. To help them respond appropriately to your needs, create a specific list of dos and don'ts. For example, ask them to support you when you set aside time to exercise or avoid second helpings at dinner.

• *Plan for challenges.* Think about situations and people that might derail your program and develop ways to cope with them. For example, if you think it will be hard to stick to your usual exercise program during exams, schedule short bouts of physical activity (such as a brisk walk) as stress-reducing study breaks.

Ask Yourself

QUESTIONS FOR CRITICAL THINKING AND REFLECTION

Think about the last time you made an unhealthy choice instead of a healthy one. How could you have changed the situation, the people in the situation, or your own thoughts, feelings, or intentions to avoid making that choice? What can you do in similar situations in the future to produce a different outcome?

5. Make a Personal Contract A serious personal contract—one that commits you to your word—can result in a better chance of follow-through than a casual, offhand promise. Your contract can help prevent procrastination by specifying important dates and can also serve as a reminder of your personal commitment to change.

Your contract should include a statement of your goal and your commitment to reaching it. The contract should also include details such as the following:

- The date you will start
- The steps you will take to measure your progress
- The strategies you will use to promote change
- The date you expect to reach your final goal

Have someone—preferably someone who will be actively helping you with your program—sign your contract as a witness.

Figure 1.7 shows a sample behavior change contract for someone who is committing to eating more fruit every day.

You can apply the general behavior change planning framework presented in this chapter to any target behavior. Additional examples of behavior change plans appear in the Behavior Change Strategy sections at the end of many chapters in this text. In these sections, you will find specific plans for quitting smoking, starting an exercise program, and making other positive lifestyle changes.

Behavior Change Contract

1. I, __Tammy Lau__, agree to _increase my consumption of fruit from_ _1 cup per week to 2 cups per day._

2. I will begin on ___10/5___ and plan to reach my goal of __2 cups__ _of fruit per day_ by __12/7__

3. To reach my final goal, I have devised the following schedule of mini-goals. For each step in my program, I will give myself the reward listed.
   I will begin to have ½ cup
   of fruit with breakfast   10/5   see movie
   I will begin to have ½ cup   10/26   new video game
   of fruit with lunch
   I will begin to substitute fruit   11/16   concert
   juice for soda 1 time per day
   My overall reward for reaching my goal will be _trip to beach_

4. I have gathered and analyzed data on my target behavior and have identified the following strategies for changing my behavior: _Keep the_ _fridge stocked with easy-to-carry fruit. Pack fruit in my backpack_ _every day. Buy lunch at place that serves fruit._

5. I will use the following tools to monitor my progress toward my final goal: _Chart on fridge door_ _Health journal_

   I sign this contract as an indication of my personal commitment to reach my goal: _____Tammy Lau_____ __9/28__
   I have recruited a helper who will witness my contract and _also increase_ _his consumption of fruit; eat lunch with me twice a week._
   _____Eric March_____   __9/28__

FIGURE 1.7 **A sample behavior change contract.**

Putting Your Plan into Action

When you're ready to put your plan into action, you need commitment—the resolve to stick with the plan no matter what temptations you encounter. Remember all the reasons you have to make the change—and remember that *you* are the boss. Use all your strategies to make your plan work. Make sure your environment is change-friendly, and get as much support and encouragement from others as possible. Keep track of your progress in your health journal and give yourself regular rewards. And don't forget to give yourself a pat on the back—congratulate yourself, notice how much better you look or feel, and feel good about how far you've come and how you've gained control of your behavior.

Staying with It

As you continue with your program, don't be surprised when you run up against obstacles; they're inevitable. In fact, it's a good idea to expect problems and give yourself time to step back, see how you're doing, regroup, and make some changes before going on. If your program is grinding to a halt, identify what is blocking your progress. It may come from one of the sources described in the following sections.

Social Influences Take a hard look at the reactions of the people you're counting on, and see if they're really supporting you. If they come up short, connect with others who will be more supportive. Finding a dedicated workout partner, for example, can renew your desire to work toward your goal.

A related trap is trying to get your friends or family members to change *their* behaviors. The decision to make a major behavior change is something people come to only after intensive self-examination. The fact that you have seen a light doesn't mean that anyone else has. You may be able to influence someone by tactfully providing facts or support, but you cannot demand more. Focus on yourself. When you succeed, you may become a role model for others.

Levels of Motivation and Commitment You won't make real progress until an inner drive leads you to the stage of change at which you are ready to make a personal commitment to the goal. If commitment is your problem, you may need to wait until the behavior you're dealing with makes you unhappier or unhealthier; then your desire to change it will be stronger. Or you may find that changing your goal will inspire you to keep going.

Choice of Techniques and Level of Effort If your plan is not working as well as you thought it would, make changes where you're having the most trouble. If you've lagged on your running schedule, for example, maybe it's because you don't like running. An aerobics class might suit you better. There are many ways to move toward your goal. Or you may not be trying hard enough. Regardless, continue to push toward your goal. If it were easy, you wouldn't need a plan.

Ask Yourself

QUESTIONS FOR CRITICAL THINKING AND REFLECTION **?**

Have you tried to change a behavior in the past, such as exercising more or quitting smoking? How successful were you? Do you feel the need to try again? If so, what would you do differently to improve your chances of success?

Stress If you hit a wall in your program, look at the sources of stress in your life. If the stress is temporary, such as catching a cold or having a term paper due, you may want to wait until it passes before strengthening your efforts. If the stress is ongoing, find healthy ways to manage it (see Chapter 2). You may even want to make stress management your highest priority for behavior change.

Procrastinating, Rationalizing, and Blaming Be alert to games you might be playing with yourself, so that you can stop them. Such games include the following:

• *Procrastinating.* If you tell yourself, "It's Friday already; I might as well wait until Monday to start," you're procrastinating. Break your plan into smaller steps that you can accomplish one day at a time. Figure out how to enjoy the activity, whether that involves doing it with music, going outdoors, adding meditation to your program, or visualizing the desired end result.

• *Rationalizing.* If you tell yourself, "I wanted to go swimming today but wouldn't have had time to wash my hair afterward," you're making excuses. When you "win" by deceiving yourself, it isn't much of a victory.

• *Blaming.* If you tell yourself, "I couldn't exercise because Dave was hogging the elliptical trainer," you're blaming others for your own failure to follow through. Blaming is a way of taking your focus off the real problem and denying responsibility for your own actions.

BEING HEALTHY FOR LIFE

Your first few behavior change projects may never go beyond the planning stage. Those that do may not all succeed. But as you begin to see progress and changes, you'll start to experience new and surprising positive feelings about yourself. You'll probably find that you're less likely to buckle under stress. You may accomplish things you never thought possible—running a marathon, traveling abroad, or finding a rewarding relationship. Being healthy takes extra effort, but the paybacks in energy and vitality are priceless.

Once you've started, don't stop. Remember that maintaining good health is an ongoing process. Tackle one area at a time, but make a careful inventory of your health strengths and weaknesses and lay out a long-range plan.

Take on the easier problems first, and then use what you have learned to attack more difficult areas. Keep informed about the latest health news and trends; research is continually providing new information that directly affects daily choices and habits.

You can't completely control every aspect of your health. At least three other factors—heredity, health care, and environment—play important roles in your well-being. After you quit smoking, for example, you may still be inhaling smoke from other people's cigarettes. Your resolve to eat better foods may suffer a setback when you have trouble finding healthy choices on campus.

But you can make a difference—you can help create an environment around you that supports wellness for everyone. You can support nonsmoking areas in public places. You can speak up in favor of more nutritious foods and better physical fitness facilities. You can provide nonalcoholic drinks at your parties.

You can also work on larger environmental challenges: air and water pollution, traffic congestion, overcrowding and overpopulation, global warming and climate change, toxic and nuclear waste, and many others. These difficult issues need the attention and energy of people who are informed and who care about good health. On every level, from personal to planetary, we can all take an active role in shaping our environment.

TIPS FOR TODAY AND THE FUTURE **✳**

You are in charge of your health. Many of the decisions you make every day have an impact on the quality of your life, both now and in the future. By making positive choices, large and small, you help ensure a lifetime of wellness.

RIGHT NOW YOU CAN:
- Go for a 15-minute walk.
- Have a piece of fruit for a snack.
- Call a friend and arrange a time to catch up with each other.
- Think about whether you have a health behavior you'd like to change. If you do, consider the elements of a behavior change strategy. For example, begin a mental list of the pros and cons of the behavior, or talk to someone who can support you in your attempts to change.

IN THE FUTURE YOU CAN:
- Stay current on health- and wellness-related news and issues.
- Participate in health awareness and promotion campaigns in your community—for example, support smoking restrictions at local venues.
- Be a role model for (or at least be supportive of) someone else who is working on a health behavior you have successfully changed.

SUMMARY

- Wellness is the ability to live life fully, with vitality and meaning. Wellness is dynamic and multidimensional. It incorporates physical, emotional, intellectual, interpersonal, cultural, spiritual, environmental, financial, and occupational dimensions.

- As chronic diseases have emerged as major health threats in the United States, people must recognize that they have greater control over, and greater responsibility for, their health than ever before.

- With new health insurance options and the Healthy People initiative, the U.S. government is seeking to achieve a better quality of life for all Americans.

- Health-related disparities that have implications for wellness can be described in the context of sex and gender, race and ethnicity, income and education, disability, geographic location, and sexual orientation and gender identity.

- Although heredity, environment, and health care all play roles in wellness and disease, behavior can mitigate their effects.

- To make lifestyle changes, you need information about yourself, your health habits, and resources available to help you change.

- You can increase your motivation for behavior change by examining the benefits and costs of change, boosting self-efficacy, and identifying and overcoming key barriers to change.

- The "stages of change" model describes six stages that people move through as they try to change their behavior: precontemplation, contemplation, preparation, action, maintenance, and termination.

- You can develop a specific plan for change by (1) monitoring your behavior by keeping a journal; (2) analyzing those data; (3) setting specific goals; (4) devising strategies for modifying the environment, rewarding yourself, and involving others; and (5) making a personal contract.

- To start and maintain a behavior change program, you need commitment, a well-developed plan, social support, and a system of rewards.

- Although you cannot control every aspect of your health, you can make a difference in helping create an environment that supports wellness for everyone.

FOR MORE INFORMATION

The internet addresses listed here were accurate at the time of publication.

Centers for Disease Control and Prevention (CDC). The CDC provides a wide variety of health information for researchers and the general public.

http://www.cdc.gov

Federal Deposit Insurance Corporation. "Money Smart for Young Adults" is a free source of information, unaffiliated with commercial interests, that includes eight modules on topics such as "borrowing basics" and "paying for college and cars."

https://www.fdic.gov/consumers/consumer/moneysmart/index.html

Federal Trade Commission: Consumer Protection—Health. Includes online brochures about a variety of consumer health topics, including fitness equipment, generic drugs, and fraudulent health claims.

http://www.ftc.gov/health

Healthfinder. A gateway to online publications, websites, support and self-help groups, and agencies and organizations that produce reliable health information.

http://healthfinder.gov

Healthy People. Provides information on Healthy People objectives and priority areas.

http://www.healthypeople.gov

MedlinePlus. Provides links to news and reliable information about health from government agencies and professional associations; also includes a health encyclopedia and information about prescription and over-the-counter drugs.

http://medlineplus.gov

National Health Information Center (NHIC). Puts consumers in touch with the organizations that are best able to provide answers to health-related questions.

http://www.health.gov/nhic/

National Institutes of Health (NIH). Provides information about all NIH activities as well as consumer publications, hotline information, and an A-to-Z listing of health issues with links to the appropriate NIH institute.

http://www.nih.gov

National Wellness Institute. Serves professionals and organizations that promote health and wellness.

http://www.nationalwellness.org

Office of Minority Health. Promotes improved health among racial and ethnic minority populations.

http://minorityhealth.hhs.gov

Office on Women's Health. Provides information and answers to frequently asked questions.

http://www.womenshealth.gov

Surgeon General. Includes information on activities of the Surgeon General and the text of many key reports on topics such as tobacco use, physical activity, and mental health.

http://www.surgeongeneral.gov

World Health Organization (WHO). Provides information about health topics and issues affecting people around the world.

http://www.who.int/en

1. I, _____, agree to _____

_____

2. I will begin on _____ and plan to reach my goal of _____

_____ by _____

3. To reach my final goal, I have devised the following schedule of mini-goals. For each step in my program, I will give myself the reward listed.

Mini-goal	Target date	Reward
_____	_____	_____
_____	_____	_____
_____	_____	_____

My overall reward for reaching my goal will be _____

4. I have gathered and analyzed data on my target behavior and have identified the following strategies for changing my behavior:

_____

_____

5. I will use the following tools to monitor my progress toward my final goal: _____

_____

_____

I sign this contract as an indication of my personal commitment to reach my goal: _____

_____

I have recruited a helper who will witness my contract and _____

_____

_____

SELECTED BIBLIOGRAPHY

American Cancer Society. 2020. *Cancer Facts and Figures–2020*. Atlanta, GA: American Cancer Society. (https://www.cancer.org/content/dam/cancer-org/research/cancer-facts-and-statistics/annual-cancer-facts-and-figures/2020/cancer-facts-and-figures-2020.pdf).

American College Health Association. 2019. *American College Health Association–National College Health Assessment IIc: Reference Group Executive Summary Spring 2019*. Hanover, MD: American College Health Association. (https://www.acha.org/documents/ncha/NCHA-II_SPRING_2019_US_REFERENCE_GROUP_EXECUTIVE_SUMMARY.pdf).

American Heart Association. 2020. *Heart Disease and Stroke Statistics*. Dallas, TX: American Heart Association. (https://www.empoweredtoserve.org/en/about-us/heart-and-stroke-association-statistics).

Bakalar, N. 2019. Air pollution may damage the brain. *The New York Times*, 25 November (https://www.nytimes.com/2019/11/25/well/mind/air-pollution-brain-dementia-alzheimer-memory.html).

Bardo, A. R., and S. M. Lynch. 2019. Cognitively intact and happy life expectancy in the United States. *The Journals of Gerontology: Series B*: gbz080 (https://doi-org.laneproxy.stanford.edu/10.1093/geronb/gbz080).

Benjamin, EJ, Muntner P, Alonso A, Bittencourt MS, Callaway CW, Carson AP, et al. 2019. Heart disease and stroke statistics—2019 update: a report from the American Heart Association. *Circulation* 139(10): e56–528.

Bennett, I. M., et al. 2009. The contribution of health literacy to disparities in self-rated health status and preventive health behaviors in older adults. *Annals of Family Medicine* 7(3): 204–211.

Bleich, S. N., et al. 2012. Health inequalities: Trends, progress, and policy. *Annual Review of Public Health* 33: 7–40.

Centers for Disease Control and Prevention. 2018. Death Rates Up for 5 of the 12 Leading Causes of Death. Press Release. (https://www.cdc.gov/media/releases/2018/p0920-death-rates-up.html).

Centers for Disease Control and Prevention. 2019. Disability Impacts All of Us. (https://www.cdc.gov/ncbddd/disabilityandhealth/infographic-disability-impacts-all.html).

Centers for Disease Control and Prevention. 2019. *Division of Diabetes Translation at a Glance*. (http://www.cdc.gov/chronicdisease/resources/publications/aag/diabetes.htm).

Centers for Disease Control and Prevention. 2020. Life Expectancy Increases in 2018 as Overdose Deaths Decline Along with Several Leading Causes of Death. Press Release. (https://www.cdc.gov/nchs/pressroom/nchs_press_releases/2020/202001_Mortality.htm).

Centers for Disease Control and Prevention. 2020. National Diabetes Statistics Report. Atlanta, GA: Centers for Disease Control and Prevention, U.S. Dept of Health and Human Services. (https://www.cdc.gov/diabetes/pdfs/data/statistics/national-diabetes-statistics-report.pdf).

Cleveland Clinic. 2020. Cleveland Clinic Study Finds Obesity as Top Cause of Preventable Life-Years Lost. News Release 2017. (https://newsroom.clevelandclinic.org/2017/04/22/cleveland-clinic-study-finds-obesity-top-cause-preventable-life-years-lost/).

Curtin, S. C., et al. 2018. Recent increases in injury mortality among children and adolescents aged 10–19 year in the United States: 1999–2016. *National Vital Statistics Reports* 67(4): 1–16.

Everett, B. G, et al. 2013. The nonlinear relationship between education and mortality: An examination of cohort, race/ethnic, and gender differences. *Population Research and Policy Review* 32(6).

Fisher, E. G., G., et al. 2011. Behavior matters. *American Journal of Preventive Medicine* 40(5): e15–e30.

Flegal, K. M., et al. 2016. Trends in obesity among adults in the United States, 2005–2014. *JAMA* 315(21): 2284–2291.

Frieden, T. R. 2016. Foreword. *MMWR* 65(Suppl.) DOI: http://dx.doi.org/10.15585/mmwr.su6501a1.

Galea, S., et al. 2011. Estimated deaths attributable to social factors in the United States. *American Journal of Public Health* 101(8): 1456–1465.

Goldman, D. 2020. Obesity, Second to Smoking as the Most Preventable Cause of US Deaths, Needs New Approaches (https://healthpolicy.usc.edu/article/obesity-second-to-smoking-as-the-most-preventable-cause-of-us-deaths-needs-new-approaches/).

Herd, P., et al. 2007. Socioeconomic position and health: The differential effects of education versus income on the onset versus progression of health problems. *Journal of Health and Social Behavior* 48(3): 223–238.

Horneffer-Ginter, K. 2008. Stages of change and possible selves: Two tools for promoting college health. *Journal of American College Health* 56(4): 351–358.

Joshi, P. K., et al. 2017. Genome-wide meta-analysis associates HLA-DQA1/DRB1 and LPA and lifestyle factors with human longevity. *Nature Communications* 8(1): 910. DOI: 10.1038/s41467-017-00934-5

Kaiser Family Foundation. October 2013. Kaiser Health Tracking Poll, unpublished estimates.

National Center for Health Statistics. 2013. Health behaviors of adults: United States, 2008–10. *Vital and Health Statistics* 10(257).

National Center for Health Statistics. 2019. Health, United States Spotlight: Racial and Ethnic Disparities in Heart Disease. Hyattsville, MD: National Center for Health Statistics. (https://www.cdc.gov/nchs/hus/spotlight/HeartDiseaseSpotlight_2019_0404.pdf).

O'Loughlin, J., et al. 2007. Lifestyle risk factors for chronic disease across family origin among adults in multiethnic, low-income, urban neighborhoods. *Ethnicity and Disease* 17(4): 657–663.

Office of Disease Prevention and Health Promotion. 2020. *Healthy People 2030 Framework*. (https://www.healthypeople.gov/2020/About-Healthy-People/Development-Healthy-People-2030/Proposed-Framework).

Pinkhasov, R. M., et al. 2010. Are men shortchanged on health? Perspective on health care utilization and health risk behavior in men and women in the United States. *International Journal of Clinical Practice* 64(4): 475–487.

Printz, C. 2012. Disparities in cancer care: Are we making progress? A look at how researchers and organizations are working to reduce cancer health disparities. *Cancer* 118(4): 867–868.

Prochaska, J. O., J. C. Norcross, and C. C. DiClemente. 1995. *Changing for Good: The Revolutionary Program That Explains the Six Stages of Change and Teaches You How to Free Yourself from Bad Habits*. New York: Morrow.

Thorpe, R. J., et al. 2008. Social context as an explanation for race disparities in hypertension: Findings from the Exploring Health Disparities in Integrated Communities (EHDIC) Study. *Social Science and Medicine* 67(10): 1604–1611.

The U.S. Burden of Disease Collaborators. 2018. The state of US health, 1990–2016: Burden of diseases, injuries, and risk factors among US States. *JAMA* 319(14): 1444–1472.

U.S. Department of Health and Human Services. 2020. *Healthy People 2020: Lesbian, Gay, Bisexual, and Transgender Health* (https://www.healthypeople.gov/2020/topics-objectives/topic/lesbian-gay-bisexual-and-transgender-health).

U.S. National Library of Medicine. 2020. Is longevity determined by genetics? (https://ghr.nlm.nih.gov/primer/traits/longevity).

Williams, D. R. 2012. Miles to go before we sleep: Racial inequities in health. *Journal of Health and Social Behavior* 53(3): 279–295.

Yudell, M., et al. 2016. Taking race out of human genetics. *Science* 351(6273): 564.

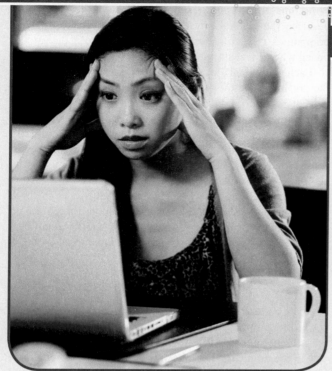

Monkey Business Images/Shutterstock

- Explain what stress is
- Describe the relationship between stress and health
- List common sources of stress
- Describe and apply techniques for managing stress

CHAPTER 2

Stress: The Constant Challenge

TEST YOUR KNOWLEDGE

1. **Which of the following events can cause stress?**
   a. Taking out a loan
   b. Failing a test
   c. Graduating from college

2. **Exercise stimulates which of the following?**
   a. Analgesia (pain relief)
   b. Birth of new brain cells
   c. Relaxation

3. **High levels of stress can impair memory and cause physical changes in the brain.**
   True or False?

4. **Which of the following can result from chronic stress?**
   a. Violence
   b. Heart attack
   c. Stroke

5. **Because eating induces relaxation, it is an excellent means of coping with stress.**
   True or False?

ANSWERS

1. **ALL THREE.** Stress-producing factors can be pleasant or unpleasant and can include physical challenges, goal achievement, and events that are perceived as negative.

2. **ALL THREE.** Regular exercise is linked to improvements in many dimensions of wellness.

3. **TRUE.** Low levels of stress may improve memory, but high stress levels impair learning and memory.

4. **ALL THREE.** Chronic—or ongoing—stress can last for years. People who suffer from long-term stress may ultimately become violent toward themselves or others. They also run a greater-than-normal risk for certain ailments, especially cardiovascular disease.

5. **FALSE.** Eating to cope with stress may lead to weight gain and to binge eating, a behavior associated with eating disorders.

ike the term *wellness, stress* is a word many people use without understanding its precise meaning. Stress is popularly viewed as an uncomfortable response to a negative event, which probably describes *nervous tension* more than the cluster of physical and psychological responses that actually constitutes stress. In fact, stress is not limited to negative situations; it is also a response to pleasurable physical challenges and the achievement of personal goals.

Whether stress is experienced as pleasant or unpleasant depends largely on the situation and the individual. Learning effective responses to stress can enhance psychological health and help prevent a number of serious diseases, and stress management can be an important part of daily life.

As a college student, you may be in one of the most stressful times of your life (see the box "The Perceived Stress Scale"). This chapter explains the physiological and psychological reactions that make up the stress response and describes how these reactions can put your health at risk. The chapter also discusses the most common sources of stress and offers methods of managing stress in your life.

WHAT IS STRESS?

In common usage, the term *stress* refers to two things: the mental states or events that trigger physical and psychological reactions (e.g., "That relationship is way too much stress"), *and* the reactions themselves (e.g., "I feel a lot of stress every time I walk into that classroom"). We use the more precise term **stressor** for a physical or psychological event that triggers physical and emotional reactions and the term **stress response** for the reactions themselves. Thoughts or feelings about an approaching event can be just as stressful as the event itself. A first date or a final exam can be a stressor that leads to sweaty palms and a pounding heart,

---

stressor Any physical or psychological event or condition that produces physical and psychological reactions.

TERMS

stress response The physical and emotional reactions to a stressor.

stress The general physical and emotional state that the stressor produces.

nervous system The brain, spinal cord, and nerves.

autonomic nervous system The part of the nervous system that controls certain basic body processes; consists of the sympathetic and parasympathetic divisions.

parasympathetic division The part of the autonomic nervous system that moderates the excitatory effect of the sympathetic division, slowing metabolism and restoring energy supplies.

sympathetic division Division of the autonomic nervous system that reacts to danger or other challenges by accelerating body processes.

---

symptoms of the stress response. We use the term **stress** to describe the general physical and emotional state that accompanies the stress response (e.g., "I take a day at the beach when I feel stressed").

Each individual's experience of stress depends on many factors, including the nature of the stressor and how it is perceived. Stressors take many different forms. Like a fire in your home, some occur suddenly and neither last long nor repeat. Others, like air pollution or quarreling parents, can continue for a long time. The memory of a stressful occurrence, such as the memory of the loss of a loved one, can itself be a stressor years after the event. Responses to stressors can include a wide variety of physical, cognitive, behavioral, and emotional changes. A short-term response might be an upset stomach or insomnia; a long-term response might be a change in your personality or social relationships.

Physical Responses to Stressors

Imagine a close call: As you step off the curb, a car careens toward you. With just a fraction of a second to spare, you leap safely out of harm's way. In that split second of danger and in the moments that follow, you experience a predictable series of physical reactions. Your body goes from a relaxed state to one prepared for physical action to cope with a threat to your life.

Two systems in your body are responsible for your physical response to stressors: the nervous system and the endocrine system. Through rapid chemical reactions affecting almost every part of your body, you are primed to act quickly and appropriately in time of danger.

The Nervous System The **nervous system** consists of the brain, spinal cord, and nerves. Part of the nervous system is under voluntary control, as when you tell your arm to reach for an orange. The part that is *not* under conscious supervision—for example, the part that controls the digestion of the orange—is the **autonomic nervous system.** In addition to digestion, it controls your heart rate, breathing, blood pressure, and hundreds of other involuntary functions.

The autonomic nervous system consists of two divisions:

- The **parasympathetic division** is in control when you are relaxed. It aids in digesting food, storing energy, and promoting growth.
- The **sympathetic division** is activated when your body is stimulated, for example, by exercise, and when you face an emergency and experience severe pain, anger, or fear.

Sympathetic nerves use the neurotransmitter norepinephrine (or *noradrenaline*) to affect nearly every organ, sweat gland, blood vessel, and muscle to enable your body to handle an emergency. In general, the sympathetic division commands your body to stop storing energy and to use it in response to a crisis.

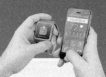

Many symptoms of excess stress are easy to notice. The following test can help you determine how much stress you have experienced in the past week.

Answer each question with a number: never = 0; almost never = 1; sometimes = 2; fairly often = 3; very often = 4.

In the past week, how often have you	NEVER	ALMOST NEVER	SOMETIMES	FAIRLY OFTEN	VERY OFTEN
1. Been upset because of something that happened unexpectedly?	0	1	2	3	4
2. Felt that you were unable to control the important things in your life?	0	1	2	3	4
3. Felt nervous and "stressed"?	0	1	2	3	4
4. *Felt confident about your ability to handle your personal problems?	0	1	2	3	4
5. *Felt that things were going your way?	0	1	2	3	4
6. Found that you could not cope with all the things you had to do?	0	1	2	3	4
7. *Been able to control irritations in your life?	0	1	2	3	4
8. *Felt that you were on top of things?	0	1	2	3	4
9. Been angered because things happened that were outside your control?	0	1	2	3	4
10. Felt difficulties were piling up so high that you could not overcome them?	0	1	2	3	4

To calculate your score, add your answers to questions 1, 2, 3, 6, 9, and 10, and subtract your answers to questions 4, 5, 7, and 8 (the questions with the asterisks). The result is your total score.

If your total score is above 14, you should take time to develop effective stress management techniques. This chapter describes many coping strategies that can aid you in dealing with college stressors. Your school's counseling center also can provide valuable support.

SOURCE: Adapted from Cohen, S., T. Kamarck, and R. Mermelstein. 1983. A global measure of perceived stress. *Journal of Health and Social Behavior*, 24: 386–396.

How the Nervous and Endocrine Systems Work Together During stress, the sympathetic nervous system triggers the **endocrine system.** This system of glands, tissues, and cells helps control body functions by releasing **hormones** and other chemical messengers into the bloodstream to influence metabolism and other body processes. The nervous system handles very short-term stress, whereas the endocrine system deals with both short-term (*acute*) and long-term (*chronic*) stress. How do both systems work together in an emergency? Higher cognitive areas in your brain decide that you are facing a threat. The nervous and endocrine systems activate adrenal glands that release the hormones **cortisol** and **epinephrine** (adrenaline). These hormones then trigger a basic set of physical reactions to stressors (as shown in Figure 2.1).

These nearly instantaneous physiological changes have been known as the **fight-or-flight reaction** but currently are called **fight, flight, or freeze**. The rapid onset of fight-or-flight reactions and the autonomic nervous system are largely driven by the neurotransmitter adrenaline. The heart accelerates, pupils dilate, and muscle tone increases. In contrast, the freeze response is more of a behavior within our awareness, along with the parasympathetic division reactions, and is driven by a different neurotransmitter. The physiological changes of the fight, flight, or freeze reaction give you the heightened reflexes and strength you need to dodge a car accident. Although these physiological changes may vary in intensity, the same basic set of reactions occurs in response to any type of stressor—positive or negative, physiological or psychological.

The Return to Homeostasis A short time after your near miss with the car, you begin to feel normal again. Once a

---

TERMS

endocrine system The system of glands, tissues, and cells that secrete hormones into the bloodstream to influence metabolism and other body processes.

hormone A chemical messenger produced in the body and transported in the bloodstream to target cells or organs for specific regulation of their activities.

cortisol A steroid hormone secreted by the cortex (outer layer) of the adrenal gland; also called *hydrocortisone*.

epinephrine A hormone secreted by the medulla (inner core) of the adrenal gland that affects the functioning of organs involved in responding to a stressor; also called *adrenaline*.

fight, flight, or freeze reaction A defense reaction that prepares a person for conflict or escape by triggering hormonal, cardiovascular, metabolic, and behavioral changes.

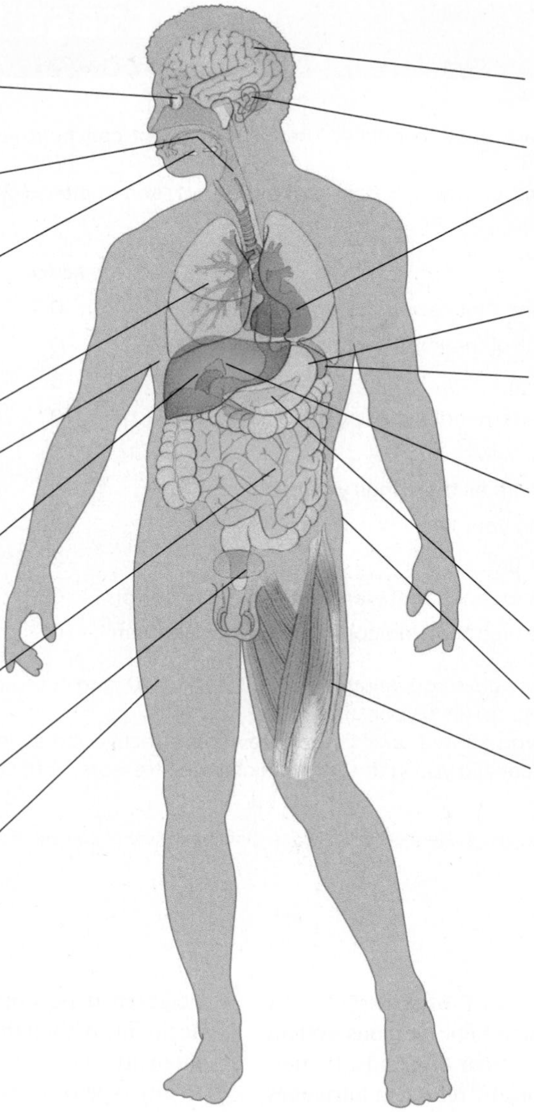

Pupils dilate to admit extra light for more sensitive vision.

Mucous membranes of nose and throat shrink, while muscles force a wider opening of air passages to allow easier airflow.

Secretion of saliva and mucus decreases; digestive activities have a low priority in an emergency.

Air passages dilate to allow more air into lungs.

Perspiration increases, especially in armpits, groin, hands, and feet, to flush out waste and cool the overheating body by evaporation.

Liver releases sugar into bloodstream to provide energy for muscles and brain.

Muscles of intestines stop contracting because digestion has halted.

Bladder relaxes. Emptying of bladder contents releases excess weight, making it easier to flee.

Blood vessels in skin and internal organs contract; those in skeletal muscles dilate. This increases blood pressure and delivery of blood to where it is most needed.

Brain releases endorphins that block any distracting pain.

Hearing becomes more acute.

Heart accelerates rate of beating. Strength of contraction increases to allow more blood flow where it is needed.

Digestion halts.

Spleen releases more red blood cells to meet an increased demand for oxygen and to replace any blood lost from injuries.

Adrenal glands stimulate secretion of epinephrine, increasing blood sugar, blood pressure, and heart rate; also spur increase in amount of fat in blood. These changes provide an energy boost.

Pancreas decreases secretions because digestion has halted.

Fat is removed from storage and broken down to supply extra energy.

Voluntary (skeletal) muscles contract throughout the body, readying them for action.

FIGURE 2.1 **Fight, flight, or freeze.** In response to a stressor, the autonomic nervous system and the endocrine system prepare the body to deal with an emergency.

stressful situation ends, the autonomic nervous system regains its balance, usually as its parasympathetic division takes command and halts the stress response. It restores **homeostasis,** a state of balance in which blood pressure, heart rate, hormone levels, and other vital functions are maintained within a narrow range of normal. Your parasympathetic nervous system calms your body, slowing a rapid heartbeat, drying sweaty palms, and returning breathing to normal. Gradually your body resumes its normal "housekeeping" functions, such as digestion and temperature regulation. Damage that may have been sustained during the stress exposure is repaired (e.g., the extra blood sugar produced to give you more energy is reabsorbed into the bloodstream rather than increasing your risk for diabetes). The day after you narrowly dodge the car, you

wake up feeling fine. In this way, your body can grow, repair itself, and acquire new reserves of energy. When the next crisis comes, you'll be ready to respond again instantly.

The Fight, Flight, or Freeze Reaction in Modern Life Fight, flight, or freeze is part of our biological heritage, a survival mechanism that has served humans well. In modern life, however, it is often absurdly inappropriate. Many of the stressors we face in everyday life—an exam, a mess left by a roommate, or a stoplight—do not require a physical response. The fight, flight, or freeze reaction prepares the body for physical action regardless of whether a particular stressor requires such a response.

People have different freeze, fight, or flight reactions to threats. Generally, a common action response to a threat is flight. But for people who are anxious or have been previously traumatized—in particular those with insecure parent–child attachments in infancy—freezing reactions are more common. People who display more aggression display fewer freezing reactions.

homeostasis A state of stability and consistency in an individual's physiological functioning. **TERMS**

Cognitive and Psychological Responses to Stressors

We all experience a similar set of physical responses to stressors (the fight, flight, or freeze reaction). These responses, however, vary from person to person and from one situation to another. People's perceptions of potential stressors—and of their reactions to such stressors—can vary greatly, depending on our cognitive and psychological framework. You may feel confident about taking exams but be nervous about talking to people you don't know. Your roommate, in contrast, may thrive in challenging social situations but may dread taking tests. Our individual ways of perceiving things play a significant role in the stress equation.

Cognitive Responses Your *cognitive appraisal* of a potential stressor is the thinking through the consequences of certain thoughts or behaviors, the processing of information. Two cognitive factors that can reduce the magnitude of the stress response are successful prediction and the perception of control. For instance, receiving a course syllabus at the beginning of the term allows you to predict the timing of major deadlines and exams. Having this predictive knowledge also allows you to exert some control over your study plans, which can help reduce the stress caused by exams.

The facts of a situation—Who? What? Where? When?—typically are evaluated fairly consistently from person to person. But evaluation with respect to personal outcome can vary: What does this mean for me? Can I do anything about it? Will it improve or worsen?

If a person perceives a situation as exceeding her or his ability to cope, the result can be negative emotions and an inappropriate stress response. If, by contrast, a person perceives a situation as a challenge that is within her or his ability to manage, more positive and appropriate responses are likely. A certain amount of stress, if coped with appropriately, can help promote optimal performance (Figure 2.2).

Looking at responses to a widespread stressor such as the coronavirus outbreak, we see that people with too much anxiety may engage in socially disruptive behaviors such as panic buying or avoiding necessary health care at hospitals or their doctors' offices for fear of contracting the virus. On the other hand, people who respond with too little anxiety may not take enough precautionary measures, such as physically distancing themselves or getting a vaccine when it becomes available.

Psychological Responses Psychological responses to stressors include cognitive ones, and they generally imply more emotion. Common psychological responses to stressors include anxiety, depression, and fear. Although emotional

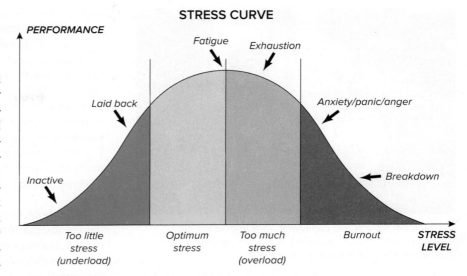

STRESS CURVE

PERFORMANCE

Fatigue
Exhaustion
Laid back
Anxiety/panic/anger
Inactive
Breakdown

Too little stress (underload)
Optimum stress
Too much stress (overload)
Burnout
STRESS LEVEL

FIGURE 2.2 **Stress level, performance, and well-being.** A moderate level of stress challenges individuals in a way that promotes optimal performance and well-being. Too little stress, and people are not challenged enough to improve; too much stress, and the challenges become stressors that can impair physical and emotional health.

SOURCE: Babson College. 2018. Stress (http://babson.edu/student-life/health-wellness/health-promotion /Pages/stress/aspx)

responses are determined in part by personality or temperament, we often moderate or learn to control them. Coping techniques that promote wellness and enable us to function at our best are discussed later in the chapter. Ineffective coping to stressors includes overeating; expressing hostility; and using tobacco, alcohol, or other drugs.

There are many factors that influence how each person responds to stress. Personality, cultural background, gender, and individual experience are important to consider when dealing with stressful situations.

PERSONALITY Some **personality** traits enable people to deal more effectively with stress. One such trait is *hardiness,* a particular form of optimism. People with a hardy personality view potential stressors as challenges and opportunities for growth and learning, rather than as burdens. They see fewer situations as stressful and react less intensely to stress than nonhardy people. Hardy people are committed to their activities, have a sense of inner purpose and an inner locus of control, and feel mostly in control of their lives.

Another psychological characteristic that prompts us to behave in a certain way is motivation. Two types of motivation have been studied that relate to stress and health. *Stressed power motivation* is associated with people who are aggressive and argumentative and who need to have power over others. One study of college students found that persons with this personality trait tend to get sick when their need for power is blocked or threatened. In contrast, people with *unstressed affiliation motivation* are drawn to others and

> **personality** The sum of behavioral, cognitive, and emotional tendencies. **TERMS**

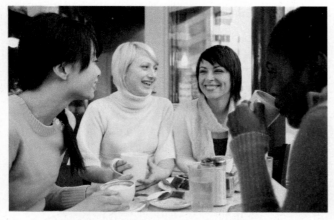

A person's emotional and behavioral responses to stressors depend on many factors, including personality, gender, and cultural background. *Fancy/Alamy Stock Photo*

want to be liked as friends. The same study of college students found that students with this trait reported the least illness. Another important personality trait—**resilience**—is especially associated with social and academic success in groups at risk for stress, such as people from low-income families and those with mental or physical disabilities. Resilient people tend to face adversity by accepting the reality of their situation, holding to a belief that life is meaningful, and being able to improvise.

Academic resilience helps college students flourish. Whether they need to bounce back from a poor grade or negative feedback, or master the art of juggling multiple academic pressures, students can learn techniques to stay and become resilient. One technique is to identify resources such as peers and counselors to lean on in times of crisis.

Contemporary research is repeatedly demonstrating that you can change some basic elements of your personality as well as your typical behaviors and patterns of thinking by using positive stress management techniques like those described later in this chapter.

CULTURAL BACKGROUND Young adults from around the world come to the United States for a higher education; most students finish college with a greater appreciation for other cultures and worldviews. The clash of cultures, however, can be a big source of stress for many students—especially when it leads to disrespectful treatment, harassment, or violence. It is important to consider that our reactions to stressful events are influenced by family and cultural background. Learning to appreciate the cultural backgrounds of other people can be both a mind-opening experience and a way to avoid stress over cultural differences.

> **resilience**   A personality trait associated with the ability to face adversity and recover quickly from difficulties.
>
> **gender role**   A culturally expected pattern of behavior and attitudes determined by a person's sex.
>
> **TERMS**

GENDER Your **gender role**—the activities, abilities, and behaviors your culture expects of you based on your sex—can affect your experience of stress. Some behavioral responses to stressors, such as crying or openly expressing anger, may be deemed more appropriate for one gender than another.

Strict adherence to gender roles, however, can limit one's response to stress and can itself become a source of stress. Gender roles can also affect one's perception of a stressor. If a man derives most of his self-worth from his work, for example, retirement may be more stressful for him than for a woman whose self-image is based on several different roles.

In her book *Overwhelmed*, Brigid Schulte describes a continuing unequal gendered division of labor: Families work more hours than they used to, but American women spend even more childraising hours than they did in the 1960s, when fewer women worked outside jobs.

Author Rachel Simmons examines how college and high school girls experience higher levels of anxiety and self-criticism than their predecessors in her 2018 book, *Enough As She Is*. Today's girls deal with pressures to do well in school and extracurricular activities while also trying to be pretty, sexy, kind, and liked by everyone in the real and virtual worlds. Social media's visual platforms, such as Instagram and Snapchat, are dominated by adolescent girls. These platforms portray effortless perfection and reward conventionally feminine expected behaviors: pleasing, performing, and looking good. This narrowing ideal of success comes at the expense of self-worth and well-being.

EXPERIENCE Past experiences can profoundly influence the evaluation of a potential stressor. If you had a bad experience giving a speech in the past, you are much more likely to perceive an upcoming speech as stressful than someone who has had positive public-speaking experiences. Effective behavioral responses, such as preparing carefully and visualizing success, can help overcome the effects of negative past experiences.

The Stress Experience as a Whole

As Figure 2.3 shows, the physical, cognitive, behavioral, and emotional symptoms of excess negative stress are distinct. But they are also intimately interrelated. The more intense the emotional response, the stronger is the physical response.

Ask Yourself

QUESTIONS FOR CRITICAL THINKING AND REFLECTION
Think of the last time you faced a significant stressor. How did you react? List the physical, cognitive, behavioral, and emotional reactions you experienced. Were the reactions appropriate to the circumstances? Did these reactions help you better deal with the stress, or did they interfere with your efforts to handle it?

Symptoms of excess stress

STRESS

PHYSICAL
- Dry mouth
- Frequent illnesses
- Gastrointestinal problems
- Headaches
- Fatigue
- High blood pressure
- Pounding heart
- Sweating

COGNITIVE
- Confusion
- Inability to concentrate
- Trouble remembering things
- Negative thinking
- Worrying
- Poor judgment

EMOTIONAL
- Anxiety
- Depression
- Edginess
- Hypervigilance
- Impulsiveness
- Irritability

BEHAVIORAL
- Sexual problems
- Social isolation
- Disrupted eating habits
- Disrupted sleep
- Irritability
- Problems communicating
- Increased use of tobacco, alcohol, or other drugs
- Crying

FIGURE 2.3 Physical, cognitive, behavioral, and emotional symptoms of excess stress.

Effective behavioral responses can lessen stress; ineffective ones only worsen it. Sometimes people have such intense responses to stressors or such ineffective coping techniques that they need professional help. More often, however, people can learn to handle stressors on their own.

STRESS AND HEALTH

Increased stress rates correspond to higher levels of physical and emotional stress symptoms: according to the American Psychological Association's 2019 Stress in America survey, 80% of respondents reported having at least one symptom of stress in the past month. In 2018, 91% of Generation Zs (the generation following Millennials, born after 1995) aged 18–21 said they had experienced at least one physical or emotional symptom due to stress in the past month compared to 74% of older adults. In 2020, self-reported stress levels increased significantly for the first time since the survey began in 2007; stress levels related to the coronavirus pandemic were even higher, particularly among parents of children under 18 and people of color. The role of stress in health is complex, but evidence suggests that stress can increase vulnerability to many ailments. Several theories have been proposed to explain the relationship between stress and disease.

The General Adaptation Syndrome

The concepts of homeostasis and adaptations to stressors came from the work of several scientists across the 20th century. The **general adaptation syndrome (GAS),** developed by biologist Hans Selye beginning in the 1930s and 1940s, is a theory that describes a universal and predictable response pattern to all stressors. It identifies an automatic self-regulation system of the mind and body that tries to return the body to a state of homeostasis after it is subjected to stress.

Some stressors, such as attending a party, are viewed as pleasant, while others, such as getting a bad grade, are viewed as unpleasant. In the GAS theory, stress triggered by a positive stressor is called **eustress;** stress triggered by a negative stressor is called **distress.** The sequence of physical responses associated with the GAS is the same for both eustress and distress and occurs in three stages (see Figure 2.4).

1. *Alarm.* The alarm stage includes the complex sequence of events brought on by the fight, flight, or freeze reaction. At this stage, the body is more susceptible to disease or injury because it is geared up to deal with a crisis. Someone in this phase may experience headaches, indigestion, anxiety, and disrupted sleeping and eating patterns.

2. *Resistance.* Under continued stress, the body develops a new level of homeostasis in which it is more resistant to disease and injury than usual. In this stage, a person can cope with normal life and added stress. However, at some point the body's resources will become depleted.

3. *Exhaustion.* The first two stages of GAS require a great deal of energy. If a stressor persists, or if several stressors occur in succession, general exhaustion sets in. This is not the sort of exhaustion you feel after a long, busy day.

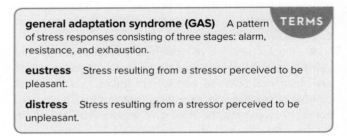

general adaptation syndrome (GAS) A pattern **TERMS** of stress responses consisting of three stages: alarm, resistance, and exhaustion.

eustress Stress resulting from a stressor perceived to be pleasant.

distress Stress resulting from a stressor perceived to be unpleasant.

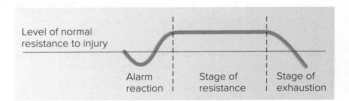

Level of normal resistance to injury

Alarm reaction | Stage of resistance | Stage of exhaustion

FIGURE 2.4 The general adaptation syndrome. During the alarm phase, the body's resistance to injury lowers. With continued stress, resistance to injury is enhanced. With prolonged exposure to repeated stressors, exhaustion sets in.

Rather, it's a life-threatening physiological exhaustion. The body's resources are depleted, and the body is unable to maintain normal function. If this stage is extended, long-term damage may result, manifesting itself in ulcers, digestive system trouble, depression, diabetes, cardiovascular problems, and/or mental illnesses.

Allostatic Load

The wear and tear on the body that results from long-term exposure to repeated or chronic stress is called the **allostatic load.** A person's allostatic load depends on many factors, including genetics, life experiences, and emotional and behavioral responses to stressors. The concept of allostatic load explains how frequent activation of the body's stress response, although essential for managing acute threats, can damage the body in the long run. For example, a student who suffers from test anxiety manages a week of exams but collapses on the weekend with a severe cold.

Although physical stress reactions may promote a new level of homeostasis (resistance stage of GAS), they also have negative effects on the body. The increased susceptibility to disease after repeated or prolonged stress may be due to effects of the stress response itself rather than to a depletion of resources (exhaustion stage of GAS). Over time, the student's allostatic load, along with susceptibility to disease, can increase. Allostatic load is generally measured through indicators of cumulative strain on several organs and tissues, especially on the cardiovascular system.

Psychoneuroimmunology

One of the most fruitful areas of current research into the relationship between stress and disease is **psychoneuroimmunology (PNI).** PNI is the study of the interactions among the nervous system, the endocrine system, and the immune system. The underlying premise of PNI is that stress, through the actions of the nervous and endocrine systems, impairs the immune system and thereby affects health.

A complex network of nerve and chemical connections exists among the nervous and the endocrine systems. In general, increased levels of cortisol are linked to a decreased number of immune system cells, or *lymphocytes*. Epinephrine appears to promote the release of lymphocytes but at the same time reduces their efficiency. Scientists have identified hormone-like substances called *neuropeptides* that appear to translate stressful emotions into biochemical events, some of which affect the immune system, providing a physical link between emotions and immune function.

Different types of stress may affect immunity in different ways. For instance, during **acute stress** (typically lasting between 5 and 100 minutes), white blood cells move into the skin, where they enhance the immune response. During a stressful event sequence, such as a personal trauma and the events that follow, however, there are typically no overall significant immune changes. Chronic (ongoing) stressors such as unemployment have negative effects on almost all functional measures of immunity. **Chronic stress** may cause prolonged secretion of cortisol (sometimes called the "antistress hormone" because it seeks to return the nervous system to homeostasis after a stress reaction) and may accelerate the course of diseases that involve inflammation, including multiple sclerosis, heart disease, type 2 diabetes, and clinical depression. In other words, this is one way that too many stress reactions over a prolonged length of time can have a negative impact on health.

Mood, personality, behavior, and immune functioning are intertwined. For example, people who are generally pessimistic may neglect the basics of health care, become passive when ill, and fail to engage in health-promoting behaviors. People who are depressed may reduce physical activity and social interaction, which may in turn affect the immune system and the cognitive appraisal of a stressor. Optimism, successful coping, and positive problem solving, by contrast, may positively influence immunity.

Health Problems and Stress

Although much remains to be learned, it is clear that people who have unresolved chronic stress in their lives or who handle stressors poorly are at risk for a wide range of health problems. In the short term, the problem might be just a cold, a stiff neck, or a stomachache. Over the long term, the problems can be more severe—cardiovascular disease (CVD), high blood pressure, impaired immune function, or a host of other problems.

Cardiovascular Disease During the stress response, heart rate increases and blood vessels constrict, causing blood pressure to rise. Chronic high blood pressure is a major cause of *atherosclerosis,* a disease in which blood vessels become damaged and caked with fatty deposits. These deposits can block arteries, causing heart attacks and strokes. The stress response can precipitate a heart attack in someone with atherosclerosis.

Certain emotional responses may increase a person's risk of CVD. As described earlier, people who tend to react to situations with anger and hostility are more likely to have heart attacks than are people with less explosive, more trusting personalities. Inflammation has been linked to stress and is a key component of the damage to blood vessels that leads to heart attacks (see Chapter 16 for more about CVD.)

> **allostatic load** The "wear and tear" on the body that results from long-term exposure to repeated or chronic stress.
>
> **psychoneuroimmunology (PNI)** The study of the interactions among the nervous, endocrine, and immune systems.
>
> **acute stress** Stress immediately following a stressor; may last only minutes or may turn into chronic stress.
>
> **chronic stress** Stress that continues for days, weeks, or longer.

TERMS

Psychological Disorders Stress contributes to many psychological problems such as depression, panic attacks, anxiety, eating disorders, and posttraumatic stress disorder (PTSD). PTSD, which afflicts war veterans, rape victims, child abuse survivors, and others who have suffered or witnessed severe trauma, is characterized by nightmares, flashbacks, and a diminished capacity to experience or express emotion. (For information about psychological health, see Chapter 3.)

Altered Immune Function Some of the health problems linked to stress-related changes in immune function include vulnerability to colds and other infections, asthma and allergy attacks, and flare-ups of chronic sexually transmitted infections such as genital herpes and HIV infection.

Headaches More than 45 million Americans suffer from chronic, recurrent headaches. Headaches come in various types but are often grouped into the following three categories:

- *Tension headaches.* Approximately 90% of all headaches are tension headaches, characterized by a dull, steady pain, usually on both sides of the head. It may feel as though a band of pressure is tightening around the head, and the pain may extend to the neck and shoulders. Acute tension headaches may last from hours to days, whereas chronic tension headaches may occur almost every day for months or even years. Ineffective stress management skills, poor posture, and

immobility are the leading causes of tension headaches. There is no cure, but the pain can sometimes be avoided and relieved with mindfulness skills (discussed later in the chapter), over-the-counter painkillers, and therapies such as massage, acupuncture, relaxation, hot or cold showers, and rest.

- *Migraine headaches.* Migraines typically progress through a series of stages lasting from several minutes to several days. They may produce a variety of symptoms, including throbbing pain that starts on one side of the head and may spread; heightened sensitivity to light; visual disturbances such as flashing lights or temporary blindness; nausea; dizziness; and fatigue. Women are more than twice as likely as men to suffer from migraines. Potential triggers include menstruation, stress, fatigue, atmospheric changes, bright light, specific sounds or odors, and certain foods. The frequency of attacks varies from a few in a lifetime to several per week. Treatment can help reduce the frequency, severity, and duration of migraines. Aerobic exercise is frequently recommended as a treatment for migraine headaches. However, the evidence for the efficacy of exercise to reduce the frequency and severity of migraine headaches is mixed. There is mild evidence that exercise may reduce stress levels, a known trigger for migraine headaches. Researchers have not been able to replicate these findings consistently, however. Several studies have failed to show exercise as an effective treatment for migraine headaches. And for some people, exercise itself can trigger migraines.

- *Cluster headaches.* Cluster headaches are severe headaches that cause intense pain in and around one eye. They usually occur in clusters of one to three headaches each day over a period of weeks or months, alternating with periods of remission in which no headaches occur. More than twice as many men as women suffer from cluster headaches. There is no known cause or cure for cluster headaches, but a number of treatments are available. During cluster periods, it is important to refrain from smoking cigarettes and drinking alcohol because these activities can trigger attacks. For more information on treating headaches and when a headache may signal a serious illness, see Appendix B.

Other Health Problems Many other health problems may be caused or worsened by excessive stress, including the following:

- Digestive problems such as stomachaches, diarrhea, constipation, irritable bowel syndrome, and ulcers
- Asthma
- Cancer
- Skin disorders
- Fibromyalgia
- Insomnia and fatigue
- Injuries, including on-the-job injuries caused by repetitive strain
- Menstrual irregularities, impotence, and pregnancy complications

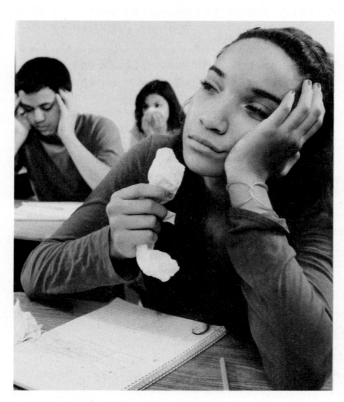

Ongoing stress has been shown to make people more vulnerable to everyday ailments, such as colds and allergies. Fuse/Somos Images/Getty Images

In addition to taking a toll on health, stress can mask underlying health problems. Here are some examples:

- Stress makes stomach ulcers worse, but eliminating a certain kind of bacteria can be an effective and simple treatment for ulcers.
- Most people have increased blood pressure when they are stressed, but if blood pressure stays high, it's better to take blood pressure lowering medications than to count on reducing your stress.
- Stress can make you feel anxious and depressed, but when these feelings are severe, you should seek out a health provider for specific therapies.

COMMON SOURCES OF STRESS

Recognizing potential sources of stress is an important step in successfully managing the stress in your life.

Major Life Changes

Any major change in your life that requires adjustment and accommodation can be a source of stress. Early adulthood and the college years are associated with many significant changes, such as moving out of the family home. Even changes typically thought of as positive—graduation, job promotion, marriage—can be stressful.

Life changes that are traumatic, such as getting fired or divorced or experiencing the death of a loved one, may be linked to subsequent health problems in some people. Personality and coping skills, however, are important moderating influences. People with strong support networks and stress-resistant personalities are less likely to become ill in response to life changes than are people with fewer resources.

Daily Hassles

Although major life changes are stressful, they seldom occur regularly. Researchers have proposed that minor problems—life's daily hassles, such as losing your keys or driving in traffic—can be an even greater source of stress because they occur much more often.

People who perceive hassles negatively are likely to experience a moderate stress response every time they face one. Over time, this can take a significant toll on health. Studies indicate that, for some people, daily hassles contribute to a general decrease in overall wellness.

College Stressors

College is a time of major changes. For many students, college means being away from home and family for the first time. Nearly all students share stresses like the following:

- *Academic stress.* Exams, grades, and an endless workload await every college student but can be especially troublesome for students just out of high school.

- *Interpersonal stress.* Most students are more than just students; they are also friends, children, employees, spouses, parents, and so on. Managing relationships while juggling the rigors of college life can be daunting, especially if some friends or family members are less than supportive.

- *Time pressures.* Class schedules, assignments, and deadlines are an inescapable part of college life. But these time pressures can be compounded drastically for students who also have job or family responsibilities.

- *Financial concerns.* The majority of college students need financial aid not just to cover the cost of tuition but also to survive from day to day while in school. For many, college life isn't possible without a job, and the pressure to stay afloat financially competes with academic and other stressors.

- *Worries about anything but especially about the future.* As college comes to an end, students face the next set of decisions: thinking about a career, choosing a place to live, and leaving the friends and routines of school behind. Students may find it helpful to go to the campus career center, where they can talk to counselors and read guides for job seekers such as *What Color Is My Parachute?* by Richard N. Bolles, first published in 1970 and updated every year.

In 2015, the Center for Collegiate Mental Health reported an increase in students' visiting counseling centers. Since then, more reports from multiple sources have shown a rise in anxiety and depression, calling attention to a surge in student stress.

In the United States, stress can be culturally perceived as a status symbol. A busy and overworked lifestyle has become an aspiration, as in the "Stress Olympics" among high school and college students. When students perceive stress as a competition for status, a complaint about it doesn't end in compassion but rather makes those not stressed feel like they are not working hard enough.

QUICK STATS

Of students who seek treatment at college and university counseling centers, **62%** report anxiety, **50%** report depression, and **44%** report stress.

—Center for Collegiate Mental Health, 2019

Job-Related Stressors

According to the Stress in America survey, work has been one of the highest-reported sources of stress for Americans. (The presidential election, mass shootings, and health care are also at the top of the list.) Tight schedules and overtime leave less time for exercising, socializing, and other stress-proofing activities. Worries about job performance, salary, job security, and interactions with others can contribute to stress. High levels of job stress are also common for people who are left out of important decisions relating to their jobs. When workers are given the opportunity to shape their job descriptions and responsibilities, job satisfaction goes up and stress levels go down.

If job-related (or college-related) stress is severe or chronic, the result can be *burnout,* a state of physical, mental, and emotional exhaustion. Burnout occurs most often in highly motivated and driven individuals who come to feel that their work is not recognized or that they are not accomplishing their goals. People in the helping professions—teachers, social workers, caregivers, police officers, and so on—are also prone to burnout. For some people who suffer from burnout, a vacation or leave of absence may be appropriate. For others, a reduced work schedule, better communication with superiors, or a change in job goals may be necessary. Improving time management skills can also help.

Social Stressors

Social networks can be real or virtual. Both types can help improve your ability to deal with stress, but any social network can also become a stressor in itself.

Real Social Networks The college years can be a time of great change in interpersonal relationships—becoming part of a new community, meeting people from different backgrounds, leaving old relationships behind. You may feel stress as you meet people of other ethnic, racial, or socioeconomic groups. You may feel torn between sticking with people who share your background and connecting with those you have not encountered before. If English is not your first language, you may face the added burden of interacting in a language with which you are not completely comfortable. All these pressures can become significant sources of stress. (See the box "Diverse Populations, Discrimination, and Stress.")

Digital Social Networks Technology can connect you with people all over the world and make many tasks easier, but it can also increase stress. The 2018 Stress in America Survey shows that social media provide a feeling of support for 55% of Generation Zs; 45% report feeling judged, and 38% report feeling bad about themselves. The Girls' Index 2017 shows that girls who spend more time using technology are much more likely to report being depressed, wanting to change their appearance, and trusting others less. Being electronically connected to work, family, and friends all the time can also impinge on your personal space, waste time, and distract you.

People who constantly check their phones and social media feeds report higher levels of overall stress than do those who do not engage with technology as often. They are also more likely to report feeling disconnected from their family as a result of technology and to report being stressed by political and cultural discussions on social media.

Environmental Stressors

Have you tried to eat at a restaurant where the food was great, but the atmosphere was so noisy that it put you on edge? This is an example of a minor environmental stressor—a condition or event in the physical environment that causes stress. Examples of more disturbing and disruptive, even catastrophic, environmental stressors include the following:

- Pandemics
- Natural disasters
- Acts of violence
- Industrial accidents
- Intrusive noises or smells

Like the noisy atmosphere of some restaurants, many environmental stressors are mere inconveniences that are easy to avoid. Others, such as pollen or construction noise, may be unavoidable daily sources of stress. For those who live in poor or violent neighborhoods, the environment can contain major stressors, and in every corner of the country today, people are exposed to disturbing news and images via the media. According to the 2019 *Stress in America* survey, mass shootings are the most common source of stress for Americans at large but also especially for minority populations.

Internal Stressors

Many stressors are found not in our environment but within ourselves, and often they are created by the ways we think and look at things. Here is one useful way to think about this: Stress is 10% what's happening and 90% how you look at it. For example, we pressure ourselves to reach goals and continually judge our progress and performance. Striving to reach goals can enhance self-esteem if the goals are reasonable. Unrealistic expectations, however, can be a significant source of stress and can damage self-esteem. Other internal

Ask Yourself

QUESTIONS FOR CRITICAL THINKING AND REFLECTION

What are the top two or three stressors in your life right now? Are they new to your life—as part of your college experience—or have you experienced them in the past? Do they include both positive and negative experiences (eustress and distress)?

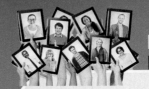

DIVERSITY MATTERS
Diverse Populations, Discrimination, and Stress

Stress is universal, but an individual's response to stress can vary depending on gender, cultural background, prior experience, and genetic factors. In diverse multiethnic and multicultural nations such as the United States, some groups face special stressors and have higher-than-average rates of stress-related physical and emotional problems. These groups include racial and ethnic minorities, the poor, those with physical or mental disabilities, and those who don't express mainstream gender roles.

Discrimination occurs when people speak or act according to their prejudices—biased, negative beliefs or attitudes toward some group. A blatant example, rising to the level of hate speech and criminal activity, is painting a swastika on a Jewish studies house or vandalizing a mosque. A more subtle example is when Middle Eastern American or African American students notice that residents in a mostly white college town tend to keep a close eye on them.

Immigrants to the United States have to learn to live in a new society. Doing so requires a balance between assimilating and changing to be like the majority, and maintaining a connection to their own culture, language, and religion. The process of acculturation is generally stressful, especially when the

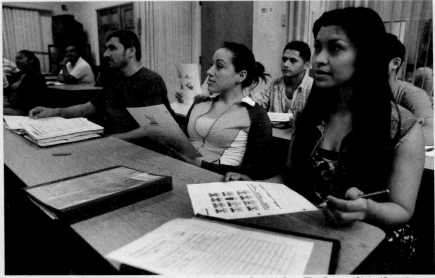

David L Ryan/The Boston Globe/Getty Images

person's background is radically different from that of the people he or she is now living among, or when people in the new community are suspicious or unwelcoming, as has recently been the case with immigrants from war-torn regions of the Middle East.

Both immigrants and minorities who have lived for generations in the United States can face job- and school-related stressors because of stereotypes and

discrimination. They may make less money in comparable jobs with comparable levels of education and may find it more difficult to achieve leadership positions.

On a positive note, however, many who experience hardship, disability, or prejudice develop effective goal-directed coping skills and are successful at overcoming obstacles and managing the stress they face.

---

stressors are emotional states such as despair or hostility, and physical states, such as chronic illness and exhaustion; each can be both a cause and an effect of unmanaged stress.

Traumatic Stressors

Traumatic stressors are extreme stressors that result from exposure to events that are life threatening and can cause bodily injury. For college-age people, the most common traumatic stressors are automobile accidents, assaults, and rape. Being the victim of or even witnessing such an event can result in posttraumatic stress disorder (PTSD). Symptoms can include obsessive thinking about what happened, flashbacks (a vivid memory of the event), and going out of your way to avoid reminders of the event. All this may be accompanied by anxiety, depression, and inability to sleep. PTSD is not something you can handle on your own. If symptoms are severe or persist, you should contact a counselor to help you (see the box "Coping with News of Traumatic Events").

MANAGING STRESS

You can control most stress in your life by taking the following steps:

- Shore up your support system.
- Improve your communication skills.
- Develop healthy exercise and eating habits.
- Learn to identify and moderate individual stressors.
- Learn mindfulness skills.

The effort required for stress management is well worth the time. People who manage stress effectively not only are healthier but also have more time to enjoy life and accomplish goals.

Social Support

Meaningful connections with others can play a key role in stress management and overall wellness. One study of college

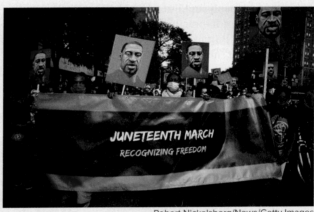

We are continually exposed to news of tragic events: shootings, natural disasters, war, terrorism, and poverty. Both experiencing trauma and observing it can result in extreme stress, requiring time and effort to recover. Such events can weaken your sense of security and create uncertainty about how the future may unfold. People react to such news in different ways, depending on their proximity to the event and how recent it was. People far from the site may suffer emotional reactions simply from watching endless coverage on television.

Responses to trauma include disbelief, shock, fear, anger, resentment, anxiety, mood swings, irritability, sadness, depression, panic, guilt, apathy, feelings of isolation or powerlessness, and many of the symptoms of excess stress. Some people affected by such violence develop posttraumatic stress disorder, a more serious condition.

In the case of the shooting rampages in 2017 at a country music festival in Las Vegas, and in 2018 at a high school in Parkland, Florida, both of which left many people dead and injured, communities mobilized quickly to respond to the expected surge in behavioral health needs generated by the attacks. Information sources and support groups were established for people grieving the loss of friends, family, neighbors, or colleagues.

Unfortunately these kinds of horrific events have been repeated numerous times in recent years. If you are becoming preoccupied with some recent disastrous event, such as a school shooting or terrorist attack, take these steps:

- Be sure you have the best information about what happened and whether a continuing risk is present. That information may be available through websites or on local radio or TV stations; it's a good idea to check your facts through multiple sources.

- Don't expose yourself to so much media coverage that it overwhelms you.

- Take care of yourself. Use the stress-relief techniques discussed in this chapter.

- Share your feelings and concerns with others. Be a supportive listener.

- If you feel able, help others in any way you can, such as by volunteering to work with victims.

- If you feel emotionally distressed days or weeks after the event, consider asking for professional help.

Robert Nickelsberg/News/Getty Images

---

students living in overcrowded apartments, for example, found that those with a strong social support system were less distressed by their cramped quarters than those who navigated life's challenges on their own. Other studies have shown that married people live longer than single people and have lower death rates from a wide range of conditions, although some studies suggest that marriage benefits men more than women.

A sense of isolation can lead to chronic stress, which in turn can increase one's susceptibility to illnesses like colds and to chronic illnesses, such as heart disease. Although the mechanism isn't clear, social isolation can be as significant to mortality rates as factors like smoking, high blood pressure, and obesity.

There is no single best pattern of social support that works for everyone. However, research suggests that having a variety of types of relationships may be important for wellness. Here are some tips for strengthening your social ties:

• *Foster friendships.* Keep in regular contact with your friends. Offer respect, trust, and acceptance, and provide help and support in times of need. Build your communication skills, and express appreciation for your friends.

• *Keep your family ties strong.* Stay in touch with the family members you feel close to. If your family doesn't function well as a support system for its members, create a second "family" of people with whom you have built meaningful ties.

• *Get involved with a group.* Do volunteer work, take a class, attend a lecture series, or join a religious group. These types of activities can give you a sense of security, a place to talk about your feelings or concerns, and a way to build new friendships. Choose activities that are meaningful to you and that include direct involvement with other people.

Volunteering

Studies show that not all giving is the same—for example, donating money does not have the same beneficial health effects as volunteering that involves personal contact. A few simple guidelines can help you get the most out of giving:

• Choose a volunteer activity that puts you in contact with people.

- Volunteer with a group. Sharing your interests with other volunteers increases social support. Volunteering seems to have the most benefits for people who also have other close relationships and social interests.
- Know your limits. Helping that goes beyond what you can handle depletes your own resources and is detrimental to your health.

Communication

Communicating in an assertive way that respects the rights of others—while protecting your own rights—can prevent stressful situations from getting out of control.

Some people have trouble either telling others what they need or saying no to the needs of others. They may suppress their feelings of anger, frustration, and resentment, and they may end up feeling taken advantage of or suffering in unhealthy relationships. At the other extreme are people who express anger openly and directly by being verbally or physically aggressive or indirectly by making critical, hurtful comments to others. Because their abusive behavior pushes away other people, they also have problems with relationships.

Better communication skills can help everyone form and maintain healthy relationships. Chapter 3 includes a discussion of anger and its impact on health and relationships. Chapter 5 discusses communication techniques for building healthy relationships.

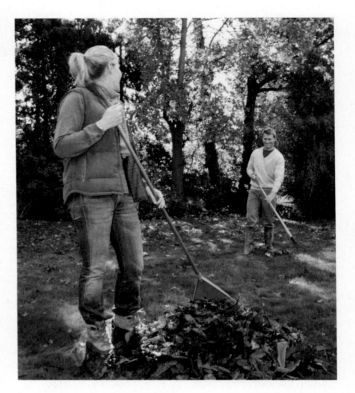

Exercise—even light activity—can be an antidote to stress. Nick Daly/Photodisc/Getty Images

Exercise

Exercise helps maintain a healthy body and mind and even stimulates the birth of new brain cells. Regular physical activity can also reduce many of the negative effects of stress. Consider the following examples:

- Taking a long walk can decrease anxiety and blood pressure.
- A brisk 10-minute walk can leave you feeling more relaxed and energetic for up to two hours.
- People who exercise regularly react with milder physical stress responses before, during, and after exposure to stressors.
- In one study, people who took three brisk 45-minute walks each week for three months reported fewer daily hassles and an increased sense of wellness.

These findings should not be surprising because the stress response mobilizes energy resources and readies the body for physical emergencies. If you experience stress and do not physically exert yourself, you are not completing the energy cycle. You may not be able to exercise while your daily stressors occur—during class, for example, or while sitting in a traffic jam—but you can be active at other times of the day. Physical activity allows you to expend the nervous energy you have built up and trains your body to more readily achieve homeostasis following stressful situations.

QUICK STATS

Nearly half of adults (44%) say they exercise to cope with stress.

—American Psychological Association, 2019

Nutrition

A healthful diet gives you an energy bank to draw from whenever you experience stress. Eating wisely also can enhance your feelings of self-control and self-esteem. Learning the principles of sound nutrition is easy, and sensible eating habits rapidly become second nature when practiced regularly. (For information about nutrition and healthy eating habits, see Chapter 13.)

For managing stress, limit or avoid caffeine. Although one or two cups of coffee a day probably won't hurt you, caffeine is a mildly addictive stimulant that leaves some people jittery, irritable, and unable to sleep. Consuming caffeine during stressful situations can raise blood pressure and increase levels of cortisol.

Although your diet affects the way your body handles stress, the reverse is also true. Excess stress can negatively affect the way you eat. Many people, for example, respond to stress by overeating; other people skip meals or stop eating altogether during stressful periods. Not only are both responses ineffective (they don't address the causes of stress), but they are also potentially unhealthy.

Time Management

Learning to manage your time can be crucial to coping with everyday stressors. Overcommitment, procrastination, and even boredom are significant stressors for many people. Try these strategies for improving your time management skills:

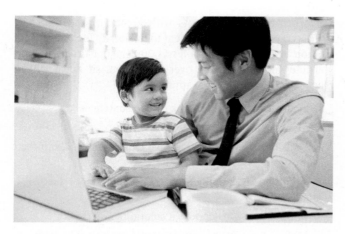

Managing the many commitments of adult life—including work, school, and parenthood—can produce a great deal of stress. Time management skills, including careful scheduling with a date book, smartphone, or tablet, can help people cope with busy days. Cathy Yeulet/123RF

• **Set priorities.** Divide your tasks into three groups: essential, important, and trivial. Focus on the first two, and ignore the third.

• **Schedule tasks for peak efficiency.** You've probably noticed you're most productive at certain times of the day (or night). Schedule as many of your tasks for those hours as you can, and stick to your schedule.

• **Set realistic goals and write them down.** Attainable goals spur you on. Impossible goals, by definition, cause frustration and failure. Fully commit yourself to achieving your goals by putting them in writing.

• **Budget enough time.** For each project you undertake, calculate how long it will take to complete. Then tack on another 10–15%, or even 25%, as a buffer.

• **Break up long-term goals into short-term ones.** Instead of waiting for large blocks of time, use short amounts of time to start a project or keep it moving.

• **Visualize the achievement of your goals.** By mentally rehearsing your performance of a task, you will be able to reach your goal more smoothly.

• **Keep track of the tasks you put off.** Analyze why you procrastinate. If the task is difficult or unpleasant, look for ways to make it easier or more fun.

• **Consider doing your least favorite tasks first.** Once you have the most unpleasant ones out of the way, you can work on the tasks you enjoy more.

• **Consolidate tasks when possible.** For example, try walking to the store so that you run your errands and exercise in the same block of time.

• **Identify quick transitional tasks.** Keep a list of 5- to 10-minute tasks you can do while waiting or between other tasks, such as watering your plants, doing the dishes, or checking a homework assignment.

• **Delegate responsibility.** Asking for help when you have too much to do is no cop-out; it's good time management. Just don't delegate the jobs you know you should do yourself.

• **Say no when necessary.** If the demands made on you don't seem reasonable, say no—tactfully, but without guilt or apology.

• **Give yourself a break.** Allow time for play—free, unstructured time when you can ignore the clock. Don't consider this a waste of time. Play renews you and enables you to work more efficiently.

• **Avoid your personal "time sinks."** You can probably identify your own time sinks—activities that consistently use up more time than you anticipate and put you behind schedule, like watching television, surfing the internet, or talking on the phone. On particularly busy days, avoid these problematic activities altogether. For example, if you have a big paper due, don't sit down for a five-minute TV break if that's likely to turn into a two-hour break. Try a five-minute walk instead.

• **Stop thinking or talking about what you're going to do, and just do it!** Sometimes the best solution for procrastination is to stop waiting for the right moment and just get started. You will probably find that things are not as bad as you feared, and your momentum will keep you going.

Cultivating Spiritual Wellness

Spiritual wellness is associated with more effective coping skills and higher levels of overall wellness. It is a very personal wellness component, and there are many ways to develop it. Researchers have linked spiritual wellness to longer life expectancy, reduced risk of disease, faster recovery, and improved emotional health. Although spirituality is difficult to study, and researchers aren't sure how or why spirituality seems to improve health, several explanations have been offered. To develop spiritual wellness, choose activities that are meaningful to you, such as the following:

• Look inward. Spend quiet time alone with your thoughts and feelings.

• Spend time in nature, experiencing continuity with the natural world.

• Notice art, architecture, and music.

• Engage in a favorite activity that allows you to express your creative side.

• Engage in a personal spiritual practice, such as prayer, meditation, or yoga.

Reach out to others:

• Share writings that inspire you.

• Practice small acts of personal kindness for people you know as well as for strangers.

• Perform community service.

Confiding in Yourself through Writing

Keeping a diary is analogous to confiding in others, except that you are confiding in and becoming more attuned to yourself. This form of coping with severe stress may be especially helpful for those who find it difficult to open up to others. Although writing about traumatic and stressful events may have a short-term negative effect on mood, over the long term, stress is reduced and positive changes in health occur. A key to promoting health and well-being through journaling is to write about your emotional responses to stressful events. Set aside a special time each day or week to write down your feelings about stressful events in your life.

Thinking and Acting Constructively

Certain ideas, beliefs, perceptions, and patterns of thinking can add to your stress level. One way to address this is through **mindfulness**, the intentional cultivation of attention in a way that is nonjudging and nonstriving. This objectivity and openness makes mindfulness an ideal way to restore a sense of balance and manage stress. Each of the following techniques can help you change unhealthy thought patterns to ones that will help you cope with stress (also see the box "Mindfulness Meditation"). As with any skill, mastering these techniques takes practice and patience.

Think back to the worries you had last week. How many of them were needless? By growing more aware of the ways you habitually think and feel, you can learn to recognize habits of mind that create distress and divest from them before they overwhelm you. Think about what you *can* control, particularly your way of looking at things. Try to stand outside of the problem, consider more effective steps you can take to solve it, and then carry them out. Remember that between a stimulus and a response there is a space, and in that space lies your freedom and power. In other words, if you can successfully recognize that a stressor is occurring, you can better control your response to it. Invest energy in considering how you may better promote the things you want individually or socially. This may mean reflecting on how you may better deal with an unpleasant person or stay focused in a class you find boring. By taking a constructive approach, you can prevent stressors from becoming negative events and perhaps even turn them into positive experiences.

Take Control   A situation often feels more stressful if you feel you're not in control of it. Time may seem to be slipping away before a big exam, for example. Unexpected obstacles may appear in your path, throwing you off course. When you feel your environment is controlling you instead of the other way around, take charge! Concentrate on what you can control rather than what you cannot, and set realistic goals. Be confident of your ability to succeed.

> **mindfulness**   The intentional cultivation of attention in a way that is nonjudging and nonstriving.   **TERMS**

Problem-Solve   Students with greater problem-solving abilities report easier adjustment to university life, higher motivation levels, lower stress levels, and higher grades. When you find yourself stewing over a problem, sit down with a piece of paper and try this approach:

1. Define the problem in one or two sentences.
2. Identify the causes of the problem.
3. Consider alternative solutions. Don't just stop with the most obvious one.
4. Weigh positive and negative consequences for each alternative.
5. Make a decision—choose a solution.
6. Make a list of tasks you must perform to act on your decision.
7. Carry out the tasks on your list.
8. Evaluate the outcome and revise your approach if necessary.

Modify Your Expectations   Expectations are exhausting and restricting. The fewer expectations you have, the more possibilities for spontaneity and joy. The more you expect from others, the more often you will feel let down. And trying to meet the expectations others have of you is often futile.

Stay Positive   If you tend to beat up on yourself—"Late for class again! You can't even cope with college! How do you expect to ever hold down a real job?"—try being kind to yourself instead. Talk to yourself as you would to a child you love: "You're a smart, capable person. You've solved other problems; you'll handle this one. Tomorrow you'll simply schedule things so you get to class with a few minutes to spare."

Practice Affirmations   One way of cultivating the positive is to systematically repeat positive thoughts, or *affirmations,* to yourself. For example, if you react to stress with low self-esteem, you might repeat sentences such as "I accept myself completely" and "It doesn't matter what others say, but what I believe." Say kinder and more loving things to yourself every day to promote more responding and less reacting.

Cultivate Your Sense of Humor   When it comes to stress, laughter may be the best medicine. It is said, "He who can laugh at himself will never cease to be amused!" Even a fleeting smile produces changes in your autonomic nervous system that can lift your spirits. A few minutes of belly laughing can be as invigorating as brisk exercise. Hearty laughter elevates your heart rate, aids digestion, eases pain, and triggers the release of endorphins and other pleasurable and stimulating chemicals in the brain. After a good laugh, your muscles go slack; your pulse and blood pressure dip below normal. You are relaxed. Cultivate the ability to laugh at yourself, and you'll have a handy and instantly effective stress reliever.

Be Kind to Yourself   Self-compassion can be a predictor of well-being. Self-compassion means being kind and

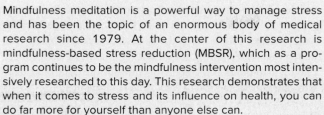

Mindfulness meditation is a powerful way to manage stress and has been the topic of an enormous body of medical research since 1979. At the center of this research is mindfulness-based stress reduction (MBSR), which as a program continues to be the mindfulness intervention most intensively researched to this day. This research demonstrates that when it comes to stress and its influence on health, you can do far more for yourself than anyone else can.

MBSR was founded by Jon Kabat-Zinn in 1979 at the University of Massachusetts Medical Center and is now offered in over 800 medical centers, hospitals, and clinics around the United States and many more hospitals and medical centers around the world, such as the Scripps Center for Integrative Medicine, Duke Integrative Medicine, and the Myrna Brind Center for Integrative Medicine at Jefferson.

MBSR classes are taught by physicians, nurses, social workers, counselors, and psychologists as well as other non-health professionals who have invested themselves in becoming MBSR teachers.

At the core of this model is a philosophy of health based on the inherent wholeness and interconnectedness of everyone and an understanding that in a very real way, no matter what health condition you are coping with, "there is more right with you than there is wrong with you." In practice, this program facilitates an active partnership in which patients or clients seeking help with stress take on significant responsibility for doing interior work to tap into their own deepest inner resources for learning, growing, and healing.

Mindfulness is both a mental state and the practices that cultivate this mental state. We cultivate this mental state by paying attention in a kind way to our mental, physical, and behavioral activities as they happen. By investing this kind of attention in ourselves and our lives, we soon discover that we all create most of our own stress, and that we can each do more than anyone else can to reduce that stress and take better care of ourselves. Here are two practices to use for stress reduction.

Mindful Breathing

You are always breathing, so this is a powerful and convenient way to become present wherever you go and in whatever you do. After you read these instructions, please close your eyes and invest 5–15 minutes in being present with your breath.

Sitting comfortably where you are right now, bring your body into a posture that is upright and supported, with a sense of balance and dignity. See if you can align your head, neck, and body in a way that is neither too rigid nor too relaxed, but somewhere in between. The intention is to be wakeful and alert, yet not tense; at ease, but not sleeping.

Bring attention to your breathing, wherever you feel it most prominently and notice the sensations of your breath coming and going as it will, in its own way and with its own pace. If your mind wanders from your breath, return to it by feeling the sensations of the breath as they come and go. Use these sensations as your way to be present, here and now, in each successive moment for the time you have set aside. Research has repeatedly demonstrated that extending this practice to 30 or 45 minutes on a regular basis significantly reduces stress and stress-related illnesses and conditions.

Walking Meditation

Find a place where you can walk and be uninterrupted by other people or traffic—if possible, in natural surroundings, like in a park. You can adapt this practice to fit yourself, whatever your circumstances are with mobility—for example, it can become a mindful-rolling practice if you rely on a wheelchair. Once you're ready, begin walking—slowly at first (as slowly as possible for about 10 minutes)—paying close attention to each step and using the sensations of each foot touching the ground as your way to be present. When you are ready, accelerate your pace, broadening your attention to take in more of your experience as you walk. In this mindful-movement practice, you may walk any distance, anywhere, at any speed that feels right for you. In the beginning, however, give yourself about 30 minutes.

The principal instruction is to be fully present in each moment you are walking rather than consumed with mind chatter or destination. Be open to the experience of your environment and notice, for example, the way clouds move or how the sunlight glistens in the trees and foliage around you. Turn toward whatever calls your attention and be with it as long as you like, stopping if you want to take a close look at a bug or flowers or to listen to the rustling of leaves. Remember, the overarching intention is to be mindful, to be in this experience of the now. In other words, shift to experiential presence and away from the usual conceptual and discursive activities of mind.

As you become more skilled in mindful awareness practice, you will be able to do this anywhere, even on a bustling college campus. If you want to pick up the speed or duration of your walk, you can make this walking practice part of a regular exercise program, and you will grow in strength and cardiovascular health as well as mindfulness.

Mindfulness is a lifetime engagement—not to get somewhere else, but to be where and as you are in this very moment, whether the experience is pleasant, unpleasant, or neutral. The more you invest in the practice, the more you draw forth and nourish the mental state of mindfulness with which you were born.

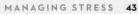

understanding to yourself when confronted with personal failings, rather than harshly judging and criticizing yourself for inadequacies and shortcomings.

Focus on What's Important   A major source of stress is trying to store too much data. Forget unimportant details (they will usually be self-evident) and organize important information. One technique you can try is to "chunk" important material into categories. If your next exam covers three chapters from your textbook, consider each chapter a chunk of information. Then break down each chunk into its three or four most important features. Create a mental outline that allows you to trace your way from the most general category down to the most specific details. This technique can be applied to managing daily responsibilities as well.

Body Awareness Techniques

Research conducted by neuroscientist Richard Davidson suggests that practicing mindfulness promotes stronger connections between the prefrontal cortex and the amygdala areas of the brain. This connection has been demonstrated to facilitate greater problem-solving skills, emotional self-regulation, and resilience.

In a recent University of California study, researchers reported that schoolteachers who took an eight-week mindfulness-based stress-reduction course were less anxious and depressed and had a greater ability to face a stressor than those in a control group.

Practicing mindfulness includes forms of meditation as well as more familiar forms of neuromuscular activities, such as yoga and tai chi.

Yoga   Hatha yoga, the most common yoga style practiced in the United States, emphasizes physical balance and breath control. It integrates components of flexibility, muscular strength and endurance, and muscle relaxation; it also sometimes serves as a preliminary to meditation. A session of yoga typically involves a series of postures, each held for a few seconds to several minutes, which involve stretching and balance and coordinated breathing. Yoga can be a powerful way to cultivate body awareness, ease, and flexibility.

Tai Chi   This martial art (in Chinese, *taijiquan*) is a system of self-defense that incorporates philosophical concepts from Taoism and Confucianism. In addition to self-defense, tai chi aims to bring the body into balance and harmony to promote health and spiritual growth. It teaches practitioners to remain calm and centered, to conserve and concentrate energy, and to manipulate force by becoming part of it—by "going with the flow." Tai chi is considered the gentlest of the martial arts. Instead of quick and powerful movements, tai chi consists of a series of slow, fluid, elegant movements, which reinforce the idea of moving *with* rather than *against* the stressors of everyday life.

Biofeedback   Biofeedback helps people reduce their response to stress by enabling them to become more aware of their level of physiological arousal. In biofeedback, some measure of stress—perspiration, heart rate, skin temperature, or muscle tension—is electronically monitored, and feedback is given using sound (a tone or music), light, or a meter or dial. With practice, people begin to exercise conscious control over their physiological stress responses. The point of biofeedback training is to develop the ability to transfer the control skills to daily life without the use of electronic equipment.

Sleep   Don't underestimate the value of a good night's sleep as a means of managing stress. Getting enough sleep isn't just good for you physically. Adequate sleep also improves mood, fosters feelings of competence and self-worth, enhances mental functioning, and supports emotional functioning. Chapter 4 will tell you more about the physiology of sleep and how you can sleep better.

Counterproductive Coping Strategies

College is a time when you'll learn to adapt to new and challenging situations and gain skills that will last a lifetime. It is also a time when many people develop counterproductive and unhealthy habits in response to stress. Such habits can last well beyond graduation.

Should You Avoid Challenging Situations?   Without the stress that goes along with accomplishing your goals and encountering new situations, your life might be very unfulfilling and boring. One theory is that for the best life, you should try to maintain a stress level that isn't too high or too low. In any case, studies show that people who have a positive attitude toward stress take the opportunity to learn about themselves and how to cope better, and they are then less likely to become anxious or depressed after stressful events.

Tobacco Use   Many young adults who never smoked in high school smoke their first cigarette in college, usually at a party or in a dorm with friends. Many smokers report that smoking helps them cope with stress by helping them relax, giving them something to do with their hands in social situations, or breaking up monotony and routine.

Cigarettes and other tobacco products contain *nicotine,* a chemical that enhances the actions of neurotransmitters. Nicotine can make you feel relaxed and even increase your ability to concentrate, but it is highly addictive. In fact, nicotine dependence itself is considered a psychological disorder. Cigarette smoke also contains substances that cause heart disease, stroke, lung cancer, and emphysema. These negative consequences far outweigh any beneficial effects, and tobacco use should be avoided. The easiest way to avoid the habit is to not start. See Chapter 12 for more about the health effects of tobacco use and for tips on how to quit.

Use of Alcohol and Other Drugs   Like nicotine, alcohol is addictive, and many alcoholics find it hard to relax without a drink. Having a few drinks might make you feel temporarily at ease, and drinking until you're intoxicated may help you forget your current stressors. However, using alcohol to deal with stress places you at risk for all the short- and long-term problems associated with alcohol abuse. It also does nothing to address the causes of stress in your life. Although limited alcohol consumption may have potential health benefits for some people, many college students have patterns of drinking that detract from wellness. For more about the responsible use of alcohol, refer to Chapter 11.

Using other psychoactive drugs to cope with stress is also usually counterproductive:

- **Stimulants,** such as *amphetamines,* can activate the stress response. They also affect the same areas of the brain that are involved in regulating the stress response.

- Use of **marijuana** causes a brief period of euphoria and decreased short-term memory and attentional abilities. Physiological effects clearly show that marijuana use doesn't cause relaxation; in fact, some neurochemicals in marijuana act to enhance the stress response, and getting high on a regular basis can elicit panic attacks. To compound this, withdrawal from marijuana may also be associated with an increase in circulating stress hormones.

- **Opioids** such as morphine and heroin can mimic the effects of your body's natural painkillers and act to reduce anxiety. However, tolerance to opioids develops quickly, and many users become dependent.

- **Tranquilizers** such as Valium and Xanax mimic some of the functions of your body's parasympathetic nervous system, and as with opioids, tolerance develops quickly, causing increased dependency and toxicity.

For more information about the health effects of using psychoactive drugs, see Chapter 10.

Unhealthy Eating Habits   The nutrients in the food you eat provide energy and substances needed to maintain your body. Eating is also psychologically rewarding. The feelings of satiation and sedation that follow eating produce a relaxed state. However, regular use of eating as a means of coping with stress may lead to unhealthy eating habits. In fact, a survey by the American Psychological Association revealed that about 25% of Americans use food as a means of coping with stress or anxiety. These "comfort eaters" are twice as likely to be obese as average Americans.

Certain foods and supplements are sometimes thought to fight stress. Carbohydrates may reduce the stress response by promoting activity of the parasympathetic nervous system; however, a high-carbohydrate diet can lead to weight gain in

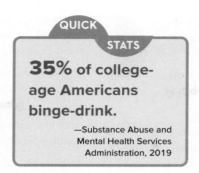

sedentary people and is not recommended as a strategy for coping with stressors. In addition, some evidence suggests that greater ingestion of carbohydrates, simple sugars, and fatty foods may be a predisposing factor for psychological distress. Many dietary supplements are marketed for stress reduction, but supplements are not required to meet the same standards as medications in terms of safety, effectiveness, and manufacturing (see Chapters 13 and 21).

Getting Help

What are the most important sources of stress in your life? Are you coping successfully with them? No single strategy or program for managing stress will work for everyone. The most important starting point for a successful stress management plan is to learn to listen to your body. When you recognize the stress response and the emotions and thoughts that accompany it, you'll be in a position to take charge of that crucial moment and handle it in a healthy way.

If the techniques discussed so far don't provide you with enough relief, you might need to look further. Excellent self-help guides can be found in bookstores or the library. Additional resources are listed in the For More Information section at the end of the chapter.

Your student health center or student affairs office can tell you whether your campus has a mindfulness-based stress-reduction program. If you are seeking social support, see if your campus offers a peer counseling program. Such programs are usually staffed by volunteer students with special training that emphasizes maintaining confidentiality. Peer counselors can guide you to other campus or community resources or can simply provide understanding.

Support groups are typically organized around a particular issue or problem. In your area, you might find a support group for first-year students; for reentering students; for single parents; for students of your race or ethnicity, religion, or national origin; for people with eating disorders; or for rape survivors. The number of such groups has increased in recent years as more and more people discover how therapeutic it can be to talk with others who share the same situation.

Short-term psychotherapy can also be tremendously helpful in dealing with stress-related problems. Your student health center may offer psychotherapy on a sliding-fee scale; the county mental health center in your area may do the same. If you belong to any type of religious organization, check to see whether pastoral counseling is available. Your physician can refer you to psychotherapists in your community. Not all therapists are right for all people, so be prepared to have initial sessions with several. Choose the one with whom you feel most comfortable.

- Job-related stress is common, particularly for employees who have little control over decisions relating to their jobs. If stress is severe or prolonged, burnout may occur.

- New and changing relationships, prejudice, and discrimination are examples of interpersonal and social stressors.

- Social support systems help buffer people against the effects of stress and make illness less likely. Good communication skills foster healthy relationships.

- Exercise, nutrition, sleep, and time management are wellness behaviors that reduce stress and increase energy.

- Developing new and healthy patterns of thinking, such as practicing problem solving, monitoring self-talk, and cultivating a sense of humor, is important for coping with stress.

- Body awareness techniques and biofeedback are useful for some people.

- Along with exercise and good nutrition, good sleep is a critical pillar of good health.

- Additional help in dealing with stress is available from self-help books, peer counseling, support groups, and psychotherapy.

SUMMARY

- When confronted with a stressor, the body undergoes a set of physical changes known as the fight, flight, or freeze reaction. The autonomic nervous system and endocrine system act on many targets in the body to prepare it for action.

- Emotional and behavioral responses to stressors vary among individuals. Ineffective responses increase stress but can be moderated or changed.

- Factors that influence emotional and behavioral responses to stressors include personality, cultural background, gender, and past experiences.

- The general adaptation syndrome (GAS) has three stages: alarm, resistance, and exhaustion.

- A high allostatic load characterized by prolonged or repeated exposure to stress hormones can increase a person's risk of health problems.

- Psychoneuroimmunology (PNI) looks at how the physiological changes of the stress response affect the immune system and thereby increase the risk of illness.

- Health problems linked to stress include cardiovascular disease, colds and other infections, asthma and allergies, flare-ups of chronic diseases, psychological problems, digestive problems, headaches, insomnia, and injuries.

- A cluster of major life events that require adjustment and accommodation can lead to increased stress and an increased risk of health problems. Minor daily hassles increase stress if they are perceived negatively.

- Sources of stress associated with college may be academic, interpersonal, time related, or financial pressures.

FOR MORE INFORMATION

American Headache Society. Provides information for consumers and clinicians about different types of headaches, their causes, and their treatment.

http://www.americanheadachesociety.org

American Psychiatric Association: Healthy Minds, Healthy Lives. Provides information about mental wellness developed especially for college students.

http://www.psychiatry.org/news-room/apa-blogs

American Psychological Association. Provides information about stress management and psychological disorders.

http://www.apa.org

http://www.apa.org/helpcenter

Association for Applied Psychophysiology and Biofeedback. Provides information about biofeedback and referrals to certified biofeedback practitioners.

http://www.aapb.org

Benson-Henry Institute for Mind Body Medicine. Provides information about stress management and relaxation techniques.

http://www.massgeneral.org

Center for Mindfulness in Medicine, Health Care, and Society (U Mass Medical School). Provides information about mindfulness-based stress reduction (MBSR) professional training, research, and resources.

http://www.umassmed.edu/cfm/

National Institute of Mental Health (NIMH). Publishes brochures about stress and stress management as well as other aspects of mental health.

http://www.nimh.nih.gov

Spirit Rock Meditation Center. A resource for meditation retreats and education in mindfulness meditation.

http://www.spiritrock.org

Do you perform as well as you should on tests? Does anxiety interfere with your ability to study effectively before a test and to think clearly in the test situation? If so, you may be experiencing test anxiety. Two effective methods can help you deal with test anxiety: systematic desensitization and success rehearsal.

Systematic Desensitization

Systematic desensitization is based on the premise that you can't feel anxiety and be relaxed at the same time.

Phase I: Constructing an Anxiety Hierarchy

Begin the first phase by thinking of 10 or more situations related to your fear, such as hearing the announcement of the test date in class, studying for the test, reading the test questions, and so on. Write each situation on an index card. On the other side, list several realistic details or prompts that will help you vividly imagine yourself actually experiencing the situation. For example, if the situation is "hearing that 50% of the final grade will be based on the two exams," the prompts might include details such as "sitting in the big lecture auditorium in Baily Hall," "taking notes in my blue notebook," and "listening to Professor Smith's voice."

Next arrange your cards in order, from least tense to most tense situation. Rate each situation on a scale of 0–100, and make sure the distances between items are fairly small and about equal. When you're sure your anxiety hierarchy is a true reflection of your feelings, number the cards.

Phase II: Learning and Practicing Muscle Relaxation

The second phase of the program involves learning to relax your muscles and to recognize when they are relaxed (see the description of progressive relaxation in this chapter). As you become proficient at this technique, you'll be able to go into a deeply relaxed state within just a few minutes. When you can do this, go on to the next phase of the program.

Phase III: Implementing the Desensitization Program

Use the quiet place where you practiced your relaxation exercises. Sit comfortably and take several minutes to relax completely, and then look at the first card, reading both the brief phrase and the descriptive prompts. Close your eyes and imagine yourself in that situation for about 10 seconds. Then put the card down and relax completely for about 30 seconds. Look at the card again, imagine the situation for 10 seconds, and relax again for 30 seconds.

At this point, evaluate your current level of anxiety about the situation on the card in terms of the rating scale you devised earlier. If your anxiety level is 10 or below, relax for two minutes and go on to the second card. If it's higher than 10, repeat the routine with the same card until the anxiety decreases.

If you have difficulty with a particular item, go back to the previous item and try it again. If you still can't visualize it without anxiety, try to construct three new items with smaller steps between them and insert them before the troublesome item.

You should be able to move through one to four items per session.

Sessions can be conducted from twice a day to twice a week and should last no longer than 20 minutes. It's helpful to graph your progress in a way that has meaning for you.

After you have successfully completed your program, you should be desensitized to the real-life situations that previously caused anxiety. If you find that you experience some anxiety in the real situations, take 30 seconds or a minute to relax completely, just as you did when you were practicing.

SUCCESS REHEARSAL

To practice this variation on systematic desensitization, take your hierarchy of anxiety-producing situations and vividly imagine yourself successfully dealing with each one. Create a detailed scenario for each situation, and use your imagination to experience genuine feelings of confidence. Recognize your negative thoughts ("I'll be so nervous I won't be able to think straight") and replace them with positive ones ("Anxiety will keep me alert so I can do a good job").

Proceed one step at a time, thinking as you go of strategies for success that you can later implement. These might include the following:

- Before the test, find out everything you can about it—its format, the material to be covered, the grading criteria. Ask the instructor for practice materials. Study in advance; don't just cram the night before. Avoid all-nighters.

- Devise a study plan. This might include forming a study group with one or more classmates or outlining what you will study, when, where, and for how long. Generate your own questions and answer them.

  - In the actual test situation, sit away from possible distractions, listen carefully to instructions, and ask for clarification if you don't understand a direction.

  - During the test, answer the easiest questions first. If you don't know an answer and there is no penalty for incorrect answers, guess. If there are several questions you have difficulty answering, review the ones you have already handled. Figure out approximately how much time you have to cover each question.

  - For true-false questions, look for qualifiers such as *always* and *never.* Such questions are likely to be false.

- Avoid worrying about past performance, how others are doing, or the negative consequences of a poor test grade. If you start to become nervous, take some deep breaths and relax your muscles completely for a minute or so.

The best way to counter test anxiety is with successful test-taking experiences. If you find that these methods aren't sufficient to get your anxiety under control, you may want to seek professional help.

American College Health Association. 2019. *American College Health Association-National College Health Assessment II: Reference Group Executive Summary Spring 2019*. Hanover, MD: American College Health Association.

American Psychological Association. 2017. *Stress in America: Coping with Change*. Washington, DC: American Psychological Association.

American Psychological Association. 2017. *Stress in America: The State of Our Nation*. Washington, DC: American Psychological Association.

American Psychological Association. 2018. *Stress in America: Generation Z*. Washington, DC: American Psychological Association (https://www.apa.org/news/press/releases/2018/stress-gen-z.pdf).

American Psychological Association. 2019. *Stress in America 2019*. Washington, DC: American Psychological Association (https://www.apa.org/news/press/releases/stress/2019/stress-america-2019.pdf).

American Psychological Association. 2020. *Stress in America: Stress in the Time of COVID-19*. Volume 1. Washington, DC: American Psychological Association (https://www.apa.org/news/press/releases/stress/2020/stress-in-america-covid.pdf).

Bartolomucci, A., and R. Leopardi. 2009. Stress and depression: Preclinical research and clinical implications. *PLoS One* 4(1): e4265.

Bellezza, S., N. Paharia, and A. Keinan. 2017. Conspicuous consumption of time: When busyness and lack of leisure time become a status symbol. *Journal of Consumer Research* 44(1): 118–138.

Burch, R. C., et al. 2015. The prevalence and burden of migraine and severe headache in the United States: Updated statistics from government health surveillance studies. *Headache* 55(1): 21–34.

Caldwell, K., et al. 2010. Developing mindfulness in college students through movement-based courses: Effects on self-regulatory self-efficacy, mood, stress, and sleep quality. *Journal of American College Health* 58(5): 433–442.

Center for Collegiate Mental Health. 2019. *2018 Annual Report* STA: 19–180.

Centers for Disease Control and Prevention. 2019. *Coping with a Disaster or Traumatic Event: Information for Individuals and Families* (http://emergency.cdc.gov/mentalhealth/general.asp).

Dallman, M. 2010. Stress-induced obesity and the emotional nervous system. *Trends in Endocrinology and Metabolism* 21(3): 159–165.

Darabaneanu, S. 2011. Aerobic exercise as a therapy option for migraine: A pilot study. *International Journal of Sports Medicine* 32(6): 455–460.

Davidson, R., and S. Begley. 2012. *The Emotional Life of Your Brain*. New York: Penguin.

Eisenberg, D., et al. 2016. Too distressed to learn? Mental health among community college students. *Wisconsin HOPE Lab*, March: 1–15.

Flory, E. S. 2019. Student stress surges: Community colleges strive to meet the increasing demand for mental health services nationwide. *Community College Journal*, August/September (https://www.ccjournal-digital.com/ccjournal/august_september_2019?pg=1#pg1).

Flugel Colle, K. F., et al. 2010. Measurement of quality of life and participant experience with the mindfulness-based stress reduction program. *Complementary Therapies in Clinical Practice* 16(1): 36–40.

Foureur, M., et al. 2013. Enhancing the resilience of nurses and midwives: Pilot of a mindfulness-based program for increased health, sense of coherence and decreased depression, anxiety and stress. *Contemporary Nurse* 45: 114–125.

Fox, S., and M. Duggan. 2013. *The Diagnosis Difference. Pew Research Internet Project* (http://www.pewinternet.org/2013/11/26/the-diagnosis-difference/).

Germer, C., R. Siegel, and P. Fulton. 2005. *Mindfulness and Psychotherapy*. New York: Guilford.

Hagenaars, M. A., M. Oitzl, and K. Roelofsa. 2014. Updating freeze: Aligning animal and human research. *Neuroscience & Biobehavioral Reviews* 47: 165–176.

Hefner, J., and D. Eisenberg. 2009. Social support and mental health among college students. *American Journal of Orthopsychiatry* 79(4): 491–499.

Hensle, A. M., et al. 2015. Religious coping and psychological and behavioral adjustment after Hurricane Katrina. *Journal of Psychology* 149(6): 630–642.

Hinkelman, L. 2017. *The Girls' Index: New Insights Into the Complex World of Today's Girls*. Columbus, OH: Ruling Our Experiences, Inc.

Hölzel, B. K., et al. 2010. Stress reduction correlates with structural changes in the amygdala. *Social Cognitive and Affective Neuroscience* 5(1): 11–17.

Hook, J. N., et al. 2010. Empirically supported religious and spiritual therapies. *Journal of Clinical Psychology* 66(1): 46–72.

Jayson, S. 2013. Who's feeling stressed? *USA Today*, February 7.

Kabat-Zinn, J. 2011. *Mindfulness for Beginners: Reclaiming the Present Moment—and Your Life*. Louisville, CO: Sounds True.

Kemeny, M. 2012. Contemplative/emotion training reduces negative emotional behavior and promotes prosocial responses. *Emoticon* [1528–3542] (12): 338–350.

Kim, B. 2014. *How the Body Works: Overview of the Nervous and Endocrine Systems* (http://drbenkim.com/nervous-endocrine-system.htm).

Manzoni, G. C., et al. 2016. Age of onset of episodic and chronic cluster headache—a review of a large case series from a single headache centre. *Journal of Headache Pain* 17: 44.

Marsh, I. C., S. W. Y. Chan, and A. MacBeth. 2018. Self-compassion and psychological distress in adolescents—a meta-analysis. *Mindfulness* 9: 1011–1027.

McGonigal, K. 2015. *The Upside of Stress*. New York: Penguin Random House.

Neff, K. D., and C. K. Germer. 2013. A pilot study and randomized controlled trial of the mindful self-compassion program. *Journal of Clinical Psychology* 69: 28–44.

Nordboe, D. J., et al. 2007. Immediate behavioral health response to the Virginia Tech shootings. *Disaster Medicine and Public Health Preparedness* 1(Suppl. 1): S31–S32.

Roddenberry, A., and K. Renk. 2010. Locus of control and self-efficacy: Potential mediators of stress, illness, and utilization of health services in college students. *Child Psychiatry and Human Development* 41(4): 353–370.

Roelofs, K. 2017. Freeze for action: Neurobiological mechanisms in animal and human freezing. *Philosophical Transactions of the Royal Society of London. Series B, Biological Sciences*, 372(1718): 20160206.

Schulte, Brigid. 2014. *Overwhelmed: Work, Love, and Play When No One Has the Time*. New York: Sarah Crichton Books.

Schwartz, G. E. 1979. Biofeedback and the behavioral treatment of disorders of disregulation. *Yale Journal of Biology and Medicine* 52(6): 581–596.

Seaward, B. L. 2018. *Managing Stress: Principles and Strategies for Health and Well-Being*. 9th ed. Burlington, MA: Jones & Bartlett Learning.

Segerstrom, S., and D. Hodgson, eds. 2019. Psychoneuroimmunology [Special Edition]. *Current Opinion in Behavioral Sciences* 28: 1–162.

Shapiro, S. L., and L. E. Carlson. 2009. *The Art and Science of Mindfulness: Integrating Mindfulness into Psychology and the Helping Professions*. Washington, DC: American Psychological Association.

Simmons, R. 2018. *Enough As She Is: How to Help Girls Move Beyond Impossible Standards of Success and Live Healthy, Happy and Fulfilling Lives*. New York: HarperCollins.

Southwick, S. M., and D. S. Charney. 2012. *Resilience: The Science of Mastering Life's Greatest Challenges*. Cambridge, UK: Cambridge University Press.

Substance Abuse and Mental Health Services Administration. 2019. *Key Substance Use and Mental Health Indicators in the United States: Results from the 2018 National Survey on Drug Use and Health* (HHS Publication No. PEP19-5068, NSDUH Series H-54). (http://www.samhsa.gov/data).

Taylor, S., et al. 2020. Development and initial validation of the COVID Stress Scales. *Journal of Anxiety Disorders* 72: 102232.

Telles, S., et al. 2009. Effect of a yoga practice session and a yoga theory session on state anxiety. *Perceptual and Motor Skills* 109(3): 924–930.

U.S. Department of Health and Human Services, National Institutes of Health. 2012. *Stress* (http://www.nlm.nih.gov/medlineplus/stress.html).

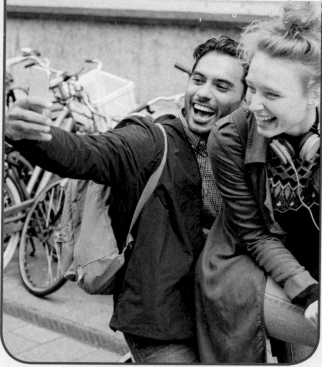
Hoxton/Sam Edwards/Getty Images

CHAPTER OBJECTIVES

- Describe what it means to be psychologically healthy
- Discuss psychological approaches you can use to face life's challenges with a positive self-concept
- Describe common psychological disorders
- Recognize the warning signs, risk factors, and protective factors related to suicide
- Summarize the models of human nature on which therapies are based
- Describe the types of help available for psychological problems

CHAPTER **3**

Psychological Health

TEST YOUR KNOWLEDGE

1. **Normality is a key component of psychological health.**
   True or False?

2. **Trying to think rationally about what bothers you won't get you very far because psychological problems are usually due to emotions, not thinking.**
   True or False?

3. **About how many American adults have a diagnosable psychological disorder during the course of a year?**
   a. 9%
   b. 19%
   c. 29%

4. **People with enough willpower can force themselves to snap out of their depression.**
   True or False?

5. **A person who attempts suicide but survives did not really intend to die.**
   True or False?

ANSWERS

1. **FALSE.** Normality simply means being close to average, and having unusual ideas or attitudes doesn't mean that a person is mentally ill.

2. **FALSE.** Research has shown that getting people to adopt more realistic attitudes and beliefs about themselves and others can alleviate depression.

3. **B.** About 46.5 million or 19% of U.S. adults have a mental illness not including substance abuse problems. The most common types of disorders are simple phobias and depression. The majority of people with psychological disorders do not receive appropriate treatment.

4. **FALSE.** Depression, a disorder strongly linked to brain chemistry, can overcome whatever willpower a person has and make it impossible for her or him to make decisions.

5. **FALSE.** A person may intend to die but miscalculate how to succeed in the attempt.

P sychological health contributes to every dimension of wellness. It can be difficult to maintain emotional, social, or even physical wellness if you are not psychologically healthy.

Psychological health, however, is a broad concept—one that is as difficult to define as it is important to understand. That is why the first section of this chapter is devoted to explaining what psychological health is. The rest of the chapter discusses a number of common psychological problems (including mental illnesses), their symptoms, and their treatments.

DEFINING PSYCHOLOGICAL HEALTH

Psychological health (or *mental health*) can be defined either negatively, as the absence of sickness, or positively, as the presence of wellness. The vast majority of people do not suffer from mental illness, yet all of us have to deal with stress, interpersonal conflicts, and difficult emotions. Psychological health refers to the extent to which we are able to function optimally in the face of these challenges, whether or not we have a mental illness.

Positive Psychology

In his book *Toward a Psychology of Being,* psychologist Abraham Maslow adopted a perspective that he called "positive psychology." Maslow developed a *hierarchy of needs* (Figure 3.1): The most important kind is the satisfaction of physiological needs; following this is a feeling of safety, a state of being loved, maintenance of self-esteem, and finally, self-actualization.

When urgent (life-sustaining) needs—such as the need for food and water—are satisfied, less basic needs take priority. Maslow's conclusions were based on his study of a group of visibly successful people who seemed to have lived, or to be living, at their fullest. He suggested that these people had fulfilled a good measure of their human potential and achieved **self-actualization.** Self-actualized people all share certain qualities:

- *Realism.* Self-actualized people know the difference between what is real and what they want. As a result, they can

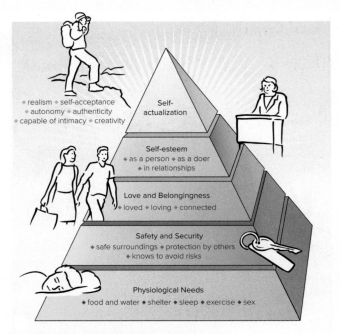

FIGURE 3.1 **Maslow's hierarchy of needs.**
SOURCE: Maslow, A. 1970. *Motivation and Personality,* 2nd ed. New York: Harper & Row.

cope with the world as it exists without demanding that it be different; they know what they can and cannot change. Just as important, realistic people accept evidence that contradicts what they want to believe.

- *Acceptance.* Self-accepting people have a positive but realistic **self-concept,** or *self-image.* They typically feel satisfaction and confidence in themselves, and thus they have healthy **self-esteem.** Self-acceptance also means being tolerant of your own imperfections—an ability that makes it easier to accept the imperfections of others.

- *Autonomy.* *Autonomous* people can direct themselves, acting independently of their social environment. **Autonomy** is more than physical independence. It is social, emotional, and intellectual independence, as well.

- *Authenticity.* Self-actualized people are not afraid to be themselves. Sometimes, in fact, their capacity for being "real" may give them a certain childlike quality. They respond in a genuine, or *authentic,* spontaneous way to whatever happens, without pretense or self-consciousness.

- *Capacity for intimacy.* People capable of intimacy can share their feelings and thoughts without fear of rejection. They are open to the pleasure of physical contact and the satisfaction of being close to others—but without being afraid of the risks involved in intimacy, such as the possibility of rejection. (Chapters 5 and 6 discuss intimacy in more detail.)

- *Creativity.* Creative people continually look at the world with renewed appreciation and curiosity. Such buoyancy can enhance creativity.

TERMS

psychological health Mental health, defined as the extent to which we are able to function optimally in the face of challenges, whether we have a mental illness or not.

self-actualization The highest level of growth in Maslow's hierarchy of needs.

self-concept The ideas, feelings, and perceptions a person has about himself or herself; also called *self-image.*

self-esteem Satisfaction and confidence in yourself; the valuing of yourself as a person.

autonomy Independence; the sense of being self-directed.

Self-actualization is an ideal to strive for rather than something most people can reasonably hope to achieve. Maslow believed it was rarely achieved. An additional adjustment we might make to Maslow's model is that it is more fluid than originally conceived: Studies have found that social reputation is so important that people will risk their safety and instead prioritize their sense of belonging when they choose to perform a disgusting or painful task rather than have negative information about them made public. For example, in one study, participants took a test that (falsely) identified them as racist. Most people opted to fully submerge their hands in a bucket of live worms or near-freezing water to stop their scores from being published. Still, Maslow's pyramid offers a model for goals to work for, whether we strive for a personal target or consider welfare policies that protect others' needs.

Influenced by the work of Abraham Maslow, psychologist Martin Seligman suggests that the goal of **positive psychology** is "to find and nurture genius and talent" and "to make normal life more fulfilling" rather than just to identify and treat illness. In other words, it means being able to define positive goals and identify concrete, measurable ways of achieving them.

According to Seligman, happiness can come to us through three equally valid dimensions:

- *The pleasant life.* This life is dedicated to maximizing positive **emotions** about the past, present, and future, and to minimizing pain and negative emotions.

- *The engaged life.* This life involves cultivating positive personality traits (such as courage, leadership, kindness, and integrity) and actively using your talents. "Engagement" also involves cultivating a capacity to "live in the moment" and immerse yourself fully in your activities.

A key to being engaged and successful in life is the positive personality trait of **emotional intelligence.** An emotionally intelligent person can identify and manage his or her own emotions and respond to the emotions of others. Psychologists and educators believe that emotional intelligence is not as rooted as abstract intelligence and that it can be learned.

- *The meaningful life.* Another road to happiness entails working with others toward a meaningful end. Many people find meaning in their connections with and service to families, friends, religious institutions, social causes, and/or work. The happiness to be found by following this path is strongest when meaning comes from more than one source.

Not everyone accepts the ideas of positive psychology—or even the concept of psychological health—because they involve value judgments that are inconsistent with psychology's scientific status. Defining psychological health requires making assumptions and value judgments about what human goals are desirable, and some people think these are matters for religion or philosophy. Positive psychology has also been criticized as promoting a shortsighted denial of reality and unwarranted optimism. In particular, therapists guided by existential philosophy believe that psychological health comes from acknowledging and accepting the painful realities of life.

What Psychological Health Is Not

We can define normal body temperature because a few degrees above or below this temperature means physical sickness, but we cannot measure psychological health this way. Your ideas and attitudes can vary tremendously without

QUICK STATS

20% of U.S. adults experience mental illness.
—National Alliance on Mental Illness, 2020

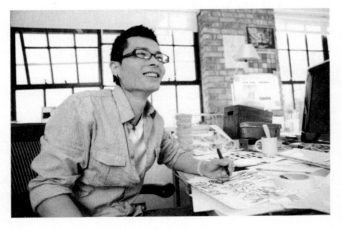

You can develop happiness in any number of ways. The keys are to focus on work and activities you enjoy and to develop a supportive network of friends and family. Ciaran Griffin/Lifesize/Getty Images

TERMS

positive psychology   The ability to define positive goals and to identify concrete, measurable ways of achieving them.

emotion   A feeling state involving some combination of thoughts, physiological changes, and an outward expression or behavior.

emotional intelligence   The capacity to identify and manage your own emotions and, where possible, the emotions of others.

impeding your ability to function well or causing you to feel emotional distress. Moreover, psychological diversity—the understanding, acceptance, and respect for how much individuals differ in psychological terms—is actually a valuable asset; encountering a wide range of ideas, lifestyles, and attitudes broadens our perspectives and helps us solve problems of the social world. Psychological health does not mean being "normal": What is considered healthy for one person may be quite different for someone else.

Seeking help for personal problems does not prove someone is psychologically unhealthy or mentally ill. Unhappy—and unhealthy—people may avoid seeking help for many reasons, and severely disturbed people may not even realize they need help.

Further, we can't say people are "mentally ill" or "mentally healthy" based solely on the presence or absence of symptoms. Consider the symptom of anxiety, for example. Anxiety can help you face a problem and solve it before it becomes too big. Someone who shows no anxiety may be refusing to recognize problems or to do anything about them. A person who is anxious for good reason may be more psychologically healthy in the long run than someone who is inappropriately calm.

Finally, we cannot judge psychological health from the way people look. All too often, a person who seems to be okay and even happy suddenly takes his or her own life. At an early age, we learn to conceal our feelings and even to lie about them. We may believe that our complaints put unfair demands on others. Although maintaining privacy about emotional pain may seem to be a virtue, it can also be an impediment to getting help.

MEETING LIFE'S CHALLENGES WITH A POSITIVE SELF-CONCEPT

Life is full of challenges—large and small. Everyone, regardless of heredity and family influences, must learn to cope successfully with new situations and new people. For emotional and mental wellness, each of us must continue to cultivate an adult identity that enhances our self-esteem and autonomy. We must also learn to communicate honestly, handle anger and loneliness appropriately, and avoid being defensive.

Growing Up Psychologically

Our responses to life's challenges influence the development of our personality and identity. Psychologist Erik Erikson proposed that development proceeds through a series of eight stages that extend throughout life. Each stage is characterized by a conflict or turning point—a time of increased vulnerability as well as increased potential for psychological growth (Table 3.1).

The successful mastery of one stage is a basis for mastering the next, so early failures can have repercussions in later life. Fortunately, life provides ongoing opportunities for mastering these tasks. For example, although the development of trust begins in infancy, it is refined as we grow older. We learn to trust some people outside our immediate family and to identify others as untrustworthy.

Developing a Unified Sense of Self   The development of an adult identity begins in adolescence; this unified sense of self can be seen in the attitudes, beliefs, and ways of

Table 3.1	Erikson's Stages of Development

AGE	CONFLICT	IMPORTANT PEOPLE	TASK
Birth–1 year	Trust vs. mistrust	Mother, father, or other primary caregiver	In being fed and comforted, developing the trust that others will respond to your needs
1–3 years	Autonomy vs. shame and self-doubt	Parents	In toilet training, locomotion, and exploration, learning self-control without losing the capacity for assertiveness
3–6 years	Initiative vs. guilt	Family	In playful talking and locomotion, developing a conscience based on parental prohibitions that are not too inhibiting
6–12 years	Industry vs. inferiority	Neighborhood and school	In school and playing with peers, learning the value of accomplishment and perseverance without feeling inadequate
Adolescence	Identity vs. identity confusion	Peers	Developing a stable sense of who you are—your needs, abilities, interpersonal style, and values
Young adulthood	Intimacy vs. isolation	Close friends, sex partners	Learning to live and share intimately with others, often in sexual relationships
Middle adulthood	Generativity vs. self-absorption	Work associates, children, community	Doing things for others, including parenting and civic activities
Older adulthood	Integrity vs. despair	Humankind	Affirming the value of life and its ideals

SOURCE: Erikson, E. 1963. *Childhood and Society.* New York: Norton.

acting that are genuinely your own. To know who you are, what you are capable of, what roles you play, and your place among your peers gives you a voice to respond to ambiguous situations. This self-identification gives a sense of your uniqueness but also appreciation for what you have in common with others. It lets you view yourself realistically and be able to assess your strengths and weaknesses without relying on the opinions of others. Identifying with some core traits also means that you can form intimate relationships with others while maintaining a strong sense of self.

Still, identity does not develop by itself. Our identities evolve as we interact with the world and make choices about what we'd like to do and whom we'd like to model ourselves after. We all experiment with different self-representations as we proceed through adolescence. We show different sides of ourselves, not just as we pass through different ages, but also from one day to the next, depending on whom we're with or the environment we're in.

Early identities are often modeled after parents and adult caregivers—or they are modeled after the opposite of parents, in rebellion against what they represent. Over time, peers, celebrities, athletes, and religious figures are added to the list of possible role models. In high school and college, people often join cliques that assert a certain identity, such as "jocks," "nerds," or "hipsters." Although much of our identity is internal—a way of viewing ourselves and the world—certain aspects of it can be external, in terms of the way we express ourselves through styles of talking and dressing, and in terms of the names given to us by other people.

Early identities are rarely permanent. A hardworking student seeking approval one year can turn into a dropout devoted to sleeping all day and partying all night the next year. At some point, however, most of us adopt a more stable, individual set of identities that ties together the experiences of childhood and the expectations and aspirations of adulthood. A unified sense of self reflects a lifelong process, and it changes as a person develops new relationships and roles.

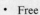

Ask Yourself

QUESTIONS FOR CRITICAL THINKING AND REFLECTION

Write down times when you felt

- Free
- Aloof
- Angry
- Generous
- Happy
- Talkative

For each moment you recall, whom were you with when you felt those ways? What had recently happened in your life? Where were you? Did you feel most "yourself" in any of those moments? Which?

Developing Values and Purpose in Your Life Erikson assigned his last two stages, *generativity versus self-absorption* and *integrity versus despair,* to middle adulthood and older adulthood, respectively. But these stages concern values that need to be addressed by young people and reexamined throughout life.

Values are criteria for judging what is good and bad, and they underlie our moral decisions and behavior. The first morality of the young child is to consider "good" to mean what brings immediate and tangible rewards, and "bad" to mean whatever results in punishment. An older child will explain right and wrong in terms of authority figures and rules. But the final stage of moral development, one that not everyone attains, is being able to conceive of right and wrong in more abstract terms such as justice and virtue.

As adults we need to assess how far we have evolved morally and what values we have adopted. Without an awareness of our personal values, our lives may be hurriedly driven forward by immediate desires and the passing demands of others. Living according to values means

- Considering your options carefully before making a choice
- Choosing among options without succumbing to outside pressures that conflict with your values
- Making a choice and acting on it rather than doing nothing

Your actions and how you justify them proclaim to others what you stand for.

Achieving Healthy Self-Esteem

Having a healthy level of self-esteem means regarding yourself—which includes all aspects of your identity—as good, competent, and worthy of love. It is a critical component of wellness.

Developing a Positive Self-Concept Ideally a positive self-concept begins in childhood, based on experiences both within the family and outside it. Children need to develop a sense of being loved and being able to give love and to accomplish their goals. If they feel rejected or neglected by their parents, they may fail to develop feelings of self-worth. They may grow to have a negative concept of themselves.

Another component of self-concept is *integration*. An integrated self-concept is one that you have made for yourself—not someone else's image of you or a mask that doesn't quite fit. Important building blocks of self-concept are the personality characteristics and mannerisms of parents, which children may adopt without realizing it. Later they may be surprised to find themselves acting like one of their parents.

values Criteria for judging what is good and bad, which underlie an individual's moral decisions and behavior. **TERMS**

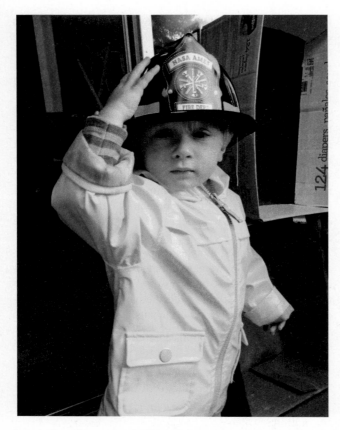

A positive self-concept begins early. The knowledge that he's loved and valued by his parents gives this toddler a solid basis for lifelong psychological health. Claire Insel

Eventually such building blocks may be reshaped and integrated into a new, individual personality.

Another aspect of self-concept is *stability*. Stability depends on the integration of the self and its freedom from contradictions. People who have gotten mixed messages about themselves from parents and friends may have contradictory self-images, which defy integration and make them vulnerable to shifting levels of self-esteem. At times they regard themselves as entirely good, capable, and lovable—an ideal self—and at other times they see themselves as entirely bad, incompetent, and unworthy of love. Neither of these extreme self-concepts allows people to see themselves or others realistically, and their relationships with other people are filled with misunderstandings and ultimately with conflict.

Meeting Challenges to Self-Esteem As an adult, you sometimes run into situations that challenge your self-concept. People you care about may tell you they don't love

you or feel loved by you, for example, or your attempts to accomplish a goal may end in failure.

You can react to such challenges in several ways. The best approach is to acknowledge that something has gone wrong and try again, adjusting your goals to your abilities without radically revising your self-concept. Less productive responses are denying that anything went wrong and blaming someone else. These attitudes may preserve your self-concept temporarily, but in the long run they keep you from meeting the challenge.

The worst reaction is to develop a lasting negative self-concept in which you feel bad, unloved, and ineffective—in other words, to become demoralized. Instead of coping, the demoralized person gives up (at least temporarily), reinforcing the negative self-concept and setting in motion a cycle of bad self-concept and failure. In people who are genetically predisposed to depression, demoralization can progress to additional symptoms, which are discussed later in the chapter.

NOTICE YOUR PATTERNS OF THINKING One method for fighting demoralization is to recognize and test the negative thoughts and assumptions you may have about yourself and others. Note exactly when an unpleasant emotion—feeling worthless, wanting to give up, feeling depressed—occurs or gets worse, to identify the events or daydreams that trigger that emotion, and to observe whatever thoughts come into your head just before or during the emotional experience. Keep a daily journal about such events.

AVOID FOCUSING ON THE NEGATIVE Imagine that you are waiting for a friend to meet you for dinner, but he's 30 minutes late. What kinds of thoughts go through your head? You might wonder what caused the delay: Perhaps he is stuck in traffic, you think, or needs to help a roommate who has the flu. This kind of reaction is healthy for several reasons:

• You aren't jumping to a conclusion or blaming your friend for a failure.

• You are being reasonable by giving your friend the benefit of the doubt.

• You avoid personalizing the situation in such a way that you feel hurt or betrayed.

By contrast, people who are demoralized tend to use all-or-nothing thinking. They overgeneralize from negative events. They overlook the positive and make negative assumptions, minimizing their own successes and magnifying the successes of others. They take responsibility for unfortunate situations that are not their fault, then jump to more negative conclusions and more unfounded overgeneralizations. Patterns of thinking that make events seem worse than they are in reality are called **cognitive distortions.**

DEVELOP REALISTIC SELF-TALK When you react to a situation, an important piece of that reaction is your **self-talk**—the statements you make to yourself inside your own mind. To pick up on our earlier example, suppose your friend is late for a dinner date. As you wait for your friend to arrive, your self-talk has a profound effect on your reaction to his lateness.

Do your patterns of thinking make events seem worse than they truly are? Substituting realistic self-talk for negative self-talk can help you build and maintain self-esteem and cope better with the challenges in your life. Here are examples of common types of distorted, negative self-talk, along with suggestions for more accurate and rational responses:

COGNITIVE DISTORTION	NEGATIVE SELF-TALK	REALISTIC SELF-TALK
Focusing on negatives	Babysitting is such a pain in the neck; I wish I didn't need the extra money so badly.	This is a tough job, but at least the money's decent and I can study once the kids go to bed.
Expecting the worst	I know I'm going to get an F in this course. I should just drop out of school now.	I'm not doing too well in this course. I should talk to my professor to see what kind of help I can get.
Overgeneralizing	My hair is a mess and I'm gaining weight. I'm so ugly. No one would ever want to date me.	I could use a haircut and should try to exercise more. This way I'll start feeling better about myself and will be more confident when I meet people.
Minimizing	It was nice of everyone to eat the dinner I cooked, even though I ruined it. I'm such a rotten cook.	Well, the roast was a little dry, but they ate every bite. The veggies and rolls made up for it. I'm finally getting the hang of cooking!
Blaming others	Everyone I meet is such a jerk. Why aren't people friendlier?	I am going to make more of an effort to meet people who share my interests.
Expecting perfection	I cannot believe I flubbed that solo. They probably won't even let me audition for the orchestra next year.	It's a good thing I didn't stop playing when I hit that sour note. It didn't seem like anyone noticed it as much as I did.
Believing you're the cause of everything	Tom and Sara broke up, and it's my fault. I shouldn't have insisted that Tom spend so much time with me and the guys.	It's a shame Tom and Sara broke up. I wish I knew what happened between them. Maybe Tom will tell me at soccer practice. At any rate, it isn't my fault; I've been a good friend to both of them.
Thinking in black and white	I thought that Mike was really cool, but after what he said today, I realize we have nothing in common.	I was really surprised that Mike disagreed with me today. I guess there are still things I don't know about him.
Magnifying events	I stuttered when I was giving my speech today in class. I must have sounded like a complete idiot. I'm sure everyone is talking about it.	My speech went really well, except for that one stutter. I'll bet most people didn't even notice it, though.

Someone who is demoralized or wrestling with a poor self-concept might immediately react with negative self-talk: "He isn't coming. It's my fault; he probably doesn't like me because I'm boring. I bet he's with someone else." In your own fight against demoralization, you may find it hard to think of a rational response until hours or days after the event that upset you. Responding rationally can be especially hard when you are having an argument with someone else, which is why people often say things they don't mean in the heat of the moment or develop hurt feelings even when the other person had no intention of hurting them.

Once you get used to noticing the way your mind works, however, you may be able to catch yourself thinking negatively and change the process before it goes too far. This approach to controlling your reactions is not the same as positive thinking—which means substituting a positive thought for a negative one. Instead you simply try to make your thoughts as logical and accurate as possible, based on the facts of the situation as you know them, and not on snap judgments or conclusions that may turn out to be false.

Demoralized people can be tenacious about their negative beliefs, making them come true in a self-fulfilling prophecy. For example, if you conclude that you are so boring that no one will like you anyway, you may decide not to bother socializing. This behavior could make the negative belief become a reality because you limit your opportunities to meet people and develop new relationships.

For additional tips on changing distorted, negative ways of thinking, see the box "Realistic Self-Talk."

Psychological Defense Mechanisms—Healthy and Unhealthy

We are always trying to manage our feelings, even if we aren't aware we are doing it. We try to manage uncomfortable feelings through what are called psychological defenses. By using defense mechanisms, we change unacceptable feelings (like shame or anger or anxiety) into ones with which we are more comfortable. Table 3.2 lists some standard **defense mechanisms.** Defense mechanisms can be healthy and adaptive—such as humor and altruism—but they can also be maladaptive. For example, it would be maladaptive to displace your anger at your teacher by yelling at your roommates because doing so doesn't help your relationship with your teacher or your roommates. The drawback of many defenses is that they make you feel better temporarily but don't address underlying causes.

Recognizing our own defense mechanisms can be difficult because they occur unconsciously. But we all have some inkling about how our minds operate. By remembering the details of conflict situations, a person may be able to figure out which defense mechanisms she or he used in successful or unsuccessful attempts to cope. Recall a psychologically stressful situation and view yourself as an objective outside observer would; now analyze your thoughts and behavior in that situation. Having insight into what strategies you typically use can lead to new, more rewarding and effective ways of coping.

Being Optimistic

Most of us have a predisposition toward optimism or pessimism. **Pessimism** is a tendency to focus on the negative and expect an unfavorable outcome; **optimism** is a tendency to emphasize the hopeful and expect a favorable outcome. Pessimists not only expect repeated failure and rejection but also accept it as deserved. They do not see themselves as capable of success and irrationally dismiss any evidence of their own accomplishments. This negative point of view is learned, typically at a young age from parents and other authority figures. Optimists, by contrast, consider bad events to be temporary and consider failure to be limited and look forward to new pursuits.

You can learn to be optimistic by recording adverse events in a diary, along with the reactions and beliefs with which you met those events. By doing so, you learn to recognize and dispute the false, negative predictions you generate about yourself, like "The problem is going to last forever and ruin

TERMS

defense mechanism A mental mechanism for coping with conflict or anxiety.

pessimism The tendency to expect an unfavorable outcome.

optimism The tendency to expect a favorable outcome.

Table 3.2	Defense and Coping Mechanisms	
MECHANISM	DESCRIPTION	EXAMPLE
Projection	Reacting to unacceptable impulses by denying their existence in yourself and attributing them to others	A student who dislikes his roommate feels that the roommate dislikes him.
Repression	Keeping an unpleasant feeling, idea, or memory out of awareness	The child of an alcoholic, neglectful father remembers only when her father showed consideration and love.
Denial	Refusing to acknowledge to yourself what you really know to be true	A person believes that smoking cigarettes won't harm her because she's young and healthy.
Displacement	Shifting your feelings about a person to another person	A student who is angry with one of his professors returns home and yells at one of his housemates.
Dissociation	Detaching from a current experience to avoid emotional distress	Rather than listen to his angry father, Beethoven composes a piece in his mind.
Rationalization	Giving a false, acceptable reason when the real reason is unacceptable	A shy young man decides not to attend a dorm party, telling himself he'd be bored.
Reaction formation	Concealing emotions or impulses by exaggerating the opposite ones	A person who dislikes children frequently buys expensive gifts for, and speaks with enthusiasm about, the children of her friends.
Substitution	Replacing an unacceptable or unobtainable goal with an acceptable one	A man in love with an unavailable partner throws himself into training for a marathon.
Acting out	Engaging in an action that makes an unacceptable feeling go away	A person who feels disrespected and devalued gets into a fight at a bar with a stranger.
Humor	Finding something funny in unpleasant situations	A student whose bicycle has been stolen thinks how surprised the thief will be when he or she starts downhill and discovers the brakes don't work.
Altruism	Serving others without expecting anything in return	A person who grew up in an upper-class neighborhood volunteers at a foundation that helps people get out of poverty.

everything, and it's all my fault." Refuting such negative self-talk frees energy for realistic coping.

Maintaining Honest Communication

Another important area of psychological functioning is communicating honestly with others. It can be very frustrating for us and for people around us if we cannot express what we want and feel.

Some people know what they want others to do but don't state it clearly because their request may be denied, which they interpret as personal rejection. Such people might benefit from assertiveness training: learning to insist on their rights and to bargain for what they want. **Assertiveness** includes being able to say no or yes depending on the situation.

Communicating your feelings appropriately and clearly is important. For example, if you tell people you feel sad, they may have various reactions. If they feel close to you, they may express an intimate thought of their own. Or they may feel guilty because they think you're implying they have caused your sadness. They may even be angry because they feel you expect them to cheer you up.

Although keeping your real thoughts and feelings to yourself may help you avoid a confrontation (or even a discussion) with someone, it is unfair because you are not really being clear about what you want.

Finding a Social Media Balance

For many (if not most) young adults, social media platforms are an important part of their social and intellectual lives. There has been concern recently about the relationship between increasing social media use and the development of psychological problems such as depression and anxiety.

Some people believe that social media use can lead to more social interaction and less loneliness, while others believe it can lead to social isolation and psychological harm. Use your own judgment when looking at how much time you spend on the internet. Is social media helping you feel connected? Or left out? Is it widening your community or keeping you from things (like getting together with people—or doing your classwork!)? Everyone needs to find a balance in their social media use for it to be healthy for them.

Dealing with Loneliness

It can be hard to strike the right balance between being alone and being with others. Some people are motivated to socialize out of a fear of being alone. If you discover how to enjoy being by yourself, you'll be better able to cope with periods when you're forced to be alone—for example, when you are no longer in a romantic relationship or when your usual friends are away on vacation.

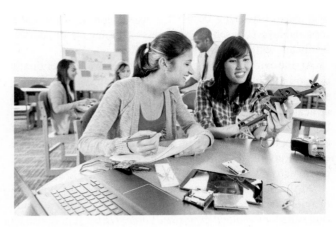

College offers many antidotes to loneliness in the forms of clubs, organized activities, sports, and just hanging out with friends. Steve Debenport/E+/Getty Images

Loneliness may come from feelings of rejection—that others are not interested in spending time with you. Before you reach such a conclusion, be sure that you give others a real chance to get to know you.

Examine your patterns of thinking: You may harbor unrealistic expectations about other people—for example, that everyone you meet must like you and, if they don't, you must be flawed. You might also consider the possibility that you expect too much from new acquaintances, and, sensing this, they start to draw back, triggering feelings of rejection. Not everyone you meet is suitable and willing to have a close or intimate relationship. Feeling pressure to have such a relationship may lead you to connect with someone whose interests and needs are remote from yours or whose need to be cared for leaves you with little time of your own. You may have traded loneliness for potentially worse problems.

Loneliness is a passive feeling state. If you decide that you're not spending enough time with people, change the situation. Decide whether scrolling through your social media feed is a way of avoiding contact with others or enhances your social life. College life provides many opportunities to meet people. If you're shy or introverted, you may have to push yourself to join a group. Look for something you've enjoyed in the past or in which you have a genuine interest.

Dealing with Anger

Anger is a part of the array of normal emotions, yet it is often confusing and difficult to deal with. Some people feel that expressing anger is beneficial for psychological and physical health. However, if angry words or actions damage relationships or produce feelings of guilt or loss of control, they do not contribute to psychological wellness. It is important to

assertiveness   Expression that is forceful but not hostile.   **TERMS**

distinguish between a destructive expression of anger and a reasonable level of self-assertiveness—standing up for yourself firmly but without aggression.

At one extreme are people who never express anger or any opinion that might offend others, even when their own rights and needs are being jeopardized. They may be trapped in unhealthy relationships or chronically deprived of satisfaction at work and at home. If you have trouble expressing your anger, consider training in assertiveness and appropriate expressions of anger to help you learn to express yourself constructively.

At the other extreme are people whose anger is explosive or misdirected—such expression of anger can signal a condition called *intermittent explosive disorder (IED)*. It may also be a symptom of a more serious problem—angry outbursts, for instance, are associated with posttraumatic stress disorder. Explosive anger may also happen during periods of intoxication with alcohol or drugs such as amphetamines or cocaine. Explosive anger or rage, like a child's tantrum, renders an individual temporarily unable to think straight or to act in his or her own best interest. During an IED episode, a person may lash out uncontrollably, hurting someone else physically or verbally, or destroying property. Anyone who expresses anger this way should seek professional help. Some studies have suggested that overtly hostile people seem to be at higher risk for heart attacks.

Managing Your Anger   If you feel explosive anger coming on, consider the following two strategies to head it off. First, try to *reframe* what you're thinking at that moment. You'll be less angry at another person if there is a possibility that his or her behavior was not intentionally directed against you. Imagine that another driver suddenly cuts in front of you. You would certainly be angry if you knew the other driver did it on purpose, but you probably would be less angry if you knew he simply did not see you. If you're angry because you've just been criticized, avoid mentally replaying scenes from the past when you received other unjust criticisms. Think about what is happening now, and try to act differently from how you would have in the past—less defensively and more analytically.

Second, until you're able to change your thinking, try to *distract* yourself. Use the old trick of counting to 10 before you respond, or start concentrating on your breathing. If necessary, cool off by leaving the situation until your anger has subsided. This does not mean that you should permanently avoid the sensitive topics. Return to the matter after you've had a chance to think clearly about it.

Dealing with Anger in Other People   Anger can be infectious, and it disrupts cooperation and communication. If someone you're with becomes very angry, respond "asymmetrically" by reacting not with anger but with calm. Try to

validate the other person by acknowledging that he or she has some reason to be angry: "I totally get that this is making you mad," or "If I were you, I'd be upset, too." This does not mean apologizing if you don't think you're to blame, or accepting verbal abuse. It means that you have considered the other's perspective and that you understand why she might be angry. Finally, if the person cannot be calmed, it may be best to disengage, at least temporarily. After a time-out, you may have better luck trying to solve the problem rationally.

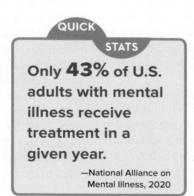

Ask Yourself

QUESTIONS FOR CRITICAL THINKING AND REFLECTION
Think about the last time you were truly angry. What triggered your anger? How did you express it? Do you typically handle your anger in the same manner? How appropriate does your anger-management technique seem?

PSYCHOLOGICAL DISORDERS

All of us have periods when we feel anxious or down or experience irrational or strange thoughts and feelings. These experiences can be normal responses to the ordinary challenges of life, but when emotions or irrational thoughts interfere with daily activities and rob us of peace of mind, they can be considered symptoms of a psychological disorder.

Psychological disorders are generally the result of many factors. Genetics, which underlies differences in how the brain processes information and experiences, are known to play an important role, especially in certain disorders such as autism, schizophrenia, and bipolar disorder. However, exactly which genes are involved, and how they alter the structure and chemistry of the brain, is still under study. A dysfunctional interaction between neurotransmitters and their receptors is associated with some psychiatric disorders (Figure 3.2). The trouble may begin when neurotransmitters (chemicals that transmit messages between nerve cells) misfire and the nerve cells do not communicate properly.

Learning and life events are important, too: Although one identical twin is often at higher risk of having a disorder if the other has it, the two don't necessarily have the same psychological disorders despite having identical genes. Some people have been exposed to more traumatic events than others, leading either to greater vulnerability to future traumas or, conversely, to the development of better coping skills. Further, what your parents, peers, and others have taught you strongly influences your level of self-esteem and how you

QUICK STATS

Only **43%** of U.S. adults with mental illness receive treatment in a given year.

—National Alliance on Mental Illness, 2020

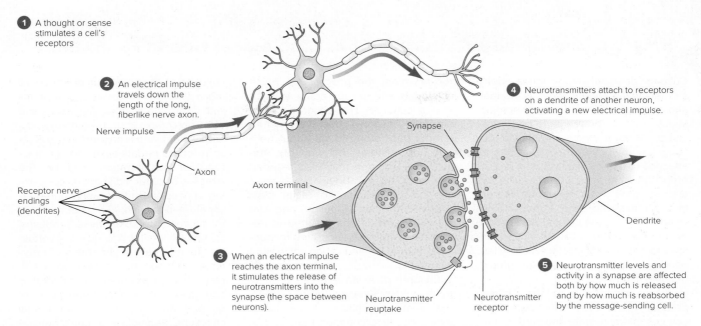

① A thought or sense stimulates a cell's receptors

② An electrical impulse travels down the length of the long, fiberlike nerve axon.

Nerve impulse

Axon

Receptor nerve endings (dendrites)

③ When an electrical impulse reaches the axon terminal, it stimulates the release of neurotransmitters into the synapse (the space between neurons).

Synapse

Axon terminal

Neurotransmitter reuptake

Neurotransmitter receptor

④ Neurotransmitters attach to receptors on a dendrite of another neuron, activating a new electrical impulse.

Dendrite

⑤ Neurotransmitter levels and activity in a synapse are affected both by how much is released and by how much is reabsorbed by the message-sending cell.

FIGURE 3.2 **Nerve cell communication.** Nerve cells (neurons) communicate through a combination of electrical impulses and chemical messages. Neurotransmitters such as serotonin and norepinephrine alter the overall responsiveness of the brain and are responsible for mood, levels of attentiveness, and other psychological states. Many psychological issues are related to problems with neurotransmitters and their receptors, and drug treatments frequently target them. For example, some antidepressant drugs increase levels of serotonin by slowing the resorption (reuptake) of serotonin.

deal with frightening or depressing life events (see the box "Ethnicity, Culture, and Psychological Health").

This section examines some of the more common psychological disorders, including anxiety disorders, mood disorders, and schizophrenia. Table 3.3 shows the likelihood of these disorders occurring during a lifetime.

Anxiety Disorders

Fear is a basic and useful emotion. Its value for our ancestors' survival cannot be overestimated. For modern humans, too, fear motivates us to protect ourselves and to learn how to cope with new or potentially dangerous situations. We consider fear to be a problem only when it is out of proportion to real danger. **Anxiety** is another word for fear, in particular, fear that is not in response to any definite threat. It becomes a disorder when it occurs almost daily or in life situations that recur and cannot be avoided, interfering with your relationships and the ability to function in social and professional situations.

Specific Phobia The most common and understandable anxiety disorder, called **specific phobia,** is a fear of something definite like lightning, a particular type of animal, or a place. Snakes, spiders, and dogs are commonly feared animals; high or enclosed spaces are often frightening places. Sometimes, but not always, these fears originate in bad experiences, such as being bitten by a snake.

Social Anxiety Disorder The 15 million Americans with **social anxiety disorder** (also known as **social phobia**) fear humiliation or embarrassment. Fear of speaking in public

is perhaps the most common phobia of this kind. Extremely shy people can have social fears in almost all social situations; this is in contrast to being introverted, which is not a psychological problem. People with these kinds of fears may not continue in school as far as they could and may restrict themselves to lower-paying jobs in which they do not have to come into contact with new people.

Panic Disorder People with **panic disorder** experience sudden unexpected surges in anxiety, accompanied by symptoms such as rapid and strong heartbeat, shortness of breath, loss of physical equilibrium, and a feeling of losing mental control. Such attacks usually begin in a person's early twenties and can lead to a fear of being in crowds or closed places or of driving or flying. Sufferers fear that a panic attack will occur in a situation from which escape is difficult (in an elevator), where the attack could be incapacitating and result in a dangerous or embarrassing loss of control (driving a car or shopping), or where no medical help would be available

anxiety Fear that is not a response to any definite **TERMS** threat.

specific phobia A persistent and excessive fear of a specific object, activity, or situation.

social anxiety disorder (social phobia) An excessive fear of being observed by others; speaking in public is the most common example.

panic disorder A syndrome of severe anxiety attacks accompanied by physical symptoms.

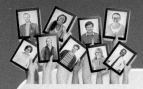

DIVERSITY MATTERS
Ethnicity, Culture, and Psychological Health

Cultures develop unique ideas about mental health—about what is normal and what is problematic, how symptoms should be interpreted and communicated, whether treatment should be sought, and whether a social stigma is attached to a particular symptom or disorder. What happens to these culturally distinct ideas when the group comes into contact with other groups? The United States is the leading destination of international migration. What specific stressors do immigrants face, having left one home for another and having now become minorities?

Asian immigrants to the United States have often come from *collectivist* cultures that anticipate and care for the needs of each other, so that individuals don't need to request support. In U.S. cultures, usually no group is expected to look after the needs of an individual; rather, individuals or their close families are responsible for seeking help for themselves. For this reason Asian immigrants appear to have more trouble than European Americans asking for explicit social support.

A hybrid identity can be greater than the sum of its parts—for example, a Mexican American is now both Mexican and American, both Spanish and English speaking—and this biculturalism can provide more options for healthy living. There is evidence that immigrants who arrive after adolescence tend to experience better mental health than adults who were born in the United States.

Although biculturalism helps bring about better mental health, sometimes younger immigrants and second-generation immigrants may be particularly vulnerable to the effects of *acculturation*, the process by which individuals and groups adapt to each other's cultures. The children of immigrants respond positively when parents pass along ideas about heritage and customs that promote ethnic pride. Children may also respond well to teachings about how to cope with discrimination and racial bias; however, too much focus on negative cultural identities has resulted in depressive symptoms, according to studies of both Asian and Latino children of immigrants.

Children of Asian and Latino immigrants, who collectively make up 77% of all immigrant children in the United States, can face common transcultural stressors, such as economic hardships and living in neighborhoods with fewer resources. Studies have found differences, however, in the ways these groups react to such stressors: Adolescent children of Chinese immigrants tended to internalize their parents' economic hardships by expressing depressive symptoms. The ones who lived in worse neighborhoods externalized, or acted outwardly toward others, through behaviors like bullying and vandalism. These behaviors then eroded positive parenting practices, including spending enough time monitoring the children.

For Mexican American adolescents, neighborhood disadvantage first influenced parenting styles negatively—undermining warm parenting or increasing harsh parenting. This change then led to the adolescents' acting out against others. These negative outcomes could be mitigated when families had more members stepping in to reciprocate responsibilities. Some children of Mexican immigrants were more likely to suffer from problems with depression, substance abuse, and birth outcomes (e.g., prematurity, low birth weight, and teen pregnancy). Reasons for the negative psychological effects of acculturation may be the stresses of cultural disparities concerning concepts of individuality, interpersonal relationships, and what it means to succeed. Despite these problems, second-generation Americans nevertheless tend to have higher rates of insurance coverage and access to health care. Their greater facility with English is correlated with higher frequencies of general physical, vision, and dental checkups. Regardless of one's generation, other factors affect immigrants' health outcomes living in the United States: education, wealth, and occupational and language skills all influence their lifestyles, as well as the policies of the government and attitudes of Americans already here.

SOURCES: Fisher, E. B. 2014. Peer support in health care and prevention: Cultural, organizational, and dissemination issues. *Annual Review of Public Health* 35: 363–383; Kim, S. Y., et al. 2018. Culture's influence on stressors, parental socialization, and developmental processes in the mental health of children of immigrants. *Annual Review of Clinical Psychology* (https://doi .org/10.1146/annurev-clinpsy-050817 -084925); Leyse-Wallace, R. 2013. *Nutrition and Mental Health*. Boca Raton, FL: CRC Press; Brick, K., et al. 2011. *Mexican and Central American Immigrants in the United States*. Washington, DC: Migration Policy Institute; Lara, M., et al. 2005. Acculturation and Latino health in the United States: A review of the literature and its sociopolitical context. *Annual Review of Public Health* 26: 367–397.

TERMS

agoraphobia   An anxiety disorder characterized by fear of being alone away from help and by avoidance of many different places and situations; in extreme cases, a fear of leaving home.

panic attack   A brief surge of overwhelming anxiety that usually resolves in an hour or less.

if needed (alone away from home). These fears can drive avoidance of potentially problematic situations, which may spread until a person is virtually housebound, a condition called **agoraphobia.** People with panic disorder can often function normally in feared situations if they are with someone they trust. Panic disorder is different from an occasional **panic attack,** which affects about 40 million American adults

Table 3.3	Prevalence of Selected Psychological Disorders among Americans

	MEN	WOMEN
DISORDER	LIFETIME PREVALENCE (%)	LIFETIME PREVALENCE (%)
Anxiety disorders*		
Specific phobia	9.9	17.5
Social anxiety disorder	11.8	14.2
Panic disorder	3.3	7.0
Generalized anxiety disorder	4.6	7.7
Obsessive-compulsive disorder	1.8	3.6
Posttraumatic stress disorder	4.0	11.7
Mood disorders		
Major depressive episode	14.7	26.1
Bipolar disorder	2.5	2.5
Manic episode	1.0	1.0
Schizophrenia	3.7	3.4

*Anxiety disorders from the National Comorbidity Survey Replication, based on DSM-IV-TR/CIDI. OCD and PTSD are no longer categorized as anxiety disorders in the DSM-5.

SOURCES: Hasin, D. S., et al. 2018. Epidemiology of adult DSM-5 major depressive disorder and its specifiers in the United States. *JAMA Psychiatry* 75(4): 336–346; Kessler, R. C., et al. Twelve-month and lifetime prevalence and lifetime morbid risk of anxiety and mood disorders in the United States. *International Journal of Methods in Psychiatric Research* 21(3): 169–184; Lee, J., et al. 2017. Bipolar I disorder. Johns Hopkins Psychiatry Guide (https://www .hopkinsguides.com/hopkins/view/Johns_Hopkins_Psychiatry_Guide/787045/all/Bipolar_I_Disorder); McGrath, J., et al. 2008. Schizophrenia: A concise overview of incidence, prevalence, and mortality. *Epidemiologic Reviews* 30: 67–76.

aged 18 and older every year. This occasional attack of overwhelming anxiety may have no obvious cause and usually resolves in an hour or less.

Generalized Anxiety Disorder A basic reaction to future threats is to worry about them. **Generalized anxiety disorder (GAD)** is a diagnosis given to people whose worries about multiple issues linger more than six months. Worries may involve family, other relationships, work, school, money, and health.

The GAD sufferer's worrying is not completely unjustified—after all, thinking about problems can result in solutions. But this kind of thinking often goes around in circles, and the more you try to stop it, the more you feel at its mercy. The end result is a persistent feeling of nervousness, often accompanied by depression.

Obsessive-Compulsive Disorder Someone diagnosed with **obsessive-compulsive disorder (OCD)** struggles with obsessions, compulsions, or both. **Obsessions** are recurrent, unwanted thoughts or impulses. Unlike the worries of GAD, they are not ordinary concerns but improbable fears, like suddenly committing an antisocial act or of having been contaminated by germs.

Compulsions are repetitive, difficult-to-resist urges to act in a certain way, usually associated with obsessions and against one's own wishes. A common compulsion is hand washing, associated with an obsessive fear of contamination by dirt.

QUICK STATS

In the USA, about **10%** of women compared with **4%** of men develop PTSD sometime in their lives.

—U.S. Department of Veterans Affairs, 2019

Other compulsions are counting and repeatedly checking whether something has been done—for example, whether a door has been locked or a stove turned off.

People with OCD feel anxious, out of control, and embarrassed. Their rituals can occupy much of their time and make them inefficient at work and difficult to live with.

Posttraumatic Stress Disorder People who suffer from **posttraumatic stress disorder (PTSD)** are reacting to severely traumatic events (defined as exposure to actual or threatened death, serious injury, or sexual vio-

TERMS

generalized anxiety disorder (GAD) An anxiety disorder characterized by excessive, uncontrollable worry about all kinds of things and anxiety in many situations.

obsessive-compulsive disorder (OCD) An anxiety disorder characterized by uncontrollable, recurring thoughts and the performing of senseless rituals.

obsession A recurrent, irrational, unwanted thought or impulse.

compulsion An irrational, repetitive, forced action, usually associated with an obsession.

posttraumatic stress disorder (PTSD) An anxiety disorder characterized by reliving traumatic events through dreams, flashbacks, and hallucinations.

lence). Trauma occurs in personal assaults (sexual assault, interpersonal violence, military combat), natural disasters (floods, hurricanes), and accidents (fires, airplane or car crashes).

Symptoms include reexperiencing the trauma in dreams and in intrusive memories, trying to avoid anything associated with the trauma, and numbing of feelings. Hyperarousal (being on edge or easily startled), sleep disturbances, and other symptoms of anxiety and depression also commonly occur. Such symptoms can last months or even years. Those whose symptoms have lasted only a month before resolving are considered to have **acute stress disorder.** PTSD symptoms often decrease over time, but up to one-third of PTSD sufferers do not fully recover. Recovery may be slower in those who have previously experienced trauma or who suffer from other ongoing psychological problems.

Treating Anxiety Disorders   Therapies for anxiety disorders range from medication to psychological interventions concentrating on a person's thoughts and behavior. Both drug treatments and cognitive-behavioral therapies are effective in panic disorder, OCD, and GAD. Specific phobias are best treated without drugs.

Attention-Deficit/Hyperactivity Disorder

Attention-deficit/hyperactivity disorder (ADHD) is one of the most common disorders of childhood and adolescence. The main features of ADHD are inattention, hyperactivity, and/or impulsivity. Because these behaviors are normally found in children, attention must be paid to the persistence and severity of the symptoms. They may go misdiagnosed for a time: An impulsive child may be labeled a "discipline problem." An inattentive child may be described as "unmotivated" or "unintelligent." A diagnosis of ADHD is made only if the individual exhibits a persistent pattern of these behaviors; the behaviors must also interfere with the individual's functioning or development, as well as negatively affect school performance, peer relationships, or behavior at home.

Inattention includes failure to pay close attention to details; tendency to make careless mistakes; trouble holding attention; failure to listen when spoken to directly; inability to follow through on or complete a task; avoidance of activities that require sustained effort; and tendency to get easily distracted. *Hyperactivity* and *impulsivity* include a tendency to fidget or squirm; inability to stay seated when expected; inability to play quietly; tendency to be high energy, to talk excessively, and to interrupt others; and inability to wait his or her turn.

To be diagnosed with ADHD, a person must have inattentive or hyperactive-impulsive symptoms of ADHD before age 12 (even if an adult at first diagnosis). There must also be evidence that the ADHD behaviors are present in two or more settings—for example, at home, school or work; with friends and family; and in other activities. Someone who can pay attention at work but is inattentive only at home usually wouldn't qualify for a diagnosis of ADHD. Additionally, it must be clear that the symptoms interfere with or reduce the quality of functioning in social, school, or work settings.

ADHD has no cure, and scientists are still working on treatments. They are using tools such as brain imaging to find ways to prevent it. The use of medications is standard for people who have ADHD and whose functioning is clearly impaired by it; however, medications are considered controversial by some who feel that ADHD is overdiagnosed in people who do not actually have it. Other important treatments include psychotherapy, education and training, and a combination of treatments.

Mood Disorders

We've all experienced sadness and feeling "down" or irritable, but sometimes these feelings can be persistent or severe and interfere with life functioning. The two main types of **mood disorder,** major depressive disorder and bipolar disorder (what used to be called manic-depression), are together the most common mental disorders in the United States.

Depression   Depression differs from person to person but includes the following symptoms that persist most of the day and last more than two consecutive weeks:

- A feeling of sadness and hopelessness or loss of pleasure in doing usual activities (anhedonia)
- Poor appetite and weight loss or, alternatively, increased eating compared to usual
- Insomnia or disturbed sleep, including sleeping more than normal
- Decreased energy
- Restlessness or, alternatively, slowed thinking or activity
- Thoughts of worthlessness and guilt
- Trouble concentrating or making decisions
- Thoughts of death or suicide

A person experiencing depression may not have all of the symptoms listed here but must have depressed mood or anhedonia (inability to experience pleasure) and at least four other symptoms. People can have multiple symptoms of depression without feeling depressed, although they usually

---

acute stress disorder   An anxiety disorder that resolves in a month or less.

attention-deficit/hyperactivity disorder (ADHD)   A disorder characterized by persistent, pervasive problems with inattention and/or hyperactivity to a degree that is not considered appropriate for a child's developmental stage and that causes significant difficulties in school, work, or relationships.

mood disorder   An emotional disturbance that is intense and persistent enough to affect normal function; two common mood disorders are depression and bipolar disorder.

TERMS

How do you know if you are depressed? Having periods of feeling down or disappointed, having trouble sleeping, or feeling uncertain about yourself does not necessarily mean that you are clinically depressed, but if these experiences start to last a while and lead to problems functioning, then you might be depressed. You should be evaluated by a professional if you've had five or more of the following symptoms for more than two weeks or if any of them prevents you from keeping up your usual routine.

When You're Depressed

_____ You feel sad or cry a lot, and it doesn't go away.

_____ You feel guilty for no reason; you feel you're no good; you've lost your confidence.

_____ Life seems meaningless, or you think nothing good is ever going to happen again.

_____ You have a negative attitude a lot of the time, or it seems as if you have no feelings.

_____ You don't feel like doing a lot of the things you used to like—music, sports, being with friends, going out, and so on—and you want to be left alone most of the time.

_____ It's hard to make up your mind. You forget lots of things, and it's hard to concentrate.

_____ You get irritated often. Little things make you lose your temper; you overreact.

_____ Your sleep pattern changes: You start sleeping a lot more or you have trouble falling asleep at night; or you wake up really early most mornings and can't get back to sleep.

_____ Your eating patterns change: You've lost your appetite or you eat a lot more.

_____ You feel restless and tired most of the time.

_____ You think about death or feel as if you're dying or have thoughts about suicide.

When You're Manic or Hypomanic

_____ You feel abnormally good or confident, like you're "on top of the world."

_____ You get unrealistic ideas about the great things you can do—things that you really can't do.

_____ Thoughts go racing through your head, you jump from one subject to another, and you talk a lot.

_____ You're starting multiple projects at the same time—doing too many things at once.

_____ You do risky things that may be out of character—spending much more money than usual, having more sex with more partners, driving recklessly, and so on.

_____ You're so energized that you don't need much sleep.

_____ You're so abnormally irritable that you can't get along at home or school or with your friends.

If you are concerned about depression or manic behavior in yourself or a friend, or if you are thinking about hurting or killing yourself, talk to someone about it and get help immediately.

experience a loss of interest or pleasure. (See the box "Are You Suffering from a Mood Disorder?")

In some cases, depression is a clear-cut reaction to a specific event, such as the loss of a loved one or a failure in school or work, whereas in other cases no trigger event is obvious. Regardless of the reason, severe symptoms should be taken seriously. Someone who has symptoms of major depression for more than two weeks, even if it is in reaction to a specific event, should consider treatment. One danger of severe depression is suicide, which is discussed later in this chapter, but the overall impact of depression on general health and ability to function, with or without suicidal thoughts, can be devastating.

The National Institutes of Health estimates that **depression** strikes nearly 6.7% of Americans annually—20% of people have it in their lifetime—making depression the most common

mood disorder. Depression affects the young as well as adults; about 14% of 12–25-year-olds suffer a major depressive episode each year. Depression tends to be more severe and persistent in blacks than in people of other races. Despite this, only about 60% of blacks affected by depression receive treatment for it. Almost twice as many women as men have serious depression. Overall, about three times as many women as men attempt suicide, but women's attempts are less likely to be lethal.

Why more women than men have depression is a matter of debate. Some experts think much of the difference is the

depression A mood disorder characterized by loss of interest, sadness, hopelessness, loss of appetite, disturbed sleep, and other physical symptoms.

TERMS

result of reporting bias: Women are more willing to admit experiencing negative emotions, being stressed, or having difficulty coping. Women may also be more likely to seek treatment. Other experts point to biologically based sex differences, particularly in the level and action of hormones. It may also be that men are more likely than women to have symptoms such as anger or irritability when they are depressed, leading them to be misdiagnosed or for the diagnosis to be missed. In addition, women's social roles and expectations often differ from those of men. Women may put more emphasis on relationships in determining self-esteem, so the deterioration of a relationship is a cause of depression that can hit women harder than men. Culturally determined gender roles are more likely to place women in situations where they have less control over key life decisions, and lack of autonomy is associated with depression.

TREATMENT OF DEPRESSION Although treatments are highly effective, only about 35% of people who suffer from depression currently seek treatment. Treatment for depression depends on its severity and on whether the depressed person is suicidal.

The best initial treatment for moderate to severe depression is probably a combination of drug therapy and psychotherapy. Newer prescription antidepressants work well, although they may need several weeks to take effect, and patients may need to try multiple medications before finding one that works well. If someone is severely depressed and at risk of suicide, hospitalization for more intensive treatment to ensure the patient's safety is sometimes necessary.

Antidepressants work by targeting key neurotransmitters in the brain, including serotonin. When you take an antidepressant, your levels of serotonin increase. This increase has been revealed to help depression and other body conditions that serotonin influences, including mood, sexual desire and function, appetite, sleep, memory and learning, temperature regulation, and some social behavior.

When women take antidepressants, they may need a lower dose than men; at the same dosage, blood levels of medication tend to be higher in women. An issue for women who may become pregnant is whether antidepressants can harm a fetus or newborn. The best evidence indicates that the most frequently prescribed types of antidepressants do not cause birth defects,

although some studies have reported withdrawal symptoms in some newborns whose mothers used certain antidepressants.

Repetitive transcranial magnetic stimulation (rTMS) is a new treatment that targets specific areas of the brain with electromagnetic pulses. rTMS treatments are usually done in 30- to 60-minute sessions five to six times per week for several weeks. It may help some patients whose depression has not responded to other medications.

Electroconvulsive therapy (ECT) is effective for severe depression when other approaches have failed, including medications and other electronic therapies. In ECT, an epileptic-like seizure is induced by an electrical impulse transmitted through electrodes placed on the head. Patients are given an anesthetic and a muscle relaxant to reduce anxiety and prevent injuries associated with seizures. ECT usually includes three treatments per week for two to four weeks.

For patients with **seasonal affective disorder (SAD)**—a type of depression—the treatment involves sitting with eyes open in front of a bright light source every morning. For patients with SAD, depression worsens during winter months as daylight hours diminish. Light therapy may work by extending the perceived length of the day and thus convincing the brain that it is summertime even during the winter months. The American Psychiatric Association estimates that 10–20% of Americans suffer symptoms that may be linked to the disorder. SAD is more common among people who live at higher latitudes, where there are fewer hours of light in winter.

Bipolar Disorder People who experience **mania,** characteristic of a severe mood disorder called **bipolar disorder,** undergo discrete periods of time when they may be restless, have excess energy or activity, feel rested with less sleep than usual, and speak rapidly. They may feel elevated (that is, much better than normal) or abnormally irritable. These feelings are often accompanied by impulsive behavior without regard for the consequences—for example, spending too much money or engaging in risky sexual activity. When such episodes are severe (requiring hospitalization, for example, or producing severe consequences), they are known as manic episodes, and the person who experiences them has what is known as *bipolar I disorder.* If such episodes of elevation or irritability are not so severe as to significantly impair functioning, they are known as *hypomanic episodes.* If hypomania alternates with periods of depression, that person is diagnosed with what is known as *bipolar II disorder.*

People with bipolar disorder typically have periods of both mania or hypomania and depression, and the periods of depression can be persistent and severe. Bipolar disorder typically begins in the late teens through the twenties. Many people with bipolar disorder also struggle with substance and alcohol abuse and anxiety. Suicide rates are high in bipolar disorders, especially early in life. This syndrome affects men and women equally.

TERMS

electroconvulsive therapy (ECT) The use of electric shock to induce brief, generalized seizures; used in the treatment of selected psychological disorders.

seasonal affective disorder (SAD) A mood disorder characterized by seasonal depression, usually occurring in winter, when there is less daylight.

mania A mood disorder characterized by excessive elation, irritability, talkativeness, inflated self-esteem, and expansiveness.

bipolar disorder A mental illness characterized by alternating periods of depression and mania.

Antimanic drugs include lithium (a salt that treats manic episodes), mood stabilizers, and antipsychotic medications. For people who have recurrent episodes of mania or depression, continued, lifelong medication treatment is recommended. Specific medications to treat bipolar depression may also be prescribed.

Schizophrenia

Schizophrenia is a devastating mental disorder that affects a person's thinking and perceptions of reality. People with schizophrenia frequently develop paranoid ideas, false beliefs (delusions), or hallucinations that they believe to be real. The disease can be severe and debilitating or so mild that it's hardly noticeable. Although people are capable of diagnosing their own depression, they usually don't diagnose their own schizophrenia because they often can't see that anything is wrong. This disorder is not rare; in fact, 1 in every 100 people has schizophrenia, most commonly starting in adolescence, which is perhaps what is most tragic and disturbing about the disease—that it starts to affect people in the prime of their lives.

Scientists are uncertain about the exact causes of schizophrenia. Researchers have identified possible chemical and structural differences in the brains of people with the disorder as well as several genes that appear to increase risk. Schizophrenia is likely caused by a combination of genetic and environmental factors that occur during pregnancy and development. For example, children born to older fathers have higher rates of schizophrenia, as do children with prenatal exposure to certain infections or medications.

Some general characteristics of schizophrenia include the following:

• **Disorganized thoughts.** Thoughts may be expressed in a vague or confusing way.

• **Disorganized or abnormal motor behavior.** There may be unexplained agitation, catatonic behavior (not moving or moving in a stereotyped, repetitive way), or "silly," childlike behavior.

• **Delusions.** People with delusions—firmly held false beliefs—may think that their minds are controlled by outside forces, that people can read their minds, that they are great personages like Jesus Christ or the queen of England, or that they are being persecuted by a group such as the CIA.

• **Auditory hallucinations.** People with schizophrenia may hear voices when no one is present. Sometimes these voices tell them to do things (like harm themselves or others), belittle and criticize them, or give them a running commentary on their thoughts and behaviors. These voices can seem very real to the person hearing them and therefore are quite terrifying.

• **Deteriorating social and work functioning.** Social withdrawal and increasingly poor performance at school or work may be so gradual that they are hardly noticed at first, but over time people suffering from the disease fall far behind their peers—and far behind others' earlier expectations.

None of these characteristics is invariably present. Some schizophrenic people are quite logical except on the subject of their delusions. Others show disorganized thoughts but no delusions or hallucinations.

A schizophrenic person needs help from a mental health professional. Suicide is a risk in schizophrenia, and expert treatment can reduce that risk and minimize the social consequences of the illness by shortening the period when symptoms are active. The key element in treatment is regular medication. Sometimes hospitalization is required temporarily to relieve family and friends.

SUICIDE

In the United States, suicide is the second leading cause of death for young people aged 10–34 and the 10th leading cause for people of all ages. In 2018, an estimated 4% of adults seriously considered suicide; 1% planned suicide, and 0.6% attempted it (see Figure 3.3 for data on suicidal

schizophrenia A psychological disorder that involves a disturbance in thinking and in perceiving reality.

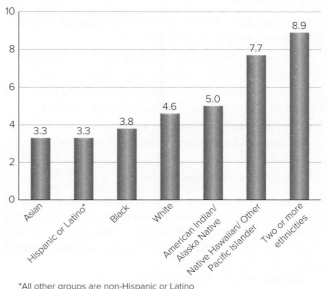

*All other groups are non-Hispanic or Latino

FIGURE 3.3 **Percentages of American adults having suicidal thoughts in the past year, by ethnicity.**

SOURCE: National Institute of Mental Health, 2019.

Table 3.4 — Myths about Suicide: Don't Be Misled

MYTH	FACT
People who really intend to kill themselves do not let anyone know about it.	This belief can be an excuse for doing nothing when someone says he or she might attempt suicide. In fact, most people who eventually follow through with suicide *have* talked about doing it.
People who made a suicide attempt but survived did not really intend to die.	This belief may be true for certain people, but people who seriously want to end their lives may fail because they misjudge what it takes. Even a pharmacist may misjudge the lethal dose of a drug.
People who succeed in suicide really wanted to die.	We cannot be sure of that either. Some people are only trying to make a dramatic gesture or plea for help but miscalculate.
People who really want to kill themselves will do it regardless of any attempts to prevent them.	Few people are single-minded about suicide even at the moment of attempting it. People who are quite determined to take their lives today may completely change their minds tomorrow.
Suicide is proof of mental illness.	Many suicides are carried out by people who do not meet ordinary criteria for mental illness, although people with depression, schizophrenia, and other psychological disorders (including substance use disorders) have a much higher than average suicide rate.
People inherit suicidal tendencies.	Certain kinds of depression that lead to suicide do have a genetic component. But many examples of suicide running in a family can be explained by factors such as psychologically identifying with family members who kill themselves, often a parent.
All suicides are irrational.	By some standards, all suicides may seem "irrational." But many people find it at least understandable that someone might want to attempt suicide—for example, when approaching the end of a terminal illness or when facing a long prison term.

thoughts). Suicide rates vary by race or ethnicity and gender: For both males and females, the suicide rate is highest among American Indians or Alaska Natives and second highest among European Americans. The suicide rate among men is about four times higher than that among women.

Suicide rarely occurs without warning signs (see Table 3.4). About 60% of people who kill themselves are depressed. The more symptoms of depression a person has, the greater the risk. A threat of suicide should be taken not only as a cry for help but also as a possible future occurrence. Here are specific warning signs:

- Any mention of dying, disappearing, jumping, shooting oneself, or other types of self-harm
- Changes in personality, including sadness, withdrawal, irritability, anxiety, fatigue, indecisiveness, or apathy
- A sudden, inexplicable brightening of mood (which can mean the person has decided to attempt suicide)
- A sudden move to give away important possessions, accompanied by statements, such as "I won't be needing these anymore"
- An increase in reckless behaviors

In addition to warning signs, certain risk factors increase the likelihood that someone will attempt suicide (see the box "Deliberate Self-Harm"). Protective factors decrease the likelihood. Risk factors and protective factors can be *intrapersonal, social/situational,* or *cultural.*

The following are key risk factors:

- A history of previous attempts
- A sense of hopelessness, helplessness, guilt, or worthlessness

- Alcohol or other substance use disorders
- Serious medical problems
- Mental disorders, particularly mood disorders such as depression and bipolar disorder
- Availability of a weapon
- Family history of suicide
- Social isolation
- A history of having been abused or neglected
- A current or past experience of being a victim of bullying, in person or online

The following are key protective factors:

- Strong religious faith or other cultural prohibition on suicide
- Connection to other people, including family that is supportive
- Engagement in treatment in which the person is getting help
- Connection with one's own children (or even pets)
- Lack of access to lethal means (guns, pills, railroad tracks)

If you are severely depressed or know someone who is, expert help from a mental health professional is essential. Don't be afraid to discuss the possibility of suicide with someone you fear is suicidal. Ask direct questions to determine whether someone seriously intends to kill himself or herself. Encourage your friend to talk and to take positive steps to improve his or her situation.

You can call the National Suicide Prevention Lifeline at 800-273-TALK (8255). Trained crisis workers are available to talk 24 hours a day, 7 days a week. If you think someone is in

In general, people want to be well and healthy and to protect themselves from harm. But many individuals—predominantly in their teens and adolescence—do deliberately harm themselves, although in a nonfatal way. A common method of self-harm involves people cutting or burning their own skin, leaving scars that they hide beneath their clothes.

Self-cutting and other self-injurious behaviors are not aesthetically motivated. Many people who engage in these behaviors report seeking the physical sensations (including pain) produced by a self-inflicted injury, which may temporarily relieve feelings of tension, perhaps through a release of endorphins.

The Center for Collegiate Mental Health's 2019 report found that self-injury among college students had risen for the past nine years in a row to nearly 29% among students receiving counseling services. In examining differences between self-injurers and noninjurers, individuals who had recently engaged in self-harm were significantly more depressed, anxious, and disgusted with themselves. Compared to noninjurers, self-injurers were roughly 4 times more likely to report a history of physical abuse and 11 times more likely to report a history of sexual abuse.

Self-injury is not the same as a suicide attempt, but individuals who repeatedly hurt themselves are more likely than the general population to kill themselves. In any case, self-injury should be taken seriously. Treatment usually includes group therapy, individual therapy, medication (e.g., antidepressants), or stress reduction and management skills. Pharmacological therapy (medication) is a common form of treatment for many psychological disorders. Medications can be very effective, but they have risks and side effects, and they do not work for all patients.

immediate danger, do not leave him or her alone. Call for help or take him or her to an emergency room.

Most communities have emergency help available, often in the form of a hotline telephone counseling service run by a suicide prevention agency.

Firearms are used in more suicides than homicides. Among gun-related deaths in the home, 83% are the result of suicide, often by someone other than the gun owner. If you learn someone at high risk for suicide has access to a gun, try to convince him or her to put it in safekeeping.

MODELS OF HUMAN NATURE AND THERAPEUTIC CHANGE

The psychological disorders discussed in this chapter can be evaluated from at least four perspectives: biological, behavioral, cognitive, and psychodynamic. Each perspective has a distinct view of human nature, which leads to distinct therapeutic approaches.

The Biological Model

The *biological model* emphasizes that the mind's activity depends entirely on an organic structure, the brain, whose composition is genetically determined. The activity of neurons, mediated by complex chemical reactions, gives rise to our most sophisticated thoughts, our most ardent desires, and our most pathological behaviors. As an organ, the brain responds well to healthy lifestyle behaviors such as maintaining a nutritious diet and exercising. When severe mental health issues arise, however, drug therapies can help.

Pharmacological Therapy The most important kind of therapy inspired by the biological model is pharmacological, or medication treatment. All medications require a prescription from a psychiatrist or other medical doctor. All have received U.S. Food and Drug Administration approval as being safe and more effective than a placebo. However, as with all pharmacological therapies, these drugs may cause side effects. For example, the side effects of widely used antidepressants range from diminished appetite to loss of sexual pleasure. In addition, a patient may have to try several drugs before finding one that is effective and has acceptable side effects. Some of the popular medications currently used for treating psychological disorders are the following:

1. *Antidepressants.* One group is called selective serotonin reuptake inhibitors (SSRIs) because of one of their actions; this group includes Prozac (fluoxetine), Paxil (paroxetine), Zoloft (sertraline), Celexa (citalopram), and Lexapro (escitalopram). Another group is called serotonin and norepinephrine reuptake inhibitors (SNRIs) and includes Effexor (venlafaxine), Pristiq (desvenlafaxine), and Cymbalta (duloxetine). Antidepressants that do not fit into these groups include Wellbutrin (bupropion), Remeron (mirtazapine), Brintellix (vortioxetine), Viibryd (vilazodone), and Fetzima (levomilnacipran). Another group is called the tricyclics because of their chemical structure; it includes Aventyl (nortriptyline) and Elavil (amitriptyline), although these medications are used only infrequently because they may have more side effects than newer antidepressants, and they can be fatal in overdose due to their effects on heart rhythms. No one antidepressant is known to be better than another, and they are often chosen based on their side effects (or lack thereof). Surprisingly, these antidepressants are as effective in treating panic disorder and certain kinds of

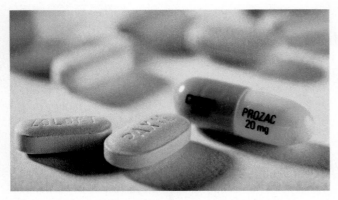

Pharmacological therapy (medication) is a common form of treatment for many psychological disorders. Medications can be very effective, but they have risks and side effects, and they do not work for all patients. Jonathan Nourok/Getty Images

chronic anxiety; some also alleviate the symptoms of OCD. For more information, see the National Institute of Mental Health's "Mental Health Medications" website at https://www.nimh.nih.gov/health/topics/mental-health-medications/index.shtml.

2. *Mood stabilizers.* Lithium carbonate, Depakote (valproic acid), and Lamictal (lamotrigine) are prescribed as mood stabilizers. They are taken to prevent mood swings that occur in bipolar disorder and schizoaffective disorder. Lamictal is used primarily to prevent depression, Depakote to prevent mania, and lithium to prevent both.

3. *Antipsychotics.* Older antipsychotics include Haldol (haloperidol) and Prolixin (fluphenazine); newer antipsychotics (sometimes called "atypical antipsychotics") are Clozaril (clozapine), Zyprexa (olanzapine), Risperdal (risperidone), Seroquel (quetiapine), Abilify (aripiprazole), Geodon (zisprasidone), Latuda (lurasidone), Rexulti (brexpiprazole), Saphris (asenapine), and Vralar (cariprazine). The drugs reduce hallucinations and disordered thinking in people with schizophrenia and delirium; some treat mania in bipolar disorder, and they have a calming effect on agitated patients.

4. *Anxiolytics (antianxiety agents) and hypnotics (sleeping pills).* One of the largest and most prescribed classes of anxiolytics is the benzodiazepines, a group of drugs that includes Valium (diazepam), Librium (chlordiazepoxide), Xanax (alprazolam), and Ativan (lorazepam). Dalmane (flurazepam), Restoril (temazepam), and Halcion (triazolam) are benzodiazepines that have been prescribed as sleeping aids, but newer non-benzodiazepine hypnotics such as Sonata (zaleplon), Ambien (zolpidem), and Lunesta (eszopiclone) are also commonly prescribed. Belsomra (suvorexant) is an orexin receptor antagonist. The neuropeptide orexin signaling system promotes wakefulness, and suvorexant suppresses it.

5. *Stimulants.* Ritalin (methylphenidate) and Adderall (dextroamphetamine and amphetamine) are most commonly used to treat ADHD in children and less often in adults. Drugs of this type are also marketed under the names Dexedrine, Concerta, Focalin, Vyvanse, Daytrana, and Metadate. An antidepressant-like drug called Strattera (atomoxetine) is used to treat ADHD, and two antihypertensive medications (medications that lower blood pressure)—Kapvay (clonidine) and Intuniv (guanfacine)—also work to treat ADHD.

Issues in Drug Therapy The discovery that many psychological disorders have a biological basis in disordered brain functioning has led to a revolution in the treatment of many disorders, particularly depression. The new view of depression as based in brain function may have also lessened the stigma attached to the condition, leading more people to seek treatment. Antidepressants are now among the most widely prescribed drugs in the United States. The development of effective drugs has provided relief for many people, but the wide use of antidepressants has also raised many questions. Critics of drug therapy ask whether the efficacy of antidepressants has been exaggerated by drug company–sponsored research, and they claim that psychological treatments of depression are usually just as good.

Research indicates that, for mild cases of depression, psychotherapy may be more effective than antidepressants. For moderate to severe depression, combined therapy appears to be significantly more effective than either type of treatment alone. Psychotherapy can provide help in managing symptoms and putting them in perspective. A therapist can provide guidance in changing patterns of thinking and behavior that contribute to the problem.

The Behavioral Model

The *behavioral model* focuses on what people do—their overt behavior—rather than on brain structures and chemistry or on thoughts and consciousness. This model regards psychological problems as "maladaptive behavior" or bad habits. When and how a person learned maladaptive behavior is less important than what makes it continue in the present.

Behaviorists analyze behavior in terms of **stimulus, response,** and **reinforcement.** The essence of behavior therapy is to discover what reinforcements keep an undesirable behavior going and then to try to alter those reinforcements. For example, if people who fear speaking in class (the stimulus) remove themselves from that situation (the response), they experience immediate relief, which acts as reinforcement for future avoidance and escape.

To change their behavior, fearful people are taught to practice **exposure**—to deliberately and repeatedly enter the feared

---

TERMS

stimulus Anything that causes a response.

response A reaction to a stimulus.

reinforcement Increasing the future probability of a response by following it with a reward.

exposure A therapeutic technique for treating fear; the subject learns to come into direct contact with a feared situation.

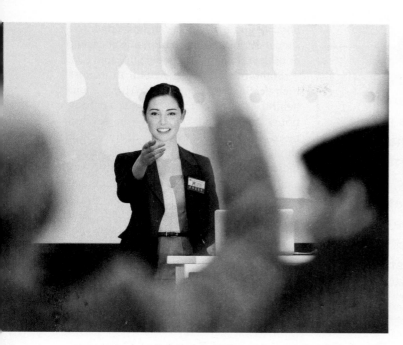

Behavioral therapy can help people overcome many kinds of fears, including that of public speaking. PeopleImages.com/Digital Vision/Getty Images

situation and remain in it until their fear begins to abate. A student who is afraid to speak in class might begin his behavioral therapy program by keeping a diary listing each time he makes a contribution to a classroom discussion, how long he speaks, and his anxiety levels before, during, and after speaking. He would then develop concrete but realistic goals for increasing his speaking frequency and contract with himself to reward his successes by spending more time in activities he finds enjoyable.

Although exposure to the real situation works best, exposure in your imagination or through the virtual reality of computer simulation can also be effective. For example, in the case of someone who is afraid of flying, a simulated scenario would likely be vivid enough to elicit the fear necessary to practice exposure techniques.

The Cognitive Model

The *cognitive model* emphasizes the effect of ideas on behavior and feeling. According to this model, behavior results from complicated attitudes, expectations, and motives rather than from simple, immediate reinforcements.

Cognitive therapy tries to expose and identify false ideas that produce feelings such as anxiety and depression. For example, a student afraid of speaking in class may harbor thoughts such as "If I begin to speak, I'll say something stupid; if I say something stupid, the teacher and my classmates will lose respect for me; then I'll get a low grade, my classmates will avoid me, and life will be hell." In cognitive therapy, these ideas will be examined critically. If the student prepares, will he or she really sound stupid? Does every sentence said have to be exactly correct and beautifully delivered, or is that an unrealistic expectation? Will classmates'

opinions be completely transformed by one presentation? Do classmates even care that much? And why does the student care so much about what *they* think? People in cognitive therapy are taught to notice their unrealistic thoughts and to substitute more realistic ones, and they are advised to repeatedly test their assumptions.

The Psychodynamic Model

The *psychodynamic model* also emphasizes thoughts. Proponents of this model, however, do not believe thoughts can be changed directly because they are fed by other unconscious ideas and impulses. Symptoms are not isolated pieces of behavior but the result of a complex set of wishes and emotions hidden by active defenses (see Table 3.2). In psychodynamic therapy, patients are strongly encouraged to speak and try to gain an understanding of the basis of their feelings toward the therapist and others. Through this process, patients gain insights that help them overcome their maladaptive patterns. Current therapies of this type tend to focus more on the present (the here and now) than on the past, and the therapist tries to facilitate self-exploration rather than providing explanations.

Evaluating the Models

Most clinicians do not subscribe to a single model but understand mental illness through a *biopsychosocial model*. This model combines many aspects of understanding the mind, recognizing that people are vulnerable to their own genetic history in an environment that includes relationships, culture, and personal idiosyncrasies. Ignoring theoretical conflicts among psychological models, therapists have recently developed pragmatic *cognitive-behavioral therapies* (CBTs) that combine effective elements of both models in a single package. For example, the package for treating social anxiety emphasizes exposure as well as changing problematic patterns of thinking (see the Behavior Change Strategy "Dealing with Social Anxiety" at the end of the chapter). Combined therapies have also been developed for panic disorder, obsessive-compulsive disorder, generalized anxiety disorder, and depression. These packages, involving 10 or more individual or group sessions with a therapist and homework between sessions, have been shown to produce significant improvement.

Drug therapy and CBTs are also sometimes combined, especially in the case of depression. For anxiety disorders, both kinds of therapy are equally effective, but the effects of drug therapy last only as long as the drug is being taken, whereas CBTs produce longer-term improvement. For schizophrenia, drug therapy is a must, but a continuing relationship with therapists who give support and advice is also indispensable.

Psychodynamic therapies have been attacked as ineffective and endless. Of course, effectiveness is hard to demonstrate for therapies that do not focus on specific symptoms. But common sense tells us that being able to open yourself up and discuss your problems with a supportive but objective person who focuses on you and lets you speak freely can enhance your sense of self and reduce feelings of confusion and despair.

Other Psychotherapies

In addition to existing forms of treatment, newer psychotherapies such as *dialectical behavior therapy* (DBT) have become available. Developed by psychologist Marsha Linehan, DBT is used to treat borderline personality disorder and chronic suicidal behavior, but it has since been expanded to treat other disorders, such as drug addiction and eating disorders. This therapy uses the principles of standard CBT by encouraging distress tolerance and acceptance of painful feelings and emotions through *mindfulness* (see Chapter 2), originally derived from Buddhist meditation and other Eastern practices. Mindfulness encourages a person to be aware of feelings rather than react to them, and to learn techniques to regulate emotions, by decreasing the intensity of emotional reactions. Mindfulness is practiced in group and individual therapy, often involving the use of workbooks and homework between sessions.

GETTING HELP

Understanding the different therapeutic models can help you decide which option might be the best fit for you. When you know you need help, it can seem overwhelming to decide where to turn. Options include self-help, peer counseling, support groups, online help, and professional help—and all of them offer distinct advantages.

Self-Help

A smart way to begin helping yourself is by finding out what you can do on your own. For example, certain behavioral and cognitive approaches can be effective because they involve developing an awareness of self-defeating actions and ideas for combating them. Start with a self-help list: being more assertive or less aggressive, depending on what's appropriate; communicating honestly; raising your self-esteem by avoiding negative thoughts, people, and actions that undermine it. Confront rather than avoid the things you fear. Although information from books in the psychology or self-help sections of

libraries and bookstores can be helpful, you should avoid any that make fantastic claims or deviate from mainstream approaches.

Some people find it helpful to express their feelings in a journal. Writing about painful experiences may provide an emotional release and can help you develop more constructive ways of dealing with similar situations in the future. Research indicates that using a journal in this way can improve physical as well as emotional wellness.

For some people, religious belief and practice may promote psychological health. Religious organizations provide a social network and a supportive community, and religious practices, such as prayer and meditation, offer a path for personal change and transformation.

Peer Counseling and Support Groups

Sharing your concerns with others is another helpful way of dealing with psychological health challenges. Just being able to share what's troubling you with an accepting, empathetic person can bring relief. Comparing notes with people who have problems similar to yours can give you new ideas about coping.

Many colleges offer peer counseling through a health center or through the psychology or education department. Volunteer students specially trained in maintaining confidentiality are usually those who offer counsel. They may steer you toward an appropriate campus or community resource or simply offer a sympathetic ear. Support groups are typically organized around a specific problem, such as eating disorders or substance abuse. There are self-help groups through online social media such as Facebook and Twitter (among many

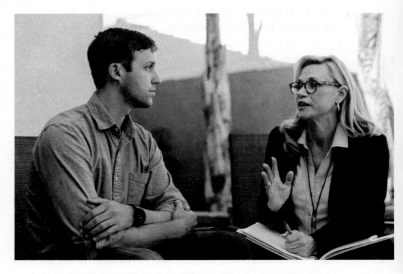

Individual therapy is just one of many approaches to psychological counseling. Tom M Johnson/Blend Images/Getty Images

Ask Yourself

QUESTIONS FOR CRITICAL THINKING AND REFLECTION

Does using computer technology and social media affect you negatively or positively? Do you fear missing out? Do you compare yourself negatively to peers? Are you more engaged with your peers than you otherwise would be? Have you accessed mental health resources or support this way?

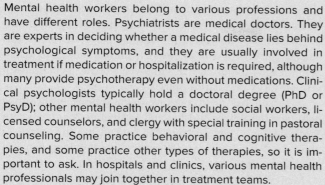

Mental health workers belong to various professions and have different roles. Psychiatrists are medical doctors. They are experts in deciding whether a medical disease lies behind psychological symptoms, and they are usually involved in treatment if medication or hospitalization is required, although many provide psychotherapy even without medications. Clinical psychologists typically hold a doctoral degree (PhD or PsyD); other mental health workers include social workers, licensed counselors, and clergy with special training in pastoral counseling. Some practice behavioral and cognitive therapies, and some practice other types of therapies, so it is important to ask. In hospitals and clinics, various mental health professionals may join together in treatment teams.

In choosing a mental health professional, financial considerations are important. Research the costs and what your health insurance will cover. City, county, and state governments may support mental health clinics for those with few financial resources. Some on-campus services may be free or offered at very little cost.

The cost of treatment is linked to how many therapy sessions will be needed, which in turn depends on the type of therapy and the nature of the problem. Getting this information before you start treatment is important. Many mental health professionals do not accept health insurance payments and only accept direct payments from patients. Psychological therapies focusing on specific problems may require weekly visits for a period of 8–24 sessions, depending on the type of therapy. Therapies based on CBT and DBT are often time limited, and your therapist can tell you how many sessions to expect. Therapies aiming for psychological awareness and personality change, such as psychodynamic therapies, can last months or years.

Deciding whether a therapist is right for you will require meeting the therapist in person. More recently, psychotherapies are offered remotely by video (by computer, tablet, or smartphone), which don't require visiting a physical office. Before or during your first meeting, find out about the therapist's background and training:

- Do they have a degree from an appropriate professional school and a state license to practice?

- Have they had experience treating problems similar to yours?

- How much will therapy cost?

You have a right to know the answers to these questions and should not hesitate to ask them. After your initial meeting, evaluate your impressions:

- Does the therapist seem like a warm, attentive person who would be able to help you and seems interested in doing so?

- Are you comfortable with the therapist's personality, values, and beliefs?

- Are they willing to talk about the techniques in use? Do these techniques make sense to you?

If you answer yes to these questions, this therapist may be satisfactory for you. If you feel uncomfortable—and you're not in need of emergency care—it's worthwhile to set up one-time consultations with one or two others before you make up your mind. Take the time to find someone who feels right for you.

Later in your treatment, evaluate your progress:

- Are you being helped by the treatment?

- If you are displeased, is it because you aren't making progress, or because therapy is raising difficult, painful issues you don't want to deal with?

- Can you express dissatisfaction to your therapist? Such feedback can improve your treatment.

The most important predictor of whether your therapy will be helpful is how much rapport you feel with your therapist *at the first session*. This has been shown to be true no matter what model of psychotherapy the therapist is practicing. You have to like your therapist and feel that she or he will be able to help you—if you do, there's a good chance that it will be helpful. If you sense that your therapy isn't working or is actually harmful, thank your therapist for her or his efforts, and find another. It's extra work for you, but it's important for your health.

---

platforms), but it is sometimes hard to be certain of their legitimacy. National organizations such as the National Alliance on Mental Illness (NAMI; nami.org) and the Depression and Bipolar Support Alliance (DBSA; dbsalliance.org) can direct you to such support.

Online Help and Apps

With advances in technology, there are more ways to access help both online and through mobile apps, but these are still very new and are not well tested or studied. The Department of Veterans Affairs has developed a series of free mobile apps to help with PTSD and insomnia, for example, among other

problems. PTSD Coach and iCBT Coach are both available to the general public. There are many others, of course, but none of them is regulated. Psychotherapy through online channels or apps is sometimes offered by secure connection to computer, tablet, or smartphone; licensed professionals also provide therapy through video chats. The use of bots to deliver help is also quite new but untested, and at this time it cannot be recommended as an alternative to professional help.

Professional Help

Sometimes trying self-help or talking to nonprofessionals is not enough, especially if you might have a mental illness.

Professional help is appropriate in any of the following situations:

- Depression, anxiety, or other emotional problems interfere seriously with school or work performance or in getting along with others.
- Suicide is attempted or is seriously considered.
- Symptoms such as hallucinations, delusions, incoherent speech, or loss of memory occur.
- Alcohol or drugs are used to the extent that they impair normal functioning much of the time or reducing their dosage leads to psychological or physiological withdrawal symptoms.

Overcoming the stigma about seeking help is a first step. In many communities and cultures, great shame and stigma are associated with talking to a mental health professional; in others, there is much less. You may someday find yourself having to overcome your own reluctance, or that of a friend, about seeking help.

Widespread education efforts seem to be reducing the stigma of getting help for psychological symptoms. The rate of college students in treatment increased from 19% in 2007 to 34% by 2017. This does not necessarily mean that more students have mental illnesses, but perhaps that the stigma surrounding mental illness (such as depression) or psychological distress may have decreased. More than 50% of students with depression now report seeking help for it in the past year. Student activism and the social acceptance of mental health illness treatment (especially through the openness of social media platforms) have likely played a role in this change. Surveys of college presidents reveal that more than 8 in 10 of them reported that improved student mental health was a priority on their campuses.

A person has many options when seeking professional help (see the box "Choosing and Evaluating Mental Health Professionals"). For students, the student health center is a great start. Pediatricians and primary care providers can also make referrals.

Many kinds of professionals are trained to evaluate people's psychological and psychiatric needs and to provide treatment. Psychotherapists come from a variety of backgrounds, including licensed social workers and family and marital therapists (with master's degrees); specially trained nurses with advanced degrees; psychologists (with doctorates); and psychiatrists, who have medical degrees and thus can prescribe medication.

Many national organizations have websites that may be useful in finding help. (See the end of this chapter under For More Information.)

TIPS FOR TODAY AND THE FUTURE

Most of life's psychological challenges can be met with self-help and everyday skills. You can take many steps to maintain your mental health.

RIGHT NOW YOU CAN:

- Take a serious look at how you've felt recently. If you have any feelings that are especially hard to handle, consider how you can get help with them.
- Think of the way in which you are most creative (an important part of self-actualization), whether it's in music, art, or whatever you enjoy. Try to focus at least an hour each week on this activity.
- Review the list of defense mechanisms in Table 3.2. Have you used any of them recently or consistently over time? Think of a situation in which you used one of those mechanisms, and determine how you could have coped with it differently.

IN THE FUTURE YOU CAN:

- Write 100 positive adjectives that describe you. This exercise may take several days to complete. Post your list in a place where you will see it often.
- Record your reactions to upsetting events in your life. Are your reactions and self-talk typically negative or neutral? Decide whether you are satisfied with your reactions and if they are healthy.

SUMMARY

- Psychological health refers to the extent to which we are able to function optimally in the face of challenges, whether we have a mental illness or not.

- Maslow's definition of psychological health centers on self-actualization, the highest level in his hierarchy of needs. Self-actualized people have high self-esteem and are realistic, inner directed, authentic, capable of emotional intimacy, and creative.

- Psychological health encompasses more than a single particular state of normality. Psychological diversity—the understanding, acceptance, and respect for how much individuals differ in psychological terms—is valuable.

- Crucial parts of psychological wellness include developing an adult identity, establishing intimate relationships, and developing values and purpose in life.

- A sense of self-esteem develops during childhood as a result of giving and receiving love and learning to accomplish goals. Self-concept is challenged every day; healthy people adjust their goals to their abilities.

- Using defense mechanisms to cope with problems can make finding solutions harder. Analyzing thoughts and behavior can help people develop less defensive and more effective ways of coping.

- A pessimistic outlook can be damaging; it can be overcome by developing more realistic self-talk.

- Honest communication requires recognizing what needs to be said and saying it clearly. Assertiveness enables people to insist on their rights and to participate in the give-and-take of good communication.

- People may be lonely if they haven't developed ways to be happy on their own or if they interpret being alone as a sign of rejection. Lonely people can take action to expand their social contacts.

- Dealing successfully with anger involves distinguishing between a reasonable level of assertiveness and gratuitous expressions of anger; heading off rage by reframing thoughts and distracting yourself; and responding to the anger of others with an asymmetrical, problem-solving orientation.

- Some people with psychological disorders have symptoms severe enough to interfere with daily living.

- Anxiety is a fear that is not directed toward any definite threat. Anxiety disorders include simple phobias, social anxiety disorders, panic disorder, generalized anxiety disorder, obsessive-compulsive disorder, and posttraumatic stress disorder.

- Depression is a common mood disorder in which a person experiences loss of interest or pleasure in things (anhedonia) in combination with at least four other symptoms. Severe depression carries a high risk of suicide, and suicidal depressed people need professional help.

- Symptoms of mania include abnormally elevated moods or abnormal irritability with unrealistically high self-esteem, little need for sleep, and rapid speech. Mood swings between mania and depression characterize bipolar disorder.

- Schizophrenia is characterized by disorganized thoughts, inappropriate emotions, delusions, auditory hallucinations, and deteriorating social and work performance.

- The biological model emphasizes that the mind's activity depends on the brain, whose composition is genetically determined. Therapy based on the biological model is primarily pharmacological.

- The behavioral model focuses on overt behavior and treats psychological problems as bad habits. Behavior change is the focus of therapy.

- The cognitive model considers how ideas affect behavior and feelings; behavior results from complicated attitudes, expectations, and motives, not just from simple reinforcements. Cognitive therapy focuses on changing a person's thinking.

- The psychodynamic model asserts that false ideas are fed by unconscious ideas and cannot be addressed directly. In psychodynamic therapy, patients speak as freely as possible in front of the therapist and try to gain an understanding of the basis of their feelings toward the therapist and others.

- Help is available in a variety of forms, including self-help, peer counseling, support groups, and therapy with a mental health professional.

FOR MORE INFORMATION

Adolescent Mental Health Initiative. Offers information on mental health issues specifically for teens.

> http://www.annenbergpublicpolicycenter.org/ahrci
> /adolescent-mental-health-initiative-book-series/

American Association of Suicidology. Provides information about suicide and resources for people in crisis.

> http://www.suicidology.org

Anxiety and Depression Association of America (ADAA). Provides information and resources related to anxiety disorders and depression.

> http://www.adaa.org

Depression and Bipolar Support Alliance (DBSA). Provides educational materials and information about support groups.

> http://www.dbsalliance.org

Mental Health America. Provides consumer information on a variety of issues, including how to find help.

> https://www.mhanational.org/

NAMI (National Alliance on Mental Illness). Provides information and support for people affected by mental illness.

> 800-950-NAMI (help line)
> http://www.nami.org

National Hopeline Network. 24-hour hotline for people who are thinking about suicide or know someone who is; calls are routed to local crisis centers.

> 800-442-HOPE
> 800-SUICIDE
> http://www.hopeline.com

National Institute of Mental Health (NIMH). Provides helpful information about anxiety, depression, eating disorders, and other challenges to psychological health.

> http://www.nimh.nih.gov

Substance Abuse and Mental Health Services Administration. A one-stop source for information and resources relating to mental health.

> http://www.samhsa.gov

U.S. Food and Drug Administration. Provides access to Medication Guides, which are paper handouts that come with many prescription drugs.

> https://www.fda.gov/drugs/drug-safety-and-availability/
> medication-guides

BEHAVIOR CHANGE STRATEGY
Dealing with Social Anxiety

Shyness is often the result of both high anxiety levels and lack of key social skills. To help overcome shyness, you need to learn to manage your fear of social situations and to develop social skills such as making appropriate eye contact, initiating topics in conversations, and maintaining the flow of conversations by asking questions and making appropriate responses.

As described in the chapter, repeated *exposure* to the source of your fear—in this case, social situations—is the best method for reducing anxiety. When you practice new behaviors, they gradually become easier and you experience less anxiety.

A counterproductive strategy is avoiding situations that make you anxious. Although this approach works in the short term—you eliminate your anxiety because you escape the situation—it keeps you from meeting new people and having new experiences. Another counterproductive strategy is to self-medicate with alcohol or drugs. Being under their influence actually prevents you from learning new social skills and new ways to handle your anxiety.

To reduce your anxiety in social situations, try some of the following strategies:

- Remember that physical stress reactions are short-term responses to fear. Don't dwell on them. Remind yourself that they will pass, and they will.

- Refocus your attention away from the stress reaction you're experiencing and toward the social task at hand. Your nervousness is much less visible than you think.

- Allow a warm-up period for new situations. Realize that you will feel more nervous at first, and take steps to relax and become more comfortable. Refer to the suggestions for deep breathing and other relaxation techniques in Chapter 2.

- If possible, take breaks during anxiety-producing situations. For example, if you're at a party, take a moment to visit the restroom or step outside. Alternate between speaking with good friends and striking up conversations with new acquaintances.

- Watch your interpretations. Having a stress reaction doesn't mean that you don't belong in the group, that you're unattractive or unworthy, or that the situation is too much for you. Think of yourself as excited or highly alert instead of anxious.

- Avoid cognitive distortions and practice realistic self-talk. Replace your self-critical thoughts with more supportive ones, such as "No one else is perfect, and I don't have to be either" or "It would have been good if I had a funny story to tell, but the conversation was interesting anyway."

- Give yourself a reality check: Ask if you're really in a life-threatening situation (or just at a party), if the outcome you're imagining is really likely (or the worst thing that could possibly happen), or if you're the only one who feels nervous (or if many other people might feel the same way).

- Don't think of conversations as evaluations. Remind yourself that you don't have to prove yourself with every social interaction. And remember that most people are thinking more about themselves than they are about you.

Starting and maintaining conversations can be difficult for shy people, who may feel overwhelmed by their physical stress reactions. If small talk is a problem for you, try the following strategies:

- Introduce yourself early in the conversation. If you tend to forget names, repeat your new acquaintance's name to help fix it in your mind ("Nice to meet you, Amelia").

- Ask questions and look for shared topics of interest. Simple, open-ended questions like "How's your presentation coming along?" or "How do you know our host?" encourage others to carry the conversation for a while and help bring up a variety of subjects.

- Take turns talking, and elaborate on your answers. Simple yes and no answers don't move the conversation along. Try to relate something in your life—a course you're taking or a hobby you have—to something in the other person's life. Match self-disclosure with self-disclosure.

- Have something to say. Expand your mind and become knowledgeable about current events and local or campus news. If you have specialized knowledge about a topic, practice discussing it in ways that both beginners and experts can understand and appreciate.

- If you get stuck for something to say, try giving a compliment ("Great presentation!" or "I love your earrings.") or performing a social grace (pass the chips or get someone a drink).

- Be an attentive listener. Reward the other person with your full attention and with regular responses. Make frequent eye contact and maintain a relaxed but alert posture. (See Chapter 5 for more on being an effective listener.)

- At first, your new behaviors will likely make you anxious. Don't give up—things *will* get easier.

SOURCES: Aron, E. 2010. *The Undervalued Self.* New York: Little, Brown; Brown, B. 2010. *The Gifts of Imperfection: Let Go of Who You Think You're Supposed to Be and Embrace Who You Are. Your Guide to a Wholehearted Life.* Center City, MN: Hazelden.

Ahmedani, Brian K. 2015. "Racial/Ethnic Differences in Health Care Visits Made Before Suicide Attempt across the United States." *Medical Care* 53(5): 430–435.

American Psychiatric Association. 2013. *Diagnostic and Statistical Manual of Mental Disorders (DSM-5),* 5th ed. Washington, DC: American Psychiatric Publishing.

American Psychiatric Association. 2015. *Mental Health* (http://www.psychiatry.org/patients-families/what-is-mental-illness).

Asselmann, E., et al. 2016. Risk factors for fearful spells, panic attacks and panic disorder in a community cohort of adolescents and young adults. *Journal of Affective Disorders* 193: 305–308.

Banks, M. V., and K. Salmon. 2013. Reasoning about the self in positive and negative ways: Relationship to psychological functioning in young adulthood. *Memory* 21(1): 10–26.

Beard, C., et al. 2010. Health-related quality of life across the anxiety disorders: Findings from a sample of primary care patients. *Journal of Anxiety Disorders* 24(6): 559–564.

Carver, C. S., M. F. Scheier, and S. C. Segerstrom. 2010. Optimism. *Clinical Psychology Review* 30(7): 879–889.

Cawood, C. D., and S. K. Huprich. 2011. Late adolescent nonsuicidal self-injury: The roles of coping style, self-esteem, and personality pathology. *Journal of Personality Disorders* 25(6): 765–781.

Center for Collegiate Mental Health. 2020. *2019 Annual Report.* Publication No. STA 20-244 (https://ccmh.memberclicks.net/assets/docs/2019-CCMH-Annual-Report_3.17.20.pdf).

Centers for Disease Control and Prevention. 2010. Attitudes toward Mental Illness—35 States, District of Columbia, and Puerto Rico, 2007. *Morbidity and Mortality Weekly Report* 59(20): 619–625.

Ferrier-Auerback, A. G., et al. 2010. Predictors of emotional distress reported by soldiers in the combat zone. *Journal of Psychiatric Research* 44(7): 470–476.

Gaynes, B. N., et al. 2014. Repetitive transcranial magnetic stimulation for treatment-resistant depression: A systematic review and meta-analysis. *Journal of Clinical Psychiatry* 75(5): 477–489.

Greenhoot, A. F., et al. 2013. Making sense of traumatic memories: Memory qualities and psychological symptoms in emerging adults with and without abuse histories. *Memory* 21(1): 125–142.

Harvard Health Publishing. 2017. What causes depression? Onset of depression more complex than a brain chemical imbalance. Harvard Medical School (https://www.health.harvard.edu/mind-and-mood/what-causes-depression).

Kirov, G. G., et al. 2016. Evaluation of cumulative cognitive deficits from electroconvulsive therapy. *British Journal of Psychiatry* 208(3): 266–270.

Klein, D. N., et al. 2013. Predictors of first lifetime onset of major depressive disorder in young adulthood. *Journal of Abnormal Psychology* 122(1): 1–6.

Kochanek, K. D., et al. 2016. Deaths: Final data for 2014. *National Vital Statistics Reports* 65(4).

Lattie, E. G., S. K. Lipson, and D. Eisenberg. 2019. Technology and college student mental health: Challenges and opportunities. *Frontiers in Psychiatry* 10: 246.

Lin, Y. R., et al. 2008. Evaluation of assertiveness training for psychiatric patients. *Journal of Clinical Nursing* 17(21): 2875–2883.

Linehan, M. M. 1993. *Cognitive-Behavioral Treatment of Borderline Personality Disorder.* New York: Guilford.

Lipson, S. K., E. G. Lattie, and D. Eisenberg. 2019. Increased rates of mental health service utilization by U.S. college students: 10-year population-level trends (2007–2017). *Psychiatric Services* 70(1): 60–63.

Merritt Hawkins. 2017. *2017 Review of Physician and Advanced Practitioner Recruiting Incentives: An Overview of the Salaries, Bonuses, and Other Incentives Customarily Used to Recruit Physicians, Physician Assistants and Nurse Practitioners.* 24th ed. Dallas, TX: Merritt Hawkins.

Molouki, S., and D. M. Bartels. 2017. Personal change and the continuity of the self. *Cognitive Psychology* 93: 1–17.

National Institute of Mental Health. 2018. *Depression* (http://www.nimh.nih.gov/health/topics/depression/index.shtml?utm_source=BrainLine.orgutm_medium=Twitter).

National Institute of Mental Health. 2019. Prevalence: Any Mental Illness (AMI) among U.S. Adults (http://www.nimh.nih.gov/health/statistics/prevalence/any-mental-illness-ami-among-us-adults.shtml).

National Institute of Mental Health. 2020. *Anxiety Disorders* (http://www.nimh.nih.gov/health/topics/anxiety-disorders/index.shtml).

Nemeroff, C. B. 2007. The burden of severe depression: A review of diagnostic challenges and treatment alternatives. *Journal of Psychiatric Research* 41(3–4): 189–206.

Oldis, M., et al. 2016. Trajectory and predictors of quality of life in first episode psychotic mania. *Journal of Affective Disorders* 195: 148–155.

Penn State Center for Collegiate Mental Health. 2016. *2015 Annual Report on Student Counseling Centers* (Publication No. STA 15–108).

Pozzi, M., et al. 2016. Antidepressants and, suicide and self-injury: Causal or casual association? *International Journal of Psychiatry in Clinical Practice* 20(1): 47–51.

Rickwood, D., and S. Bradford. 2012. The role of self-help in the treatment of mild anxiety disorders in young people: An evidence-based review. *Psychology Research and Behavior Management* 5: 25–36.

Rosenthal, B. S., and W. C. Wilson. 2012. Race/ethnicity and mental health in the first decade of the 21st century. *Psychological Reports* 110(2): 645–662.

Rothwell, J. D. 2009. *In the Company of Others: An Introduction to Communication,* 3rd ed. New York: McGraw Hill.

Schatzberg, A. F., J. O. Cole, and C. DeBattista. 2010. *Manual of Clinical Psychopharmacology,* 7th ed. Washington, DC: American Psychiatric Publishing.

Seligman, M. E. P. 2008. Positive health. *Applied Psychology: An International Review* 57, 3–18.

Simon, G. 2009. Collaborative care for mood disorders. *Current Opinion in Psychiatry* 22(1): 37–41.

Singh, N. N., et al. 2007. Individuals with mental illness can control their aggressive behavior through mindfulness training. *Behavior Modification* 31(3): 313–328.

Soeteman, D., M. Miller, and J. J. Kim. 2012. Modeling the risks and benefits of depression treatment for children and young adults. *Value in Health* 15(5): 724–729.

Substance Abuse and Mental Health Services Administration. 2019. *Key Substance Use and Mental Health Indicators in the United States: Results from the 2018 National Survey on Drug Use and Health* (HHS Publication No. SMA PEP19-5068, NSDUH Series H-54). Rockville, MD: Center for Behavioral Health Statistics and Quality, Substance Abuse and Mental Health Services Administration (https://www.samhsa.gov/data/).

Thurber, C. A., and E. A. Walton. 2012. Homesickness and adjustment in university students. *Journal of American College Health* 60(5): 415–419.

Turner, B. J., A. L. Chapman, and B. K. Layden. 2012. Intrapersonal and interpersonal functions of nonsuicidal self-injury: Associations with emotional and social functioning. *Suicide & Life-Threatening Behavior* 42(1): 36–55.

U.S. Department of Health and Human Services. 2014. Results from the 2013 National Survey on Drug Use and Health: Mental Health Findings. Substance Abuse and Mental Health Services Administration. Rockville, MD: Center for Behavioral Health Statistics and Quality.

U.S. Department of Veterans Affairs. 2019. How Common Is PTSD in Adults? https://www.ptsd.va.gov/understand/common/common_adults.asp

Verhaak, P. F., et al. 2009. Receiving treatment for common mental disorders. *General Hospital Psychiatry* 31(1): 46–55.

Vonasch, A. J., et al. 2017. Death before dishonor: Incurring costs to protect moral reputation. *Social Psychological and Personality Science* (https://doi.org/10.1177/1948550617720271).

Williams, D., et al. 2007. Prevalence and distribution of major depressive disorder in African Americans, Caribbean blacks, and non-Hispanic whites. *Archives of General Psychiatry* 64: 305–315.

Williams, J. 2014. Inside the *New York Times Book Review* "My Age of Anxiety." *New York Times,* January 24, 2014.

Design Elements: Assess Yourself icon: Aleksey Boldin/Alamy Stock Photo; Diversity Matters icon: Rawpixel Ltd/Getty Images; Wellness on Campus icon: Rawpixel Ltd/Getty Images; Take Charge icon: VisualCommunications/Getty Images; Critical Consumer icon: pagadesign/Getty Images.

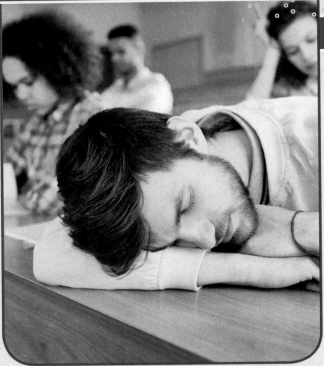

SeventyFour/Shutterstock

CHAPTER 4

CHAPTER OBJECTIVES

- Identify the three stages of sleep
- Understand how to apply good sleep habits
- Explain the health-related benefits of sleep and the consequences of disrupted sleep
- Understand changing sleep needs throughout the life span
- List common sleep disorders, their symptoms, and their treatments
- Understand your patterns of sleepiness and alertness throughout the day
- Understand sleep disrupters and how to reduce their effects

Sleep

TEST YOUR KNOWLEDGE

1. During sleep, the brain shuts down and remains inactive until awakening.
   True or False?

2. Adults need less and less sleep as they age.
   True or False?

3. Insufficient sleep is associated with which of the following conditions:
   a. Depression
   b. Obesity
   c. Cardiovascular disease

4. Staying awake for 20 hours impairs cognition to an extent comparable with a blood alcohol level of
   a. 0.02%
   b. 0.04%
   c. 0.08%

5. Humans are biologically programmed to be awake during the day and to sleep at night.
   True or False?

ANSWERS

1. **FALSE.** The brain is highly active during sleep, strengthening important neural connections vital to memory, learning, and creative thinking.

2. **FALSE.** Adults need 7–9 hours of sleep each night throughout their lifetime. For many people, however, the ability to attain this much sleep each night becomes more difficult with age.

3. **ALL THREE.** Insufficient sleep is associated with psychiatric disorders, metabolism, and cardiovascular diseases.

4. **C.** Going without sleep for 20 hours is comparable to being legally drunk in most states.

5. **TRUE.** Those who work night shifts and sleep during the day are more prone to certain diseases and disorders.

We spend almost one-third of our lives asleep, but few of us understand what sleep is for and why it is necessary for our health. Since we are mostly unconscious during sleep, it is not uncommon to feel that we could be better off if we did not need sleep, and it can be tempting to cut back on sleep to make more time for entertainment or work. As we learn more about how sleep promotes all aspects of our health, however, we see that sleep is as vital as nutrition and physical fitness.

SLEEP BIOLOGY

Sleep affects almost all systems of the body, including the respiratory, cardiovascular, endocrine, gastrointestinal, urinary, and nervous systems. When we fall asleep, our heart rate and respiratory rates slow, our blood pressure drops, and our body temperature declines. Our consciousness is also profoundly changed during sleep. We are less responsive to the surrounding environment, and we experience fantastical dreams.

Sleep Stages

Even though we are not conscious when we are sleeping, our brains are still active. Sleep is divided into distinct stages characterized by different patterns of electrical brain activity. The way these patterns come together is called *sleep architecture*, and it changes over the course of the life span.

Brain activity during sleep is typically measured by a monitoring device called an **electroencephalogram (EEG).** During wakefulness, when a person is quietly resting with eyes closed, the EEG shows a pattern called the alpha rhythm. This pattern is characterized by regular brain waves that occur 8–10 times per second. These brain waves change, and different parts of the brain are activated or suppressed as a person progresses through the three stages of sleep.

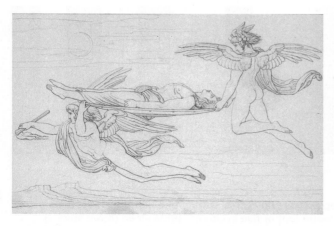

Sleep's resemblance to the loss of consciousness at the end of life was portrayed in Greek mythology. Sleep and death were personified by twin brothers Hypnos and Thanatos. akg-images/Newscom

NREM Sleep The first three stages of sleep are grouped together as **non–rapid eye movement (NREM) sleep**. The purpose of NREM sleep remains mysterious, but theories suggest that it improves neural connections; it also facilitates information processing and cell restoration and repair. As we move through the stages of sleep, brain waves grow larger and slower. Resting with eyes closed produces an EEG pattern called the alpha rhythm. Stage I and II sleep produce theta waves. In the deepest stage of sleep, Stage III, delta waves are even slower, like large waves in the ocean (see Figure 4.1).

STAGE I Stage I is a short transitional phase from wakefulness to sleep. It is light sleep, easily disturbed by outside stimuli. Sometimes it is hard to differentiate between a person's awake state and Stage I. Someone who wakes from this stage may not even be aware they had fallen asleep. In Stage I, the eyes may move slowly back and forth (not to be confused with rapid eye movement sleep, described below); respiration

electroencephalogram (EEG) A monitoring device that records brain activity. **TERMS**

non–rapid eye movement (NREM) sleep Of two main sleep phases, the phase that constitutes three substages, including one with the deepest sleep and with slow-wave brain activity.

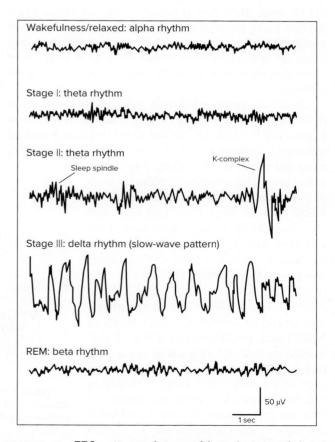

Wakefulness/relaxed: alpha rhythm

Stage I: theta rhythm

Stage II: theta rhythm

Sleep spindle

K-complex

Stage III: delta rhythm (slow-wave pattern)

REM: beta rhythm

50 μV

1 sec

FIGURE 4.1 EEG patterns change with each stage of sleep.

grows more regular than during wakefulness; and muscles relax and may twitch.

STAGE II Deeper than Stage I but still a light sleep is Stage II. In Stage II sleep, the heart rate slows and body temperature drops. The EEG shows bursts of brain activity called *sleep spindles* and *k-complexes*. Lasting one or two seconds, these waves appear only during NREM sleep, and they occur most often in Stage II. These bursts represent the brain working to remain asleep during occurrences of external stimuli, such as a noise in the room. But in this stage of sleep, sensory stimuli from the environment can no longer reach the higher-level brain centers, meaning people are not as responsive. If awakened, people in Stage II are more likely to know they had been asleep.

STAGE III Stage III is the deepest stage of sleep and the one most necessary for feeling well rested upon waking. It is also believed to be the stage that supports the most restorative functions, such as rejuvenating actions like synthesizing proteins or managing stress. The length of this stage increases after physical exercise or extended periods without sleep.

In this **slow-wave sleep,** or deep sleep, it is difficult for us to wake up quickly and, if awakened, we may at first be confused for several minutes. Parts of the brain associated with memory, learning, and other cognitive functions can become active during Stages II and III.

REM Sleep
The final stage of sleep is **rapid eye movement (REM) sleep**. REM sleep is named for periods during which the eyes under closed lids move quickly, similar to a person who is awake. This is when most dreaming occurs. Although it can be difficult to wake people from REM sleep, once awake they are usually oriented to their surroundings and not confused.

Unlike the synchronized brain waves of NREM sleep, in REM sleep the brain exhibits electrical activity that is indistinguishable from that of a person who is awake and engaged in complex thinking. Some regions of the brain are up to 30% more active during REM sleep than during wakefulness. This is especially evident in parts of the brain that are related to emotions. Blood pressure, respiration, and heart rate also rise in REM. Muscles in the limbs, however, are actively inhibited by the brain so that the body is prevented from moving during dreaming, a form of paralysis.

Sleep Cycles
When people fall asleep, they first cycle through the three stages of NREM sleep, possibly repeating Stage II after completing Stage III. This is followed by a period of REM sleep, which is always a final stage in the sleep cycle. From beginning to end, the sequence lasts about 90 minutes, and then the cycle repeats (Figure 4.2). During one night of sleep, a person may go through four to five cycles, but the cycles differ some-

what over the course of the night. The periods of slow-wave sleep are longer in the first part of the night, and the periods of REM are longer in the last part of the night; confusional awakening and sleepwalking are therefore more likely to occur during this time. Because people have more REM sleep in the last part of the night, that is when dreaming most often occurs.

Natural Sleep Drives

One key for understanding both how sleep can be disrupted and how it can be improved is to understand the natural biological sleep drives. There are two major biological sleep drives: the circadian rhythm and the homeostatic sleep drive.

Circadian Rhythm
The **circadian rhythm** is the sleep-and-wake pattern coordinated by the brain's master internal clock, the **suprachiasmatic nucleus (SCN)**. The SCN controls the sleep–wake cycle not only of the brain but also of the

> **TERMS**
>
> **slow-wave sleep** Characteristic patterns of electrical brain activity measured by the electroencephalogram (EEG) during the deepest stage of sleep, Stage III.
>
> **rapid eye movement (REM) sleep** One of two main phases of sleep, the final phase of a sleep cycle, when most dreaming occurs and eyes rapidly move under closed eyelids. Brain activity increases to levels equal to or greater than those during waking hours, and blood pressure, respiration, and heart rates rise.
>
> **circadian rhythm** The body's sleep-and-wake pattern coordinated by the brain's master internal clock, the suprachiasmatic nucleus (SCN).
>
> **suprachiasmatic nucleus (SCN)** Master clock that sets and controls the sleep–wake cycle, sending signals to the brain and to every cell in every organ of the body.

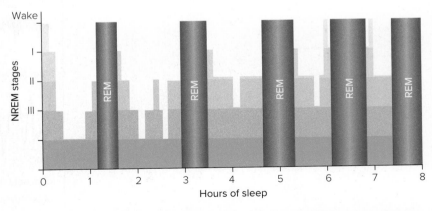

FIGURE 4.2 **Sleep stages and cycles. During one night of sleep, the sleeper typically goes through four or five cycles of NREM sleep (three stages) followed by REM sleep.**

SOURCE: Krejcar, O., J. Jirka, and D. Janckulik. 2011. Use of mobile phones as intelligent sensors for sound input analysis and sleep state detection. *Sensors* 11(6): 6037–6055.

entire body. Every cell in every organ has a sleep–wake cycle, DNA machinery that produces an internal clock; and the SCN synchronizes all of them. It also regulates the timing of hundreds of other biological processes, including hunger and thirst, sexual behavior, body temperature, and emotions. The power of the circadian system for many different aspects of biology is being increasingly recognized, and the 2017 Nobel Prize in Physiology was awarded to Jeffrey Hall, Michael Rosbash, and Michael Young, scientists who helped explain the genetic mechanisms underlying clock timing on the cellular level (see Figure 4.3).

Night is our circadian rest phase, and though we are physically inactive during sleep, our bodies are repairing cells, removing toxins, and consolidating memory. Insufficient sleep at night greatly hinders the body from accomplishing these life-sustaining tasks. Interestingly, not everyone shares the same physiological clock times. The average clock time is about 24 hours.

CIRCADIAN RHYTHM VARIATION Are you a "night owl" or a "morning lark"? Genetics plays a role. Larks perform better in the morning, but tire earlier in the day and are more sensitive to sleep loss. Owls perform better in the evening and handle sleep loss better. But because they don't grow sleepy until later in the evening, and social obligations often come early in the day, the sleep needs of night owls are often difficult to attain. Many of us fall somewhere in between these two types.

Throughout the day, we also encounter external stimuli that can influence our master clock. Some of us are more sensitive to these "time-givers," called **zeitgebers,** so it is important to be aware of how they can affect sleep quality,

needs, and behavior. There are many zeitgebers, including activity, exercise, and eating, but the strongest and most important is light.

LIGHT Light has a direct connection to the SCN master clock via specific cells in the eye. Instead of processing vision, these cells send impulses directly to the SCN to allow it to measure light. If we are exposed to light in the morning at a certain time on a regular basis, this exposure signals the SCN that it should set the internal clock to wake around that time. This allows us to develop sleep habits that are naturally regulated.

But exposure to light can also reinforce unhealthy behavior. For example, if we are regularly exposed to it late at night, then the SCN will reset itself, shifting our sleep and wake periods to occur later. This is because the body responds to light in the evening by delaying the sleep phase. In contrast, when we are exposed to light in the morning, our body resets to an earlier clock time and earlier wake time, advancing the sleep phase.

If your goal is advancing the sleep phase, the early-morning light exposure needs to occur about two hours prior to your usual wake time, and not before. For example, let's say you usually get up at 10:00 a.m. You stay up late with the light

> **zeitgebers** Phenomena that can influence and reset the body's master clock, such as light, activity, exercise, and eating. Light directly affects cells in the eye to send signals directly to the SCN to measure outside light. **TERMS**

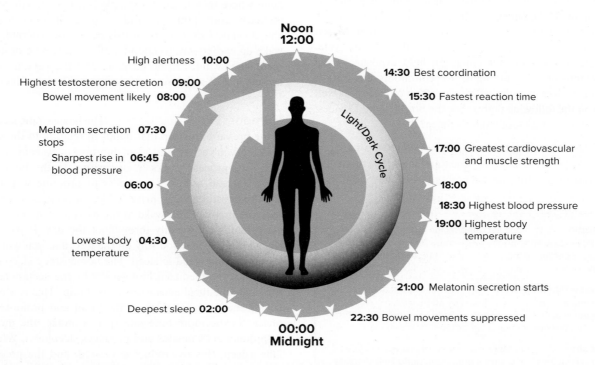

FIGURE 4.3 **The circadian clock of a person who wakes up in the morning and sleeps at night.**

SOURCE: School of Biological Sciences, Royal Holloway University of London, Matthew Ray/EHP

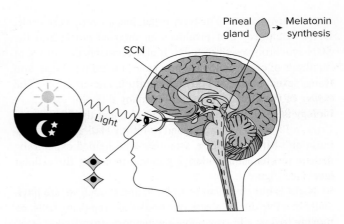

Ask Yourself

QUESTIONS FOR CRITICAL THINKING AND REFLECTION

Do you ever use a device right before going to sleep? Do you ever wake up at night to check your phone? How could you change your digital behavior to improve your sleep?

FIGURE 4.4 **Light coming into the eye is conveyed via the SCN to the pineal gland, which produces melatonin.**

SOURCE: Tan, Du-Xian, L. C. Manchester, Lorena Fuentes-Broto, S. D. Paredes, and Russel Reiter. (2011). Significance and application of melatonin in the regulation of brown adipose tissue metabolism: Relation to human obesity. *Obesity Review* 12(3): 167–188.

on, and even though a 6:00 a.m. light gets you out of bed, your sleep phase the following evening is still delayed. That 6:00 a.m. light hit you too early, and you will still not feel like sleeping at an early bedtime.

A light exposure that would cause a morning reset of sleep time would be between 8:00 and 9:00. This exposure would advance your sleep phase, so that you feel like waking up a little earlier the next day. Interestingly, the reversal point at which the effect of light changes the SCN coincides with the time when body temperature is lowest.

Another mechanism involving the SCN detects the loss of light at the end of the day. When natural light fades at dusk, an impulse is conveyed via the SCN to the pineal gland in the brain to produce **melatonin,** which signals to systems that are involved in preparation for sleep (see Figure 4.4). People who are blind often have problems with sleep because they lack the visual light signals that help synchronize circadian rhythms.

To strengthen the circadian rhythm, it can help to get good light exposure in the morning and throughout the day and to reduce exposure to light at night. The challenge is that, day and night, we are exposed to abundant sources of artificial light, which undermine our reliance on the sun's natural 24-hour cycle. Electronics compound our unnatural light exposure, especially by introducing blue light. We commonly use backlit electronic devices at night, which can affect our sleep, as well as sleep on the following nights. See the box "Digital Devices: Help or Harm for a Good Night's Sleep?"

CIRCADIAN RHYTHM DISRUPTIONS Anyone who has traveled to another time zone is probably familiar with jet lag, which occurs when the internal body clock is set to a different

> **QUICK STATS**
>
> **The best time to take a nap is between 1:00 and 2:30 p.m.**
>
> —The Better Sleep Council, 2018

time from that of a new environment. People with jet lag commonly experience difficulty falling asleep and waking up at appropriate times. It can also cause nausea and loss of appetite, which is related to the gastrointestinal system's being out of sync with the new time zone.

But jet lag is not the only disrupter of the circadian rhythm. Some people have habits that cause their internal body clocks to be set at a time that is different from the time zone where they live. An example is a person who stays up regularly until 4:00 a.m. and sleeps until noon, a pattern called *delayed sleep phase*. If this person occasionally has to wake up earlier—say, to attend a morning lecture or appointment—the switch can be difficult, and the person may feel unwell, just like a person with jet lag will feel dysfunctional.

Homeostatic Sleep Drive The **homeostatic sleep drive** is the pressure to sleep that builds in relation to the amount of sleep you've had and your duration of wakefulness. The circadian process works in opposition to the homeostatic drive, instead arousing networks to promote wakefulness. The homeostatic sleep drive is like an hourglass that turns over the moment you wake in the morning: the pressure for sleep builds up steadily throughout the day. If you do not sleep all night, and you stay up the next day, you will feel an ever-increasing need to sleep. The homeostatic sleep drive is thought to be mediated biologically by the accumulation of the neurochemical **adenosine** in the brain. This is a by-product of energy metabolism in the brain and promotes sleep onset. So the more time one spends awake, the more this by-product accumulates and produces sleepiness. When one falls asleep, this by-product is cleared, and the pressure to sleep is reduced. Naps in the afternoon will clear adenosine and reduce feelings of sleepiness during the day, but they

> **TERMS**
>
> **melatonin** A hormone secreted by the pineal gland, especially in response to darkness and in inverse proportion to the amount of light received by the retina. It helps control sleep-and-wake cycles and circadian rhythms.
>
> **homeostatic sleep drive** Pressure to sleep that builds the longer one is awake, mainly driven by adenosine, a neurochemical that accumulates in the brain. Sleep clears the adenosine, thereby reducing the pressure to sleep.
>
> **adenosine** An important neurochemical that accumulates during wakefulness, and after a prolonged period will mediate sleepiness.

Many apps are promoted as sleep aids and trackers. Can they really improve sleep? Or can using digital devices hurt the body's natural sleep cycles?

Digital Devices and Sleep

Before we look at sleep apps, let's consider how your use of digital devices can negatively affect your sleep. Tablets, smartphones, and computers emit blue light, which impedes the release of melatonin, a hormone that affects sleep and wake cycles. In one study, researchers compared the sleep of people who read an e-book on a backlit digital device in the hours before bedtime with that of people who read a print book. Those who read the backlit digital book had reduced melatonin release and therefore took longer to fall asleep and were less alert the next morning.

Does heavy texting affect sleep? Psychologist Karla Murdock reported that texting was a direct predictor of sleep problems among first-year students in a study that examined links among interpersonal stress, text-messaging behavior, and three indicators of college students' health: burnout, sleep problems, and emotional well-being.

Murdock and other sleep experts suggest turning off your screens. Use them less during the day and also when preparing to sleep at night. If you have trouble relaxing and transitioning to sleep in the evenings, shut down all your devices an hour or more before you intend to sleep.

Digital Aids for Relaxation

Now that you are resting in the dark, why would you consider using a sleep app or digital tracker? Ironically, a smartphone may help you get to sleep.

Many free and low-cost apps provide aids for relaxation and for improving sleep. Some include music, white noise, or nature sounds (e.g., wind, rain, waves, or songbirds). Others offer specific techniques, such as guided meditation or breathing exercises, to promote relaxation to aid in falling asleep. Experiment to find the aids that work best for you.

Digital Sleep Trackers

More complicated technologies try to track and analyze sleep. Many are based on movement detectors inside smartphones. Others work with sensors attached to your mattress or pillow that estimate the amount and type of sleep you get based on your movements during the night. These apps may generate detailed graphs of your sleep quality and may time your wake-up alarm to go off at the point in your sleep cycle when you will feel the most refreshed. Some apps also include a sound recorder, which detects sleep talking, snoring, and other noises, providing further information about nighttime sleep behavior.

In addition to smartphone apps, specialized fitness wristbands such as those by Fitbit include sleep trackers. These rely on wearable movement detectors. Some incorporate heart-rate data as well, but evidence is meager that adding heart-rate data to movement data improves the accuracy of results. Certain fitness-focused wearables may combine sleep and exercise data to provide an overall picture of an individual's activity over the course of a day.

Apps and devices may be popular, but no current consumer technology can match a sleep lab when it comes to detecting sleep stages or diagnosing specific sleep disorders such as sleep apnea. If you enjoy the features of an app or wearable tracker, go ahead and use them, but don't rely on an app to diagnose the presence or absence of a serious sleep problem. One good effect of using a sleep tracker is simply the greater focus it places on sleep.

SOURCES: Chang, A. M., et al. 2015. Evening use of light-emitting eReaders negatively affects sleep, circadian timing, and next-morning alertness. *Proceedings of the National Academy of Sciences* 112(4): 1232–1237; Bhat, S., et al. 2015. Is there a clinical role for smartphone sleep apps? Comparison of sleep cycle detection by a smartphone application to polysomnography. *Journal of Clinical Sleep Medicine,* February 3; Gradisar, M., et al. 2013. The sleep and technology use of Americans. *Journal of Clinical Sleep Medicine* 9(12): 1291–1299; Behar, J., et al. 2013. A review of current sleep screening applications for smartphones. *Physiological Measurement* 34(7): R29–R46; Lewis, J. G. 2013. Sleep cycle app: Precise, or placebo? *Mind Read: Connecting Brain and Behavior* (http://www.nature.com/scitable/blog/mind-read/sleep_cycle_app_precise_or); Murdock, K. K. 2013. Texting while stressed: Implications for students' burnout, sleep, and well-being. *Psychology of Popular Media Culture* 2(4): 207-221; Ritterband, L. M., et al. 2009. Efficacy of an Internet-based behavioral intervention for adults with insomnia. *Archives of General Psychiatry* 66: 692–698.

may also reduce the pressure to sleep at night. Different people may have stronger or weaker homeostatic sleep pressure systems. Someone with insomnia, who has a problem falling asleep or staying asleep, might benefit from trying to increase sleep pressure and strengthen the homeostatic sleep drive. This can be done by setting a reasonably early wake time every morning and avoiding naps during the day, allowing enough wake time for the sleep drive to increase.

Caffeine blocks the homeostatic sleep drive by blocking adenosine receptors in the brain. If you have problems falling asleep, reduction of caffeine can be very important. It is important to bear in mind that caffeine can have effects for up to 24 hours; even if consumed in the morning, it can disrupt nighttime sleep. (See Figure 4.5.)

How the Two Systems Work Together   The homeostatic sleep drive and the circadian system interact in a complex process of mutual opposition. The pressure to sleep generated by the homeostatic sleep drive is directly related to how much sleep we've gotten and how long we've been

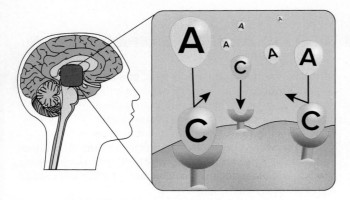

FIGURE 4.5 **Caffeine blocks adenosine in the brain and delays the homeostatic sleep drive.**

awake. The alerting signals generated by the circadian clock, however, are not influenced by time asleep or awake, but instead occur each day at the same time. These two sleep-regulating forces work independently of one another, although they are broadly aligned to promote sleep and wakefulness.

CHANGES IN SLEEP BIOLOGY ACROSS THE LIFE SPAN

Sleep rhythms and needs change throughout our lives. Babies need the most sleep and may sleep up to 19 hours per day. As you can see from Figure 4.6, the number of sleep hours we need generally declines until adulthood, at which point most people need between 7 and 9 hours of sleep. Teenagers typically need 8–10 hours of sleep nightly, but surveys of adolescents across the world make it clear that most teenagers get much less than the recommended amount. Some teens may try to restore their sleep deficit on the weekends, which can be a regular pattern, but even so, teenagers are often sleep deprived during the week.

It is important to realize that the requirement for sleep depends on the individual. Genetics plays a role in how much sleep we need. Carriers of specific genes may be so-called short sleepers, who need only 4 to 6 hours of sleep per night to prevent sleep deprivation. Other individuals need 9 or 10 hours of sleep to feel their best.

How much sleep we each need is up to each of us to figure out. But the optimal amount of sleep, for most people, should fall within the ranges recommended by sleep research.

Changes in Circadian Rhythm

Among the most prominent changes with respect to sleep patterns during the life span are circadian rhythm changes. Children need to go to bed quite a bit earlier than adults, and this should be reinforced by adults. Sufficient sleep schedules reduce problems with attention and learning as well as behaviors that occur in sleep-deprived children.

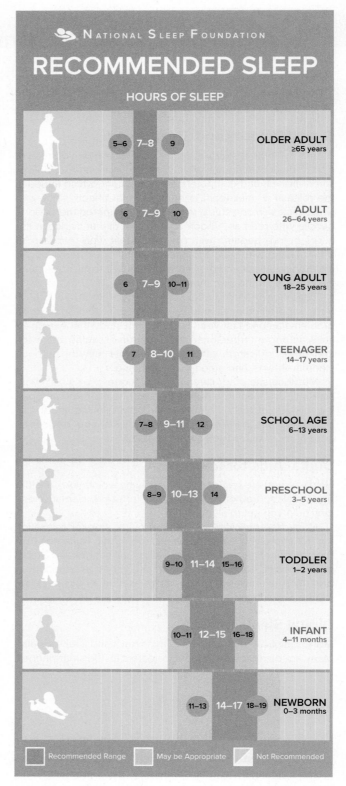

FIGURE 4.6 **Sleep needs change over the course of the life span.**

SOURCE: National Sleep Foundation

During adolescence and young adulthood, there is a change in circadian rhythm, so that teenagers may not feel sleepy until late at night and have a natural drive to sleep longer in the morning. Like children and adults, sufficient sleep provides adolescents with cognitive and emotional benefits—specifically, it can positively affect grades and mood and reduce risk-taking behavior. Both high school and college students show a sleep deficit of 1–3 hours on school nights. Then they sleep much longer and later on weekends. College students tend to go to bed 75 minutes later than high school students. In a large study of college students, almost one-third reported poor sleep. According to the study's criteria, however, almost two-thirds were getting poor sleep—less than 7 hours of sleep per night and more than 30 minutes of time to fall asleep.

School start times often force students to rise during their biological night—their circadian period scheduled for sleep—and this results in serious sleep deprivation. Sleep is especially important during adolescence because parts of the brain in charge of higher-order thinking, problem solving, reasoning, and good judgment are still developing. School districts that have implemented later start times, allowing teens more sleep and biologically appropriate wake times, found a decrease in tardiness, absences, dropout rates, school nurse visits, and car accidents and improved alertness and behavior in class, better grades, and higher standardized testing scores.

A recent RAND Corporation study has estimated that delaying school start times until 8:30 a.m. would create a $9 billion economic gain for the country, primarily by greater lifetime earnings realized through better school performance—and by the reduction in car accidents caused by drowsy teens. Despite these gains, logistics and scheduling hurdles, as well as attitudes that mistakenly associate toughness and discipline with sleep duration, have prevented most school districts from implementing later start times. California will become the first state in the country to mandate 8:30 a.m. or later high school start times, with the law going into effect July 2022.

In our twenties, our circadian rhythms shift away from the night-owl tendency so that we experience earlier sleep and wake times.

Sleep Cycles, Age, and Gender

As we age, the duration and quality of our sleep decrease. Children are the hardest to rouse. Their increased amount of slow-wave sleep and greater threshold for transitioning from sleep to wakefulness may explain why sleepwalking is more common in children. Sleepwalking happens during slow-wave sleep, when the transition from sleep to wakefulness does not happen easily.

By our late twenties, we enter less into deep sleep. By our late forties, 60–70% of deep sleep is gone. By age 70, it has decreased 80–90%, and by age 74 it may be completely absent. Still, not all older adults suffer the same degree of sleep disruption. There are, for example, differences among the sexes: women over the age of 70 show much less disruption and impairment in slow-wave sleep than men over 70.

As we get older, we wake up more easily. The elderly generally wake up more often during the night because they are in lighter stages of sleep. They have lost a lot of the deep sleep stage and so are more sensitive to external stimuli. The shift to earlier sleep and wake times, combined with sleep debt and reduced deep sleep, can cause inadvertent napping too late in the day, which can in turn prevent sleep when it is attempted at bedtime. Their regressed circadian rhythm prevents catch-up sleep in the morning and leads to more sleepiness during the day.

Age not only reduces the time spent in restorative sleep, it also diminishes the number, the amplitude, and the intensity of deep-sleep brain waves. Scientists don't yet know if reduced slow-wave sleep is a response to less physical activity and learning, or an indication that the brains of older adults lose the ability to sustain the slow, coordinated brain activity of deep sleep. Reduced or absent slow-wave sleep may also be linked to neurodegeneration. Due to their tendency to awaken more easily, older people should be aware of factors that can disrupt sleep at night.

Women in general report more symptoms of sleeplessness and are more likely to be diagnosed with insomnia; men report more snoring and are more likely to be diagnosed with **sleep apnea,** repeated involuntary breathing pauses during sleep. One reason women may notice changes in their sleep patterns is hormones. During the menstrual cycle, some women may experience increased sleepiness or disrupted sleep. Progesterone levels rise during the second half of the menstrual cycle, promoting sleep, but drop just before the cycle begins, causing sleep difficulty. During pregnancy, extra weight and the position of the fetus can make sleep difficult. During menopause, many women have additional sleep problems, such as hot flashes. Awareness of these changes in sleep can help women cultivate strategies to ensure that they meet their sleep needs, despite these hormonal influences.

Ask Yourself

QUESTIONS FOR CRITICAL THINKING AND REFLECTION

Can you think of a time you had an early class and had difficulty focusing? Did you make adjustments to your schedule? What other actions improved the way you felt?

sleep apnea The involuntary, repeated interruption of normal breathing during sleep, caused by blocked airways (for example, throat or trachea) or faulty brain signaling to muscles that support breathing. **TERMS**

SLEEP AND ITS RELATION TO HEALTH

Sleep directly influences our moods, creativity, and ability to learn, and it has an impact on immune function and longevity. College students who sleep enough hours and sleep efficiently have faster reaction times, higher grades, more optimism, and higher energy levels. They suffer less daytime sleepiness, a lower risk of traffic accidents, and fewer mental health complaints.

Mood and Depression

Depression and anxiety are common; most people will experience them at some point in their lives. Sleeping difficulty, especially insomnia, is often also present in people struggling with depression or mood disorders. Research shows that the risk for depression rises with insomnia, even when people were not depressed when sleep troubles began. Recent studies have also shown that when patients with depression specifically treat sleep problems, their depression also improves, even if the treatments are not medicinal. One explanation for this link is that the neurochemical changes associated with sleep problems make people more vulnerable to depression.

It is probably apparent to most people that a night of poor sleep can make them irritable the next day. This effect can compound over the course of many days or weeks. Lack of sleep can also affect emotions, making people more volatile and disinhibited, which can lead to behaviors people might regret or decisions that are not carefully thought out. In adolescence and young adulthood, risk-taking behaviors have been shown to increase with insufficient sleep.

Sometimes sleep problems are correlated with suicide risk, especially among young adults. A study of 438 female college students reports an important association between insomnia and suicidal thoughts. Other studies of college students found an association between nightmares and suicidal thoughts. Some students classified as suicidal also reported taking sleep medications and often feeling too cold while sleeping. Being aware of the connections between mood and sleep, and prioritizing sleep health, can contribute to better mental health.

Dementia

One major disease that can affect memory as we get older is dementia. Dementia is so common that up to 20% of us are likely to develop memory problems as we age. This is a devastating disease, but it turns out that better sleep may help prevent us from developing mild cognitive impairment and dementia. Studies in mice have revealed that there are changes in the fluid that surrounds the brain during sleep, such that the flow around the nerve cells or the cerebrospinal fluid increases by 90% in the tissues of the brain while we sleep. It appears that this increase in flow allows

Ask Yourself ?

QUESTIONS FOR CRITICAL THINKING AND REFLECTION

Can you remember a time when you were sleep deprived and did something you regretted? How did you feel that day?

for by-products of nerve metabolism to clear out. These by-products include proteins such as amyloid, which can accumulate in the brain during the day and have been associated with the development of Alzheimer's disease, a form of dementia. The fluid-clearance system in the brain, called the glymphatic system, processes the waste from the brain. Without sleep, this system does not clear as efficiently. Epidemiological studies and cohort studies in humans provide further evidence that poor sleep, and particularly sleep disruption at night, increases the risk for dementia or causes it to develop earlier.

Athletic Performance

Because performance can be improved by changing our sleep habits, professional sports teams and athletes have started hiring sleep consultants. One researcher studying competitive college swimmers observed that after adhering to a more rigid sleep schedule, students performed their personal bests. The research was more formally developed to evaluate college basketball players, and it showed that shooting accuracy and sprint times improved after several weeks of instituting a 10-hour sleep schedule.

The amount of sleep is not the only influential factor: Circadian rhythms also affect performance. A study of 40 years of NFL games compared West Coast versus East Coast teams who were playing on the opposite coast. Crossing time zones, especially with longer flights, increases fatigue and jet lag for most athletes. But the real disadvantage hits the East Coast teams playing night games on the West Coast. They consistently performed poorly due to circadian factors that kick in by the game's end, around 2:00 a.m. on their body clocks. Nighttime exercise also disrupts sleep schedules by delaying athletes' sleep onset.

Among a number of other sleep-related physiological factors that affect performance are hormones. Growth hormones and testosterone, for example, are released during sleep, and their levels are reduced with sleep loss. When, for the purposes of a study, male college students restricted their sleep to only 4 hours and 48 minutes for a week, their daytime testosterone levels decreased 10–15%—the same amount expected after aging 11 more years. The lowest levels occurred at 2:00 p.m. and 10:00 p.m., when it is likely their homeostatic sleep drive increased. Testosterone is important for muscular health, stamina, and energy, so sleep has a significant impact on men's health.

Finally, sleep is vitally important for intense skills training. Sleep can help consolidate the motor learning required to make new techniques more efficient and automated. For example, getting a night's sleep after learning to press a sequence on the keyboard enhanced study participants' speed and accuracy on the computer. Some studies have shown that there is only one opportunity to take advantage of this. If you do not get enough sleep the first night after learning, getting extra sleep on subsequent nights will not result in skills improvement.

Musculoskeletal Pain

Poor sleep can increase our risk for developing body pain and create a lower pain threshold. If someone is suffering from body pain, it is especially worthwhile to screen for sleep disorders. Improving a patient's sleep can improve pain symptoms. One challenge to this approach is that pain can interfere with sleep, creating a feedback loop; however, in some patients it may be easier to address sleep problems, which can ease pain symptoms and, in turn, lead to better sleep.

Obesity and Weight Management

We eat more and gain more weight when we don't get enough sleep. Obesity is a big public health problem in the United States, and many more people who are not obese are overweight (see Chapter 15). Healthy eating habits and exercise are necessary for maintaining a healthy weight, and attention to sleep is also helpful. Ghrelin and leptin, hormones that regulate appetite, are affected by sleep. Ghrelin rises when we have not eaten, increasing appetite. Leptin rises after we eat, reducing hunger and making us feel full. When people are sleep deprived, leptin levels are 20–30% lower. Meanwhile, ghrelin levels can increase 20–30%.

The link between increased obesity and sleep deprivation has been documented in multiple longitudinal studies of children and young adults who experience reduced sleep time. Other studies have shown that reward centers in the brain are activated more by food stimuli when people are sleep deprived, an effect associated with increased sugar and fat intake. Other related consequences of sleep deprivation further compound the effects on weight gain. People who are sleep deprived tend to be more fatigued, which makes them more sedentary. It's no coincidence that increased use of electronic media—a sedentary activity—is associated with weight gain.

Cardiovascular Disease

The connection between sleep and cardiovascular disease has been studied extensively. The strongest connection is between sleep apnea, which is prevalent in people who snore, and hypertension (abnormally high blood pressure). One of the largest studies showed that people with mild sleep apnea had twice the risk of developing hypertension in the next four years, while those with moderate or severe apnea had three times the risk.

Hypertension is particularly worrisome because it is directly related to risks of other cardiac disorders, such as coronary artery disease, heart attacks, and strokes. In addition to causing hypertension, sleep apnea directly promotes inflammatory pathways that are thought to further contribute to the buildup of plaques that narrow the arteries of the heart and brain. Cardiac arrhythmias, including atrial fibrillation, which is a major risk factor for stroke, can also be promoted by sleep apnea.

People who sleep less or who have insomnia also appear to have increased cardiovascular risk. In men with insomnia and sleep duration of less than six hours, there was an increased risk of mortality over 14 years of 400%. If these men also had hypertension, the risk rose to 700%. A study of more than 6000 people showed that insomnia in midlife led to a threefold greater risk of mortality over 13–15 years. How helpful are sleep medications? Because sleeping pills generally inhibit neural activity and do not produce natural sleep, it is best to avoid them if possible. Several large studies suggest that the use of sleep medications is associated with a higher mortality risk.

Diabetes

Diabetes is also a common condition, and it increases the risk for other disorders, including cardiovascular diseases. According to the Centers for Disease Control and Prevention (CDC), prediabetes is present in over one-third of people aged 18 or older and in nearly half of people 65 or older. Diabetes mellitus is also listed as the seventh most common cause of death in the United States. While obesity is by far the major risk factor for the development of diabetes after childhood, sleep can affect the risk of diabetes as well. In studies of short sleep duration, the risk for type 2 diabetes was shown to rise, especially in men. Men with short sleep durations had twice the risk for developing diabetes. In another series of studies in which people were asked about their sleep quality, those who reported problems falling asleep or staying asleep had a 50% increased risk for developing diabetes.

When sleep apnea goes untreated, people appear to have problems with glucose regulation also seen in diabetes. In young, healthy people, when slow-wave sleep was disrupted by low-grade noise, even when the total sleep time remained the same, the ability of insulin to regulate glucose was impaired.

Public Health Impact

Because we consistently underestimate how sleep deprived we are, we risk our own and others' lives without realizing it. One misconception is that we can recover from missed sleep with one or two good nights' rest. But even three nights of recovery sleep does not bring us back to full functioning. How many errors are committed on the road, in the skies, or while controlling hazardous materials because the operator falls asleep? What can we do about this?

You can notice a sleep deficit with the following signs: difficulty getting out of bed in the morning and missed alarm clocks, an ability to fall back asleep at 10:00 or 11:00 a.m., an inability to feel alert before noon without caffeine, grogginess that lasts more than a half hour after waking or continues after the natural circadian post-lunch dip, and a tendency to fall asleep while reading or watching a movie. Frequent movement during sleep as recorded by a wearable device can indicate awakenings and fragmented sleep you may not even be aware of and can thus be an indication of sleep debt. While brief naps at certain times of the day can renew alertness, the ability to fall asleep during the day can also be a sign of sleep debt.

Auto Accidents Do not get behind the wheel without enough sleep. In driving simulations, study participants who slept only four hours a night drove off the road six times more often than people who had slept eight hours. The number of errors committed by the sleep-deprived matched the number committed by another group of participants who had slept eight hours but were legally drunk. A fourth group, both sleep-deprived and drunk, drove off the road almost 30 times more than the rested, sober group. This means that the combination of alcohol and sleep deprivation are exponentially lethal; unfortunately, people tend to drink alcohol at nighttime, when sleep pressure is greatest.

In many states, driving while sleepy is considered driving while impaired, and people can be fully liable for the consequences (see Chapter 22). The National Highway Traffic Safety Administration conservatively estimates that sleepiness accounts for 72,000 traffic accidents per year. The CDC, which believes much drowsy driving is underreported, estimates sleep-deprived drivers are responsible for nearly 6000 fatal crashes each year.

A **microsleep,** or momentary lapse in concentration, can last just a few seconds. That brief moment, however, is time enough to fatally crash your vehicle. During a microsleep, your brain loses perception of the outside world. You lose sight, your eyelids closing partially or all the way, and you lose control of your motor skills. Most of the time you don't even realize you've had a microsleep.

People who are most at risk for falling asleep driving are those who regularly get less than seven hours of sleep. They include young people aged 18–29 and men slightly more often than women. Other candidates are parents with small children, shift workers, people who have accumulated sleep debt, or those who have other untreated sleep disorders such as sleep apnea or insomnia. Although they can occur at any

time, the peak period for drowsiness-related accidents is 4:00 to 6:00 a.m. Sleepiness can increase when people take substances such as muscle relaxants, antihistamines, cold medicines, or alcohol.

The good news is that accidents due to sleepiness can be prevented. First and foremost, it is important to ensure adequate sleep time and avoid extremes of sleep deprivation and ensure that any disorder of sleep, like sleep apnea, is properly treated. If you feel drowsy while driving, it is best to immediately pull over and stop driving.

You can prepare for an anticipated period of sleep deprivation by napping. Studies found that pilots who napped early in the evening before a red-eye flight could protect themselves from lapses in concentration that are so dangerous in the last 90 minutes of the flight. Caffeine can provide a short-term burst of alertness if needed, but it shouldn't be used excessively because it can promote sleep deprivation. Open windows and sufficient noise from a radio for stimulation may help. It is always important to remember that only a few seconds of losing consciousness on the road can lead to tragedy, and the best course of action is always to stop driving when drowsy.

Workplace Accidents Workplace accidents and even major environmental disasters have been attributed to human error that was related to sleepiness. Such errors contributed to the 1989 *Exxon Valdez* oil spill in Alaska, the 1986 Chernobyl nuclear disaster in the Soviet Union, the 1979 Three Mile Island nuclear disaster in the United States, and even the 1986 space shuttle *Challenger* disaster, each of which was related to sleep-deprived workers. The U.S. Navy has reevaluated the schedules of crews to ensure they get enough sleep while at sea. Sleep deprivation is a suspected cause of at least four major incidents in 2017 alone that resulted in the deaths of 17 sailors.

GETTING STARTED ON A HEALTHY SLEEP PROGRAM

This chapter attempts to show some ways sleep can affect our health and well-being, which helps highlight the reasons that it can be important to prioritize sleep health.

Step I: Take an Inventory

Use the sleep questionnaire in the Assess Yourself box to get a general idea of whether you are getting enough sleep. You can then use the sleep diary (Figure 4.7) for a closer look at your sleep habits. Most people can identify several issues that might be improved. Especially if you have trouble falling asleep or staying asleep, this list should be scrutinized.

microsleep a momentary lapse in which some parts of the brain lose consciousness **TERMS**

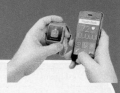

Here is a brief questionnaire to help you reflect on your sleep habits and patterns.

Directions: For each description, choose the number under the heading (Usually, Sometimes, Rarely, Never) that corresponds most closely to your experience. Notice that the numbers vary in each column.

	USUALLY	SOMETIMES	RARELY	NEVER
1. I sleep soundly.	1	2	3	4
2. I feel that I get enough sleep.	1	2	3	4
3. I go to bed at about the same time each night.	1	2	3	4
4. I engage in a stimulating activity just before bedtime.	4	3	2	1
5. I drink coffee a few hours before bedtime.	4	3	2	1
6. My snoring wakes me up.	4	3	2	1
7. I take a nap during the day.	4	3	2	1
8. I feel sleepy during the day.	4	3	2	1
9. I fall asleep reading or watching TV.	4	3	2	1
10. I wake up more than once during the night.	4	3	2	1
11. I have difficulty falling asleep.	4	3	2	1
12. I wake up feeling rested.	1	2	3	4
13. I remember that I had dreams when I wake up.	1	2	3	4
14. I have a problem waking in the morning.	4	3	2	1
15. I drink alcohol a few hours before or near to bedtime.	4	3	2	1
16. I look at the clock several times before getting up.	4	3	2	1
17. I have to get up to use the bathroom.	4	3	2	1
18. I take medication to sleep.	4	3	2	1
19. If I wake up during the night, I have trouble going back to sleep.	4	3	2	1
20. I feel sleep deprived.	4	3	2	1

Scoring

To calculate your score, total the numbers you selected. The result is your total score.

If your score is above 40 you should track your sleep in Figure 4.7. This chapter describes many coping strategies that can help you improve the quality of your sleep. Your school's counseling center can also provide valuable support.

Step II: Identify Sleep Disrupters

Sleep disrupters are factors that interfere with the ability to fall asleep or stay asleep that can usually be corrected if they are targeted specifically. Some of them might seem simple or trivial, but they can have marked effects over time on your sleep.

> **sleep disrupters** Factors that interfere with the ability to fall asleep or stay asleep that can usually be corrected if they are targeted specifically. Examples are caffeine, reflux, nasal congestion, cough, urination, anxiety or stress, pain, and environmental factors, among others. **TERMS**

SLEEP DISRUPTER CHECKLIST

- Do I have symptoms of apnea or risk for apnea (snoring or gasping even if healthy weight)?
- Do I have symptoms of restless leg syndrome, or do I kick in my sleep frequently?
- Do I have frequent rhinitis or nasal congestion?
- Do I have reflux?
- Do I often have to get up to use the bathroom at night?
- Do I have discomfort or pain at night?
- Is there something in the bedroom that wakes me up at night?

Sleep Diary

	Name							
Complete in the Morning	Today's date (include month/day/year):	**Mon**	**Tues**	**Wed**	**Thurs**	**Fri**	**Sat**	**Sun**
	Time I went to bed last night: Time I woke up this morning: No. of hours slept last night:							
	Number of awakenings and total time awake last night:							
	How long I took to fall asleep last night:							
	How awake did I feel when I got up this morning? 1—Wide awake 2—Awake but a little tired 3—Sleepy							
Complete in the Evening	Number of caffeinated drinks (coffee, tea, cola) and time when I had them today:							
	Number of alcoholic drinks (beer, wine, liquor) and time when I had them today:							
	Naptimes and lengths today:							
	Exercise times and lengths today:							
	How sleepy did I feel during the day today? 1—So sleepy had to struggle to stay awake during much of the day 2—Somewhat tired 3—Fairly alert 4—Wide awake							

FIGURE 4.7   **A sleep diary can help you discover your sleep pattern.**

SOURCE: National Heart, Lung, and Blood Institute (NHLBI)

Disrupters   There are certain medical and health conditions that can physiologically affect sleep. Other, outside disrupters can come from the environment.

REFLUX   Reflux, a common hidden sleep disrupter, occurs when a small amount of fluid from the acidic contents of the stomach rises into the esophagus, irritating the upper airway. This can cause impaired sleep quality and awakenings. Reflux is worsened by caffeine, chocolate, and mint, which cause the muscle that closes the stomach opening (the gastroesophageal sphincter) to relax. Most people have experienced reflux symptoms, which can also be more common at night when lying down.

Even babies and small children can have reflux that pauses their breathing and disrupts sleep. One sign of reflux can be a dry cough at night or a hoarse voice during the day, even when there is no sensation of acid. For anyone suffering disrupted sleep, it is worthwhile to consider avoiding food and fluid for at least three hours before bedtime. Take vitamins, medicines, or supplements during the day so they do not aggravate reflux problems at night.

NASAL CONGESTION AND COUGH   Many people suffer from allergies that cause a runny or stuffy nose. Even when mild, this can lead to changes in breathing at night and cause sleep disruption. Measures that can be taken to reduce this problem include having anti-allergy pillow covers and ensuring clean bedsheets. There are also nasal saline sprays, and if needed, over-the-counter nasal anti-inflammatory steroid types of medications. It is important not to take medications that have ephedrine on a long-term basis since these can worsen nasal congestion. Nasal saline and nasal steroid sprays do not cause these problems. If nasal obstruction is more severe, it can sometimes be beneficial to discuss this with an ear, nose, and throat specialist. Coughing can cause sleep disruption at night. Common causes of coughing at night are postnasal drip, asthma, and reflux. It is best to avoid using cough suppressants if possible. It is generally better to find and treat the cause of the cough.

URINATION   People can be awakened by needing to use the bathroom at night. One simple remedy can be to avoid all fluids in the three hours prior to bedtime.

ANXIETY AND STRESS   Stress and worry can make sleeping more difficult. (See Chapter 2 to learn about how to manage stress.) Daytime exercise can be helpful for reducing stress and may reduce anxiety at night. It is important not to engage in stimulating or stressful activities right before bed. Students are often studying and working in the evening, and it can be better to stop these about an hour before bedtime to have a "wind-down" period. To avoid having to deal with problems left until nighttime, set aside some time during the day to allow for planning. Meditation and other relaxation strategies in the evening can also help to clear one's mind before bedtime.

PAIN   Pain can be a significant sleep disrupter. Lack of sleep can worsen pain symptoms. There are some commonsense interventions that may be helpful in alleviating pain at night. Replace the mattress if it promotes pain. Pillows should be of appropriate thickness for optimal neck positioning. Mattress toppers, including the memory foam type, may be beneficial for joint pain. Be cautious with pain medications (see the box "Sleep-Improving and Sleep-Disrupting Medications"). If concerns with urination, anxiety and stress, or pain persist, consult with a health care provider.

THE BEDROOM   To sleep well, you need a physical environment that is comfortable and does not interfere with normal physiological sleep processes. Ideal room temperature is warm enough for a person to be comfortable but cool enough to allow body temperature to decline as a person falls asleep. Some people tend to have cold feet or hands before going to bed, and for those people it may be beneficial to take a bath or be adequately warmed before getting into bed. A bedroom should also be quiet and dark, without television and pets. Pets should generally be trained to stay off the bed, though good sleepers may like to have them in the bedroom.

TOO MUCH CAFFEINE   If you have problems falling or staying asleep, you should consider the possibility that caffeine is interfering with sleep. When you try to fall asleep at night, you may have enough sleep pressure to do so quickly; however, as your sleep pressure is relieved, the effects of caffeine consumed earlier in the day may grow more pronounced. It is important to be aware of the many hidden sources of caffeine and the variability in caffeine content in these sources (Table 4.1). It pays to scrutinize all the beverages that you may consume and to consider whether you should be having chocolate at night.

NEXT STEPS

- Sleep log—keep a sleep diary to discover your sleep pattern. It is best when doing the sleep diary to fill it out just once per day following the night of sleep. The sleep time should be an estimate and does not have to be exact, since it is best not to have any clocks visible at night in the bedroom.

Table 4.1	Caffeine Content of Common Beverages and Chocolate	
FOOD	SERVING SIZE	CAFFEINE (MG)
Coffee, Starbucks, brewed	8 fl. oz	160
Coffee, regular, brewed	8 fl. oz	130
Frappuccino beverage, Starbucks	9.5 fl. oz	115
Red Bull	8.3 fl. oz	80
Ice cream, coffee	8 fl. oz	50–80
Espresso, Starbucks	1 fl. oz	75
Vault	12 fl. oz	70
Mountain Dew	12 fl. oz	55
Tea, regular, brewed	8 fl. oz	50
Tea, latte, Starbucks Tazo Chai	8 fl. oz	50
Espresso, regular	1 fl. oz	40
Coca-Cola/Pepsi, regular, flavored, diet	12 fl. oz	35–40
Tea, fruited, Snapple	8 fl. oz	20
Dark chocolate, Hershey's	1.45 oz	20
Milk chocolate, Hershey's	1.55 oz	10
Sprite/7-Up	12 fl. oz	0

SOURCE: Insel, P., et al. 2021. *Nutrition*. 7th ed. Burlington, MA: Jones & Bartlett Learning.

- Choose some principles to implement or sleep disrupters to target.
- Which sleep disrupters did you identify as potential problems?

Step III: Improve Sleep Fitness

In general, once sleep disrupters have been addressed, improving sleep often comes down to consolidating sleep or identifying the best sleep window for your biological rhythms, and as much as possible trying to adhere to that optimal frame for obtaining good sleep.

Lack of Sleep   Daytime sleepiness is a major problem for college students. It can act as a roadblock to good grades, wellness, and achieving the optimal college experience, which is a foundation for later independence, employment, and social well-being.

Barring a major sleep disorder, you will not fall asleep playing basketball, weeding a garden, or painting a house. But remove the physical exertion, and sleep can occur rapidly—especially if your brain and body are yearning for much more than you are getting. Dull sedentary situations—e.g., warm rooms, boring classes, long drives, alcohol—do not cause but rather unmask feelings of sleepiness; they are therefore a good sign that your waking hours are impaired by a sleep deficit.

It's important to understand that the physiological tendency to sleep has only one primary cause, which is the

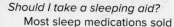

WELLNESS ON CAMPUS:
Sleep-Improving and Sleep-Disrupting Medications

Should I take a sleeping aid?

Most sleep medications sold over the counter contain diphenhydramine (the active ingredient in Benadryl) or a similar antihistamine product. Histamine is a normal wake-promoting neurochemical in the brain, so antihistamines will tend to induce sleepiness. Over-the-counter sleep aids (Tylenol PM, Advil PM) contain twice the amount of diphenhydramine found in most allergy medications. These can slow down cognitive function and cause forgetfulness—they should rarely be taken on a regular basis. Melatonin is an over-the-counter medicine with relatively few side effects, making it a better choice than diphenhydramine and cetirizine. Taking a low dose several hours before bedtime mimics the natural release of the melatonin that occurs at dusk. If possible, prescription sleep medications should be avoided. They have been associated with a variety of problems, including sleepwalking, incoordination and falls, sleep-eating, car accidents, and in some studies, dementia and earlier mortality. These are generally not intended for long-term use, and studies have shown that nonmedicinal interventions are as effective and have longer-term benefits without the side effects of prescription medications.

Alcohol and Tobacco

Some people think that an alcoholic drink at night helps with sleep. Although alcohol may help with sleep onset in some people, most find that it has a negative effect later in the night, resulting in nighttime awakenings and poor-quality sleep. Even if people are not aware of this overnight, they will feel the effects the next day. Alcohol also worsens sleep-related breathing disorders.

Tobacco also has adverse effects on sleep. Tobacco is a stimulant and can directly interfere with sleep. In heavier users, it also has withdrawal effects that can wake them up.

Medications

Many medications cause insomnia or interfere with sleep, and other medications cause sleepiness. If you are having trouble sleeping and are taking medications prescribed by a doctor, it may be important to review these medications to ensure that none is responsible for the sleep difficulty or increased sleepiness. For medications that can promote insomnia, it might be helpful to discuss alternative medications that cause less sleep disruption or to discuss dosing these at earlier times of the day. Medications that cause sleepiness should be taken later in the day.

Common medications that may cause insomnia include many antidepressants, beta-blockers for high blood pressure, steroid medications, and over-the-counter medications labeled for daytime use. In susceptible people, medications for thyroid disorders or attention disorders can reduce sleep quality if these are taken in the afternoon or evenings.

Pain medications can also be bad for sleep. Opioids, in particular, cause a large number of problems, including addiction and sleep disruption. These medications negatively affect breathing and cause sleep apnea.

Opioids also directly cause sleepiness in almost 75% of people. Muscle relaxants can also affect respiration at night and can cause considerable sleepiness. While these may be prescribed for short periods, there are almost always alternatives.

ever-building pressure to sleep exerted by the homeostatic sleep drive. Knowing this, we won't be tempted to blame our sleepiness on the factors just discussed. With adequate and quality sleep, and little sleep debt, alertness, energy, motivation, and optimal functioning should continue throughout the day.

If your drowsiness is related to insufficient sleep, start by thinking about your baseline sleep needs. People are different in terms of how much sleep they need. Start with a trial of simply increasing the time that is allowed for sleep to see what amount provides you with optimal functioning. This is the type of exercise that was instituted in some of the studies of athletes that led to better athletic performance, but increasing sleep time has also been shown to enhance school performance. To implement a 9- or 10-hour sleep opportunity, first identify a consistent time to wake up that would allow enough time to meet obligations in the morning. Depending on your sleep needs, even trying to ensure an 8-hour sleep opportunity might change your life.

In people who do not have a delayed sleep phase or insomnia, a nap might help compensate for some sleep loss. Several college campuses now have napping centers to give college students a place to get extra sleep during the day. College students may also compensate for lost sleep by allowing for longer sleep times on the weekends. Bear in mind that in some people this can contribute to sleep problems like delayed sleep phase, insomnia, or post-weekend jet-lag-like symptoms.

Social Jet Lag If you are someone who regularly sleeps until noon on the weekends, it may be difficult to sleep when you are trying to get up and ready for the work or school week, which for most people is on Sunday night. The weekend schedule may also cause difficulty getting up and functioning well on Monday. For some, this may not be a problem. For others, it can cause weekdays to go off the natural circadian schedule.

This turnabout can lead to a jet-lag type of feeling throughout the week. When a circadian rhythm is out of sync be-

Common to young adults and college students is the delayed sleep phase. As teenagers, our circadian rhythm shifts forward, so we naturally stay up later than our parents. As we age into young adults, or even middle-aged adults, our schedule gradually slides back to bedtimes somewhere around 10:00 or 11:00 p.m. In this transition time, we can nevertheless get into the habit of staying up too late—and have great difficulty getting up in the morning. People who have a biologically based night-owl tendency are more likely to fall into this pattern. A variety of tactics can be used to get us our optimal amounts of sleep.

1. Bedtime Goal

A bedtime goal can be calculated by figuring out what your individual sleep need is. It may be helpful to identify a time in your life when you felt you were sleeping well and were able to function and engage well during the day with less difficulty getting up. Once you consider how many hours of sleep you were getting at that time, you can set up a goal sleep time frame. If you function best with 8.5 hours of sleep and have to get up at 7:00 a.m., then the goal bedtime might be 10:30. People with delayed tendencies should be realistic about setting an attainable schedule.

No matter your schedule, think about how to strengthen your circadian rhythm to help you get sleepy around the goal bedtime. Delayed-type people tend to eat late at night, so it is important to count back three hours before your intended bedtime to try to finish eating. Similarly, physical activity should occur during the day and not in the evening.

2. Winding Down

You should give yourself a wind-down time of about an hour before bedtime. During this time, avoid engaging with work, electronic devices, or any negative mental activity; instead this time might be spent arranging things in the house or setting things up to make yourself ready for the next morning when people are typically less alert. Some people find that taking a low dose of melatonin a few hours before their wind-down time is helpful.

3. Getting an Early Start

It is helpful to get good sunlight in the early part of the day, to start the circadian period. Also, it may be helpful to eat a snack or a light breakfast to start the circadian clock.

Strengthening the circadian rhythm will not be effective if a reasonably consistent wake time is not also adhered to. In a person with delayed sleep phase tendencies it can be especially important not to let the wake time drift later, since that will also make it harder to fall asleep that night. Keeping the wake times in a set range will help reinforce the realignment of the circadian rhythm.

4. Limit Caffeine and Napping

A few things can sabotage progress on counteracting delayed sleep phase tendencies. These include caffeine—people with delayed sleep phase can be sensitive to caffeine because it will block the buildup of sleep pressure, and if keeping a set bedtime continues to be a problem, it is worth trying to taper off the use of caffeine, including in the morning.

As discussed earlier, if delayed sleep phase continues to be a problem, consider the potential negative effect of napping. Naps absorb the sleep pressure that accumulates during the day, in the natural homeostatic sleep drive. If a nap is necessary, it is better to take it before 2:00 p.m. and limit it to 20 minutes.

tween the weekdays and weekends, the effects can be profound. Remember that every cell in the body and every organ has a circadian rhythm, and when these are not in sync, people can experience not only sleepiness but also nausea, changes in mood, and changes in alertness and in their ability to learn, think, and work. In general, it may be better to avoid sleeping late two days in a row or sleeping much later than usual. For those people with insomnia or delayed sleep phase tendencies, it may be especially important to avoid changing your wake time too much on the weekends, even if you stay up a little later in the evening.

SLEEP DISORDERS

Although many of us can attribute the lack of sleep to long workdays and family responsibilities, as many as 70 million Americans suffer from chronic sleep disorders—medical conditions that prevent them from sleeping well. Some of the most common ones are described in the sections that follow.

Chronic Insomnia

Many people have trouble falling asleep or staying asleep—a condition called **insomnia.** About 30% of U.S. adults have some symptoms of insomnia, and as many as 10% suffer from pure insomnia.

Insomnia Symptoms   People with insomnia who do not have circadian rhythm issues or a sleep disrupter typically do not feel sleepy in the daytime because they tend to have a

> **insomnia**   A sleep problem involving the inability to fall or stay asleep.   **TERMS**

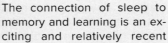

WELLNESS ON CAMPUS:
Learning While Sleeping

The connection of sleep to memory and learning is an exciting and relatively recent area of sleep science research. Around 100 years ago, the first sleep-memory experiments asked their subjects to learn a list of nonsense syllables. The researchers found that when the subjects slept after learning the list, they could recall more syllables than if they stayed awake. In a Harvard study, students learned to navigate a complex maze. Some napped for 90 minutes; others stayed awake. When the students tried to solve the maze again, only the few who dreamed about it during their naps did better. These results suggest that dreaming may reactivate and reorganize recently learned material, which would help memory and boost performance.

How does sleeping help us learn? Our memories develop in three stages: encoding, consolidating, and retrieving. When we first experience information, it is encoded, or converted from sensory stimuli into a representation stored in the area of the brain called the hippocampus. When we then sleep, some of the newly encoded memories are consolidated, or stabilized in the cerebral cortex, where they become more permanent. The information we recently learned is selected to be rehearsed and becomes more ingrained and available for later retrieval, or reactivation.

Some studies indicate that NREM sleep is especially important for learning of certain types, like learning a new motor sequencing task or learning new word associations. But REM sleep might be better for other types of learning consolidation and problem solving. Researchers gave 77 participants a list of creative problems in the morning. Everyone was asked to think about solutions, and half of the participants took a nap before being tested.

All the nappers were monitored during sleep. Only those who took longer naps entered REM sleep, which occupied about 14 minutes of the 73-minute naps. NREM napping did not boost creative problem solving, but people who entered REM sleep enhanced their performance by nearly 40%, as compared with both non-nappers and NREM nappers. The improvement was specific for problems that were introduced before napping; rather than simply boosting alertness and attention, REM sleep allowed the brain to work creatively on problems posed before sleep.

When sleep is disrupted, we can develop problems with attention, which can interfere with learning. Children and young adults who have trouble sleeping at night are especially prone to developing problems during the day—not so much that they are sleepy, but that they have trouble focusing their attention. One study looked at sleep apnea in first graders who were performing at or below the 10th percentile. Among the group who screened positive for sleep apnea, some followed a treatment plan. In the next grade, those children who were treated increased their performance to the 50th percentile; those who did not receive treatment remained at or below the 10th percentile.

Pulling all-nighters does not help grades and learning. Subjects who stayed awake 35 hours managed performances on memory tests that would earn them the equivalent of two letter grades lower than subjects who had slept.

SOURCES: Puller, K. A., and D. Oudielle. 2018. Sleep learning gets real. *Scientific American* 319(5): 27–31; Harvard Men's Health Watch. 2012. Learning while you sleep: Dream or reality. Harvard Health Publishing, Harvard Medical School (https://www.health.harvard.edu/staying-healthy/learning-while-you-sleep-dream-or-reality); Hershner, S. D., and R. D. Chervin. 2014. Causes and consequences of sleepiness among college students. *Nature and Science of Sleep* 6: 73–84; Vorster, A. P., and J. Borna. 2015. Sleep and memory in mammals, birds and invertebrates. *Neuroscience & Biobehavioral Reviews* 50: 103–119.

higher arousal tendency. That is, they have trouble sleeping not only at night, but also in the day (even though they may feel fatigued). A person is considered to have chronic insomnia if sleep disruption occurs at least three nights per week and lasts at least three months.

Insomnia Treatment Behavioral intervention and treatment of insomnia rely on addressing sleep disrupters or circadian rhythm factors. Examples of sleep disrupters are caffeine, reflux, congestion, cough, urination, anxiety or stress, pain, and environmental factors, among others. Even if those are not the sole reason for sleeplessness, it is helpful to treat those first or at least simultaneously; otherwise an insomnia treatment is unlikely to succeed. Most people can overcome insomnia by discovering the cause of poor sleep and taking steps to remedy it. If your insomnia lasts more than six months and interferes with daytime functioning, you should probably talk to a sleep specialist in a medical center. Sleeping pills are not recommended for chronic insomnia because they can be habit-forming; they also lose their effectiveness over time.

SLEEP ROUTINE If you suffer from insomnia, changing your sleep schedule can bring relief. Counterintuitively, the core behavioral approach for treating insomnia is based on shortening the sleep period slightly and setting a very strict sleep window. Go to bed at the same time every night and, more important, get up at the same time every morning, seven days a week, regardless of how well you slept. This increases the homeostatic pressure to drive sleep onset (a longer time to build up sleepiness in the day) and also sets a consistent wake time and sleep time to establish circadian synchrony. When the sleep-window approach fails, it's usually because people tend to go to bed earlier than their sleep frame bedtime, or they sleep later in the morning. Sleep restriction or consolidation approaches to treating insomnia are very effective.

Another important component of a sleep routine is that naps during the day need to be limited. Typically naps should be limited to 20 minutes and taken before 2:00 p.m. Because the sleep-window treatment is meant to produce sleepiness, naps should be taken only if absolutely necessary. Daytime sleepiness means the treatment is working! It can be tempting to try to stock up on sleep, but there are no biological benefits to oversleeping. In fact, it can extend your homeostatic sleep drive and delay your sleep phase, leading to another bout of insomnia.

Some mindset tips are useful. If you find yourself lying in bed, unable to fall asleep, that is okay. Disregard occasional setbacks and remember that light dozing or daydreaming have restorative value. You do not need to be completely unconscious, as long as you are relaxed. If you get anxious and start to worry, you might need to leave the bedroom and engage in a quiet activity to relax again. It is better to return to the bedroom when you feel sleepy again. Finally, it is important not to look at the clock. Try to forget about time once you are in bed.

ENVIRONMENTAL AND OTHER FACTORS After addressing your sleep patterns, turn your attention to other factors that influence your sleep. First, create a healthy sleep environment. While sleeping, keep your space quiet, dark, and at a comfortable temperature. Use your bed only for sleep; don't eat, read, study, or watch television there. This helps you associate your bed with sleep, which can support your routine.

Exercise every day, but not too close to bedtime. Your metabolism takes up to six hours to slow down after exercise, so you may feel more awake during that time.

Everyone is different with respect to how they respond to caffeine, but people who are light sleepers can be much more sensitive. As bedtime approaches, relax with a bath, a book, music, or relaxation exercises. Try to avoid screen-based technology to limit your exposure to blue light.

PROFESSIONAL HELP If sleep problems persist, visit your physician for help. If you take any medications (prescription or not), ask if they interfere with sleep. If you and your physician cannot identify potential problems, ask for a referral to a sleep specialist. You may be a candidate for a sleep study—an overnight evaluation of your sleep pattern that can uncover sleep-related disorders.

Restless Leg Syndrome

Restless leg syndrome (RLS) is an important sleep disrupter to identify because it is common and may be treatable with some simple interventions. RLS affects about 5% of the adult population and can affect as many as 25% of pregnant women. People are more susceptible to developing it if they have a family member who has it, and as many as 50% of people with RLS can identify another family member who has similar symptoms.

> **QUICK STATS**
> People with insomnia are **28%** more likely to develop type 2 diabetes.
> —American Academy of Sleep Medicine, 2019

Restless Leg Syndrome Symptoms RLS is characterized by a feeling of discomfort or body tension, often affecting the legs (the exact kind of discomfort can vary from person to person; it is often a feeling of something crawling under the skin, but it can be an ache, a tingling feeling, or a deep or sharp pain). The symptoms are related to the time of day, and they happen more in the evening or when lying down at night. Symptoms are helped by walking around or moving the legs, and they are worsened by sitting still, like during long airplane or car rides. RLS can be associated with small kicking movements during the night while sleeping that can cause arousals, even if one is not aware of them. If the person is awakened, the symptoms can make it harder to fall back to sleep.

Restless Leg Syndrome Treatment Simple measures that help RLS include getting more exercise during the day, avoiding all caffeine, stretching legs and muscles before bedtime, and ensuring that iron levels are in the middle range. Certain substances such as diphenhydramine (Benadryl), a common ingredient in over-the-counter sleeping pills (e.g., Tylenol PM, Advil PM), paradoxically worsen this symptom and can worsen sleep. Medications can sometimes be needed to treat RLS when the behavioral interventions and elimination of triggers have not been successful. In cases that are resistant to these types of interventions, a health care provider may need to offer specialized expertise for treatment.

Sleep Apnea

Sleep apnea is probably the most common disrupter of sleep. The risk for sleep apnea increases with age, and up to 50% of people may have sleep apnea after age 65. In younger and middle-aged groups, the rate is approximately 10–15%. Like RLS, sleep apnea can run in families, and if a person is a loud snorer with sleep problems, or has a primary relative with these symptoms, that person should probably seek evaluation.

> **TERMS**
> **restless leg syndrome (RLS)** A sleep disrupter characterized by a feeling of discomfort or body tension, often affecting the legs.

Sleep Apnea Symptoms The disorder is usually caused by a narrowed airway that gets more obstructed when sleeping, causing short, repeated breathing pauses (see Figure 4.8). Major medical problems, including high blood pressure, heart attack, and stroke, are associated with sleep apnea. It also has a negative impact on diabetes and increases the risk of work-related and automobile accidents. In children, if untreated, it can lead to poorer school performance and attention problems. Although sleep apnea is most common when people are overweight, it can affect people of any weight.

Not all people with sleep apnea are sleepy during the day, nor do all people realize that their sleep is disrupted, because they have become accustomed to it. Moderate to loud

> **narcolepsy** A rare neurological disorder characterized by excessive daytime sleepiness, sleep paralysis, and sudden loss of muscle control.
>
> **TERMS**

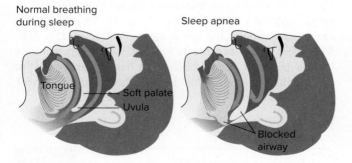

Normal breathing during sleep

Sleep apnea

Tongue

Soft palate

Uvula

Blocked airway

FIGURE 4.8 **Sleep apnea.** Sleep apnea occurs when soft tissues surrounding the airway relax, "collapsing" the airway and restricting airflow.

snoring and a family history for sleep apnea should make one consider checking for this possibility even in the absence of symptoms.

Interestingly, many people with sleep apnea are aware of having insomnia, but they do not complain of breathing problems or snoring.

Sleep Apnea Treatment Sleep apnea is treatable, and treatment can have a major impact on quality of life and daytime function while also reducing associated risks. There are a number of treatments for sleep apnea, ranging from lifestyle adjustments to medical devices. Lifestyle changes include weight loss, sleeping on your side, quitting smoking, and using nasal sprays or allergy medicines to keep nasal passages open at night. Medical interventions include removal of the tonsils or adenoids, oral appliances, or continuous positive airway pressure (CPAP) nasal masks and machines. Dental devices, which are inserted mouthpieces, can be worn at night to adjust the position of the lower jaw. A CPAP machine has a mask that fits over the mouth and/or the nose and gently blows air into the throat, keeping it open. As sleep apnea has become increasingly recognized, it has become more and more common to see people bringing their CPAP machines onto airplanes or to hotels.

Narcolepsy

Narcolepsy is a rare disorder that affects about 1 in 2000 people and appears between the ages of 10 and 20. The condition comes from a gene mutation in the brain and cannot be passed down from parent to child. Its symptoms include excessive daytime sleepiness, sleep paralysis, and sudden loss of muscle control.

Narcolepsy Symptoms When narcoleptic people feel sleepy in the daytime, it can come as an overwhelming urge to sleep while driving, working, or eating—very inconvenient times. At nighttime, they do not sleep well. And in the transition to waking, the paralysis that we all experience during REM lingers for people with narcolepsy: Instead of the brain releasing them from paralysis at just the right time, they may have difficulty talking or moving. Gradually the paralysis wears off. The third symptom, called *cataplexy*, is a sudden loss of muscle control that might be noticeable in slurred speech, a jaw dropping, or legs buckling. The cataplexy can be triggered by strong emotions like laughing hard or getting startled. In these moments, a narcoleptic person may collapse into a body paralysis.

Narcolepsy Treatment Unfortunately, treatments for narcolepsy are few and ineffective. The disorder is rare enough that drug companies have not found it profitable to invest much research in drug therapies. But patients can take a drug called Provigil to help them stay awake during the day and antidepressants to help suppress REM sleep and thus the paralysis characteristic of the other two symptoms.

SUMMARY

- Sleep affects almost all systems of the body, including respiratory, cardiovascular, endocrine, gastrointestinal, urinary, and nervous systems.

- Sleep occurs in two main phases: rapid eye movement (REM) sleep and non-rapid eye movement (NREM) sleep, which constitutes three stages. A sleeper goes through several cycles of NREM and REM sleep each night. Each stage is characterized by different patterns of electrical brain activity as measured by the electroencephalogram (EEG) and accomplishes different functions.

- Two main natural forces drive us toward sleep—the homeostatic sleep drive and the circadian rhythm. Homeostatic sleep drive is driven by a neurochemical that promotes sleep onset, adenosine, which accumulates in the brain as a by-product of energy the brain uses. The drive is strengthened by a reasonable wake–sleep schedule without naps and caffeine.

- Circadian rhythm is the sleep and wake pattern coordinated by the brain's master internal clock, the suprachiasmatic nucleus (SCN). The SCN sets and controls—synchronizes—the sleep-wake cycle of the brain and of every cell in every organ of the body. The rhythm can be disrupted by jet lag and irregular sleep practices, as well as by substances such as caffeine and alcohol. Our circadian rhythm is most strongly influenced by light exposure, as well as by activity, exercise, and eating—zeitgebers that can reset our wake-sleep clocks. Good light exposure in the morning and daytime and reduced exposure to light at night strengthen the rhythmic effects.

- Sleep rhythms and needs change with aging. In the teen years, a delayed sleep phase develops, and other circadian rhythms change. Adults consistently need 7-9 hours of sleep per night. As we age, however, the amount of overall sleep and the amount of deep sleep we get diminish. Differences in sleep arousal evolve throughout life.

- Sleep is important for mental health, mood, creativity and learning, and physical health. It promotes longevity and diminishes the risk for the emergence of major diseases. Poor-quality or insufficient sleep has been associated with a number of health problems and impairments—heart disease, high blood pressure, depression, earlier death, increased risk for dementia, weight gain, poorer glucose control, increased risk for accidents, reduced motivation and attention, and increased irritability or hyperactivity. Improving your sleep can combat our national public epidemic of sleep deprivation.

- Lack of sleep has a great impact on stress. In someone who is suffering from sleep deprivation (not getting enough sleep over time), mental and physical processes deteriorate steadily. A sleep-deprived person experiences headaches, feels irritable, cannot concentrate, and is prone to forgetfulness. Poor-quality sleep has long been associated with stress and depression.

- Drowsiness slows your reaction time and lessens your ability to pay attention and make good decisions. People who are most at risk for falling asleep while driving include young adults aged 18-29. Researchers estimate that drowsy driving is responsible for more than 70,000 crashes, 40,000 injuries, and as many as 7500 deaths per year. Accidents due to sleepiness are preventable.

- As many as 70 million Americans suffer from chronic sleep disorders—medical conditions that prevent them from sleeping well. Very common sleep disorders are chronic insomnia, trouble falling asleep or staying asleep; restless leg syndrome, and sleep apnea, repeated stops in breathing for short periods—frequently 20 to 40 seconds—while asleep. They can all be treated, some through lifestyle changes.

- Sleep disrupters are specific factors that interfere with the ability to fall or stay asleep that can usually be corrected if they are targeted specifically. These include caffeine, reflux, nasal congestion, cough, urination, anxiety or stress, pain, environmental factors such as room temperature and lighting, electronic devices, alcohol, tobacco, medications, among others.

- Sleep time has to be tailored to the individual, and then reasonable practices can be developed that improve quality of sleep: supporting natural sleep rhythms and drives, creating a good sleep environment, and avoiding substances and events that disrupt sleep.

- You can take control of your sleep by monitoring your sleep habits (keeping a sleep diary to identify your schedule and the best hours for adequate sleep), tracking your eating and exercise behaviors, and noting any medical conditions that might interfere, and then setting goals and identifying strategies for improving sleep behaviors.

- Chronic insomnia, repeated disrupted sleep that lasts for months, is very common and affects an estimated 10% of the population. Behavioral intervention and treatment is based on shortening the sleep period slightly and setting a very strict sleep window—denying

LAB EXERCISES
Sleep Case Scenarios

These cases by no means exhaust the many patterns of sleep issues people may face, and most people can encounter some of these various problems at different times. Being aware of how to troubleshoot sleep problems can help you take charge of your sleep-related health and know when to seek further help when a problem becomes more persistent.

Case 1. I have trouble falling asleep at night.

Some potential remedies: (1) Cut down and eliminate all sources of caffeine—even in the morning. (2) Avoid all daytime naps or at least limit these to 20 minutes before 2:00 p.m. (may set an alarm). (3) Avoid bright lights and electronic activities in the hour before bedtime, and remove clocks or devices that tell the time from the bedroom. It is best if cell phones are charged outside of the bedroom. (4) Increase bright light exposure in the morning. (5) Avoid exercising in the evening. (6) Set bedtime late enough to allow for sleep drive to accumulate (an appropriate bedtime might be 11:00 p.m. or later for some people). (7) Set wake time early enough so that there is enough time to develop sleep need over the day. (8) Ensure that you are not accidentally dozing before bedtime and using up the sleep drive that helps you fall asleep (you can try to sit in less comfortable chairs or be more active in the evenings if this is the case).

Case 2. I have several episodes of waking up during the night.

(1) Ensure that you are not drinking or eating in the three hours before bedtime. (2) Do you have any nasal allergies? Treatment of these may improve sleep continuity. (3) Have you been drinking any caffeine during the day? Caffeine can cause wakeups during the night after the sleep drive has worn off, and eliminating caffeine can help. (4) Do you have a family history of apnea, or are you a snorer? Is there a possibility you might have apnea? (5) Are there factors in the environment waking you up? Noise? Is the temperature too hot? Are there pets in the bedroom? (6) Did you drink alcohol before going to bed?

Case 3. I have trouble waking up in the morning.

(1) Do you have different times that you wake up on different days—for example, do you wake up much later on the weekend and much earlier on certain days of the week? If so, you may be putting your body through a frequent jet-lag experience, and keeping your wake times closer to one another from day to day may be helpful to keep your circadian rhythm in sync. (2) Are you getting enough sleep? Do you need to wind down earlier? (3) Do your bedtimes tend to get later and later? You may need to anchor your circadian rhythm with more light in the morning. (4) Are there sleep disrupters at night that are disturbing your sleep (see Case 2)?

Case 4. I am too sleepy in the daytime.

(1) Are you getting enough sleep at night? This problem may be helped by increasing your sleep time. You may be a naturally long sleeper and need more sleep time. (2) Is nighttime sleep disrupted by snoring, possible apnea, reflux, nasal congestion, noise, or other factors so that you are not getting enough continuous sleep at night even though you are in bed? (3) Are you taking medications that can worsen sleepiness? (4) Do most of your problems with sleepiness occur in the morning, and might you have problems outlined in Case 3?

sleep outside that time constraint—to slightly sleep-deprive the person. That in turn has the effect of "kickstarting" the natural physiological sleep rhythms.

- While a good effect of using a digital sleep tracker is the greater focus it places on sleep, no consumer technology can equal the ability of a sleep lab to detect sleep stages or diagnose specific sleep disorders.

- General benefits of adequate sleep:

  Improves memory of recently learned information

  Washes waste from the brain that can contribute to mild cognitive impairment

  Addressing a sleep disorder may improve inattention symptoms and learning capacity

  Helps optimize athletic performance

  Positively affects appetite regulation factors ghrelin and leptin

  Improves mood and stamina against depression

- The good news is that with more knowledge about sleep and the factors that affect it, people can improve their sleep and, in turn, their health. Along with exercise and good nutrition, good sleep is a critical pillar of good health.

FOR MORE INFORMATION

American Academy of Sleep Medicine. Advocates research and advocacy to improve sleep health.

> https://aasm.org/

American Sleep Association. Advances the medical specialty of sleep medicine.

> https://www.sleepassociation.org

Centers for Disease Control and Prevention. Seeks to raise awareness about the problems connected to insufficient sleep and related disorders.

> https://www.cdc.gov/sleep/index.html

Choose Sleep. Aims to increase awareness about the risks of sleep disorders and the importance of sleep.

> http://www.choosesleep.org

Healthy Sleep. An education resource offered by Harvard Medical School Division of Sleep Medicine.

> http://healthysleep.med.harvard.edu/portal/

National Institutes of Health. Supports research about key health topics, including sleep.

> http://www.nih.gov

National Sleep Foundation. Provides information about sleep and how to overcome sleep problems such as insomnia and jet lag.

https://www.sleepfoundation.org/

SELECTED BIBLIOGRAPHY

AAA Foundation for Traffic Safety. 2018. *Prevalence of Drowsy Driving Crashes: Estimates from a Large-Scale Naturalistic Driving Study.* AAA Foundation for Traffic Safety.

Baroni, A., et al. 2018. Impact of a sleep course on sleep, mood and anxiety symptoms in college students: A pilot study. *Journal of American College Health* 66(1): 41–50.

Becker, S. P., et al. 2018. Sleep in a large, multi-university sample of college students: Sleep problem prevalence, sex differences, and mental health correlates. *Sleep Health* 4(2): 174–181.

Becker, S. P., et al. 2018. Sleep problems and suicidal behaviors in college students. *Journal of Psychiatric Research* 99: 122–128.

Berry, J. D., et al. 2012. Lifetime risks of cardiovascular disease. *New England Journal of Medicine* 366: 321–329.

Cappuccio, F. P., et al. 2010. Quantity and quality of sleep and incidence of type 2 diabetes: A systematic review and meta-analysis. *Diabetes Care* 33(2): 414–420.

Centers for Disease Control and Prevention. 2020. *Diabetes Home* (www.cdc.gov/diabetes/data/statistics/statistics-report.html).

Centers for Disease Control and Prevention. 2019. *Drowsy Driving: Asleep at the Wheel.* CDC Features (www.cdc.gov/features/dsdrowsydriving/index.html).

Chaput, J-P., C. Dutil, and H. Sampasa-Kanyinga. 2018. Sleeping hours: What is the ideal number and how does age impact this? *Nature and Science of Sleep* 10: 421–430.

Dement, W. 2006. *The Stanford Sleep Book.* Stanford, CA: Author.

Fein, A. S., et al. 2013. Treatment of obstructive sleep apnea reduces the risk of atrial fibrillation recurrence after catheter ablation. *Journal of the American College of Cardiology* 4: 300–305.

Gozal, D. 1998. Sleep-disordered breathing and school performance in children. *Pediatrics.* 102: 616–620.

Greer, S. M., A. N. Goldstein, and M. P. Walker. 2013. The impact of sleep deprivation on food desire in the human brain. *Nature Communications* 4: 2259.

Hauser, C., and I. Kwai. 2019. California tells schools to start later, giving teenagers more sleep. *The New York Times,* 14 October (https://www.nytimes.com/2019/10/14/us/school-sleep-start.html).

Ingraham, C. 2017. Letting teens sleep in would save the country roughly $9 billion a year. *The Washington Post,* September 1 (https://www.washingtonpost.com/news/wonk/wp/2017/09/01/letting-teens-sleep-in-would-save-the-country-roughly-9-billion-a-year/?utm_term=.28c0b499742c).

Karni, A., et al. 1994. Dependence on REM sleep of overnight improvement of a perceptual skill. *Science* 265: 679–682.

Kripke, D. F. 2016. Mortality risk of hypnotics: Strengths and limits of evidence. *Drug Safety* 39: 93–107.

Lewis, P. 2013. *The Secret World of Sleep.* New York: St. Martin's Press.

Luckhaupt, S. E. 2012. Short sleep duration among workers—United States, 2010. *Morbidity and Mortality Weekly Report* 61(6): 281–285.

Mah, C. D., et al. 2011. The effects of sleep extension on the athletic performance of collegiate basketball players. *Sleep* 34(7): 943–950.

Mander, B. A., J. R. Winer, and M. P. Walker. 2017. Sleep and human aging. *Neuron* 94(1): 19–36.

Marin, J., et al. 2005. Long-term cardiovascular outcomes in men with obstructive sleep apnoea-hypopnoea with or without treatment with continuous positive airway pressure: An observational study. *Lancet* 365: 1046–1053.

National Highway Traffic Safety Administration. 2017. *Asleep at the Wheel: A National Compendium of Efforts to Eliminate Drowsy Driving.* U.S. Department of Transportation (https://www.nhtsa.gov/sites/nhtsa.dot.gov/files/documents/12723-drowsy_driving_asleep_at_the_wheel_031917_v4b_tag.pdf).

National Institute of Neurological Disorders and Stroke. 2017. *Brain Basics: Understanding Sleep.* Patient & Caregiver Education (www.ninds.nih.gov/Disorders/Patient-Caregiver-Education/Understanding-Sleep).

National Sleep Foundation. 2018. *Sleep in America Poll 2018* (https://www.sleepfoundation.org/wp-content/uploads/2018/03/Sleep-in-America-2018_prioritizing-sleep_1.pdf?x26987).

National Sleep Foundation. *2005 Adult Sleep Habits and Styles* (http://sleepfoundation.org/sleep-polls-data/sleep-in-america-poll/2005-adult-sleep-habits-and-styles).

National Sleep Foundation. *2008 Sleep, Performance and the Workplace* (http://sleepfoundation.org/sleep-polls-data/sleep-in-america-poll/2008-sleep-performance-and-the-workplace).

Nielsen, L. S., K. V. Danielsen, and T. I. A. Sørensen. 2011. Short sleep duration as a possible cause of obesity: Critical analysis of the epidemiological evidence. *Obesity Reviews* 12: 78–92.

Peppard, P. E., et al. 2000. Prospective study of the association between sleep-disordered breathing and hypertension. *New England Journal of Medicine* 342: 1378–1384.

Sivertsen, B., S. Pallesen, N. Glozier, et al. 2014. Midlife insomnia and subsequent mortality: The Hordaland health study. *BMC Public Health* 14: 720.

Steiner, S., et al. 2008. Impact of obstructive sleep apnea on the occurrence of restenosis after elective percutaneous coronary intervention in ischemic heart disease. *Respiratory Research* 9: 50.

Stickgold, R. 2005. Sleep-dependent memory consolidation. *Nature* 437(27): 1272–1278.

Stickgold, Robert, LaTanya James, and J. Allan Hobson. 2000. Visual discrimination learning requires sleep after training. *Nature Neuroscience* 3(12): 1237–1238.

Taylor, D. J., et al. 2013. Epidemiology of insomnia in college students: Relationship with mental health, quality of life, and substance use difficulties. *Behavior Therapy* 44(3): 339–348.

Vgontzas A. N., D. Liao, S. Pejovic, et al. 2009. Insomnia with objective short sleep duration is associated with type 2 diabetes: A population-based study. *Diabetes Care* 32(11): 1980–1985.

Vgontzas A. N., D. Liao, S. Pejovic, et al. 2010. Insomnia with short sleep duration and mortality: The Penn State cohort. *Sleep* 33: 1159–1164.

Vgontzas, A. N., J. Fernandez-Mendoza, D. Liao, and E. O. Bixler. 2013. Insomnia with objective short sleep duration: The most biologically severe phenotype of the disorder. *Sleep Medicine Reviews* 17: 241–254.

Vitale, K. C., et al. 2019. Sleep hygiene for optimizing recovery in athletes: Review and recommendations. *International Journal of Sports Medicine* 40(08): 535–543.

Vyazovskiy, V. V., and A. Delogu. 2014. NREM and REM sleep: Complementary roles in recovery after wakefulness. *The Neuroscientist* 20(3): 203–219.

Walker, M. 2017. *Why We Sleep: Unlocking the Power of Sleep and Dreams.* New York: Scribner.

Williamson, A. M., and Anne-Marie Feyer. 2000. Moderate sleep deprivation produces impairments in cognitive and motor performance equivalent to legally prescribed levels of alcohol intoxication. *Occupational and Environmental Medicine* 57(10): 649–655.

Wolfson, A. R., and M. A. Carskadon. 1998. Sleep schedules and daytime functioning in adolescents. *Child Development* 69(4): 875–887.

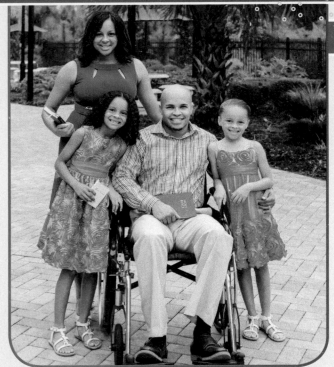
Lokibaho/Getty Images

CHAPTER 5

CHAPTER OBJECTIVES

- Explain the qualities that help people develop and maintain intimate relationships
- Explain elements of healthy and productive communication
- Describe types of love relationships as well as singlehood
- Discuss the benefits and challenges of marriage
- Describe challenges and rewards of family life

Intimate Relationships and Communication

TEST YOUR KNOWLEDGE

1. **Which of the following is the most helpful when expressing anger?**
   a. Speaking very softly
   b. Letting everything out in the moment while it is still fresh
   c. Bringing up past complaints
   d. Framing the problem with how you feel rather than what the other person has done

2. **Affordable child care is available to most families who want it.**
   True or False?

3. **About what percentage of children today live with both their father and mother, who are married to each other?**
   a. 45%
   b. 65%
   c. 85%

4. **It is normal, and therefore healthy, to have unequal social relationships in a family.**
   True or False?

ANSWERS

1. **D.** Framing the problem by expressing how you feel rather than what the other person has done avoids a personal attack that could escalate the argument.

2. **FALSE.** Child care costs exceed $20,000 per year in 22 U.S. states. Unlike other wealthy countries, few U.S. workplaces with significant numbers of employees offer on-site child care.

3. **B.** 65%. About 21% live with a solo mother, 4% with a solo father. Others surveyed live with cohabiting parents, stepparents, or no parents.

4. **FALSE.** As children, many of us might have observed and assumed that unequal family interactions, such as those between a husband and wife, were normal. By today's standards, however, they could be considered unhealthy.

We are born needing others. Our survival as a species has always relied on our ability to form strong mutual attachments, cherish each other, provide mutual economic, social, and emotional support, and create social groups, like families or villages, to raise children and produce the next generation of humans. As individuals, throughout each stage of life, we seek out others. Who do I want to be with, be like, have listen to me? How do I navigate the relationships I am thrown into by circumstance and those that I choose? Relationships are held together by a variety of factors. Those relationships we consider closest—family, friends, spouses, sexual partners—are healthiest when we can both give and receive love. Love in its many forms is the wellspring from which much of life's meaning and delight flow.

DEVELOPING INTERPERSONAL RELATIONSHIPS

Successful relationships often depend on a belief in ourselves and the people around us. Can I trust myself to say what I really think or feel, or do I depend on a façade that lets me get by for the moment?

Psychologist Carl Rogers described three conditions that characterize healthy relationships: genuineness, empathy, and unconditional positive regard. *Genuineness* refers to honest and accurate communication of thoughts and feelings. *Empathy* refers to stepping into another's shoes and trying to understand someone else's position regardless of personal feeling. And more than just an intellectual experience, *empathy* also implies vicariously experiencing the feelings and emotions of others. *Unconditional positive regard* is the ability to experience another person without judgment and negative feelings. In the development of children's self-concept, those raised in an environment of unconditional positive regard have the opportunity to realize their full potential. Those raised in an environment of conditional positive regard feel worthy only if they match conditions (what Rogers described as conditions of worth) that have been laid down for them by others.

Rogers suggests that when a person takes the risk to share something very personal and it is not received and not understood, it can be a deflating and lonely experience. We must be willing to share our ideas, feelings, time, and needs and to recognize what others want to give us in return. Just as important is the relationship we develop with ourselves—that is, how we generally feel about ourselves, a principal element we bring to all our relationships.

Self-Concept, Developing from Childhood

Building successful relationships with others requires having a healthy relationship with yourself. This means being able to soothe yourself, manage your emotions, and feel comfortable with your own company. These factors allow us to love and respect others.

Our identity and sense of self begins to form in childhood, through the relationships we have with our caregivers. As adults, we are more likely to feel that we are basically lovable, and to view ourselves as worthwhile people who can trust others, if we had the following experiences as babies and children:

- We felt loved, valued, accepted, and respected.
- Adults responded to our needs in appropriate ways.
- Adults gave us the freedom to play, explore, and develop a sense of being separate individuals.

These conditions encourage us to develop a positive self-concept and healthy self-acceptance, and they contribute to a basic self-confidence that helps us navigate life's inevitable challenges.

Gender Role and Communication In early childhood we learn to take on a **gender role**—the activities, abilities, and other characteristics our culture considers appropriate for our biological sex.

From almost day one of our lives, we receive cultural messages about what it means to be male or female, what capacities, behaviors, clothing, even colors, are for boys versus girls. As is discussed in Chapter 6, sex and gender are not the same thing. Gender roles are cultural creations rather than biological facts, and there is tremendous cross-cultural variability in the meanings assigned to being female or male. Not all cultures have only two gender roles; some have three or four.

Since gender roles are cultural inventions, an individual's natural abilities, preferences, likes and dislikes, personality characteristics, or internal sense of self (gender identity) may not match their assigned gender role. This can cause problems in societies, like our own, which traditionally discouraged gender role crossing or have powerful cultural or religious beliefs that gender roles are ordained by God or deeply rooted in nature (biology).

Over the past decades, in the United States and elsewhere, traditional cultural expectations about gender have been changing. For example, the so-called traditional division of labor, with the male provider role and mother at home caring for the children, is a relatively recent invention found in large, hierarchical societies. Even in the United States, some women, especially single and poorer married women, have always worked outside the home. Today, however, women make up almost half of the total labor force and, like men, consider job/career a central part of their lives.

The enormous growth of research on gender has challenged other cultural beliefs. We now know that U.S. gender stereotypes, such as males being more "logical" and females more

> **gender role** The activities, abilities, and characteristics deemed culturally appropriate for us based on our sex.
> **TERMS**

"emotional," are neither universal nor biologically real, but reflect long-standing European-Judeo-Christian cultural-religious ideology.

Studies have shown that girls do not necessarily play more cooperatively or less competitively than boys and that gender behaviors that previously seemed so ingrained can be changed depending on the messages children receive from caregivers, mass media, and other **socializing** influences.

You may have heard that men and women in the United States speak different languages or have different communicative styles that can lead to misinterpretation and even conflict. But while we can find variations in speech styles of some men and women, the research on gendered communication reveals a more complex reality.

For example, girls in early adolescence often start using their voices so that in one moment they speak in a low pitch and in the next a high one. Boys, by contrast, decrease their range in pitch, sounding relatively monotone. These represent cultural ways that adolescents differentiate their genders, preparing to participate in what Penelope Eckert calls a heterosexual market. They speak differently in order to fit in socially and eventually find a mate. So there is no gene for gendered language. We learn how to communicate in gendered ways, just as we learn other aspects of our culture's gender roles. But we can decide how we want to communicate based on any particular situation.

---

socialization   The process of learning to behave in a way that is acceptable to society.

attachment   The emotional tie between an infant and his or her caregiver or between two people in an intimate relationship.

TERMS

Attachment   Where do we learn how to relate to others? Psychologists have suggested that our adult styles of affection and loving are based on the type of **attachment** we established in infancy with our mother, father, siblings, or other primary caregivers. According to this view, people who are secure in their intimate relationships as adults probably had a secure, trusting, mutually satisfying attachment to their parents or caregivers. Securely attached people find it relatively easy to get close to others, and they don't worry excessively about being abandoned or others' getting too close. They feel that other people accept them and are generally well intentioned.

People who run from relationships may have experienced an "anxious/avoidant" attachment as children. In this type of attachment, a parent's responses were either engulfing or abandoning. Anxious/avoidant adults feel uncomfortable being close to others and seek escape from another's control. They're distrustful and fearful of becoming dependent on and intimate with their partners.

Individuals who endured distant and aloof attachments as children can still establish satisfying relationships later in life. Human beings can be resilient and flexible. And cultures vary in their ways of expressing attachment and intimacy. We have the capacity to change our ideas, beliefs, and behaviors. We can learn ways to raise our self-esteem and become more trusting, accepting, and appreciative of others and ourselves. We can acquire the communication and conflict resolution skills needed to maintain successful relationships. Although it helps to have a good start in life, it may be even more important to begin again, right from where you are.

Nonsexual Intimate Relationships: Family, Friends, Peers

In childhood, we often develop close relationships with people outside our immediate family, such as adult caregivers in our home or at a child care center or teachers at our school. Extended family—grandparents, aunts, uncles, cousins—play an important role in many people's lives, not just as caregivers but also in social and emotional ways.

Peer relationships also are influential in our growth. Cousins, along with siblings, may be our earliest and primary companions. Attending school, camp, and after-school activities brings us in intense contact with more peers. Through these encounters, we learn about the complexities of human relationships, positive and negative. But we also learn about tolerance, sharing, trust,

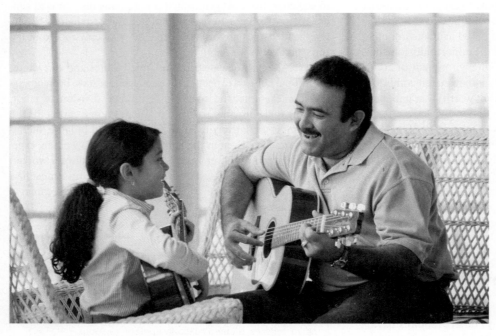

The type and strength of our attachment to our caregivers can affect other relationships throughout our lives. Ariel Skelley/Blend Images LLC

and other aspects of successful intimate peer relationships, including friendships.

Healthy friendships usually include the following characteristics:

• **Companionship** is the good feeling you have when you're with someone else. Friends are usually relaxed and happy when together. They typically share common values and interests. But friends can also be tense and unhappy with each other. Even on bad days, we support our friends as we would want them to support us.

• **Respect.** Good friends respect each other's feelings and opinions and work to resolve their differences without demeaning or insulting each other.

• **Acceptance.** Friends accept each other "warts and all." They feel free to be themselves and express their feelings honestly without fear of ridicule or criticism.

• **Help.** Friends know they can rely on each other in times of need. Help may include sharing time, energy, and material goods.

• **Trust.** Friends will not intentionally hurt each other. They feel safe confiding in one another.

• **Loyalty.** Friends can count on one another. In conflicts, friends will stand up for their partner rather than join the opposition.

• **Mutuality.** Friends retain their individual identities, but close friendships are characterized by a sense of mutuality—"what affects you affects me." Friends share the ups and downs in each other's lives.

• **Reciprocity.** Friendships are reciprocal. There is give-and-take between friends and mutual exchange of joys and burdens.

Intimate sexual partnerships are like friendships in many ways. But in addition to sexual desire and expression, there is often a greater demand for exclusiveness and deeper levels of caring. Friends are often more accepting and less critical than lovers, perhaps because their expectations differ. Friendships may be more stable and longer lasting. Like other intimate relationships, friendships bind society together, providing people with emotional support and buffering them from stress.

Love, Sex, and Intimacy

Love is one of the most basic and profound human emotions. Most of us first experience intense love in our families. As we grow older, we expand our love circle, even to people we don't know, like celebrities. We seem to love to love. Love can encompass opposites: affection and anger, excitement and boredom, stability and change, bonds and freedom. Love cannot give us complete happiness, but it can give our lives more meaning.

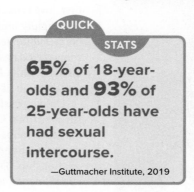

QUICK STATS

65% of 18-year-olds and **93%** of 25-year-olds have had sexual intercourse.
—Guttmacher Institute, 2019

As adults, our love relationships may be intertwined with sexuality. Most religious traditions have considered marriage the only acceptable context for sexual activity, particularly for females. Many religions also traditionally viewed having children as the goal of marriage rather than love or sexual pleasure.

Today, in the United States and elsewhere, many people reject these ideas and rely on other norms and values to make sexuality-related decisions. According to Gallup and other surveys, the proportion of adults who view sex between an unmarried man and woman as morally acceptable increased from 29% in 1972 to 69% in 2017. Guttmacher Institute reports the average age in the United States for first sex is now 18. At the same time, the age at which we first marry keeps rising, currently around 28 for females, 30 for males. Clearly, for more and more people, engaging in a sexual relationship and getting married are separate decisions.

Some religious communities worry that premarital sex (along with changing gender roles) and same-sex marriage threaten what they call "traditional family values." Young people have taken "chastity" vows as a way of upholding these traditions. Some doctors report they have been asked to provide "virginity" tests for young women. And in some schools, comprehensive sex education has been replaced with "abstinence only" programs.

Almost half of young people experience a romantic or dating relationship before age 18, although most do not involve sexual intercourse. Scholars have found that the quality of these early relationships strongly predicts our well-being as adults, including the likelihood of experiencing major depression, low self-esteem, and suicide attempts. Schools are starting to incorporate relationship issues, including how to negotiate safe sex practices or say no to sex, into their comprehensive sex education programs. Interestingly, among high school students, the percentage having had sexual intercourse actually declined from 2013 to 2017, from 47% to 40%. Yet there is a clear need for more counseling about all aspects of intimate sexual partnerships. Regardless of their views on premarital sex, most Americans see love, sex, and commitment as closely linked. Love reflects the positive factors that draw people together and sustain their relationship. It includes trust, caring, respect, loyalty, interest in the other, and concern for their well-being. Sex intensifies the relationship, bringing excitement, passion, fascination, and pleasure. Commitment, including responsibility, reliability, honesty, faithfulness, and making long-term plans, contributes stability, which helps maintain a relationship. According to psychologist Robert Sternberg, different stages and types of love reflect different combinations of *intimacy*, *passion*, and *commitment* (Figure 5.1). Relationships based on two or three are more likely to survive than those based on only one.

Other elements can be identified as features of intimate-sexual-romantic love, such as euphoria, preoccupation,

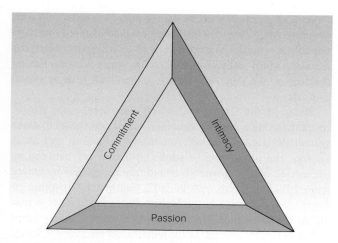

FIGURE 5.1 **The triangular theory of love.**

idealization or devaluation of the loved one, and so on, but these elements tend to be temporary. They often fade or deepen into something more substantial. As relationships progress, the central aspects of love and commitment increase in importance.

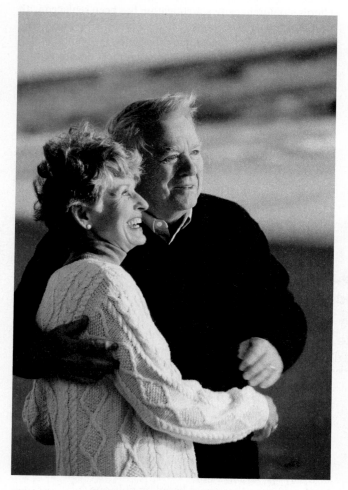

Although passion and physical intimacy often decline with time, other aspects of a relationship—such as commitment—tend to grow as the relationship matures. Francisco Cruz/Purestock/SuperStock

Researchers suggest that gender plays a role in attitudes toward sexual intimacy. Although many men report that their most erotic sexual experiences occur in the context of a love relationship, studies find that men separate love from sex more easily than women do. Women more often view sex as an expression of an intimate relationship. This probably reflects deeply internalized cultural gender roles and our history of shaming females who pursue sex purely for pleasure.

Yet more people (females as well as males) now believe you can have satisfying sex without love, whether with friends, acquaintances, or strangers, unpaid or paid. Although sex with love remains an important norm in our culture, in practice the two are increasingly pursued separately (see the box "Hooking Up").

The Pleasure and Pain of Love Experiencing intense love has confused and tormented lovers throughout history. Artists, writers, and popular culture all describe a tumultuous state of excitement, subject to wildly fluctuating feelings of joy and despair. Lovers lose their appetite, can't sleep, and think of nothing but the loved one. Is this happiness? Misery? Both?

The contradictory nature of passionate love can be understood by recognizing that human emotions have two components: physiological arousal and an emotional impetus for the arousal. Although experiences like attraction and sexual desire are pleasant, extreme excitement can be disturbing. For this reason, passionate love may be too intense for some people to enjoy. Over time, the physical intensity and excitement tend to diminish. When this happens, pleasure may actually increase.

The Transformation of Love Human relationships change over time, and love relationships are no exception. At first, love is likely to be characterized by high levels of passion and rapidly increasing intimacy. Passion decreases as we become habituated to it and to the person. The diminishing of romance or passionate love can be experienced as a crisis in a relationship. If a more lasting love fails to emerge, the relationship will likely break up.

Unlike passion, commitment does not necessarily diminish over time. Commitment brings stability to a relationship but also helps partners overcome its inevitable ups and downs. Committed partners put effort and energy into their relationship. They make time to indulge their partners, give compliments, and resolve conflict when it arises. To many people, commitment is the most important part of a relationship. When intensity diminishes, partners often discover a more enduring love. They can now move from absorption in each other to a relationship that includes external goals and projects, family, and friends. In this kind of intimate, more secure love, satisfaction comes not just from the relationship but from achieving other creative goals, such as work, home improvements, child rearing, or travel. Successful relationships transform passion into an intimate love based on closeness, caring, and the promise of a shared future.

Challenges in Relationships

Although love makes an intimate relationship easier to begin and maintain, obstacles and challenges inevitably arise. Even in the best of circumstances, a loving relationship will be tested. Partners enter a relationship with diverse needs, desires, backgrounds, and ways of handling inter personal problems. These differences may emerge only at times of change or stress. Relationship challenges can relate to commitment, expectations, competitiveness, jealousy, and self-disclosure.

What Opportunities Do Our Relationships Offer?

We have relationships for many reasons: companionship, emotional connections, erotic expression, children, financial support, and social pressure. But are we fully conscious of the motivations for our choices of intimate partners? Do these relationships repeat issues and conflicts from our past—or offer a way to heal and grow beyond these early-life problems? Some experts suggest that, as adults, we unconsciously recreate relationships with others that replay the dramas of childhood. In doing so, we attempt to work through problems from the past.

We may unconsciously play the part of our younger selves—or the part of another person (such as a parent or a sibling)—with the new emotional figure in our lives. We often hope to get emotionally what we failed to get as children. But we can also use past positive models to provide nurturing behaviors in current relationships.

Problems in relationships don't always signal incompatibility. Sometimes they reflect issues that are emotionally difficult because of past hurtful experiences. The good news is that relationship problems can provide a potential path to growth, as individuals and as couples. A man who feels he doesn't receive enough love from his partner (and didn't from his parents) may benefit from cultivating additional close relationships rather than hoping for complete satisfaction from one person. A woman who feels the need for more independence in a relationship (which she didn't have growing up) may learn how to cope with intimacy and gradually experience closeness without becoming fearful.

Ultimately the healthiest relationships are those that allow us to feel secure even when we are apart. Developmental psychologists suggest that the healthiest infants can be comforted by their caregivers without feeling overwhelmed and can be apart from their caregivers without feeling abandoned. Knowing when to comfort and when to let go can be a critical part of any relationship.

Psychologist Carl Rogers suggests that relationships in which we can be open, nonjudgmental, expressive, and understood offer us the greatest chance to grow, develop our potential, and experience the best life has to offer. We can help ourselves and others by offering and asking for love and compassion. We can free ourselves from the past by going where we are afraid to go in our intimate relationships, and then going there with our partners.

Honesty and Openness

At the beginning of a relationship most of us prefer to present ourselves in the most favorable light. Although sharing thoughts and feelings can be emotionally risky, honesty is necessary in an intimate relationship. Over time, you and your partner will learn more about each other and feel more comfortable sharing. In fact, intimate familiarity with your partner's life is a key characteristic of successful long-term relationships.

Emotional Intelligence

Recent research shows that classical IQ measures only a few, rather narrow, components of what we call human intelligence. To function well in life requires a wide range of abilities, including self-awareness, self-discipline, empathy, the ability to understand others' perspectives, and to communicate effectively—in short, what some have called *social* or *emotional* intelligence.

Psychologists Peter Salovey and John D. Mayer define emotional intelligence as "the subset of social intelligence that involves the ability to monitor one's own and others' feelings and emotions, to discriminate among them and to use this information to guide one's thinking and actions." The key to developing emotional intelligence lies in cultivating *mindfulness*—the ability to dispassionately observe thoughts and feelings as they occur (see Chapter 2). When we observe emotions without judging or immediately acting on them, we can make more measured, wise, and skillful responses. These skills can be particularly helpful when we are in an argument or a conflict with someone with whom we have a close relationship.

Mindfulness can be cultivated by being attentive to the operation of our minds, slowing our lives so we can make detailed observations, and staying in the moment as we go about our day-to-day activities. Although we cannot always control external events, we can discipline, focus, and train our minds. Practicing mindfulness and developing emotional intelligence will improve your sense of self and the quality of your relationships, and it may produce the peace of mind that many people find so elusive. (To rate your current level of emotional intelligence, see the box "Are You Emotionally Intelligent?")

Unequal or Premature Commitment

When one person in an intimate partnership becomes more serious about the relationship than the other, feelings are bound to be hurt. Sometimes a couple makes a premature commitment, and then one partner has second thoughts. Eventually both partners recognize that something is wrong, but each is afraid to tell the other. It may be painful but necessary to resolve this conflict by stepping up and saying, "We have a problem. Can we have an honest talk about it?" Such problems usually can be resolved only by honest and sensitive communication.

Unrealistic Expectations

Each partner brings hopes and expectations to a relationship. Some may be unrealistic,

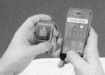

ASSESS YOURSELF
Are You Emotionally Intelligent?

Below are the behavioral habits of emotional intelligence. As you read these, rate yourself on each habit. Is this a habit you practice

Always?	Usually?	Sometimes?	Seldom?	Almost Never?
5 points	4 points	3 points	2 points	1 point

Behavioral Habit	Score
1. I respect other people and their feelings	
2. I can easily identify my feelings	
3. I take responsibility for own emotions	
4. I can maintain control of my emotions	
5. I find it easy to validate others' feelings and values	
6. I do not rush to judge or label other people and situations	
7. I do not try to manipulate, criticize, blame, or overpower others	
8. I challenge my habitual responses and am willing to try considered alternatives	
9. I live in the present, learn from experiences, and do not carry negative feelings forward	

Scoring:

40–45 = You have a high level of emotional maturity, awareness, and control. You have a positive and inspiring impact on others.

35–39 = You have a higher than average level of emotional intelligence. Concentrate on self-awareness and control, and developing increased empathy for others.

27–34 = You have a baseline awareness of what emotional intelligence is. Be alert for opportunities to increase levels of self-awareness and empathy toward others, and to refine responses.

9–26 = Now that you're aware of emotional intelligence, monitor your emotions and their impact on you and others. Notice how your behavior affects others and get feedback on how to modify behavior that provokes a defensive response.

SOURCE: Donna Earl, 2003. www.DonnaEarlTraining.com. Donna Earl is a business educator who provides workshops on Emotional Intelligence. Used by permission.

unfair, and ultimately damaging to the relationship. These include the following:

• *Expecting your partner to change.* Your partner may have certain behaviors that you like, and others that annoy you. It's okay to discuss them, but it's unfair to demand that your partner change to meet all of your expectations. Accept the differences between your ideal and reality.

• *Assuming that your partner has all the same opinions, priorities, interests, and goals as you.* Don't assume that you think or feel the same way about everything—or that you must if the relationship is to succeed. Agreement on key issues (such as whether to have children or to get married if you are single) is important, but differences can enhance a relationship as long as partners understand and respect each other's points of view.

• *Believing a relationship will fulfill all your personal, financial, intellectual, and social needs.* Expecting a relationship to fulfill all your needs places too much pressure on your partner and on your relationship, and it will lead to disappointment. For your own well-being, it's important to maintain some degree of autonomy and self-sufficiency.

Competitiveness If one partner feels compelled or entitled to compete and win—traditionally the male over the female in a patriarchal culture—it can detract from the sense of connectedness, equality, and mutuality between partners. The same can be said for a perfectionistic need to always be right and win every argument.

If competitiveness is a problem for you, ask yourself if your need to win is more important than your partner's feelings or the future of your relationship. Try noncompetitive activities

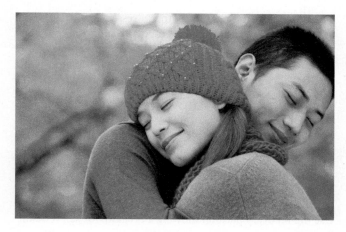
Supportiveness is a sign of commitment and compassion and is an important part of any healthy relationship. FangXiaNuo/E+/Getty Images

or an activity where you are a beginner and your partner excels. Accept that your partner's views may be just as valid and important to them as your own views are to you.

Balancing Time Together and Apart You may enjoy time together with your partner, but it is healthy to also spend time alone or with family and friends. Interpreting this as rejection or a lack of commitment can damage the relationship. Talk with your partner about your expectations and what time apart and together means to you. Consider your partner's feelings carefully, and try to reach a compromise that satisfies both of you.

Differences in expectations can mirror differences in ideas about emotional closeness. Any romantic relationship requires giving up some autonomy in order to develop as a couple. But remember that people are not all the same in their needs for distance and closeness in a relationship.

Jealousy Jealousy is the angry, painful response to a partner's real, imagined, or possible involvement with something outside the relationship, like a person or activity. Some people (and cultures) believe that the existence of jealousy proves the existence of love, but jealousy is often a sign of insecurity or possessiveness.

In its extreme forms, jealousy can destroy a relationship by its attempts at control. Jealousy is a factor in the violence in dating relationships among both high school and college students. An abusive spouse often uses jealousy to justify violence. Since physical violence in heterosexual intimate relationships, whether within or outside marriage, is primarily by males against female partners, traditional gender roles may be underlying factors.

People with a healthy level of self-esteem and people who do not feel entitled to control their partners are less likely to feel jealous. When jealousy occurs in a relationship, it's important for the partners to communicate clearly with each other. In this sense, jealousy can offer partners the chance to look closely at issues like possessiveness; insecurity; low self-

esteem; and feelings of entitlement, control, and dominance. This can strengthen the relationship.

Supportiveness Another key to successful relationships is the ability to ask for and give support. Partners need to know that they can count on each other during difficult times.

Unhealthy Intimate Relationships

Should we be able to recognize an unhealthy relationship? Not necessarily. We may never have experienced healthy relationships in our own family or social community. Families tend to mirror the types of social interactions characteristic of the broader culture or society to which they belong. Most major societies, until recently, were hierarchical, authoritarian, and stratified by class. Most social relationships were unequal, dominant-subordinate ones.

Interactions between individuals of very unequal status often differ significantly from those between equals. Those with authority and power can enforce their will on others ("get their way"), with or without discussion or agreement. Criticism can be one means to prevail. They can choose to abuse, verbally and even physically, those in subordinate positions.

Hierarchical relationships have traditionally characterized families in the United States and elsewhere, with status based on generation, age, kinship relationship, and gender. In its patriarchal form, the oldest male is the head of the family with legal authority over other members, male and female. Family social interactions, such as those between husband and wife, father and son, eldest son and younger son, often still display patterns typical of unequal social relationships. For many of us, these are what we observed and internalized as children and learned to think of as normal. By today's standards, however, they might be considered unhealthy. Today parents try to give children a voice and some agency in decisions that affect them. This is because contemporary ideas of healthy intimate relationships assume that they are egalitarian, that partners consider themselves equals, with shared rights and authority. They also are characterized by mutual respect, reciprocity, collaboration, and consensus building.

Examples of unhealthy relationships are those that are physically or emotionally abusive or that involve extreme dependency by one or both partners. According to the Centers for Disease Control and Prevention, almost 1 in 11 female and 1 in 15 male high school students report that their romantic relationship involved physical violence in the past year. The proportion is higher among those with less education and income, perhaps because they experience more stress and have been exposed to fewer models of healthy relationships.

Another vulnerable group are women, who are more likely than men to experience childhood abuse from caregivers and family members, and later, from romantic (intimate) partners. These events can make it harder to form healthy relationships and marriages in adulthood. Low-income, low-education women, especially with children, face additional difficulties because they tend to prioritize having children earlier over attaining higher education goals.

If your relationship lacks love and respect and places little value on the time you and your partner have spent together, it may be time to get professional help or to end the partnership. Further, if your relationship is characterized by communication styles that include criticism, contempt, and defensiveness, you also need to seek help, especially if you or your partner come from families with unhealthy communication patterns. Many health plans, such as Kaiser Permanente, offer couples communication classes. Sometimes, despite efforts by one or both partners to repair these destructive patterns, the relationship may not be salvageable. Consider these questions:

- Do you and your partner have more negative than positive experiences and interactions?
- Are there old hurts that you or your partner cannot forgive?
- Do you feel disrespected or unloved?
- Do you find it increasingly hard to feel positive feelings of affection for your partner?
- Does it feel as if your relationship has been a waste of time?
- Do you, and your partner, recognize your own roles in creating and solving the relationship problems?

Spiritual leaders suggest that relationships are unhealthy when one or both partners feel a deadening of their sense of spontaneity, potential for inner growth and joy, and connection to their spiritual life. There are negative physical and mental consequences of being in an unhappy relationship. Although breaking up is painful and difficult, it is ultimately better than living in a toxic relationship.

Ending a Relationship

Even when a couple starts out with the best of intentions, an intimate relationship may not last. Some breakups happen quickly following direct action by one or both partners, but many occur over an extended period as the couple goes through a cycle of separation and reconciliation.

If you are involved in a breakup, the following suggestions may help make the ending easier:

- *Give the relationship a fair chance before breaking up.* If it's still not working, you'll know you did everything you could.

- *Be fair and honest.* If you're initiating the breakup, don't try to make your partner feel responsible.

- *Be tactful and compassionate.* You can leave the relationship without deliberately damaging your partner's self-esteem. Emphasize your mutual incompatibility, and admit your own contributions to the problem.

- *If you are the rejected person, give yourself time to resolve your anger and pain.* Mobilize your coping resources, including social support and other stress management techniques. You may go through a process of mourning the relationship, experiencing disbelief, anger, sadness, and finally acceptance. Remember that there are many people with whom you can potentially have an intimate relationship.

- *Recognize the value in the experience.* Honor the feelings that you shared with your partner by validating the relationship as a worthwhile experience. Ending a close relationship can teach you valuable lessons about your needs, preferences, strengths, and weaknesses. Reflect on the experience and use your insights to increase your chance of success in your next relationship.

Use the recovery period following a breakup for self-renewal. Redirect more attention to yourself, and reconnect with people and areas of your life that were neglected during your relationship. Time will help heal the pain of the loss.

Finally, be aware of the impulse to "rebound" quickly into another relationship. Although it may mute the pain of a breakup, forming a relationship in order to avoid feeling pain is not a good strategy. Too often, rebound relationships fail because they were designed to be "lifeboats" or because one or both partners is not truly ready for another intimate relationship.

COMMUNICATION

A key to developing and maintaining healthy intimate relationships is good communication. Most of the time we don't think about communicating; we simply talk and behave normally. But when problems arise—when we feel others don't understand us or when someone accuses us of not listening—we become aware of our limitations or, more commonly, what we think are other people's limitations. Miscommunication creates frustration and distances us from those closest to us.

Nonverbal Communication

Even when we're silent, we're communicating. We send messages when we look at someone or look away, lean forward or sit back, smile or frown. Especially important forms of nonverbal communication in the United States are touch, eye contact, and proximity. If someone we're talking to touches our hand or arm, looks into our eyes, and leans toward us when we talk, we get the message that the person is interested in us and cares about what we're saying. If a person keeps looking around the room while we're talking or takes a step backward, we get the impression the person is uninterested or wants to end the conversation.

The ability to interpret nonverbal messages correctly is important to the success of relationships. It's also important, when sending messages, to make sure our body language agrees with our words. When our verbal and nonverbal messages don't correspond, we send a mixed message.

Attunement, or tuning in to each other's tone of voice, is important. More than any other cue, tone of voice can convey most accurately a person's emotional state. Our effectiveness at connecting or reconnecting emotionally with another depends on the accuracy of our attunement. Effective attunement recreates a healthy child-caregiver connection, or it provides a connection that was lacking during childhood.

How we feel when communicating with another can give the listener important data about the speaker. If "out of nowhere" we begin to feel sad, anxious, or angry, these may be emotional states the other person is communicating. An example would be feeling sad when communicating with a grieving friend.

Digital Communication and Our Social Networks

Social media enable us to communicate more rapidly, but some experts question whether this capability is undermining interpersonal relations and our ability to relate to others in person. Some evidence suggests the opposite is true: Surveys by the Pew Internet and American Life Project found that technology users had larger and more diverse discussion networks and were just as involved in their communities as people who communicate face-to-face. Many young adults (aged 18–29 years) who were in a serious relationship reported feeling closer to their spouse or partner due to online or text-message conversations. Some said they were able to resolve arguments that they couldn't face-to-face.

Recent research suggests the relationship between social media and mental health goes in both directions. Social media can impact the well-being of users; but poor mental health, such as depressive symptoms, also predicts more frequent use of social media. The critical question is really what users are doing on social media, and the content to which they are being exposed, not the amount of time spent.

Social media create diverse forms of communication. The brief immediacy of a tweet is very different from an extended conversation over Skype. But people often use a tweet to communicate something too complicated for anything other than Skype.

Some observers worry that technologies alter the nature of the social environment and the size and makeup of social networks. Facebook, for example, facilitates relationships with people we have shared interests with but may never meet in person. As it becomes more common for family members to live apart and as online communication evolves, the face-to-face aspects of relationships may become less significant, but perhaps more valued.

Social media do provide some advantages. They allow for instant and easy communication with others across the globe. They enable long-distance connections; reconnections with important people from our past; and affiliations with others who share similar (sometimes rare) identities, interests, and experiences. They allow teenagers (and others) to experiment with new behaviors, such as flirting, or assume new identities in a relatively risk-free environment.

But they also make it easier to communicate impulsively, such as sending angry or threatening messages, stalking, posting embarrassing pictures of peers or ex-partners, or pursuing new partners while in a supposedly monogamous relationship. Some people even end intimate relationships online. Electronic bullying (and "shaming") is a significant problem among pre-college students and has led to several suicides. In 2017, almost 15% of high school students reported being electronically bullied. These figures were significantly higher for females (19.7%) than for males (9.9%) and higher for Euro-Americans than for African Americans or Latinx. Similar levels of bullying were reported in previous years.

Using social media while avoiding the pitfalls requires being mindful of how these technologies can influence communication and relationships. In addition to the capacity for impulsive communication, here are other problem areas online:

- *Missing nonverbal cues such as body language and tone of voice.* A comment or joke intended as playful may instead come off as critical or harsh.

- *Promoting an idealized version of oneself.* Since we control our online image (to a degree), many of us promote a version that involves only the most flattering photos and happiest moments. Doing so can have a serious downside if the gap between one's "real" and online lives becomes too large, or maintaining the image becomes too consuming.

- *Spying.* In the past, people who suspected their partners of cheating had to follow them or hire detectives to see what they were doing. These days, it is as easy as checking statuses and messages, which makes it more tempting to invade a partner's privacy when feeling suspicious or insecure.

- *Checking one's phone rather than staying present.* How often have you seen a couple at a restaurant, and both of them are checking their phones rather than engaging in conversation? Social media can be great tools, but only when they don't replace experiencing life in the moment.

- *Publicizing more areas of one's life.* Messages, photos, and status updates are often accessible to large numbers of people, making it important to think carefully about what information to share on social media. Sometimes people in a relationship differ dramatically in their ideas about what should be public versus private, so this is an important topic for discussion. Any potentially embarrassing or intimate (e.g., nude) photos should never be posted without the permission of those in the photo.

Communication Skills

Three skills essential to good communication in relationships are self-disclosure, listening, and feedback:

• *Self-disclosure* involves revealing personal information that we ordinarily wouldn't reveal due to the risk involved. It usually increases feelings of closeness and moves the relationship to a deeper level of intimacy. Friends often confide in each other, sharing feelings, experiences, hopes, and disappointments. Married couples sometimes feel less need to share, making unwarranted assumptions because they think that they already know everything about each other.

• *Listening* requires that we spend more time and energy trying to fully understand another person's "story" and less time judging, evaluating, blaming, advising, analyzing, or trying to control. Empathy, warmth, respect, and genuineness are qualities of skillful listeners. Attentive listening encourages friends or partners to share more and, in turn, to be attentive listeners. To connect with other people and develop real emotional intimacy, listening is essential.

• *Feedback,* a constructive response to another's self-disclosure, is the third key to good communication. Giving positive feedback means acknowledging that the friend's or partner's feelings are valid—no matter how upsetting or troubling—and offering self-disclosure in response. If, for example, your partner discloses unhappiness about your relationship, it is more constructive to say that you're concerned or saddened by that and want to hear more about it than to get angry, blame, try to inflict pain, or withdraw. Self-disclosure and feedback can open the door to change, whereas other responses block communication and change. (For tips on improving your skills, see the box "Guidelines for Effective Communication.")

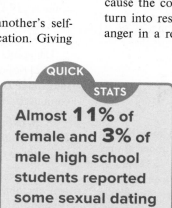

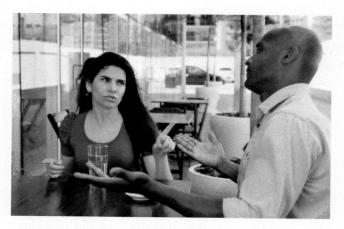

Conflict is an inevitable part of any intimate relationship. How can we resolve our conflicts in constructive ways? DMEPhotography/Getty Images

Conflict and Conflict Resolution

Conflict is normal in intimate relationships. No matter how close two people become, they remain separate individuals with their own needs, desires, past experiences, and ways of seeing the world. In fact, the closer the relationship, the more differences and the more opportunities for conflict.

Although conflict may suggest that the relationship is deepening, if it is not handled constructively, conflict can damage—and ultimately destroy—the relationship. Consider the guidelines discussed here, but remember that different couples communicate in different ways around conflict. Gender, family and cultural background, education, and income level are among factors that influence how we experience and deal with conflict.

Conflict is often accompanied by anger—a natural emotion—but one that can be difficult to handle, especially for those who haven't learned to channel it in a constructive way. If we express anger aggressively, we risk creating distrust, fear, and distance. If we act out our anger, we can cause the conflict to escalate. If we suppress anger, it may turn into resentment and hostility. The best way to handle anger in a relationship is to recognize it as a symptom of something that requires attention and needs to be addressed. When angry, partners should exercise restraint so as not to become abusive. It is important to express anger skillfully and not in a way that is out of proportion to the issue at hand. The best time to express yourself is when you are not boiling over with strong emotions.

The sources of conflict for couples change over time but revolve, at least on the surface, primarily around issues of finances, sex, children, in-laws, and household responsibilities. Issues of power, authority, and challenges to traditional gender roles are often deeper roots of conflict. Although there are numerous theories on and approaches to conflict resolution, these fundamental strategies can be helpful:

1. *Clarify the issue.* Take responsibility for thinking through your feelings and discovering what's really bothering you. Agree that one partner will speak first and have the chance to speak fully while the other listens. Then reverse the roles. Try to understand your partner's position fully by repeating what you've heard and asking questions to clarify or elicit more information. Agree to talk only about the topic at hand and not get distracted by other issues. Sum up what your partner has said.

2. *Find out what each person wants.* Ask your partner to express their desires. Don't assume you know what your partner wants, and don't speak for them.

3. *Determine how you both can get what you want.* Brainstorm to come up with a variety of options.

4. *Decide how to negotiate.* Work out a plan for change. Be willing to compromise, and avoid trying to "win."

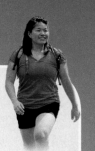

Getting Started

• When you want to have a serious discussion with your partner, choose a private place and a time when you won't be interrupted or rushed. Avoid having important conversations via text or other media.

• Face your partner and maintain eye contact. Use nonverbal feedback to show that you are interested and involved.

Being an Effective Speaker

• State your concern or issue as clearly as you can.

• Use "I" statements rather than statements beginning with "you." When you use "I" statements, you take responsibility for your feelings. "You" statements are often blaming or accusatory and will probably get a defensive or resentful response. The statement "I feel unloved," for example, sends a clearer, less blaming message than the statement "You don't love me."

• Focus on a behavior, not the whole person. Be specific about the behavior you like or don't like. Avoid generalizations beginning with "you always" or "you never." Such statements make people feel defensive.

• Make constructive requests. Opening your request with "I would like" keeps the focus on your needs rather than your partner's supposed deficiencies.

• Avoid blaming, accusing, and belittling. Even if you are right, you have little to gain by putting your partner down. When people feel criticized or attacked, they are less able to think rationally or solve problems constructively.

• Set up your partner for success. Tell your partner what you would like to have happen in the future; don't wait for him or her to blow it and then express anger or disappointment.

Being an Effective Listener

• Provide appropriate nonverbal feedback (nodding, smiling, making eye contact, and so on).

• Don't interrupt.

• Listen reflectively. Don't judge, evaluate, analyze, or offer solutions (unless asked to do so). Your partner may just need to sort out his or her feelings. By jumping in to "fix" the problem, you may cut off communication.

• Don't offer unsolicited advice. Giving advice implies that you know more about what a person needs to do than she or he does; therefore, it often evokes anger or resentment.

• Clarify your understanding of what your partner is saying by restating it in your own words and asking if your understanding is correct. "I think you're saying that you would feel uncomfortable having dinner with my parents and that you'd prefer to meet them in a more casual setting. Is that right?" This type of specific feedback prevents misunderstandings and helps validate the speaker's feelings and message.

• Be sure you are really listening, not off somewhere in your mind rehearsing your reply. Try to tune in to your partner's feelings and needs as well as the words. Accurately reflecting the other person's feelings and needs is often a more powerful way of connecting than just reframing his or her thoughts.

• Let your partner know that you value what they are saying and want to understand. Respect for the other person is the cornerstone of effective communication.

---

5. **Solidify the agreements.** If necessary, go over the plan and write it down, to ensure that you both understand and agree to it.

6. **Review and renegotiate.** Decide on a time frame for trying out your plan, and set a time to discuss how it's working. Make adjustments as needed.

To resolve conflicts, partners must feel safe in voicing disagreements. They have to trust that the discussion won't get out of control, that they won't be abandoned, and that their vulnerability won't be taken advantage of. Partners should follow some basic ground rules when they argue, such as avoiding ultimatums, resisting the urge to give the silent treatment, refusing to "hit below the belt," and not using sex to smooth over disagreements.

When you argue, maintain a spirit of goodwill and avoid being harshly critical or contemptuous. Remember—you care about your partner and want things to work out. See the disagreement as a difficulty that the two of you have together rather than as something your partner does to you. Finish serious discussions on a positive note by expressing your respect and affection for your partner and your appreciation for having been listened to. If you and your partner find that you argue again and again over the same issue, it may be better to stop trying to resolve that problem and instead come to accept the differences between you, or part ways if the differences are intolerable.

PAIRING AND SINGLEHOOD

Alternatives to the old model of marriage are increasingly popular. Cohabitation, divorce, and singlehood have become common. Same-sex marriage is now legal in all 50 states, and the concept of family is expanding. Multiple marriages, polymorphy (three-or-more-person relationships), blended families, and nonkinship-based families are examples of new creative intimate social arrangements.

Choosing a Partner

Studies have shown that most people pair with someone who

- Lives in the same geographic area
- Comes from a similar racial, ethnic, and socioeconomic background
- Has a similar educational status
- Leads a lifestyle like theirs
- Has (what they think is) the same level of physical attractiveness as themselves

Once the euphoria of romantic love winds down, personality traits, behaviors, and socioeconomic status become more significant in how partners view each other. The emphasis shifts to basic values and future aspirations regarding career, family, and children. At some point, they decide whether the relationship feels viable and is worthy of their continued commitment.

Perhaps the most important question for potential mates to ask is, "How much do we have in common?" Although differences add interest to a relationship, similarities increase its chance of success. Differences in values, religion, race, ethnicity, cultural background, socioeconomic status, and beliefs about gender and sexuality can produce strains. But acceptance and communication skills go a long way toward making a relationship work, no matter how different the partners.

Dating

Every culture has certain criteria and rituals for finding and choosing mates. Historically, families played a major role in selecting spouses, sometimes explicitly, as in arranged marriages, or more informally, through casual references to unacceptable future spouse characteristics (e.g., other races, religions, ethnic groups). Often parents used family and social networks to find "suitable" mates for their children. And people married at an early age.

Arranged marriage by families is still the norm today in many parts of the world. Such marriages tend to be stable and permanent. With the rise in education and the age of marriage, potential spouses now have a greater say in the marriage. They may meet and get to know each other before consenting. But premarital dating, in the sense we think of it today, is a relatively new phenomenon and far from universal.

Nevertheless, American cultural norms of romantic love and personal choice in courtship and mate selection have an enormous appeal globally. Themes of romantic love and finding one's soul mate permeate popular culture (movies, music, videos, TV) and consumer marketing around the world. But in the United States, as elsewhere, the popularity of dating services and online matchmaking suggests that people want help finding a suitable partner.

Dating is still a common way to find a romantic partner. In recent years, new innovations such as speed dating enable participants to meet a large number of people for short periods of time in a single, highly organized session. It is an efficient way of screening for attraction. Casual group dates

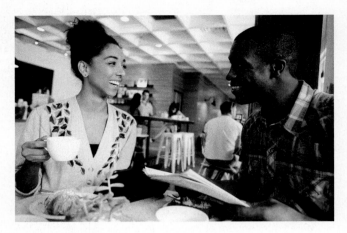

Physical attraction plays a strong role in the initial choosing of a partner. People tend to gravitate toward others who share similar characteristics, such as appearance, race, ethnicity, education, and socioeconomic background. monkeybusinessimages/Getty Images

allow people to get to know each other without the pressure of being on a "date." Two people may begin to spend more time together, within and outside the group. If sexual involvement develops, it is more likely to be based on friendship, respect, and common interests than on gender role expectations. Such relationships may lead to marriage. In contrast, some teenagers and young adults are turning to *hooking up*—casual sexual activity without any relationship commitment. For more about this trend, see the box "Hooking Up."

Online Dating and Relationships

Until 2013, probably since the earliest days of mating, the most popular way to meet a potential mate was through family and friends. Over the past few years, online dating has continued to grow, and it has now surpassed all other ways to date. For one, the sets of people available to meet are larger than friend connections. These numbers are especially valuable for people searching for something hard to find, like particular qualities in others, or non-heterosexual orientations. With millions of singles using dating sites that let them describe in detail what they are seeking, the internet can increase a person's chance of finding a good match.

Another benefit of connecting online is freedom from your family, friends, and even candidate dating partners. Connecting with others online allows people to communicate in a relaxed way, try out different personas, and share things they normally would not reveal face-to-face. You can set your own pace and start and end relationships at any time. If they don't pass initial filters, it is easier to block unwanted dates before meeting in person.

Some people, however, misrepresent themselves, pretending to be older or younger or even of a different sex than they really are. Investing time and emotional resources in such relationships can be painful. In rare cases, online romances become dangerous or even deadly (see Chapter 22 for information on cyberstalking).

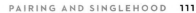

Hooking up—having casual sexual encounters with acquaintances or strangers with no commitment or investment in an emotionally intimate relationship—may be a current trend among teenagers and young adults. Although casual sex is not new, the difference today is that hooking up is said to be the main form of sexual activity for some people, as opposed to sexual activity within a relationship. Some data indicate that more than 80% of college students have had at least one hookup experience. If dating occurs at all, it happens after people have had sex and become a couple.

Hooking up is said to have its roots in the changing social and sexual patterns of the 1960s. Since then, changes in college policies have contributed to the shift, such as the move away from colleges acting *in loco parentis* (in the place of parents), the trend toward coed dorms, a trend toward getting married at a later age, and the availability of dating apps. The availability of effective contraception and access to legal abortion have also allowed women to explore their sexuality without past fears of pregnancy. Hooking up addresses the desire for "instant intimacy" but also protects the participants from the risk or responsibility of emotional involvement.

Because hooking up is often fueled by alcohol, it is associated with sexual risk taking and negative health effects, including the risk of acquiring a sexually transmitted infection. Those aged 15–24 account for half of STI cases in the United States. Hooking up can also have adverse emotional and mental health consequences, including sexual regret and psychological distress.

Due to these and other concerns, a backlash against hooking up has taken place on some college campuses. In some cases, individuals are deciding they don't want to be part of the hookup culture. In other cases, groups and organizations have formed to call for a return to traditional dating or at least some middle ground between dating and hooking up.

However, recent studies question whether hookup culture is actually anything new. Results from the General Social Survey, which explores attitudes and behaviors around a wide variety of issues, suggest that millennials are actually less sexually active than previous generations. If that's true, then how did the idea of hookup culture become so widespread? First, we tend to look at the past with rose-colored glasses and thus imagine the "good old days" when people had sex only in the context of committed relationships. Second, young people have a tendency to assume (incorrectly) that all their peers are having sex—that everyone around them is hooking up, except for them. Third, people who aren't the norm (that is, outliers who are having outrageous amounts of sex) are the ones who tend to get media attention, since they provide a more titillating story.

SOURCES: Carpenter, L., and J. DeLamater, eds. 2012. *Sex for Life: From Virginity to Viagra, How Sexuality Changes Throughout Our Lives.* New York: New York University Press, pp. 128–144; CDC. 2017. STDs in adolescents and young adults (https://www.cdc.gov/std/stats16/adolescents.htm). Garcia, J. R., et al. 2013. Sexual hook-up culture. *Monitor on Psychology* 44(2): 60; Wade, L. 2017. *American Hookup: The New Culture of Sex on Campus.* New York: W. W. Norton.

Because people online reveal only what they want to, users may see idealized versions of online partners. If your online friend seems perfect, take that as a warning sign. You may search for perfection, find fault quickly, and not give people a chance; conversely, you may act on impulse with insufficient information.

Relationship sites also remove an important and powerful element from the process: chemistry and in-person intuition. Much of our communication is transmitted through body language, tone, and even scent. Consider these questions. Are you comfortable disclosing personal information about yourself? Is there a balance in the amount of time spent talking by each of you? Is the other person respecting your boundaries? Just as in face-to-face dating, online relationships require you to use common sense and to trust your instincts.

If you pursue an online relationship, these guidelines may help you have a positive experience and stay safe:

• Choose a site that fits with your own relationship goals. Some sites are primarily geared for hookups—that is, arranging meetings for casual sex—whereas others aim to facilitate classic dating relationships. Inspect each site thoroughly before registering or providing any information about yourself. If you aren't comfortable with a site's content or purpose, close your web browser and clear out its cache and its store of cookies.

• Know what you are looking for as well as what you can offer someone else. If you are looking for a relationship that is not just physical, make that clear. Find out the other person's intentions.

• Don't post photos unless you are completely comfortable with potential consequences (e.g., they might be downloaded by others).

• Don't give out personal information, including your real full name, school, or place of employment, until you feel sure that you are giving the information to someone who is trustworthy.

• Set up a second email account for sending and receiving dating-related emails.

> **QUICK STATS**
> Almost **40%** of heterosexual couples meeting in 2017 met online
> —Rosenfeld, Thomas, and Hausen, 2019

- If someone does not respond to a message, don't take it personally. There are many reasons why a person may not pursue the connection. Don't continue to send messages to an unresponsive person; doing so could lead to an accusation of stalking.

- Before deciding whether to meet an online contact in person, consider talking over the phone.

- Don't agree to meet someone face-to-face unless you feel comfortable about it. Always meet initially in a public place—a museum, a coffee shop, or a restaurant. Consider bringing along a friend to increase your safety, and let others know where you will be.

- At the same time, don't let too much time pass exchanging messages: It's important to discover your compatibility in person.

If you pursue online relationships, don't let them interfere with your other personal relationships and social activities. To support your emotional and personal wellness, use the Internet to widen your circle of friends, not shrink it.

Sexual Orientation and Gender Identity in Relationships

People demonstrate great diversity in their emotional and sexual attractions (see Chapter 6). **Sexual orientation** refers to a pattern of emotional and sexual attraction to persons of the same sex or gender, a different sex or gender, or more than one sex or gender. The term **queer** has emerged to describe sexual orientations other than **heterosexual/straight.** Some people prefer an umbrella word that includes a range of potential sexual orientations such as "gay," "lesbian," "bisexual," "questioning," "cisgender," or "fluid." Categories are human inventions and can be disrupted, as we see happening today with sexual orientation and gender categories. *Queer* is originally a pejorative term that has been reclaimed by some LGBT communities. The terminology of sex-gender is complex and constantly changing. Sometimes we're not sure what terms to use for ourselves or for other people. The best approach is usually to respect and use, when possible, the identity or label people choose for themselves.

Regardless of sexual orientation, most people look for love in a committed relationship. In this sense, queer couples are similar to straight couples. Like any intimate relationship, queer partnerships provide intimacy, passion, and security. However, there are some significant differences. Same-sex partnerships tend to be more egalitarian (equal) than heterosexual partnerships, probably because they are not bound by traditional gender roles. Same-sex couples put greater emphasis on partnership. Most reject the heterosexual sexual division of labor with "wife" or "husband" roles. Domestic responsibilities are shared or divided, and both partners contribute financially or are self-supporting.

Same-sex couples also experience challenges related to their sexual orientation, especially if they come from families, religions, or communities that do not accept alternatives to heterosexuality. Sexual minorities often deal with social hostility, ambivalence, or simple discomfort with their relationships, in contrast to the social approval and rights given to heterosexual couples (see the box "Marriage Equality"). **Homophobia,** which is fear or hatred of homosexuals, can be obvious, as in the case of violence or discrimination. Or it can be subtler, as in stereotypical portrayals of same-sex couples in the media. Societal and

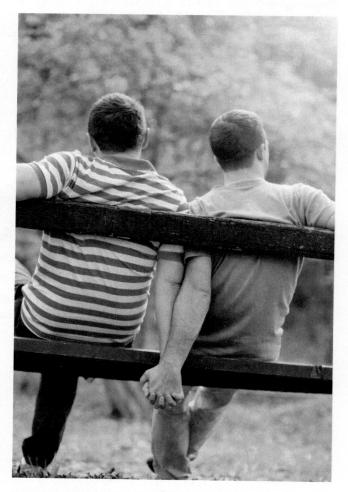

Same-sex partnerships still constitute a minority of the population, but they have become more visible than they used to be. Pekic/Getty Images

TERMS

sexual orientation A consistent pattern of emotional and sexual attraction based on biological sex; it exists along a continuum that ranges from exclusive heterosexuality (attraction to people of the other sex) through bisexuality (attraction to people of both sexes) to exclusive homosexuality (attraction to people of one's own sex).

queer Sexual orientations other than heterosexual/straight.

heterosexual/straight Attraction to people of the other sex.

homophobia Fear or hatred of homosexuals.

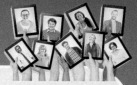

In its legal definitions, marriage is an institution in which couples derive legal and economic rights and responsibilities from state and federal statutes. The U.S. Government Accountability Office says more than 1000 federal laws make distinctions based on marriage. Marital status affects many aspects of life, such as Social Security benefits, federal tax status, inheritance, and medical decision making.

The push for legal recognition of same-sex partnerships has gone on for decades. Supporters of same-sex marriage rights have met opposition at the local, state, and federal levels, in both the public and private sectors. However, support for marriage equality has increased rapidly in the past several years. In 2001, Americans opposed marriage equality by a 57% to 35% margin, but in 2017, a majority of Americans (63%) found gay relationships morally acceptable. In 2013, the U.S. Supreme Court ruled that the federal government must recognize same-sex marriages performed by states that allow them, and in 2015, it declared all state bans on same-sex marriage unconstitutional.

Couples in which one or both partners are transgender are affected by this ruling as well, but only if their legal gender classifies them as a same-sex couple at the time of their marriage. Heterosexual transgender couples were generally able to marry previous to this ruling, so long as they were legally man-and-woman at the time of the marriage.

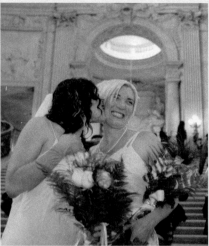

Eric Risberg/AP Images

What are benefits of marriage for same-sex couples?

- Health insurance and retirement benefits for employees' spouses

- Social Security benefits for spouses, widows, and widowers

- Support and benefits for military spouses, widows, and widowers

- Joint income tax filing and exemption from federal estate taxes

- Immigration protections for binational couples

- Rights to creative and intellectual property

- Protection from some types of employment discrimination (e.g., getting fired for marrying a same-sex spouse)

Marriage also matters in terms of child rearing. Children who grow up with married parents benefit because their parents' relationship is recognized by law and receives legal protections. Additionally, spouses are generally entitled to joint child custody and visitation should the marriage end in divorce. They also bear an obligation to pay child support.

Finally, marriage can have an impact on emotional well-being. Research shows that married people tend to live longer, have higher incomes, engage less frequently in risky behaviors, have a healthier diet, and have fewer psychological problems than unmarried people. Finally, studies show that denying same-sex couples the right to marry has a negative impact on their mental health. The long-term impact of marriage equality is not yet known, but it is likely to benefit the legal, economic, and emotional well-being of millions of Americans.

SOURCES: Shah, Dayna K. 2004. Letter to Senator Bill Frist (http://www.gao.gov/new.items/d04353r.pdf); Marriage Equality FAQ: Frequently Asked Questions about the Supreme Court's Marriage Ruling (https://marriageequalityfacts.org/); News Service. 2017. Americans Hold Record Liberal Views on Most Moral Issues Gallup Poll Social Series: Values and Beliefs (news.gallup.com/poll/210542/americans-hold-record-liberal-views-moral-issues.aspx); Gonzales, G. 2014. Same-sex marriage—A prescription for better health. *New England Journal of Medicine* 370: 1373–1376; Wight, R. G. 2013. Same-sex legal marriage and psychological well-being: Findings from the California Health Interview Survey. *American Journal of Public Health* 103(2): 339–346.

personal sources of rejection often take their toll, especially among young people, and easily accessible sources of support are essential. Many communities offer support groups for same-sex partners and families to help them build social networks.

See Chapter 6 for more information about sexual orientation, gender identity, and sexual behavior.

Singlehood

Research shows that a growing percentage of American adults are single. In 2018, according to the U.S. Census, approximately half of all adults over age 15 were married. The remaining 50%, or about 131 million people, were single. Of course, not all singlehood is voluntary. Being single includes people who are no longer married, are divorced or widowed, or have never married. In 2018, about 10% were divorced, which is not always both partners' choice. And many singles have partners with whom they may also live.

But singlehood is becoming a popular alternative to marriage. And the "never married" group is getting larger and older. While the Pew Research figures are slightly higher for males than females, other studies find that many women, like men, no longer feel that marriage is essential to a fulfilling life. According to *Singular Magazine*, a magazine for singles, there is even an annual week in September called Unmarried and Single Americans Week that celebrates single life.

Several factors contribute to the growing number of singles. One is a much more positive view toward singlehood. Education and careers are delaying the age at which young people marry. More young people are living with their parents as they complete their education, seek jobs, pay off debts, and strive for financial independence. As cohabitation has gained acceptance, many singles simply live with partners rather than marry. High divorce rates also create more singles. People who have experienced divorce may be more open to remaining single. Finally, as our life span increases, our chances of becoming single through divorce or the death of our spouse also increases. Among those 65 or older, only 44% of females and 70% of males are currently married. The rest are single.

Being single, however, does not mean living without intimate relationships. Single people date, enjoy active and fulfilling social lives, and have a variety of sexual experiences and relationships. Other advantages of being single, especially for those without children, include more opportunities for personal and career development, fewer family obligations, and more freedom and control over life choices. Disadvantages include less companionship, potential loneliness, and sole responsibility for one's life (home, health, economic situation, recreation, etc.). Living on one income, especially in today's economy and housing market, can be a challenge for anyone, but particularly for lower-income workers and for women who, on average, earn less than men. Singles, both men and women, may experience discrimination because of their marital status and social pressure to get married.

How enjoyable and valuable single life is depends on several factors. These include whether it is by choice; the quality of one's social relationships, standard of living, and job; how comfortable one is with being alone; and how resourceful and energetic the person is about creating an interesting and fulfilling life.

Living Together

Living together, or cohabitation, is one of the most dramatic social changes of the past few decades. Both attitudes and behavior have changed. A 2019 Pew Research Center study, "Marriage and Cohabitation in the United States," found that more adults (ages 18–44) have now lived with a romantic partner than have ever been married. Most Americans now find cohabitation acceptable even if the couple has no plans to marry. While young people are most likely to hold these views (78% of 18–29-year-olds), a majority in all age groups agree.

Several factors are involved in this change, including greater acceptance of sex outside of marriage, the availability of contraceptives, more emphasis on career development, and a desire to delay marriage and children. Financial concerns, such as student debt burden and skyrocketing housing costs, also play a role. In the Pew Study, about 40% of those who were cohabiting (versus married) cited financial considerations and "convenience" as important reasons for moving in with their partners. In addition, many people have experienced divorce in their own families or marriages. They may be wary of making a marriage commitment without living together first.

Cohabitation provides many of the benefits of marriage: a steady intimate, romantic, and sexual partner; companionship; and an opportunity to develop greater intimacy through learning, compromising, and sharing. In the Pew study, love and companionship were the two major reasons couples gave for cohabiting, as well as for marrying.

Are there advantages to living together and not marrying? For one thing, it may give both partners a greater sense of autonomy. Not bound by the social rules and expectations of marriage, partners may find it easier to experiment with living arrangements that match their identities, interests, and abilities. For some couples, cohabitation is a chance to try out the relationship before assuming legal entanglements. If things don't work out, it may be easier to leave. Researchers previously believed that cohabiting before marriage led to higher divorce rates, but a 2014 study by the Council on Contemporary Families found that what has a greater impact on relationship longevity is the age at which couples first cohabit or marry. Those who wait until at least age 23 to marry or cohabit have the best relationship outcomes.

According to the Pew study, almost half of U.S. adults say that living together before marriage increases the chance of its success. Among married couples in the study who had lived with their spouses before marriage, 66% said they initially viewed cohabitation as a step toward marriage. Younger people are much more likely than older people to view cohabitation as increasing the chances of a successful marriage.

A majority of Americans, according to Pew Research, also say that cohabiting couples can raise children as well as married couples. Significantly, over half of cohabiting adults ages 18 to 44 are raising children; and about one-third of these are the couples' own children (versus just one partner's).

Of course, living together unmarried has drawbacks. The legal protections of marriage are often absent, such as health insurance benefits and property and inheritance rights. These can be serious if the couple has children or if partners become ill or are aging. Married couples, especially with

> **QUICK STATS**
>
> **About a quarter of cohabiters say that wanting to test their relationship was a major reason why they decided to move in with their partner.**
>
> —Pew Research Center, 2019

only one earner, receive substantial tax benefits from filing jointly. Couples may feel social or family pressure to marry or otherwise change their living arrangements. The general trend, however, is toward legitimizing nonmarital partnerships; for example, some employers, communities, and states now extend benefits and legal rights to registered unmarried domestic partners.

Not everyone is comfortable with the trend toward cohabitation. As on many social issues, religious affiliation makes a difference. In the Pew Report, only a third of Euro-American evangelical Protestant Christians and less than half of African American Protestants find cohabitation without marriage acceptable. Far fewer (33% of Christians versus 59% of nonreligious people) say cohabiting couples can raise children as well as married couples. These attitudes reflect broader concerns many people, especially evangelical Christians, have about the breakdown of "traditional" (Christian) forms of family, gender, and sexuality.

MARRIAGE

Marriage has been both challenged and transformed over the past decades. At the same time, it remains very popular, even among those who choose to cohabit. For many same-sex couples, marriage has a connotation and symbolism that is not attainable through cohabitation or *domestic partnership*. Marriage, though it varies enormously across cultures, seems to be universal in human societies. It addresses many basic human and societal needs. Social, political, economic, reproductive, sexual, and other considerations often guided marriage choices in the past, such as raising children or forming an economic unit. Today people in the United States marry more for personal, emotional, and companionship reasons.

The Benefits of Marriage

The primary functions and benefits of marriage are those of any intimate relationship: affection, personal affirmation, companionship, sexual fulfillment, and emotional growth. Marriage also provides a setting in which to raise children, although an increasing number of couples choose not to have children. For those with children, more are choosing to raise them without being married, either by themselves, with a partner, or with the help of parents or other family members.

With or without children, commitments to long-term relationships are motivated by a desire for close, intimate, even lifelong companions as well as some insurance for later years. Research also indicates that marriage contributes to health and well-being, particularly for men but

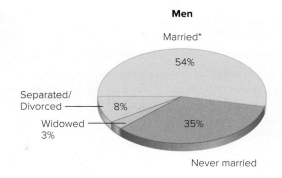

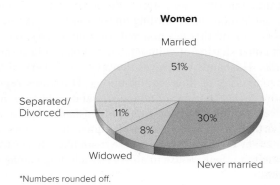

FIGURE 5.2 **Marital status of the U.S. adults aged 15 and over, 2019.**

SOURCE: U.S. Census Bureau. 2019. Historical Marital Status Tables (https://www.census.gov/data/tables/time-series/demo/families/marital.html).

for women as well. Married couples tend to have more daily social interactions, which are associated with reduced risk for dementia and harmful lifestyle behaviors. Married people live longer and survive cancer and other diseases more often.

Issues and Trends in Marriage

Traditional marriage roles have undergone profound changes. Most married couples today have two working spouses. The vast majority of married heterosexual families (over 80%) no longer follow a traditional "male as the provider" model.

According to the Bureau of Labor Statistics, a majority of married mothers, even with small children, participated in the labor force: Approximately three-fourths were employed full time.

Today's husbands participate more in domestic and child rearing activities, particularly when wives are employed. Sometimes there is no choice, as when a mother's work schedule makes it impossible to drive her children to school or to prepare meals. But many men have been exposed to new, shared models of family responsibilities and are willing to help out, especially when asked explicitly.

> **QUICK STATS**
>
> In the United States, the median age at first marriage is 30 for men and 28 for women—the highest in history.
> —U.S. Census Bureau, 2018

At the same time, old patterns die slowly when it comes to boring, tedious, unrewarding household tasks. A recent Pew study found that few married (or cohabiting) couples report equal sharing of child-related or household responsibilities. Husbands and wives, however, have very different perceptions of their contributions. Husbands report far more "equal sharing" of housework and child care than do wives. As for managing finances, husbands and wives have virtually opposite views, with almost half of men reporting they do the most. Wives are more likely to say they do more than their spouse in all areas, including managing finances.

The Pew study also finds that married couples who report more equally shared responsibilities are more satisfied with their arrangements. This suggests, as do other studies, that a more egalitarian sexual division of labor contributes to greater marital satisfaction.

Other recent trends include couples marrying later, choosing not to marry, or remarrying. Second and third marriages and later life unions are becoming more common, including among long-term family friends whose spouses have died.

Although most people marry for love, love is not enough to make a successful marriage. Relationship problems can become magnified rather than solved by marriage. The following appear to be the best predictors of a happy marriage:

- The partners have realistic expectations about their relationship.
- Each feels good about the personality of the other.
- Partners develop friendships with other couples.
- They communicate well.
- They have effective ways of resolving conflicts.
- They agree on religious/ethical values.
- They have an egalitarian role relationship.
- They have a good balance of individual versus joint interests and leisure activities.

Once married, couples must provide each other with emotional support, negotiate and establish marital roles, establish domestic and career priorities, handle their finances, make sexual adjustments, manage boundaries and relationships with their extended family, and participate in the larger community.

Separation and Divorce

Divorce has become quite common in the United States, a dramatic change from 60 years ago, when both religious and civil society strongly discouraged or even prohibited divorce. At that time, "incompatibility" was generally not considered legal grounds for divorce; instead extreme situations, such as adultery, abandonment, or insanity had to be proven. Attitudes have changed enormously, and dissolution of marriage is now the decision of the couple. There is an increasing emphasis on "no fault," nonadversarial approaches to divorce, using mediators to handle the process, reducing the role of lawyers and the court system.

Current estimates are that about 40 to 50% of first marriages will end in divorce. Approximately 20% of first marriages end within five years, and nearly half do not last beyond 20 years. For those who remarry, divorce rates are higher for subsequent marriage.

High divorce rates in the United States (Figure 5.3) may partially reflect our high expectations for emotional fulfillment and satisfaction in marriage. Young people often receive harmful and unrealistic messages about marriage through movies and other media. But we also may no longer embrace the concept of marriage as permanent, regardless of the quality of the relationship. This may partially explain why divorce rates are rising among older couples, many married for decades.

The process of divorce usually begins with an emotional separation. Often one partner is unhappy and looks for a more satisfying relationship. Dissatisfaction increases until the unhappy partner decides they can no longer stay. Physical separation follows, although it may take longer for the relationship to be over legally and then emotionally.

Divorce can be one of the greatest stress-producing events in life. Many men and women experience turmoil, depression, and lowered self-esteem during and after divorce. People may experience separation distress and loneliness for about a year and then begin a recovery period of one to three years. During this time they gradually construct a postdivorce identity, along with a new pattern of life. Most people are surprised at how long it takes to recover from divorce.

Children are especially vulnerable to the trauma of divorce, and counseling can help them adjust to the change. However, recent research finds that children who spend substantial time with both parents are usually better adjusted than those in sole custody and are as well adjusted as their peers from intact families. Coping with divorce is difficult for children at any age, including adult children.

Some couples have tried to relieve this stress through creative living arrangements. For example, instead of children moving between parents, children stay in their original residence. Each parent takes turn staying at "home" with the children. Or divorced parents will set up households within a few blocks of each other, making it easier for children to see each parent.

Despite the distress of separation and divorce, the negative effects are usually balanced sooner or later by the

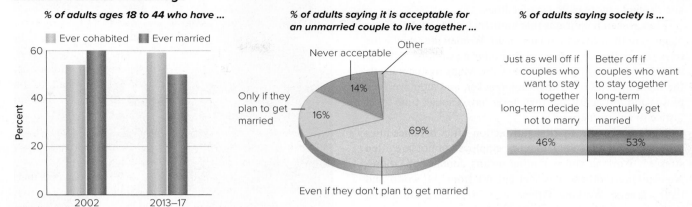

Amid Changes in Marriage and Cohabitation, Wide Acceptance of Cohabitation, Even as Many Americans See Societal Benefits in Marriage

FIGURE 5.3 **Wide acceptance of cohabitation, even as many Americans see societal benefits in marriage.**

SOURCE: Pew Research Center, 2019 (https://www.pewsocialtrends.org/2019/11/06/marriage-and-cohabitation-in-the-u-s/psdt_11-06-19_cohabitation-00-010/).

possibility of finding a more suitable partner, constructing a new life, and developing new aspects of one's self. One result of the high divorce and remarriage rate is a growing number of merged families, either informally or legally, as stepfamilies.

FAMILY LIFE

American families are very different today from families decades ago. In the 1960s, most people married first and then had children. Then, 88% of children under the age of 18 lived with both parents; in 2018, it was 65%. Over the same time period, the proportion of children living with a single mother nearly tripled, from 8% to 23%, and the percentage living with only their father increased from 1% to 4.4%. An additional 3.2% of children currently live with other relatives.

Becoming a Parent

Few new parents are prepared for the job of parenting. In the past, people learned about parenting by observing their own parents, extended family members, neighbors and others in their community. Today, with smaller and more dispersed families, few of us have much direct experience. Fortunately, a slew of books and articles are available which, along with parenting classes, help us prepare for the parenting experience. Family members, especially mothers, aunts, and sisters, can be helpful. In some U.S. ethnic groups, it is normal for the new mother's mother to come and stay with her before and after the birth, sometimes for several months. And more and more fathers (or other close men) are participating in the birthing and post-birthing process. Single mothers increasingly draw upon their own family members, friends, and other parenting networks to assist in the birth and post-birth transition. And more local groups and health organizations

are offering post-birth parenting assistance, such as "Mommy and Me" classes.

Nevertheless, few people are fully prepared for the daunting responsibility of caring for a new infant, yet they literally must assume the role overnight. Apart from the basics of holding, feeding, changing diapers, and putting a newborn down to sleep, there is the more complex process of learning to differentiate a cry of hunger from a cry of pain or fear. Or discerning whether a rash or slight fever is normal or requires a call to a health provider. No wonder the birth of the first child is one of the most stressful transitions for any couple.

Even those heterosexual couples committed to an egalitarian relationship can easily slip into traditional marital roles after the arrival of a new baby. Ideally, if both parents have jobs with paid parental leave, or are able to work part-time, they could participate equally, or nearly equally, in caring for the new infant. Even breastfeeding by the birth mother can be a joint activity whether or not breast milk is pumped and saved. Both mothers and fathers learn and become more confident in their parenting skills. This lays the groundwork for shared parenting and eliminates the typical gender gap in parenting "skills" that arises because only one parent, usually the mother, is doing the initial parenting.

The same structures that divide Americans into different social strata make it difficult for many parents to achieve an ideal balance. The United States is far behind other wealthy, industrialized countries when it comes to parental leave, especially paid parental leave, and especially for fathers. Bureau of Labor Statistics data show that in 2018, only 17% of civilian workers had access to paid family leave, which includes parental leave. Overall, private industry lags behind state and local government, except for companies with over 500 workers. And the Bureau of Labor Statistics data exclude agricultural and domestic workers, who rarely have family leave of any type. Unpaid family leave is far more common.

Unlike other wealthy countries, few U.S. workplaces with significant numbers of employees offer on-site child care, even those, like medical centers, with mostly female workforces.

Apple's new $5 billion "Spaceship" campus in Cupertino, California, has virtually everything an employee could desire...except on-site child care facilities.

Most research indicates that mothers have to make greater changes in their lives than fathers do. Women are usually the ones who make job changes, either quitting work or reducing work hours to stay home with the baby. Many mothers juggle the multiple roles of mother, homemaker, and employer/employee and feel guilty that they never have enough time to do justice to any of these roles.

Not surprisingly, marital satisfaction often declines after the birth of the first child. Parents, employed or not, are often stressed. Working and parenting means double obligations. Nonworking mothers may feel cut off from the world and their careers. Working fathers can experience additional stress from suddenly becoming the sole earner. Some husbands have difficulty sharing their wife's attention with the baby, especially if they are less involved in parenting.

But marital dissatisfaction after the baby is born is not inevitable. Couples who successfully weather the stresses of a new baby are reported to have these characteristics in common:

1. They had developed a strong relationship before the baby was born.

2. They had planned to have the child.

3. They communicate well about their feelings and expectations.

4. They accept the need to share household and child care responsibilities and have worked out concrete strategies for doing so.

Parenting

No one action or decision (within limits) will determine a child's personality or development. Instead the *parenting style,* or overall approach to parenting, is most important. Parenting styles vary according to how parents approach each of the following:

• *Demandingness* encompasses the use of discipline and supervision, the expectation that children act responsibly and maturely, and the direct reaction to disobedience.

• *Responsiveness* refers to the parents' warmth and intent to facilitate independence and self-confidence in their child by being supportive, connected, and understanding of their child's needs.

Several parenting styles have been identified. Each style emerges according to the parents' balance of demandingness and responsiveness. Here are some examples:

• *Authoritarian* parents are high in demandingness and low in responsiveness. They give orders and expect obedience, giving little warmth or consideration to their children's special needs.

• *Authoritative* parents are high in both demandingness and responsiveness. They set clear boundaries and expectations,

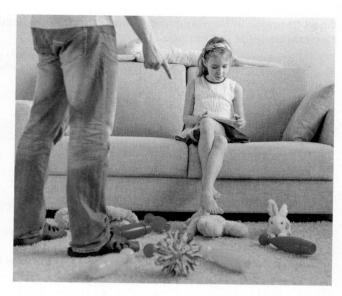

Setting clear boundaries, holding children to high expectations, and responding with warmth to children's needs are all positive parenting strategies. Dmitri Ma/Shutterstock

but they are also loving, supportive, and attuned to their children's needs.

• *Permissive* parents are high in responsiveness and low in demandingness. They do not expect their children to act maturely but instead allow them to follow their own impulses. They are very warm, patient, and accepting, and they are focused on not stifling their child's innate creativity.

• *Uninvolved* parents are low in both demandingness and responsiveness. They require little from their children and respond with little attention, frequency, or effort. In extreme cases, this style of parenting might reach the level of child neglect.

Children's Temperaments   Every child has a tendency toward certain moods or ways of reacting, that is, a particular temperament that appears in infancy and persists into childhood. *Some children* are normally happy and content and have regular sleeping and eating habits. They are adaptable and not easily upset. Others are fussier, more fearful in new situations or with strangers, and have irregular sleeping and feeding habits. They are easily upset and often hard to soothe.

Some are initially fearful but then warm up and adapt easily to new situations and people. Children's temperaments, or personalities, are influenced by family and community circumstances. And as children grow older, socialization processes, such as those in schools, shape individual temperaments along culturally appropriate lines. Margaret Mead's classic anthropological research revealed how profoundly cultures affect individual temperaments.

Sometimes a child's temperament may not match that of its parents or other caretakers. For example, a parent who expects a quick response to a request may have trouble adjusting to a child who is naturally slow to respond. Pediatrician W. Thomas Boyce argues in his 2019 book, *The Orchid and the Dandelion,* that children fall into two categories: dandelions can easily adapt and thrive almost anywhere, whereas orchids are sensitive and "psychologically unprotected." But given the right environment and understanding, orchids can become something extraordinary.

Parenting and the Family Life Cycle   At each stage of the family life cycle, the relationship between parents and children changes. And with those changes come new challenges. The parents' initial responsibility to a baby is to ensure its physical well-being around the clock. As babies grow into toddlers and begin to walk and talk, they begin to take care of some of their own physical needs. For parents, the challenge at this stage is to strike a balance between giving children the freedom to explore and setting limits that will keep them safe and secure. As children grow into adolescents, parents need to give them increasing independence and be willing to let them risk success or failure on their own.

Marital satisfaction for most couples tends to decline during their children's school years. Reasons include the financial and emotional pressures of a growing family and the increased job and community responsibilities of parents in their thirties, forties, fifties, and even sixties. Many parents also start assuming greater responsibility for their own aging parents, producing the so-called Sandwich Generation. If the children have all left home, parents have more time to focus on each other. If adult children continue to live at home or return home, marital satisfaction can decrease, but, according to some research, perhaps only if coresidence is not the norm or is due to the children having problems living on their own.

Single Parents

Single parenthood, like singlehood, is becoming increasingly common. According to the 2018 data from the U.S. Census Bureau, there are nearly 25 million children living with only one parent (Figure 5.4). As we saw earlier, more parents are reversing the traditional family life cycle, with the baby coming before the marriage. Sometimes the single parent is a teenage mother, although rates of teenage pregnancy have declined significantly in recent years. Economic difficulties can be substantial, especially for those with little education or job skills or from poorer families. On the other hand, some single parents are professional women who for various reasons choose to have a baby on their own, through sperm donors or adoption. If they are well-established in their careers and in a solid financial position, they can find nannies or other child care arrangements while they continue in their professions.

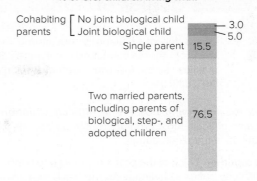

Diversity in Family Living Arrangements
% of U.S. children living with:

Cohabiting parents — No joint biological child — 3.0
— Joint biological child — 5.0
Single parent — 15.5

Two married parents, including parents of biological, step-, and adopted children — 76.5

FIGURE 5.4   **Living arrangements for American families with children under age 18.**
SOURCE: U.S. Census Bureau. 2018. America's Families and Living Arrangements: 2018

QUICK STATS

4% of American children live in a home where neither parent is present.
—U. S. Census Bureau, 2019

Single parents, especially those without partners, may experience conflicting demands of being both father and mother and the difficulty of satisfying their own needs for adult companionship and affection. Having strong family or other social networks, however, can greatly ease the demands of single parenting.

Research about the effect on children of growing up in a single-parent family is inconclusive. Evidence suggests that educational level and financial resources of parents, whether one or two, and the quality of the relationships among children, parents, and other caretakers are the most important factors in children's well-being. Two-parent families are not necessarily better if one of the parents spends little time relating to the children or is physically or emotionally abusive. Extended families have traditionally played a significant role in child rearing cross-culturally and within some U.S. communities. They can offer enormous support for single parents.

Stepfamilies/Blended Families

Single parenthood is often a transitional stage: About three of four divorced women and about four of five divorced men will remarry. If either partner brings children into the new family unit, a stepfamily (or *blended family*) is formed.

The American Psychological Association recommends three key issues to consider.

1. **Financial and living arrangements.** Couples who share most of their finances have reported greater family satisfaction than those working from individual accounts. Moving to a home that is new for everyone can create a feeling of a shared, level playing field. However, children sensitive to transition and change benefit from as much continuity as possible.

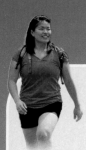

Life is full of challenges, but strong families work together to meet those challenges. Strong families use the following strategies to deal with life's difficulties:

- **Look for something positive in difficult situations.** No matter how difficult, most problems teach us lessons that we can draw on in future situations.

- **Pull together.** Think of the problem not as one family member's difficulty but as a challenge for the family as a whole.

- **Get help outside the family.** Call on extended family members, supportive friends, neighbors, colleagues, members of your religious community, and health care and community professionals.

- **Listen and empathize.** Offer each other nonjudgmental support.

- **Use rituals for bonding and healing.** A ritual could include a memorial event, a tradition that the family repeats each year on a significant date or for a holiday, or a shared daily meal or time for conversation.

- **Be flexible.** Crises often force family members to learn new approaches to life or take on different responsibilities. Each person needs time to heal from challenges at their own pace.

- **Give each other space.** Respect family members' need for privacy and alone time.

- **Focus on the big picture and set priorities.** Getting caught up in details rather than the essentials can make people edgy, even hysterical.

- **Take care of each other.** We often forget that we are biological beings. Like kindergartners, we need a good lunch and time to play. We need to have our hair stroked, a hug, or a nap.

- **Validate each other.** Offer appreciation and praise.

- **Create a life full of meaning and purpose.** We all face severe crises in life; they're unavoidable. Sometimes it helps to focus on others, to offer service to the community. Giving of ourselves brings richness and dignity to our lives despite the troubles we endure.

- **Actively meet challenges head-on.** Life's disasters do not go away when we look in another direction.

- **Go with the flow to some degree.** Sometimes we are relatively powerless in the face of a crisis. Simply saying to ourselves that things will get better with time can be useful.

- **Be prepared in advance for life's challenges.** Healthy family relationships are like an ample bank balance: If our relational accounts are in order, we will be able to weather life's most difficult storms—together.

SOURCES: Binghamton University Counseling Center. n.d. Dealing with crisis and trauma events. American Academy of Experts in Traumatic Stress (http://www.aaets.org/article164.htm); Olson, D. H., and J. DeFrain. 2007. *Marriages and Families: Intimacy, Diversity, and Strengths,* 6th ed. New York: McGraw Hill Education. Copyright © 2007.

2. **Resolving feelings and issues from the previous marriage.** Old hurts and patterns can resurface, for both adults and children, if not worked out. Hearing that a parent plans to remarry can sadden a child who hoped her parents might reconcile.

3. **Parenthood.** Couples should discuss the role that the stepparent will take with the new spouse's children. Stepparents should first take on a role more akin to friend or "camp counselor," rather than disciplinarian. Younger children, those under age 10, are usually more accepting of a new adult in the family than are adolescents.

Stepfamilies can be very different from primary families, although a lot depends on the age of children and the nature of their relationships with prior and new family members. It's important for the other parent, outside the stepfamily, to continue regular visits and maintain a good relationship with the children so that they don't feel abandoned. Seeing a psychologist can help everyone in the family. It may take two to four years for a new stepfamily to adjust to living together.

Stepfamilies may find it difficult to duplicate the emotions and relationships of a primary family. Research has shown that healthy stepfamilies are less cohesive but more adaptable than healthy primary families; they have a greater capacity to allow for individual differences and accept that biologically related family members will have emotionally closer relationships. Stepfamilies gradually gain a sense of being a family as they build a history of shared daily experiences and major life events.

Successful Families

Family life can be extremely challenging. A strong family is not a family without problems; it's a family that copes successfully with stress and crisis (see the box "Strategies of Strong Families").

An excellent way to build strong family ties is to develop family rituals and routines, repeated activities that have meaning for family members. Families with regular routines and rituals have healthier children, more satisfying marriages, and stronger family relationships. Some common routines identified in research studies are dinnertime, a regular bedtime, and household chores; common rituals include birthdays, holidays, and weekend activities. Family routines may even serve as protective factors, balancing out potential risk factors associated with single-parent families and families with divorce and remarriage. Incorporating a regular family mealtime into a family's routine allows parents and children to develop closer relationships and leads to better parenting, healthier children, and better school performance.

Experts have proposed seven major characteristics of strong American families:

1. **Commitment.** The family is very important to its members, and members take their responsibilities seriously. Everyone knows they are loved, valued, and special to each other.

2. **Appreciation.** Family members care about one another and express their appreciation. They don't wait for special occasions to celebrate each other.

3. **Communication.** Family members spend time listening to one another and enjoying each other's company. They talk through disagreements and attempt to solve problems.

4. **Time together.** Family members do things together—often simple activities that don't cost money. They put down their devices and their work, and they focus on each other.

5. **Spiritual wellness.** The family promotes sharing, love, and compassion for other human beings.

6. **Stress and crisis management.** When faced with illness, death, marital conflict, or other crises, family members pull together, seek help, and use other coping strategies to meet challenges.

7. **Affectionate physical contact.** People of all ages need hugs, cuddles, and caresses for their emotional health and to demonstrate caring and love for one another.

It may surprise some people that members of strong families are often seen at counseling centers. They know that the smartest thing to do in some situations is to get help.

Ask Yourself

QUESTIONS FOR CRITICAL THINKING AND REFLECTION

Do you think of your own family as successful? In what ways could your family relationships improve? Are you comfortable talking to your family about these issues?

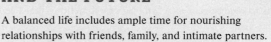

TIPS FOR TODAY AND THE FUTURE

A balanced life includes ample time for nourishing relationships with friends, family, and intimate partners.

RIGHT NOW YOU CAN:

- Seek out an acquaintance or a new friend and arrange a coffee date to get to know the person better.
- Call someone you love and tell them how important the relationship is to you. Don't wait for a crisis.

IN THE FUTURE YOU CAN:

- Think about the conflicts you have had in the past with your close friends or loved ones and consider how you handled them. Decide whether your conflict management methods were helpful. Using the suggestions in this chapter and Chapter 3, determine how you could better handle similar conflicts in the future.
- Think about your prospects as a parent. What kind of example have your parents set? If you don't already have children, how do you feel about having them in the future? What can you do to prepare yourself to be a good parent?

SUMMARY

- Healthy intimate relationships are an important component of the well-being of both individuals and society. Many intimate relationships are held together by love.

- Successful relationships begin with a positive sense of self and reasonably high self-esteem. Personal identity, gender roles, and attachment styles, all rooted in childhood experiences, contribute to this sense of self.

- Characteristics of friendship include companionship, respect, acceptance, help, trust, loyalty, mutuality, and reciprocity.

- Love, sex, and commitment are closely linked ideals in intimate relationships. Love includes trust, caring, respect, and loyalty. Sex brings excitement, fascination, and passion to the relationship. Commitment contributes stability, which helps maintain a relationship.

- Common challenges in relationships relate to issues of self-disclosure, commitment, expectations, competitiveness, balance of time together and apart, and jealousy. Gender roles, especially traditional gender roles, influence each of these.

- Partners in successful relationships have strong communication skills and support each other during difficult times. Social media can both ease and undermine communication in relationships.

- The keys to good communication in relationships are self-disclosure, listening, and feedback.

- Conflict is inevitable in intimate relationships; partners need to find ways to negotiate their differences. Conflict is often accompanied by anger, and the best way to handle anger in a relationship is to recognize it as a symptom of something that needs to be addressed.

- People usually choose partners like themselves (except on gender). If partners are very different, acceptance and good communication skills are especially necessary to maintain the relationship.

- Most Americans find partners through dating or getting together in groups. Internet sites that match people can expand dating options and create positive experiences as long as safety precautions are taken. Cohabitation is a growing social pattern that allows partners to get to know each other intimately without being married.

- Same-sex partnerships are similar to heterosexual partnerships, with some differences. Same-sex couples put greater emphasis on partnership than on role assignment, and they may experience social hostility or ambivalence rather than approval of their partnerships.

- Singlehood is a growing lifestyle in our society. Advantages include autonomy, greater variety in intimate partners, and more freedom to make and pursue life choices; disadvantages include greater possibility of economic hardship, sole responsibility for a household, and lack of guaranteed companionship.

- Marriage fulfills many functions for individuals and society. It can provide people with affection, affirmation, and sexual fulfillment; a context for child rearing; and the promise of lifelong companionship.

- Love isn't enough to ensure a successful marriage. Partners must be realistic, feel good about each other, have communication and conflict resolution skills, share values, and balance their individual and joint interests.

- When problems can't be worked out, people often separate and divorce. Divorce can be traumatic for all involved, especially children, but the negative effects are usually balanced in time by positive ones.

- At each stage of the family life cycle, relationships change. Marital satisfaction may be lower during the child-rearing years and higher later.

- Many families today are single-parent families. The quality of the caretaker relationships and the parents' education level and financial resources are the most important factors in children's well-being.

- Stepfamilies, also referred to as blended families, are formed when single, divorced, or widowed people remarry and create new family units. Stepfamilies gradually gain more of a sense of being a family as they build a history of shared experiences.

- Important qualities of successful families include commitment to the family, appreciation of family members, communication, physical affection, time spent together, spiritual wellness, sharing of responsibilities, and effective methods of dealing with stress.

FOR MORE INFORMATION

For resources in your area, check your campus directory for a counseling center or peer counseling program, or search online.

American Association for Marriage and Family Therapy. Provides information about a variety of relationship issues and referrals to therapists.

http://www.aamft.org

American Psychological Association. Offers general and specific advice about how to navigate marriage, divorce, and family life.

https://www.apa.org

Association for Couples in Marriage Enrichment (ACME). Promotes activities to strengthen marriage; a resource for books, tapes, and other materials.

http://www.bettermarriages.org

The Blended Family Podcast. Conversations with real parents in blended families about their strategies for making things work.

http://www.blendedfamilypodcast.com

Conflict Resolution Information Source. Provides links to a broad range of internet resources for conflict resolution. Information covers interpersonal, marital, family, and other types of conflicts.

http://www.crinfo.org

Family Education Network. Provides information about education, safety, health, and other family-related issues.

http://www.familyeducation.com

The Gottman Institute. Includes tips and suggestions for relationships and parenting, including an online relationships quiz.

http://www.gottman.com

Parents Without Partners (PWP). Provides educational programs, literature, and support groups for single parents and their children. Search the online directory for a referral to a local chapter.

Pew Research Center. Surveys Americans about issues and attitudes and analyzes publications in mass media and social science research.

http://www.pewresearch.org

U.S. Census Bureau. Provides current statistics on births, marriages, and living arrangements.

http://www.census.gov

U.S. Government Accountability Office. Acts like a "congressional watchdog," investigating how the federal government spends taxpayer money.

http://www.gao.gov

See also the listings for Chapters 3 and 9.

SELECTED BIBLIOGRAPHY

American College Health Association. 2017. *American College Health Association–National College Health Assessment II Fall 2017 Reference Group Data Report.* Hanover, MD: American College Health Association.

Bishop, R. 2017. Here are Apple's child care benefits. *The Outline* (https://theoutline.com/post/1623/here-are-apple-s-child-care-benefits?zd=3&zi=122pwsu5).

Boyce, W. T. 2019. *The Orchid and the Dandelion.* New York: Alfred A. Knopf.

Centers for Disease Control and Prevention. 2018. Youth Risk Behavior Surveillance—United States, 2017. *MMWR Surveillance Report* 67(22-8) (https://www.cdc.gov/healthyyouth/data/yrbs/pdf/trendsreport.pdf).

Centers for Disease Control and Prevention. 2020. *Preventing Teen Dating Violence* (https://www.cdc.gov/violenceprevention/intimatepartnerviolence/teendatingviolence/fastfact.html).

Davis, E. M., K. Kim, and K. L. Fingerman. 2018. Is an empty nest best? Coresidence with adult children and parental marital quality before and after the Great Recession. *The Journals of Gerontology: Series B* 73(3): 372–381.

DePaulo, B. 2017. Is it true that single women and married men do best? Sex differences in marriage and single life: Still debating after 50 years. *Psychology Today* (https://www.psychologytoday.com/us/blog/living-single/201701/is-it-true-single-women-and-married-men-do-best).

Denworth, L. 2019. Social media has not destroyed a generation. *Scientific American*, November, 46–49 (https://www.scientificamerican.com/article/social-media-has-not-destroyed-a-generation/).

Eckert, P., and S. McConnell-Ginet. 2013. *Language and Gender*, 2nd ed. New York: Cambridge University Press.

Federal Interagency Forum on Child and Family Statistics. 2015. *America's Children: Key National Indicators of Well-Being, 2015*. Washington, DC: U.S. Government Printing Office.

Goleman, D. 1995. *Emotional Intelligence: Why It Can Matter More Than IQ*. New York: Bantam Books.

Goodwin, M. H. 2006. *The Hidden Life of Girls: Games of Stance, Status, and Exclusion*. Oxford, UK: Blackwell.

Guttmacher Institute. 2019. Fact Sheet: Adolescent Sexual and Reproductive Health in the United States (https://www.guttmacher.org/fact-sheet/american-teens-sexual-and-reproductive-health).

Hancock, J. T., et al. 2019. Social Media Use and Well-Being: A Meta-Analysis, *69th Annual International Communication Association Conference*, Washington, D.C.

Kirschenbaum, H., and V. Henderson. 1989. *The Carl Rogers Reader*. Boston: Houghton Mifflin.

Mead, M. 1928. *Coming of Age in Samoa*. New York: William Morrow & Co.

Mernitz, S. E., and C. Kamp Dush. 2016. Emotional health across the transition to first and second unions among emerging adults. *Journal of Family Psychology* 30(2): 233–244.

Mukhopadhyay, C. C., and T. Blumenthal. "Gender and Sexuality." *In Perspectives: An Open Invitation to Cultural Anthropology*, 2nd ed.,
ed. N. Brown, T. McIlwraith, and L. Tubelle de González. *The Society for Anthropology in Community Colleges* (http://perspectives.americananthro.org/).

National Center for Health Statistics. 2019. National Survey of Family Growth (https://www.cdc.gov/nchs/data/factsheets/factsheet_nsfg.pdf).

Pew Research Center. 2019. Marriage and Cohabitation in the U.S. (https://www.pewsocialtrends.org/2019/11/06/marriage-and-cohabitation-in-the-u-s/psdt_11-06-19_cohabitation-00-010/).

Rogers, C. R. 1961. *On Becoming a Person*. Boston: Houghton Mifflin.

Rosenfeld, M. J., R. J. Thomas, and S. Hausen. 2019. Disintermediating your friends: How online dating in the United States displaces other ways of meeting. *Proceedings of the National Academy of Sciences of the United States of America* 116 (36): 17753–17758.

Salovey, P., et al., eds. 2004. *Emotional Intelligence: Key Readings on the Mayer and Salovey Model*. Port Chester, NY: Dude Publishing.

Schlagel, D. 2019. *Our Modern Blended Family: A Practical Guide*. Emeryville, CA: Rockridge Press.

Schoen, R., et al. 2007. Family transitions in young adulthood. *Demography* 44(4): 807–820.

Simpson, D. M., N. D. Leonhardt, and A. J. Hawkins. 2018. Learning about love: A meta-analytic study of individually-oriented relationship education programs for adolescents and emerging adults. *Journal of Youth and Adolescence* 47(3): 477–489.

Sommerlad, A., et al. 2018. Marriage and risk of dementia: Systematic review and meta-analysis of observational studies. *Journal of Neurology, Neurosurgery, and Psychiatry* 89: 231–238.

Tannen, D. 1994. *Gender and Discourse*. New York: Oxford University Press.

Twenge, J. M., R. A. Sherman, and B. E. Wells. 2015. Changes in American adults' sexual behavior and attitudes. *Archives of Sexual Behavior* 44: 2273.

U. S. Bureau of Labor Statistics. 2019. Access to paid and unpaid family leave in 2018. *The Economics Daily* (https://www.bls.gov/opub/ted/2019/access-to-paid-and-unpaid-family-leave-in-2018.htm).

U. S. Bureau of Labor Statistics. 2019. Employment Characteristics of Families Summary (https://www.bls.gov/news.release/famee.nr0.htm).

United States Census Bureau. 2018. America's Families and Living Arrangements: 2018 (https://www.census.gov/data/tables/2018/demo/families/cps-2018.html).

- Describe the structure and function of human genital-sexual anatomy
- Explain the role of hormones in sexual and genital development
- Describe how the body functions during sexual activity
- Explain the range of gender roles and sexual orientations
- Explain the development and varieties of sexual behavior

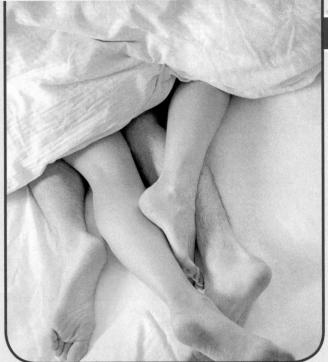

Tim Hawley/Getty Images

CHAPTER 6

Sex and Your Body

TEST YOUR KNOWLEDGE

1. Although testosterone is the primary male hormone, it is also produced in women.
   True or False?

2. Which of the following physical conditions are associated with erectile dysfunction ("impotence")?
   a. Smoking
   b. Being above average weight
   c. Physical inactivity
   d. High blood pressure

3. Calcium supplements may reduce symptoms of premenstrual syndrome (PMS) in some women.
   True or False?

4. There are only two sexes.
   True or False?

ANSWERS

1. **TRUE.** Testosterone is produced in small amounts by a woman's ovaries.

2. **ALL FOUR.** 70–80% of cases of erectile dysfunction are thought to involve physical factors.

3. **TRUE.** Other self-help strategies for PMS include getting exercise, reducing stress, eating a diet rich in complex carbohydrates, and avoiding alcohol and caffeine.

4. **FALSE.** The term *intersex* describes a person not easily assigned a category male or female.

The phrase human **sexuality** refers to a complex and interconnected group of *physical-biological* characteristics as well as *learned* behaviors that we acquire from our families, communities, and other social organizations, such as religious and political institutions. Sexuality includes our assigned sex and expressed gender, along with sex-specific anatomy and physiology, sexual functioning and practices, and social and sexual interactions with others. Our sense of who we are is powerfully influenced by sexuality, and because sexuality is so multifaceted, it should be thought of as a spectrum of identities and behaviors rather than as a binary system.

Basic information about the body, sexual functioning, sexual identity, and sexual behavior is vital to sexual wellness. Understanding the facts gives us a better basis for evaluating the messages we get about our bodies. With these facts we can also then make choices that promote our individual and collective well-being.

SEXUAL ANATOMY

Despite their different appearances, sex organs develop from the same anatomical structures and fulfill many of the same functions. **Gonads** (ovaries and testes) produce **germ cells** and sex hormones. Germ cells are called **ova** (eggs) in people who are assigned female at birth and **sperm** in people who are assigned male. Ova and sperm are the basic units of reproduction.

From Binary to Spectrum

The term *sex* is often understood as a binary: that is, that people are either one *or* the other. At birth we are assigned one of these two sexes—male and female—based on the appearance of our genitals. Doctors use visual examination or ultrasound images to make an assignment. Although male and female are the terms familiar, 1 out of 1500 people cannot be accurately categorized by either of these words; such people are currently described as **intersex**. There is a wide variety of intersex conditions, and some initially go undetected because of genitals that do not appear to differ from the norm.

Parents and doctors of visibly intersex infants sometimes use surgery to assign these children to a particular sex, but many adults who have undergone such procedures are now calling for an end to these early surgeries so that people with intersex conditions can choose what sex is right for them, on their own time. In 2017, Germany began to legally recognize a third sex category, making it easier for parents and doctors to assign a sex to these children. Nepal, India, Pakistan, Bangladesh, Germany, New Zealand, and Australia, as well as some U.S. states, all legally recognize a third option for people who do not consider themselves either male or female.

Our bodies, and how we understand them, are widely diverse. In order to present information that pertains to the majority of the population, however, this chapter primarily uses the words *male, female, man, woman, boy,* and *girl.* We recognize that these words do not represent the totality of sex and gender variation in the world—at the same time, these social categories are hard to dismantle (see the box "Transforming Bodies, Transforming Language").

Female Sex Organs

The external sex organs (genitals) of people assigned female at birth are collectively called the **vulva** (Figure 6.1a). Commonly confused with the vagina, the vulva includes the *mons pubis, labia majora* and *minora,* clitoris, and urethral and vaginal openings. The *mons pubis,* a rounded mass of fatty tissue over the pubic bone, becomes covered with hair during puberty. Below it are two paired folds of skin called the *labia majora* (outer lips) and the *labia minora* (inner lips). Enclosed within these folds are the *clitoris,* the opening of the urethra, and the opening of the vagina. The *labia majora* vary widely in size, color, shape, and overall appearance, and they often play a significant role in sexual sensation.

The **clitoris** is highly sensitive to stimulation and, for many people, plays an important role in sexual arousal and orgasm. The clitoris consists of 8000 nerve endings concentrated in the glans, or head. The clitoris may be externally visible between the labia. It extends internally into the anterior wall of the vagina (Figure 6.1b). Inside the clitoris, spongy, erectile tissue fills with blood during sexual excitement, creating engorgement of the genitals. The clitoral hood, or **prepuce,** covers the glans and is formed from the upper portion of the inner lips. For many trans men (people assigned female at birth who now identify as men), the clitoris can function like a penis during sexual activity.

The female **urethra** is a duct that transports urine directly from the urinary bladder to its opening between the clitoris and

---

TERMS

sexuality A dimension of personality shaped by biological, psychosocial, and cultural forces and concerning all aspects of sexual behavior and feelings.

gonads The primary organs that produce germ cells and sex hormones; the ovaries and testes.

germ cells Sperm and ova (eggs).

ovum A germ cell produced by an ovary; can combine with a germ cell called a *sperm* to create what will become an embryo; plural, ova. Also called an egg.

sperm A germ cell produced by a testis; if combined with an ovum, it can produce what will become an embryo.

intersex A condition in which a person is born with genitals, chromosomes, gonads, and hormones that cannot be classified as either male or female.

vulva The external female genitals, or sex organs.

clitoris A highly sensitive genital structure located on the vulva; its only known function is to contribute to sexual pleasure.

prepuce The foreskin of the clitoris or penis.

urethra The duct that carries urine from the bladder to the outside of the body.

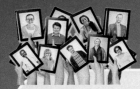

DIVERSITY MATTERS
Transforming Bodies, Transforming Language

People who are gender nonconforming refer to themselves in a variety of ways. Cisgender people—those whose gender identity aligns with their sex assigned at birth—and institutions that ask for personal information may not recognize the wide sex and gender diversity that describes our population. Schools, health organizations, or the criminal justice system—essentially all forms we fill out—demand that we make a binary decision about who we are.

Binary System

Female	Male
Girl	Boy
XX	XY
Vagina	Penis

As we understand better that sex and gender are varied concepts, in which people fit a spectrum rather than neatly into one of two categories, we can also adapt our language.

Pronouns

If you don't know what pronoun to use when talking with someone, just ask! Transgender and nonbinary people report encountering others—classmates, health care professionals, members of the public, family members—who refuse to call them by their preferred name or gender pronoun. This

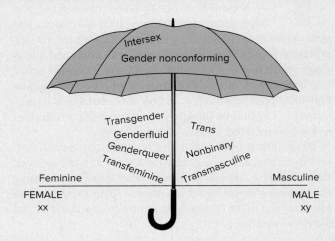

Now we are evolving toward acceptance of a spectrum of sexual identities.

denial is called *misgendering*. A common set of pronouns used by gender nonconforming people is they/them/their. For example: "Have you met Jordan? They are studying economics and are close to finishing their degree."

SOURCES: Lee, C. 2019. Welcome, singular "they." *APA Style Blog* (https://apastyle.apa.org/blog/singular-they); Levin, D. 2019. The fluidity of gender, language and the 'human experience.' *The New York Times*, 30 June; Schilt, K., and D. Lagos. 2017. The development of transgender studies in sociology. *Annual Review of Sociology* 43: 425–443.

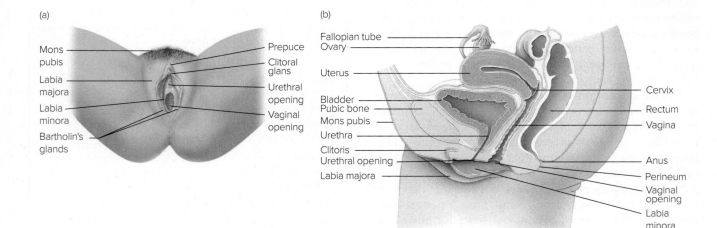

FIGURE 6.1   (a) An external view of the vulva. (b) An internal view of the pelvis.

the opening of the vagina. Most women have a much shorter urethra than do men and, as a result, some women are more susceptible to urinary tract or bladder infections (UTIs). All people should make it a habit to urinate after sexual activity to cleanse this tube. In addition, fluids apparently expelled through the female urethra during sexual activity can resemble ejaculate. It is similar to the fluid that comes from the male prostate gland.

The **vagina** is a passage that leads to the internal sexual organs and can be used for **sexual intercourse,** or coitus. It is the canal through which a baby travels during vaginal delivery and through which menstrual fluid is expelled from the uterus. Located about 1–2 inches inside the vagina is the Gräfenberg- or *G-spot*. This region overlays the root of the clitoris and can be highly sensitive. Projecting into the upper part of the vagina is the **cervix,** which is the opening of the **uterus** (sometimes called *womb*) where a fertilized egg is implanted and develops into a *fetus*. A pair of **fallopian tubes** (or *oviducts*) extends from the top of the uterus. The end of each oviduct surrounds an **ovary** and guides the mature ovum down into the uterus.

Male Sex Organs

For people assigned male at birth, the external sex organs are called the penis and scrotum (Figure 6.2a). The **penis** comprises a glans and a shaft. Also known as the head, the glans is typically the most sensitive part of the penis. The shaft extends from the head to the body of the penis and is made up of spongy tissue that can become engorged with blood during sexual excitement, causing the organ to enlarge and become erect.

The **scrotum** is a pouch that contains a pair of sperm-producing gonads, called **testes.** Because sperm production is an extremely heat-sensitive process, the scrotum's ability to regulate the temperature of the testes is important. The scrotum maintains the testes at a temperature approximately 5°F below that of the rest of the body—that is, at about 93.6°F. In

hot temperatures, the muscles in the scrotum relax and the testes move away from the heat of the body. Regular self-exams of the testes are important for detecting unusual growths, which could be cancerous. The best place to do this is in the shower because it is warm and the scrotal sac will hang farther away from the body.

The penile urethra is a tube that runs through the entire length of the penis and carries both urine and **semen** (sperm-carrying fluid) to the opening at the tip of the penis. The **Cowper's glands** are two small structures flanking the urethra. During

TERMS

vagina The canal leading from the vulva to the uterus. The location of the G-spot.

sexual intercourse Sexual relations involving penetration of the genitals or anus; also called coitus.

cervix The opening of the uterus in the upper part of the vagina.

uterus The hollow, thick-walled, muscular organ in which a fertilized egg might develop and where menstrual blood collects each month.

fallopian tube A duct that guides a mature ovum from the ovary to the uterus; also called an *oviduct*.

ovaries Paired glands that produce ova (eggs) and sex hormones; one of two types of gonads.

penis The genital structure consisting of a glans, shaft, and spongy tissue that often becomes engorged with blood during sexual excitement. The basis for assigning a male sex at birth.

scrotum The loose sac of skin and muscle fibers that contains the testes.

testis The site of sperm production; plural, *testes*. Also called *testicle*.

semen The fluid that carries sperm out of the penis during ejaculation.

Cowper's gland A small organ that produces preejaculatory fluid from the penis.

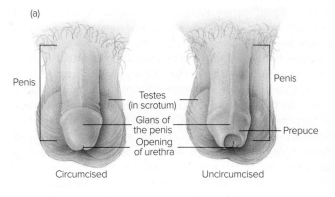

(a)

Penis · Testes (in scrotum) · Glans of the penis · Opening of urethra — Circumcised

Penis · Prepuce — Uncircumcised

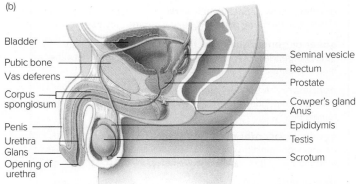

(b)

Bladder · Pubic bone · Vas deferens · Corpus spongiosum · Penis · Urethra · Glans · Opening of urethra

Seminal vesicle · Rectum · Prostate · Cowper's gland · Anus · Epididymis · Testis · Scrotum

FIGURE 6.2 **(a) An external view of the penis and scrotum. (b) An internal view of the pelvis.**

Ask Yourself

QUESTIONS FOR CRITICAL THINKING AND REFLECTION

What are your personal views on circumcision? What are your views about other forms of genital cutting? Who or what has influenced those opinions? Are the bases of your views cultural, moral, or medical? If you had a child, would you want their genitals altered?

sexual arousal, these glands excrete a clear, mucous-like fluid that appears at the tip of the penis. This preejaculatory fluid is thought to help lubricate the urethra to facilitate the passage of sperm and flush out any urine remaining in the tube. The release of preejaculatory fluid is an involuntary reflex and may contain sperm. This means that, for penile-vaginal coitus, withdrawal of the penis before ejaculation is not a reliable form of contraception. It is also possible to contract a sexually transmitted infection (STI)—in the mouth, anus, or vagina—from preejaculatory fluid.

Sperm production—at a rate of approximately 400 million per day—begins at about age 14. Sperm then take the following journey:

1. Sperm are produced inside a maze of tiny, tightly packed tubules within the testes. As they begin to mature, sperm flow into a single storage tube called the **epididymis,** which lies on the surface of each testis.

2. Sperm move from each epididymis into another tube—called the **vas deferens.**

3. The two *vasa deferentia* eventually merge into a pair of **seminal vesicles,** whose secretions provide nutrients for the sperm. The sperm then pass through an organ called the **prostate gland,** where they pick up a milky fluid and become semen.

4. On the final stage of their journey, sperm flow into the **ejaculatory ducts.** Although urine and semen share a common passage, they are prevented from mixing together by muscles that control their entry into the urethra.

The smooth, rounded tip of the penis is the highly sensitive **glans,** an important component in sexual arousal. The glans is partially covered by the foreskin, or prepuce, a retractable fold of skin that can be removed by **circumcision.** Circumcision is common in the United States, but rates vary widely among cultural groups and in other parts of the world.

GENDER ROLES AND SEXUAL ORIENTATION

Your *gender role* is everything you do in your daily life—including dress, speech patterns, and mannerisms—that expresses the gender with which you identify. Parents often choose gender-specific names, clothes, and toys for their children, and children may model their own behavior after their same-gender parent. Family and friends create an environment that teaches children how to act appropriately as a girl, boy, or other gender. Teachers, television, books, and even strangers model these gender roles. The concept of gender roles is intertwined with—but not the same as—that of sexual orientation.

Gender Roles

In general, **gender** is distinct from sex in that it refers to how people identify and feel about themselves, rather than the body parts and sexual organs they have. For example, a person who was assigned male because of a penis may feel more like a girl or a woman than a man. They may also feel like neither, and identify as **queer, genderqueer, nonbinary** or **gender nonconforming.** Some people who feel masculine or feminine but whose sex does not match their gender refer to themselves as **transgender.** The language we have for naming trans or nonbinary gender roles is limited. Nonbinary gender terms can be confusing because their definitions may overlap, or they may describe or omit subtle differences; some definitions are not agreed upon, and all will likely continue to evolve with time and usage. While some of these words may seem new, the people and behaviors they refer to have always been a part of humanity, and they have been recognized by cultures around the world for millennia. The wide diversity of terms reflects the many ways we can feel about our gender.

TERMS

epididymis   A storage duct for maturing sperm, located on the surface of each testis.

vas deferens   A tube that carries sperm from the epididymis through the prostate gland to the seminal vesicles; plural, *vasa deferentia.*

seminal vesicle   A tube leading from the vas deferens to the ejaculatory duct; secretes nutrients for the sperm.

prostate gland   A reproductive organ that produces some of the fluid in semen, which helps to transport and nourish sperm.

ejaculatory duct   A tube that carries mature sperm to the urethra so that they can exit the body upon ejaculation.

glans   The head of the penis or the clitoris.

circumcision   Surgical removal of the foreskin of the penis.

gender   How people identify and feel about themselves, rather than the body parts and sexual organs they have.

queer or **genderqueer**   A term describing people who question gender categories and who may not identify as either a man or woman, or as straight or gay.

nonbinary   A gender identity that cannot be described in traditional categories and actively questions or refuses the male/female binary.

gender nonconforming   An alternative term describing people who question gender categories and who do not dress or identify as either a man or a woman.

transgender   A term describing an individual whose bodily sex and gender assignment differ from their own gender identity.

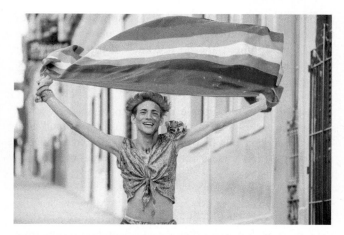

It is important that colleagues refer to transgender people by their preferred pronouns. Pollyana Ventura/Getty Images

Transgender individuals may be heterosexual, homosexual, bisexual, or asexual, or they may have a combination of sexual orientations. They may identify based on the gender they feel like—a woman, man, both, or neither—or based on who they feel attracted to, love, or want to have sex with. Over 20 countries have legally recognized and awarded rights, to varying degrees, to transgender individuals. In some places, this includes being able to formally identify as neither male nor female.

Some people use the term **androgyny** to describe the state of being neither overtly male or female. Androgynous adults are less gender stereotyped in their thinking; in how they look, dress, and act; in how they divide work in the home; in how they think about jobs and careers; and in how they express themselves sexually. Many people now use the term *nonbinary* to describe a person with these beliefs and practices.

The term **cisgender** describes people who feel that the sex they were assigned at birth (typically male or female), and the gender they were raised with as a result, aligns with the way they feel about themselves. A cisgender woman, for example, would likely have been born with a vulva, clitoris, and vagina, would have been raised as a girl, and would go on to experience herself as a woman.

Transexual is a term that describes transgender people who seek sex reassignment. This involves hormonal treatments to induce secondary sex characteristics such as breasts or facial hair, and/or surgery to change the appearance and function of the genitals or breasts. People who were assigned male at birth and fully transition to being a woman are sometimes called male-to-female transexuals. People assigned female who undergo surgery and procedures to become men are likewise sometimes called female-to-male transexuals. Many people who undergo these procedures prefer the term *transgender*.

Not all transgender people desire surgical or hormonal treatment, but they often still wish to live in a gender different from the one that aligned with their birth sex assignment. These people might also use the terms *trans woman* (man-to-woman transition) or *trans man* (woman-to-man transition).

In contrast, the term **transvestite** refers to a person, usually a cisman, who enjoys wearing clothing identified with another gender (usually a woman). Cross-dressing covers a broad range of behaviors, from wearing one article of clothing associated with another gender in a private location to wearing an entire outfit in public. Though once thought to be gay men, the majority of transvestites are heterosexual (straight) married men.

Transgender children may, from an early age, show intense and persistent distress about their assigned sex and associated gender and may view themselves as another sex and gender. Some of these children may be diagnosed with *gender dysphoria*, and some may be given medications to delay the bodily changes associated with puberty.

Gender roles vary from one time to another. The acceptance in mainstream culture of men wearing "man-buns" and women playing aggressive sports points to how gender expectations have changed over time. They also vary from one society to another. In Denmark today, for example, both parents, regardless of gender, may share 32 weeks of parental leave, sometimes with full pay. In the United States, no federal provision for paternity leave exists, and mothers are provided only 12 weeks of unpaid maternity leave at most. These disparities powerfully communicate the beliefs these societies hold regarding the roles men and women should play, in parenthood and elsewhere.

Sexual Orientation

Sexual orientation refers to who you are drawn to emotionally, romantically, and sexually. It exists along a continuum that ranges from exclusive heterosexuality (attraction only to people of another gender) through bisexuality (attraction to people of "both" genders) to exclusive homosexuality

androgyny The state of being neither overtly male nor female.

TERMS

cisgender A term that describes individuals whose initial sex and gender assignment align with their personal gender identity.

transexual A transgender person who undergoes sex reassignment, which involves hormonal treatments to induce secondary sex characteristics such as breasts or facial hair, and/or surgical alteration of the genitals.

transvestite A term for people, usually men, who enjoy wearing clothing identified with another gender.

(attraction only to people of your same gender) to **asexuality** (lack of sexual attraction to others). The terms *straight* and *gay* are often used to refer to heterosexuals and homosexuals, respectively, and female homosexuals are also referred to as *lesbians*. As mentioned earlier, in recent years the term *queer* has been reclaimed as a self-identifier by some elements of the gay community as well as by people who do not identify with conventional gender categories. Some people refer to themselves as **pansexual**, meaning that they are attracted to people of all gender identities—queer, nonbinary, trans, straight, gay, or however an individual defines themselves.

Sexual orientation involves feelings and self-concept, and individuals may or may not express their sexual orientation in their behavior. In national surveys, about 3.9% of men and 5.1% of women identify themselves as LGBT (lesbian, gay, bisexual, and transgender). Gauging the accuracy of these estimates is difficult because people may not tell the truth in surveys that probe sensitive and private aspects of their lives. In addition, our expressed sexual orientations may be quite different from our actual sexual practices. For example, some people identify as heterosexual, but most of their sexual partners may be of their own gender. Sexual orientation is also not the same as gender identity. A transgender person, for example, may be heterosexual or homosexual, or have a different orientation.

Heterosexuality   A majority of people are heterosexual. Heterosexual relationships usually include all of the behavior and relationship patterns described in Chapter 5: dating, engagement, living together, and marriage.

Homosexuality   Though homosexuality has existed throughout recorded history and currently exists in all parts of the world, attitudes toward homosexuality vary tremendously. In some cultures, homosexual behavior is fully accepted; in others, it is tolerated but not encouraged. In some societies, homosexuality is illegal and can be punished severely, even by death. Homosexual individuals are as varied and different from one another as heterosexuals are. Just like heterosexuals, lesbians and gay men may be in long-term, committed relationships, or they may date different people. As of 2019, same-gender couples could marry in 30 countries, including the United States.

Bisexuality   Because many experts believe that human sexuality exists on a spectrum, they also believe that many of us are potentially bisexual. However, only a relatively small number of people are attracted equally to both ends of the

gender spectrum. In the United States, approximately 3% of the population identify as bisexual. Some observers think bisexuals are confused and do not know if they like men or women; however, most bisexuals are clear they like *both* men and women.

Asexuality   Some people do not experience or express any sexual desire, though they may form intimate and even romantic attachments. Though previously deemed a problem, asexuality is now understood as another sexual orientation. (More on this below.)

The Origins of Sexual Orientation   Many theories try to account for the development of sexual orientation. At this time, most experts agree that sexual orientation results from multiple genetic, hormonal, cultural, social, and psychological factors. The majority of experts agree that conscious choice is not usually a factor in whether someone is gay, straight, or queer.

Some scientists, however, continue to look for genetic markers associated with sexual orientation in males. Twin studies are one way of looking at the genetic contribution to sexual identity. Identical twins share the same DNA, so if sexual orientation were entirely genetically determined, we would expect that if one identical twin were homosexual, the other would be as well. But studies of many identical male twins show that if one twin is gay, there is only a 50–52% chance that the other twin will have the same sexual orientation. When we consider fraternal twins, who share fewer genes, the chances decrease to 22%. Two adopted children, who share an environment but no genetic makeup, have an 11% chance of both being gay. According to these studies, the less genetic makeup two family members share, the less likely that, if one is gay, the other will be as well. Not all scientists who study this issue come to the same conclusions, however, and it is more difficult to make a genetic connection when looking at females, suggesting that female sexuality may differ from male sexuality. These studies provide evidence that our genes, while not wholly responsible for our sexual orientation, may contribute to it.

Many psychological theories have been proposed to explain the development of heterosexual or homosexual sexual orientation. Researchers have looked at how much contact children have with different genders, at the types of relationships children have with their parents, and at family dynamics. Early negative experiences with heterosexuality or positive experiences with homosexuality have also been proposed as possible influences. The significant growth of single-parent families over the past 40 years has not been accompanied by large shifts in sexual orientation among Americans, so it is unlikely that family dynamics or early learning experiences are strong factors in determining sexual orientation. In addition, parents' sexual orientations have little impact on children's sexual orientations. Studies of children raised by gay or lesbian parents show that these children's ultimate sexual orientations are similar to those of children raised by heterosexual parents. In addition, most people who identify as gay or lesbian had heterosexual parents.

TERMS

asexual   A person who does not experience sexual desire or arousal. Asexuality is a sexual orientation and not a sexual dysfunction.

pansexual   The term used to describe people who are attracted to all genders, including nonbinary, genderqueer, and transgender identities.

HORMONES AND THE REPRODUCTIVE LIFE CYCLE

The hormones produced by the ovaries or testes have a major influence on the development and function of the genital-sexual organs—and even the brain—throughout life.

All people produce testosterone, estrogens, and progestogens; however, the quantities differ across assigned sexes. The dominant sex hormones made by the testes are called **androgens,** the most active of which is *testosterone.* Testes also produce estrogen and progesterone, but at lower levels. Hormones produced by the ovaries belong to two groups: **estrogens** and **progestogens.** The ovaries also produce a small amount of testosterone. **Adrenal glands** also produce sex hormones in all people.

Sex hormones are regulated by the **pituitary gland,** located at the base of the brain. This gland in turn is controlled by hormones produced by the **hypothalamus** in the brain.

Differentiation of the Embryo

How do we become what is eventually called a girl or a boy? All human cells typically contain 23 pairs of chromosomes (Figure 6.3). In 22 of the pairs, the two partner chromosomes match. But in the 23rd pair, one comes from the mother and one from the father; these are called the **sex chromosomes.** Ovaries contribute an X and testes an X or a Y. People who are designated female typically have an XX chromosomal pair; people who are designated male have an XY pair. This is established at the moment of conception.

Variations in chromosomal and hormonal patterns can occur, making it more challenging to classify some babies as male or female. The two most common disorders of sex chromosomes—also known as intersex conditions—are Klinefelter syndrome and Turner syndrome. Klinefelter syndrome, a condition in which a person assigned male at birth carries two or more X chromosomes in addition to a Y chromosome, occurs in about 1 in 1000 babies and causes infertility and atypical genitalia. People with Turner syndrome, which occurs in about 1 in 2500 babies assigned female at birth, have only a single complete X chromosome. Because of these variations, people with intersex conditions often need technological assistance if they wish to have children, and they can sometimes have other medical problems.

For people without intersex conditions, the chromosomal combinations of XX and XY dictate whether the undifferentiated gonads become ovaries or testes. In an XY combination, the gonads will likely become testes and produce the male hormone **testosterone.** Testosterone circulates throughout the body and causes the undifferentiated reproductive structures to develop into a penis and scrotum. If the chromosomal arrangement is XX, the gonads become ovaries and the genital structures develop into a vagina, clitoris, and labia. Some researchers believe that this process, often referred to as *sexual differentiation,* is influenced solely by the presence or absence of testosterone. Others, however, believe that the relationships

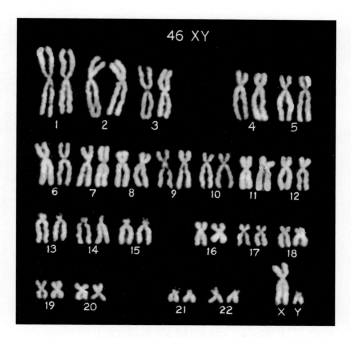

FIGURE 6.3   A typical set of chromosomes. The first 22 pairs are matched, but the last pair (the sex chromosomes) does not match, indicating the person carrying these chromosomes will have a penis and scrotum and will likely be assigned male. Biophoto Associates/Photo Researchers/Science Source

among chromosomes, genes, and hormones are far more complex, and that intersex conditions are a natural variation of these complicated processes. Testosterone is produced by all people, not just men.

> **androgens**   Sex hormones that are produced by the testes.   **TERMS**
>
> **estrogens**   A class of sex hormones, produced by the ovaries, that bring about sexual maturation at puberty and maintain ovarian and other sexual-reproductive functions.
>
> **progestogens**   A class of sex hormones, produced by the ovaries, that sustain reproductive and other sexual functions.
>
> **adrenal glands**   Endocrine glands, located over the kidneys, that produce sex hormones.
>
> **pituitary gland**   An endocrine gland at the base of the brain that produces hormones and regulates the release of hormones—including sex hormones—by other glands.
>
> **hypothalamus**   A region of the brain above the pituitary gland whose hormones control the secretions of the pituitary; also involved in the control of many bodily functions, including hunger, thirst, temperature regulation, and sexual functions.
>
> **sex chromosomes**   The X and Y chromosomes, which contribute to genital development, hormone secretion and, thus, the sex that we are assigned at birth.
>
> **testosterone**   The hormone responsible for the development of the penis, scrotum, and related secondary sex characteristics at puberty, such as deepened voice and growth of facial and body hair.

Exposure to hormones also influences development of the brain. Some research has suggested that males perform better than females at tasks requiring spatial skills, and that females perform better than males on tests of verbal skills. Proponents of this research suggest that the reason males sometimes perform better at spatial skills is that androgens are involved. For example, genetic (XX) females exposed to androgens in utero (such as those with an XY twin) might sometimes perform better at spatial skills, and genetic males deprived of these hormones do worse. There are many criticisms of this research, however, because it is very difficult to separate the ways that boys and girls—even infants—are treated by people from the effects of biological hormones on their abilities. Research in this area also tends to focus on non-intersex and non-transgender people, leading to results that might overemphasize binary differences among sexes and genders.

What is important to consider is that each person is a combination of biological, environmental, and cultural events. Biology acts on the cells in the body, including the brain. The physical and social environment then shapes this biological foundation to produce unique individuals.

Sexual Maturation

Although humans are typically sexually differentiated at birth, sex-based differences are accentuated at **puberty,** the period during which the reproductive system matures, secondary sex characteristics develop, and bodies begin to appear more distinctive (while still sharing many features). The changes of puberty are primarily induced by testosterone, estrogen, and **progesterone.**

Puberty in Females The first signs of puberty usually appear between the ages of 8 and 12. Physical changes include breast development, often followed by a rounding of the hips and buttocks. As breasts develop, hair appears in the pubic region and later in the underarms. A general increase in growth rate often follows between ages 9 and 15.

The Menstrual Cycle A major landmark of puberty for most young women is the onset of the **menstrual cycle,** the

> **puberty** The period of biological maturation during adolescence; in this stage of development, the individual becomes capable of sexual reproduction.
>
> **progesterone** A sex hormone that regulates the menstrual cycle and sustains pregnancy. The active ingredient in many long-acting forms of contraception.
>
> **menstrual cycle** The monthly ovarian cycle, regulated by hormones; in the absence of pregnancy, menstruation occurs.
>
> **menarche** The first menstrual period, which is typically experienced during adolescence.
>
> **menses** The portion of the menstrual cycle characterized by menstrual flow (bleeding).
>
> **TERMS**

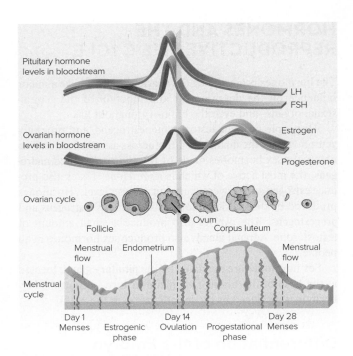

FIGURE 6.4 **The menstrual cycle.**

monthly ovarian cycle that leads to menstruation (loss of blood and tissue lining the uterus) in the absence of pregnancy. The timing of **menarche** (the first *menstrual period*) varies with several factors, including race/ethnicity, genetics, and nutritional status. The typical range for the onset of menstruation is wide; some girls experience menarche as young as 9 or 10, and others when they are 16 or 17 years old. The current average age of menarche in the United States is around 12½ years of age. Two hundred years ago, the average age of menarche was closer to 17 years. The earlier onset of menarche today is likely due to nutritional factors. When age at menarche is examined worldwide, studies show that menarche tends to come later to girls who live in relative poverty with diets lacking in protein and calories. Early menarche has been shown to correlate with higher than average weight, which may explain the current trend in the United States. Because it is the biological norm for people born with female sex organs to menstruate, girls should check with a health care provider if their menstrual cycle does not begin during their adolescence. Although it might be normal, it might also indicate an intersex condition or another problem, including pregnancy.

The day of the onset of bleeding is considered to be day 1 of the menstrual cycle. For the purposes of our discussion, a cycle of 28 days will be used as a model; however, normal cycles vary in length from 21 to 35 days. The menstrual cycle consists of the following four phases (Figure 6.4):

1. *Menses.* During **menses,** characterized by the menstrual flow (bleeding from the uterus), blood levels of hormones from the ovaries and the pituitary gland are relatively low. This phase of the cycle usually lasts from day 1 to about day 5.

2. *Estrogenic phase.* The estrogenic phase begins when bleeding ceases and the pituitary gland begins to produce follicle-stimulating hormone (FSH) and luteinizing hormone (LH). Under the influence of FSH, an egg-containing ovarian **follicle** begins to mature, producing increasingly higher amounts of estrogen. Stimulated by estrogen, the **endometrium** (the uterine lining) thickens with large numbers of blood vessels and uterine glands.

3. *Ovulation.* A surge of a potent estrogen called *estradiol* from the follicle causes the pituitary gland to release a large burst of LH and a smaller amount of FSH. The high concentration of LH stimulates the developing follicle to release its ovum. This event is known as **ovulation.** After ovulation, the follicle is transformed into the **corpus luteum,** which produces progesterone and estrogen. Ovulation theoretically occurs about 14 days prior to the onset of menstrual flow, with the window of greatest fertility occurring from a few days before ovulation to about one day after. This information has been used to attempt to predict the most fertile time during the menstrual cycle for fertility treatments and natural family planning methods (see Chapter 7). However, a recent study showed that even women with regular menstrual cycles often have unpredictable ovulation, and they can actually be fertile on any day of the month, including during menstruation. The "window of fertility" is especially unpredictable in teenagers and women who are approaching menopause.

4. *Progestational phase.* During the progestational phase of the cycle, the amount of progesterone secreted from the corpus luteum increases and remains high until the onset of the next menses. Under the influence of estrogen and progesterone, the endometrium continues to develop, preparing itself to support a fertilized ovum. If pregnancy occurs, the fertilized egg produces a hormone called human chorionic gonadotropin (hCG), which maintains the corpus luteum. Thus levels of ovarian hormones remain high and the uterine lining is preserved, preventing menses. hCG is the hormone detected by pregnancy tests.

If pregnancy does not occur, the corpus luteum degenerates, and estrogen and progesterone levels gradually fall. Below certain hormonal levels, the endometrium can no longer be maintained, and it begins to slough off, initiating menses. As the levels of ovarian hormones fall, a slight rise in LH and FSH occurs, and a new menstrual cycle begins.

Menstrual Problems   Menstruation is a normal biological process, though physical or emotional symptoms associated with the menstrual cycle are common. Many people experience menstrual cramps, the severity of which tends to vary from cycle to cycle. **Dysmenorrhea,** discomfort associated with menstruation, can include any combination of the following symptoms: lower abdominal cramps, backache, vomiting, nausea, bloating, diarrhea, headache, and fatigue. Many of these symptoms can be attributed to uterine muscular contractions caused by chemicals called *prostaglandins.* Nonsteroidal anti-inflammatory drugs (NSAIDs) such as ibuprofen often relieve dysmenorrhea by blocking the effects of prostaglandins. Oral contraceptives are also effective in reducing dysmenorrheal symptoms in most women. Some people also obtain relief from rest, acupuncture, and other nonmedical treatments.

Many people experience transient emotional symptoms prior to the onset of their menstrual flow. Depending on their severity, these symptoms may be categorized along a continuum: **premenstrual tension**, **premenstrual syndrome (PMS)**, and **premenstrual dysphoric disorder (PMDD).** Premenstrual tension symptoms are mild and may include negative mood changes and physical symptoms such as abdominal cramping and backache. More severe symptoms are classified as PMS; very severe symptoms that impair normal daily and social functioning are classified as PMDD. All three conditions share a definite pattern. Symptoms appear prior to the onset of menses and disappear within a few days after the start of menstruation. Premenstrual tension is quite common, PMS affects about 1 in 5 women, and PMDD affects fewer than 1 in 10 women.

Symptoms associated with PMS and PMDD can include breast tenderness, water retention (bloating), headache, fatigue, insomnia or excessive sleep, appetite changes, food cravings, irritability, anger, increased

---

TERMS

follicle   A saclike structure within the ovary, in which an egg (ovum) matures.

endometrium   The lining of the uterus.

ovulation   The release of a mature egg (ovum) from an ovary.

corpus luteum   The part of the ovarian follicle left after ovulation; secretes estrogen and progesterone during the second half of the menstrual cycle.

dysmenorrhea   Painful or problematic menstruation.

premenstrual tension   Mild physical and emotional changes associated with the time before the onset of menses.

premenstrual syndrome (PMS)   A condition characterized by physical discomfort, psychological distress, and behavioral changes that begin after ovulation and cease when menstruation begins.

premenstrual dysphoric disorder (PMDD)   A severe form of PMS, characterized by symptoms serious enough to interfere with daily activities and relationships.

interpersonal conflict, depression, anxiety, tearfulness, inability to concentrate, social withdrawal, and the sense of being out of control or overwhelmed.

These conditions are especially tricky to research because the symptoms overlap with many other conditions, and they are also normal responses to stress, which is common. Most researchers agree that PMS is probably caused by a combination of hormonal, neurological, genetic, dietary, psychological, and social factors.

The following strategies provide relief for many women with premenstrual symptoms, and all of them can contribute to a healthy lifestyle at any time:

- *Limit salt intake.* Salt promotes water retention and bloating.
- *Exercise.* Women who exercise may experience fewer symptoms before and after menstrual periods.
- *Don't use alcohol or tobacco.* Alcohol and tobacco may aggravate certain symptoms of PMS and PMDD.
- *Eat a nutritious diet.* Choose a low-fat diet rich in complex carbohydrates from vegetables, fruits, and whole grains. Get enough calcium, and minimize your intake of sugar and caffeine.
- *Relax and sleep.* Stress reduction is always beneficial, and stressful events can trigger PMS symptoms. Try relaxation techniques during the premenstrual time and be sure to get sufficient sleep (7-8 hours per night). Orgasms, including those from **masturbation,** can also help reduce stress and relieve cramping. Most importantly, there is no need to be embarrassed about premenstrual or menstrual difficulties, as they are part of normal bodily processes.

If you suffer persistent premenstrual symptoms, keep a daily diary to track the types of symptoms, their severity, and their correlation with your menstrual cycle. Some people find help after being evaluated by a health care provider.

Selective serotonin reuptake inhibitors (SSRIs), such as Prozac and Zoloft, are sometimes used to treat PMS and PMDD. Until recently, women using SSRIs took the medication throughout the entire menstrual cycle, but taking the medication during just the progestational phase of the cycle is effective in some women. However, these medications are not without side effects, and they may negatively affect sexual functioning—specifically causing low desire as well as difficulty with arousal and attaining orgasm.

Other drug treatments for PMS and PMDD include certain oral contraceptives, diuretics to minimize water retention, and NSAIDs such as ibuprofen. A number of vitamins, minerals, and other dietary supplements have also been studied for PMS relief. Only one supplement, calcium, has been shown to provide relief in rigorous clinical studies; several others show promise, but more research is needed.

> **masturbation** Self-stimulation for the purpose of sexual arousal and orgasm. **TERMS**

Finally, another problem related to menstruation, albeit indirectly, is toxic shock syndrome. Although rare, occurring in 0.8 to 3.4 per 100,000 in the United States, this condition has been associated with highly absorbent tampons, especially if used more than 48 hours. These tampons have now been taken off the market, reducing the incidence of this problem even further.

Puberty in Males Testicular growth usually begins at about age 10 or 11 (Figure 6.5). The penis also begins to grow at this time, reaching adult size by about age 18. Pubic hair starts to develop as the genitals begin increasing in size, and underarm and facial hair gradually appear. Hair later develops on the chest, back, and abdomen. Facial hair often continues to get thicker and darker for several years after puberty. The voice deepens as a result of the lengthening and thickening of the vocal cords. Body hair and breasts are not always mutually exclusive, and some boys with chest and facial hair will also develop small amounts of breast tissue, a condition called *gynecomastia.* This is very normal, usually decreases after puberty, and can sometimes be associated with being of higher than normal weight.

Boys grow taller for about six years after the first signs of puberty, with a rapid period of growth about two years after puberty starts. Largely because of the influence of testosterone, muscle development and bone density are much greater in males than in females. By adulthood, and on average, men have one and a half times the lean body mass of women and nearly half the body fat. However, many individual men and women fall outside these averages.

Aging and Human Sexuality

Despite the changes in sexual functioning that can accompany aging, sexuality and sensuality can continue to be a source of great satisfaction throughout the life course. A recent study of sexuality in older Americans found that three-fourths of 57- to 64-year-olds were sexually active (defined as having had at least one sexual partner in the past year). Half of people aged 65–74 and about one-fourth aged 75–85 remained sexually active. People who are able to remain healthy and physically active are much more likely to continue to be sexually active in their older years. Other people gain satisfaction from redefining what it means to be "sexually active" as they age or their level of ability changes.

Menopause Ovaries eventually stop releasing eggs and producing hormones, usually between the ages of 45 and 55.

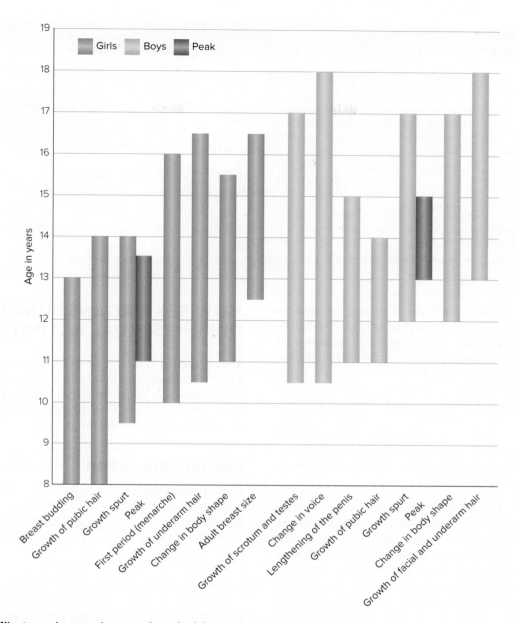

FIGURE 6.5 **Milestones in sexual maturation of adolescents.**

SOURCE: *The Merck Manual Home Health Handbook,* Online Version. © 2019 Merck Sharpe & Dohme Corp., a subsidiary of Merck & Co., Inc., Whitehouse Station, NJ, USA (https://www.merckmanuals.com/home/children-s-health-issues/growth-and-development/physical-growth-and-sexual-maturation-of-adolescents?query=sexual%20maturation).

When this happens, a person enters **menopause,** the cessation of menstruation (Table 6.1). For some people the associated drop in hormone production causes troublesome symptoms. The most common of these is the hot flash, a sensation of warmth rising to the face from the upper chest, with or without perspiration and chills. During a hot flash, skin temperature can rise by more than 10 degrees. Other menopausal symptoms include vaginal dryness, low libido (sexual desire), painful intercourse, night sweats, insomnia, thinning of head hair, and mood changes. Osteoporosis—decreasing bone density—can develop, making older women more vulnerable to fractures.

As a result of decreased estrogen production during menopause, the vaginal walls thin, and lubrication in response to sexual arousal can diminish. Sexual intercourse may become painful. Hormonal treatment or the use of lubricants during intercourse can minimize these problems.

Cross-cultural studies comparing Japanese with North American women dispel the idea that hot flashes and other meno-

> **menopause** The cessation of menstruation, occurring gradually between the ages of 45 and 55.

Table 6.1	Reproductive Aging in Women	
AGE*	SIGNS & SYMPTOMS—WHAT'S HAPPENING	STAGE OF REPRODUCTION
9–15	First period; variable menstrual cycles	Menarche; beginning reproductive years
16–30	Regular menstrual cycle; fertility peaking	Reproductive years
31–42	Regular menstrual cycle; fertility progressively declining	Reproductive years
Early 40s	Lengths of menstrual cycle vary increasingly	Menopausal transition
Late 40s–early 50s	Two or more skipped periods; hot flashes, irritability, and sleep disturbance; bone loss begins ·	Menopausal transition
45–55	Final period (i.e., no period for 12 months)	Menopause
50s and beyond	Vaginal dryness, bone loss. Hot flashes can persist (for a few women, into their 60s and 70s).	Postmenopause

*Women vary a great deal in the ages at which they go through these stages. The average length of menopause and the transition leading up to it is 4 years, but for some women symptoms may last only a few months, and for others, 10 years.

SOURCE: American Society for Reproductive Medicine. 2012. *Reproductive Aging in Women* (http://www.reproductivefacts.org).

pausal reactions are universal. A diet of fish and vegetables; an exercise regimen of cycling, walking, or farming; and cultural ideas about the meaning of bodily changes positively affected the Japanese experience of menopause among the women studied.

In Western medicine, doctors once regularly prescribed estrogen to relieve a host of symptoms in a regimen called hormone replacement therapy, or HRT. However, a reanalysis of the data on potential side effects, which include cardiovascular disease, blood clots, and breast cancer, has resulted in more individualized approaches, such as low-dose estrogen, which treats specific symptoms of menopause and carries a reduced risk of side effects.

Andropause   Testosterone production decreases between the ages of 35 and 65, resulting in what is sometimes referred to as *male menopause* or *andropause*. Some experts prefer the term *aging male syndrome* because the process is much more gradual than menstrually defined menopause. Symptoms vary widely, but include loss of muscle mass, increased fat mass, decreased sex drive, erectile problems, depressed mood, irritability, difficulties with concentration, increased urination, loss of bone mineral density, and sleep difficulties. For some, carefully prescribed testosterone replacement therapy can help with these symptoms.

As some men get older, they depend on more direct physical stimulation for sexual arousal, take longer to achieve an erection, and find it more difficult to maintain one. Orgasmic contractions may also be less intense. Prescription medications can increase blood flow to the penis, resulting in firmer and more predictable erections.

Conception and pregnancy can occur well into middle age. Due to changes in both eggs (which are all present at birth and released monthly as part of the menstrual cycle) and sperm (which is produced throughout one's lifetime), however, fertility begins to decrease at about age 40. Indeed, the pregnancy rate drops to 50% for heterosexual couples when a man is over age 35, regardless of the woman's age. Children conceived by parents over age 40 are also more likely to have a disability, including autism, schizophrenia, and Down syndrome.

HOW SEX ORGANS FUNCTION DURING SEXUAL ACTIVITY

Sexual function is largely based on stimulus and response. Erotic stimulation leads to sexual arousal (excitement), which may culminate in the intensely pleasurable experience of orgasm. Pleasure comes from engaging the entire body and mind, which often includes the genitals.

Sexual Stimulation

Physical stimuli excite us directly; some people believe psychological stimuli—thoughts, fantasies, desires, perceptions—excite us even more. Regardless of the source, all stimulation has a physical basis, to which the brain gives meaning.

Physical Stimulation   Physical stimulation comes through the senses: We are aroused by things we see, hear, taste, smell, and feel. Sexual stimuli frequently come from other people, but they may also come from books, images, songs, social media, films, fantasies, or our own bodies.

An obvious and effective means of physical stimulation is touching. Even though culturally defined practices and individual preferences vary, most sexual encounters eventually involve some form of touching with hands, lips, and body surfaces. For some people, including those with physical disabilities, these encounters may also involve prosthetics or other technological objects. Kissing, caressing, fondling, and hugging are as much a part of sexual encounters as they are a part of expressing affection.

Some of the most intense stimulation involves the genitals; the clitoris and the glans of the penis are particularly sensitive. Other highly responsive areas—sometimes called erogenous zones—include the vaginal opening and labia, nipples, breasts, insides of the thighs, buttocks, anal region, scrotum, lips, armpits, and earlobes. Often, what determines a sexual response is not *what* is touched but how, for how long, and by whom. Talking explicitly about sex is also very arousing to some people, both before and during sexual activity.

Psychological Stimulation Sexual arousal also has an important psychological component, regardless of the nature of the physical stimulation. Fantasies, memories, and mood can all generate sexual excitement. Erotic thoughts may be linked to an imagined person or situation or to a sexual experience from the past. Fantasies may involve activities a person may not wish to experience in reality, sometimes because they're dangerous, frightening, or forbidden.

Arousal is also powerfully influenced by emotions and attitudes about sex. How you feel about sex and the person or people you are with, and how they feel about you, matter tremendously in how sexually responsive you are likely to be. Even the most direct forms of physical stimulation carry emotional overtones. Kissing, caressing, and fondling express affection and caring. The emotional charge they give to a sexual interaction plays a significant role in sexual arousal—for some, as significant as the purely physical stimulation achieved by touching.

The Sexual Response Cycle

Researchers disagree about whether the sexual response cycle differs across sex and gender, and some note that gender roles affect patterns of arousal and excitement. For example, stereotypes of aggressive masculinity and passive femininity can affect how people respond sexually. Two physiological mechanisms explain most genital and bodily reactions during sexual arousal and orgasm (Figure 6.6): **vasocongestion** and muscular tension. Vasocongestion is the engorgement of tissues that results when more blood flows into an organ than is flowing out. Thus the penis and the clitoris become erect on the same principle that makes a garden hose become stiff when the water is turned on. Increased muscular tension culminates in rhythmic muscular contractions during orgasm.

There are several models of human sexual response, most of which are variations on the one described here. Some researchers include the feeling of desire as an integral part of the model, others describe gendered differences, and some don't center orgasm as the culminating experience of sexual activity. In this model, developed by William Masters and Virginia Johnson in 1966, four phases characterize the sexual response cycle:

1. ***The excitement phase.*** The clitoris, labia, and vaginal walls become engorged with blood. Tension increases in the vaginal muscles, and the vaginal walls become moist with lubricating fluid. The penis becomes erect as its tissues become engorged with blood. The testes expand and are pulled upward within the scrotum.

2. ***The plateau phase.*** This is an extension of the excitement phase during which reactions become more marked. The uterus rises, causing the inner one-third of the vaginal canal (closest to the cervix) to lengthen and "tent" open near the cervix while the outer one-third of the vagina (closest to the opening) swells, and vaginal lubrication increases. The penis becomes harder, and the testes become larger.

3. ***The orgasmic phase.*** In this phase, sometimes called **orgasm,** rhythmic contractions occur along the vagina,

penis, urethra, prostate gland, seminal vesicles, and muscles in the pelvic and anal regions. These involuntary muscular contractions can lead to two types of ejaculation: semen, which consists of sperm cells from the testes and secretions from the prostate gland and seminal vesicles, from the penis; and fluid from a woman's urethra, known as female ejaculation.

4. ***The resolution phase.*** All changes initiated during the excitement phase are reversed. Excess blood drains from tissues, the muscles in the region relax, and the genital structures return to their unstimulated states. Following ejaculation, the penis and scrotum are subject to a *refractory period* during which more stimulation will not lead to physiological arousal.

More general physical reactions accompany the genital changes in these four phases. Beginning with the excitement phase, nipples become erect, breasts begin to swell, and the skin of the chest becomes flushed (this is more visible in people with lighter skin); these changes are more marked in women. The heart rate doubles by the plateau phase, and respiration becomes faster. During orgasm, breathing becomes irregular and the person may moan or cry out. A feeling of warmth leads to increased sweating during the resolution phase. Deep relaxation and a sense of well-being pervade the body and the mind as the brain chemicals dopamine and oxytocin are released during the response cycle.

Reactions during the sexual response cycle may be somewhat sex-specific. For instance, the female excitement phase may lead directly to orgasm, or orgasmic and plateau phases may be fused. Male orgasm is typically marked by the ejaculation of semen. Women do not experience a refractory period and may immediately experience one or more orgasms.

Sexual Problems

Both physiological and psychological factors can interfere with sexual functioning. Many diseases specifically affect the sex organs. Any illness that affects your general health is likely to also affect your ability to function sexually. These problems may be due to physical problems, psychological issues, or a combination of both. The absence of sexual desire is not—in and of itself—a problem, unless a person wants to feel desire. Asexuality is not an illness.

Common Sexual Health Problems

• *Vaginitis* (inflammation of the vagina) is a common problem that can be caused by a variety of organisms: *Candida* (yeast infection), *Trichomonas* (trichomoniasis), and the overgrowth

> **vasocongestion** The accumulation of blood in tissues and organs by more blood flowing into an area than flowing out.
>
> **orgasm** The discharge of accumulated sexual tension with characteristic genital and bodily manifestations and a subjective sensation of intense pleasure; may include ejaculation.
>
> **TERMS**

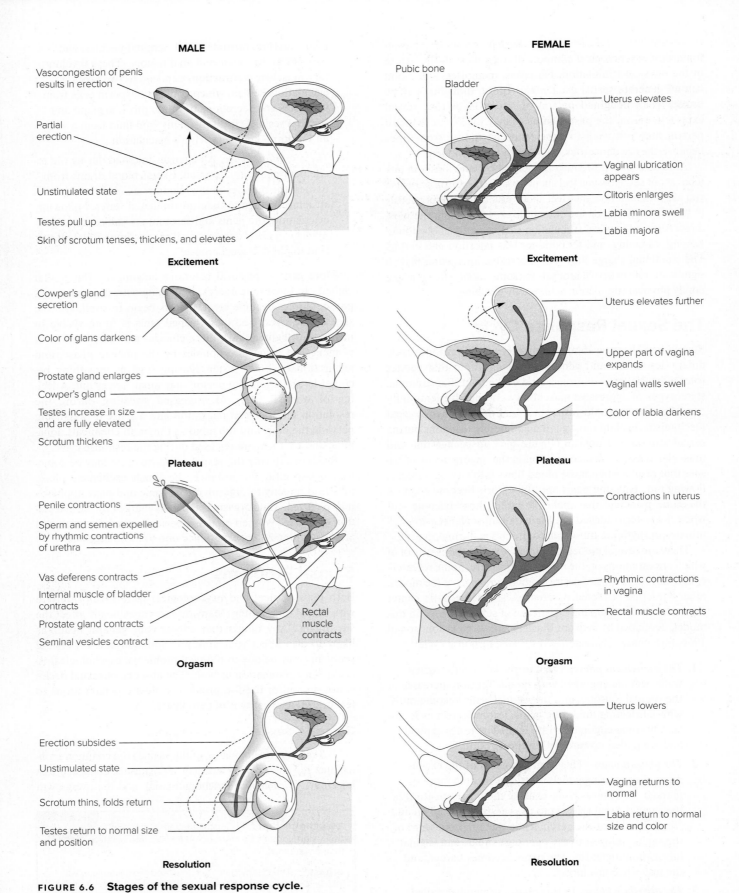

MALE

Vasocongestion of penis results in erection

Partial erection

Unstimulated state

Testes pull up

Skin of scrotum tenses, thickens, and elevates

Excitement

Cowper's gland secretion

Color of glans darkens

Prostate gland enlarges

Cowper's gland

Testes increase in size and are fully elevated

Scrotum thickens

Plateau

Penile contractions

Sperm and semen expelled by rhythmic contractions of urethra

Vas deferens contracts

Internal muscle of bladder contracts

Prostate gland contracts

Seminal vesicles contract

Rectal muscle contracts

Orgasm

Erection subsides

Unstimulated state

Scrotum thins, folds return

Testes return to normal size and position

Resolution

FEMALE

Pubic bone

Bladder

Uterus elevates

Vaginal lubrication appears

Clitoris enlarges

Labia minora swell

Labia majora

Excitement

Uterus elevates further

Upper part of vagina expands

Vaginal walls swell

Color of labia darkens

Plateau

Contractions in uterus

Rhythmic contractions in vagina

Rectal muscle contracts

Orgasm

Uterus lowers

Vagina returns to normal

Labia return to normal size and color

Resolution

FIGURE 6.6   Stages of the sexual response cycle.

of a variety of bacteria (bacterial vaginosis). Symptoms include vaginal discharge, vaginal irritation, and pain during vaginal penetration. Vaginitis is treated with a variety of topical and oral medications. (See Chapters 18 and 19 for more information about infection and sexually transmitted infections.)

- **Vulvodynia,** or chronic and unexplained vulvar pain, affects 15–18% of women in the United States. Women describe this pain as "burning," "knifelike," and "raw." Because the condition is hard to talk about, people with symptoms may wait five or more years for a diagnosis and appropriate treatment. Women of color may wait even longer.

- **Endometriosis** is the growth of endometrial-like tissue outside the uterus. It occurs most often during childbearing years. Pain in the lower abdomen and pelvis is the most common symptom. Painful premenstrual intercourse may occur. Endometriosis can cause serious problems if left untreated because endometrial tissue can scar and partially or completely block the oviducts, making it difficult or even impossible to become pregnant. Endometriosis is treated with medication and/or surgery.

- **Pelvic inflammatory disease (PID)** is an infection of the uterus, oviducts, or ovaries caused when microorganisms spread to these areas from the vagina. Approximately 50–75% of PID cases are caused by sexually transmitted infections. (See Chapter 19.)

- **Dyspareunia,** or painful intercourse, which is more common in women, has many possible causes. Infection, lack of lubrication, endometriosis, past sexual trauma, fear of penetration, menopause, and scarring due to childbirth are a few common reasons for pain during intercourse. For some people, *vaginismus* (the involuntary contractions of pelvic muscles) makes vaginal penetration difficult to impossible. This condition may also include discomfort with inserting a tampon or finger, or during a pelvic exam.

Dyspareunia and vaginismus are treated first by diagnosing and treating any underlying physical cause of the problem. The use of generous amounts of lubricant during sexual activity is important. Sexual therapy for vaginismus often involves gradual desensitization techniques including the use of dilators. Dilators range in size and are inserted into the vagina in order to relax the vaginal muscles, to stop the involuntary spasms and to help the vagina to gradually stretch. Some people with this condition receive injections of botulinum toxin, a chemical that paralyzes and can therefore help to relax the muscles of the pelvis.

- **Prostatitis** is an inflammation or infection of the prostate gland. Prostatitis can be acute (sudden) or chronic (gradual and long lasting). The symptoms of *acute bacterial prostatitis* may include fever, chills, flulike symptoms, pain in the lower back or groin, problems with urination, and painful ejaculation. Acute prostatitis is treated with antibiotics. It is potentially serious, so anyone with these symptoms needs to seek immediate medical attention. *Chronic prostatitis* is more common after age 40 and can be caused by infection or inflammation of the prostate. It is sometimes difficult to diagnose and treat. (See Chapter 17 for more information about prostate and testicular cancer.)

- **Testicular cancer** occurs most commonly in men in their twenties and thirties. A rare cancer, it has a very high cure rate if detected early. Every man should perform testicular self-exams regularly for lumps and abnormalities (see Chapter 17).

- **Epididymitis** is an inflammation of the epididymis (the coiled tube located on the top and back of each testicle). The most common cause of epididymitis is infection, often sexually transmitted. Symptoms include tenderness over the testicle, swelling, fever, and pain with ejaculation. The treatment is antibiotics.

- **Testicular torsion** occurs when the spermatic cord, which supplies blood to the testicle, becomes twisted. Decreased blood flow to the testicle causes severe, sudden pain, and if not treated quickly, it can cause permanent damage to the testicle. Testicular torsion is most common in adolescents and young men. It can be associated with trauma to the testicle, but it can occur spontaneously. Testicular pain should be evaluated by a medical professional promptly; sudden, severe pain is a medical emergency.

Sexual Dysfunctions The term **sexual dysfunction** encompasses disturbances in sexual desire, performance, or satisfaction. Many physical conditions and drugs can interfere with sexual functioning. Psychological causes and relationship problems can be important factors as well. Sexual satisfaction is highly individual, so only you can determine if some aspect of your sexuality is creating a problem for you or your partner.

COMMON SEXUAL DYSFUNCTIONS **Erectile dysfunction (ED;** previously called *impotence*) is the inability to achieve or maintain a penile erection sufficient for sexual penetration. And though the condition is most commonly associated with advancing age, erectile dysfunction can occur at any time in a person's life. Indeed, recent studies suggest that rates of ED are increasing among men under 40 years of age. **Premature ejaculation** (ejaculation before or just after penetration) is also common, especially at younger ages. **Delayed ejaculation** is the inability to ejaculate after an erection is achieved. If any of these problems is persistent or bothersome, a number of possible treatments can be explored. In addition, some people experience occasional difficulty achieving an erection or ejaculating because of excessive alcohol consumption, drug use (including prescriptions), fatigue, or stress.

TERMS

sexual dysfunction A disturbance in sexual desire, performance, or satisfaction that causes distress.

erectile dysfunction The inability to achieve or maintain a penile erection sufficient for sexual activity.

premature ejaculation Involuntary orgasm before or shortly after the penis enters the vagina, mouth, or anus; ejaculation that takes place sooner than desired.

delayed ejaculation The inability to ejaculate when you wish to during sexual activity.

The search for substances that can enhance sexual function and pleasure probably began long before recorded history. A large variety of herbal and animal-derived concoctions reputedly improve sexual function, including ginseng, raw oysters, bear gallbladder, rhinoceros horn, and tiger penis. Although research has shown that none of these products works, people continue to sell them, sometimes at extremely high prices, to gullible buyers. The demand for exotic animal parts has contributed to the endangerment of some of these species.

Several sex enhancement products have been shown to contain potentially dangerous ingredients. For example, the FDA has cautioned against many dietary supplements sold as "all natural" sexual enhancement products. Some of these supplements contain compounds the same as or very similar to those found in prescription drugs for erectile dysfunction such as Viagra, despite their claims of being herbal or "all natural." No mention of these compounds is found on these supplements' labels, although many of them contain full- or even double-strength doses of these drugs.

The FDA is concerned that these falsely labeled products could have dangerous or even lethal side effects, especially when used by people who take drugs that contain nitrates. Nitrates are commonly found in drugs used to treat heart disease and high blood pressure. Nitrates cause blood vessels to dilate, as do prescription drugs used to treat erectile dysfunction. When the two types of drug are used together, blood pressure can plummet, potentially resulting in fainting, falls, heart attacks, or strokes.

People with heart disease who take nitrates are usually instructed not to take Viagra-like medications, so they may be especially tempted to try sexual enhancement products that are marketed as "natural" or "herbal." Other types of nitrate compounds, such as amyl nitrate, are used as recreational drugs (sometimes called "poppers") and can be dangerous when combined with Viagra-like drugs.

Another potentially dangerous group of products includes male sex hormones such as testosterone and DHEA (dehydroepiandrosterone). Side effects of these hormones include acne, testicular atrophy, infertility, enlarged breasts, baldness, and accelerated growth of preexisting prostate cancer. Nonprescription hormone products sold on the internet are of particular concern because the FDA does not monitor dietary supplements for strength, purity, quality, effectiveness, or safety.

Another example of a potentially unsafe product sold on the internet for sexual improvement is yohimbine, an extract of tree bark. It is marketed as a dietary supplement for low libido, erectile dysfunction, and female sexual problems. Nonprescription forms of yohimbine are not monitored by the FDA. The FDA does regulate a prescription form (yohimbine hydrochloride). Yohimbine can cause blood pressure changes and rapid or irregular heartbeat.

SOURCES: Spar, M. D., and G. E. Muñoz, eds. 2014. *Integrative Men's Health*. New York: Oxford University Press; Mayo Clinic. 2013. *Yohimbine* (Oral Route) (http://www.mayoclinic.com/health/drug-information/DR601453); U.S. Food and Drug Administration. 2020. Tainted Sexual Enhancement Products. https://www.fda.gov/drugs/medication-health-fraud/tainted-sexual-enhancement-products.

In addition to penile dysfunctions, sexual problems can involve a lack of desire to have sex, the failure to become physically aroused and/or lubricated even when sex is desired, the inability to have an orgasm (**orgasmic dysfunction**), or pain during sex. All these problems can have physical and psychological components. Factors such as hormonal birth control, menopause, and antidepressants can negatively affect sexual functioning. Psychological and social issues such as relationship difficulties, family stresses, depression, shame, guilt, religious prohibitions, and past sexual trauma are all frequent causes of sexual dysfunction for all genders.

Orgasmic dysfunction has been the subject of a great deal of discussion over the years, as people debated the nature of nonpenile orgasms. Women are far more likely to achieve orgasm from stimulation to the clitoris, through self-stimulation, manual stimulation with a partner, oral sex, or use of a vibrator than through penile-vaginal intercourse alone. Because many straight couples do not engage in some practices that might lead to female orgasm (cunnilingus, for example), and because women are sometimes discouraged from masturbating, many women believe they have an orgasmic dysfunction when a simple behavior change might lead to success.

In general, the inability to experience orgasm is a problem only if a person considers it to be one.

CAUSES OF SEXUAL DYSFUNCTION The first step for those who suspect they may be experiencing a sexual dysfunction is to have a physical examination. This exam should evaluate overall health and explore a possible medical cause for the dysfunction. Sexual health problems can be related to *systemic diseases*—illnesses like diabetes, heart disease, or poor immune function that can affect organs throughout the body. Smoking, alcoholism, and excess weight can also lead to erectile dysfunction and other sexual problems. Sexual difficulties are frequently the first sign of serious health problems because any disease that affects the cardiovascular, nervous, or endocrine system is likely to have an impact on sexual functioning. This possibility of an underlying medical condition is one reason why people should think twice before buying treatments online (see the box "Sex Enhancement Products"). Up to 80% of all erectile problems are thought to be due to physical factors, particularly

> **orgasmic dysfunction** The inability to experience orgasm, despite engaging in the types of stimulation that would typically lead to one.

TERMS

vascular problems involving restriction of blood flow. Smoking affects blood flow in the genitals (and throughout the body) and is an independent risk factor for erectile dysfunction. Being of higher than average weight is a risk factor for cardiovascular problems, and can also affect hormonal balance.

Alcohol and many prescription and nonprescription drugs can inhibit sexual response. In particular, antidepressant drugs (especially SSRIs) are believed to cause sexual dysfunction in up to 50% of people. Sometimes drugs are used to counteract the side effects of antidepressants.

Other common medications that can inhibit sexual response include certain drugs that treat high blood pressure. If optimum sexual functioning is a concern for you, ask your health care provider if there is a medication that can treat your condition that will not lead to sexual side effects.

TREATING SEXUAL DYSFUNCTION Most forms of sexual dysfunction, particularly erectile dysfunction, are treatable. Drugs like Viagra (sildenafil citrate) work by enhancing the effects of nitric oxide, a chemical that relaxes smooth muscles in the penis. The relaxed muscles increase blood flow and allow a natural erection to occur in response to sexual stimulation. The medications are generally safe, but they should not be used by people with a high risk of heart attack or stroke. They are effective in about 70% of users, but there are potential side effects, including headaches, indigestion, facial flushing, back pain, visual and hearing disturbances, and changes in blood pressure.

The use of erectile dysfunction drugs between the ages of 18 and 45 has risen dramatically—possibly because some people use them for recreational rather than medical reasons. The drugs may cut the refractory period in those who do not have erectile dysfunction; younger men may also be using them to cope with performance anxiety or the effects of other drugs, such as antidepressants.

Although these drugs are not approved by the FDA for use by women, a growing number of women are trying them to help increase blood flow to the genitals, which is necessary for arousal and orgasm. Recent studies have shown that these drugs can sometimes help women with sexual dysfunction caused by the use of antidepressants.

Other treatments for erectile dysfunction are available. Prostaglandin E1 (Alprostadil) dilates blood vessels and can be injected into the penis or placed into the tip of the penis as a tiny suppository about the size of a grain of rice. It works by relaxing the smooth muscles lining the blood vessels in the penis. There are also vacuum devices that pull blood into the penis, and in cases where other treatments are unsuccessful, penile implants can be used. Exercise may also help improve erectile function, especially exercises that target the muscles of the pelvic floor.

For those experiencing erectile dysfunction and low testosterone, hormone replacement therapy is an option. Testosterone replacement is a typical course of treatment when testosterone levels are lower than normal. Symptoms of low testosterone include low libido, fatigue, anemia, increased body fat, reduced muscle mass, and mild depression.

Many people with no obvious physical disorder have sexual problems because of psychological and social issues. Too often sexual difficulties are treated with drugs when nondrug

Ask Yourself

QUESTIONS FOR CRITICAL THINKING AND REFLECTION

What do you think about using medication to treat sexual dysfunction? What alternatives do you think should be considered before trying medication? Do you think the general public is appropriately educated about the side effects of such products? In your opinion, would the potential benefits of such products outweigh the risks? Who do you think is most qualified to determine if someone has a sexual dysfunction?

strategies may be more appropriate. Psychosocial causes of dysfunction include troubled relationships, a lack of sexual skills, ineffective stimulation, religious prohibitions, particular attitudes and beliefs, anxiety, shame, prior experiences, and psychosexual trauma such as sexual abuse or **rape.** Some sexual problems are the result of rigid gender roles that can lead men to believe they need to be the sexual aggressor, women to believe they should remain passive, and genderqueer people to believe that they are sexually abnormal or deviant. None of these beliefs is based in biological or social fact. Many of these problems can be addressed through sex therapy or counseling. A therapist can promote open discussion between partners and suggest specific techniques.

Premature ejaculation is an example of a common sexual problem that often responds well to nondrug therapy. On average, men typically ejaculate between 2 and 10 minutes after penetration and thrusting begin, but most men periodically ejaculate more quickly. Several nondrug techniques are frequently helpful for people who habitually ejaculate sooner than they would like. Kegel exercises, which strengthen and improve control of the pelvic muscles, as well as practicing masturbation to extend arousal, are often helpful. Certain antidepressants delay ejaculation and are sometimes prescribed for this purpose.

Women who seek treatment for orgasmic dysfunction often have not learned what types of stimulation will excite them and bring them to orgasm. Most sex therapists treat this problem by teaching patients about their own anatomy and sexual responses, and encouraging them to experiment with masturbation, focusing on the clitoris, until they experience orgasm. Vibrators can be helpful devices during masturbation or intercourse. Previously taboo, they are now both common and easy to obtain from stores and online retailers that specialize in "sex positive" approaches. Once someone can masturbate to orgasm, they can transfer this learning to other sexual behaviors including those with a partner. Because women are not socialized to masturbate, they may have a more difficult time learning this set of behaviors.

Substances being tested for the treatment of female sexual dysfunction include prostaglandin creams and testosterone

rape A criminal offense defined in most states as **TERMS** forcible sexual relations with a person against that person's will or when a person is incapable of providing consent to sexual activity.

patches. Testosterone replacement is currently being used off-label to treat low desire in women because there has not been an FDA testosterone approved for women. A prostaglandin cream that improves blood flow to the clitoris is currently being developed and may be available to treat sexual arousal disorder in the future. Other options are a vibrator and a device that creates suction over the clitoris to increase blood flow and sensitivity.

In 2015, a drug called Addyi (flibanserin) was introduced as a treatment for hypoactive sexual desire disorder specific to women. The FDA approved the drug after two previous rejections and a lot of controversy. Some were eager to have access to a "pink Viagra," but opponents argued that it had more risks than benefits. Unlike erectile dysfunction drugs, flibanserin must be taken every day, cannot be mixed with alcohol, and can lead to dizziness and even unconsciousness in users. Detractors further argue that a decreased desire for sex is a more complicated problem than erectile dysfunction (which is a matter of restoring blood flow to the penis) and that a pill will provide false reassurance to women who might benefit more from education, behavioral changes, or therapy. Clinical studies showed that the drug helped 10–12% of users, who averaged 0.5 more "sexual events" per month than nonusers. Researchers who study sexual assault and coercion are also concerned about young women using a drug that, especially when mixed with alcohol, can lead to unconsciousness, compromising the user's ability to refuse unwanted sex.

SEXUAL BEHAVIOR

A wide variety of behaviors stem from sexual impulses, and sexual expression takes a variety of forms. For some people, the most basic aspect of sexuality is reproduction; for others, sex is more about fun and pleasure. In general, sexual excitement and satisfaction are aspects of sexual behavior separate from reproduction, and the intensely pleasurable sensations of arousal and orgasm are some of the strongest motivators for human sexual behavior. People are infinitely varied in the ways they seek to experience erotic pleasure.

Not all people experience sexual pleasure in the same way. *Asexual* is the term used to describe people who do not experience sexual desire but who may still enjoy being in romantic and other close relationships. Some asexual people, called demisexuals, experience sexual attraction only to people with whom they feel an intimate or loving bond. Asexuality refers to a lack of sexual desire, but not necessarily an avoidance of sexual behavior. Celibacy and abstinence are not the same thing as asexuality: many asexual people engage in sexual activity with the people they love and feel close to, and many people who experience sexual feelings and desire choose to practice celibacy, for religious and other reasons.

The Development of Sexual Behavior

Sexual behavior is a product of many factors, including genetics, physiology, psychology, and social and cultural

influences. Our behavior is shaped by the interplay of our biological predispositions and our life experiences.

Gender, Sexuality, and the Mass Media Many of our ideas about sexuality and gender roles are shaped by the mass media, including social media. Media images of sexuality can be as influential as family in shaping individuals' sexual attitudes and behaviors. Yet these images are often unrealistic and help perpetuate sexual stereotypes in our society. For example, the mass media rarely portray people negotiating safer sex or asking for explicit consent. Nor are they likely to show sex in its less glamorous forms: STIs, unwanted pregnancy, boring or "bad" sex, or struggles over how to define and interpret consent, all of which are normal aspects of sexuality.

Childhood Sexual Behavior The capacity for genital response is present at birth. Ultrasound studies suggest that penile erections can occur in utero, and both penile erections and vaginal lubrication are possible during infancy (though not all babies will experience them). Many children will discover this capacity as they grow. Sexual behaviors emerge gradually; self-exploration and touching the genitals are common forms of play and have been observed among infants as young as six months. These behaviors often lead to more deliberate forms of masturbation, with or without orgasm.

Children are also likely to explore their playmates' genitals, often as part of games such as "playing house" or "playing doctor." By age 12, 40% of boys have engaged in sex play. The peak exploration age for girls is 9, by which time 14% have had such experiences.

Adolescent Sexuality A person who has experienced puberty is on their way to becoming a biological adult. But in psychological and social terms, it can take 5–10

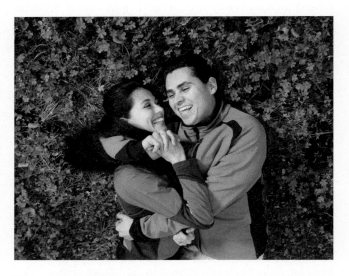

The mass media often portray young Americans as sexual athletes, who frequently engage in casual sex with many partners. Such characters are seldom shown discussing safer sex practices. John M Lund Photography Inc/Getty Images

more years to attain full adult status. This discrepancy between biological and social maturity creates considerable confusion over what constitutes appropriate sexual behavior during adolescence. Most countries have laws regarding the age at which someone is deemed old enough to make the decision to have sexual intercourse, sometimes referred to as the "age of consent." In the United States, this age varies between 16 and 18, depending on the state.

Sexual fantasies and dreams become more common and explicit in adolescence than at earlier ages, often as an accompaniment to masturbation. Some research suggests that masturbation is the most common sexual activity in which teenagers engage, and that there are fewer gender differences in masturbation habits in younger populations. Once puberty is reached, orgasm in boys is accompanied by ejaculation. Teenagers of all genders have orgasmic dreams. When they involve penile ejaculation, they are called **nocturnal emissions** ("wet dreams").

Sexual activity refers to more than intercourse and includes a variety of behaviors and stimulation. Sexual interaction during adolescence often takes place between peers in the context of dating or partying. Sexual intimacy is often expressed through kissing, caressing, and stimulating the breasts and genitals. Although these activities lead to arousal, they don't always result in orgasm.

According to a recent report, just over 40% of high school students have "ever had" sexual intercourse, a drop from just over 53% in 1993. Rates for premarital sex vary considerably from one group to another, based on racial, ethnic, educational, socioeconomic, religious, geographic, and many other factors. First-time intercourse is affected by these same factors, alongside psychological readiness, fear of consequences, being in love, religious affiliation, sexual orientation, gender identity and expression, going steady, peer pressure, and the desire to act like an adult, gain popularity, or rebel. Family relationships and attitudes toward sex also influence teen sexual behavior. Additionally, teen perceptions of what is "normal" among peers strongly influences choices about sex. Fears of pregnancy and the pressure to maintain one's virginity lead many teenagers to engage in forms of oral and anal sex that they do not believe are "real" sex. Girls especially are pressured to preserve their virginity, often for religious reasons. These behaviors can have emotional and social consequences because they can generate many of the same feelings of intimacy, rejection, and confusion that come with penetrative intercourse. Medical consequences are also possible without adequate precautions in the form of safer sex practices, which can lead to sexually transmitted infections.

Beginning in childhood, sex play involves members of various sexes and genders. Same-gender attractions, with or without sexual encounters, are common in adolescence and are not always necessarily related to adult sexual orientation. Many adult gay men and women, however, recall same-gender attractions in childhood.

Adult Sexuality Early adulthood is a time when people make important life choices—a time of increasing responsibility in terms of interpersonal relationships and family life. The average age at marriage in the United States is almost 30 for men and 28 for women. According to the Kinsey Institute, men are typically sexually active for 10 years before getting married, and women for 8 years. Today more people in their twenties believe that becoming sexually experienced rather than preserving virginity is an important prelude to selecting a mate. (See the box "Questions to Ask before Engaging in a Sexual Relationship.")

Films, television, social media, and other sources project the image that everyone is having sex, with many partners. The reality is likely far more complicated, and recent research suggests that young people especially are having less sex than ever. Individual motivations for engaging in sexual activities change with age. Younger men state that they engage in sex for physical reasons, whereas women of the same age state that they engage in sex for emotional reasons. As men and women get older, their motives change; men more often engage in sex for emotional reasons, and women more often for physical reasons. This is to say that people of all kinds have sex for all kinds of reasons, all of which make sense to them at the time.

Sexuality in Illness and Disability Any disease or disability that affects mobility, well-being, self-esteem, or body image has the potential to affect sexual expression. People with chronic diseases or disabilities often have special needs regarding their sexual behavior. They may also confront the perception that they are asexual or have lost themselves as the sexual person they once knew. Sexuality is integral, however, and disabilities should not be interpreted as a permanent obstacle to having and enjoying sexual experiences. In a society organized around able-bodied people, disabled people will likely benefit from resources designed to help them learn more about how their disability and sexual behaviors affect one another.

nocturnal emission Orgasm and ejaculation (wet dream) during sleep.   TERMS

Ask Yourself

QUESTIONS FOR CRITICAL THINKING AND REFLECTION

How did your romantic and sexual relationships (or lack thereof) during adolescence influence how you felt about yourself? What influenced your beliefs about what sex would be like? Were your first sexual experiences what you expected? What misconceptions did you have about sex during adolescence? When and how were they corrected? Whether you are straight, gay, lesbian, or asexual, how and when did you become aware of your sexual orientation?

Who Am I Sexually Attracted To?

• What are the characteristics that usually attract me to someone in a physical way?

• How comfortable am I with the people I find sexually attractive? What would I change if I could? Do I feel safe when I am with them?

• Are the people I am usually sexually attracted to the same types of people as those I consider having a long-term, stable relationship with? Why or why not?

What Sexual Behaviors Are Comfortable for Me Right Now?

• What has influenced my comfort level with these behaviors?

• What am I not entirely comfortable with, but would be willing to experiment with in order to please a partner? What level of trust would I need to establish with that partner in order to proceed? What would we need to talk about ahead of time?

• What exactly do I say in order to make my comfort level clear to my partner? What do I do if my partner tries to push me beyond my comfort level?

How Can I Express My Sexual Needs, Desires, and Concerns to a Potential Sexual Partner?

• When would be the best time to talk about these needs, desires, and concerns?

• How do I start the conversation?

• What will I do if my needs are not being met or my concerns are not taken seriously?

What Preparations Do I Need to Make in Order to Engage in the Safest Sex Possible?

• If I am engaging in heterosexual sexual activity, and I do not wish to reproduce, I need to obtain birth control. Have I consulted a health professional to figure out the best method of birth control for myself and my partner? Do I know how to employ this method correctly? Have we discussed what we plan to do if a pregnancy occurs?

• If I am engaging in any type of sexual activity with a partner, I need protection from sexually transmitted infections. Have I consulted a health professional to figure out the best method of STI protection for myself and my partner? Do I know how to employ this method correctly? Have I discussed with my partner their sexual history, including information about risky behavior and STIs? Do I understand the ways that sexual behaviors transmit these infections?

• What do I need from my partner in order to ensure that I feel emotionally safe before, during, and after our sexual behavior together?

• Do I engage in any behaviors that cause me to participate in sexual activity that I wouldn't otherwise be comfortable with, such as excessive drinking or drug use? What do I need to do in order to reduce or eliminate these behaviors?

• Do I make sure that the people I am being sexual with are actively consenting to the behaviors? Do I understand what constitutes sexual consent? Do I understand that I need to stop what I'm doing if the other person asks me to or is not communicating active and willing consent?

• Do I have trusted friends and adults with whom I can discuss my sexual concerns, questions, and relationships? If not, how can I go about finding those people so that I don't have to figure all of this out on my own or overly rely on a romantic partner?

Varieties of Human Sexual Behavior

Some sexual behaviors are aimed at self-stimulation only, whereas other practices involve interaction with one or more partners. Some people feel sexual but choose not to express it, and some people do not feel any form of sexual desire (asexuality).

Health considerations and religious and moral beliefs may lead some people to celibacy, particularly until marriage or until an acceptable partner appears. Many people use the related term *abstinence* to refer to the avoidance of just one sexual activity—penetrative intercourse.

Autoeroticism   The most common sexual behavior for humans is masturbation. Masturbation is one form of **autoeroticism;** another is **erotic fantasy,** or creating imaginary experiences that range from fleeting thoughts to elaborate scenarios. Orgasms originate in our brain as it gives meaning to stimulation and pleasure. Using functional MRI (fMRI) scans to map orgasms in the brain, researchers at Rutgers University found that at the time of orgasm every part of our brain is engaged. No other activity produces the same brain response.

Masturbation involves manually stimulating the genitals, rubbing them against objects, or using stimulating devices such as vibrators or masturbation sleeves. Although commonly associated with adolescence, masturbation is

	TERMS
autoeroticism Behavior aimed at sexual self-stimulation.	
erotic fantasy Sexually arousing thoughts and daydreams.	

practiced by many adults. It may be used as a substitute for sexual activity or it may include a partner. Research has shown that up to 94% of men and up to 85% of women in the United States have masturbated and that gender differences in masturbation habits are lower in more liberal countries. Women especially find that if they are stimulating their clitoris during penetration with a partner, they are more likely to experience orgasm. Masturbation can give a person control over the pace, time, and method of sexual release and pleasure and, when practiced, can help people better understand what they desire during sex with other people.

Touching and Foreplay   For many people, touching is integral to sexual experiences, whether in the form of massage, kissing, fondling, or holding. The entire body surface is a sensory organ, and touching almost anywhere can enhance intimacy and sexual arousal. Touching can convey a variety of messages, including affection, comfort, and a desire for further sexual contact.

During arousal, many partners manually and orally stimulate each other by touching, stroking, and caressing their partner's genitals. People vary greatly in their preferences for the type, pace, and vigor of such **foreplay.** Working out the details to accommodate each other's pleasure is a key to enjoying these activities. Direct communication about preferences can enhance sexual pleasure and protect both partners from physical and psychological discomfort and abuse. There is no correct order in which to engage in sexual activity, and these behaviors can also be engaged in instead of or after penetrative intercourse.

Oral-Genital Stimulation   **Cunnilingus** (the stimulation of the vulva and vagina with the lips and tongue) and **fellatio** (the stimulation of the penis with the mouth) are common practices. Oral sex may be practiced either as part of foreplay or as a sex act culminating in orgasm. Although prevalence varies in different populations, 90% of men, 88% of women, and more than 50% of teens report that they have engaged in oral sex. A recent study showed that more teens aged 15–19 had engaged in oral sex than had engaged in vaginal intercourse. The most common reasons given for postponing vaginal-penile intercourse were avoidance of pregnancy, the desire to remain technically a virgin, and the mistaken belief that STIs cannot be transmitted via oral sex. Some studies show that straight people who report having oral sex are usually talking about fellatio and not cunnilingus, and many women report that male partners are reluctant to orally stimulate their genitals. Denied this stimulation, some women find it difficult to have regular orgasms during straight encounters.

Like all acts of sexual expression between two people, oral sex requires the cooperation and consent of both partners. If they disagree about its acceptability, they need to discuss their feelings and try to reach a mutually accommodating solution.

Anal Intercourse   About one-third of women and men report having ever engaged in anal sex. Some people find they are able to achieve orgasm through receptive anal sex. Males who are being penetrated, either by a penis, finger, or sex toy,

by a person of any gender, may find this induces orgasm because stimulation to the prostate may cause an ejaculation. This stimulation is often referred to as "milking the prostate" or prostate massage.

Because the anus is composed of delicate tissues that tear easily with friction, anal intercourse can be one of the riskiest of sexual behaviors for the transmission of HIV and other STIs. If people are monogamous or use barrier devices such as condoms, the risk becomes lower. The use of condoms is highly recommended for anyone engaging in anal sex. Special care and precaution should be exercised if anal sex is practiced—cleanliness, lubrication, and gentle entry at the very least. Because bacteria normally present in an anus can cause vaginal infections, as well as urinary tract infections, anything inserted into the anus should not subsequently be put into a vagina unless it has been washed thoroughly.

Sexual Intercourse   Men and women engage in vaginal intercourse for a variety of reasons, including to fulfill sexual and psychological needs and to reproduce. Among adults aged 18–44, 92% of men and 94% of women report having had penile-vaginal intercourse. The most common heterosexual practice involves the man inserting his erect penis into the woman's lubricated vagina after sufficient arousal.

Much has been written on how to enhance pleasure through various coital techniques, positions, and practices. Key factors in physical readiness for coitus include vaginal lubrication, penile erection, and psychological readiness (being aroused and receptive).

Sexual Coercion   The use of force and coercion in sexual relationships is one of the most serious problems in human interactions. The most extreme manifestation of **sexual coercion**—forcing a person to submit to another's sexual desires—is rape, but it occurs in many subtler forms, such as sexual harassment. The Rape, Abuse, and Incest National Network (RAINN) is an excellent resource for anyone wanting to learn more about how to resist and respond to sexually coercive situations and relationships.

Commercial Sex

Conflicting feelings about sexuality are apparent in the attitudes of Americans toward commercial sex—prostitution and sexually oriented media. Although prostitution (sex work) is illegal in most of the United States, and it faces some social disapproval, it is understood by many sexuality scholars and activists to be a legitimate type of work and economic exchange.

TERMS

foreplay   Kissing, touching, and any form of oral or genital contact.

cunnilingus   Oral stimulation of the vulva, clitoris, and vagina.

fellatio   Oral stimulation of the penis.

sexual coercion   The use of physical or psychological force or intimidation to make a person submit to sexual demands.

Ask Yourself

What do you consider to be appropriate sexual behavior? What behaviors do you think are inappropriate or wrong? What experiences have shaped your views of such behaviors? Have they changed in the past five years? What do you think they will be like five years from now?

Pornography

Pornography (*porn*) is readily available and widely viewed in our society, although many people are concerned about its ubiquitous nature and its blurring with popular culture. A major problem in identifying pornographic material is that people and communities differ about what is obscene, as obscenity is typically a judgment by someone who finds it offensive. Child pornography—showing children who are under age 18 naked and/or in sexual settings—is illegal in all parts of the United States.

Some people argue that adults who want to view pornographic materials in the privacy of their own homes should be allowed to do so. Others feel that the exposure to explicit sexual material can lead to delinquent or criminal behavior, such as rape or the sexual abuse of children. Currently there is no reliable evidence that pornography by itself leads to violence or rape, and debate is likely to continue. Many people distinguish between so-called soft-core and hard-core types of pornographic materials. Soft-core porn, often marketed to couples, typically includes an apparently loving couple having sex in a relaxed setting. There is mutual kissing and touching, and both partners are shown as having a positive experience. In hard-core porn, there is usually less mutual touching, and the focus is on penile penetration and ejaculation. Hard-core porn sometimes explicitly depicts sexual violence and exploitation. Hard-core porn materials tend to be the focus of more debate and disagreement, because many people feel that it prioritizes the male sexual experience. Though straight sex is most commonly depicted, all gender identities and sexual orientations can be found in pornography.

Online Porn and Cybersex

The appearance of thousands of sexually oriented websites has expanded the number of people with access to pornography, and it has made it more difficult for authorities to enforce laws regarding porn. People who might have hesitated to buy magazines or rent videos in person can now access sexually explicit materials online, anonymously, and often free of charge. Of special concern is the increased availability of child pornography, which previously could be acquired only with great difficulty and at great legal risk. Online porn is now a multibillion-dollar industry.

In addition to (or instead of) viewing porn online, hundreds of thousands of people also use the internet to engage in **cybersex**, or *virtual sex*. Cybersex is erotic interaction between people who are communicating over the internet. People can engage in cybersex in many ways, such as by visiting sexually oriented websites, joining cybersex chat rooms, participating in videoconferences via web cams, or even exchanging email or text messages (sexting). Participants may have sexually explicit discussions, share private photographs, or engage in fantasy role-playing online. Many cybersex participants report feeling some degree of sexual excitement; some masturbate while viewing erotic images online or engaging in sexual chat. Online sex is an excellent way for people who have difficulty meeting partners to meet others and maintain relationships. It is also, for many people, a fun and novel way of expressing their sexuality.

Although many people view cybersex as a safe form of sexual expression, it is not without problems. It can be addictive, and some cybersex addicts report spending more than 50 hours a week online for sexual purposes. People who become addicted may become isolated, perform poorly at work or school, and have trouble with their interpersonal relationships.

"Sexting," sending provocative photos via mobile devices, has also become popular, sometimes with serious consequences. Images can end up being widely shared and can even appear on social media. These images can haunt individuals years later if they are viewed by potential employers or partners. Some teens have found themselves charged with child pornography and have even faced jail time as a result of forwarding a sexually explicit photo of an underage person to a friend. Teens who have found pictures of themselves engaging in sexual activity posted or shared online have faced adverse effects. Some have even committed suicide. Posting "revenge porn"—when an ex-partner widely shares nude or sexually explicit images that were initially meant only for the couple—is an increasingly serious problem, especially for women. In 2019, a U. S. congresswoman resigned after being subjected to revenge porn by an ex-husband.

Prostitution

The exchange of sexual services for money is **prostitution,** also called **sex work.** Sex workers may be any age or gender; the buyer is nearly always a man, white, middle class, middle-aged, and married. Sex work is illegal in the United States, except in parts of Nevada.

Purchasing sex can offer someone physical release without having to confront some of the more complicated aspects of sex: commitment, an expectation of intimacy, or a fear of rejection. Some people patronize prostitutes in order to have sex with a different type of partner than usual or to engage in a type of sex in which their usual partner is uninterested.

TERMS

pornography The depiction of sexual activities in pictures, writing, film, or other material with the intent to arouse.

cybersex Erotic interaction between people who are not in physical contact, conducted over a network such as the internet; also called *virtual sex.*

prostitution/sex work The exchange of sexual services for money or goods.

To talk with your partner about sexuality, follow the general suggestions for effective communication in Chapter 5. Getting started may be the most difficult part. Some people feel more comfortable if they begin by initiating a discussion about why people are so uncomfortable talking about sexuality. Talking about sexual histories—how partners first learned about sex or how family and cultural background influenced sexual values and attitudes—is another way to get started. Reading about sex can also be a good beginning: Partners can read an article or book and then discuss their reactions.

Be honest about what you feel and what you want from your partner. Cultural and personal obstacles to discussing sexual subjects can be difficult to overcome, but self-disclosure is important for successful relationships. Research indicates that when one person openly discusses attitudes and feelings, partners are more likely to do the same. If your partner seems hesitant to open up, try asking open-ended or either/or questions: "Where do you like to be touched?" or "Would you like to talk about this now or wait until later?"

If something is bothering you about your sexual relationship, choose a good time to initiate a discussion with your partner. Be specific and direct but also tactful. Focus on what you actually observe rather than on what you think the behavior means. "You didn't touch or hug me when your friends were around" is an observation. "You're ashamed of me around your friends" is an inference about your partner's feelings. Try focusing on a specific behavior that concerns you rather than on the person as a whole—your partner can change behaviors but not their entire personality. For example, you could say, "I'd like you to take a few minutes away from studying to kiss me" instead of "You're so caught up in your work, you never have time for me."

If you are going to make a statement that your partner may interpret as criticism, try mixing it with something positive: "I love being with you, but I feel annoyed when you. . . ." If your partner says something that upsets you, an aggressive response may make you feel better in the short run, but it will not help the communication process or the quality of the relationship.

If you want to say no to some sexual activity, say no unequivocally. Don't send mixed messages. If you are afraid of hurting your partner's feelings, offer an alternative if it's appropriate: "I am uncomfortable with that. How about . . .?"

If you're in love, you may think that the sexual aspects of a relationship will work out magically without discussion. However, partners who never talk about sex deny themselves the opportunity to increase their closeness and improve their relationship.

Finally, it is never necessary to experience these thoughts, concerns, or feelings alone. Identify trusted friends and adults from whom you can seek advice and support if and when sex and sexuality issues feel especially challenging.

Sex workers come from a variety of backgrounds, and, like everyone who participates in the labor force, they are economically (rather than sexually) motivated. Many people who have sex for money lack the skills and education to engage in other forms of work, and they view their bodies as their most marketable asset. Many, though not all, report having been sexually abused as children; some begin as runaways who are escaping abusive homes and turn to sex work as a way to survive. Queer and transgender people who have had to leave homes that do not accept their identities sometimes engage in sex work to support themselves. This is sometimes referred to as "survival sex."

Although many sex workers routinely use condoms with their clients, HIV infection and other STIs are still a concern. The rate of HIV infection among sex workers and their clients can be as high as 25–50%, though rates vary drastically according to country, gender/sex of sex workers and clients, and the legal and public health systems that might regulate these practices. Some argue that making sex work legal could lessen the problems for both clients and sex workers.

Responsible Sexual Behavior

Healthy sexuality is an important part of adult life. It can be a source of pleasurable experiences and emotions and an important part of intimate partnerships. But there are potential consequences to most sexual behavior, including pregnancy, STIs, social embarrassment, and emotional changes in relationships. Every sexually active person should be aware of these consequences and accept responsibility for them. Consider the following with your partners:

Open, Honest Communication Each person needs to clearly indicate what sexual involvement means to them. Does it mean love, fun, a permanent commitment, or something else? The intentions of each person should be clear. For strategies on talking about sexual issues with your partner, see the box "Communicating about Sexuality."

Agreed-On Sexual Activities No one should pressure or coerce or force anyone to be sexual. Sexual behaviors should be consistent with the sexual values, preferences, and comfort level of all partners. Everyone has the right to refuse sexual activity at any time, including married couples, and including after sexual behavior has begun. Sexual activity should be explicitly and enthusiastically consented to by all people involved; the absence of a stated "no" does not indicate clear and enthusiastic consent to sexual activity. Some state legislatures and U.S. universities are considering adopting a "yes means yes" standard of consent for sexual activities.

Sexual Privacy Intimate relationships involving sexual activity are based on trust, and that trust can be violated if partners reveal private information about the relationship to others; this includes disseminating images that were shared privately. Sexual privacy also involves respecting other people—not engaging in activities in the presence of others that would make them uncomfortable. The question of how to handle bringing a partner back to a shared dorm room is a situation that many college students must address. Roommates should be respectful of one another and discuss the situation in advance to avoid embarrassing encounters.

Safe Sex Sexual partners should be aware of and practice safe sex to guard against STIs and unwanted pregnancies. Many sexual behaviors carry the risk of STIs, including HIV infection. Partners should be honest about their health and any medical conditions and work out a plan for protection.

Contraception Use If pregnancy is not desired, contraception should be used during penile-vaginal intercourse. Both partners need to take responsibility for protecting against unwanted pregnancy. Partners should discuss contraception before sexual involvement begins. (See Chapter 7.)

Sober Sex The use of alcohol or drugs in sexual situations increases the risk of unplanned, unprotected sexual activity. Such consequences are particularly true for young adults, many of whom binge-drink during social events.

Binge drinking also increases the risk of sexual assault. RAINN estimates that 11.2% of college students experience rape or sexual assault through physical force, violence, or incapacitation; college-aged women are almost five times as likely as men to be forced into an unwanted sexual experience. Unfortunately, a cycle then ensues for some of these women: those with a history of sexual assault are more likely to drink heavily. Approximately 30% of underage college women engage in such heavy episodic drinking, and women under age 21 also bear the highest risk for sexual assault in college. Alcohol and drugs impair judgment and should not be used in association with sexual activity. Be honest with yourself; if you need to drink in order to engage in sexual activities, it may be a good idea to rethink your social life and relationships. This can be facilitated by talking with a trusted friend or a professional counselor. Someone who is intoxicated cannot legally consent to sex.

Aside from the dangers of mixing alcohol and sex, alcohol typically impairs sexual performance. Although alcohol may lower sexual inhibition and make people more likely to attempt a sexual encounter, too much alcohol makes it difficult to achieve or keep an erection, decreases vaginal lubrication, and makes orgasm more difficult to achieve. Chronic overuse of alcohol reduces testosterone, ultimately causing erectile dysfunction, infertility, and body changes such as enlarged breasts in men. Women who overuse alcohol often experience menstrual abnormalities and decreased sexual function. Similarly, cigarette smoking has a powerful negative effect on sexual function, primarily because it decreases blood flow to the genitals.

TIPS FOR TODAY AND THE FUTURE

A healthy sexual life is built on acceptance of yourself and good communication with your partners.

RIGHT NOW YOU CAN:

- Deal with any sexual question or problem you've been avoiding. A good place to start is by talking with your health care provider, counselor, or other trusted adult. Don't be afraid or embarrassed to ask questions.
- Articulate to yourself exactly what your beliefs are about sexual relationships. Consider whether you are acting in accordance with your values. Your beliefs may be different from those of your partners, parents, family, and caregivers.
- If you're in a sexual relationship, consider the information you and your partner have shared about sex. Are you comfortable that you know enough about each other to have a safe and healthy sexual relationship? Consider also what you have learned, in school and via other sources. Do you have adequate and accurate information to make the best choices? Where can you go to acquire more or better information?

IN THE FUTURE YOU CAN:

- If you're in a sexual relationship, or if you plan to begin one, open (or reopen) a dialogue about sex. Make time to talk at length about the responsibilities and consequences of a sexual relationship. You can also do this regularly with trusted friends and adult mentors.

Ask Yourself

QUESTIONS FOR CRITICAL THINKING AND REFLECTION

If you are sexually active or plan to become active soon, how open have you been in communicating with your partner? Are you aware of your partner's feelings about sex and about their comfort level with certain activities? Do you and your partner share the same views on contraception, STI prevention, and ethical issues about sex?

SUMMARY

- The external sex organs of people who are assigned female at birth are referred to as the vulva. This includes the clitoris, the highly sensitive genital structure that plays an important role in sexual arousal and orgasm because of its high concentration of nerve endings.

- The vagina leads to the internal sex organs known as the uterus, oviducts or fallopian tubes, and ovaries.

- The external sex organs of people assigned male at birth are the penis and the scrotum. The glans of the penis is an important site of sexual arousal because of the high concentration of nerve endings.

- Via the urethra, the penis is connected to internal structures called the testes, epididymis, vasa deferentia, seminal vesicles, Cowper's gland, ejaculatory duct, and prostate gland.

- Some gender characteristics are biologically influenced, and others are defined more strongly by society. Children learn traits and behaviors traditionally deemed appropriate for particular sexes and genders.

- In general, gender is distinct from sex in that the former refers to how people identify and feel about themselves, rather than the body parts and sexual organs they have.

- A person's sexual orientation can be heterosexual, homosexual, bisexual, asexual, pansexual, or queer. Possible influences include genetics, hormonal factors, and early childhood experiences.

- Language is always changing, and the terms evolving for nonbinary gender and sexualities reflect a wide diversity in behavior and biological makeup.

- The fertilizing sperm influences the sex of the individual. Genes on the Y chromosome initiate the process of sexual differentiation in the embryo. Some infants are born without a clear chromosomal, genital, or hormonal indication of a male or female status. Many of these children, who are referred to as intersex, are surgically or medically monitored throughout their sexual development. Many intersex people choose to forego genital or other surgeries that would align them with either the male or female sex.

- Hormones initiate the changes that occur during puberty: The reproductive system matures, and secondary sex characteristics develop, increasing the number of visible sex-linked differences.

- The menstrual cycle has four phases: menses, the estrogenic phase, ovulation, and the progestational phase.

- The ovaries gradually cease to function with age. Menopause signals the end of menstruation and reproductive capacity. Testosterone production also gradually decreases with age.

- Sexual activity is based on stimulus and response. Stimulation may be physical or psychological. A lack of sexual feelings in response to stimuli may indicate a problem or may indicate that a person is asexual.

- Vasocongestion and muscle tension are the primary physiological mechanisms of sexual arousal.

- The sexual response cycle developed by Masters and Johnson has four stages: excitement, plateau, orgasm, and resolution. There are other models of sexual response, and some include desire as a stage.

- Physical and psychological problems can interfere with sexual functioning.

- Treatment for sexual dysfunction first addresses any underlying medical conditions and then looks at psychosocial problems.

- The ability to respond sexually is present at birth. Sexual behaviors emerging in childhood include self-exploration, masturbation, erections, vaginal lubrication, and possibly orgasm.

- Although puberty defines biological adulthood, people can take 5–10 more years to reach social maturity.

- Human sexual behaviors include celibacy, fantasy, masturbation, touching, cunnilingus, fellatio, anal intercourse, and coitus.

- To evaluate whether an atypical sexual behavior is problematic, experts consider the issues of consent between partners and whether the behavior results in physical or psychological harm.

- Pornography and sex work are examples of the commercialization of sex.

- Responsible sexuality includes open, honest communication; consent to sexual activities; sexual privacy; contraception use; safe sex practices; sober sex; and the taking of responsibility for consequences.

FOR MORE INFORMATION

American Association of Sexuality Educators, Counselors, and Therapists (AASECT). Certifies sex educators, counselors, and therapists and provides listings of local therapists dealing with sexual problems.

http://www.aasect.org

American Psychological Association: Answers to Your Questions about Transgender People, Gender Identity, and Gender Expression. Offers question-and-answer format sections on transgender and homosexuality.

http://www.apa.org/topics/sexuality/transgender.aspx

The Asexuality Visibility and Education Network (AVEN). Provides information and forums for people who identify as, are in relationships with, or want to know more about asexuality.

http://www.asexuality.org/home/

Center for Young Women's Health. Includes information about topics such as menstruation, gynecological exams, eating disorders, body piercing, and sexual health.

http://www.youngwomenshealth.org

Children Now: Talking with Kids. Provides advice for parents about talking with children about difficult issues, including sex, relationships, and STIs.

https://www.childrennow.org/talkingwithkids/

The Food and Drug Administration. The Tainted Sexual Enhancement Products page lists products that have been found to contain hidden drug ingredients; in 2019 alone, there were 37 public health warnings.

https://www.fda.gov/drugs/medication-health-fraud/tainted -sexual-enhancement-products

The Guttmacher Institute. A leading research and policy organization committed to advancing sexual and reproductive health and rights in the United States and globally. They provide a wealth of information and resources about sexual and reproductive health.

http://www.guttmacher.org

The Kinsey Institute for Research in Sex, Gender, and Reproduction. One of the oldest and most respected institutions doing research on sexuality.

http://www.kinseyinstitute.org

National Center for Health Statistics. Provides a report on national survey data on sexual behavior, sexual attraction, and sexual identity in the United States.

http://www.cdc.gov/nchs/data/nhsr/nhsr110.pdf

National Institutes of Health, National Cancer Institute. Features an extensive directory and library on prostate cancer, including treatment and prevention options, recent research advances, and current clinical trials.

http://www.cancer.gov/types/prostate

The New View Campaign. This group questions the routine practice of cosmetic labial surgeries and challenges the "medicalization" of female sexual problems.

http://www.newviewcampaign.org

Rape, Abuse, and Incest National Network (RAINN). This group provides information, counseling, and support for those concerned about sexual abuse, rape, and incest.

http://www.rainn.org

Sexuality Information and Education Council of the United States (SIECUS). Provides information about many aspects of sexuality and has an extensive library and numerous publications.

http://www.siecus.org

Trans Student Educational Resources. Pursues a trans-friendly education system and a set of resources for the public and trans activists.

https://www.transstudent.org/

SELECTED BIBLIOGRAPHY

American Academy of Pediatrics, Task Force on Circumcision. 2012. Technical report: Male circumcision. *Pediatrics* 130(3): e756–785.

American College Health Association. 2009. *American College Health Association–National College Health Assessment II: Reference Group Executive Summary Fall 2009.* Linthicum, MD: American College Health Association.

American Congress of Obstetricians and Gynecologists. 2020. Elective Female Genital Cosmetic Surgery Number 795 (https://www.acog.org /clinical/clinical-guidance/committee-opinion/articles/2020/01/elective -female-genital-cosmetic-surgery).

American Psychological Association. 2020. *Transgender People, Gender Identity and Gender Expression* (http://www.apa.org/topics/lgbt/transgender).

American Psychological Association. 2008. *Sexual Orientation & Homosexuality* (http://www.apa.org/topics/lgbt/orientation).

American Psychological Association. 2020. *Answers to Your Questions about Individuals with Intersex Conditions* (http://www.apa.org/topics/lgbt /intersex).

Appleton, S. 2018. Premenstrual syndrome: Evidence-based evaluation and treatment. *Clinical Obstetrics and Gynecology* 61(1): 52–61.

Balter, M. 2015. Can epigenetics explain homosexuality puzzle? *Science* 350(6257): 148.

Basson, R. 2000. The female sexual response: A different model. *Journal of Sex & Marital Therapy* 26(1): 51–65.

Bogaert, A. F. 2006. Biological versus nonbiological older brothers and men's sexual orientation. *Proceedings of the National Academy of Sciences* 103(28): 10771–10774.

Bogle, K. 2008. *Hooking Up: Sex, Dating and Relationships on Campus.* New York: New York University Press.

Brewer, G., and C. Hendrie. 2011. Evidence to suggest that copulatory vocalizations in women are not a reflexive consequence of orgasm. *Archives of Sexual Behavior* 40(3): 559–564.

Centers for Disease Control and Prevention. 2020. *Healthy Youth–Sexual Risk Behaviors* (http://www.cdc.gov/HealthyYouth/sexualbehaviors /index.htm).

Centers for Disease Control and Prevention. 2019. *Human Papillomavirus* (http://www.cdc.gov/hpv/index.html).

Centers for Disease Control and Prevention. 2019. *Prostate Cancer* (http:// www.cdc.gov/cancer/prostate/index.htm).

Centers for Disease Control and Prevention. 2018. Youth Risk Behavior Surveillance System, United States, 2017. *MMWR Surveillance Summaries* 67(8) (https://www.cdc.gov/healthyyouth/data/yrbs/pdf/2017/ss6708.pdf).

Compton, D'L. and Tristan Bridges. 2019. 2018 Update on the US LGB Population. *Inequality by (Interior) Design* blog, April 12. (https:// inequalitybyinteriordesign.wordpress.com/2019/04/12/2018-gss-update -on-the-u-s-lgb-population/).

Copen, C. E., A. Chandra, and I. Febo-Vazquez. 2016. Sexual behavior, sexual attraction, and sexual orientation among adults aged 18–44 in the United States: Data from the 2011–2013 National Survey of Family Growth. *National Health Statistics Report* No. 88. Hyattsville, MD: National Center for Health Statistics.

Crooks, R., and K. Baur. 2014. *Our Sexuality.* Belmont, CA: Wadsworth/ Cengage Learning.

Dewitte, M., et al. 2015. Sex in its daily relational context. *Journal of Sexual Medicine* 12(12): 2436–2450.

Driemeyer, W., et al. 2017. Masturbation experiences of Swedish senior high school students: Gender differences and similarities. *The Journal of Sex Research* 54(4-5): 631–641.

Erickson-Schroth, L. ed. 2014. *Trans Bodies, Trans Selves.* Oxford, UK: Oxford University Press.

Gades, N. M., et al. 2005. Association between smoking and erectile dysfunction: A population-based study. *American Journal of Epidemiology* 161(4): 346–351.

Garcia-Falgueras, A., and D. Swaab. 2010. Sexual hormones and the brain: An essential alliance for sexual identity and sexual orientation. *Pediatric Endocrinology* 17: 22–35.

Gilmore, A. K., and K. E. Bountress. 2016. Reducing drinking to cope among heavy episodic drinking college women: Secondary outcomes of a web-based combined alcohol use and sexual assault risk reduction intervention. *Addictive Behaviors* 61: 104–111.

Grant, Jamie M., et al. 2011. *Injustice at Every Turn: A Report on the National Transgender Survey.* Washington, DC: National Center for Transgender Equality and National Gay and Lesbian Task Force (http://www .thetaskforce.org/injustice-every-turn-report-national-transgender -discrimination-survey/).

Hock, R. R. 2012. *Human Sexuality.* Upper Saddle River, NJ: Pearson.

Iveniuk, J., C. O'Muircheartaigh, and K. A. Cagney. 2016. Religious influence on older Americans' sexual lives: A nationally representative profile. *Archives of Sexual Behavior* 45(1): 121–131.

Joannides, P. 2013. *Guide to Getting It On.* Waldport, OR: Goofy Foot Press.

Jordan-Young, R. M. 2010. *Brain Storm: The Flaws in the Science of Sex Differences.* Cambridge, MA: Harvard University Press.

Julian, K. 2018. Why are young people having so little sex? *The Atlantic*, December. (https://www.theatlantic.com/magazine/archive/2018/12/the -sex-recession/573949/).

Kaplan, Helen. 1979. *Disorders of Sexual Desire (and Other New Concepts and Techniques in Sex Therapy).* Bruner Meisel University.

Kaschak, E., and L. Tiefer, eds. 2001. *A New View of Women's Sexual Problems.* New York: Routledge.

Kelly, G. F. 2013. *Sexuality Today,* 11th ed. New York: McGraw Hill.

Labuski, C. 2015. *It Hurts Down There: The Bodily Imaginaries of Female Genital Pain.* Albany: State University of New York Press.

Lindau, S. T., and N. Gavrilova. 2010. Sex, health, and years of sexually active life gained due to good health. *British Medical Journal* 340: c810.

Mayo Clinic. 2020. *Premenstrual Syndrome* (http://www.mayoclinic.com /health/premenstrual-syndrome/DS00134/DSECTION=lifestyle-and home-remedies).

Mayo Clinic. 2020. *Erectile Dysfunction* (http://www.mayoclinic.org/-diseases -conditions/erectile-dysfunction/symptoms-causes/syc-20355776).

McKee, R., & W. J. Taverner. 2013. *Taking Sides: Clashing Views on Controversial Issues in Human Sexuality,* 13th ed. New York: McGraw Hill.

Meston, C., and D. Buss. 2009. *Why Women Have Sex: Understanding Sexual Motivation.* New York: Henry Holt.

National Center for Health Statistics. 2010. *Trends in Circumcision among Newborns* (http://www.cdc.gov/nchs/data/hestat/circumcisions /circumcisions.htm).

National Institutes of Health, National Cancer Institute. 2013. *Prostate Cancer* (http://www.cancer.gov/cancertopics/types/prostate).

National Women's Health Network. *Top Ten Things to Know about Addyi* (https://www.nwhn.org/wp-content/uploads/2015/10/NWHN_Addyi _Fact_Sheet_P2.pdf).

Newport, F. 2018. In U.S., estimate of LGBT population rises to 4.5%. (https://news.gallup.com/poll/234863/estimate-lgbt-population-rises .aspx?g_source=link_NEWSV9&g_medium=TOPIC&g _campaign=item_&g_content=In%2520U.S.%2c%2520Estimate%2520of %2520LGBT%2520Population%2520Rises%2520to%25204.5%2525).

Pacik, P. T. 2009. Viewpoint: Botox treatment for vaginismus. *Plastic & Reconstructive Surgery* 124(6): 455e–456e.

Padilla, M. 2007. *Caribbean Pleasure Industry: Tourism, Sexuality, and AIDS in the Dominican Republic.* Chicago: University of Chicago Press.

Ross, A., and H. W. Shoff. 2019. *Toxic Shock Syndrome.* StatPearls Publishing, National Center for Biotechnology Information (https://www.ncbi .nlm.nih.gov/books/NBK459345/).

Sample, I. 2011. Female orgasm captured in series of brain scans. *Guardian,* November 14, p. 9.

Savage, Dan. 2012. *It Gets Better.* New York: Penguin Books.

Slaughter, A.-M. 2015. *Unfinished Business: Women Men Work Family.* New York: Random House.

Wawer, M. J., et al. 2009. Circumcision in HIV-infected men and its effect on HIV transmission to female partners in Rakai, Uganda: A randomised controlled trial. *Lancet* 374(9685): 229–237.

WebMD. 2014. *Menopause and Hormone Replacement Therapy* (http://www .webmd.com/menopause/guide/menopause-hormone-therapy?page=2).

Wilcox, A. J., et al. 2000. The timing of the "fertile window" in the menstrual cycle: Day-specific estimates from a prospective study. *British Medical Journal* 321(7271): 1259–1262.

Williams Institute. 2016. *How Many Adults Identify as Transgender in the United States?* (https://williamsinstitute.law.ucla.edu/wp-content/uploads /How-Many-Adults-Identify-as-Transgender-in-the-United-States.pdf).

World Health Organization. 2020. *Female Genital Mutilation* (http://www .who.int/mediacentre/factsheets/fs241/en/).

World Health Organization. 2020. *Male Circumcision for HIV Prevention: Publications.* (http://www.who.int/hiv/pub/malecircumcision/en/).

Yarber, W. L., et al. 2012. *Human Sexuality: Diversity in Contemporary America,* 8th ed. New York: McGraw Hill.

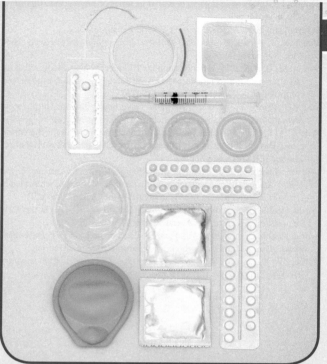

CHAPTER OBJECTIVES

- Explain how contraceptives work
- Describe the types of long-acting and short-acting reversible contraceptives and how they work
- Explain approaches to emergency contraception
- Explain the types of permanent contraception
- Discuss key interpersonal and educational issues related to contraception
- Choose a contraceptive method that is right for you

CHAPTER **7**

Contraception

TEST YOUR KNOWLEDGE

1. **Which of the following contraceptive methods offers the best protection against pregnancy?**
   a. Oral contraceptives
   b. Male condoms
   c. Diaphragm with spermicidal foam
   d. Long-acting reversible contraception (IUDs and implants)

2. **Sperm can survive only about 24 hours inside a woman's body.**
   True or False?

3. **Hand lotion and baby oil are good condom lubricants.**
   True or False?

4. **Worldwide, which of the following is the most commonly used contraceptive method?**
   a. Oral contraceptives
   b. Sterilization
   c. Condoms
   d. Diaphragms

5. **Emergency contraception (Plan B One-Step) is now available without a prescription to anyone.**
   True or False?

ANSWERS

1. **D.** Long-acting reversible contraception is the most effective at preventing pregnancy.

2. **FALSE.** Sperm usually live about 72 hours within the woman's body but can live up to six or seven days.

3. **FALSE.** Only water-based lubricants such as K-Y Brand Jelly or Astroglide should be used as condom lubricants. Any product that contains mineral oil can cause latex condoms to disintegrate.

4. **B.** Worldwide, sterilization is the most popular method of contraception. Although male sterilization is less expensive and less prone to complications, female sterilization is far more common.

5. **TRUE.** Plan B One-Step can be purchased by anyone without a prescription. Other forms of emergency contraception, for example, Next Choice One Dose, can also be purchased without a prescription but only by people aged 17 and older.

For thousands of years, people have used **birth control** to manage **fertility** and prevent unwanted pregnancies. Records dating to the fourth century BCE describe foods, herbs, drugs, douches, and sponges used to prevent **conception**—the fusion of an ovum and a sperm that creates a fertilized egg, or *zygote*. Early attempts at **contraception** (the act of blocking conception through a device, substance, or method) followed the same principle as many modern birth control methods.

Today people can choose from many types of **contraceptives** to avoid unwanted pregnancies. *Modern* contraceptives—that is, female and male sterilization, oral hormonal pills, intrauterine devices (IUDs), male and female condoms, injectables, implants, vaginal barrier methods, and emergency contraception—are much more predictable and effective than in the past. They are also more predictable and effective than *traditional* or *natural* methods of contraception, which include rhythm (periodic abstinence); withdrawal; and the lactational amenorrhea method, based on the fact that breast milk production causes lack of menstruation.

How effective is contraception at preventing pregnancy? Of all unintended pregnancies, only 5% occur in women who use contraception consistently (Figure 7.1). In addition to being more effective, contraception is also now more available, at least to certain populations. With the implementation of the Affordable Care Act, privately insured women in the United States pay fewer dollars for their birth control.

Worldwide, however, the situation is quite different. People in many countries have little access to contraceptive information and supplies. Among worldwide pregnancies between 2010 and 2014, an estimated 44% were unintended. The highest rate occurred in the Caribbean and East Africa and the lowest rates in North America and Europe. Notably, of all industrialized nations, the United States has one of the highest teen pregnancy rates, though rates have been dropping since the 1990s, and even more so since the Great Recession in 2007. Because many men's and especially women's lives are significantly affected by unplanned child rearing and because the option of abortion is becoming more restricted, the problem of unplanned, unwanted pregnancies is more serious than the numbers show.

The United Nations reports that in 2019 about 45% of contraceptive users relied on either sterilization or intrauterine devices; still, a shift has occurred over the past 20 years away from sterilization and toward injectables (hormonal shots given every three months) and male condoms. These shifts reflect an increase in contraceptive usage in sub-Saharan African countries, where injectables are more common. In North America and Europe, the most used contraceptives are the pill, the male condom, and IUDs.

In addition to preventing pregnancy, the barrier methods of contraception play an important role in protecting against **sexually transmitted infections (STIs).** (Chapter 19 provides a comprehensive overview of STIs, a term replacing *sexually transmitted diseases,* or *STDs.*) Informing yourself about the realities and risks and making responsible decisions about sexual and contraceptive behavior can be critical to lifelong wellness.

HOW CONTRACEPTIVES WORK

To understand how contraception works, you must first understand the process required for contraception. Sperm must survive the acidic environment of the vagina and pass through the thickened cervical mucus at the entrance to the uterus. The sperm must then travel into the fallopian tube to meet an unfertilized ovum (egg). As long as hormones have supported the process of ovulation, ovaries release one egg each month into one of the fallopian tubes. Once fertilization occurs in the fallopian tube and a zygote is formed, the zygote must then travel back down the fallopian tube to implant within the endometrium (the lining of the inside of the uterus).

Contraception can work at each of the points along this pathway by preventing sperm from entering the vagina or passing through the cervix, by preventing ovulation, by blocking the fallopian tubes, or by altering the endometrium to prevent implantation of a fertilized egg.

Effective approaches to contraception include the following:

• **Barrier methods** work by physically blocking the sperm from reaching the egg. Condoms are the most popular method based on this principle.

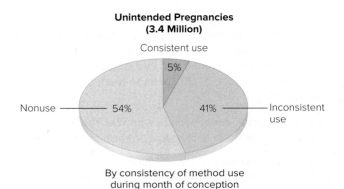

Unintended Pregnancies (3.4 Million)

Consistent use 5%

Nonuse 54%

Inconsistent use 41%

By consistency of method use during month of conception

FIGURE 7.1 **The number of unintended pregnancies in relation to contraception use.**

SOURCES: Guttmacher Institute. 2018. Contraceptive use in the United States. (https://www.guttmacher.org/fact-sheet/contraceptive-use-united-states).

TERMS

birth control The practice of managing fertility and preventing unwanted pregnancies.

fertility The ability to reproduce.

conception The fusion of ovum and sperm, resulting in a fertilized egg, or *zygote*.

contraception The prevention of conception through the use of a device, substance, or method.

contraceptive Any agent or method that can prevent conception.

sexually transmitted infection (STI) Any of several contagious infections contracted through intimate sexual contact.

barrier method A contraceptive that acts as a physical barrier, blocking sperm from uniting with an egg.

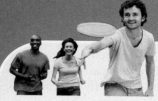

WELLNESS ON CAMPUS
Contraception Use and Pregnancy among College Students

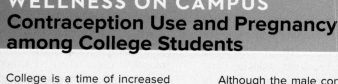

College is a time of increased sexual activity for many young adults. Those who were sexually active in high school may engage with more sexual partners or in riskier behaviors once they enter college; those who abstained from intercourse during high school may begin to explore their sexuality once they enter this new environment.

This greater and newfound sexual activity among young women, especially, is often discussed in popular media and in scientific literature in terms of danger: increased risk for STIs and mental health and other problems. But studies have shown that young adults who avoid sexual activity may be deprived of opportunities for positive sexual experiences. To combat this negative focus surrounding women, research institutions such as the American Psychological Association and the Centers for Disease Control and Prevention encourage a new emphasis on women's comfort and happiness in their sexual activities. Sexual exploration in a variety of relationship contexts (e.g., experiencing more than one relationship) is also increasingly seen as an important part of a young woman's sexual health.

With more sexual partners and exploration, it becomes important for all partners to discuss safety and risks. Young adults tend to prefer romantic relationships to hookups, even during college. But if a committed romantic partner is not available, then casual sex may be perceived as acceptable in the short term. Over 50% of undergraduates reported engaging in sexual activity with an uncommitted partner.

Concerns about STIs and pregnancy are on the minds of many students. Male condoms were the most commonly used contraceptive, with about 65% of men using this method; women who used a contraceptive at last intercourse reported using the pill (51% of the time), IUDs (16%), and implants (9%). Of note, the withdrawal method was used by 30% of respondents; this method neither protects against STIs nor reliably prevents pregnancy.

Although the male condom is effective at preventing the transmission of a wide variety of STIs and the oral contraceptive pill is a highly effective form of contraception when used as directed, they must be used together to provide simultaneous protection against both pregnancy and STIs. This is particularly important for couples who are not in a long-term, mutually monogamous relationship. However, surveys show that college students use a male condom plus another form of contraception only about 45% of the time.

Around 1% of college women report having become pregnant in the prior year, many unintentionally. A disproportionate number of these pregnancies occur in students attending community colleges; recent data indicate that 10% of female dropouts at community colleges were due to unplanned births—as were 7% of all community college dropouts.

The consequences of pregnancy among college students can be significant. For example, studies have demonstrated that 60% of women who became pregnant while attending community college subsequently dropped out. Those who continue their education face added expenses and stress. Given the importance of education in achieving long-term career and financial goals, the implementation of effective contraception during the college years can have a significant impact on the lives of young women. Unfortunately, only 42% of students report that their college provided any information about pregnancy prevention.

SOURCES: Kaestle, C. E., and L. M. Evans. 2018. Implications of no recent sexual activity, casual sex, or exclusive sex for college women's sexual well-being depend on sexual attitudes. *Journal of American College Health* 66(1): 32–40; Hamilton, K. M., et al. 2019. Nonmedical use of prescription drugs during sexual activity as a predictor of condom use among a sample of college students. *Journal of American College Health* 67(5): 459–468; American College Health Association. 2019. American College Health Association-National College Health Assessment II: Reference Group Data Report. Spring 2019. Silver Spring, MD: American College Health Association (https://www.acha.org/documents/ncha/ncha-ii_spring_2019_us_reference_group_data_report.pdf).

TERMS

hormonal method   A contraceptive that alters the biochemistry of a woman's body, preventing ovulation and making it more difficult for sperm to reach an egg if ovulation does occur.

intrauterine device method   A form of contraception that prevents the sperm from reaching the egg through chemical or hormonal changes.

natural method   An approach to contraception that does not use drugs or devices; requires avoiding intercourse during the menstrual cycle when an egg is most likely to be present at the site of conception and the risk of pregnancy is greatest.

surgical method   Sterilization to permanently prevent the transport of sperm or eggs to the site of conception.

• **Hormonal methods,** such as oral contraceptives (birth control pills), alter the biochemistry of the body, preventing ovulation (the release of the egg) and producing changes that make it more difficult for the sperm to reach the egg if ovulation does occur.

• **Intrauterine device methods** prevent the sperm from reaching the egg through chemical or hormonal changes.

• **Natural methods** of contraception are based on the fact that the egg and the sperm have to be present at the same time for fertilization to occur; intercourse is avoided around the time of ovulation.

• **Surgical methods**—female and male sterilization—permanently prevent the union of sperm and eggs.

All contraceptive methods have advantages and disadvantages that make them appropriate for some people but not for others, and the best choice during one period of life may not be the best in another (see the box "Contraception Use and Pregnancy among College Students"). Factors that may affect the choice of method include effectiveness, convenience, cost, reversibility, side effects and risks, and protection against STIs. This chapter helps you sort through these factors to decide which contraceptive method is best for you.

Contraceptive effectiveness is determined partly by the reliability of the method itself—the failure rate if it were always used exactly as directed ("perfect use"). Effectiveness is also determined by user characteristics, including fertility of the individual, frequency of intercourse, and how consistently and correctly the method is used. This "typical use" **contraceptive failure rate** is based on studies that directly measure the percentage of unintended pregnancies in the first year of contraceptive use. For example, the 7% failure rate of oral contraceptives means 7 out of 100 typical users will become pregnant in the first year. This failure rate is likely to be lower for women who are consistently careful in following instructions and higher for those who are frequently careless; the "perfect use" failure rate of oral contraceptives is 0.3%.

Another measure of effectiveness is the **continuation rate**—the percentage of people who continue to use the method after a specified period of time. This measure is important because many unintended pregnancies occur when a method is stopped and not immediately replaced with another. Thus a contraceptive with a high continuation rate would be more effective at preventing pregnancy than one with a low continuation rate. A high continuation rate also indicates user satisfaction with a particular method.

Contraception is often divided into categories, or tiers, based on efficacy. Figure 7.2 offers a graphic depiction of these tiers along with the typical use effectiveness ratings and tips on how to improve efficacy.

> **QUICK STATS**
>
> **Contraception designed for women (e.g., female sterilization, IUDs, and pills) accounts for most contraceptive use worldwide.**
>
> —United Nations, 2019

> **TERMS**
>
> **contraceptive failure rate**   The percentage of women using a particular contraceptive method who experience an unintended pregnancy in the first year of use.
>
> **continuation rate**   The percentage of people who continue to use a particular contraceptive after a specified period of time.
>
> **long-acting reversible contraception (LARC)**   Intrauterine devices and implant methods of contraception, which last for several years, earn high satisfaction rates, and reduce rates of unintended pregnancy and abortion compared to other methods.
>
> **intrauterine device (IUD)**   A device inserted into the uterus as a contraceptive.

LONG-ACTING REVERSIBLE CONTRACEPTION

Long-acting reversible contraception (LARC) consists of intrauterine devices (IUDs) and implants. These methods of contraception give very high satisfaction rates and decrease instances of unintended pregnancy and abortion more than other methods. The Academy of Medicine and the American College of Obstetricians and Gynecologists advocate for expanded access to LARC methods for all appropriate candidates, including adolescents and women who have not yet given birth.

Intrauterine Devices (IUDs)

An **intrauterine device (IUD)** is a small plastic object placed in the uterus as a contraceptive. Five different IUDs are now available in the United States. The Copper T-380A (also known as ParaGard) provides protection for up to 12 years. Hormonal IUDs Mirena, Liletta, Kyleena, and Skyla release small amounts of progestin (a synthetic progesterone) and remain effective for three to five years.

Current evidence suggests that ParaGard works primarily by preventing fertilization. This IUD contains copper, which is thought to cause biochemical changes in the uterus that affect the movement of sperm and eggs. If fertilization does occur, ParaGard may also interfere with the implantation of fertilized eggs in the uterine lining. The hormonal IUDs also work primarily by preventing fertilization. As a result of the slow release of very small amounts of progestin, the cervical mucus thickens, and sperm are unable to swim up to an egg.

An IUD must be inserted and removed by a trained professional. It can be inserted at any time during the menstrual cycle, as long as the woman is not pregnant. The device is threaded into a sterile inserter that is introduced through the cervix; a plunger pushes the IUD into the uterus. IUDs have two threads attached that protrude from the cervix into the vagina so that a woman can feel them to make sure the device is in place. These threads are trimmed so that only 1-1½ inches remain in the upper vagina (Figure 7.3).

Advantages   Intrauterine devices are highly reliable and are simple and convenient to use, requiring no attention. They do not require the woman to anticipate or interrupt sexual activity. IUDs have only local effects and tend to be very safe, including for women with complex medical problems. The long-term expense of using an IUD is also low. The main advantage is their low failure rate: Less than 1% of women using IUDs will get pregnant. In the absence of complications, they are also fully reversible, meaning that fertility is restored as soon as the IUD is removed.

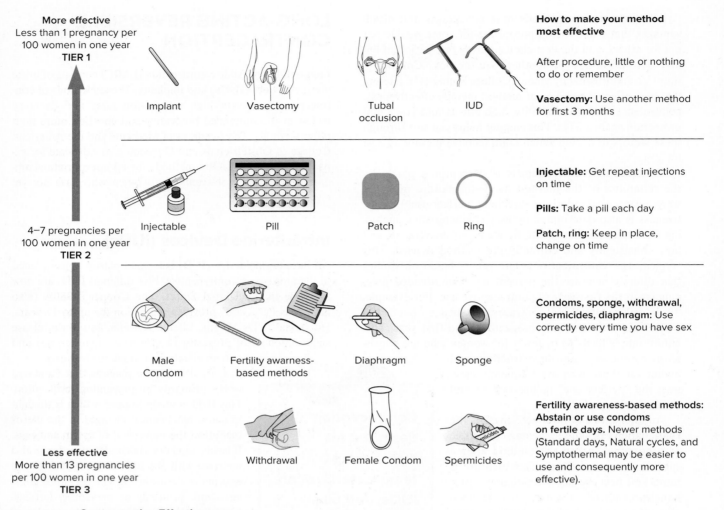

More effective
Less than 1 pregnancy per 100 women in one year
TIER 1

Implant   Vasectomy   Tubal occlusion   IUD

How to make your method most effective

After procedure, little or nothing to do or remember

Vasectomy: Use another method for first 3 months

4–7 pregnancies per 100 women in one year
TIER 2

Injectable   Pill   Patch   Ring

Injectable: Get repeat injections on time

Pills: Take a pill each day

Patch, ring: Keep in place, change on time

Less effective
More than 13 pregnancies per 100 women in one year
TIER 3

Male Condom   Fertility awarness-based methods   Diaphragm   Sponge

Condoms, sponge, withdrawal, spermicides, diaphragm: Use correctly every time you have sex

Withdrawal   Female Condom   Spermicides

Fertility awareness-based methods: Abstain or use condoms on fertile days. Newer methods (Standard days, Natural cycles, and Symptothermal may be easier to use and consequently more effective).

FIGURE 7.2 Contraceptive Effectiveness.

SOURCE: Trussell, J. et al. 2018. Efficacy, safety, and personal considerations. In R. A. Hatcher, et al., eds. *Contraceptive Technology*, 21st ed. New York, NY: Ayer Company Publishers, Inc.

Hormonal IUDs have the added advantage of greatly decreasing blood flow during menstruation, and they are often used as a treatment for excessive bleeding. In fact, after a year of using Mirena, menstrual bleeding is decreased by about 90%. Mirena generally reduces menstrual cramps and is often prescribed for that reason. The Mirena IUD has also been shown to prevent endometrial cancer (in the lining of the uterus) and even reverse the endometrial changes that precede endometrial cancer. ParaGard has been shown to decrease the risk of endometrial cancer, but the reasons for this are less clear. Women who are breastfeeding can use IUDs.

Disadvantages The IUD offers little to no protection against STIs. Most IUD side effects are limited to the genital tract. Side effects differ between the types of IUD. Heavy menstrual flow and increased menstrual cramping sometimes occur with ParaGard, whereas hormonal IUDs cause a reduction in bleeding and cramping. Spontaneous expulsion of the IUD happens to 3% of women within the first year, most

commonly during the first months after insertion. In rare cases, an IUD can puncture the uterine wall and migrate into the abdominal cavity.

A serious but rare complication of IUD use is pelvic inflammatory disease (PID). Most pelvic infections among IUD users occur shortly after insertion, are relatively mild, and can be treated successfully with antibiotics. Early and adequate treatment is critical—a lingering infection can lead to tubal scarring and subsequent infertility.

For many years, IUD use was not recommended for women who had never had a child. However, extensive research now reveals that the IUD is a safe and highly effective contraceptive in this patient population and therefore can be recommended.

IUDs are not suitable for women with suspected pregnancy, large tumors of the uterus, other anatomical abnormalities, or unexplained bleeding; Mirena is also not to be used in women with certain hormonally responsive cancers. Early IUD danger signals include abdominal pain, fever,

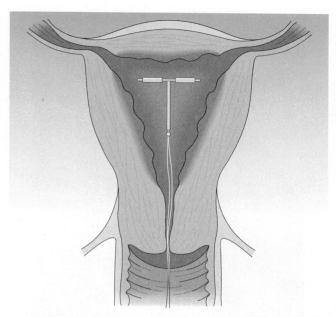

FIGURE 7.3   An IUD (Copper T-380A, or ParaGard) properly positioned in the uterus.

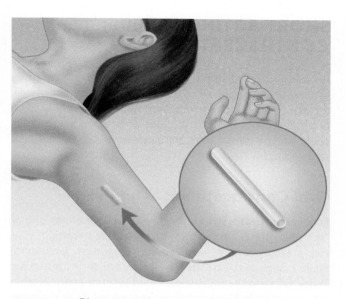

FIGURE 7.4   Placement of contraceptive implant. The Implanon/Nexplanon implant device has to be placed and removed by a trained medical professional.

chills, foul-smelling vaginal discharge, and unusual vaginal bleeding. A change in string length may also be a sign of a problem.

Because of the relatively high up-front costs associated with the IUDs, including the cost of the device as well as the practitioner's insertion fee, the IUD is typically most cost-effective for women who desire contraception for at least six months. The percentage of the cost covered by insurance plans varies greatly.

Effectiveness   The typical first-year failure rate of IUDs is 0.8% for ParaGard, 0.5% for Skyla, and 0.2% for Mirena, Liletta, and Kyleena. Effectiveness can be increased by periodically making sure that the device is in place and by using a backup method for the first week of IUD use. If pregnancy occurs, the IUD may need to be removed to safeguard the woman's health and to maintain the pregnancy; removal depends on the location of the IUD with respect to the pregnancy. If an IUD must be left in place during pregnancy, there is an increased risk of complications.

Contraceptive Implants

Contraceptive implants are placed under the skin of the upper arm and deliver a small but steady dose of progestin over a period of years. One implant, called Nexplanon, is available in the United States, though other brands are available in other countries. Nexplanon is a single implant effective for four years and is considered to be one of the most effective forms of contraception (Figure 7.4).

The progestin in implants has several contraceptive effects. It causes hormonal shifts that may inhibit ovulation and affect development of the uterine lining. The hormone also thickens the cervical mucus, inhibiting the movement of sperm. Contraceptive implants are best suited for women who wish to have continuous, highly effective, and long-term protection against pregnancy.

Advantages   Contraceptive implants are highly effective, with a failure rate of less than 1%. After insertion of the implants, no further action is required; contraceptive effects are reversed quickly upon removal. Because implants contain no estrogen, they carry a lower risk of certain side effects, such as blood clots (venous thromboembolism) and other cardiovascular complications. Menstrual bleeding tends to decrease but becomes irregular. Women who are breastfeeding can use Nexplanon.

Disadvantages   An implant provides little to no protection against STIs. Although the implants are barely visible, their presence may bother some women. Only specially trained practitioners can insert or remove the implants. The up-front costs associated with the implant, including the cost of the device as well as the practitioner's fees, can be significant; therefore, the device is cost-effective only for users desiring more than six months of contraception.

Common side effects of contraceptive implants are menstrual irregularities, including longer menstrual periods, spotting between periods, or having no bleeding at all. The menstrual cycle usually becomes more regular after one year of use. Less common side effects include headaches, weight gain, breast tenderness, nausea, acne, and mood swings.

Effectiveness   The overall failure rate for Nexplanon is estimated at about 0.05%. It is one of the most effective methods of contraception and also one of the most discreet.

SHORT-ACTING REVERSIBLE CONTRACEPTION

A variety of hormonal and barrier methods fall into the group of short-acting reversible contraceptives. For these methods, the user must take action on a daily, weekly, or monthly basis, or at the time of intercourse. Such short-acting methods include, among others, oral contraceptives, skin patches, and vaginal rings.

Oral Contraceptives: The Pill

Oral contraceptives (OCs), also known as *birth control pills* or "the pill," prevent pregnancy by preventing ovulation. Pills give a steady level of estrogen and progestins, laboratory-made compounds that are closely related to progesterone. Today OCs are the most widely used form of contraception among unmarried women and are second only to sterilization among married women.

In addition to preventing ovulation, the pill also inhibits the movement of sperm by thickening the cervical mucus. In the rare event that ovulation does occur, the pill alters the rate of ovum transport by means of its hormonal effects on the fallopian tubes, and it may prevent implantation by changing the lining of the uterus.

The Combination Pill The most common type of OC is the *combination pill,* which contains varying amounts of estrogen and progestin. Traditionally each one-month packet contained a three-week supply of "active" pills that combine varying types and amounts of estrogen and progestin, as well as a one-week supply of "placebo" pills that do not contain hormones. Increasingly, however, combination pills are offering different schedules, including 24 active pills and 4 placebo pills, and 84 active pills and 7 placebo pills. During the time in which no hormones are taken, "your placebo week," a light menstrual period occurs. The newer schedules allow a decreased frequency of menstrual periods. However, a side effect of these extended-cycle regimens is unpredictable light bleeding (known as *spotting*).

The Minipill A much less common type of OC is the *minipill,* a small dose of a synthetic progesterone taken every day of the month. Because the minipill contains no estrogen, it has fewer side effects and health risks, but it is less effective and is associated with more irregular bleeding patterns. Additionally, it must be taken at the same time every day to maintain efficacy. It is sometimes prescribed for women who are breastfeeding or have medical problems that make it unsafe for them to take estrogen.

> **oral contraceptive (OC)** Hormone compounds (made of estrogen and progestins) in pill form that prevent conception by preventing ovulation; also called the *birth control pill* or "the pill." **TERMS**

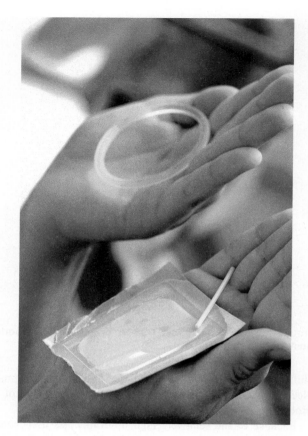

Reversible hormonal contraceptives are available in several forms. Shown here are the patch, the ring, and an implant. Phanie/Science Source

How Oral Contraceptives Are Used A woman is usually advised to start the first cycle of pills with a menstrual period to increase effectiveness and eliminate the possibility of unsuspected pregnancy. But if pregnancy has been ruled out, the pill can be started immediately, that is, at any time during the cycle. A backup contraceptive method, such as condoms, should also be used during the first week. The woman must take one pill every day. Taking a few pills just prior to having sexual intercourse does not provide effective contraception. Linking pill taking to part of their regular routine, such as teeth brushing, helps many women remember to take their pills the same time every day.

During the first cycle or two, hormonal adjustments may cause slight bleeding between periods. This spotting is considered normal.

Ask Yourself

QUESTIONS FOR CRITICAL THINKING AND REFLECTION

Do you think the onus of contraception should fall equally on both partners? What can each partner do to enable the safest outcome? How could you begin a conversation about contraception while keeping you and your partner comfortable?

Table 7.1	Risks of Contraception, Pregnancy, and Abortion	
CONTRACEPTION		**RISK OF DEATH**
Oral contraceptives		
Nonsmoker		
Ages 15–34		1 in 1,667,000
Ages 35–44		1 in 33,300
Smoker		
Ages 15–34		1 in 57,800
Ages 35–44		1 in 5,200
IUDs		1 in 10,000,000
Barrier methods, spermicides		None
Fertility awareness–based methods		None
Tubal ligation		1 in 66,700
PREGNANCY		**RISK OF DEATH**
Pregnancy		1 in 6,900
ABORTION		**RISK OF DEATH**
Spontaneous abortion		1 in 142,900
Medical abortion		1 in 200,000
Surgical abortion		1 in 142,900

SOURCE: Hatcher, R. A., et al. *Contraceptive Technology*, 20th revised ed. 2011, Ardent Media.

Advantages Oral contraceptives are fairly effective in preventing pregnancy and are much less risky than pregnancy (see Table 7.1). The majority of women who get pregnant while using the pill get pregnant because the pills were not taken as directed. The typical one-year failure rate is 7%. The pill is relatively simple to use and does not hinder sexual spontaneity. Most women also appreciate the predictable regularity of periods, as well as the reduction in cramps and blood loss. Women who have significant problems associated with menstruation may benefit from menstrual suppression with extended-cycle OCs. Finally, the pills are reversible, and fertility returns shortly after stopping the pill.

Medical advantages include a decreased incidence of benign breast disease, acne, iron-deficiency anemia, ectopic pregnancy, colon and rectal cancer, endometrial cancer, and ovarian cancer. Women who have ever taken the pill have a 30% lower risk of endometrial cancer, and those who use the pill long term (more than five years) reduce their risk even further. The risk of ovarian cancer drops by 30% for women using the pill, and up to 50% with long-term use (five years or more); some doctors recommend OC use as a preventive measure for women at high genetic risk for ovarian cancer. Some studies have shown that OCs also reduce the risk of colorectal cancer by 15% to 20% in current and recent users.

QUICK STATS

The percentage of teenagers who report having ever had sexual intercourse is less than **50%** and has declined over the past 25 years by **14%** for females and **22%** for males.

—Centers for Disease Control and Prevention, 2017

OC use reduces dysmenorrhea (painful periods), endometriosis, and polycystic ovary syndrome. Health care providers prescribe OCs to treat other medical problems such as menstrual migraine, adenomyosis, and heavy perimenopausal bleeding.

Disadvantages Although simple to ingest, remembering to take a pill every single day can be challenging. Furthermore, OCs do not protect against STIs. In some studies, OCs have been associated with increased risk of cervical chlamydia. If you are using the pill, you should also be using condoms regularly (an exception could be if you have a long-term, mutually monogamous relationship with an uninfected partner).

The hormones in birth control pills influence many tissues in the body and can lead to a variety of side effects, most of which are minor. The majority of women do not experience any side effects associated with OC use. Among women who experience problems with OCs, the most common issue is bleeding during midcycle (called *breakthrough bleeding*), which is usually slight and tends to disappear after a few cycles. Morning nausea and swollen breasts may appear during the first few months of OC use, although these side effects are uncommon with the low-dose pills in current widespread use. Other side effects can include depression, nervousness, changes in sex drive, dizziness, generalized headaches, migraine, and vaginal discharge. Acne may develop or worsen when women take OCs, but most women find their acne improves when they take the pill. In fact, OCs are frequently prescribed as a treatment for acne.

Research shows that currently used low-dose OCs do not, on average, cause weight gain. Most women experience no change in their weight while taking OCs; a small percentage lose weight, and an equally small percentage gain weight while taking OCs. The myth that OCs cause women to gain weight is actually dangerous because many unintended pregnancies result when women avoid taking OCs due to unfounded fear of weight gain.

Another myth about OCs is that they cause cancer. Actually, taking the pill greatly reduces a woman's risk for endometrial and ovarian cancers. A small increase in breast cancer risk has been found for hormonal contraception: for every 8000 users of hormonal contraception, an additional one case of breast cancer occurs. Similarly, an increased risk of cervical cancer is not large enough to outweigh benefits or change recommendations for the use of the combination pill.

Serious OC side effects have been reported in a small number of women. These include blood clots, stroke, and heart attack, concentrated mostly in older women who smoke or have a history of circulatory disease. Recent studies have shown no increased risk of stroke or heart attack for healthy, young, non-

CRITICAL CONSUMER
Obtaining a Contraceptive from a Health Clinic or Physician

If you are considering a method of contraception that requires a prescription or professional fitting or insertion, you'll need to go to a health clinic or a physician to get it. Many of the female contraception methods—including hormonal methods, IUDs, diaphragms, and cervical caps—require at least an initial professional visit. An exception is that several states have passed laws allowing some pharmacists to provide hormonal methods without a prescription; for example, California (pills, patches, injections) and Oregon (pills, patches). Similar laws exist in Colorado, Hawaii, Idaho, Maryland, New Mexico, Utah, West Virginia, and the District of Columbia.

The thought of visiting a physician's office or health clinic to discuss and obtain contraception makes many people nervous. Remember that the people in the office are health care professionals who will not pass moral judgment on you. They are dedicated to meeting your health care needs. Knowing what to expect can help you get more from your visit.

Before Your Visit

Prepare for a successful visit by doing the following:

1. If possible, discuss with your partner how you can share the time and money costs of the contraception.

2. Pull together your personal and family medical history. Make sure it's accurate and up to date.

3. Review the section in this chapter titled "Which Contraceptive Method Is Right for You?" Carefully consider each topic, and discuss it with your partner if that would be helpful.

4. Write down any questions you have. Decide what you need to learn about your contraceptive options.

5. If you have questions about sexually transmitted infections or other aspects of sexuality, write those down, too.

6. If you like, plan to have your partner, a friend, or a family member accompany you to your appointment.

7. Remember that the more honest you are with your health care provider, the more helpful the advice can be.

During Your Visit

When you arrive, you'll probably be asked to fill out forms detailing your background and medical history. A physician or staff member will then review the various contraceptive methods with you and answer your questions. She or he can help you evaluate the key factors affecting your choice of method, including health risks, lifestyle factors, cost, and protection against STIs. Blood and urine samples may be taken for lab tests.

The Physical Exam

Your physical exam will probably include a check of your breasts, external genitals, and abdomen, plus a Pap test and possible screening for certain STIs. The exam will help ensure that you can safely use the contraceptive method you have chosen, as well as protect your overall health. If this is your first pelvic exam or you feel nervous or uncomfortable, tell the clinician, and ask her or him to explain each step of the examination.

For the pelvic exam, you will be asked to lie on your back on an examination table, with your feet in stirrups and your knees bent and spread apart. The exam doesn't usually hurt. An instrument called a *speculum* will be inserted into the vagina to hold it open so that the clinician can look at the cervix and vaginal walls. For the Pap test, the clinician will scrape some cells from the cervix and place them on a glass slide. These cells will be analyzed for any signs of cancer. You may feel a slight pressure while the cells are collected. The clinician will also check your internal organs by placing two gloved fingers into the vagina and the other hand on the lower abdomen. They will palpate (examine by touching) the uterus and ovaries to check for any abnormalities.

If you're getting a diaphragm or a cervical cap that is available in multiple sizes, you will be fitted for it at this time. The clinician will probably try different sizes to find the best fit and then will show you how to insert and remove it.

Following Your Exam

After your exam, a health care worker will provide you with your contraceptive, arrange for a further appointment (if necessary), or give you a prescription. Make sure you know exactly how to use the method you've chosen. Written instructions and information should be available. Be sure to ask for a phone number you can call if you have questions later—and don't forget to return to your health care provider for other health care and screenings.

SOURCE: Kaiser Family Foundation. 2020. Birth control (https://healthy.kaiserpermanente.org/health-wellness/birth-control); National Alliance of State Pharmacy Associations. 2019. Pharmacist Prescribing: Hormonal Contraceptives (https://naspa.us/resource/contraceptives/).

---

smoking women on lower-dosage pills. OC users may be slightly more prone to high blood pressure, gallbladder disease, and, very rarely, benign liver tumors.

Birth control pills are not recommended for women with a history of blood clots (or a close family member with unexplained blood clots at an early age), heart disease or stroke, migraines with changes in vision, any form of cancer or liver tumor, or impaired liver function. Women with certain other health conditions or behaviors, including migraines without changes in vision, high blood pressure, cigarette smoking, and sickle-cell disease, require close monitoring when taking the pill.

When deciding whether to use OCs, each woman needs to weigh the benefits against the risks. To make an informed decision, she should begin by getting advice from a health care professional (see the box "Obtaining a Contraceptive from a Health Clinic or Physician").

Effectiveness Oral contraceptive effectiveness varies substantially because it depends so much on individual factors. If taken as directed, the failure rate is as low as 0.3%. However, the typical user has a 7% failure rate. The continuation rate for OCs also varies; the average rate is 67% after one year. Besides forgetting to take the pill, another reason for OC failure is poor absorption of the drug due to vomiting or diarrhea, or to interactions with other medicines (including certain antibiotics, antiseizure medications, and the commonly used herb St. John's wort).

Contraceptive Skin Patch

The contraceptive skin patch, Ortho Evra, is a thin, 1¾-inch square patch that slowly releases an estrogen and a progestin into the bloodstream. The contraceptive patch prevents pregnancy in the same way as combination OCs, following a similar schedule. Each patch is worn continuously for one week and is replaced on the same day of the week for three consecutive weeks. The fourth week is patch-free, allowing a woman to have her menstrual period.

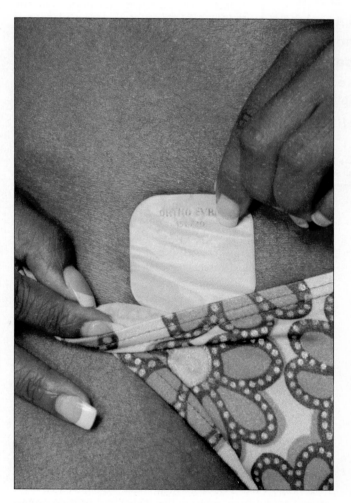

The contraceptive skin patch can be worn on several different parts of a woman's body; it remains on during bathing or swimming. Bob Pardue - Medical Lifestyle/Alamy Stock Photo

The patch can be worn on the upper outer arm, abdomen, buttocks, or upper torso (excluding the breasts); it is designed to stick to skin even during bathing or swimming. If a patch should fall off for more than a day, the U.S. Food and Drug Administration (FDA) advises starting a new four-week cycle of patches and using a backup method of contraception for the first week. Patches should be discarded according to the manufacturer's directions to avoid leakage of hormones into the environment.

Advantages Because the patch provides the same combination of hormones as a combined birth control pill, the advantages are similar. The medical benefits of the patch include, but are not limited to, lighter, less painful menses; decreased risk of uterine and ovarian cancers; decreased anemia; and the ability to control your cycle. With both perfect and typical use, the patch is as effective as OCs in preventing pregnancy. Compliance seems to be higher with the patch than with OCs, probably because the patch requires weekly instead of daily action.

Disadvantages Like other hormonal contraceptives, the patch doesn't protect against STIs. Patch users should also use condoms for STI protection unless they are in a long-term monogamous relationship with an uninfected partner. Minor side effects are similar to those of OCs, although breast discomfort may be more common in patch users. Some women also experience skin irritation around the patch. More serious complications are thought to be similar to those of OCs, including an increased risk of side effects among women who smoke. However, because Ortho Evra exposes users to higher doses of estrogen than most OCs, patch use may further increase the risk of blood clots. Recent studies show conflicting results regarding the risk of blood clots, but it is possible that the risk is slightly higher with the patch compared to low-dose OCs.

Effectiveness With perfect use, the patch's failure rate is very low (0.3%) in the first year of use. The typical failure rate is approximately 7%, similar to that of the oral contraceptive pill. Failure rates have been shown to be higher in women weighing more than 198 pounds.

Vaginal Contraceptive Ring

The NuvaRing is a vaginal ring that is molded with a mixture of progestin and estrogen. The two-inch ring slowly releases hormones and maintains blood hormone levels comparable to those found with OC use. The ring prevents pregnancy in the same way as OCs. A woman inserts the ring anytime during the first five days of her menstrual cycle and leaves it in place for three weeks. During the fourth week, when the ring is removed, her next menstrual cycle occurs. A new ring is then inserted seven days later. Rings should be discarded according to the manufacturer's directions to avoid leakage of hormones into the environment. Backup contraception must

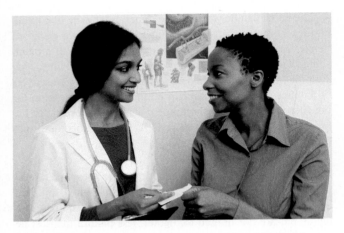

A careful explanation by a health care professional will help this young woman choose a contraceptive method that is right for her.
bikeriderlondon/Shutterstock

be used for the first seven days of the first ring use or if the ring has been removed for more than three hours.

Advantages The NuvaRing offers one month of protection with no daily or weekly action required. It does not require a fitting by a clinician, and exact placement in the vagina is not critical as it is with a diaphragm. Because the ring provides the same combination of hormones as a combined birth control pill, the advantages are similar. The medical benefits of the ring include, but are not limited to, lighter, less painful menses; decreased risk of uterine and ovarian cancer; decreased anemia; and the ability to control your cycle.

Disadvantages The NuvaRing provides no protection against STIs. Side effects are roughly comparable to those seen with OC use, except for a lower incidence of nausea and vomiting. Other side effects may include vaginal discharge, vaginitis, and vaginal irritation. Medical risks also are similar to those found with OC use.

Effectiveness As with the pill and patch, the perfect use failure rate is around 0.3%. The ring's typical use failure rate is similar to the pill's at 7%.

Injectable Contraceptives

Hormonal contraceptive injections were first developed in the 1960s. The first injectable contraceptive approved for use

> **QUICK STATS**
>
> More than **99%** of women aged 15–44 who have ever had sexual intercourse have used at least one contraceptive method.
>
> —National Center for Health Statistics, 2018

in the United States was Depo-Provera, which uses long-acting progestins. Injected into the arm or buttocks, Depo-Provera is usually given every 12 weeks, although it may provide effective contraception for a few weeks beyond that. The product prevents pregnancy by inhibiting ovulation.

Advantages Injectable contraceptives are highly effective and require little action on the part of the user. Because the injections leave no trace and involve no ongoing supplies, injectable contraceptives allow women almost total privacy in their decision to use contraception. Depo-Provera has no estrogen-related side effects.

Disadvantages Injectable contraceptives provide no protection against STIs. A woman must visit a health care facility every three months to receive the injections. The side effects of Depo-Provera are similar to those of implants: Menstrual irregularities are the most common, and after one year of using Depo-Provera many women have no menstrual bleeding at all. Weight gain is a common side effect. After discontinuing the use of Depo-Provera, women may experience temporary infertility for up to 12 months, making it less ideal for women who plan on conceiving in the near future.

Depo-Provera also has a unique risk: It can cause a reduction in bone density, especially in women who use it for an extended period. The rate of decline in bone density is most rapid in the first two years of use, but the good thing is that the bone density begins to increase shortly after discontinuation. Women who use Depo-Provera are advised to do weight-bearing exercise and ensure an adequate intake of dietary calcium. Due to conflicting data, the FDA states that women should use Depo-Provera as a long-term contraceptive (longer than two years, for example) only if other methods are inadequate. However, multiple gynecologic associations believe that the benefits of this highly effective contraception outweigh the theoretical risks, and continuation should not be denied due to concerns regarding bone density.

Effectiveness The perfect use failure rate is 0.2% for Depo-Provera. With typical use, the failure rate increases to 4% in the first year of use.

Male Condoms

The **male condom** is a thin sheath designed to cover the penis during sexual intercourse. Most brands available in the United States are made of latex, although condoms made of polyurethane and polyisoprene are also available. Condoms prevent sperm from entering the vagina and provide protection against most STIs. Condoms are the most widely used barrier method and the third most popular of all contraceptive

> **male condom** A thin sheath that covers the penis during sexual intercourse; used for contraception and to prevent STI transmission.
>
> **TERMS**

methods used in the United States, after the pill and female sterilization.

Condom sales have increased dramatically in recent years, primarily because they are the only method of contraception that provides substantial protection against HIV infection as well as some protection against other STIs. At least one-third of all male condoms are bought by women. This figure will probably increase as more women assume the right to insist on condom use. Many couples combine various contraceptives, using condoms for STI protection and another contraceptive method for greater protection against pregnancy.

The man or his partner must put the condom on the penis before it is inserted into the vagina because the small amounts of fluid that may be secreted unnoticed prior to **ejaculation** often contain sperm capable of causing pregnancy. The rolled-up condom is placed over the head of the erect penis and unrolled down to the base of the penis, leaving a half-inch space (without air) at the tip to collect semen (Figure 7.5). Some brands of condoms have a reservoir tip designed for this purpose. Uncircumcised men must first pull back the foreskin of the penis. Partners must be careful not to damage the condom with fingernails, rings, or other rough objects.

Many condoms are prelubricated with water-based or silicone-based lubricants. These lubricants make the condom more comfortable and less likely to break. Many people find that using extra, non-oil-based lubricant can be helpful. Prelubricated condoms are also available containing the **spermicide** nonoxynol-9, the same agent found in many of the contraceptive creams that women use. However, spermicidal condoms are no more effective than condoms without spermicide. They cost more and have a shorter shelf life than most other condoms. Further, condoms with nonoxynol-9 have been associated with urinary tract infections in women and, if they cause tissue irritation, an increased risk of HIV transmission.

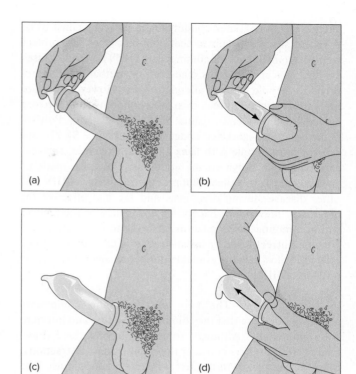

FIGURE 7.5 Use of the male condom. (a) Place the rolled-up condom over the head of the erect penis. Hold the top half-inch of the condom (with air squeezed out) to leave room for semen. (b) While holding the tip, unroll the condom onto the penis. Gently smooth out any air bubbles. (c) Unroll the condom down to the base of the penis. (d) To avoid spilling semen after ejaculation, hold the condom around the base of the penis as the penis is withdrawn. Remove the condom away from your partner, taking care not to spill any semen.

Water-based lubricants such as K-Y Brand Jelly or Astroglide can be used as needed. Any products that contain mineral or vegetable oil—including baby oil, many lotions, regular petroleum jelly, cooking oils (corn oil, shortening, butter, and so on), and some vaginal lubricants and antifungal or anti-itch creams—should not be used with latex condoms. Such products can cause latex to start disintegrating within 60 seconds, thus greatly increasing the chance of condom breakage. (Polyurethane is not affected by oil-based products.)

When the man loses his erection after ejaculating, the condom loses its tight fit. To avoid spilling semen, the condom must be held around the base of the penis as the penis is withdrawn. If any semen is spilled on the vulva, sperm may find their way to the uterus.

Advantages Condoms are easy to purchase and are available without prescription or medical supervision. In addition to being free of medical side effects (other than occasional

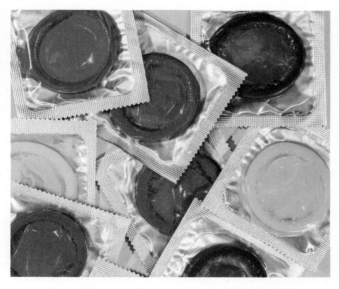

Condoms come in a variety of sizes, textures, and colors. mikroman6/Getty Images

ejaculation An abrupt discharge of semen from the penis during sexual stimulation.

spermicide A chemical agent that kills sperm.

TERMS

allergic reactions), latex condoms help protect against STIs. A recent study determined that condoms may also protect women from human papillomavirus (HPV), which causes cervical cancer. Condoms made of polyurethane are appropriate for people who are allergic to latex. However, they are more likely to slip or break than latex condoms and therefore may give less protection against STIs and pregnancy. Polyisoprene condoms, marketed under the brand name SKYN, are safe for most people with latex allergies, stretchier, and less expensive than polyurethane condoms. Condoms made of lambskin are also available but permit the passage of HIV and other disease-causing organisms and are less effective for pregnancy prevention. Except for abstinence or intercourse within a monogamous relationship with an uninfected partner, the correct and consistent use of latex male condoms offers the most reliable available protection against the transmission of HIV.

Disadvantages The two most common complaints about condoms are that they diminish sensation and interfere with spontaneity. Although some people find these drawbacks serious, others consider them only minor distractions. Many couples learn to creatively integrate condom use into their sexual practices. Indeed, condom use can be a way to improve communication and share responsibility in a relationship.

Effectiveness During the first year of typical condom use among 100 users, approximately 13 pregnancies will occur. And even with perfect use, the first-year failure rate is about 2%. At least some pregnancies happen because the condom is removed carelessly after ejaculation. Some may also occur because of breakage or slippage. Other contributing factors include poorly fitting condoms, insufficient lubrication (which increases the risk of breakage), excessively vigorous sex, and improper storage. (Because heat destroys rubber, latex condoms should not be stored for long periods in a wallet or a car's glove compartment.) To help ensure quality, condoms should not be used past their expiration date or more than five years past their date of manufacture (two years for those with spermicide).

If a condom breaks or is removed carelessly, a woman can reduce the risk of pregnancy by immediately using an emergency contraceptive (discussed later in the chapter). The most common cause of pregnancy that condom users experience is either occasionally not using a condom at all or delaying use until after preejaculatory fluid (which may contain sperm) has already entered the vagina.

Female Condoms

The female condom is a clear, stretchy, disposable pouch with two rings that can be inserted into a woman's vagina. It was designed as an alternative to the male condom because the woman can control its use. It can be inserted up to eight hours before intercourse, so it need not interfere with the moment.

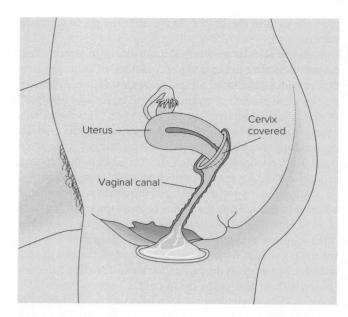

FIGURE 7.6   **The female condom properly positioned.**

The one-size-fits-all condom, called the FC2, consists of a soft, loose-fitting, nonlatex rubber sheath with two flexible rings (Figure 7.6). The ring at the closed end is inserted into the vagina and placed at the cervix much like a diaphragm. The ring at the open end remains outside the vagina. The female condom protects the inside of the vagina and part of the external genitalia.

The manufacturer strongly recommends practicing inserting the female condom several times before actually using it for intercourse. Most women find that it is easy to use after they have practiced inserting the FC2 several times. The FC2 comes prelubricated with a silicone lubricant, but extra lubricant or a spermicide can be used if desired. As with male condoms, users need to take care not to tear the condom during insertion or removal. Following intercourse, the woman should remove the condom before standing up. By twisting and squeezing the outer ring, she can prevent the spilling of semen. A new condom should be used for each act of sexual intercourse. A female condom should not be used with a male condom because tearing is more likely to occur.

Advantages For many women, the greatest advantage of the female condom is the control it gives them over contraception and STI prevention. (Partner cooperation is still important, however.) Female condoms can be inserted up to eight hours before sexual activity and are thus less disruptive than male condoms. Because the outer part of the condom covers the area around the vaginal opening as well as the base of the penis during intercourse, it offers potentially better protection against genital warts or herpes. The synthetic rubber pouch can be used by people who are allergic to latex. Because the material is thin and pliable, there is little loss of sensation. The FC2 is generously lubricated and the material conducts heat well, increasing comfort and natural feel during intercourse.

When used correctly, the female condom should theoretically provide protection against HIV transmission and STIs comparable to that of the latex male condom. However, in research involving typical users, the female condom was slightly less effective in preventing pregnancy and STIs. Effectiveness improves with careful practice and instruction.

Disadvantages The female condom is unfamiliar to most people and requires practice to learn to use it effectively. The outer ring of the female condom, which hangs visibly outside the vagina, may be bothersome to some couples. During coitus, both partners must take care that the penis is inserted into the pouch, not outside it, and that the device does not slip inside the vagina. Female condoms, like male condoms, are made for one-time use. A single female condom costs about three to four times as much as a single male condom. Female condoms are harder to find than male condoms. Some pharmacies do not currently carry them. You can buy the FC2 at Planned Parenthood and online (see http://www.fc2.us.com/).

Effectiveness The typical first-year failure rate of the female condom is 21%. For women who follow instructions carefully and consistently, the failure rate is considerably lower—about 5%. Female condoms rarely break during use, but slippage occurs in nearly 10% of users. Having emergency contraception available is recommended.

Diaphragm with Spermicide

Before oral contraceptives were introduced, about 25% of all American couples who used any form of contraception relied on the **diaphragm.** Many diaphragm users subsequently switched to the pill or IUDs, and therefore the device is rarely used now. However, the diaphragm still offers advantages that are important to some couples.

The diaphragm is a dome-shaped cup of silicone with a flexible rim. When correctly used with spermicidal cream or jelly, the diaphragm covers the cervix, blocking sperm from the uterus. There are two diaphragms available in the United States: the Milex, which comes in two styles and multiple sizes, and the single-size Caya.

Diaphragms are available in the United States only by prescription. Because of individual anatomical differences among women, the round Milex diaphragm must be carefully fitted by a trained clinician to ensure both comfort and effectiveness. The fit should be checked with each routine annual medical examination, as well as after childbirth, abortion, abdominal or pelvic surgery, or a weight change of more than 10 pounds. Caya comes in only one size and does not require fitting; it is oval in shape and designed to fit most women. Caya is contoured for easier use and includes grip "dimples" on the sides to help with insertion and a small dome to aid in removal of the device.

A diaphragm should be used with spermicidal jelly or cream on the diaphragm before inserting it and checking its place-

ment (Figure 7.7). If more than six hours elapse between the time of insertion and the time of intercourse, additional spermicide must be applied. The diaphragm must be left in place for at least six hours after the last act of coitus to give the spermicide enough time to kill all the sperm. With repeated intercourse, a condom should be used for additional protection.

To remove the diaphragm, the woman hooks the front rim (Milex) or small removal dome (Caya) down from the pubic bone with one finger and pulls it out. After each use, a diaphragm should be washed with mild soap and water, rinsed, patted dry, and examined for holes or cracks. Defects would most likely develop near the rim and can be spotted by looking at the diaphragm in front of a bright light. A diaphragm should be stored in its case.

Advantages Diaphragm use is less intrusive than male condom use because a diaphragm can be inserted up to six hours before intercourse. Its use can be limited to times of sexual activity only, and it allows for immediate and total reversibility. The diaphragm is free of medical side effects (other than rare allergic reactions) and increased risk of urinary tract infection.

Disadvantages Diaphragms must always be used with a spermicide, so a woman must keep both of these supplies with her whenever she anticipates sexual activity. Diaphragms require extra attention because they must be cleaned and stored with care to preserve their effectiveness. Some women cannot wear a diaphragm because of their vaginal or uterine anatomy. In other women, diaphragm use can cause bladder infections and may need to be discontinued if repeated infections occur.

Diaphragms have also been associated with a slightly increased risk of **toxic shock syndrome (TSS),** an occasionally fatal bacterial infection. To reduce the risk of TSS, a woman should wash her hands carefully with soap and water before inserting or removing the diaphragm, should not use the diaphragm during menstruation or when abnormal vaginal discharge is present, and should never leave the device in place for more than 24 hours.

Effectiveness The diaphragm's effectiveness depends on its proper use. The typical failure rate is 17% during the first year of use. The main causes of failure are incorrect insertion, inconsistent use, and inaccurate fitting. If a diaphragm slips during intercourse, a woman should use emergency contraception.

> **TERMS**
>
> **diaphragm**   A contraceptive device consisting of a flexible, dome-shaped cup that covers the cervix and prevents sperm from entering the uterus.
>
> **toxic shock syndrome (TSS)**   A bacterial disease usually associated with tampon use, and sometimes diaphragm use; symptoms include fever, rash, nausea, headache, dizziness, confusion, fainting, sore throat, cough, and abdominal pain.

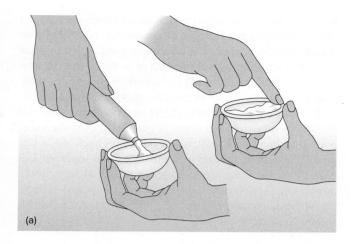

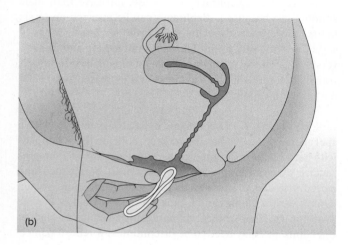

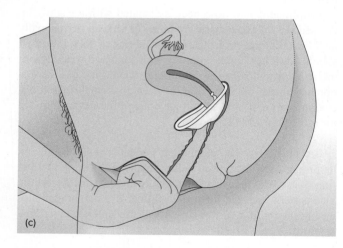

FIGURE 7.7 **Use of the diaphragm.** Wash your hands with soap and water before inserting the diaphragm. It can be inserted while squatting, lying down, or standing with one foot raised. (a) Place about a tablespoon of spermicidal jelly or cream in the concave side of the diaphragm, and spread it around the inside of the diaphragm and around the rim. (b) Squeeze the diaphragm into a long, narrow shape between the thumb and forefinger. Insert it into the vagina, and push it up along the back wall of the vagina as far as it will go. For the Caya, use the grip nubs to fold and grasp the device during insertion. (c) Check its position to make sure the cervix is completely covered and that the front rim of the diaphragm is tucked behind the pubic bone.

Cervical Cap

The **cervical cap,** another barrier device, is a small flexible cup that fits snugly over the cervix and is held in place by suction. This cervical cap is a clear silicone cup with a brim around the dome to hold spermicide and trap sperm, and a removal strap over the dome. It comes in three sizes and must be fitted by a trained clinician. It is used like a diaphragm, with a small amount of spermicide placed in the cup and on the brim before insertion. The cervical cap is reusable but must be replaced annually.

Advantages Advantages of the cervical cap are similar to those associated with diaphragm use. It is an alternative for women who cannot use a diaphragm because of anatomical reasons or recurrent urinary tract infections. The cap fits tightly, so it does not require backup condom use with repeated intercourse. It may be left in place for up to 48 hours.

Disadvantages Along with most of the disadvantages associated with the diaphragm, difficulty with insertion and removal is more common for cervical cap users. Because there may be a slightly increased risk of TSS with prolonged use, the cap should not be left in place for more than 48 hours.

Effectiveness Studies indicate that the average failure rate for the cervical cap is 17% for women who have never had a child and 32% for women who have had a child.

Contraceptive Sponge

The **contraceptive sponge** is a round, absorbent device that fits snugly over the cervix. The sponge is made of polyurethane and is presaturated with the same spermicide used in contraceptive creams and foams. The spermicide is activated when moistened with a small amount of water just before insertion. The sponge, which can be used only once, acts as a barrier and a spermicide and absorbs seminal fluid.

Advantages The sponge offers advantages similar to those of the diaphragm and cervical cap. In addition, sponges can be obtained without a prescription or professional fitting, and they may be safely left in place for 24 hours without the addition of spermicide for repeated intercourse. Most women and men find the sponge to be comfortable and unobtrusive during sex.

Disadvantages Reported disadvantages include difficulty with removal and an unpleasant odor if the sponge is

cervical cap A small flexible cup that fits over the cervix; used with spermicide. **TERMS**

contraceptive sponge A contraceptive device about two inches in diameter that fits over the cervix and acts as a barrier and spermicide and absorbs seminal fluid.

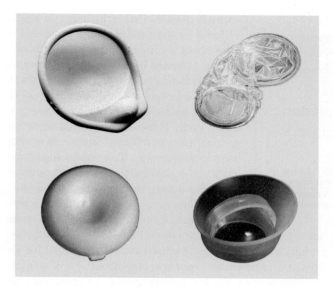

Many contraceptive methods work by blocking sperm from entering the cervix. While not as widely used as the hormonal methods, the barrier methods shown here (clockwise from top left)—Caya diaphragm, female condom, cervical cap, and sponge—are important options for some couples. Phanie/Alamy Stock Photo; Phanie/Alamy Stock Photo; Christopher Kerrigan/McGraw Hill; Jill Braaten/McGraw Hill

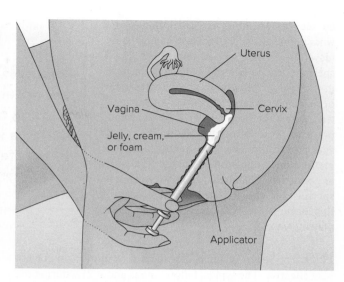

FIGURE 7.8   The application of vaginal spermicide.

left in place for more than 18 hours. Allergic reactions, such as irritation of the vagina, are more common with the sponge than with other spermicide products, probably because the overall dose of spermicide contained in each sponge is significantly higher than that used with other methods. (A sponge contains 1000 milligrams of spermicide compared with the 60–100 milligrams present in one application of other spermicidal products.) If irritation of the vaginal lining occurs, the risk of yeast infections and STIs (including HIV) may increase. The sponge is a single-use device and must be thrown away after each use. Additionally, the sponge cannot be used during menstruation.

Because the sponge has also been associated with toxic shock syndrome, the same precautions must be taken as those described for diaphragm use. A sponge user should be especially alert for symptoms of TSS when the sponge has been difficult to remove or was not removed intact.

Effectiveness   The typical effectiveness of the sponge is the same as that of the diaphragm (14% failure rate during the first year of use) for women who have never experienced childbirth. For women who have had a child, however, the failure rate rises to 27%. One possible explanation is that the sponge's size may be insufficient to adequately cover the cervix after childbirth. The user should carefully check the expiration date on each sponge because shelf life is limited.

Vaginal Spermicides

Spermicidal compounds developed for use with a diaphragm have been adapted for use without a diaphragm by combining them with a bulky base. Foams, creams, jellies, suppositories, and films are all available. Spermicides alone are not very effective methods of contraception, so most people use them in combination with a barrier method, such as a condom. Foam is sold in an aerosol bottle or a metal container with an applicator that fits on the nozzle. Creams and jellies are sold in tubes with an applicator that can be screwed onto the opening of the tube (Figure 7.8).

Foams, creams, and jellies must be placed deep in the vagina near the cervical entrance and must be inserted no more than 60 minutes before intercourse. After an hour, their effectiveness is reduced drastically, and a new dose must be inserted. Another application is also required before each repeated act of coitus.

The spermicidal suppository is small and easily inserted like a tampon. Because body heat is needed to dissolve and activate the suppository, it is important to wait at least 15 minutes after insertion before having intercourse. The suppository's spermicidal effects are limited in time, and coitus should take place within one hour of insertion. A new suppository is required for every act of intercourse.

The vaginal contraceptive film (VCF) is a paper-thin two-inch square of film that contains spermicide. It is folded over one or two fingers and placed high in the vagina, as close to the cervix as possible. In about 15 minutes the film dissolves into a spermicidal gel that is effective for up to one hour. A new film must be inserted for each act of intercourse.

Advantages   The use of vaginal spermicides is relatively simple and can be limited to times of sexual activity. They are readily available in most drugstores and do not require a prescription or a pelvic examination. Spermicides allow complete and immediate reversibility, and the only medical side effects are occasional allergic reactions.

Disadvantages   When used alone, vaginal spermicides must be inserted shortly before intercourse, so their use may be seen as an annoying disruption. Some women find the slight increase in vaginal fluids after spermicide use unpleasant. Also, spermicides can alter the balance of bacteria in the vagina. Because this may increase the occurrence of yeast infections and urinary tract infections, women who are especially prone to these infections may want to avoid spermicides. Also, this contraception method does not protect against STIs such as gonorrhea, chlamydia, or HIV. Overuse of spermicides can irritate vaginal tissues; if this occurs, the risk of HIV transmission may increase.

Effectiveness   Vaginal spermicides on their own are not very effective. The typical failure rate is about 21% during the first year of use. Spermicide is generally recommended only in combination with other barrier methods or as a backup to other contraceptives. Emergency contraceptives provide a better backup than spermicides, however.

Abstinence, Fertility Awareness, and Withdrawal

Millions of people worldwide do not use any of the contraceptive methods described earlier because of religious convictions, cultural prohibitions, poverty, or lack of information and supplies. If they use any method at all, they are likely to use one of the following relatively "natural" methods of attempting to prevent conception.

Abstinence   The decision not to engage in sexual intercourse for a chosen period of time, or **abstinence,** has been practiced throughout history for a variety of reasons. Until relatively recently, many people abstained because they had no other contraceptive measures. Concern about possible contraceptive side effects, STIs, and unwanted pregnancy may be factors. For others, the most important reason for choosing abstinence is a moral one, based on cultural or religious beliefs or strongly held personal values.

Fertility Awareness–Based Methods   Women who practice a **fertility awareness–based method** of contraception abstain from intercourse during the fertile phase of their menstrual cycle. Ordinarily only one egg is released by the ovaries each month, and it lives about 24 hours unless it is fertilized. Sperm deposited in the vagina may be capable of fertilizing an egg for up to six or seven days, so conception can theoretically occur only during six to eight days of any menstrual cycle. However, predicting which six to eight days is difficult. Studies show that even in women who have regular menstrual cycles, it is possible to become pregnant at any time during the menstrual cycle. Any woman for whom pregnancy would be a serious problem should not rely on these methods alone because the failure rate is high—up to 23% each year. Fertility awareness–based methods are not recommended for women who have very irregular cycles—about 15% of all menstruating women. Further, fertility awareness–based methods offer no protection against STIs. Some women use fertility awareness in combination with a barrier method to reduce their risk for unwanted pregnancy.

Calendar methods are based on the idea that the average woman releases an egg 14–16 days before her period begins. To avoid pregnancy, she should abstain from intercourse for about eight days during her cycle, beginning several days before and during the time that ovulation is most likely to occur. However, in one recent study only about 10% of women with regular 28-day cycles actually ovulated 14 days before the next period. The situation is complicated further by the fact that many women have somewhat or very irregular cycles; calendar methods are extremely unreliable for these women.

Temperature methods are based on the knowledge that a woman's body temperature drops slightly just before ovulation and rises slightly after ovulation. A woman using the temperature method records her basal (resting) body temperature (BBT) every morning before getting out of bed and before eating or drinking anything. Once the temperature pattern is apparent (usually after about three months), the unsafe period for intercourse can be calculated as the interval from day 5 (day 1 is the first day of the period) until three days after the rise in BBT.

The *mucus method* (or Billings method) is based on changes in the cervical secretions throughout the menstrual cycle. During the estrogenic phase, cervical mucus increases and is clear and slippery. At the time of ovulation, some women can detect a slight change in the texture of the mucus and find that it is more likely to form an elastic thread when stretched between thumb and finger. After ovulation, these secretions become cloudy and sticky and decrease in quantity. Infertile, safe days are likely to occur during the relatively dry days just before and after menstruation. One problem that may interfere with this method is that vaginal infections, vaginal products, or medication can also alter the cervical mucus.

Withdrawal   In **withdrawal,** or *coitus interruptus,* the male removes his penis from the vagina just before he ejaculates. Withdrawal has a high failure rate because the male has to

---

abstinence   Avoidance of sexual intercourse; a method of contraception.

fertility awareness–based method   A method of preventing conception based on avoiding intercourse during the fertile phase of a woman's cycle.

withdrawal   A method of contraception in which the man withdraws his penis from the vagina prior to ejaculation; also called *coitus interruptus.*

TERMS

Table 7.2 — Contraceptive Methods and STI Protection

METHOD	LEVEL OF PROTECTION
Hormonal methods	Do not protect against HIV or STIs in lower reproductive tract; may increase risk of cervical chlamydia; provide some protection against PID.
IUD	Does not protect against STIs.
Latex, polyisoprene, or polyurethane male condom	Best method for protection against STIs (if used correctly); does not protect against infections from lesions that are not covered by the condom. (Lambskin condoms do not protect against STIs.)
Female condom	Slightly less reduction of STI risk than that of male condom; may provide extra protection for external genitalia.
Diaphragm, sponge, or cervical cap	Provides some protection against cervical infections and PID. Diaphragms, sponges, and cervical caps should not be relied on for protection against HIV.
Spermicide	Modestly reduces the risk of some vaginal and cervical STIs; does not reduce the risk of HIV, chlamydia, or gonorrhea. If vaginal irritation occurs, infection risk may increase.
Fertility awareness–based methods	Do not protect against STIs.
Sterilization	Does not protect against STIs.
Abstinence	Complete protection against STIs (as long as all activities that involve the exchange of body fluids are avoided).

overcome a powerful biological urge. Further, because preejaculatory fluid may contain viable sperm, pregnancy can occur even if the man withdraws prior to ejaculation. Sexual pleasure is often affected because the man must remain in control and the sexual experience of both partners is interrupted.

The failure rate for typical use is about 22% in the first year. Withdrawal does not protect against STIs.

Combining Methods

Couples can choose to combine the preceding methods in a variety of ways, both to add STI protection and to increase contraceptive effectiveness. For example, condoms are strongly recommended along with hormonal contraception whenever there is a risk of STIs (Table 7.2). For many couples, and especially for women, the added benefits far outweigh the extra effort and expense of using multiple methods.

EMERGENCY CONTRACEPTION

Emergency contraception (EC) refers to postcoital methods—those used after unprotected sexual intercourse. An emergency contraceptive may be appropriate if a regularly used method has failed (for example, if a condom breaks) or if unprotected sex has occurred. Sometimes called the "morning-after pill," emergency contraceptives are designed only for emergency use and should not be relied on as a regular birth control method; other methods of birth control are more effective.

When emergency contraceptives were first approved by the FDA, opponents feared that they might act as an **abortifacient**—preventing implantation of a fertilized egg,

theoretically causing abortion. However, recent evidence indicates that emergency contraceptives do not interrupt an established pregnancy. Next-day or after-sex pills work primarily by inhibiting or delaying ovulation and by blocking the transport of sperm and eggs.

Plan B One-Step, Next Choice One Dose, and Ella are now in common use and are more effective, with fewer side effects, than older methods of EC. If taken within 24 hours after intercourse, emergency contraceptives may prevent as many as 75–95% of expected pregnancies. Overall they reduce pregnancy risk by about 89%. They are most effective if initiated in the first 12 hours, but they can be taken up to 120 hours (five days) after unprotected intercourse. Possible side effects include nausea, stomach pain, headache, dizziness, and breast tenderness. If a woman is already pregnant, these pills will not interfere with the pregnancy. Current emergency contraceptives are considered very safe.

Plan B One-Step is available over the counter (no prescription required) for everyone. Next Choice One Dose is available for persons 17 and older. To buy an emergency contraceptive, you need to ask for it at the pharmacy counter. It is recommended that you call ahead to make sure your pharmacy has EC on hand. The vast majority of pharmacies, especially the larger chains, currently carry emergency contraceptives. Ella is available only by prescription.

> **QUICK STATS**
>
> **The FDA approval of emergency contraception is one of the greatest achievements in women's health.**
> —U.S. Department of Health and Human Services, 2019

> **TERMS**
>
> **emergency contraception (EC)** A birth control method used after unprotected sexual intercourse has occurred.
>
> **abortifacient** An agent or substance that induces abortion.

Some clinicians advise women to keep a package of emergency contraceptives on hand in case their regular contraception method fails or they have unprotected intercourse. Research has found that ready access to emergency contraception increases the rate of use and decreases the time to use. It does not result in less unprotected sex or STIs.

Intrauterine devices can also be used for emergency contraception. If inserted within five days of unprotected intercourse, the Copper T ParaGard IUD (discussed earlier) is even more effective than pills for emergency contraception. It has the added benefit of providing up to 12 years of contraception.

PERMANENT CONTRACEPTION

Sterilization is permanent, and it is highly effective at preventing pregnancy. At present it is tied with the pill as the most commonly used contraceptive method in the United States and is by far the most common method used worldwide. It is especially popular among couples who have been married 10 or more years and have had all the children they intend to have. Sterilization does not protect against STIs.

An important consideration in choosing sterilization is that, in most cases, it cannot be reversed. Although the chances of restoring fertility are being increased by modern surgical techniques, such operations are costly, and pregnancy can never be guaranteed.

Many studies indicate that male sterilization is preferable to female sterilization for a variety of reasons. The overall cost of a female procedure is about four times that of a male procedure, the surgery itself is more complex, and women are much more likely than men to experience complications following the operation. Further, feelings of regret after sterilization seem to be more prevalent in women than in men. Before performing the procedure, most physicians require a thorough discussion with anyone considering sterilization.

Male Sterilization: Vasectomy

The procedure for male sterilization, **vasectomy,** involves severing the vasa deferentia, two tiny ducts that transport sperm from the testes to the seminal vesicles. After surgery, the testes continue to produce sperm, but the sperm are absorbed into the body. Because the testes contribute only about 10% of the total seminal fluid, the actual quantity of ejaculate is

sterilization Surgically altering the reproductive system to prevent pregnancy. Vasectomy is the procedure in males; tubal sterilization or hysterectomy is the procedure in females.

vasectomy The surgical severing of the ducts that carry sperm to the ejaculatory duct.

TERMS

reduced only slightly. Hormone production from the testes continues with very little change, and secondary sex characteristics are not altered.

Vasectomy is ordinarily performed in a physician's office and takes about 30 minutes. A local anesthetic is injected into the skin of the scrotum. Small incisions are made at the upper end of the scrotum where it joins the body, and the vas deferens on each side is exposed, severed, and tied off or sealed by electrocautery. Some doctors seal each of the vasa with a plastic clamp, which is the size of a grain of rice. The incisions are then closed with sutures, and a small dressing is applied (Figure 7.9). Pain and swelling are usually slight and can be relieved with ice compresses and a scrotal support. Bleeding and infection occasionally develop but can be treated easily. After the procedure most men can return to work in two days.

Men can have sex after vasectomy as soon as they feel no discomfort, usually after about a week. However, another method of contraception must be used for at least three

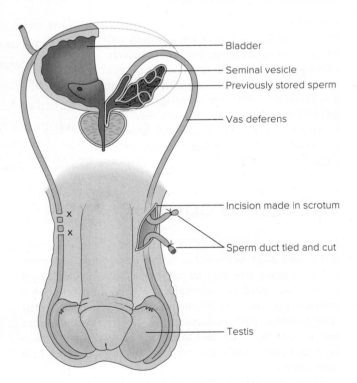

FIGURE 7.9 **Vasectomy.** This surgical procedure involves severing the vasa deferentia, thereby preventing sperm from being transported and ejaculated.

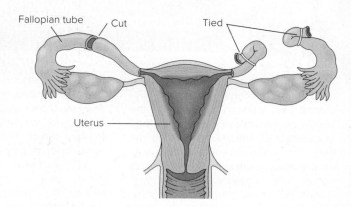

Ask Yourself

QUESTIONS FOR CRITICAL THINKING AND REFLECTION

What are your personal views on sterilization? Do you think it could be an option for you one day? Do you believe people should forgo considering sterilization until they have reached a certain point in their lives? When does sterilization become the best option?

months after vasectomy because sperm produced before the operation may still be present in the semen. Microscopic examination of a semen sample, called *semen analysis*, is required to confirm that sperm are no longer present in the ejaculate. Most doctors recommend having the first semen analysis about three months after surgery and a second test to confirm the results sometime in the future. Studies show that many men fail to complete follow-up testing after vasectomy. Fortunately, unintended pregnancies following vasectomy are rare, even when follow-up procedures are ignored.

Vasectomy is highly effective. In a small number of cases, a severed vas rejoins itself. The overall failure rate for vasectomy is 0.15%. Vasectomy costs $400 to $1000 in the United States and is covered by Medicaid in most states and by many private insurance companies.

About one-half of vasectomy reversals are successful, though this rate can vary significantly depending on the number of years since the initial surgery. In at least half of all men who have had vasectomies, the process of absorbing sperm (instead of ejaculating it) results in antisperm antibodies that may interfere with later fertility. Vasectomy reversal costs between $5,000 and $15,000 in the United States.

Female Sterilization

The most common method of female sterilization involves severing or blocking the oviducts, thereby preventing eggs from reaching the uterus, and sperm from entering the fallopian tubes. Ovulation and menstruation continue, but the unfertilized eggs are released into the abdominal cavity and absorbed. Hormone production by the ovaries and secondary sex characteristics are generally not affected.

Tubal sterilization (also called *tubal ligation*) is most commonly performed by a method called **laparoscopy.** A laparoscope, a camera containing a small light, is inserted through a small abdominal incision, and the surgeon looks through it to locate the fallopian tubes. Instruments are passed either through the laparoscope or through a second small incision, and the two fallopian tubes are sealed off with ties or staples or by electrocautery (Figure 7.10). General anesthesia is usually used. The operation takes about 30 minutes, and women can usually leave the hospital two to four hours after surgery. Tubal sterilization can also be performed shortly after a vaginal delivery through a small incision, or in the case of cesarean section during the same surgery.

FIGURE 7.10 **Tubal sterilization.** This procedure involves severing or blocking the fallopian tubes, thereby preventing eggs from traveling from the ovaries to the uterus. It is a more complex procedure than vasectomy.

Although tubal sterilization is riskier than vasectomy, with a rate of minor complications of about 6–11%, it is the more common procedure. Potential problems include bowel injury, wound infection, and bleeding. Serious complications are rare, and the death rate is low.

The failure rate for tubal sterilization is about 0.5%. When pregnancies occur, an increased percentage of them are ectopic (occurring outside the uterus). Ectopic pregnancy is dangerous and can even cause death, so any woman who suspects she might be pregnant after having tubal sterilization should seek medical help. Because successful reversal rates are low and the procedure is costly, female sterilization should be considered permanent.

A form of incision-free female sterilization has also become available. This procedure can be performed with local anesthetic in a doctor's office and has a short recovery time. Called the Essure system, it consists of tiny springlike metallic implants that are inserted through the vagina and into the fallopian tubes, using a special catheter. Within three months, scar tissue forms over the implants, blocking the tubes. A backup method must be used until a test shows that the tubes are occluded. Placement of the device doesn't require an incision or general anesthesia, and recovery time is quicker than that following tubal sterilization. Only clinicians with specialized training and equipment can perform this procedure.

Hysterectomy, removal of the uterus, is the preferred method of sterilization for only a small number of women, usually those with preexisting menstrual or other uterine problems. Because of the risks involved, hysterectomy is not

tubal sterilization Severing or blocking the oviducts to prevent eggs from reaching the uterus; also called *tubal ligation*.

TERMS

laparoscopy Examining the internal organs by inserting a small camera through an abdominal incision.

hysterectomy Total or partial surgical removal of the uterus.

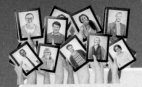

Even in ideal circumstances, raising children is challenging. Although birth control was inadequate well into the 1960s, people today have a wide range of choices for effective contraception. Why, then, when the stakes are so high, do so many unintended pregnancies occur? Why doesn't everyone who wishes to prevent pregnancy use contraception consistently? Here are some of the reasons.

A complex mix of factors relating to financial status, gender, age, culture, history, and policy can create barriers to effective contraception. For intrauterine devices, the cost for the medical exam, the IUD, the insertion of the IUD, and follow-up visits to a health care provider can range up to $1300, depending on health insurance. This cost may deter some candidates. In heterosexual couples, women tend to bear the brunt of the costs. When partners share in these burdens, it becomes easier to overcome them.

Another deterrent is family culture. A cofounder of the Women of Color Sexual Health Network, Bianca Laureano, writes about barriers young women may face when their parents or guardians do not believe in birth control. Laureano herself grew up in a Puerto Rican family who advised her that birth control kills Puerto Rican women.

Young women who are being closely monitored by families that distrust birth control cannot wear a visible patch, nor use a method that requires visits to a physician, especially if a parent or guardian attends their physical exams. They must also continue having a menstrual cycle, so they cannot use Depo-Provera, which, in some cases, causes menstrual bleeding to stop.

In other cases, some young people do not want a contraceptive method that requires them to remember to take a pill each day (oral birth control pills) or to touch their genitals (for example, the NuvaRing).

Oral contraceptive pills are still the most widely used form of contraception. The people who use them most are women who are younger, white (more so than Hispanic or black women), and more educated. Long-acting reversible contraception (LARC) methods, such as implants and IUDs, are very effective but have faced opposition. Historically, some doctors have discouraged younger women from using them. Now they have been shown to be safe, both in research and in the increased numbers of sexually active women aged 15–44 using IUDs successfully.

Still, women of color contend with an additional history of medical mistrust; some observers are concerned that campaigns targeting "at-risk" women focus too much on minority, poor, and young women. In her book *Exposing Prejudice: Puerto Rican Experiences of Language, Race, and Class*, Bonnie Urciuoli presents a history of U.S. policies toward Puerto Rican immigrants, which included controlling their population through sterilization, enforced contraception, and migration. In *Killing the Black Body*, Dorothy Roberts describes the experiences of black women throughout U.S. history—from being forced to bear children during slavery to having their fertility controlled by modern-day welfare policies. Thus, having less access to these methods is not the only reason women of color might avoid them.

In recent decades, contraception use has increased and teen pregnancies have decreased. However, with government actions and public debates curtailing access to contraception and general reproductive rights, we still have ways to go to equalize the burden of contraception and embrace its protective safeguards.

SOURCES: England, P., et al. 2016. Why do young, unmarried women who do not want to get pregnant contracept inconsistently? Mixed-method evidence for the role of efficacy. *Socius: Sociological Research for a Dynamic World* 2; Roberts, D. 1997. *Killing the Black Body: Race, Reproduction, and the Meaning of Liberty*. New York: Pantheon; Sweeney, M. M., and R. Kelly Raley. 2014. Race, ethnicity, and the changing context of childbearing in the United States. *Annual Review of Sociology* 40: 539–558; Urciuoli, B. 1996. *Exposing Prejudice: Puerto Rican Experiences of Language, Race, and Class*. Boulder, CO: Westview; Kaiser Family Foundation. 2019. Oral Contraceptive Pills (https://www.kff.org/womens-health-policy/fact-sheet/oral-contraceptive-pills/); Ome, M. 2020. The surprisingly fraught question of who pays for birth control. *The Atlantic*, 19 February.

recommended as a form of contraception unless the woman has a disease of the uterus or the uterus has been damaged, and future surgery appears inevitable.

ISSUES IN CONTRACEPTION

The subject of contraception is closely tied to several issues that receive a lot of attention in the United States, such as premarital sexual relations, gender and ethnic differences, and sexuality education for teens (see the box "Barriers to Contraceptive Use").

When Is It OK to Begin Having Sexual Relations?

Americans have a wide range of opinions on this issue: only after marriage; when 18 years or older; when in a loving, stable relationship; when the partners have completed their education or could support a child; whenever both partners feel ready and are using protection against pregnancy and STIs.

As the average age of first marriage increases (currently ages 27 for women and 29 for men), young people typically experience a decade or more between puberty and marriage,

Many people have a difficult time talking about contraception with a potential sex partner. How should you bring it up? And whose responsibility is it? Talking about the subject may be embarrassing at first, but imagine the possible consequences of not talking about it. An unintended pregnancy or an STI could profoundly affect you for the rest of your life. Talking about contraception is one way of showing that you care about yourself, your partner, and your future.

Before you talk with your partner, explore your own thoughts and feelings. Find out the facts about different methods of contraception, and decide which one you think would be most appropriate for you. If you're nervous about having this discussion with your partner, it may help to practice with a friend.

Pick a good time to bring up the subject. It makes sense to have this discussion before you start having sex, but even if you've already had intercourse with your partner, it's important to be on the same page about contraception. A time when you're both feeling comfortable and relaxed will improve your chances of having a good discussion. Tell your partner what you know about contraception and how you feel about using it, and talk about what steps you both need to

take to get and use an appropriate method. Listen to what your partner has to say, and try to understand his or her point of view. You may need to have more than one discussion, and it may take some time for both of you to feel comfortable with the subject.

If you want your partner to be involved but he or she isn't interested in talking about contraception, you may want to enlist the support of a friend, family member, or health care provider to help you make and implement decisions about contraception.

If you have been involved in hooking up with people you don't know well and are not having an ongoing relationship with, discussions about contraception may seem unrealistic. At a minimum, refuse to have sex with anyone who won't use a condom. If you are a woman, purchase emergency contraception ahead of time, and don't hesitate to use it. Both men and women should carefully consider the risks involved in hooking up. Remember that no contraceptive method can completely protect you from the potential consequences of being intimate with a person you do not know well.

making sex outside marriage and sex with multiple partners more likely. As a result, decisions about sexual activity, contraception, and STI prevention become even more important for young people (see the box "Talking with a Partner about Contraception").

Contraception and Gender Differences

Couples engaging in sexual intercourse who are nonmonogamous, or have not been tested for STIs, or do not want to get pregnant should share the burden of contraception. Men and women should both discuss and research options and share the responsibility of acquiring and using protection. For one, it takes time, money, and effort to research contraception options, visit a doctor, get refills, and—with the pill—remember to take it. When partners share in these burdens, it becomes easier to overcome them. This makes it more likely that contraceptives and protection against STIs will be used.

Some ways men can and do share this burden are: paying half the cost of a partner's contraceptives, accompanying partners to doctor visits, setting reminders for partners to take the pill, providing condoms, and if the decision has been made never to have children, undergoing vasectomy. Often, though, the burden has fallen on women.

One reason for this disproportionate burden is that women face potentially greater consequences from sexual

activity, risking pregnancy and long-term effects from STIs. Whereas men may suffer only local and short-term effects from the most common diseases (not including HIV infection), women face an increased risk of cervical cancer or pelvic infection with associated infertility from these same STIs. In addition, women are more likely than men to contract HIV from an infected partner. Women may also have accepted more responsibility for contraception because more methods are available to them. (Scientists have tried to develop a hormonal contraceptive for males for many years; it would work by suppressing testosterone to lower sperm production.)

But another powerful reason for the imbalance of responsibility stems from a social imbalance in gendered relationships. Attitudes are more punitive toward women and place much greater responsibility and blame on them when an unintended pregnancy occurs. This double standard—shaming women but praising men who pursue sexual pleasure—still exists in the United States and elsewhere. Even medical professionals in family planning clinics frame contraception as the woman's responsibility.

One Commonwealth Fund study showed that women in the United States have a harder time getting needed health care than women in other high-income countries do. Among 11 high-income countries, women in the United States had the highest rate of maternal mortality because of complications from pregnancy or childbirth. Although the Affordable Care Act made strides in insurance coverage for contraception, the Trump administration tried to overturn this progress, filing petitions with the Supreme Court. The administration worked against efforts to ensure that women could receive contraception, abortion, and information under the Title X program about pregnancy options and how to safely get health care services such as abortion.

Research on college-age and younger people have found that women are less likely than men to use condoms. Women can face more difficulties in purchasing and carrying condoms; they have reported feeling too embarrassed to buy condoms and initiate condom use. A percentage worry about the impact of condom use on sexual pleasure or comfort.

Nearly 20 million new STIs occur annually in the United States, and almost half of these new infections occur among individuals aged 15–24. Over half of college students report not using a condom or another protective barrier during sexual intercourse within the past month. Unprotected sex and multiple sex partners is often more likely to occur after alcohol and drug use.

Although there is substantial public support for reproductive rights and easy access to birth control, many voters and voices in the American media do not support them. This lack of support has also meant a general lack of education. Studies suggest an increased focus on specific college populations to help develop more tailored sexual education campaigns on campuses, with an emphasis on the importance of safe sexual protection practices and shared responsibility.

Sexuality and Contraception Education for Teenagers

Sexuality education and pregnancy prevention programs for teenagers are an important issue. Opinion in the United States is sharply divided on this subject, but the medical data are clear. Certain groups are concerned that more sexuality education and especially the availability of contraceptives will lead to more sexual activity and promiscuity. However, countless studies have shown this is not the case.

Research shows that teens not yet sexually active do not start having sex sooner as a result of attending comprehensive sex education programs. Conversely, most studies show that abstinence-only school programs do not reduce the number of teens who are having sex, and they also lead to decreased rates of contraception use. The American Academy of Pediatrics also supports the provision of factual, comprehensive sexual education in all schools as part of a standard curriculum.

Ask Yourself

QUESTIONS FOR CRITICAL THINKING AND REFLECTION

Do you feel your sexual education up to this point in your life has been complete? Do you feel it has prepared you to have a healthy, safe, and responsible sexual life?

Although a great deal of focus has been placed on HIV and STI prevention, the nearly 195,000 yearly U.S. teenage pregnancies are a serious public health problem and warrant much greater national attention. Although past federal programs have funded organizations that provide factual information about STIs and pregnancy prevention to teens, the Trump administration did not prioritize the issue of teen pregnancy and cut funding.

WHICH CONTRACEPTIVE METHOD IS RIGHT FOR YOU?

The process of choosing and using a contraceptive method can be complex and varies from one couple to another. Each person must consider many variables in deciding which method is most acceptable and appropriate for her or him. Key considerations include those listed here. (To help make a choice that's right for you, take the quiz in the box "Which Contraceptive Method Is Right for You and Your Partner?")

1. *The implications of an unplanned pregnancy and the efficacy of the method.* Many teens and young adults fail to consider how their lives would be affected by an unexpected pregnancy. People who choose to be sexually active but would be negatively affected by an unplanned pregnancy need to use an effective means of birth control and use it consistently.

2. *Health risks.* When considering any contraceptive method, determine whether it may pose a risk to your health. However, most women are candidates for most, if not all, methods of contraception. Pregnancy carries significant health risks that are generally much greater than the risks of contraception.

3. *STI risk.* STIs are another potential consequence of sex. In fact, several activities besides vaginal intercourse (such as oral and anal sex) can put you at risk for an STI. Condom use is of critical importance whenever any risk of STIs is present, even if you are using another contraceptive method to prevent pregnancy. This is especially true whenever you are not in an exclusive, long-term relationship.

4. *Convenience and comfort level.* The most convenient methods are the LARC methods (IUDs and implants) that do not require any work on the part of the user. Most women using hormonal methods also rank them high in convenience. If forgetting to take pills is a problem for you, a vaginal ring, contraceptive patch, implant, or injectable method may be a good alternative. For those who choose a barrier method, condoms are the most common. The diaphragm, cervical cap, contraceptive sponge, female condom, and spermicides can be inserted before intercourse begins, unlike condoms, which must be put on the erect penis.

5. *Type of relationship.* Barrier methods require more motivation and sense of responsibility from *each* partner

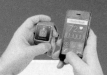

If you are sexually active, you need to use the contraceptive method that works best for you. The following questions will help you sort out factors that affect your choice and pick an appropriate contraceptive method. Answer yes or no for each statement.

_____ 1. I like sexual spontaneity and don't want to be bothered with contraception at the time of sexual intercourse.

_____ 2. I need a contraceptive immediately (today).

_____ 3. It is very important that I (or my partner) do not become pregnant now.

_____ 4. I want a contraceptive method that will protect me and my partner against sexually transmitted infections.

_____ 5. I prefer a contraceptive method that requires the cooperation and involvement of both partners.

_____ 6. I have sexual intercourse frequently.

_____ 7. I have sexual intercourse infrequently.

_____ 8. I am forgetful or have a variable daily routine.

_____ 9. I have more than one sex partner.

_____ 10. I have (or my partner has) heavy periods with cramps.

_____ 11. I prefer a method that requires little or no action or bother on my part.

_____ 12. I am (or my partner is) a nursing mother.*

_____ 13. I want the option of conceiving immediately after discontinuing contraception.

_____ 14. I want a contraceptive method with few or no side effects.

_____ 15. I want a very effective contraceptive method that requires no work on my part (or my partner's part) for at least three years.

If you answered yes to these statements:	These contraceptive methods may be a good choice for you:
1, 3, 6, 10, 12, 13	Oral contraceptives
1, 3, 6, 8, 10, 13	Contraceptive patch, vaginal ring
1, 3, 6, 8, 10, 11, 12	Injectable contraceptive (Depo-Provera)
1, 3, 6, 8, 10, 11, 12, 15	Contraceptive implant (Nexplanon)
1, 3, 6, 8, 10, 11, 12, 13, 14, 15	IUD (Mirena, Liletta, Kyleena, Skyla)
1, 3, 6, 8, 11, 12, 13, 14, 15	IUD (ParaGard)
2, 4, 5, 7, 9, 12, 13, 14	Condoms (male and female)
2, 5, 7, 12, 13, 14	Vaginal spermicides and sponge
5, 7, 12, 13, 14	Diaphragm and spermicide, cervical cap

*Progestin-only hormonal contraceptives (the minipill and Depo-Provera injections) are safe for use by nursing mothers; contraceptives that include estrogen are usually not recommended.

than hormonal methods do. When the method depends on the cooperation of one's partner, assertiveness is necessary, no matter how difficult. This is especially true in new relationships, when condom use is most important.

6. **Ease and cost of obtaining and maintaining each method.** Investigate the costs of different methods. In July 2020, the U.S. Supreme Court upheld the Trump administration's regulation that allows employers with religious or moral objections to opt out of contraception coverage. Remember that your student health clinic probably provides family planning services, and many communities have low-cost family planning clinics, such as Planned Parenthood.

7. **Religious or philosophical beliefs.** For some people, abstinence and/or fertility awareness–based methods may be the only permissible contraceptive methods.

8. **Potential noncontraceptive benefits.** Women with dysmenorrhea, irregular periods, acne, endometriosis, severe premenstrual syndrome (PMS), and other medical problems may benefit from using a particular method of contraception. Be sure to discuss these issues with your health care provider so that you can take advantage of the noncontraceptive benefits associated with many methods of birth control.

Whatever your needs, circumstances, or beliefs, *do* make a choice about contraception. Contraception is an area in which taking charge of your health has immediate and profound implications for your future. The method you choose today won't necessarily be the one you'll want to use your whole life or even next year. But it should be one that works for you right now.

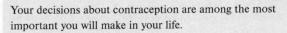

TIPS FOR TODAY AND THE FUTURE

Your decisions about contraception are among the most important you will make in your life.

RIGHT NOW YOU CAN:

- If you're sexually active, consider whether you are confident that you're doing everything possible to prevent an unwanted pregnancy.
- If you're sexually active, discuss your contraceptive method with your partner. Make sure you are using the method that works best for you.
- Work with your partner to choose a backup contraceptive method to use in case your primary method isn't effective enough. Consider keeping an emergency contraceptive on hand in case of a slip-up.

IN THE FUTURE YOU CAN:

- Talk to your physician about contraception and get his or her advice on choosing the best method.
- Occasionally discuss your contraceptive method with your partner to make sure it continues to meet your needs. A change in health status or lifestyle may make a different form of contraception preferable in the future.

SUMMARY

- Barrier methods of contraception physically prevent sperm from reaching the egg; hormonal methods are designed to prevent ovulation, fertilization, and/or implantation; and surgical methods permanently block the movement of sperm or eggs to the site of conception.

- The choice of contraceptive method depends on effectiveness, convenience, cost, reversibility, side effects, risk factors, protection against STIs, and noncontraceptive benefits. Measures of effectiveness include failure rate and continuation rate.

- Hormonal methods may include a combination of estrogen and progestins, or progestins alone. Hormones may be delivered via pills, patch, vaginal ring, IUD, implants, or injections.

- Hormonal methods prevent ovulation, inhibit the movement of sperm, and affect the uterine lining so that implantation is prevented.

- IUDs and implants can provide very effective long-term (3–12 years) contraception and are especially useful for women who want contraception for at least six months.

- Male condoms are simple to use, are immediately reversible, and provide STI protection; female condoms can be inserted hours before intercourse.

- The diaphragm, cervical cap, and contraceptive sponge cover the cervix and block sperm from entering; all need to be used with or contain spermicide.

- Vaginal spermicides come in the form of foams, creams, jellies, suppositories, and film.

- So-called natural methods include abstinence, withdrawal, and fertility awareness; the latter are based on avoiding intercourse during the fertile phase of a woman's menstrual cycle. These methods are significantly less effective than other options.

- Combining methods can increase contraceptive effectiveness and help protect against STIs. The most common combination is a hormonal method, such as the birth control pill, combined with condoms.

- The most commonly used emergency contraceptive, Plan B One-Step, is available without a prescription.

- Vasectomy—male sterilization—involves severing the vas deferens. Female sterilization involves severing or blocking the oviducts so that the egg cannot reach the uterus.

- Issues to be considered in choosing a contraceptive include the individual health risks of each method, the implications of an unplanned pregnancy, STI risk, convenience and comfort level, type of relationship, the cost and ease of obtaining and maintaining each method, and religious or philosophical beliefs.

FOR MORE INFORMATION

Bedsider.Org Provides information on all methods of contraception. Describes how to use a method, typical side effects, cost, and how to get the method.

    https://bedsider.org/

Emergency Contraception website. Provides extensive information and hotline about emergency contraception; sponsored by the Office of Population Research at Princeton University.

    http://ec.princeton.edu and 888-NOT-2-LATE

Guttmacher Institute. Provides reproductive health research, policy analysis, and public education.

    http://www.guttmacher.org

It's Your Sex Life. Provides information about sexuality, relationships, contraceptives, and STDs; geared toward teenagers and young adults. Provided by the Kaiser Family Foundation and MTV.

    http://www.itsyoursexlife.com

Kaiser Family Foundation: Women's Health Policy: Contraception. Provides information and reports focused on how policies affect reproductive health care and access to contraceptives.

    http://kff.org/other/womens-health-policy-contraception/

Managing Contraception. Provides brief descriptions and tips for using many forms of contraception. Features a detailed survey to help with contraceptive choices.

    http://www.managingcontraception.com

Next Choice One Dose. Shows pharmacies in your area that carry this EC product, which is slightly less expensive than Plan B One-Step.

    http://www.mynextchoiceonedose.com

Plan B One-Step. Contains a card you can print and hand to the pharmacist as an easy way to request EC.

    http://www.planbonestep.com

Planned Parenthood Federation of America. Provides information on family planning, contraception, and abortion and offers counseling services.

http://www.plannedparenthood.org

See also the listings for Chapters 6, 8, 9, and 19.

SELECTED BIBLIOGRAPHY

Abma, J. C., and G. M. Martinez. 2017. Sexual activity and contraceptive use among teenagers in the United States, 2011-2015. *National Health Statistics Reports* 4. Hyattsville, MD: National Center for Health Statistics.

American Cancer Society. 2018. *Can Ovarian Cancer Be Prevented?* (https://www.cancer.org/cancer/ovarian-cancer/causes-risks-prevention/prevention.html).

American Cancer Society. 2020. *Risk Factors for Cervical Cancer* (https://www.cancer.org/cancer/cervical-cancer/causes-risks-prevention/risk-factors.html).

American College Health Association. 2019. American College Health Association-National College Health Assessment II: Reference Group Data Report. Spring 2019. Silver Spring, MD: American College Health Association (https://www.acha.org/documents/ncha/NCHA-II_SPRING_2019_US_REFERENCE_GROUP_DATA_REPORT.pdf).

Anawalt, B. D. 2007. Update on the development of male hormonal contraceptives. *Current Opinion in Investigational Drugs* 8(4): 318-323.

Bearak, J., et al. 2018. Global, regional, and subregional trends in unintended pregnancy and its outcomes from 1990 to 2014: Estimates from a Bayesian hierarchical model. *The Lancet Global Health* (6)4: PE380-E389.

Bitzer, J., and J. A. Simon. 2011. Current issues and available options in hormonal contraception. *Contraception* 84(4): 342-356.

Brohet, R. M., et al. 2007. Oral contraceptives and breast cancer risk in the international BRCA 1/2 carrier cohort study: A report from EMBRACE, GENEPSO, GEO-HEBON, and the IBCCS Collaborating Group. *Journal of Clinical Oncology* 25(25): 3831-3836.

Burke, A. E. 2011. The state of hormonal contraception today: Benefits and risks of hormonal contraceptives: Progestin-only contraceptives. *American Journal of Obstetrics and Gynecology* 205(4): S14-S17.

Centers for Disease Control and Prevention. 2019. *Contraception* (https://www.cdc.gov/reproductivehealth/contraception/index.htm).

Centers for Disease Control and Prevention. 2019. *About Teen Pregnancy* (https://www.cdc.gov/teenpregnancy/about/index.htm).

Cha, A. E. 2018. Nine organizations sue Trump administration for ending grants to teen pregnancy programs. *The Washington Post*, February 15 (https://www.washingtonpost.com/news/to-your-health/wp/2018/02/15/planned-parenthood-sues-trump-administration-for-ending-grants-to-teen-pregnancy-programs/).

Chamley, L. W., and G. N. Clarke. 2007. Antisperm antibodies and conception. *Seminars in Immunopathology* 29(2): 169-184.

Cook, L. A., et al. 2007. Vasectomy occlusion techniques for male sterilization. *Cochrane Database of Systematic Reviews*, April 18 (2): CD003991.

Cremer, M., and R. Masch. 2010. Emergency contraception: Past, present and future. *Minerva Ginecologica* 62(4): 361-371.

Critical Trials Arena. 2019. *Phase I Trial of Male Birth Control Pill Reveals Positive Results* (https://www.clinicaltrialsarena.com/news/trial-11-beta-mntdc/).

Daniels, K., and J. C. Abma. 2018. Current contraceptive status among women aged 15-49: United States, 2015-2017. *NCHS Data Brief*, No 327. Hyattsville, MD: National Center for Health Statistics (https://www.cdc.gov/reproductivehealth/contraception/index.htm).

Dehlendorf, C., et al. 2011. Race, ethnicity and differences in contraception among low-income women. *Perspectives on Sexual and Reproductive Health* 43(3): 181-187.

Fine, P., et al. 2010. Ulipristal acetate taken 48-120 hours after intercourse for emergency contraception. *Obstetrics and Gynecology* 115: 257-263.

Guttmacher Institute. 2018. *Global, Regional, and Subregional Trends in Unintended Pregnancy and Its Outcomes from 1990 to 2014: Estimates from a Bayesian Hierarchical Model* (https://www.guttmacher.org/article/2018/03/unintended-pregnancy-and-its-outcomes-global-regional-and-subregional-trends-1990).

Guttmacher Institute. 2018. *Unintended Pregnancy Rates Declined Globally 1990-2014* (https://www.guttmacher.org/news-release/2018/unintended-pregnancy-rates-declined-globally-1990-2014).

Hannaford, P. C., et al. 2010. Mortality among contraceptive pill users: Cohort evidence from Royal College of General Practitioners' Oral Contraception Study. *British Medical Journal*. doi: 10.1136/bmj.c927.

Hatcher, R. A., et al. 2011. *Contraceptive Technology*, 20th ed. New York: Bridging the Gap Foundation.

Jick, S. S., et al. 2010. Postmarketing study of Ortho Evra and levonorgesterol oral contraceptives containing hormonal contraceptives with 30 mcg of ethinyl estradiol in relation to nonfatal venous thromboembolism. *Contraception* 81(1): 16-21.

Kossler, K., et al. 2011. Perceived racial, socioeconomic and gender discrimination and its impact on contraceptive choice. *Contraception* 84(3): 273-279.

Leung, V. W., et al. 2010. Mechanisms of action of hormonal emergency contraceptives. *Pharmacotherapy* 30(2): 158-168.

Livingston, G., and D. Thomas. 2019. Why is the teen birth rate falling? *Fact Tank: News in the Numbers* (https://www.pewresearch.org/fact-tank/2019/08/02/why-is-the-teen-birth-rate-falling/).

Lopez, L. M., et al. 2011. Hormonal contraceptives for contraception in overweight or obese women. *Obstetrics and Gynecology* 116(5): 1206-1207.

Lopez, L. M., et al. 2011. Steroidal contraceptives: Effect on bone fractures in women. *Cochrane Database of Systematic Reviews*, July 6 (7): CD006033.

Lyus, R., et al. 2011. Use of the Mirena LNG-IUS and ParaGard CuT380A intrauterine devices in nulliparous women. *Contraception* 81(5): 367-371.

Macmillan, C. 2019. *Setting the Record Straight on Contraception Misconceptions* (https://www.yalemedicine.org/stories/best-birth-control-options/).

Mansour, D., et al. 2011. Fertility after discontinuation of contraception: A comprehensive review of the literature. *Contraception* 84(5): 465-477.

McNicholas, C., et al. 2015. Use of the etonogestrel implant and levonorgestrel intrauterine device beyond the U.S. Food and Drug Administration-approved duration. *Obstetrics & Gynecology* 125(3): 599-604.

Meirik, O., and T. M. Farley. 2007. Risk of cancer and the oral contraceptive pill. *British Medical Journal* 335(7621): 621-622.

Meyer, J. L., et al. 2011. Advance provision of emergency contraception among adolescent and young adult women: A systematic review of the literature. *Journal of Pediatric and Adolescent Gynecology* 24(1): 2-9.

Michielsen, D., and R. Beerthuizen. 2010. State-of-the-art of non-hormonal methods of contraception: IV. Male sterilization. *European Journal of Contraception and Reproductive Health Care* 15(2): 136-149.

Mohamad, A. M., et al. 2011. Combined contraceptive ring versus combined oral contraceptive. *International Journal of Gynecology and Obstetrics* 114(2): 145-148.

National Alliance of State Pharmacy Association. 2019. *Pharmacist Prescribing: Hormonal Contraceptives* (https://naspa.us/resource/contraceptives/).

National Cancer Institute. 2018. *Oral Contraceptives and Cancer Risk* (https://www.cancer.gov/about-cancer/causes-prevention/risk/hormones/oral-contraceptives-fact-sheet).

National Center for Health Statistics. 2018. *National Survey of Family Growth: Contraception* (http://www.cdc.gov/nchs/nsfg/key_statistics/e.htm#contraception).

Planned Partenthood. 2020. *Title X: The Nation's Program for Affordable Birth Control and Reproductive Health Care* (https://www.plannedparenthoodaction.org/issues/health-care-equity/title-x).

Ramasamy, R., and P. N. Schlegel. 2011. Vasectomy and vasectomy reversal: An update. *Indian Journal of Urology* 27(1): 92-97 (http://www.ncbi.nlm.nih.gov/pmc/articles/PMC3114592/).

Richardson, A. R., and F. N. Maltz. 2012. Ulipristal acetate: Review of the efficacy and safety of a newly approved agent for emergency contraception. *Clinical Therapeutics* 34(1): 24–36.

Sedgh, G., S. Singh, and R. Hussain. 2014. Intended and unintended pregnancies worldwide in 2012 and recent trends. *Studies in Family Planning* 45(3): 301–314.

Sedgh, G., et al. 2015. Adolescent pregnancy, birth, and abortion rates across countries: Levels and recent trends. *Journal of Adolescent Health.* 56(2): 223–230.

United Nations, Department of Economic and Social Affairs, Population Division. 2019. *Contraceptive Use by Method 2019: Data Booklet* (ST/ESA/SER.A/435) (https://www.un.org/en/development/desa/population/publications/pdf/family/ContraceptiveUseByMethodDataBooklet2019.pdf).

U.S. Department of Health and Human Services. 2019. *Approval of Emergency Contraception* (https://www.womenshealth.gov/30-achievements/19).

Van Vliet, H. A., et al. 2011. Triphasic versus monophasic oral contraceptives for contraception. *Cochrane Database of Systematic Reviews*, November 9 (11): CD:003553.

Whittaker, P. G., et al. 2007. Characteristics associated with emergency contraception use by family planning patients: A prospective cohort study. *Perspectives on Sexual and Reproductive Health* 39(3): 158–166.

Winner, B., et al. 2012. Effectiveness of long-acting reversible contraception. *New England Journal of Medicine* 366(21): 1998–2007.

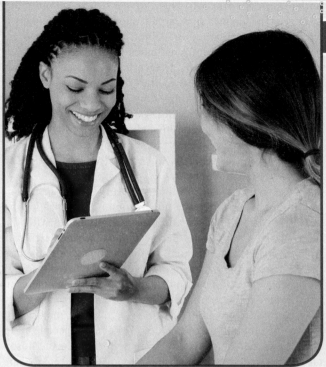

Rocketclips, Inc./Shutterstock

CHAPTER OBJECTIVES

- Summarize the history of abortion in the United States since the 19th century
- Discuss basic facts about abortion and the decision to have one
- Explain the methods of abortion
- Explain postabortion care
- Describe the legal restrictions placed on abortion in the United States
- Explain the current debate over abortion

Abortion

TEST YOUR KNOWLEDGE

1. **What is the most common emotional response of women after an abortion?**
   a. Guilt or regret
   b. Indifference
   c. Acceptance

2. **About what percentage of abortions in the United States take place in the first three months of pregnancy?**
   a. 70%
   b. 80%
   c. 90%

3. **At what point during pregnancy is a fetus generally considered to become viable, meaning it can survive outside the womb?**
   a. 3 months
   b. 6 months
   c. 8 months

4. **A majority of Americans are in favor of the right to a legal abortion in at least some circumstances.**
   True or False?

5. **Although abortion has been legal in the United States since 1973, a majority of American women have limited access to it.**
   True or False?

ANSWERS

1. **C.** Research suggests that over 95% of women who have an abortion believe that it was the right decision for them. Emotions immediately after an abortion may be positive or negative, such as relief, happiness, regret, guilt, sadness, or anger, but the intensity of the emotion fades with time.

2. **C.** Over 90% of all U.S. abortions take place in the first three months of pregnancy; more than 60% take place in the first two months.

3. **B.** Today most clinicians define this point as 23–24 weeks of gestation (about 6 months).

4. **TRUE.** According to a 2019 Gallup poll, 78% of Americans thought abortion should be legal at least under some circumstances; of those, 25% thought it should be legal under any circumstance.

5. **TRUE.** Currently 43 states prohibit abortion after a certain point in pregnancy. In addition, many women live in areas with no abortion providers, which limits their access. Other state-based restrictions pose additional barriers.

While techniques to end pregnancy have changed over time, the practice of abortion goes back thousands of years. In the United States, until the 19th century, abortion was largely a private affair without any government or professional oversight. Women who conceived at times in their lives when having a child was unacceptable either ended the pregnancy themselves or sought help from midwives or apothecaries. Abortion services were advertised in the newspapers and provided by individuals of varying medical competence. During this time, without any regulation or standards, having an abortion was often dangerous or ineffective, resulting in physical harm or having a child.

ABORTION IN THE UNITED STATES SINCE THE 19TH CENTURY

The first anti-abortion campaign was launched in the mid-19th century, and physicians were at the forefront of this movement. They intended to raise the standard of abortion care, mandating that abortions should be performed only by physicians in a hospital setting for health conditions that were life-threatening. Consequently, most abortion care became criminalized because it did not meet these narrow criteria. For instance, it became illegal for a family who could not afford another child to ask a midwife to perform an abortion at home. Instead, the pregnant woman would need to be admitted to the hospital by a physician, which was expensive, and demonstrate that she needed an abortion to save her life. Unfortunately, the techniques used by physicians in hospitals to terminate pregnancies were not necessarily safer than techniques used by nonphysicians in the community.

The new policies criminalizing much of abortion care greatly limited the supply of abortion services, but the demand did not change. This is because the rate of unintended pregnancies did not change as women and men had few options to prevent pregnancy, and available methods of contraception were much less effective than the methods we have today. Many women did not have a serious medical condition to justify an abortion or could not pay for an abortion in the hospital. Consequently, thousands of women who sought to end their pregnancies had no choice but to seek illegal abortions. In desperation, many found themselves using the services of unskilled individuals in unsanitary conditions and suffered injury, subsequent infertility, or death.

By the mid-20th century, the medical profession started to recognize the harms of criminalizing abortion. Also during this time, women's status improved as they entered the labor force and demanded a say over reproductive decisions and access to safe abortion. Abortion was legalized in the United States in 1973 with the landmark Supreme Court decision in *Roe v. Wade,* determining with the following language that abortion is a fundamental right under the due process clause of the 14th Amendment: "Right of privacy . . . is broad enough to encompass a woman's decision whether or not to terminate her pregnancy. . . . The decision vindicates the right of the physician to administer medical treatment according to his professional judgment up to the points where important state interests provide compelling justifications for intervention." This meant that doctors were no longer limited to perform abortions for medical indications only—the reason for an abortion was up to the woman and her doctor within certain constraints such as how far along the woman was in her pregnancy.

Subsequently, legalization of abortion allowed significant improvements in its safety and technique. From a public health perspective, legalization of abortion ranks with the discovery of antibiotics in decreasing the overall death rate from abortion complications. New technologies expanded the provision of abortion in clinics rather than in hospitals exclusively, lowering cost and improving access for women nationwide. As a result, the abortion care we have today looks very different from pre–*Roe v. Wade*: The majority of women who obtain abortions do so in clinics specialized in abortion care. Abortions are rarely performed in the hospital as they once were, and it has become an extremely safe and effective process.

In terms of safety, the evolution of abortion care in the United States is overall a great success and has influenced abortion care worldwide; however, it is not without challenges. The biggest problem created by the current model is the separation of abortion care from other reproductive health care services. Few women turn to their primary care physicians or obstetricians/gynecologists to end a pregnancy, although they obtain other reproductive health services from these providers. Most clinicians in women's health do not offer abortion services even though they could, by investing minimal effort to upgrade their skills. Some clinicians abstain for personal reasons, but a majority are not able to provide abortions even if they want to because institutional rules or logistics make it extremely difficult or impossible to do so. Restricting abortion care to abortion clinics has perpetuated stigma for women seeking abortion and clinicians who perform them, implying that abortion is somehow different from other reproductive services. Furthermore, it has made abortion clinics vulnerable to attacks by extremist individuals and groups that oppose abortion. Since the early 1990s there has been an increase in violence against abortion providers and abortion clinics, including vandalism, bombing, arson, and shootings, some of which have been fatal.

Using the legal system to restrict abortion has become an important strategy in state and national politics by groups opposed to abortion and has shifted the conversation away from the area of health and the status of women in society. Over the past 40 years, some federal and many state laws have tested the limits of *Roe v. Wade* by making it more difficult for a woman to obtain an abortion.

UNDERSTANDING ABORTION

The word **abortion** generally refers to a pregnancy ending. A **spontaneous abortion,** also called a miscarriage, is a pregnancy that ends on its own; it may be an emotionally trying event for some women and their families, and often experienced as a loss.

About 15% of pregnant women experience spontaneous abortions, which occur most frequently during the first trimester. Generally, chromosomal abnormalities lead to an abnormal pregnancy that is incompatible with life and that the body ultimately detects and ends. **Induced abortion,** or pregnancy termination, is a pregnancy that is intentionally ended. The rest of this chapter focuses on induced abortion.

U.S. Abortion Statistics

The decision to have an abortion may be complex or straightforward depending on the circumstances of one's life at that time, and is usually in the context of an unintended pregnancy.

An **unintended pregnancy** includes pregnancies that are (1) *mistimed,* meaning that a woman or couple wanted to conceive but at a later date or (2) *unwanted,* meaning that a woman or couple did not want to conceive at all. Mistimed pregnancies account for 60% of unintended pregnancies, a larger percentage than unwanted pregnancies. Those who do not use contraception at all or do not use contraception consistently or correctly are at greatest risk of having an unintended pregnancy. More than half of women with unintended pregnancies continue their pregnancies and give birth. The remainder of women with unintended pregnancies have either an induced abortion or a miscarriage in relatively equal proportions.

About 900,000 abortions are performed in the United States each year, making abortion the most common procedure that women of reproductive age undergo. In fact, one in five women has an abortion by age 30, making it very likely that each of us knows someone who has had one.

Some argue that if abortion were illegal or significantly restricted, fewer women would have abortions, assuming that a lower abortion rate is a socially desirable goal. History, however, challenges this idea, because women determined to end their pregnancies find a way to have an abortion whether it is legal or not. What criminalizing abortion does is remove important protections for women. In the United States, studies show that legalization did not increase abortions. Researchers estimate that about 800,000 illegal abortions were performed annually in the years before *Roe v. Wade.* The number of legal abortions rose after 1973, reaching a peak in the early 1980s and then declining steadily; the rate in 2017 was the lowest since 1973 (Figure 8.1). Stricter laws that limit access to abortion do not appear to be responsible for the drop, as the decrease has occurred across the nation and not just in states with the most significant restrictions. Pregnancy and birth rates have also declined, most likely due to increased access to and use of contraception to prevent unintended pregnancy. Moreover, the timing of abortions has shifted to earlier in pregnancy, with over 90% taking place within the first 13 weeks.

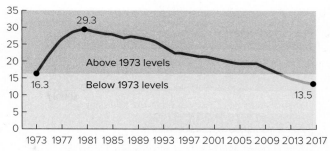

No. of abortions per 1,000 women aged 15–44

FIGURE 8.1 **The U.S. abortion rate reached a historic low in 2017.**

SOURCE: Guttmacher Institute. September 2019. Induced abortion in the United States (https://www.guttmacher.org/fact-sheet/induced-abortion-united-states).

Personal and Social Indicators Several personal and social indicators are commonly given as reasons for terminating a pregnancy (Figure 8.2). These reasons include lack of financial resources; interference with the woman's work, educational aspirations, or ability to care for their children; reluctance to become a single mother; or problems in a relationship. Younger women who become pregnant often report that they are unprepared for the transition to motherhood, whereas older women regularly cite that a pregnancy would interfere with their responsibility to their existing children.

Women who have abortions represent various ages, religions, races, and levels of education. Poverty has been identified as a key factor leading to an abortion. In 2014, 75% of women undergoing an abortion were poor or low income by federal standards.

Fetal and Maternal Indicators Women or couples with a planned pregnancy may ultimately decide to end it if they learn that the fetus has a significant abnormality. Most abortions performed for fetal anomalies occur in the second trimester because fetal problems are typically discovered at this time through genetic testing or a detailed ultrasound.

Due to risks to their own health, pregnant women with serious medical conditions sometimes need to end their pregnancies. These conditions might include severe high blood pressure, a lung disease called pulmonary hypertension, severe kidney disease, advanced diabetes, and severe cardiac disease. Some conditions that already exist can worsen in pregnancy and permanently compromise a woman's health after pregnancy. If she knows that her health is at

> **TERMS**
>
> **abortion** A pregnancy ending.
>
> **spontaneous abortion** Also known as *miscarriage* or *pregnancy loss*; a pregnancy that ends on its own.
>
> **induced abortion** An ongoing pregnancy that is ended deliberately; synonymous with pregnancy termination.
>
> **unintended pregnancy** A mistimed (wrongly timed) or unwanted (not desired at all) pregnancy.

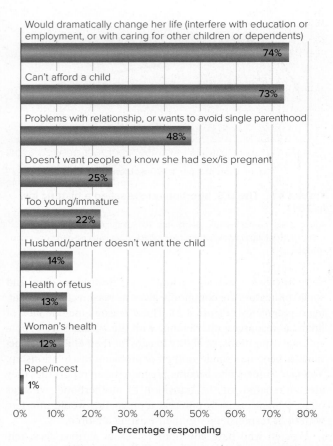

Would dramatically change her life (interfere with education or employment, or with caring for other children or dependents)
74%

Can't afford a child
73%

Problems with relationship, or wants to avoid single parenthood
48%

Doesn't want people to know she had sex/is pregnant
25%

Too young/immature
22%

Husband/partner doesn't want the child
14%

Health of fetus
13%

Woman's health
12%

Rape/incest
1%

0% 10% 20% 30% 40% 50% 60% 70% 80%
Percentage responding

FIGURE 8.2   The reasons women have abortions. Researchers asked women to describe their reasons for deciding to have an abortion.

SOURCE: Finer, L. B., et al. 2005. Reasons U.S. women have abortions. Quantitative and qualitative perspectives. *Perspectives on Sexual and Reproductive Health* 37(3): 110–118.

risk, ending the pregnancy before the fetus becomes **viable** (able to survive outside the womb) may prevent a life-threatening problem.

Personal Considerations for the Woman

For the pregnant woman with an unintended or abnormal pregnancy, the decision about how to proceed is not political, especially as she attempts to weigh the many short- and long-term ramifications for all those who are directly concerned. If she continues the pregnancy, how will her life change by having a child? Can she become a mother to this child? If she has other children, how will another child affect them? How does she feel about adoption? What are her long-term feelings likely to be? (The box "The Adoption Option" addresses some of these questions.) If she ends the pregnancy, does she

viable   Able to survive outside the uterus.   **TERMS**

Ask Yourself

QUESTIONS FOR CRITICAL THINKING AND REFLECTION

Suppose one of your friends has an unplanned pregnancy and does not know what to do. How would you begin discussing how she feels and what options are available to her? What kind of support would you be willing to offer?

feel like it contradicts her own moral or religious beliefs, and if so, can these be reconciled? What are her partner's feelings about having this child? If he is unsupportive, does she have the social and emotional resources to raise the child without him? If she is young, what will be the effects on her own growth? Will she be able to continue with her educational and personal goals? What about the ongoing financial responsibilities?

Personal Considerations for the Man

Men are often involved in the decision-making process with their partners, and they may experience a range of emotions similar to those felt by women. Men may also accompany their partners during the abortion process. Accompaniment may reflect an effort to share responsibility for the pregnancy as well as to provide emotional and practical support by providing transportation or helping to pay for the abortion. Supporting each other through the abortion process may strengthen their relationship. In some instances, men disagree with the woman's decision, and they may try to control the outcome of the pregnancy or may be abusive. Many abortion facilities are sensitive to creating a safe space for women in such situations.

METHODS OF ABORTION

Abortion can be extremely safe. To put it into perspective, it is safer than childbirth. It is usually performed at an outpatient clinic or doctor's office rather than a hospital, and women go home shortly after the visit. The technique used to end the pregnancy depends on how far along a woman is in her pregnancy. Ultrasound (a device that shows an image of the developing fetus) is the most accurate way to determine this. If an ultrasound is not available, the date of the woman's last period and a gynecologic exam provide an estimate.

First-Trimester Abortion

As noted earlier, 90% of abortions in the United States take place in the first trimester. Women who are up to 2.5 months pregnant can choose between taking pills or having a procedure to end the pregnancy. Women who are 2.5–3.5 months pregnant undergo a procedure.

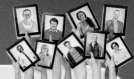

Before abortions were legal, women with unintended pregnancies had the legal options of becoming a parent or pursuing adoption. Before 1979, about 9% of babies born to never-married women were relinquished for adoption, and in the mid-1990s to early 2000s, the number dropped to 1%. This decline may be due to a variety of factors, including an easing of the social stigma of single parenthood. A drop in adoption rates in the 1970s probably reflected an increase in the abortion rate following the 1973 legalization of abortion. Since 1990, however, adoption rates have remained steady, whereas the abortion rate has declined, indicating that overall, women are not choosing abortion over adoption.

Many children who are adopted are adopted by a relative or foster parent. Adoptions in which the child is not related to an adoptive parent(s) are more common among those with higher levels of income and educational attainment.

The decision to go through an unintended pregnancy and then give the baby to another family may be emotionally difficult. Adoption is permanent: The adoptive parents will raise the child and have legal authority for his or her welfare. Many people can help a pregnant woman consider her options, including her partner; friends; family members; a professional counselor; a family planning clinic; or family services, social services, or adoption agencies. A counselor should always be respectful and willing to discuss all three options—continuing the pregnancy and becoming a parent, arranging an adoption, or ending the pregnancy.

Adoptions can be open or closed, also known as confidential. In a confidential adoption, the birth parents and the adoptive parents never know each other. Adoptive parents receive any information that might help them take care of the child. A later meeting between the child and birth parents is possible

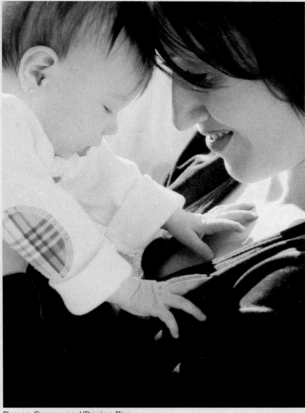

Darren Greenwood/Design Pics

in confidential adoption; laws vary by state, but in many, information about birth parents and adopted individuals can be released if both parties consent (visit childwelfare.gov for additional information).

In an open adoption, the birth parents and adoptive parents know something about each other. The levels of openness range from reading a brief description of prospective adoptive parents to meeting them and sharing full information. Birth parents may also be able to stay in touch with the family by visiting, calling, or writing. In all states, a mother can work with a licensed child placement (adoption) agency. It may also be possible to work directly with an adopting couple or their attorney; this is called a private or independent adoption.

A woman who places the child for adoption should also consider the reaction and rights of the biological father. A woman can choose to have an abortion without the consent or knowledge of the father, but once the baby is born, the father has certain rights. These rights vary from state to state, but at a minimum, most states require that the biological father be notified of the adoption. In some states, the biological father may be able to take the child even if the mother prefers that the child go to an adoptive family. Working with an adoption agency can help a person navigate the laws in each particular state. Throughout the adoption process, the mother should make sure she has the help she needs and that she carefully considers all her options.

SOURCES: Child Welfare Information Gateway. 2014. *Are You Pregnant and Thinking about Adoption?* (https://www.childwelfare.gov/pubs/f _pregna/f_pregna.pdf); Child Welfare Information Gateway. 2005. *Voluntary Relinquishment for Adoption: Numbers and Trends* (https://www.childwelfare.gov/pubs/s_place.pdf); Fisher, A. P. 2003. Still "not quite as good as having your own"? Toward a sociology of adoption. *Annual Review of Sociology* 29: 335–361.

Medical Abortion   **Medical abortion,** also known as *medication abortion* or *abortion pill*, entails taking two medications, mifepristone and misoprostol. Medical abortion is not the same as emergency contraception, also known as the "morning-after pill." Emergency contraception is designed to

> **medical abortion**   A method of ending an early first trimester pregnancy by taking two sets of pills: mifepristone and misoprostol. Misoprostol may be taken at home or in another nonmedical setting.   **TERMS**

prevent pregnancy, whereas medical abortion *ends* an already existing pregnancy.

Women who have a medical abortion take mifepristone in a doctor's office and then go home. They take the second medication, misoprostol, on their own. This second medication causes period-like cramps and causes the pregnancy tissue to pass out of the body, usually within 4 hours but up to 48 hours. The amount of bleeding is similar to that of a heavy period or miscarriage. Women return to see their provider 1–2 weeks later and have an ultrasound or a serum pregnancy test to confirm they are no longer pregnant. Medical abortion successfully ends pregnancies 95–97% of the time. If the woman continues to be pregnant, she may repeat the medications or undergo an aspiration procedure.

Aspiration Abortion   **Aspiration abortion** is another way to end a pregnancy in the first trimester. It is also known as "suction abortion," or dilation and curettage (D&C). This is a procedure performed in a medical facility (usually in an outpatient clinic and rarely in a hospital) by a trained provider. The woman is usually awake, and the procedure is done through the vagina exclusively (no cut on the abdomen). The provider dilates the cervix (opening to the uterus) and inserts a slender tube (called a cannula or suction curette) into the uterus, which is attached to a vacuum device, and removes the pregnancy (Figure 8.3). The procedure may cause strong cramps and usually takes fewer than 10 minutes. Women undergoing the procedure receive a powerful oral or intravenous pain medication in addition to a numbing medication administered vaginally. The cramping subsides once the procedure is over. Women return home the same day—typically within 30 minutes to an hour after the pain medication has worn off.

Aspiration abortions are successful 98% of the time. Many women receive contraception such as an intrauterine device right after the abortion is completed, saving them an extra visit and protecting them from future pregnancy.

Medical vs. Aspiration Abortion in the First Trimester   Some women may have the option of selecting either medical or aspiration abortion to end a first-trimester pregnancy. A number of women feel that medical abortion allows them to take more control of the process and gives them more privacy than an aspiration abortion. Additionally, some women feel it is a more "natural" process

> **QUICK STATS**
>
> **Over a third of abortions at 8 weeks' gestation or less involve taking medications.**
>
> —CDC, 2019

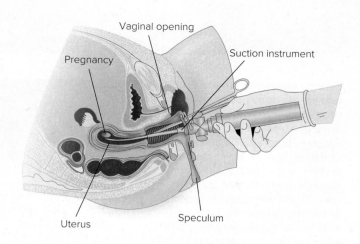

FIGURE 8.3   Suction curettage. This procedure takes 5–10 minutes and can be performed until the end of the first trimester of pregnancy.

because it mimics a miscarriage. It is also a noninvasive alternative to aspiration abortion because no instruments are introduced into the uterus. Most women who select a medical abortion are satisfied with this method.

A downside of medical abortion is that it takes longer to complete, typically at least 24 hours from the time the first pill is taken to the time the pregnancy passes, whereas an aspiration abortion takes about 10 minutes for the entire procedure. Side effects of one of the medications, misoprostol, include nausea, vomiting, diarrhea, fever, and abdominal pain for some women. Women undergoing a medical abortion are typically given additional medications to help with these symptoms. Medical abortion also generally requires more clinic visits, and there is a small risk of failure, which would then require another round of medications or an aspiration procedure. Vaginal bleeding is often more prolonged and in a few cases heavier than with aspiration abortion. The financial cost to the patient is generally about the same.

Second-Trimester Abortion

About 10% of abortions take place in the second trimester (between three and six months of pregnancy). Women who have an abortion at this stage in pregnancy may do so for a variety of reasons: They recognized they were pregnant later in the pregnancy; they had a difficult time finding a facility to have an abortion; they felt conflicted about ending the pregnancy and needed more time to decide; they discovered that the fetus had problems; or they became sick themselves, making it difficult or dangerous to continue the pregnancy. The approach to ending a second-trimester pregnancy depends on where the woman goes for care and how far along she is.

Some medical facilities offer termination of pregnancy by inducing labor with medications, a process called

> **aspiration abortion (D&C)**   A vaginal procedure **TERMS** to end a first-trimester pregnancy that involves aspiration of the uterus; also known as *suction abortion, suction curettage,* or *dilation and curettage.*

Ask Yourself

QUESTIONS FOR CRITICAL THINKING AND REFLECTION

How may restrictive abortion laws increase the number of women who have second-trimester abortions? Do these laws affect poor women differently than they do more affluent women? What about the variation among states in abortion laws and number of providers?

?

induction abortion. Other facilities offer surgery called **dilation and evacuation (D&E),** the most common method of second-trimester pregnancy termination in the United States. While similar to a first-trimester abortion, a D&E may take longer, and women typically receive stronger pain medications. Dilation and evacuation is typically done as outpatient surgery, but a woman may need to visit the health care provider or clinic the day before to take medications or begin the process of dilating the cervix. Under general or regional anesthesia, the fetus is surgically removed from the uterus through the vagina, and suction is used to remove any remaining tissue; women can usually go home the same day. Soreness and cramping may occur for a day or two after the procedure, and some bleeding may last for 1–2 weeks. Second-trimester pregnancy termination is also very safe.

POSTABORTION CONSIDERATIONS

The recovery after an abortion is rapid, usually lasting a few days, and most women do not need to significantly modify their everyday activities as part of recovery. Abortion does not cause infertility, jeopardize a woman's ability to have children in the future, compromise her reproductive organs, or increase her chances of cancer. The incidence of immediate problems following an abortion (infection, bleeding, trauma to the cervix or uterus, and incomplete abortion requiring repeat curettage) is rare. The potential for problems is reduced significantly by a woman's good health, early timing of the abortion, use of the suction method compared to an older technique using sharp curettage, performance by a well-trained clinician, and the availability and use of prompt follow-up care.

Problems related to infection can be minimized through preabortion testing and treatment for gonorrhea, chlamydia, and other infections. Also, women are given antibiotics at the time of the procedure to decrease the likelihood of infection. Postabortion danger signs are as follows:

- Fever above 100°F
- Abdominal pain or swelling, cramping, or backache
- Abdominal tenderness (to pressure)
- Prolonged or heavy bleeding
- Foul-smelling vaginal discharge
- Vomiting or fainting

Possible Emotional Effects

Is there a risk that women who have an abortion face long-term mental health consequences? Would they be better off by having the child instead? The Turnaway Study was designed to answer these questions. It recruited pregnant women between 2008 and 2010 across the United States who wanted to end their pregnancies. It compared women who successfully had an abortion to women who were "turned away" because the medical facilities where they sought care deemed their pregnancies to be too far along. (Medical facilities and state laws determine limits for performing procedures and vary widely. Women who got an abortion and those who were turned away were similarly far along in their pregnancies.) The study found that a person's feelings toward an unintended pregnancy and feelings toward having an abortion are mixed—many women felt regret about an unwanted pregnancy and felt that the decision to have an abortion was the right decision for them.

Most women who were denied an abortion gave birth and adjusted to motherhood, happy to have that child. Nine percent of the women pursued adoption. Rates of mental health problems were not higher in women who had an abortion compared to women who gave birth or vice versa. This shows that abortion does not typically lead to mental health problems. The most profound measurable effect in the women who were denied an abortion and had a child was economic. They had four times greater odds of ending up below the federal poverty level and three times greater odds of being unemployed compared to women who had abortions, despite having similar socioeconomic status before the pregnancy. As many women predict when making a decision to have an abortion, having a child significantly strains their resources.

LEGAL RESTRICTIONS ON ABORTION

In 1973 in the landmark case of *Roe v. Wade,* the U.S. Supreme Court made abortion legal in every state in the United States. To replace the restrictions most states still imposed at that time, the justices devised new standards to govern abortion decisions. They divided pregnancy into three parts, or *trimesters,* giving a woman less choice about abortion as her pregnancy advances toward full term. According to *Roe v. Wade,* in the first trimester, the abortion decision must be left

---

induction abortion A method to end a second-trimester pregnancy by administering medications to induce labor and delivery of a fetus.

dilation and evacuation (D&E) A vaginal procedure to end a second-trimester pregnancy that involves surgical removal of the pregnancy from the uterus.

TERMS

to the judgment of the pregnant woman and her physician. During the second trimester, similar rights remain up to the point when the fetus becomes viable. Today most clinicians define this point as 24 weeks of gestation. When the fetus is considered viable, a state may regulate and even bar all abortions except those considered necessary to preserve the mother's life or health.

Three years after *Roe v. Wade,* Congress passed the Hyde Amendment, which prevents the use of federal funds (such as Medicaid) to pay for an abortion unless the pregnancy arises from incest or rape or if the woman's life is endangered. In practice, this amendment affects women who rely on Medicaid to pay for medical services. They must pay out of pocket for abortion-related care, and if they are unable to pay or they take too long to raise funds, they may be compelled to continue their pregnancies. Concerns have been raised that a two-tiered system has been created—one for women with means to pay for an abortion and another for those without.

Since 1973, many campaigns have been waged to overturn the *Roe v. Wade* decision, whereas other campaigns have tried to strengthen the rights provided by the decision. Although abortion remains legal throughout the United States, subsequent rulings by the Supreme Court, starting with *Planned Parenthood of Southeastern Pennsylvania v. Casey* (1992), have allowed states to regulate abortion throughout pregnancy as long as no "undue burden" is imposed on women seeking these services. (Figure 8.4 shows the availability of clinics offering abortions for women in different states.) The following are examples of restrictive laws that exist on the state level:

- ***Physician and hospital requirements.*** Forty states require an abortion to be performed by a licensed physician. Nineteen

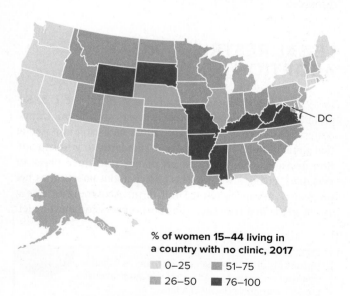

% of women 15–44 living in a country with no clinic, 2017

- 0–25
- 26–50
- 51–75
- 76–100

FIGURE 8.4 **In 25 states, the majority of women live in a county with no abortion clinic**

SOURCE: Jones, R. K., E. Witwer, and J. Jerman. 2019. Abortion incidence and service availability in the United States, 2017. Guttmacher Institute, New York.

states require an abortion to be performed in a hospital after a specified point in the pregnancy, and 17 states require the involvement of a second physician after a specified point.

Studies show that other medical professionals such as nurse practitioners, nurse-midwives, and physician assistants can safely provide abortions. Permitting other providers to perform abortions expands access to abortion. Abortion is held to the same safety standards as all other medical treatments in the United States, and additional regulation is not necessary.

- ***State-mandated counseling.*** Eighteen states mandate that, before an abortion, women have counseling that includes information on at least one of the following: the purported link between abortion and breast cancer (5 states), the ability of a fetus to feel pain (13 states), or long-term mental health consequences for the woman (8 states).

- ***Refusal.*** Forty-five states allow individual health care providers to refuse to participate in an abortion.

Such laws are problematic because there is no standard to meet to show that refusal is on moral grounds ("conscientious") rather than on the basis of political beliefs, stigma, inaccurate understanding of medical evidence, personal inconvenience, or other reasons. Furthermore, if a medical professional refuses, there are no systems in place to ensure that a woman still gets the care she is seeking.

There is no evidence to suggest that abortions lead to breast cancer or have other long-term consequences for women, as discussed earlier in this chapter. Furthermore, there is no biological evidence that a fetus feels pain.

- ***Waiting periods.*** Twenty-seven states require a woman seeking an abortion to wait a specified period of time, usually 24 hours, between the time she receives counseling and when the procedure is performed.

Strong evidence suggests that women have made up their minds to have an abortion prior to seeking an abortion and that it is not a decision taken lightly. Mandating a waiting time creates an extra hurdle to having an abortion and is not founded on a medical explanation.

- ***Parental involvement.*** Thirty-seven states require some type of parental involvement in a minor's decision to have an abortion. Twenty-six states require one or both parents to consent to the procedure.

Parental involvement has not been shown to protect minors as purported and may cause harm when a minor has abusive parents or is pregnant as a result of incest. Such regulation may also motivate a minor to travel out of state to get an abortion. These restrictions do not improve communication between minors and their parents because most minors already tell their parents they are having an abortion when they feel it is safe to do so. In general, mandatory delay laws like waiting periods and parental involvement have been found to delay access to abortion, resulting in abortions at later gestational ages.

Since the composition of the U.S. Supreme Court became more conservative in 2018, some states have passed laws to ban abortions in the first trimester or early in the second trimester, directly challenging *Roe v. Wade.* Examples include

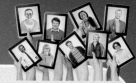

The top four causes of pregnancy-related deaths in the world are hemorrhage, infections, pregnancy-induced hypertension, and unsafe abortion. Unsafe abortions account for 13% of maternal deaths globally. An unsafe abortion is a procedure performed by a person without the appropriate training or in a setting that does not conform to minimal medical standards. Of all induced abortions performed in industrialized countries, 1% are performed unsafely, in contrast to the 56% in developing countries. The wide majority of these unsafe abortions (98%) occur in developing countries with restrictive abortion laws and limited access to family planning and abortion services. Of the women who survive unsafe abortion, 5 million suffer long-term health complications such as injuries to the genitals, reproductive organs, intestines, and bladder—injuries that result in infertility, incontinence, and chronic pain.

Anti-Abortion Laws

Many countries with strict anti-abortion laws have high abortion-related complications because women undergo abortions in secret and in unsafe conditions. Romania provides a stark example of how a ban on abortion can have devastating effects on a nation. Nicolae Ceaușescu came into power in 1965 and enforced pronatalist policies affecting contraception and abortion. Abortion was illegal unless the woman's life was endangered; one of the parents had a

dangerous hereditary illness; the woman was over 40 years old; the woman had at least four children who were in her care; or the pregnancy was a result of rape or incest.

During this time, contraceptives were neither manufactured nor imported. Thus one's ability to prevent pregnancy or end pregnancy was extremely limited, resulting in a drop in abortion rates and a rise in birth rates. After two years, the police stopped intensely monitoring physicians and patients, and abortion rates rose. Although some women could afford an illegal abortion, the most economically disadvantaged women attempted abortions themselves.

During the Ceaușescu regime, Romania had the highest recorded maternal mortality ratio in Europe: 170 maternal deaths per 100,000 births, 87% of which were attributed to abortion complications. Ceaușescu was executed in 1989, and the new government repealed the restrictive abortion law. By 1990, the proportion of maternal deaths due to unsafe abortion dropped to 69%. By 2006, the abortion-related mortality ratio was becoming more comparable to those in other European countries.

Other Considerations

The way laws are interpreted can be just as critical as the existence of laws. For example, in some countries that allow abortion for mental health reasons, the law is interpreted to allow the major-

ity of women seeking abortions to obtain them. The attitudes and beliefs of the medical community also influence the availability of abortion services. In Nigeria, for example, many physicians perform abortions despite legal bans because the medical community believes in the need for safe abortion services. In contrast, major medical associations in Poland and Ireland have adopted guidelines that are stricter than their countries' laws.

The number and location of abortion providers and the cost of abortion services also influence the true availability of abortion in a particular country, regardless of the procedure's legal status. Opposition to abortion among some physicians and communities has left parts of the United States, Austria, and Germany without abortion providers, even though abortion is legal in all three countries. In contrast, policies in Denmark go beyond just permitting safe abortion to ensuring that services are widely available. There, each county must have at least one hospital with the capability of providing abortion services, and the services are free.

SOURCES: Benson, J., et al. 2011. Reductions in abortion-related mortality following policy reform: Evidence from Romania, South Africa and Bangladesh. *Reproductive Health*; Guttmacher Institute. 2017. *In Brief: Facts on Induced Abortion Worldwide* (http://www.guttmacher.org/fact-sheet/induced-abortion-worldwide); Singh, S., et al. 2009. Abortion Worldwide: *A Decade of Uneven Progress*. New York: Guttmacher Institute.

---

prohibiting all abortions as early as at conception or after a fetal heart rate can be detected by ultrasound, which happens before many women know they are pregnant (around 6 weeks). These laws have not gone into effect due to ongoing litigation.

In contrast, in recent years, some states have passed laws in support of abortion rights and access. Some examples include protecting access to abortion clinics, allowing clinicians other than physicians to perform abortions, and requiring public and private health insurance to cover abortion services. For example, California has all of these laws supportive of abortion, and in 2019 the state enacted a law requiring public universities to provide medical abortion in

their health centers. It was the first state in the country to pass such a law. On June 29, 2020, the U.S. Supreme Court blocked a Louisiana law that would have resulted in only one doctor in the state being qualified to perform abortions.

THE PUBLIC DEBATE ABOUT ABORTION

Abortion is one of the most polarized and politicized issues of our times and has been since the 1960s (see the box "Abortion around the World"). Americans have been willing to self-identify as "pro-life" or "pro-choice," though most hold middle-ground views and do not fall neatly into one of these two categories. A percentage of this middle-ground group instinctively feels that the fetus gains increasing human value as a pregnancy advances. In this view, first-trimester abortion is acceptable, but later-term abortion should be performed only when the mother's health is in jeopardy.

Pro-life groups oppose abortion on the basis of their belief that life begins at conception. They believe that the fertilized egg must be afforded the same rights as a human being. This view holds that any woman who has sexual intercourse knows that pregnancy is a possibility; therefore, should she willingly have intercourse and get pregnant, she is morally obligated to carry the pregnancy through. For women who feel they are unable to raise a child, pro-life groups encourage adoption.

Pro-choice groups support the view that the decision to continue or end a pregnancy is a personal matter and that a woman should not be compelled to carry a pregnancy to term if she does not want to have a child. This view holds that distinctions must be made between the stages of fetal development, that the fetus is part of the pregnant woman, and that she has priority over it. Members of this group argue that pregnancy can result from contraceptive failure or other factors out of a couple's control. (All contraceptive methods except abstinence have the potential for failure.) When pregnancy occurs, pro-choice supporters believe that the most moral decision possible must be determined according to each situation and that, in some cases, greater injustice could result if abortion were not an option.

Opinions about abortion have remained generally consistent over time. Although nearly half of Americans feel that abortion is morally wrong, an overwhelming majority supports legal availability of abortion services in some circumstances (see Figure 8.5). Most Americans oppose governmental regulation of women's reproductive decisions and also feel that paying for an abortion should be an individual's responsibility. Most do not support the use of public funds to help poor women obtain abortions; they also do not support the inclusion of abortion benefits in a national basic health care plan.

Although the most vocal groups in the abortion debate tend to paint a black-or-white picture, most Americans view abortion as a complex issue and prefer to focus on preventive strategies. Because the most common reason for abortion is unintended pregnancy, more effort should be dedicated to sex education and access to effective contraception. Also, more effort should be dedicated to creating a society with policies that make it easier to raise a child. Examples of such policies include parental leave,

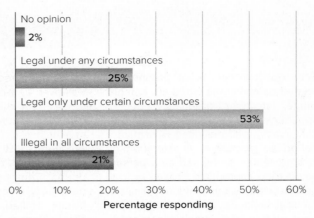

FIGURE 8.5 **Public opinion about abortion.**

SOURCE: Gallup Inc. 2019. "Abortion." *In Depth: Topics A to Z.* Gallup Inc. (http://www.gallup.com/poll/1576/abortion.aspx).

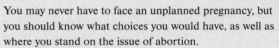

About one in four American women has an abortion before she turns 45.

—Jones and Jerman, 2017

child care programs for working parents, and reduced costs for education and health care. This broader approach expands reproductive rights to include economic, social, and health rights and describes the principles of the reproductive justice movement.

TIPS FOR TODAY AND THE FUTURE

You may never have to face an unplanned pregnancy, but you should know what choices you would have, as well as where you stand on the issue of abortion.

RIGHT NOW YOU CAN:

- Examine your feelings about the possibility of becoming a parent, especially if it were to happen unintentionally.
- Consider your views on the morality of abortion, and under which circumstances it would be acceptable to you.

IN THE FUTURE YOU CAN:

- If you are sexually active or plan to become sexually active, talk to your partner about the possibility of pregnancy. How would you proceed? Do you share similar views and feelings, or do they differ? How would you resolve conflicts about this issue?
- If you are sexually active, reexamine your contraceptive method and make sure you are using this method correctly and consistently. Become familiar with emergency contraception in case your method fails or you forget to use it. Remember that, aside from abstinence, no method of contraception is 100% effective.

SUMMARY

- From the first anti-abortion campaigns of the mid-19th century, through the landmark *Roe v. Wade* Supreme Court decision of 1973, which legalized abortion in the United States, through the heated debate that continues today, abortion is a health issue that has also become politicized.

- Abortion generally refers to a pregnancy ending. In medical terms there are two distinct types of abortion: *spontaneous abortion* and *induced abortion*. A spontaneous abortion is a pregnancy that ends on its own and is referred to as *miscarriage* or *pregnancy loss*. Induced abortion is an ongoing pregnancy that is ended deliberately.

- Couples confronted with an unplanned pregnancy have the option of continuing the pregnancy and becoming parents, placing the child for adoption, or having an abortion.

- Unintended pregnancy (mistimed or unwanted) is the most common reason women have an abortion. Abortion is the most common procedure that women of reproductive age undergo.

- Most induced abortions take place in the first trimester of pregnancy. Methods include taking medications or undergoing an aspiration procedure. Both methods are extremely safe, safer than childbirth, and complications are rare. Complications are less likely if a woman has overall good health and has an abortion earlier in pregnancy.

- Second-trimester abortions are less common than first-trimester abortions and occur when women discover they are pregnant later in the pregnancy, have decreased access to abortion services, need more time to decide, or learn that their health may be compromised by continuing the pregnancy or that the fetus has significant problems.

- Women's and men's emotional responses after an abortion include relief, happiness, regret, guilt, sadness, or anger; the strongest feelings usually occur immediately after the abortion. Research suggests that over 95% of women who have an abortion believe that it was the right decision for them.

- The 1973 *Roe v. Wade* Supreme Court case legalized abortion in all states and devised new standards to govern abortion decisions; based on the trimesters of pregnancy, it limited a woman's choices as her pregnancy advanced. Although the Supreme Court continues to uphold its 1973 decision, later rulings gave states further power to regulate abortion. Many state regulations have decreased women's access to abortion services.

- The controversy between pro-life and pro-choice viewpoints focuses on the issue of when life begins. Pro-life groups believe that a fertilized egg is a human life from the moment of conception and that a woman is obligated to carry a pregnancy to term. Pro-choice groups distinguish between stages of fetal development and argue that the fetus does not have an equal status to the pregnant woman and that the woman should make the final decision regarding her pregnancy. Most Americans are not completely pro-life or pro-choice but fall somewhere on the spectrum.

- Overall, public opinion in the United States supports legal abortion in at least some circumstances and opposes overturning *Roe v. Wade*.

FOR MORE INFORMATION

American Congress of Obstetricians and Gynecologists: Induced Abortion. Provides medical information about abortion methods.

http://www.acog.org/Patients/FAQs/Induced-Abortion

Child Welfare Information Gateway. A clearinghouse of information about many aspects of child rearing, including adoption.

http://www.childwelfare.gov

Gallup Poll. A company that conducts public opinion polls. Abortion is one topic routinely polled.

http://www.gallup.com/poll/1576/abortion.aspx

Guttmacher Institute. Publishes books and fact sheets about reproductive health issues; its journal, *The Guttmacher Policy Review,* provides timely analysis of national reproductive health policy debates.

http://www.guttmacher.org

MedlinePlus: Abortion. Managed by the U.S. National Library of Medicine and the National Institutes of Health, this site provides a list of informational resources about various aspects of abortion.

http://www.nlm.nih.gov/medlineplus/abortion.html

National Abortion and Reproductive Rights Action League. Provides information about the politics of the pro-choice movement. Also provides information about the abortion laws and politics in each state.

http://www.prochoiceamerica.org

National Abortion Federation. Provides information and resources on medical and political issues relating to abortion; managed by health care providers.

http://www.prochoice.org

National Adoption Center. A national agency focused on finding adoptive homes for children with special needs or who are currently in foster care.

http://www.adopt.org

National Right to Life Committee. Provides information about pregnancy continuation and the politics of the pro-life movement.

http://www.nrlc.org

Planned Parenthood Federation of America. Provides information about family planning, contraception, and abortion and provides counseling services.

http://www.plannedparenthood.org

See also the listings for Chapters 6, 7, and 9.

SELECTED BIBLIOGRAPHY

Advancing New Standards in Reproductive Health. Turnaway Study (http://www.ansirh.org/research/turnaway.php).

Altshuler, A. L., et al. 2016. Male partners' involvement in abortion care: A mixed methods systematic review. *Perspectives on Sexual and Reproductive Health* 48(4): 209–219.

Altshuler, A. L., et al. 2017. A good abortion experience: A qualitative exploration of women's needs and preferences in clinical care. *Social Science & Medicine* 191:109–116.

Altshuler, A., H. Gerns Storey, and S. Prager. 2015. Exploring abortion attitudes of US adolescents and young adults using social media. *Contraception* 91(3): 226–233.

American College of Obstetricians and Gynecologists. 2015. *Frequently Asked Questions: Induced Abortion* (http://www.acog.org/Patients/FAQs/Induced-Abortion).

Barnes, R. 2020. Supreme Court strikes down restrictive Louisiana abortion law that would have closed clinic. *The Washington Post*, 29 June (https://www.washingtonpost.com/politics/courts_law/supreme-court-louisiana-abortion-law-john-roberts/2020/06/29/6f42067e-ba00-11ea-8cf5-9c1b8d7f84c6_story.html).

Biggs, M., A. H. Gould, and D. G. Foster. 2013. Understanding why women seek abortions in the U.S. *BMC Women's Health* 13(1): 29.

Boonstra, H., et al. 2006. *Abortion in Women's Lives*. New York: Guttmacher Institute (https://www.guttmacher.org/report/abortion-womens-lives).

Cates, W., D. A. Grimes, and K. F. Schulz. 2004. The public health impact of legal abortion: 30 years later. *Perspectives on Sexual and Reproductive Health* 35(1): 25–28.

Charles, V., et al. 2008. Abortion and long-term mental health outcomes: A systematic review of the evidence. *Contraception* 78(6): 436–450.

Cohen, S. A. 2007. New data on abortion incidence, safety illuminate key aspects of worldwide abortion debate. *Guttmacher Policy Review* 10(4): 2–5.

Curtin S. C., J. C. Abma, and K. Kost. 2015. 2010 pregnancy rates among U.S. women (http://www.cdc.gov/nchs/data/hestat/pregnancy/2010_pregnancy_rates.htm).

Donovan, M. 2017. In real life: Federal restrictions on abortion coverage and the women they impact. *Guttmacher Policy Review* 20: 1–7.

Ely, G. E., and C. N. Dulmus. 2010. Disparities in access to reproductive health options for female adolescents. *Social Work in Public Health* 25(3): 341–351.

Finer L. B., and K. Kost. 2011. Unintended pregnancy rates at the state level. *Perspectives on Sexual and Reproductive Health* 43(2): 78–87.

Finer, L. B., and M. R. Zolna. 2016. Declines in unintended pregnancy in the United States, 2008–2011. *New England Journal of Medicine* 374(9): 843–852.

Fisher, A. P. 2003. Still "not quite as good as having your own"? Toward a sociology of adoption. *Annual Review of Sociology* 29: 335–361.

Foster, D. G., et. al. 2018. Socioeconomic outcomes of women who receive and women who are denied wanted abortions. *American Journal of Public Health*. DOI:10.2105/AJPH.2017.304247

Freedman, L. 2010. *Willing and Unable. Doctors' Constraints in Abortion Care*. Nashville, TN: Vanderbilt University Press.

Fritz, M. A., and L. Speroff, eds. 2010. *Clinical Gynecologic Endocrinology and Infertility*, 8th ed. Philadelphia: Lippincott Williams & Wilkins.

Grimes, D. A. 2006. Estimation of pregnancy-related mortality risk by pregnancy outcome, United States, 1991 to 1999. *American Journal of Obstetrics and Gynecology* 194(1): 92–94.

Grimes, D. A., et al. 2006. Unsafe abortion: The preventable pandemic. *Lancet* 368: 908–919.

Guttmacher Institute. 2019. *Fact Sheet: Induced Abortion in the United States* (https://www.guttmacher.org/fact-sheet/induced-abortion-united-states).

Guttmacher Institute. 2019. *State Policy Updates. Major Developments in Sexual & Reproductive Health* (https://www.guttmacher.org/state-policy/explore/state-funding-%ADabortion-under-medicaid).

Guttmacher Institute. 2019. *Fact Sheet: Unintended Pregnancy in the United States* (https://www.guttmacher.org/fact-sheet/unintended-pregnancy-united-states)

Harris, L. H. 2012. Recognizing conscience in abortion provision. *The New England Journal of Medicine* 367(11): 981–983.

Jatlaoui, T. C., et al. 2019. Abortion surveillance—United States, 2016. *MMWR Surveillance Summaries* 68(SS-11): 1–41.

Jerman, J., R. K. Jones, and T. Onda. 2016. *Characteristics of U.S. Abortion Patients in 2014 and Changes Since 2008*. New York: Guttmacher Institute (https://www.guttmacher.org/report/characteristics-us-abortion-patients-2014).

Joffe, C. 1995. *Doctors of Conscience. The Struggle to Provide Abortion before and after* Roe v. Wade. Boston, MA: Beacon.

Jones, R. K., and J. Jerman. 2017. Characteristics and circumstances of U.S. women who obtain very early and second-trimester abortions. *PLoS ONE* 12(1): e0169969.

Jones, R. K. et al. 2019. *Abortion Incidence and Service Availability in the United States, 2017*. New York: Guttmacher Institute (https://www.guttmacher.org/report/abortion-incidence-service-availability-us-2017).

Kulier, R., et al. 2011. Medical methods for first trimester abortion. *Cochrane Database Systematic Review* 11: CD002885.

Lie, M. L., S. C. Robson, and C. R. May. 2008. Experiences of abortion: A narrative review of qualitative studies. *BMC Health Services Research* 8(1): 150.

Major, B., et al. 1998. Personal resilience, cognitive appraisals, and coping: An integrative model of adjustment to abortion. *Journal of Personality and Social Psychology* 74(3): 735–752.

Major, B., et al. 2008. *Report of the APA Task Force on Mental Health and Abortion*. Washington, DC: American Psychological Association, pp. 1–107 (http://www.apa.org/pi/women/programs/abortion/mental-health.pdf).

National Abortion Federation. 2009. *Management of Unintended and Abnormal Pregnancy. Comprehensive Abortion Care*. Oxford, UK: Blackwell Publishing.

Raymond, E. G., and D. A. Grimes. 2012. The comparative safety of legal induced abortion and childbirth in the United States. *Obstetrics and Gynecology* 119(2.1): 215–219.

Riddle, J. 1999. *Eve's Herbs: A History of Contraception and Abortion in the West*. Cambridge, MA: Harvard University Press.

Rocca, C., et al. 2015. Decision rightness and emotional responses to abortion in the United States: A longitudinal study. *PLoS ONE* 10(7): e0128832.

Ross, L., and R. Solinger. 2017. *Reproductive Justice: A New Vision for the 21st Century*. Oakland: University of California Press.

Sedgh, G., J. et al. Alkema. 2016. Abortion incidence between 1990 and 2014: Global, regional, and subregional levels and trends. *Lancet* 388(10041): 258–267.

Smith, T. W., and J. Son. 2013. *Final Report. Trends in Public Attitudes toward Abortion*. NORC, University of Chicago (http://www.norc.org/PDFs/GSS_abortion2013_final.pdf).

SteelFisher, G. K., and J. M. Benson. 2010. Attitudes about abortion. In *American Public Opinion and Health Care* (pp. 264–291), ed. R. M. Blendon, R., et al. Washington, DC: CQ Press.

Stoll, B. J., et al. 2015. Trends in care practices, morbidity, and mortality of extremely preterm neonates, 1993–2012. *JAMA* 314(10): 1039–1051.

Upadhyay, U. D., et al. 2014. Denial of abortion because of provider gestational age limits in the United States. *American Journal of Public Health* 104(9): 1687–1694.

Ventura, S. J., et al. 2014. Estimated pregnancy rates and rates of pregnancy outcomes for the United States, 1990–2008. *National Vital Statistics Reports* 60(7): 1–22.

Weitz, T. A., et al. 2013. Safety of aspiration abortion performed by nurse practitioners, certified nurse midwives, and physician assistants under a California legal waiver, *American Journal of Public Health* 103(3): 454–461.

World Health Organization. 2011. *Unsafe Abortion: Global and Regional Estimates of the Incidence of Unsafe Abortion and Associated Mortality in 2008*, 6th ed., pp. 1–67 (http://whqlibdoc.who.int/publications/2011/9789241501118_eng.pdf).

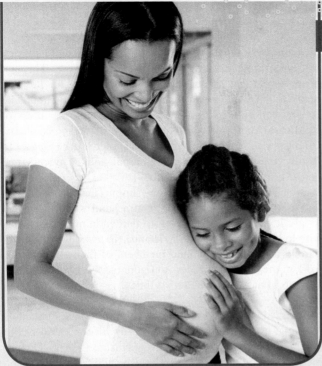

Monkey Business Images/Shutterstock

- List key issues to consider when preparing for parenthood
- Explain the principles of fertility and infertility
- Describe the physical and emotional changes related to pregnancy
- Identify the stages of fetal development
- Explain the importance of good prenatal care
- Understand potential complications of pregnancy
- Describe the choices and processes related to childbirth

CHAPTER **9**

Pregnancy and Childbirth

TEST YOUR KNOWLEDGE

1. A pregnancy is considered "high risk" under which of the following conditions:
   a. The mother is over age 35
   b. The mother is under age 20
   c. The father is over age 35
   d. The father is under age 20

2. A fertilized egg is called a *blastocyst*.
   True or False?

3. Before conception and in the early weeks of pregnancy, adequate intake of which of the following nutrients can reduce the risk of spina bifida and other neural tube defects in the baby?
   a. Iron
   b. Folic acid
   c. Calcium

4. Which theory might explain sudden infant death syndrome?
   a. The child was exposed to tobacco.
   b. The child slept on its stomach.
   c. The child had a brain abnormality.
   d. The child slept with fluffy pillows.

ANSWERS

1. **A AND B.** A woman's age is considered a high-risk factor for pregnancy.

2. **FALSE.** A fertilized egg is called a *zygote*. A *blastocyst* is the next stage of development after zygote.

3. **B.** Daily consumption of a minimum of 400 mg of folic acid from fortified foods and supplements is recommended for all reproductive-age women who intend to get pregnant to reduce the risk of spina bifida and other neural tube defects in their future child.

4. **ALL OF THE ABOVE.** Sudden infant death syndrome (SIDS), a sudden and unexpected death of a child less than 1 year of age, may result from any of these conditions.

Deciding whether to become a parent is one of the most important choices you will ever make. Yet many people approach this decision with only a vague notion of what is involved in pregnancy and childbirth.

The more you know about conception, embryology, pregnancy, prenatal care, childbirth, and parenting, the better able you will be to make informed decisions about them.

PREPARATION FOR PARENTHOOD

Before you decide whether or when to become a parent, you should consider your suitability and readiness. If you elect to have a child, there are actions you can take before the pregnancy begins to help ensure a healthy outcome for all.

Deciding to Become a Parent

Some issues are relevant for everyone who is considering parenthood; others apply only to women.

Health and Age   Generally speaking, healthier women tend to have more trouble-free pregnancies and healthier babies. Women considering motherhood should see their physicians for complete medical checkups to catch problems that can interfere with pregnancy or childbirth. For example, high blood pressure, diabetes, renal disease, cardiac disease, and rheumatologic disorders may require ongoing attention. If uncontrolled, these health problems can pose life-threatening dangers to a mother or child.

A mother's age can also be a factor in pregnancy and childbirth. Teenagers and women over age 35 have a higher incidence of certain problems that can affect the health of both mother and baby. In fact, most experts classify a pregnancy as "high risk" if the mother is a teenager or over age 35, especially if it is her first pregnancy.

Emotional Wellness   Just as they need to be physically prepared, parents also need to be emotionally ready to have a child. A new baby is totally helpless and relies on adults for everything. For parents, emotional preparedness means being strong and stable enough to handle the responsibility and being mature enough to give up certain freedoms in order to care for a child.

Relationships   The stress and expense of child rearing can strain any relationship, even a healthy one. Through open, honest discussion, partners should make sure they are ready to take the step of having a child. Both should be equally committed to parenthood and agree on matters of child care, housework, and other day-to-day responsibilities. Couples with relationship problems should work together to resolve their issues—with professional help, if necessary—before adding a child to the mix.

New parents also need a strong support network of friends and family members who can lend a hand when things get tough. It can be easy, however, to burden family and friends with too many requests for assistance. To avoid this problem, parents-to-be should include members of their support network in the planning process to figure out who will be able to help, in what ways, and at what times.

Financial Circumstances   Parenthood is financially draining, even for families with steady incomes and health insurance. According to a 2017 report from the U.S. Department of Agriculture, a two-parent, two-child family will spend between $9330 and $23,380 per year per child, depending on where they live, subsidies, and the family's income level, to raise each child to age 18. Expenses increase significantly with each additional child.

If you plan to have a child, you should be prepared financially—especially during the first few years, when the costs of diapers, furniture, pediatrician visits, and other necessities quickly add up. All told, the average estimated expense to raise a child from birth through age 17 is $233,610 for a middle-income married-couple family with two children.

Child care is an important expense to plan for, especially when both parents are working or in school full time. The cost and availability of such services can be a factor in determining whether parents can pursue their future plans. According to a 2019 report from Child Care Aware, the yearly day care costs for an infant vary widely, from $5760 in Mississippi to $24,081 in Washington, DC. Nationwide, families spend 11-36% of their income on child care.

Preconception Care

The birth of a healthy baby depends in part on the mother's overall wellness *before* conception. The U.S. Public Health Service recommends that all women receive health care to help them prepare for pregnancy. **Preconception care** should include an assessment of health risks, the promotion of healthy lifestyle behaviors, and any treatments necessary to

> ## QUICK STATS
> **Over 125,000 babies were born to mothers aged 40 and over in 2017.**
> —National Center for Health Statistics, 2018

preconception care   Health care in preparation for pregnancy.   **TERMS**

reduce risk. Following are some of the issues, tests, and treatments parents-to-be may encounter in preconception care:

- **Preexisting conditions.** Medical conditions such as diabetes, cardiac and renal disease, epilepsy, asthma, psychiatric disease, and anemia can cause problems during pregnancy. Such conditions should be treated and monitored throughout pregnancy.

- **Medications.** Some medications and dietary supplements harm the **fetus,** so a pregnant woman may need to change medications or stop taking certain drugs.

- **Prior pregnancies.** Problems with previous pregnancies or deliveries—such as miscarriage, premature birth, or delivery complications—may be due to treatable physical conditions.

- **Age.** A woman's age may place her at risk for certain problems during pregnancy. A pregnant teenager, for example, may require special nutrition to meet her own growing body's needs and those of her baby.

- **Tobacco, alcohol, and caffeine use.** These substances can harm a developing fetus. Exposure to tobacco smoke may also harm the developing newborn. Women who smoke and drink should stop before becoming pregnant. Women who are pregnant or trying to conceive should limit their caffeine intake.

- **Infections.** A woman who has any type of infection should be treated for the infection before getting pregnant to avoid passing infections to the baby. This is good advice for men, too, to avoid transmitting an infection to their partners. A woman may need to be vaccinated against hepatitis B, rubella (German measles), varicella (chicken pox), and other communicable diseases if she is at risk for them. Testing for tuberculosis and some sexually transmitted infections (STIs), including HIV, can ensure treatment prior to pregnancy.

- **Diet.** Good nutrition is essential to a healthy pregnancy. Nutritional counseling can help a woman create a plan for healthful eating before and during pregnancy. Diet is especially important for any woman with special nutritional needs or an eating disorder, or who is overweight or obese. Physicians commonly prescribe prenatal vitamin supplements to pregnant women. A woman of childbearing age needs extra folic acid to prevent neural tube defects in any future children she may have. Folic acid is part of a prenatal vitamin but can also be found in fortified foods such as enriched breakfast cereals, breads, and pastas.

- **Multiple births.** If twins or multiple births run in a woman's family, she is more likely to have multiple births, too. Multiple births are also more prevalent in mothers who are obese, over age 40, of African descent, or using certain reproductive technologies (such as in vitro fertilization) to become pregnant.

- **Genetic disorders.** If either partner has a family history of any genetic disorders, genetic counseling may be in order before pregnancy. Genetic testing can determine whether the mother or father is a carrier for a specific disease. With counseling, a couple can decide how best to deal with the possibility of transferring a disease to a child. Members of some ethnic groups are at higher risk for genetic disorders. For more information about such disorders, see the box "Ethnicity and Genetic Disease."

Additional evaluation may be recommended for prospective parents who have recently traveled outside the United States; work with chemicals, radiation, or toxic substances; participate in physically demanding activities or occupations; or face significant psychosocial risks, including homelessness, an unsafe home environment, or mental illness.

UNDERSTANDING FERTILITY AND INFERTILITY

Conception is a complex process. Although many couples conceive easily, others face a variety of difficulties.

Conception

The process of conception begins with the union of the nucleus of an egg cell (ovum) and the nucleus of a sperm cell—a process called **fertilization** (Figure 9.1). Every month during a woman's fertile years, her body prepares itself for conception and pregnancy. In one of her ovaries, an egg matures and is released from its follicle. The egg, about the size of a fine grain of sand, travels through an oviduct, or fallopian tube, to the uterus in three to four days. The endometrium, which is the lining of the uterus, has already thickened

Ask Yourself

QUESTIONS FOR CRITICAL THINKING AND REFLECTION

If you don't have children now, do you plan to have them someday? Have you thought about the skills and qualities that make a good parent? Given what you know about yourself today, do you think you would be a good parent? What skills or qualities do you think you would need to develop?

?

fetus The developmental stage of a human from the ninth week after conception to the moment of birth. **TERMS**

fertilization The initiation of biological reproduction; the union of the nucleus of an egg cell with the nucleus of a sperm cell.

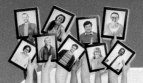
Genes carry the instructions that develop individual traits, including disease risks, in every human being. Many conditions, such as obesity or asthma, involve multiple genes and environmental influences. Some uncommon diseases, such as *sickle-cell disease* or *cystic fibrosis,* can be traced to a mutation in a single gene.

Children inherit one set of genes from each parent. If only one copy of an abnormal gene is necessary to produce a disease, it is called a *dominant* gene. Diseases caused by dominant genes seldom skip a generation; anyone who carries the gene will probably be affected by the disease.

If two copies of an abnormal gene (one from each parent) are necessary for a disease to occur, the gene is called *recessive.* Many diseases caused by recessive genes occur disproportionately in certain racial or ethnic groups where gene pools are smaller. If both parents are carriers, each of their children will have about a 25% chance of developing the disease.

The following list describes common conditions with proven genetic links in certain populations. If your family history includes any of these conditions, genetic tests and counseling can help assess the risk to your prospective children.

• **Hemochromatosis** ("iron overload") affects about 1 in 200 people. At highest risk are people of Northern European (especially Irish), Mediterranean, and Hispanic descent. In hemochromatosis, the body absorbs and stores up to 10 times the normal amount of iron. If untreated, the disease can cause organ failure and death.

Early symptoms are often vague and include weakness, lethargy, darkening of the skin, and joint pain. Treatment involves reducing iron stores by removing blood from the body (a process known as phlebotomy or "bloodletting").

• **Tay-Sachs disease,** another recessive disorder, occurs in about 1 in 3000 Jews of Eastern European ancestry (Ashkenazi Jews), as well as those of French Canadian and Cajun ancestry. People with Tay-Sachs disease cannot

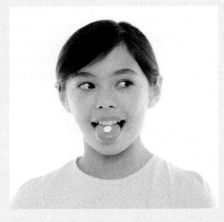

Gene therapy can happen with a pill that corrects a gene mutation such as occurs in cystic fibrosis. Science Photo Library/Getty Images

properly metabolize fatty acids. As a result, the brain and other nerve tissues deteriorate, often in childhood. Affected children show weakness in their movements and eventually develop blindness (by age 12–18 months) and seizures. This disease is fatal, and death usually occurs by age 6. No effective treatment is currently available.

• **Cystic fibrosis** affects 1 in 3000 Caucasians; about 1 in 28 carry one copy of the cystic fibrosis gene. In cystic fibrosis, essential pancreatic enzymes are deficient, which means the body cannot properly absorb nutrients. Thick mucus impairs functioning in the lungs and intestinal tracts of people with this disease. Cystic fibrosis is often fatal in early childhood, but treatments are increasingly effective in reducing symptoms and prolonging life. In some cases, symptoms do not appear until early adulthood. In 2016, the median predicted survival improved to 47.7 years from a median in the 1990s of 29.4 years due to a number of medical advances, including lung transplantation, inhaled antibiotics, and gene modulator therapies.

• **Sickle-cell disease** occurs in about 1 of every 500 African American births and in 1 of every 36,000 Hispanic American births. In this disease, red blood cells, which carry oxygen to the body's tissues, change shape under conditions of stress; the normally disc-shaped cells

become sickle-shaped. The altered cells carry less oxygen and can block small blood vessels. The resulting painful condition is called *sickle-cell crisis.* People who inherit one gene for sickle-cell disease (about 1 in 12 African Americans) experience only mild symptoms; those with two genes become severely, often fatally, ill.

• **Thalassemia** is a blood disease found most often among Italians, Greeks, and to a lesser extent, African Americans and Asians. When inherited from one parent, this form of anemia is mild; when two genes are present, the disease is severe and can cause fetal death.

Children with this condition require repeated blood transfusions, eventually resulting in a damaging iron buildup and the need for treatments that bind and remove excess iron. In severe cases, stem cell transplants from the bone marrow of a compatible sibling can be used. If thalassemia is treated early and aggressively, disease-free survival can approach 90%. However, not all affected individuals have an eligible donor. New interventions—such as genetic engineering, in utero stem cell transplantation, and umbilical cord blood donor-led transplantation—offer promise.

• **Canavan disease,** or aspartoacylase deficiency, was first identified in the early 1900s. It causes a spongy degeneration of myelin nerve fibers in infancy and affects as many as 1 in 6400 Ashkenazi Jews. The condition presents by approximately 3 months of age and causes loss of muscle tone, which progresses to spasticity and seizures. Several treatments are under investigation, but most cases are treated with supportive care. Children with Canavan disease usually do not live beyond age 10.

• **Familial dysautonomia,** a progressive sensorimotor neuropathy, is seen in 1 in 3700 Ashkenazi Jews. Clinically, infants show signs of decreased muscle tone and poor feeding with development of chronic lung disease and reflux. Those affected further develop hypertension. Treatment involves supportive and symptomatic therapies.

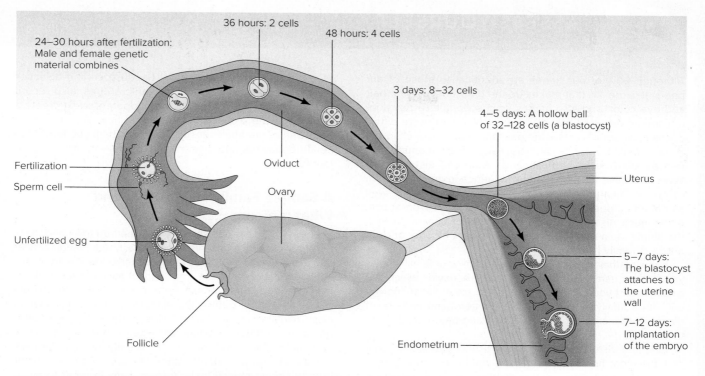

24–30 hours after fertilization:
Male and female genetic
material combines

36 hours: 2 cells

48 hours: 4 cells

3 days: 8–32 cells

4–5 days: A hollow ball
of 32–128 cells (a blastocyst)

Oviduct

Ovary

Fertilization

Sperm cell

Unfertilized egg

Follicle

Uterus

Endometrium

5–7 days:
The blastocyst
attaches to
the uterine
wall

7–12 days:
Implantation
of the embryo

FIGURE 9.1   Fertilization and early development of the embryo.

for the implantation of a **fertilized egg,** that is, a *zygote*. If the egg is not fertilized, it lasts about 24 hours and then disintegrates. The woman's body then sheds the uterine lining during menstruation.

Fertilization   Sperm cells are produced in the testes and ejaculated from the penis into the vagina during sexual intercourse (except in cases of artificial insemination or assisted reproduction; see the section "Treating Infertility"). Sperm cells are much smaller than eggs. The typical ejaculate contains millions of sperm, but only a few complete the journey through the uterus and up the fallopian tube to the egg. Many sperm cells do not survive the vagina's acidic environment.

Once through the cervix and into the uterus, many sperm cells are diverted to the wrong oviduct or get stuck along the way. Of those that reach the egg, only one will penetrate its hard outer layer. As sperm approach the egg, they release enzymes that soften this outer layer. Enzymes from hundreds of sperm must be released in order for the egg's outer layer to soften enough to allow one sperm cell to penetrate. The first sperm cell that bumps into a spot that is soft enough can swim into the egg cell. It then fuses with the nucleus of the egg, and fertilization occurs. The sperm's tail, its means of locomotion, is left behind on the egg's outer membrane, while the sperm's head is inside the egg. The egg then undergoes chemical change that makes it impenetrable to other sperm.

The ovum carries the hereditary characteristics of the mother and her family; sperm cells carry the hereditary characteristics of the father and his family. Each egg or sperm cell contains 23 chromosomes, each of which contains **genes,** which are packages of biochemical instructions for the developing baby. Genes provide the blueprint for a unique individual based on the functional and health characteristics of his or her ancestors (see the box "Creating a Family Health Tree").

Upon fertilization, the zygote undergoes cell division and the growth process begins. The zygote continues to divide as it travels through the oviduct. When it reaches the uterus, the cluster of 32–128 cells (now called a *blastocyst*) attaches to the uterine wall. Soon it becomes implanted in the endometrium and becomes an embryo.

Twins   In the usual course of events, one egg and one sperm unite to produce one fertilized egg and one baby. But if the ovaries release two eggs during ovulation and both eggs are fertilized, twins develop. These twins will be no more

> **fertilized egg**   The egg after penetration by a sperm; a *zygote*.
>
> **gene**   The basic unit of heredity; a section of a chromosome containing biochemical instructions for making a particular protein.

TERMS

ASSESS YOURSELF
Creating a Family Health Tree

Although 99% of our genes are identical to those of our peers, it is the 1% that makes up the differences in our hair and eye color, and also makes us susceptible to developing certain diseases and disorders. We inherit these differences from our parents—and pass them on to our children. In fact, heredity is the primary cause for uncommon illnesses such as hemophilia and sickle-cell disease. Researchers have found a genetic influence in many common disorders, including obesity and heart disease as well as diabetes, depression, asthma, alcohol and drug abuse, Alzheimer's disease, and certain forms of cancer. In fact, the single most reliable indicator for future alcohol or drug abuse is family history.

Knowing that a specific disease runs in your family allows you to seek early screening and modify behavior, which can greatly affect your long-term health. For example, an individual with a family history of high cholesterol and early heart disease can increase physical activity and pay special attention to diet.

Inherited diseases tend to show distinct patterns. In general, the more first-degree relatives you have with a genetically transmitted disease, the greater your risk. However, nongenetic factors—such as health habits—play an important role. Signs of strong hereditary influence include early onset of a disease, appearance of the disease largely or exclusively on one side of the family, onset of the same disease at the same age in more than one relative, and development of the disease despite good health habits.

You can put together a simple family health tree by compiling a few key facts about your primary relatives: siblings, parents, aunts and uncles, and grandparents. Those facts include the dates of birth, major diseases, health-related conditions and habits, and, for deceased relatives, the ages

at death as well as the causes. Because certain diseases are more common in particular ethnic groups, also record the ethnic background of each grandparent. Next create a tree, using the example as a guide. Show your tree to a physician or genetic counselor, who can help you target the health behaviors and screening tests that are most important for you.

A Sample Family Health Tree and What It Means

Penny is a 25-year-old woman who prepared this family tree. She has a strong family history of breast and ovarian cancer that developed early in life on her mother's side. Based on this information, her physician may suggest earlier breast screening or genetic testing for mutations in the *BRCA* genes to help gauge her risk of getting the disease. She also has several close relatives on her father's side of the family who were obese and suffered from high cholesterol and heart attacks at early ages. These risk factors significantly increase Penny's chance of having a heart attack. As such, Penny and her brother should modify their lifestyles early in order to avoid high cholesterol and prevent obesity later.

As the family tree shows, Penny's paternal grandmother also died of breast cancer—but at the age of 88. Because this case happened late in life, the heritable risk on the paternal side is not as likely. A paternal grandmother is also a more distant relative than a mother or sister (first-degree relative).

By examining your family's health history, you can make important decisions about lifestyle, screening, and counseling. In Penny's case, such decisions have an impact not only on her, but also on her daughters.

SOURCES: Centers for Disease Control and Prevention. 2019. *Family Health History* (https://www.cdc.gov/genomics/famhistory/index.htm); Hobson, K. 2009. "Why and how to put together a family history." *US News & World Report*, 30 July; Hulick, P. 2016. "Genetic testing: Reason to gather your family health history." *US News & World Report*, 21 December..

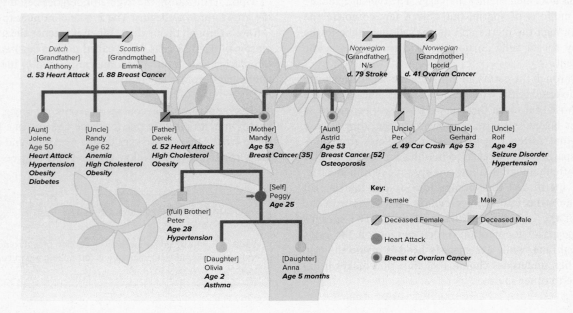

alike than siblings from different pregnancies because each will have come from a different fertilized egg. Twins who develop this way are referred to as **fraternal (dizygotic) twins;** they may be the same sex or different sexes. About 70% of twins are fraternal.

Twins can also develop from the early division of a single fertilized egg into two cells that develop separately. Because these babies share all genetic material, they will be **identical (monozygotic) twins.**

Two or more fetuses in the same pregnancy is called *multiple gestation*, and this leads to a *multiple birth*. The most serious complication of multiple births is preterm delivery (delivery before the fetuses are adequately mature). The higher the number of fetuses a woman carries, the earlier in gestation she will deliver. This leads to higher rates of complications due to prematurity.

Infertility

Thirteen percent of the U.S. population (about 2 million couples) will seek infertility services due to difficulty conceiving. **Infertility** is defined as the inability to conceive after trying for a year or more. Infertility affected about 9% of American women of reproductive age (15–49 years) in the United States. Although the focus is often on women, one-fourth of the factors contributing to infertility are male, and in one-third (35%) of infertile couples, both partners have problems. Therefore, it is important that both partners be evaluated.

Female Infertility   One-third of cases of female infertility usually result from one of two key causes—tubal blockage (14%) or failure to ovulate (21%). An additional one-third of cases of female infertility are due to anatomical abnormalities, benign growths in the uterus, thyroid disease, and other uncommon conditions; the remaining 28% of cases are unexplained.

Blocked oviducts are most commonly the result of *pelvic inflammatory disease (PID)*, a serious complication of several STIs. Most cases of PID are associated with untreated cases of chlamydia or gonorrhea, both of which can occur without symptoms. Tubal blockages can also be caused by prior surgery or by *endometriosis*, a condition in which endometrial (uterine) tissue grows outside the uterus. Tubal blockage increases the risk of infertility and ectopic pregnancy, where the embryo develops outside the uterus.

Age also affects fertility. Beginning at around age 30, a woman's fertility naturally begins to wane. Age is probably the main factor in ovulation failure. Exposure to toxic chemicals, cigarette smoke, or radiation also appears to reduce fertility, as do genetic factors identifiable in your family history (see the box "Creating a Family Health Tree").

Male Infertility   Male infertility accounts for about one quarter of infertile couples. The leading causes of male infer-

tility can be divided into four main categories: hypothalamic pituitary disease (1-2%), testicular disease (30-40%), disorders of sperm transport or posttesticular disorders (10-20%), and unexplained (40-50%). Some acquired disorders of the testes can lead to infertility, such as damage from the following causes:

- Drug use (large doses of marijuana, for example, cause lower sperm counts and suppress reproductive hormones)
- Radiation
- Infection, such as from having had mumps as a child
- Environmental toxins
- Hyperthermia, such as from prolonged hot tub use
- Smoking

Treating Infertility   The cause of infertility can be determined for about 72-85% of infertile couples. Most cases of infertility are treated with conventional medical therapies. Surgery can repair oviducts, remove endometriosis, and correct anatomical problems in men and women. Fertility drugs can help women ovulate but may cause multiple births. If these conventional treatments don't work, couples can turn to **assisted reproductive technology (ART)** techniques, as described in the following sections. According to CDC data published in 2018, about 1.8% of births in the United States are the result of ART treatments.

Most infertility treatments are expensive and emotionally draining, with a live birth occurring in about a third of cases. Some infertile couples choose not to try to have children, whereas others turn to adoption. Couples will need to balance the risks of age-related infertility with the competing demands of careers and academics.

INTRAUTERINE INSEMINATION   Male infertility can sometimes be overcome by collecting and concentrating the man's sperm and introducing the semen by syringe into a woman's vagina or uterus, a procedure known as **artificial (intrauterine) insemination.** To increase the probability of success, the woman is often given fertility drugs to induce ovulation prior to the insemination procedure. The sperm can be provided by

> **QUICK STATS**
>
> **13%** of women aged 15–49 have used infertility services.
>
> —Centers for Disease Control and Prevention, 2016

---

fraternal (dizygotic) twins   Twins who develop from separate fertilized eggs; such twins are not genetically identical.

identical (monozygotic) twins   Twins who develop from the division of a single zygote; such twins are genetically identical.

infertility   The inability to conceive after trying for a year or more.

assisted reproductive technology (ART)   Advanced medical techniques used to treat infertility.

artificial (intrauterine) insemination   The introduction of sperm into the vagina by artificial means.

TERMS

the woman's partner or a donor. Donor sperm are also used by single women and lesbian couples who want to conceive using artificial insemination. The success rate is about 5–20%. The wide range is due to age-related influences.

IVF A surgical technique used to overcome infertility, **in vitro fertilization (IVF)** involves surgically removing mature eggs from a woman's ovary and pairing the harvested eggs with sperm outside the woman's body (*in vitro*), in a laboratory dish. If eggs are successfully fertilized, one or more of the resulting embryos are inserted into the woman's uterus. The remaining embryos can then be frozen for future use.

There are disadvantages to IVF. Success rates determined by live birth rates vary from about 4% to 40% depending on the woman's age. It costs more than 15,000 per procedure and may require five or more attempts to produce one live birth. IVF also increases the chance of twins or triplets, which in turn increases the risk of premature birth and maternal complications, including pregnancy-related hypertension and diabetes.

GESTATIONAL CARRIER A *gestational carrier* is a fertile woman who agrees to carry a fetus for an infertile couple. The gestational carrier agrees to be artificially inseminated by the father's sperm or to undergo IVF with the couple's embryo, to carry the baby to term, and to give it to the couple at birth. In return, the couple pays her for her services and medical costs. As of 2016, approximately 3% of all ART in the United States is performed through gestational carriers.

Emotional Responses to Infertility Couples who seek treatment for infertility have often already confronted the possibility of not being able to become biological parents. Many infertile couples feel they have lost control over a major facet of their lives. They may lose perspective on the rest of their lives as they focus more and more on the reasons for their infertility and on treatment. Infertile couples may need to set their own limits on how much treatment they are willing to undergo.

Ask Yourself

QUESTIONS FOR CRITICAL THINKING AND REFLECTION
What are your views on infertility treatments? Do you feel treatment is appropriate, or do you think infertile couples should adopt children? If you were faced with a diagnosis of infertility, what would you consider doing?

TERMS

in vitro fertilization (IVF) Combining eggs and sperm outside the body and inserting one or more fertilized eggs into the uterus.

trimester One of the three 3-month periods of pregnancy.

Support groups for infertile couples can provide help in this difficult situation, but there are few easy answers to infertility. If treatment is unsuccessful, couples need to mourn the loss of the children they will never bear. They need to make a decision about their future—whether to pursue alternate plans or further treatment, or to adjust to childlessness and go on with their lives.

PREGNANCY

Pregnancy is usually discussed in terms of **trimesters**—three periods of about three months (or 13 weeks) each. During the first trimester, the mother experiences a few physical changes and some fairly common symptoms. During the second trimester, often the most peaceful time of pregnancy, the mother gains weight, looks noticeably pregnant, and may experience a general sense of well-being if she is happy about having a child. The third trimester is the hardest for the mother because she must breathe, digest, excrete, and circulate blood for herself and the growing fetus. The weight of the fetus, the pressure of its body on her organs, and its increased demands on her system cause discomfort and fatigue and may make the mother increasingly impatient to give birth.

Changes in the Woman's Body

Hormonal changes begin as soon as an egg is fertilized, and for the next nine months the woman's body nourishes the fetus and adjusts to its growth (Figure 9.2).

Early Signs and Symptoms Early recognition of pregnancy is important, especially for women with medical conditions or nutritional deficiencies. The following symptoms are not absolute indications of pregnancy, but they are reasons to visit a gynecologist, and maybe take a home pregnancy test (see the box "Home Pregnancy Tests"):

• *A missed menstrual period.* When a fertilized egg implants in the uterine wall, the endometrium is retained to nourish the embryo. A woman who misses a period after having intercourse may be pregnant.

• *Slight bleeding.* Following implantation of the fertilized egg into the endometrial lining, a slight bleed occurs in about 14% of pregnant women. Because this happens about when a period is expected, about two weeks after ovulation, the bleeding is sometimes mistaken for menstrual flow. It usually lasts only a few days.

• *Nausea.* Between 50% and 90% of pregnant women feel increased nausea, probably in reaction to surging levels of progesterone and other pregnancy hormones. Although this nausea is often called *morning sickness,* some women have it all day long. It frequently begins during the 6th week and disappears by the 12th week. In some cases it continues throughout the pregnancy.

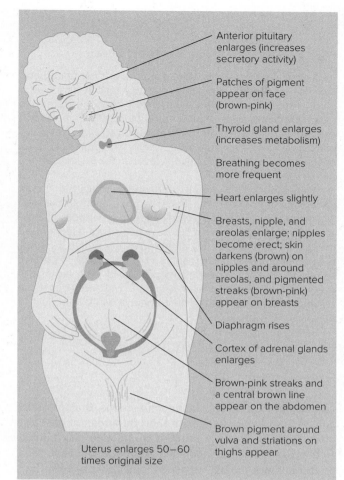

Anterior pituitary enlarges (increases secretory activity)

Patches of pigment appear on face (brown-pink)

Thyroid gland enlarges (increases metabolism)

Breathing becomes more frequent

Heart enlarges slightly

Breasts, nipple, and areolas enlarge; nipples become erect; skin darkens (brown) on nipples and around areolas, and pigmented streaks (brown-pink) appear on breasts

Diaphragm rises

Cortex of adrenal glands enlarges

Brown-pink streaks and a central brown line appear on the abdomen

Brown pigment around vulva and striations on thighs appear

Uterus enlarges 50–60 times original size

FIGURE 9.2 Physiological changes during pregnancy.

- *Breast tenderness.* Some women experience breast tenderness, swelling, and tingling, usually described as different from the tenderness experienced before menstruation.

- *Increased urination.* Increased frequency of urination can occur soon after the missed period.

- *Sleepiness, fatigue, and emotional upset.* These symptoms result from hormonal changes. Fatigue can be surprisingly overwhelming in the first trimester but usually improves significantly around the third month of pregnancy.

The first reliable physical signs of pregnancy can be distinguished about four weeks after a woman misses her menstrual period. Increased uterine growth and blood flow contribute to softening of the uterus just above the cervix, called *Hegar's sign,* and a bluish discoloration to the cervix and labia minora, termed *Chadwick's sign.*

Four weeks after a woman misses her menstrual period, she is considered to be about eight weeks pregnant because pregnancy is calculated from the time of a wom-

an's last menstrual period rather than from the time of fertilization. The uterine lining buildup in the two weeks before fertilization is part of the gestation cycle, and the timing of ovulation and fertilization is often difficult to determine. Although a woman should see her physician to determine her due date, due dates can be approximated by subtracting three months from the date of the last menstrual period and then adding seven days. For example, a woman whose last menstrual period began on September 20 would have a due date of about June 27.

Continuing Changes in the Woman's Body The most obvious changes during pregnancy occur in the reproductive organs. During the first three months, the uterus enlarges to about three times its nonpregnant size, but it still cannot be felt in the abdomen. By the fourth month, it is large enough to make the abdomen protrude. By the seventh or eighth month, the uterus pushes up under the rib cage, which makes breathing slightly more difficult. The breasts enlarge and are sensitive; by week 8, they may tingle or throb. The pigmented area around the nipple, called the *areola,* darkens and broadens. The hormones of pregnancy also contribute to hyperpigmentation and broadening of the nipple, and for some women, hyperpigmentation may show in the face or the midline of the abdomen.

Other changes are going on as well. Early in pregnancy, the muscles and ligaments attached to bones begin to soften and stretch. The joints between the pelvic bones loosen and spread, making it easier to have a baby but harder to walk. The circulatory system becomes more efficient to accommodate higher blood volume, and the heart pumps more rapidly. Much of the increased blood flow goes to the uterus and placenta (the organ that exchanges nutrients and waste between mother and fetus). The kidneys become highly efficient, removing waste products from fetal circulation and producing large amounts of urine by midpregnancy.

The average weight gain during a healthy pregnancy is 27.5 pounds, although actual weight change varies with the individual. Table 9.1 shows the weight gains recommended by the Institute of Medicine based on a woman's prepregnancy weight. About half of the weight gain is directly related to the baby (to the placenta, for example); the rest accumulates over the woman's body as fluid and fat. As the woman's skin stretches, small breaks may occur in the elastin fibers of the lower layer of skin, producing *stretch marks* on her abdomen, hips, breasts, or thighs.

Changes during the Later Stages of Pregnancy By the end of the sixth month, the increased needs of the fetus place a burden on the mother's lungs, heart, and kidneys. Her back may ache from the pressure of the baby's weight and from having to throw her shoulders back to keep her balance while standing (Figure 9.3). Her body

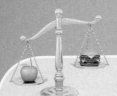

CRITICAL CONSUMER
Home Pregnancy Tests

Women have access to a variety of over-the-counter home pregnancy tests today, but generally speaking, these tests all work in the same way to determine whether a woman is pregnant. Pregnancy tests are designed to detect the presence of the hormone **human chorionic gonadotropin (hCG)**, a hormone produced by the implanted fertilized egg, which is discussed in this chapter. Because the placenta releases hCG, the hormone can be detected in a woman's urine or blood when she is pregnant.

Although home pregnancy tests have become extremely accurate since their introduction in 1975, not all tests behave equally. A sensitive test will give a "positive" result with very low levels of hCG and can identify pregnancies earlier. A less sensitive test may not give an accurate result until hCG levels are much higher. Most kits will reliably detect 97% of pregnancies one week after a missed period.

Two types of home pregnancy tests are available—those that require the test strip to be dipped into urine, and those that require the user to urinate directly onto the test strip.

A clinical blood test is more accurate but not necessarily more sensitive than a home pregnancy test. A quantitative blood test, usually called a *beta hCG test*, measures the exact number of units of hCG in the blood. This type of test can detect even the most minimal level. Labs vary in what is considered a positive pregnancy test. Common cutoffs for positive are 5, 10, and 25 units. A level under 5 is considered negative.

Women need to use home pregnancy test kits with a clear understanding of their limitations. If you're comfortable waiting, a sensitive test taken a week after your period is due will almost certainly give you accurate results. If you elect to take the test as early as the day after you've missed your period, remember that a negative result isn't 100% certain. A positive result may mean either a viable pregnancy or a pregnancy destined to end shortly after it began. With either of those results, you should plan to test again a week later, just to be sure.

Table 9.1	Recommended Weight Gain during Pregnancy

STATUS (BMI)*	WEIGHT GAIN (POUNDS)
Underweight (<18.5)	28–40
Normal (18.5–24.9)	25–35
Overweight (25–29.9)	15–25
Obese (>30)	11–20

*BMI, or body mass index, allows comparison of body weight across different heights. (See Chapter 15 to calculate BMI.)

retains more water, perhaps up to three extra quarts of fluid. Her hands, legs, ankles, or feet may swell, and she may be bothered by leg cramps, heartburn, or constipation. Despite discomfort, both her digestion and her metabolism are working at top efficiency.

Near term, the uterus prepares for childbirth with a series of preliminary contractions, called **Braxton Hicks contractions.** Unlike true labor contractions, Braxton Hicks contractions are irregular with short duration; they are also often painless. To the mother, a contraction may initially feel only as though her abdomen is hard to the touch.

In the ninth month, increased joint laxity coupled by a softening cervix allows the baby to settle deeper into the

human chorionic gonadotropin (hCG) A hormone produced by a fertilized egg that can be detected in the urine or blood of the mother shortly after conception.	**TERMS**

Braxton Hicks contractions   A pattern of late-pregnancy uterine contractions that are irregular in timing, short in duration, and painless and do not result in labor.

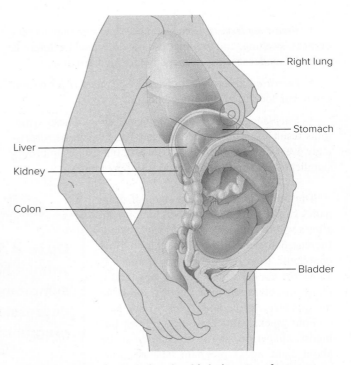

Right lung
Stomach
Liver
Kidney
Colon
Bladder

FIGURE 9.3   **The fetus during the third trimester of pregnancy.**

FIGURE 9.4   **A chronology of milestones in prenatal development.**

pelvis. This process, called **lightening,** produces a visible change in the mother's abdominal profile. Pelvic pressure increases, and pressure on the diaphragm lightens. Breathing becomes easier; urination becomes more frequent. Sometimes, after a first pregnancy, lightening does not occur until labor begins.

Emotional Responses to Pregnancy

Rapid changes in hormone levels can cause a pregnant woman to experience unpredictable emotions. A large part of pregnancy is beyond the woman's control—her changing appearance, her energy level, and possibly her variable moods. Some women may need extra support and reassurance to stay on an even keel. Hormonal changes can also make women feel exhilarated and euphoric, although for some women such moods are temporary.

Like the physical changes that accompany pregnancy, emotional responses also change as the pregnancy develops. During the first trimester, the pregnant woman may fear that she may miscarry or that the child will not be normal. Education about pregnancy and childbirth and support from her partner, friends, relatives, and health care professionals are important antidotes to these fears.

During the second trimester, the pregnant woman can feel early fetal movements, and worries about miscarriages usually begin to diminish. She may look and feel happy and be delighted as her pregnancy begins to show. However, she may also worry that her increasing size makes her unattractive. Reassurance from her partner, family, and other support systems can ease these fears.

The third trimester is the time of greatest physical stress during the pregnancy. A woman may find that her physical abilities are limited by her size. Because some women feel physically awkward and sexually unattractive, they may experience periods of depression. But many also feel a great deal of happy excitement and anticipation. The fetus may already be looked on as a member of the family, and both parents may begin talking to the fetus and interacting with it by patting the mother's belly.

FETAL DEVELOPMENT

Now that we've seen what happens to the mother's body during pregnancy, let's consider the development of the fetus (Figure 9.4).

---

lightening   A process in which the uterus sinks down because the baby's head settles into the pelvic area.   **TERMS**

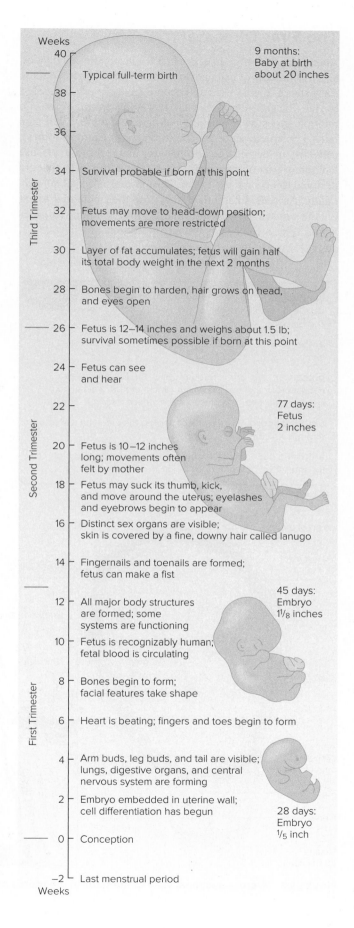

Weeks

40 — Typical full-term birth   9 months:
                                               Baby at birth
                                               about 20 inches

Third Trimester

38 —

36 —

34 — Survival probable if born at this point

32 — Fetus may move to head-down position;
     movements are more restricted

30 — Layer of fat accumulates; fetus will gain half
     its total body weight in the next 2 months

28 — Bones begin to harden, hair grows on head,
     and eyes open

26 — Fetus is 12–14 inches and weighs about 1.5 lb;
     survival sometimes possible if born at this point

24 — Fetus can see
     and hear

Second Trimester

22 —   77 days:
                                               Fetus
                                               2 inches

20 — Fetus is 10–12 inches
     long; movements often
     felt by mother

18 — Fetus may suck its thumb, kick,
     and move around the uterus; eyelashes
     and eyebrows begin to appear

16 — Distinct sex organs are visible;
     skin is covered by a fine, downy hair called lanugo

14 — Fingernails and toenails are formed;
     fetus can make a fist

12 — All major body structures   45 days:
     are formed; some   Embryo
     systems are functioning   1 1/8 inches

First Trimester

10 — Fetus is recognizably human;
     fetal blood is circulating

8 — Bones begin to form;
    facial features take shape

6 — Heart is beating; fingers and toes begin to form

4 — Arm buds, leg buds, and tail are visible;
    lungs, digestive organs, and central
    nervous system are forming

2 — Embryo embedded in uterine wall;
    cell differentiation has begun   28 days:
                                              Embryo
                                              1/5 inch

0 — Conception

−2 — Last menstrual period

Weeks

The First Trimester

About 30 hours after an egg is first fertilized, the cell divides, and this process of cell division repeats many times. In these early stages, these cells can become any type of cell needed by the growing embryo. We call this ability to transform into multiple types of tissues *pluripotency*. While every cell contains a complete set of genetic instructions (chromosomes), cells that are destined to become liver tissue, for example, use a different part of the genetic instructions from cells that are destined to become eye tissue. This process is called *differentiation*. As cells differentiate, they lose their potential to act on the unused genetic information they contain. In other words, once a cell begins to take on features of a liver cell, it can no longer transform to eye tissue.

> **TERMS**
>
> **blastocyst**   The stage of embryonic development, days 4–7, before the cell cluster becomes the embryo and placenta.
>
> **embryo**   The stage of development between blastocyst and fetus; about weeks 2–8.
>
> **placenta**   The organ through which the fetus receives nourishment and empties waste via the mother's circulatory system; after birth, the placenta is expelled from the uterus.
>
> **umbilical cord**   The cord connecting the placenta and fetus, through which nutrients pass.
>
> **amniotic sac**   A membranous pouch enclosing and protecting the fetus; also holds amniotic fluid.

On about the fourth day after fertilization, the cluster of rapidly developing cells arrives in the uterus as a **blastocyst,** a mostly hollow sphere of between 32 and 128 cells. The blastocyst attaches to the uterine wall on the sixth or seventh day, allowing for implantation into the nourishing uterine lining.

The blastocyst becomes an **embryo** by about the end of the second week after fertilization. The inner cells of the blastocyst separate into three layers. The innermost layer becomes the digestive and respiratory systems; the middle layer becomes muscle, bone, blood, kidneys, and sex glands; and the outer layer becomes the skin, hair, and nervous tissue.

The outermost shell of cells becomes the supporting structures of the pregnancy: the **placenta, umbilical cord,** and **amniotic sac** (Figure 9.5). A network of blood vessels called *chorionic villi* eventually forms the placenta. The human placenta allows a two-way exchange of nutrients and waste materials between the mother and the fetus. The placenta brings oxygen and nutrients to the fetus and transports waste products out. The placenta does not provide a perfect barrier between the fetal circulation and the maternal circulation, however. Some genetic information is exchanged, and certain substances, such as alcohol as well as most vitamins, nutrients, sugar, and oxygen, pass freely from the maternal circulation through the placenta to the fetus.

The period between weeks 2 and 9 is a time of rapid differentiation and change. All major body structures are formed during this time, including the heart, brain, liver, lungs, and sex organs. Eyes, nose, ears, arms, and legs also

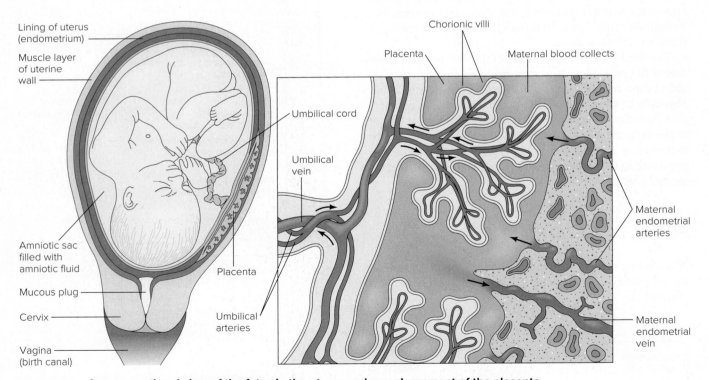

FIGURE 9.5   A cross-sectional view of the fetus in the uterus and an enlargement of the placenta.

appear. Some organs begin to function, as well; the heart begins to beat, and the liver starts producing blood cells. Because body structures are forming, the developing organism is vulnerable to damage from environmental influences such as drugs and infections.

By the end of the second month, the fetal brain sends out impulses that coordinate the functioning of its other organs. The embryo is now a fetus, and further changes will be in the size and refinement of working body parts. In the third month, the fetus becomes active. By the end of the first trimester, at 13 weeks, the fetus is about an inch long and weighs less than one ounce.

The Second Trimester

To grow during the second trimester, to about 14 inches and 1.5 pounds, the fetus requires large amounts of food, oxygen, and water, which come from the mother through the placenta. All body systems are operating, and the fetal heartbeat can be heard with a stethoscope. By the fourth or fifth month, the mother can detect early fetal movements that may feel like "flutters." A fetus born at 24–26 weeks has a better than 50% chance of survival. The age at which survival is possible depends on the development of lung tissue, which completes a critical step in weeks 24–26 of pregnancy. Prior to 23 weeks, survival without significant impairment is rare, occurring in 3–15% of cases.

The Third Trimester

The fetus gains most of its birth weight during the last three months of the pregnancy. Some of the weight is brown fat under the skin that insulates the fetus and supplies food. *Brown fat* is a special fat rich with blood supply that is found in hibernating mammals and newborns and is associated with protection against hypothermia. This is an important consideration because babies are often too small to generate much of their own heat and are too weak to move away from cold areas. The fetus also takes in other nutrients; about 85% of the calcium and iron the mother consumes goes into the fetal bloodstream.

The fetus also needs the immunity supplied by antibodies in the mother's blood during the final three months. The antibodies protect the fetus against many of the diseases to which the mother has acquired immunity.

Diagnosing Fetal Abnormalities

About 2–4% of babies are born with a major birth defect. Information about the health and sex of a fetus can be obtained prior to birth through prenatal testing.

Noninvasive Screening Tests Maternal blood testing can be used to help identify fetuses with neural tube defects, Down syndrome, and other anomalies. Traditionally, blood is taken from the mother at 16–19 weeks of preg-

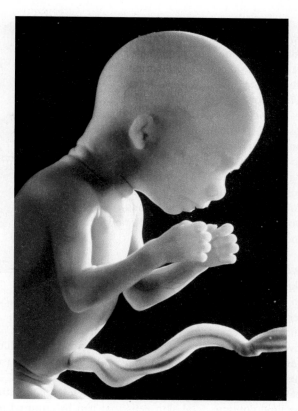

At the beginning of the third trimester, the fetus is growing rapidly, weighs about 2½ pounds, and measures about the size of a cantaloupe. The fetus is typically active and can suck its thumb, blink, frown, and turn its head. Tissuepix/Science Source

nancy and analyzed for four hormone levels—human chorionic gonadotropin (hCG), unconjugated estriol, alpha-fetoprotein (AFP), and inhibin-A. These four hormone levels, the **quadruple marker screen (QMS)**, can be compared to appropriate standards, and the results are used to estimate the probability that the fetus has particular anomalies. This type of test is a screening test rather than a diagnostic test; in the case of abnormal QMS results, parents may choose further testing such as an amniocentesis or ultrasonography.

First-trimester screening for Down syndrome combines ultrasound evaluation of the nuchal translucency (the thickness of the back of the fetus's neck) with maternal blood testing. This test can be done between the 10th and 14th weeks of pregnancy. Combining this screening with serum testing at 16 weeks helps avoid more invasive screening tests. If results indicate an increased risk of abnormality, further diagnostic studies such as amniocentesis can be done for confirmation.

---

quadruple marker screen (QMS) A measurement of four hormones, used to assess the risk of fetal abnormalities.

TERMS

A newer noninvasive screening test, **cell-free DNA**, uses small fragments of fetal DNA identified in the maternal serum typically after 10 weeks of pregnancy. Currently, this DNA is used primarily to identify chromosomal disorders, such as Down syndrome, in women with elevated risk for *aneuploidy* (an abnormal number of chromosomes in the fetus) including in pregnant women over age 35. Cell-free DNA can also identify the baby's sex chromosomes, meaning parents can learn the baby's sex as early as the 10th week of pregnancy. With time and further research, this tool has tremendous potential to revolutionize prenatal testing for rare inherited conditions.

Invasive Diagnostic Tests Chorionic villus sampling (CVS) is a diagnostic test that can be performed in weeks 10 through 12 of pregnancy for high-risk women or women with abnormal screening results. This procedure involves removing a tiny section of the chorionic villi, which contain fetal cells that can be analyzed. For later diagnosis, **amniocentesis** is typically performed between 16 and 22 weeks and removes fluid from around the developing fetus. The fluid contains fetal skin cells that can be cultured for analysis. This analysis can include genetic analyses for chromosomal disorders but also for some genetic diseases, like Tay-Sachs disease. Because the genetics are known, the sex of the fetus can also be determined. Invasive testing carries a slight risk (a 0.1–0.7% chance of miscarriage).

Ultrasonography Ultrasonography (also called *ultrasound*) uses high-frequency sound waves to create a visual image of the fetus in the uterus. Ultrasound can show the fetus's position, size, and gestational age, and it can identify the presence of certain anatomical problems. Ultrasound can also be used to determine the sex of the fetus.

Genetic Counseling Genetic counselors explain the results of the various tests so that parents can understand their implications. If a fetus is found to have a defect, it may be carried to term, undergo termination, or in rare instances,

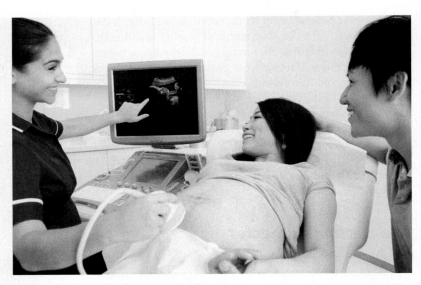
Ultrasonography provides information about the position, size, and physical condition of a fetus in the uterus. Monkey Business Images/Shutterstock

receive treatment while still in the uterus. Results of most current screening tests are not available until after week 12 of pregnancy.

THE IMPORTANCE OF PRENATAL CARE

Adequate prenatal care—as described in the following sections—is essential to the health of both mother and baby. All physicians recommend that women start getting regular prenatal checkups as soon as they become pregnant. Typically this means one checkup per month during the first eight months and then one checkup per week during the final month. About 75% of pregnant women begin receiving adequate prenatal care by the fourth month of pregnancy; about 3.5% wait until the last trimester or receive no prenatal care at all.

Regular Checkups

In the woman's first visit to her obstetrician, she will be asked for a detailed medical history and receive a complete physical exam. Her obstetrician will note any hereditary conditions that may assume increased significance during pregnancy. The tendency to develop gestational diabetes (diabetes during pregnancy only), for example, can be inherited; appropriate treatment during pregnancy reduces the risk of serious harm.

She returns for regular checkups throughout the pregnancy, during which her blood pressure and weight gain are measured, her urine is analyzed, and the fetus's size and position are monitored. Regular prenatal visits give the mother a chance to discuss her concerns and be assured that everything is proceeding normally. Physicians, midwives, health educators, and teachers of childbirth classes can provide the mother with valuable information.

> **TERMS**
>
> **cell-free DNA** Fetal genetic material in the maternal blood supply, used to assess the risk of fetal genetic conditions, especially for fetuses already identified as having elevated risk.
>
> **chorionic villus sampling (CVS)** Surgical removal of a tiny section of placental villi to be analyzed for genetic defects.
>
> **amniocentesis** A process in which amniotic fluid is removed and analyzed to detect possible birth defects.
>
> **ultrasonography** The use of high-frequency sound waves to view the fetus in the uterus; also known as *ultrasound*.

Blood Tests

A blood sample is taken during the initial prenatal visit to determine blood type and detect possible anemia or Rh incompatibilities. The **Rh factor** is a blood protein. If an Rh-positive father and an Rh-negative mother conceive an Rh-positive baby, the baby's blood will be incompatible with the mother's blood. If some of the baby's blood enters the mother's bloodstream during delivery, she will develop anti-Rh antibodies just as she would toward a virus. If she has subsequent Rh-positive babies, the circulating antibodies in the mother's blood, passing through the placenta, will destroy the fetus's red blood cells, possibly leading to jaundice, anemia, or death. This condition is completely preventable with a serum called *Rh-immune globulin,* which coats Rh-positive cells as they enter the mother's body and prevents her immune system from recognizing them and forming antibodies. Rh-immune globulin is given to Rh-negative mothers in the third trimester and again after the birth if the baby is found to be Rh-positive.

Blood may also be tested for evidence of hepatitis B, syphilis, rubella immunity, thyroid problems, and, with the mother's permission, HIV infection.

Prenatal Nutrition

A nutritious diet throughout pregnancy is essential for both the mother and her unborn baby. Not only does the baby get all its nutrients from the mother, but it also competes with her for nutrients not sufficiently available to meet both their needs. When a woman's diet is low in iron or calcium, the fetus receives most of it, and the mother may become deficient in the mineral. To meet the increased nutritional demands of her body, a pregnant woman shouldn't just eat more; she should make sure that her diet is nutritionally adequate.

To maintain her own health and help the fetus grow, a pregnant woman typically needs to consume about 250–500 extra calories per day. Breastfeeding an infant requires even more energy—about 500 or more calories per day. To ensure that she's getting enough calories and nutrients, a pregnant woman should talk to her physician or a registered dietician about her dietary habits and determine what changes she should make.

Supplements can help boost the levels of nutrients available to mother and child, helping with fetal development while ensuring that the mother doesn't become nutrient-deficient. Pregnant and lactating women, however, should not take supplements without the advice of their physicians because some vitamins, such as vitamin A, can be harmful if taken in excess. Pregnant women also should not take herbal dietary supplements without consulting a physician.

Two vitamins—vitamin D and folate—are particularly important to pregnant women. Pregnant women who do not get enough vitamin D are more likely to deliver low-birth-weight babies. Chronic vitamin D deficiency has been linked to other health problems, including heart disease.

If a woman does not get the recommended daily amount of folate, both before and during pregnancy, her child has an increased risk of neural tube defects, including spina bifida. Anyone capable of becoming pregnant should get at least 400 micrograms (0.4 milligram) of folic acid (the synthetic form of folate) daily from fortified foods or supplements, and also from folate occurring naturally in other foods. Pregnant women should get 1000 micrograms (1 milligram) every day.

Another food both pregnant and lactating women should eat is fish high in omega-3 fatty acids. Consuming 8-12 ounces of a variety of seafoods per week reduces the mother's risk for hypertensive disorders and a preterm birth; seafood also improves cognitive and language development in children.

Food safety is another special dietary concern for pregnant women because foodborne pathogens can be especially dangerous to them and their unborn children. Germs and parasites such as *Listeria monocytogenes* and *Toxoplasma gondii* are both particularly worrisome. To avoid them, pregnant women should avoid eating undercooked and ready-to-eat meats (such as hot dogs and pre-packaged deli meats) and should wash produce thoroughly before eating it. Pregnant women should also follow the FDA's recommendations for consumption of fish and seafood.

Avoiding Drugs and Other Environmental Hazards

Everything the mother ingests may eventually reach the fetus in some proportion. In addition to the food the mother eats, the drugs she takes and the chemicals she is exposed to affect the fetus. Some drugs harm the fetus but not the mother because the fetus is in the process of developing and because the proper dose for the mother is a proportionately massive dose for the fetus.

During the first trimester, when the major body structures are forming rapidly, the fetus is extremely vulnerable to environmental factors such as viral infections, radiation, drugs, and other **teratogens,** any of which can cause **congenital malformations,** or birth defects. As most organs are developing during the first trimester, exposures are of special concern during this critical window. The rubella (German measles) virus, for example, can cause congenital malformation of nerves supplying the eyes and ears in the first trimester, leading to blindness or deafness, but exposure to it later in the pregnancy does no damage. For example, excess retinoic acid (vitamin A) exposure can lead to spontaneous abortion and fetal malformations such as microcephaly and cardiac anomalies. Women who are taking medications known to cause birth defects must take care to avoid pregnancy.

> **TERMS**
>
> **Rh factor** A protein found in blood; Rh incompatibility between a mother and fetus can jeopardize the fetus's health.
>
> **teratogen** An agent or influence that causes physical defects in a developing fetus.
>
> **congenital malformation** A physical defect existing at the time of birth, either inherited or caused during gestation.

Alcohol   Alcohol is a potent teratogen. Although 1 in 10 pregnant women reports an alcohol exposure at some point, getting drunk just one time during pregnancy may be enough to cause damage in a fetus. A high level of alcohol consumption during pregnancy is associated with spontaneous miscarriage and stillbirth. Fetuses born to mothers who have consumed alcohol are at risk for **fetal alcohol syndrome (FAS)**. A baby born with FAS is likely to be characterized by mental impairment, a small head and body size, unusual facial features, congenital heart defects, defective joints, impaired vision, and abnormal behavior patterns. Researchers doubt that any level of alcohol consumption is safe during pregnancy.

Tobacco   About 10% of all women smoke during pregnancy; another 18% are exposed to secondhand and thirdhand smoke. Pregnant women who smoke should be counseled to quit, and all pregnant women should avoid places where people smoke. Smoking is a preventable risk factor associated with miscarriage, low birth weight, preterm birth, infant death, and other pregnancy complications that may occur via direct damage to genetic material. Nicotine, the active ingredient in cigarette smoke, impairs oxygen delivery to the fetus and leads to faster fetal heart rates and reduced fetal breathing.

Babies born to women who smoke during pregnancy have poorer lung function at birth. After delivery, exposure to second-hand smoke increases the infant's susceptibility to pneumonia, bronchitis, and sudden infant death syndrome (SIDS). Up to 34% of SIDS cases have been attributed to tobacco use. If a mother who smokes breastfeeds, her infant will be exposed to tobacco chemicals through breast milk.

Caffeine   Caffeine, a powerful stimulant, puts both mother and fetus under stress by raising the level of the hormone epinephrine. Caffeine also reduces the blood supply to the uterus. One study found that consuming the amount of caffeine in five or more cups of coffee a day doubled the risk of miscarriage. Coffee, colas, strong black tea, and chocolate are high in caffeine, as are some over-the-counter medications. A pregnant woman should limit her caffeine intake to no more than the equivalent of two cups of coffee per day.

Drugs   Some prescription drugs, such as some blood pressure medications, can harm the fetus, so they should be used only under medical supervision. Antidepressant use in pregnancy can lead to withdrawal symptoms in newborns after delivery. Newborns may become fussy, with high-pitched, irritable cries, and develop difficulty feeding. In rare cases, a mother's antidepressant use has been associated with persistent pulmonary hypertension in the infant. The antidepressant paroxetine has been shown to cause fetal cardiac defects. Medications to prevent seizures are associated with birth defects such as neural tube defect and cleft palate. Both prescription and over-the-counter drugs should be used only under a physician's direction. Large doses of vitamin A, for example, can cause birth defects.

Recreational drugs, such as cocaine, can increase the risk of miscarriage, stillbirth, growth abnormalities, major birth defects, and placental bleeding. Marijuana is associated with preterm birth and stillbirth. Methamphetamine use is associated with underweight babies.

Infections   Infections, including those that are sexually transmitted, are another serious problem for the fetus. The most common cause of life-threatening infections in newborns is group B streptococcus (GBS), a bacterium that can cause pneumonia, meningitis, and blood infections. As 25–30% of all pregnant women are carriers of GBS, screening at 36 weeks of pregnancy is recommended. A carrier or a woman who develops a fever during labor will be given intravenous antibiotics at the time of labor to reduce the risk of passing GBS to her baby.

In 2015, reports emerged about an outbreak of Zika virus among pregnant women in northern Brazil. Infection was associated with poor head growth in newborns (microcephaly). Since then, the mosquito-transmitted virus has spread throughout much of South America and Central America. Such cases in the United States remain incredibly rare. Symptoms include headache, muscle and joint pains, rash, and eye redness.

At present, it appears that 4–5% of cases will result in pregnancy loss or an associated birth defect. CDC guidelines recommend preventive measures such as wearing long-sleeve shirts, using mosquito repellant, and, for all pregnant women, avoiding travel to areas with current outbreaks. Because Zika can be transmitted sexually, the CDC also suggests that couples use condoms or abstain from sexual activity if the man might have been exposed to Zika and if his sex partner is pregnant or could become pregnant.

STIs   Syphilis is preventable and curable. In pregnancy, untreated syphilis has a high rate of transmission to the fetus, resulting in severe adverse outcomes: stillbirth in 40% of cases, premature delivery, neonatal infection, fetal growth restriction, and congenital anomalies. Long-term consequences

> **QUICK STATS**
>
> About **1%** of school-aged children in the United States have symptoms of fetal alcohol syndrome.
>
> —Centers for Disease Control and Prevention, 2015

> **TERMS**
>
> **fetal alcohol syndrome (FAS)**   A combination of birth defects caused by excessive alcohol consumption by the mother during pregnancy.

include deafness and neurologic impairment. Penicillin is the best treatment for syphilis.

Both chlamydia and gonorrhea are associated with increased risk for miscarriage and preterm birth. These conditions are particularly insidious because they cause nonspecific symptoms, so up to 85% of women delay seeking medical care. Gonorrhea is a major cause of blindness among newborns, and chlamydia can cause newborn pneumonias. Because 50% of women with gonorrhea are also infected with chlamydia, detected cases should also be screened for both.

All pregnant women should be tested for hepatitis B, a virus that can pass from the mother to the infant at birth. Babies born to mothers with chronic hepatitis B should receive both the vaccine and protective antibodies (hepatitis B immune globulin) at birth.

Herpes simplex virus (HSV) can cause harm to newborns. It may damage the baby's eyes, skin, and brain, leading to death. Genital herpes can be transmitted to the baby if the mother is actively shedding virus at the time of delivery. In women with evidence of a genital outbreak, babies should be delivered by cesarean section to decrease the risk to the fetus. Women with a history of genital herpes should be prescribed suppressive therapy with acyclovir in the last month of pregnancy. A primary outbreak of herpes can be dangerous if it occurs during pregnancy because the virus may pass through the placenta to the fetus. For this reason, it is important to know if the pregnant woman or her partner has a history of herpes.

Nearly 90% of children diagnosed with human immunodeficiency virus (HIV) will have acquired it through pregnancy, birth, or breastfeeding. Although shared needles from intravenous drug use can transmit HIV, most women acquire HIV/AIDS through heterosexual contact. The CDC therefore recommends routine testing for all pregnant women. Antiviral drugs, given to an HIV-infected mother during pregnancy and delivery and to her newborn immediately following birth, reduce the rate of HIV transmission from mother to infant from 25% to less than 2%.

Environmental factors affecting fetal or infant development are summarized in Table 9.2.

Prenatal Activity and Exercise

Physical activity during pregnancy contributes to mental and physical wellness (see the box "Physical Activity during Pregnancy"). Women can continue working at their jobs until late in their pregnancy, provided the work isn't so physically demanding that it jeopardizes their health. At the same time, pregnant women need more rest and sleep to maintain their own well-being and that of the fetus.

Kegel exercises, to strengthen the pelvic floor muscles, are recommended for pregnant women. These exercises are performed by alternately contracting and releasing the muscles used to stop the flow of urine. Each contraction should be held for about five seconds. Kegel exercises should be done several times a day for a total of about 50 repetitions daily.

Prenatal exercise classes are valuable because they teach exercises that tone the body muscles involved in birth, especially those of the abdomen, back, and legs. Toned-up muscles aid delivery and help the body regain its nonpregnant shape afterward.

Table 9.2	Environmental Factors Associated with Problems in a Fetus or Infant
AGENT OR CONDITION	**POTENTIAL EFFECTS**
Accutane (acne medication)	Small head, mental impairment, deformed or absent ears, heart defects, cleft lip and palate
Alcohol	Unusual facial characteristics, small head, heart defects, mental impairment, defective joints
Chlamydia	Eye infections, pneumonia
Cigarette smoking	Miscarriage, stillbirth, low birth weight, respiratory problems, sudden infant death
Cocaine	Miscarriage, stillbirth, low birth weight, small head, and other major birth defects
Cytomegalovirus (CMV)	Small head, mental impairment, blindness
Diabetes (insulin-dependent)	Malformations of the brain, spine, and heart
Gonorrhea	Eye infection leading to blindness if untreated
Herpes	Brain damage, stillbirth
HIV infection	Impaired immunity, stillbirth
Lead	Reduced IQ, learning disorders
Marijuana	Impaired fetal growth, stillbirth
Mercury	Brain damage
Propecia (hair loss medication)	Abnormalities of the male sex organs
Radiation (high dose)	Small head, growth and mental impairment, multiple birth defects
Rubella (German measles)	Malformation of eyes or ears causing deafness or blindness; small head; mental impairment
Syphilis	Fetal death and miscarriage, prematurity, physical deformities
Tetracycline	Pigmentation of teeth, underdevelopment of enamel
Vitamin A (excess)	Miscarriage; defects of the head, brain, spine, and urinary tract
Zika	Microcephaly

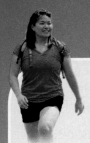

TAKE CHARGE
Physical Activity during Pregnancy

Most pregnant women benefit from moderate-intensity physical activity. It is recommended that healthy women get at least 2.5 hours of moderate aerobic activity per week during pregnancy and the postpartum period.

Maintaining a regular routine of physical activity throughout pregnancy can help a mother-to-be stay healthy and feel her best. Regular exercise can improve posture and decrease common pregnancy-related discomforts, such as backaches and fatigue. There is also evidence that physical activity may prevent gestational diabetes, relieve stress, and build stamina that can be helpful during labor and delivery.

A woman who was physically active before pregnancy should be able to continue her favorite activities in moderation, except for those that carry a risk of trauma, or unless there is a medical reason to reduce or stop exercise.

The American Congress of Obstetricians and Gynecologists (ACOG) offers advice regarding exercise during pregnancy. For example, downhill skiing or contact sports such as ice hockey, boxing, or soccer place pregnant women at risk for falls or abdominal trauma and should be avoided. Hot yoga and hot Pilates place the fetus at risk for overheating and are not recommended. In general, experts encourage low-impact aerobic activities such as walking or swimming over high-impact exercise. Physicians and pregnant women alike have concerns about exercise intensity. A good rule of thumb is never to exercise more than allows you to comfortably talk with a friend. If a pregnant woman is out of breath while exercising, she should slow down! Experts also recommend proper hydration and dressing to avoid overheating.

A woman who has never exercised regularly can safely start an exercise program during pregnancy after consulting with her health care provider. A routine of regular walking is considered safe. ACOG recommends that any pregnant woman who exercises should stop if she experiences any of the following warning signs:

- Vaginal bleeding
- Increased shortness of breath
- Dizziness
- Headache
- Pain in the chest or calves
- Regular painful contractions
- Decreased fetal movement
- Leakage of amniotic fluid

For detailed information about physical activity, see Chapter 14.

SOURCES: American College of Obstetricians and Gynecologists. 2015. Committee Opinion No. 650: Physical activity and exercise during pregnancy and the postpartum period. *Obstetrics and Gynecology* 126(6): 1326–1327; U.S. Centers for Disease Control and Prevention. 2020. *Physical Activity Basics: Healthy Pregnant or Postpartum Women* (https://www.cdc.gov/physicalactivity/basics/pregnancy/index.htm).

Preparing for Birth

Childbirth classes are almost a routine part of the prenatal experience for both mothers and fathers today. These classes typically teach the details of the birth process as well as relaxation techniques to help deal with the discomfort of labor and delivery. The mother learns and practices a variety of techniques so that she will be able to choose what works best for her during labor when the time comes. The father or her partner typically acts as a coach, supporting her emotionally and helping her with her breathing and relaxing. He or she remains with the mother throughout labor and delivery, even when a cesarean section is performed.

ectopic pregnancy A pregnancy in which the embryo develops outside the uterus, usually in an oviduct.

TERMS

COMPLICATIONS OF PREGNANCY AND PREGNANCY LOSS

Complications can arise in pregnancy for myriad reasons: *maternal diseases and exposures* such as diabetes, hypertension, or tobacco use; *placental factors,* including abruption or placenta previa; or *fetal conditions* such as genetic conditions like Down syndrome or cystic fibrosis. Each complication benefits from early diagnosis, counseling, and, if possible, corrective action.

Ectopic Pregnancy

In an **ectopic pregnancy,** the fertilized egg implants and begins to develop outside the uterus, usually in an oviduct (Figure 9.6). As the limited space of the oviduct cannot accommodate the rapid growth of a fertilized egg, ectopic pregnancies pose high risk of emergent bleeding through tubal rupture. Although ectopic pregnancies account for only 2% of all pregnancies, they contribute to 6% of all maternal deaths.

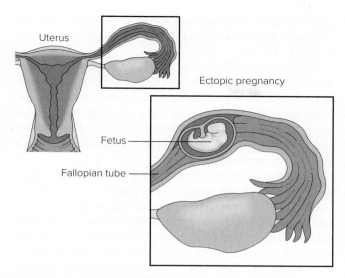

Uterus

Ectopic pregnancy

Fetus

Fallopian tube

FIGURE 9.6 Ectopic pregnancy in a fallopian tube.

Ectopic pregnancies usually occur because of occlusion (blockage) of the fallopian tube, most often as a result of pelvic inflammatory disease, although smoking also increases a woman's risk for ectopic pregnancy. The embryo may spontaneously abort, or the embryo and placenta may continue to expand until they rupture the fallopian tube. Sharp pain on one side of the abdomen or in the lower back, usually in about the seventh or eighth week of pregnancy, may signal an ectopic pregnancy, and there may be irregular bleeding. If bleeding from a rupture is severe, the woman may go into shock, characterized by low blood pressure, a fast pulse, weakness, and loss of consciousness.

Ectopic pregnancy is considered an emergency and may require surgical removal of the embryo and the fallopian tube to save the mother's life. If diagnosed early, before the fallopian tube ruptures, ectopic pregnancy can often be treated successfully without surgery using the chemotherapy drug methotrexate.

Spontaneous Abortion

A spontaneous abortion, or miscarriage, is the termination of pregnancy before the 20th week. Most miscarriages—about 60%—are due to chromosomal abnormalities in the fetus. Certain occupations that involve exposure to chemicals or radiation may increase the likelihood of a spontaneous abortion.

Vaginal bleeding (spotting) is usually the first sign that a pregnant woman may miscarry. She may also develop pelvic cramps, and her symptoms of pregnancy may disappear. Mild cramping, however, is common in pregnancy and is usually not associated with miscarriage.

One miscarriage doesn't mean that later pregnancies will be unsuccessful, and about 70–90% of women who miscarry eventually become pregnant again. About 1% of women suffer three or more miscarriages, possibly because of anatomical, hormonal, genetic, or immunological factors.

Stillbirth

The terms *fetal death, fetal demise, stillbirth,* and *stillborn* all refer to the delivery of a fetus that shows no signs of life. Each year over 3 million stillbirths occur worldwide. In the United States, the stillbirth rate is a little more than 6 in 1000. Risk factors for stillbirth include smoking, advanced maternal age, obesity, multiple gestations, and chronic disease. Race is also a factor; black women have twice as many stillbirths as white women. Although some observers attribute the increased risk for stillbirth among black women to the corresponding increased risk of preterm delivery, other reasons for race-based health care disparities may include poor access to care, infection, and the combined effects of racism and poverty.

Preeclampsia

One in 25 pregnancies in the United States will be complicated by **preeclampsia**, a condition characterized by elevated blood pressure and the appearance of protein in the urine. Left untreated, preeclampsia will worsen over time, resulting in symptoms including headache, right upper-quadrant abdominal pain, vision changes, increased swelling, and weight gain. The most significant potential complications of preeclampsia are seizures, liver and kidney damage, bleeding, fetal growth restriction, and fetal death.

Outside the United States, preeclampsia is a leading cause of maternal and fetal complications. The incidence is related to race and ethnicity as well as to environmental factors and family history. Women with preeclampsia without severe features may be monitored closely outside of the hospital. More severe cases may require hospitalization for close medical management and early delivery.

Placenta Previa

In **placenta previa,** the placenta either completely or partially covers the cervical opening, preventing the mother from delivering the baby vaginally. As a result, the baby must be delivered by cesarean section. This condition occurs in 1 in 250 live births. Risk factors include prior cesarean delivery, multiple pregnancies, intrauterine surgery, smoking, multiple gestations, and advanced maternal age. The first indication of previa not detected by ultrasound is often painless bright red vaginal bleeding with or without contractions. Previa is the attributed cause of 20% of bleeding in the third trimester.

preeclampsia   A condition of pregnancy characterized by high blood pressure and protein in the urine.

TERMS

placenta previa   A complication of pregnancy in which the placenta covers the cervical opening, preventing the mother from delivering the baby vaginally.

Placental Abruption

In **placental abruption,** a normally implanted placenta separates prematurely from the uterine wall. Patients experience abdominal pain, vaginal bleeding, and uterine tenderness. This causes 30% of all bleeding in the third trimester. The condition also increases the risk of fetal death. The risk factors for developing a placental abruption are maternal age, smoking, cocaine use, multiple gestation, trauma, preeclampsia, hypertension, and premature rupture of membranes.

Gestational Diabetes

During gestation, about 7–18% of all pregnant women develop **gestational diabetes mellitus (GDM),** in which the body loses its ability to use insulin properly. In these women, diabetes occurs only during pregnancy. The condition stems from the secretion of placental hormones: growth hormone, cortisol, placental lactogen, and progesterone. GDM arises when pancreatic function is not sufficient to overcome the insulin resistance created by these pregnancy-related hormones. Women diagnosed with GDM have an increased risk of developing type 2 diabetes later in life. It is important to accurately diagnose and treat GDM because it can lead to preeclampsia, polyhydramnios (increased levels of amniotic fluid), large fetuses, birth trauma, operative deliveries, perinatal mortality, and neonatal metabolic complications.

All women in pregnancy are therefore advised to test for GDM, which is a simple and straightforward procedure. The woman will be asked to drink a sugary beverage. After a set period of time in which she consumes nothing else, her glucose level is assessed. If the body processes the sugars normally, insulin should drive the sugar out of the bloodstream and into other compartments such as muscle, brain, and liver. After an hour, the blood sugar should be low. In the case of GDM, the body is relatively insulin-resistant and the sugars remain high. GDM is usually treated by diet and exercise modification, and sometimes medication.

Preterm Labor and Birth

When a pregnant woman goes into labor before the 37th week of gestation, she is said to experience *preterm labor.* Preterm labor is one of the most common reasons for hospitalizing pregnant women, but verifying true preterm labor can be difficult, and stopping it is even harder. About 30–50% of preterm labors resolve themselves, with the pregnancy continuing to full term.

Preterm birth is the leading direct cause of newborn death, accounting for about one-third of all infant deaths. Preterm birth is also the main risk factor for newborn illness and death from other causes, particularly infection. Babies born prematurely appear to be at a higher risk of long-term health and developmental problems, including delayed development and learning problems.

Currently, the underlying causes for preterm labor remain poorly identified and require further research. Established risk factors for preterm birth include lack of prenatal care, smoking, drug use, stress, personal health history, infections or illness during pregnancy, obesity, exposure to environmental toxins, a previous preterm birth, and the carrying of multiple fetuses. However, only about half the women who give birth prematurely have any known risk factors.

Labor Induction

If pregnancy continues well beyond the baby's due date, it may be necessary to induce labor artificially. This is one of the most common obstetrical procedures and is typically offered to pregnant women who have not delivered and are 7–14 days past their due dates.

Low Birth Weight and Premature Birth

A **low-birth-weight (LBW)** baby is one that weighs less than 5.5 pounds at birth. LBW babies may be **premature** (born before the 37th week of pregnancy) or full-term. Babies who are born small even though they're full-term are referred to as *small-for-gestational-age* babies. Low birth weight affected 8.3% of babies born in the United States in 2017. About half of all cases are related to teenage pregnancy, cigarette smoking, poor nutrition, and poor maternal health. Other maternal factors include drug use, stress, depression, and anxiety. Adequate prenatal care is the best way to prevent LBW.

Full-term LBW babies have fewer problems than premature infants. Even mild prematurity increases an infant's risk of dying in the first month or year of life. Premature infants are subject to respiratory problems and infections. They may have difficulty eating because they may be too small to suck a breast or bottle, and their swallowing mechanism may be underdeveloped. As they get older, premature infants may have problems such as learning difficulties, behavior problems, poor hearing and vision, and physical awkwardness.

TERMS

placental abruption A complication of pregnancy in which a normally implanted placenta separates prematurely from the uterine wall.

gestational diabetes mellitus (GDM) A form of diabetes that occurs during pregnancy.

low birth weight (LBW) Weighing less than 5.5 pounds at birth, often the result of prematurity.

premature Born before the 37th week of pregnancy.

Ask Yourself

QUESTIONS FOR CRITICAL THINKING AND REFLECTION

Do you know anyone who has lost a child to miscarriage, stillbirth, or a birth defect? If so, how did they cope with their loss? What would you do to help someone in this situation?

Infant Mortality and SIDS

The U.S. rate of **infant mortality,** the death of a child at less than 1 year of age, is near its lowest point ever—5.8 deaths for every 1000 live births as of 2017; however, that number remains far higher than rates in most of the developed world. Poverty and inadequate health care are key causes, with rates rising in poorer communities and lowest in areas of wealth. The infant mortality rate among African Americans is 2.4 times higher than that among Euro-Americans.

Forty-six percent of infant deaths are due to one of three leading factors: congenital abnormalities, prematurity/low birth weight, or **sudden infant death syndrome (SIDS).** SIDS is defined by a sudden and unexpected death of a child less than 1 year of age not explained by thorough investigation including autopsy. An estimated 1363 babies died of SIDS in 2017, the latest year for which statistics are available.

Prior to the 1990s, parents often put their babies to sleep on their stomachs, and the rate of SIDS was 3.5 per 1000. In 1994, however, evidence supported the introduction of the "Back to Sleep" campaign, which suggested that putting babies to bed on their backs rather than on their stomachs significantly reduces the risk of SIDS. Research suggests that abnormalities in the brain stem, the part of the brain that regulates breathing, heart rate, and other basic functions, underlie the risk for SIDS. Risk is increased greatly for infants with these innate differences if they are exposed to environmental risks such as tobacco smoke, alcohol, substance use, and, most important, sleeping stomach-side down. Because infants developmentally change how they sleep between 2 and 4 months of age, this is a time period of particular risk. Additionally, suffocation risk increases with the presence of many items common to cribs: fluffy pillows, mattresses, or plush toys. Therefore, current recommendations are to place babies to sleep back down, on a firm sleep surface, without soft bedding, plush toys, or additional clothing that might cause overheating. Several studies have found that the use of a pacifier significantly reduces the risk of SIDS.

Coping with Loss

Parents form a deep attachment to their children even before birth, and those who lose an infant before or during birth usually experience deep grief. Initial feelings of shocked disbelief and numbness may give way to sadness, anger, crying spells, and preoccupation with the loss. Physical sensations such as tightness in the chest or stomach, loss of appetite, and sleeplessness may also occur. For the mother, physical exhaustion and hormone imbalances can compound the emotional and physical stress.

Experiencing the pain of loss is part of the healing process. Use of support groups or professional counseling is often helpful. Planning the next pregnancy, with a physician's input, can be an important step toward recovery, but often a couple is physically fertile before either has emotionally healed from the loss. Subsequent pregnancies are often marked by anxiety or renewed grief.

CHILDBIRTH

By the end of the ninth month of pregnancy, most women are tired of being pregnant; both parents are eager to start a new phase of their lives. Most couples find the actual process of birth to be an exciting and positive experience.

Choices in Childbirth

Ninety-eight percent of babies in the United States in 2017 were delivered in hospitals. Less than 2% of births occur in freestanding birth centers where the environment may feel more comfortable while still remaining close to the medical resources of a hospital.

Many mothers-to-be are accompanied in the delivery room by a labor companion, called a *doula.* A doula is a woman who either has been through childbirth or has experience with birth. She stays with the laboring woman and provides support, information, and advocacy. Supportive labor companions may improve labor progress by reducing maternal anxiety. Studies suggest that the presence of a knowledgeable doula may shorten the duration of labor, increase the rate of spontaneous vaginal birth, and reduce the use of narcotic painkillers, forceps delivery, and cesarean birth.

Health care providers will need to assess maternal and fetal health and make decisions together with prospective parents about appropriate care providers and delivery location.

Labor and Delivery

The birth process occurs in three stages (Figure 9.7). **Labor** begins when hormonal changes in both the mother and the baby cause strong, rhythmic uterine **contractions**. These contractions exert pressure on the cervix and cause the lengthwise muscles of the uterus to pull on the circular muscles around the cervix, causing effacement (thinning) and dilation (opening) of the cervix. The contractions also pressure the baby to descend into the mother's pelvis, if it hasn't already. The entire process of labor and delivery usually takes between 2 and 36 hours, depending on the size of the baby, the baby's position in the uterus, the size of the mother's pelvis, the strength of the uterine contractions, the number of prior deliveries, and other factors. The

infant mortality   The death of a child at less than **TERMS** 1 year of age.

sudden infant death syndrome (SIDS)   The sudden death of an apparently healthy infant during sleep.

labor   The act or process of giving birth to a child, expelling it with the placenta from the mother's body by means of uterine contractions.

contraction   Shortening of the muscles in the uterine wall, which causes effacement and dilation of the cervix and assists in expelling the fetus.

length of labor is generally shorter for second and subsequent births.

The First Stage of Labor   The first stage of labor averages 13 hours for a first birth, although there is wide variation among women. It begins with cervical effacement and dilation and continues until the cervix is completely dilated. Contractions usually last about 30 seconds and occur every 15–20 minutes at first. They occur more often later. The prepared mother relaxes as much as possible during these contractions to allow labor to proceed without being blocked by tension. Early in the first stage, a small amount of bleeding may occur as a plug of slightly bloody mucus that blocked the opening of the cervix during pregnancy is expelled. In some women, the amniotic sac ruptures and the fluid rushes out; this is sometimes referred to as "breaking water."

The last part of the first stage of labor, called **active labor,** is characterized by strong and frequent contractions, much more intense than in the early stages of labor. Contractions may last 60–90 seconds and occur every 1–3 minutes. During active labor the cervix opens completely, to a diameter of about 10 centimeters. When the head of the fetus is flexed forward, to present its smallest diameter, it measures 9–10 centimeters. Therefore, a completely dilated cervix should permit the passage of the fetal head.

The Second Stage of Labor   The second stage of labor is the "pushing phase." It begins with the cervix completely dilated to 10 cm and ends with the delivery of the baby. With uterine contractions and maternal pushing, the baby descends through the bones of the pelvis, past the cervix, and into the vagina, which it stretches open. Some women find this the most difficult part of labor; others find that the contractions and bearing down bring a sense of relief. The baby's head and body turn to fit through the narrowest parts of the passageway, and the soft bones of the baby's skull move together and overlap as it is squeezed through the pelvis. When the top of the head appears at the vaginal opening, the baby is said to be *crowning*.

As the head of the baby emerges, the physician or midwife will check to ensure that the umbilical cord is not around the neck. With a few more contractions, the baby's shoulders and body emerge. As the baby is squeezed through the pelvis, cervix, and vagina, amniotic fluid in the lungs is forced out by the pressure on the baby's chest. Once this pressure is released as the baby emerges from the vagina, the chest expands and the lungs fill with air for the first time. The baby will appear wet and often is covered with a cheesy substance called *vernix*. The baby's head may be oddly shaped at first, due to the molding of the soft plates of bone during birth, but it usually takes on a more rounded appearance within 24 hours.

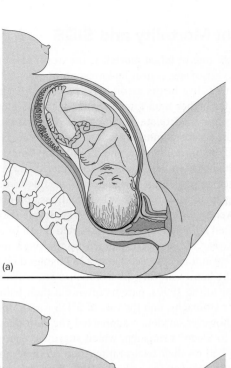
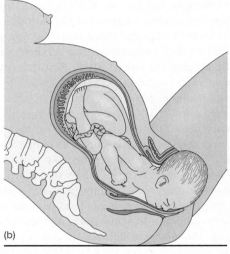
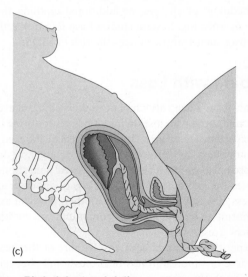

FIGURE 9.7   Birth: labor and delivery. (a) The first stage of labor contractions cause effacement and dilation; (b) the second stage of labor: delivery of the baby; (c) the third stage of labor: expulsion of the placenta.

> **active labor**   The last part of the first stage of labor, during which the cervix becomes fully dilated; characterized by intense and frequent contractions.
>
> **TERMS**

The Third Stage of Labor   In the third stage of labor, the uterus continues to contract until the placenta is expelled. This stage usually takes 5–30 minutes. The entire placenta must be expelled; if part remains in the uterus, it may cause bleeding and infection. Breastfeeding soon after delivery helps control uterine bleeding because it stimulates secretion of a hormone that makes the uterus contract.

The baby's physical condition is assessed with the **Apgar score,** a formalized system for assessing the baby's physical condition and whether medical assistance is needed. Heart rate, respiration, color, reflexes, and muscle tone are rated individually with a score of 0–2, and a total score between 0 and 10 is given at 1 and 5 minutes after birth. A score of 7–10 at 5 minutes is considered normal. Most newborns are also tested for 29 specific disorders, some of which are life-threatening. The American Academy of Pediatrics endorses these tests, but they are not routinely performed in every state.

Pain Relief during Labor and Delivery   Women vary in how much pain they experience in childbirth. First babies are typically the most challenging to deliver because the birth canal has never stretched to this extent before. It is recommended that women and their partners learn about labor and what kinds of choices are available for pain relief. Childbirth preparation courses are a good place to start, and communicating with one's obstetrician or midwife is essential to assessing pain relief options. Pain can be modified by staying active in labor, laboring in water, and using breathing and relaxation techniques, including hypnosis.

Medical pain relief can come in the form of intravenous narcotics, which are short-acting and can be used only in early labor. If a baby is born under the influence of narcotics, it can appear floppy and without vigor. The most commonly used medical intervention for pain relief is the *epidural injection*. This procedure involves placing a thin plastic catheter between the vertebrae in the lower back. Medication that reduces the transmission of pain signals to the brain is given through this catheter. Regional anesthetic drugs are given in low concentration to minimize weakening of the leg muscles so that the mother can push effectively during the birth. The advantage of the epidural is that the medication is used in low amounts in the confined space of the spinal column, protecting the fetus from the effect of the medication. The mother is awake and is an active participant in the birth.

Local anesthesia is available for repair of any tear or **episiotomy** (a surgical incision of the perineum to allow easier delivery of the baby) if the mother has not used an epidural for the labor.

Cesarean Delivery   In a **cesarean section,** the baby is removed through a surgical incision in the abdominal wall and uterus. Cesarean sections are necessary when a baby can't be delivered vaginally—for example, if the baby's head is bigger than the mother's pelvis or if the baby is not head down at the time of labor. If the mother has a serious health condition such as high blood pressure, a cesarean may be safer for her than labor and a vaginal delivery. Cesareans are more common among women who are overweight or have diabetes. Other reasons for cesarean delivery include abnormal or difficult labor, fetal distress, and the presence of a dangerous infection like herpes that can be passed to the baby during vaginal delivery.

Repeat cesarean deliveries are also very common. In 2017, 87.8% of American women who had had one child by cesarean had subsequent children delivered the same way. Although the risk of complications from a vaginal delivery after a previous cesarean delivery is low, there is a small (1%) risk of serious complications for the mother and baby if the previous uterine scar opens during labor (uterine rupture). For this reason, women and their physicians may choose to deliver by elective repeat cesarean.

Cesarean section is the most common hospital procedure performed in the United States. High rates have prompted health officials to examine ways to reduce cesarean sections, leading to a successful reduction over the past years. The safest mode of delivery for both mother and baby in an uncomplicated pregnancy is a vaginal delivery. Like any major surgery, cesarean section carries a longer recovery period and additional risks. Most cesarean deliveries are performed with regional anesthetic, which permits the mother to remain awake for the surgery with her partner present.

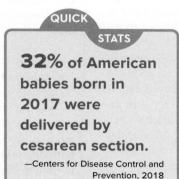

QUICK STATS

32% of American babies born in 2017 were delivered by cesarean section.

—Centers for Disease Control and Prevention, 2018

Ask Yourself

QUESTIONS FOR CRITICAL THINKING AND REFLECTION

If you are a woman, what are your views on labor and delivery options? If you have a child in the future, which facility, delivery, and pain management options do you think you would prefer? If you are a man, what are your views on participating in delivery? What steps do you think could be taken to help new mothers at home? In the workplace?

TERMS

Apgar score   A formalized system for assessing a newborn's need for medical assistance.

episiotomy   An incision made in the perineum to widen the vaginal opening to facilitate birth and prevent uncontrolled tearing during delivery.

cesarean section   A surgical incision through the abdominal wall and uterus, performed to deliver a fetus.

The Postpartum Period

The **postpartum period,** a stage of about three months following childbirth, is a time of critical family adjustments. Parenthood begins literally overnight, and the transition can cause considerable stress.

Following a vaginal delivery, mothers usually leave the hospital within one or two days (after a cesarean section, they usually stay an additional day). Uterine contractions will occur from time to time for several days after delivery, especially during nursing, as the uterus begins to return to its prebirth size. It usually takes six to eight weeks for a woman's reproductive organs to return to their prebirth condition. She will have a bloody discharge called *lochia* for three to six weeks after the birth.

Within the first few days after birth, a baby will undergo screening for certain genetic conditions such as sickle-cell disease; the mandated tests vary by state. The baby's head—if somewhat cone-shaped following a vaginal delivery—will become more rounded within a few days. It takes about a week for the umbilical cord stump to shrivel and fall off. Regular infant checkups for health screenings and immunizations usually begin when the infant is only a few weeks old.

Breastfeeding **Lactation,** the production of milk, begins about three days after childbirth. Prior to that time (sometimes as early as the second trimester), **colostrum** is secreted by the nipples. Colostrum contains antibodies that help protect the newborn from infectious diseases; it is also high in protein.

The American Academy of Pediatrics recommends breastfeeding exclusively for six months, then in combination with solid food until the baby is one year of age, and then for as long after that as a mother and baby desire. Currently only 22.3% of U.S. mothers breastfeed exclusively for six months. Human milk is perfectly suited to the baby's nutritional needs and digestive capabilities, and it supplies the baby with antibodies. Breastfeeding decreases the incidence of infant infection and diarrhea and appears to decrease diabetes and childhood obesity.

Breastfeeding is beneficial to the mother as well. It stimulates contractions that help the uterus return to normal more rapidly, contributes to postpregnancy weight loss, and may reduce the risk of breast and ovarian cancers. Nursing also provides a sense of closeness and emotional well-being for mother and child. Avoiding formula is cost saving and good for the environment. For women who want to breastfeed but who have problems, help is available from support groups, books, or lactation consultants and health care providers.

Some women find breastfeeding difficult due to physical or social problems. Some do not have enough milk or the milk will not circulate properly. Sometimes babies refuse to nurse at the breast. Tenderness or infection of the nipples can also be a constraint. If a woman has an illness or requires drug treatment, she may have to bottlefeed her baby because drugs and infectious agents may show up in breast milk. Working mothers encounter varying degrees of support from their employers.

An advantage to bottlefeeding is that it is easier to tell how much milk an infant is taking in, and bottlefed infants tend to sleep longer. Bottlefeeding also allows the father or other caregiver to share in the nurturing process. Both breastfeeding and bottlefeeding can be part of loving, secure parent-child relationships.

When a mother doesn't nurse, menstruation usually begins within about 10 weeks. Breastfeeding can prevent the return of menstruation for six months or longer because the hormone prolactin, which aids milk production, suppresses hormones vital to the development of mature eggs. However, ovulation—and pregnancy—can occur before menstruation returns, so breastfeeding is not a reliable contraceptive method. If the mother becomes pregnant while still nursing, she needs to make sure that she is receiving adequate nutrition because the energy requirement for both breastfeeding and gestating is immense. With proper counseling, breastfeeding can continue until near delivery.

Postpartum Depression The physical stress of labor, blood loss, fatigue, decreased sleep, fluctuating postpartum hormone levels, and anxieties of becoming a new parent all contribute to emotional instability postpartum. About 50–80% of new mothers experience "baby blues," characterized by episodes of sadness, weeping, anxiety, headache, sleep disturbances, and irritability. A mother may feel lonely and anxious about caring for her infant.

About 9–16% of new mothers experience **postpartum depression.** Postpartum depression is characterized by a prolonged period of anxiety, guilt, fear, or self-blame; these feelings prevent the new mother from normal participation in everyday life or the normal care of her newborn. Those close to the affected woman may fear for the well-being of the mother or those in her care. Fortunately, postpartum depression can be prevented and treated effectively. Women with a history of depression or depression during pregnancy can benefit from early referral to an appropriate mental health care provider. Rest is a key component of recovery. The mother's support system should offer to take on important responsibilities to allow the mother to rest and recover, as well as encourage her to continue outside interests and share her concerns with a professional who can assess the need for medical therapy.

Some men also seem to get a form of postpartum depression, characterized by anxiety about their changing roles and

---

TERMS

postpartum period   The period of about three months after delivering a baby.

lactation   The production of milk.

colostrum   A yellowish fluid secreted by the mammary glands around the time of childbirth until milk comes in, about the third day.

postpartum depression   An emotional low that may be experienced by the mother following childbirth.

- Factors to consider when deciding if and when to have a child include physical health and age, financial circumstances, and existing relationships.

- Preconception care examines factors such as preexisting medical conditions, current medications, ages of the parents, lifestyle behaviors, infections, nutritional status, and family history of genetic disease.

- Fertilization is a complex process culminating when a sperm penetrates the membrane of the egg released from the woman's ovary.

- Infertility affects about 8.8% of the reproductive-age population of the United States. The leading causes of infertility in women are blocked oviducts and ovulation disorders. Exposure to toxins, injury to the testicles, and infection can cause infertility in men.

- Early signs and symptoms of pregnancy include a missed menstrual period; slight bleeding; nausea; breast tenderness; increased urination; fatigue and emotional upset; and a softening of the uterus just above the cervix.

- During pregnancy, the uterus enlarges until it pushes up into the rib cage; the breasts enlarge and may secrete colostrum; the muscles and ligaments soften and stretch; and the circulatory system, lungs, and kidneys become more efficient.

- The fetal anatomy is almost completely formed in the first trimester and is refined in the second; during the third trimester, the fetus grows and gains most of its weight, storing nutrients in fatty tissues.

- Prenatal tests available include ultrasound and both noninvasive screening and invasive diagnostic testing such as amniocentesis or chorionic villus sampling.

- Health care during pregnancy includes a complete history and physical, followed by regular checkups for blood pressure monitoring, weight gain, and serial assessment of fetal growth.

- Important elements of prenatal care include good nutrition; avoidance of drugs, alcohol, tobacco, infections, and other harmful environmental agents or conditions; and regular physical activity.

- Pregnancy usually proceeds without major complications. Problems that can occur include ectopic pregnancy, spontaneous abortion, preeclampsia, low birth weight, and preterm birth. The loss of a fetus or infant is deeply felt by most parents, who need time to grieve and heal.

- Couples preparing for childbirth may have many options to choose from, including type of practitioner and facility.

- The first stage of labor begins with contractions that exert pressure on the cervix, causing effacement and dilation. The second stage begins with complete cervical dilation and ends when the baby is delivered. The third stage of labor is expulsion of the placenta.

feelings of inadequacy. Both mothers and fathers need time to adjust to their new roles as parents.

Attachment   Another feature of the postpartum period is the development of attachment—the strong emotional tie that grows between the baby and the adult who cares for the baby. Parents can foster secure attachment relationships in the early weeks and months by responding sensitively to the baby's true needs. Parents who respond appropriately to the baby's signals of gazing, looking away, smiling, and crying establish feelings of trust in their child. They feed the baby when she's hungry, for example; respond when she cries; interact with her when she gazes, smiles, or babbles; and stop stimulating her when she frowns or looks away. A secure attachment relationship helps the child develop and function well socially, emotionally, and mentally.

TIPS FOR TODAY AND THE FUTURE

Preparing for parenthood starts long before pregnancy; it includes making sound choices in all the areas of wellness.

RIGHT NOW YOU CAN:

- Take some time to think about whether you really *want* to have children. Cut through the cultural, societal, family, and personal expectations that may stand in the way of making the decision you really want to make.

- Think of one thing your mother or father did as a parent that you particularly liked; if you become a parent, consider how you can be sure to do the same thing for your children.

- Think of one thing your mother or father did as a parent that you particularly disliked; if you become a parent, consider how you can be sure to avoid doing the same thing.

IN THE FUTURE YOU CAN:

- Make behavioral changes that can improve your prospects as a parent. For example, you may need to adopt healthier eating habits or start exercising more consistently.

- If you want to be a parent someday, start looking at the many sources of information about pregnancy, childbirth, and parenting. This is a good idea for all parties involved.

Ask Yourself

QUESTIONS FOR CRITICAL THINKING AND REFLECTION

What are some early signs or symptoms of depression? Consider ways you might start a conversation about depression or help a new mother find access to help. What kinds of things might you say or do?

- During the postpartum period, the mother's body begins to return to its prepregnancy state, and she may begin to breastfeed. Both mother and father must adjust to their new roles as parents as they develop a strong emotional bond with their baby.

FOR MORE INFORMATION

American Academy of Pediatrics. Provides evidence-based information on all aspects of parenting from birth on.

> https://www.aap.org/en-us/Pages/Default.aspx

American Congress of Obstetricians and Gynecologists (ACOG). Provides written materials relating to many aspects of preconception care, pregnancy, and childbirth.

> http://www.acog.org

American Society for Reproductive Medicine. Provides up-to-date information on all aspects of infertility.

> http://www.asrm.org

Babycenter.org. Contains information and personal stories about all phases of pregnancy and birth.

> http://www.babycenter.org/pregnancy

California Department of Public Health Newborn Screening Branch, Genetic Disease Screening Program. Provides information about newborn screening tests for specific types of diseases: metabolic, endocrine, hemoglobin, and cystic fibrosis. Early identification and treatment can prevent mental retardation and/or life-threatening illness.

> http://cdph.ca.gov/nbs

Centers for Disease Control and Prevention, National Center on Birth Defects and Developmental Disabilities. Provides information about a variety of topics related to birth defects, including fetal alcohol syndrome and the importance of folic acid.

> http://www.cdc.gov/ncbddd

Eunice Kennedy Shriver National Institute of Child Health and Human Development. Provides information about reproductive and genetic problems; sponsors the "Safe to Sleep" campaign to fight SIDS.

> http://www.nichd.nih.gov/sts

Health Resources and Services Administration (HRSA): Maternal and Child Health. Provides publications, videos, and other resources relating to maternal, infant, and family health.

> http://www.mchb.hrsa.gov

International Childbirth Education Association (ICEA). Supports family-centered maternity care by providing training for educators and health care providers who promote freedom to make decisions based on knowledge of alternatives.

> http://www.icea.org

International Council on Infertility Information Dissemination. Provides information about current research and treatments for infertility.

> http://www.inciid.org

March of Dimes. Provides public education materials about many pregnancy-related topics, including preconception care, genetic screening, diet and exercise, and the effects of smoking and drinking during pregnancy.

> http://www.marchofdimes.com

Mayo Clinic Health Information. Provides information on most aspects of health issues and care, including pregnancy.

> http://www.mayoclinic.com

Resolve. Provides information, support, and referrals for people facing infertility.

> http://www.resolve.org

U.S. Department of Health and Human Services: Surgeon General's My Family Health Portrait. Offers publications and an online tool for building a Family Health Portrait.

> https://phgkb.cdc.gov/FHH/html/index.html

SELECTED BIBLIOGRAPHY

American Pregnancy Association. 2020. *Depression during Pregnancy* (http://americanpregnancy.org/pregnancy-health/depression-during-pregnancy/).

Angelucci, E., et al. 2014. Hematopoietic stem cell transplantation in thalassemia major and sickle cell disease: Indications and management recommendations from an international expert panel. *Haematologica* 99(5): 811–820.

Centers for Disease Control and Prevention. 2015. Fetal alcohol syndrome among children aged 7–9—Arizona, Colorado, and New York, 2010. *Morbidity and Mortality Weekly Report* 64(03): 54–57.

Centers for Disease Control and Prevention. 2019. *Breastfeeding Report Card United States, 2018* (http://www.cdc.gov/breastfeeding/data/reportcard.htm).

Centers for Disease Control and Prevention. 2016. *STDs during Pregnancy—Fact Sheet (Detailed)* (http://www.cdc.gov/std/pregnancy/stdfact-pregnancy-detailed.htm).

Centers for Disease Control and Prevention. 2018. *One Test Two Lives. HIV Screening for Prenatal Care* (https://www.cdc.gov/actagainstaids/campaigns/ottl/faq.html).

Centers for Disease Control and Prevention, American Society for Reproductive Medicine, Society for Assisted Reproductive Technology. 2018. *2016 Assisted Reproductive Technology National Summary Report.* Atlanta (GA): U.S. Department of Health and Human Services.

Centers for Disease Control and Prevention. 2020. *Zika and Pregnancy* (https://www.cdc.gov/pregnancy/zika/index.html).

Child Care Aware of America. 2019. *Parents and the High Cost of Child Care: 2019 Report.* Appendix 1 (https://usa.childcareaware.org/advocacy-publicpolicy/resources/research/costofcare/).

Dietary Guidelines Advisory Committee. 2020. *Scientific Report of the 2020 Dietary Guidelines Advisory Committee: Advisory Report to the Secretary of Agriculture and the Secretary of Health and Human Services.* U.S. Department of Agriculture, Agricultural Research Service, Washington, DC.

Institute of Medicine and National Research Council. 2009. *Weight Gain during Pregnancy: Reexamining the Guidelines.* Washington, DC: National Academies Press (http://www.nap.edu/catalog/12584.html).

Ismail, S., et al. 2010. Screening, diagnosing and prevention of fetal alcohol syndrome: Is this syndrome treatable? *Developmental Neuroscience* 32(2): 91–100.

Kochanek, K. D., et al. 2019. Deaths: Final data for 2017. *National Vital Statistics Reports* 68(9). Hyattsville, MD: National Center for Health Statistics.

Lino, M., et al. 2017. *Expenditures on Children by Families, 2015.* U.S. Department of Agriculture, Center for Nutrition Policy and Promotion. Miscellaneous Publication No. 1528-2015.

MacDorman, M. F., and E. Declercq. 2019. Trends and state variations in out-of-hospital births in the United States, 2004-2017. *Birth* 46(2): 279-288.

MacKenzie, T., et al. 2014. Longevity of patients with cystic fibrosis in 2000 to 2010 and beyond: Survival analysis of the Cystic Fibrosis Foundation patient registry. *Annals of Internal Medicine* 161(4): 233-241.

Martin, J. A., et al. 2018. Births: Final data for 2017. *National Vital Statistics Reports* 67(8). Hyattsville, MD: National Center for Health Statistics.

May, P., et al. 2014. Prevalence and characteristics of fetal alcohol spectrum disorders. *Pediatrics* 134: 855-866.

National Center for Health Statistics. 2019. *Infertility* (https://www.cdc.gov/nchs/nsfg/key_statistics/i_2015-2017.htm#infertility).

Ottaviani, G. 2014. *Crib Death—Sudden Infant Death Syndrome (SIDS): Sudden Infant and Perinatal Unexplained Death: The Pathologist's Viewpoint.* Berlin: Springer International.

Rysavy, M. 2015. Between-hospital variation in treatment and outcomes in extremely preterm infants. *New England Journal of Medicine* 372: 1801–1811.

Sibai, B. M. 2011. Disparity in the rate of eclampsia and adverse pregnancy outcome from eclampsia: A tale of two countries. *Obstetrics & Gynecology* 118(5): 976-977.

Snowden, J. M. 2015. Planned out-of-hospital birth and birth outcomes. *New England Journal of Medicine* 373(27): 2642–2653.

Sunderam, S., et al. 2019. Assisted reproductive technology surveillance—United States, 2016. *MMWR Surveillance Summaries* 68(No. SS-4):1–23.

U.S. Preventive Services Task Force. 2017. Screening for preeclampsia: U.S. Preventive Services Task Force recommendation statement. *JAMA* 317(16):1661–1667.

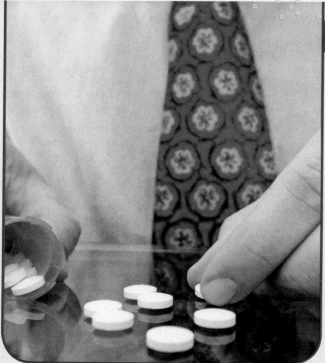
RBFried/iStock/Getty Images

CHAPTER OBJECTIVES

- Define and discuss addiction
- Explain factors that contribute to drug use and misuse and addiction
- List risks associated with drug misuse
- Understand how drugs affect the body
- List and describe the effects of the six major groups of psychoactive drugs
- Outline ways to prevent drug-related problems

CHAPTER **10**

Drug Use and Addiction

TEST YOUR KNOWLEDGE

1. **Addictions always involve drugs that cause physical withdrawal symptoms when a person stops taking them.**
   True or False?

2. **Of the following drugs, which is the most widely used among college-age Americans?**
   a. Crystal meth
   b. Hallucinogens
   c. Marijuana

3. **Caffeine use can produce physical dependence.**
   True or False?

4. **Which of the following drugs is most addictive?**
   a. Marijuana
   b. Nicotine
   c. LSD

5. **All herbal or synthetic recreational drugs are legal.**
   True or False?

ANSWERS

1. **FALSE.** Both assertions in this statement are wrong. Addiction does not always involve a drug; when it does, addiction is not defined by physical withdrawals.

2. **C.** Marijuana ranks first, followed (in order) by hallucinogens and crystal methamphetamine. Alcohol remains by far the most popular drug among college-age Americans.

3. **TRUE.** Regular users of caffeine develop physical tolerance, needing more caffeine to produce the same level of alertness. Many users experience withdrawal symptoms when they reduce their caffeine intake.

4. **B.** Nicotine is the most addictive.

5. **FALSE.** The U.S. Drug Enforcement Administration has banned some of these "designer drugs" or certain chemicals within them.

The use of **drugs** for both medical and social purposes is widespread in the United States (Table 10.1). Many Americans believe that every problem has or should have a chemical solution. When feeling tired, many turn to caffeine or other stimulants; for insomnia, sleeping pills; for anxiety, prescription medication, alcohol, or other sedative drugs. Advertisements, social pressures, and the human desire for quick solutions to difficult problems all contribute to the prevailing wishful view that drugs can ease all pain. But benefits often come with the risk of harmful consequences, and drug use can—and in many cases does—pose serious or even life-threatening risks.

This chapter introduces the concepts of addiction and misuse, and then focuses on the major classes of misused drugs, their effects, their potential for addiction and impairment, and other issues related to their use. Alcohol and nicotine—two of the most widely used and most problematic psychoactive drugs—are discussed in Chapters 11 and 12.

ADDICTION

Aside from death, the most serious drug-related risks are addiction and impairment of daily activities. The drugs most often associated with addiction and impairment are **psychoactive drugs**—those that alter a person's perception, mood, behavior, or consciousness. In the short term, psychoactive drugs can cause **intoxication,** a state in which, sometimes, unpredictable physical and emotional changes occur. People who are intoxicated may experience potentially serious changes in physical functioning. Their emotions and judgment may be affected in ways that lead to uncharacteristic and unsafe behavior. Recurrent drug use can have profound physical, emotional, and social effects.

What Is Addiction?

Today scientists view **addiction** as a chronic disease that involves disruption of the brain's systems related to reward, motivation, and memory. Dysfunction in these systems leads to biological, psychological, and social effects associated with pathologically pursuing pleasure or relief by substance use and other behaviors—despite adverse consequences to the person addicted. Addiction is a chronic (ongoing, relapsing) condition that causes compulsive substance use despite harmful consequences.

Addiction involves craving and the inability to recognize significant risk or other problems with behaviors, interpersonal relationships, and emotional responses. Like other chronic conditions, addiction often involves cycles of relapse and remission. Without treatment, addiction is progressive and can result in disabling or deadly health consequences.

TERMS

drug Any chemical other than food intended to affect the structure or function of the body.

psychoactive drug A drug that can alter a person's consciousness or experience.

intoxication The state of being mentally affected by a chemical (literally, a state of being poisoned).

addiction A chronic disease that disrupts the brain's system of motivation and reward, characterized by a compulsive desire and increasing need for a substance or behavior, and by harm to the individual and/or society.

VITAL STATISTICS

Table 10.1	Nonmedical Drug Use among Americans, 2018 (percent using in past month)		
	YOUNG ADULTS AGED 18–25	YOUTHS AGED 12–17	ALL AMERICANS AGED 12 AND OVER
ILLICIT DRUGS	23.9	8.0	11.7
Marijuana* and hashish	22.1	6.7	10.1
Cocaine	1.5	0.0	0.7
Heroin	0.2	0.0	0.1
Hallucinogens	1.7	0.6	0.5
Ecstasy	0.7	0.2	0.3
Inhalants	0.4	0.7	0.2
Methamphetamine	0.3	0.1	0.4
NONMEDICAL USE OF PSYCHOTHERAPEUTICS	3.7	1.3	2.0
Pain relievers	1.4	0.6	1.0
Tranquilizers	1.2	0.3	0.6
Stimulants	1.7	0.5	0.6
Sedatives	0.1	0.0	0.1

*See the section titled "Marijuana and Other Cannabis Products" for information about the legal status of marijuana.

SOURCE: SAMHSA Center for Behavioral Health Statistics and Quality. 2019. *Results from the 2018 National Survey on Drug Use and Health.* Retrieved from https://www.samhsa.gov/data/sites/default/files/cbhsq-reports/NSDUHDetailedTabs2018R2/NSDUHDetailedTabs2018.pdf.

Although addiction is most often associated with drug use, many experts now extend the concept of addiction to other behaviors. Looking at the nature of addiction and a range of addictive behaviors can help us understand similar behaviors when they involve drugs. **Addictive behaviors** are habits that have gotten out of control, with resulting negative effects on a person's health. The loss of control is expressed as an unrelenting pursuit of a physical or psychological reward through substance use or behaviors, such as gambling, despite unwanted consequences.

The American Psychiatric Association (APA) introduces the category of behavioral addictions, which includes gambling disorder, in the *Diagnostic and Statistical Manual of Mental Disorders (DSM-5)*, the standard classification system used by mental health professionals. Another addictive behavior, internet addiction, is not part of the *DSM-5*, but the *DSM-5* recommends that it be studied further. Internet gaming disorder involves excessive use of internet games that interferes with daily functioning.

Although experts now agree that addiction is more fully defined by behavioral characteristics, they also agree that changes in the brain may underlie addiction. One such change is **tolerance,** in which the body adapts to a drug so that the initial dose no longer produces the original emotional or psychological effects. To achieve the same high, the user requires larger and larger doses. The concept of addiction as a disease based in identifiable changes to the brain has led to many advances in the understanding and treatment of drug addiction.

The view that addiction is based in our brain chemistry does *not* imply that people are not responsible for their addictive behavior. Many experts believe it is inaccurate and counterproductive to think of all bad habits and excessive behaviors as diseases. All addictions involve an initial voluntary step, and other factors such as lifestyle, personality traits, and environmental factors play key roles in the development of addiction.

Diagnosing Substance Misuse and Addiction

It is important to note that you do not have to be addicted to a drug to suffer its serious consequences—in many cases you only have to misuse it once. **Substance misuse** is the use of a substance inconsistent with medical or legal guidelines. Misuse is a broad concept and can include the use of illegal drugs, prescription drugs in greater-than-prescribed amounts, another person's prescription drug, or even excessive use of a legal substance like alcohol. The situation in which a person takes prescribed painkillers to get high would be considered drug *misuse*. Any drug misuse carries the risk of serious and life-threatening effects.

In the *DSM-5*, the APA provides criteria for diagnosing problems associated with habitual drug use. Classifying a person as having a substance use disorder is not as simple as applying a label; instead, an individual is classified based on symptoms ranging from mild to severe.

Addiction is a psychological or physical dependence on a substance or behavior that produces undesirable, negative consequences. According to the APA, people with addiction are focused on a particular drug or behavior to the point that it takes over their lives; they use the substance or engage in the behavior compulsively despite knowing it will cause them problems.

The 11 *DSM-5* criteria for a substance use disorder are listed here, grouped in four categories. The severity of the disorder is determined by the number of criteria a person meets:

- 2–3 criteria indicate a mild disorder.
- 4–5 criteria point to a moderate disorder.
- 6 or more criteria are evidence of a severe disorder.

Impaired Control

1. *Taking the substance in larger amounts or over a longer period than was originally intended.*
2. *Expressing a persistent desire to cut down on or regulate substance use, but being unable to do so.*
3. *Spending a great deal of time getting the substance, using the substance, or recovering from its effects.*
4. *Craving or experiencing an intense desire or urge to use the substance.*

Social Problems

5. *Failing to fulfill major obligations at work, school, or home.*
6. *Continuing to use the substance despite having persistent or recurrent social or interpersonal problems caused or worsened by the effects of its use.*
7. *Giving up or reducing important social, school, work, or recreational activities because of substance use.*

Risky Use

8. *Using the substance in situations in which it is physically hazardous to do so.*
9. *Continuing to use the substance despite the knowledge of having persistent or recurrent physical or psychological problems caused or worsened by substance use.*

addictive behavior Compulsive behavior that is both rewarding and reinforcing and is often pursued to the marginalization or exclusion of other activities and responsibilities.

TERMS

tolerance Lower sensitivity to a drug or substance so that a given dose no longer exerts the usual effect and larger doses are needed.

substance misuse or abuse The use of any substance in a manner inconsistent with legal or medical guidelines; may be associated with adverse social, psychological, or medical consequences; the use may be intermittent and with or without tolerance and physical dependence.

Drug Effects

10. *Developing tolerance to the substance.* When a person requires increased amounts of a substance to achieve the desired effect or notices a markedly diminished effect with continued use of the same amount, he or she has developed tolerance to the substance.

11. *Experiencing withdrawal.* In someone who has maintained prolonged, heavy use of a substance, a drop in its concentration within the body can result in unpleasant physical and cognitive **withdrawal** symptoms. Withdrawal symptoms vary for different drugs. For example, nausea, vomiting, and tremors are common withdrawal symptoms in people dependent on alcohol, opioids, or sedatives.

The latest version of the *DSM* dropped the past distinction between *dependence* and *abuse* in diagnosing drug-related disorders; however, both terms are still used in other contexts. The term *abuse* is slowly falling out of favor because of its potential to shame people who misuse drugs, which can keep them from seeking help. Replacement terms include *misuse*, *disorder*, and *dependence*. Note that physical dependence, in a narrow sense, can be a normal bodily response to the use of a substance. For example, regular coffee drinkers may experience caffeine withdrawal symptoms if they reduce their intake. Does this mean they have a substance use disorder? Not necessarily. The National Institute specifies that more criteria, such as compulsive use, are required to qualify for substance abuse and **dependence**. A person who regularly takes prescribed low-dose opioids for chronic pain can suffer withdrawals and therefore physical dependence without exhibiting signs of an addictive disorder.

In this chapter we refer to the *DSM-5* definition of **substance use disorders** (which combines the concepts of *abuse* and *dependence*), but we also recognize the terms *dependence, abuse,* and *addiction,* which are commonly used in mental health literature.

The Development of Addiction

We all engage in activities that are potentially addictive. An addiction often starts when a person does something to bring pleasure or avoid pain. The activity may be drinking a beer, using the internet, playing the lottery, or shopping. If it works, the person is likely to repeat it. Reinforcement leads to an increasing dependence on the behavior. Tolerance—caused by physical changes to brain cells and reward pathways in the brain—develops, and the person needs more of the substance or behavior to feel the expected effect. Eventually the behavior becomes a central focus of the person's life, and other areas such as school performance or relationships deteriorate. The behavior no longer brings pleasure, but repeating it is necessary to avoid withdrawal, which is the physical and mental pain that results from going without it. Something that started as a seemingly innocent way of feeling good has triggered physiological changes in the brain that create a behavioral prison.

Although many common behaviors are potentially addictive, most people who engage in them do not develop problems. This is because the development of an addiction includes factors such as personality, lifestyle, heredity, the social and physical environment, and the nature of the substance or behavior in question. For addiction to develop, these diverse factors must work together in a certain way. For example, narcotic painkillers like morphine, fentanyl, and oxycodone have a high potential for physical addiction. Genetic factors make some individuals much more likely to develop dependence and addiction. Other factors—family, social, or cultural—play a role in determining if and at what age someone starts taking them. Like other addictions, opioid addiction often begins with a voluntary and seemingly inconsequential "yes or no" choice that spirals out of control.

Behavioral Addictions

For some people, behaviors unrelated to drugs can become addictive. Such behaviors can include eating, gambling, and playing video games. Any substance or activity that becomes the focus of a person's life at the expense of other needs and interests should be a sign there is a problem. Like substance addictions, behavioral or nondrug addiction symptoms also meet *DSM-5* criteria of craving, loss of control over the behavior, tolerance, withdrawal, and a repeating pattern of recovery and relapse. Behavioral addictions also promote changes in the brain similar to those changes associated with misuse of and addiction to alcohol, nicotine, or other drugs.

Compulsive Gambling About 1% of adult Americans are compulsive (pathological) gamblers, and another 2% are "problem gamblers." Sixty-five percent of pathological gamblers commit crimes to support their gambling addiction. The suicide rate of compulsive gamblers is 20 times higher than that of the general population.

Characteristic behaviors involved in a gambling disorder include preoccupation with gambling, unsuccessful efforts to quit, using gambling to escape problems, and lying to family members to conceal the extent of gambling.

---

withdrawal Physical and psychological symptoms **TERMS** that follow the interrupted use of a drug on which a user is physically dependent; symptoms may be mild or life threatening.

dependence Frequent or consistent use of a drug or behavior that makes it difficult for the person to get along without it; the result of physiological and/or psychological adaptation that occurs in response to the substance or behavior; typically associated with tolerance and withdrawal but can also be based solely on behavioral factors such as compulsive use.

substance use disorder A cluster of symptoms involving cognitive, bodily, and social impairment related to the continued use of a substance; a single disorder measured on a continuum from mild to severe.

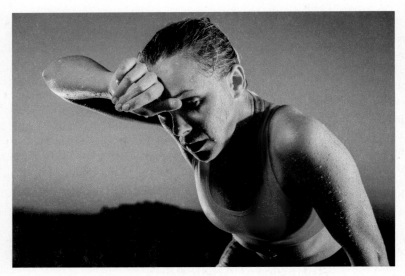

When taken to an extreme, even healthy activities such as exercise can become addictive. Erik Isakson/Blend Images LLC

Video Game Disorder Characteristic behaviors include preoccupation with internet games, loss of interest in other activities, using gaming to relieve anxiety or guilt, and risking opportunities or relationships due to time spent gaming. The disorder is separate from gambling disorder and differs from general use of social media or the internet.

Compulsive Exercising When taken to a compulsive level, even healthy activity can turn into harmful addictions. For example, compulsive exercising is now recognized as a serious departure from normal behavior. Compulsive exercising is often accompanied by more severe psychiatric disorders such as anorexia nervosa and bulimia (see Chapter 15). Traits often associated with compulsive exercising include an excessive preoccupation and dissatisfaction with body image, use of laxatives or vomiting to lose weight, and development of other obsessive-compulsive symptoms.

Work Addiction People who are excessively preoccupied with work are often called *workaholics*. Work addiction, however, is based on a set of specific symptoms, including an intense work schedule, the inability to limit your own work schedule, the inability to relax when away from work, and failed attempts to reduce work intensity.

Work addiction typically coincides with a well-known risk factor for cardiovascular disease—personality traits of competitiveness, ambition, drive, time urgency, restlessness, hyper-alertness, and hostility. (See Chapter 16.)

Sex Addiction Behaviors associated with sex addiction include an extreme preoccupation with sex, a compulsion to have sex repeatedly in a brief period of time, a great deal of time and energy spent looking for partners, sex used as a means of relieving painful feelings, and a reduced control over sexual behaviors despite the experience of negative emotional, personal, and professional consequences.

Pornography addiction, often grouped under sex addiction, is characterized by excessive viewing of pornography, using it to avoid negative feelings, needing it to be increasingly more stimulating (tolerance), feeling distress when it is stopped (withdrawal), and continuing with it despite unwanted consequences. These behaviors may result in physical problems such as erectile dysfunction, psychological problems such as preoccupation with sexual thoughts, and social consequences such as losing interest in person-to-person sexual contact, difficulty becoming aroused, and emotional detachment.

Compulsive Buying or Shopping A compulsive buyer repeatedly gives in to the impulse to buy more than they need or can afford. Compulsive spenders often buy luxury items rather than daily necessities, even though they are usually distressed by their behavior and its social, personal, and financial consequences. Some experts link compulsive shopping with neglect or abuse during childhood; it also seems to be associated with eating disorders, depression, and bipolar disorder.

Internet Addiction In the years since the internet became widely available, millions of Americans have become compulsive internet users—as many as one out of eight people fits this description; among college students, approximately one of seven. There is also a growing preoccupation with social media, mobile devices, and general screen time. Researchers are studying cell-phone behavior in the population as a whole as well as among its heaviest users—those under age 20. Although smartphones can be a source of addictive behavior, compulsive cell-phone use is associated with motivations and types of users that differ from those of compulsive computer use. (See the box "Is Internet Use a Problem for You?")

WHY PEOPLE USE AND MISUSE DRUGS

Using drugs to alter consciousness is an ancient and universal pursuit. People have used alcohol for celebration and intoxication for thousands of years. In the 19th century, chemists began extracting the active chemicals from medicinal plants, such as morphine from the opium poppy and cocaine from the coca leaf. This activity was the beginning of modern **pharmacy,** the art of compounding drugs, and of **pharmacology,** the science and study of drugs. It was also the start of the era of human-made psychoactive drugs, from codeine to methamphetamine, which continues to the present.

> **pharmacy** The art of compounding drugs from various substances.
>
> **pharmacology** The science and study of drugs.
>
> **TERMS**

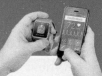
To assess the extent to which your internet use is creating problems in your life, answer the following questions using this point scale:

Not Applicable   0
Rarely   1 point
Occasionally   2 points
Frequently   3 points
Often   4 points
Always   5 points

_____ 1. How often do you find that you stay online longer than you intended?

_____ 2. How often do you neglect household chores to spend more time online?

_____ 3. How often do you prefer the excitement of the internet to intimacy with your partner?

_____ 4. How often do you form new relationships with fellow online users?

_____ 5. How often do others in your life complain about the amount of time you spend online?

_____ 6. How often do your grades or schoolwork suffer because of the amount of time you spend online?

_____ 7. How often do you check your email before something else that you need to do?

_____ 8. How often does your job performance or productivity suffer because of the internet?

_____ 9. How often do you become defensive or secretive when someone asks you what you do online?

_____ 10. How often do you block out disturbing thoughts about your life with anticipation of internet activities?

_____ 11. How often do you find yourself anticipating when you will go online again?

_____ 12. How often do you fear that life without the internet would be boring, empty, and joyless?

_____ 13. How often do you snap, yell, or act annoyed if someone bothers you while you are online?

_____ 14. How often do you lose sleep due to late-night log-ins?

_____ 15. How often do you feel preoccupied with the internet when offline or fantasize about being online?

_____ 16. How often do you find yourself saying "just a few more minutes" when online?

_____ 17. How often do you try to cut down on the amount of time you spend online and fail?

_____ 18. How often do you try to hide how long you've been online?

_____ 19. How often do you choose to spend more time online over going out with others?

_____ 20. How often do you feel depressed, moody, or nervous when you are offline, which goes away once you are back online?

Add the points associated with your responses to get your final score. The higher your score, the more problems your internet usage is causing you. Here's a general scale to help you evaluate your score:

- 0–30 points: No problematic internet usage.

- 31–49 points: You are an average online user. If your score exceeds 40 points, you may surf the web a bit too long at times, but you have control over your usage.

- 50–79 points: You are experiencing occasional or frequent problems because of the internet. You should consider their full impact on your life.

- 80–100 points: Your internet usage is causing significant problems in your life. You should evaluate the impact of the internet on your life and start thinking about how to address the problems.

SOURCE: Adapted from Netaddiction.com. *Internet Addiction Test* (http://netaddiction.com/internet-addiction-test/). Accessed February 20, 2016. Reprinted by permission of Dr. Kimberly S. Young.

Drug misuse expanded in America during the 1960s and 1970s, reaching a peak in 1979. Rates then declined until the early to mid-1990s, when drug misuse rates began to rise in certain age groups. The rate of twelfth graders vaping marijuana increased significantly by 21% between 2018 and 2019. The second most commonly misused drug in recent years has been prescription pain relievers. Besides marijuana and opioids, the use of many other drugs has remained steady, well below peak levels of the 1990s and early 2000s.

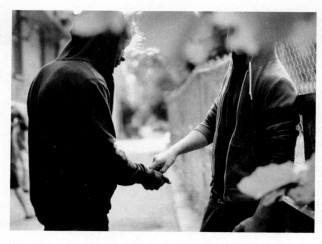

For people who are unemployed or otherwise deprived of traditional sources of livelihood, drug sales provide access to an income in an alternative economy. Marie-Reine Mattera/Getty Images

The Allure of Drugs

The main factors in the initial use of drugs are availability and peer influence. Some people use drugs because they want to alter their mood—they want to feel a euphoric high, or they are in pursuit of a spiritual experience. Others use drugs as a way to escape boredom, anxiety, depression, feelings of worthlessness, or other distressing symptoms. They use drugs to cope with the difficulties they experience in life. For people living in poverty, many of these reasons for using drugs are magnified. They may be dealing with dangerous environments, unstable family situations, severe financial stress, and lack of access to mental health services. Further, the buying and selling of drugs provide access to an unofficial alternative economy that may seem like an opportunity for success.

A group of people with easy access to drugs is health care professionals. Their access affords them more opportunities to misuse drugs and therefore puts them at a higher risk. Other susceptible groups are people genetically predisposed to a particular substance and people who were exposed to drugs in the womb. Those exposed before birth may have an increased risk of using drugs later in life.

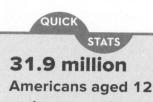

QUICK STATS

31.9 million
Americans aged 12 and over used an illicit drug in the past 30 days; this averages to about 1 in 10 Americans.

—Substance Abuse and Mental Health Services Administration, 2018

reason, one-third of people with psychological disorders also have a substance use disorder.

Whether suffering from dual disorders or not, people with addictive disorders usually have a distinct preference for a particular addictive behavior. They also often have problems with impulse control and self-regulation and tend to be risk takers.

Drug misuse and addiction occur at all income and education levels, among all ethnic groups, and across all age groups (see the box "Drug Use among College Students"). Even if a person is not predisposed to addiction nor afforded many opportunities to experiment with drugs, casual or recreational use of them can lead to addiction. Some drugs are more likely than others to lead to addiction (Table 10.2).

Risk Factors for Drug Misuse and Addiction

Can some people use psychoactive drugs without becoming addicted? The answer seems to lie in a combination of physical, psychological, and social factors. Research indicates that some people may be born with a brain chemistry or metabolism that makes them more vulnerable than others to addiction.

The causes and course of an addiction vary, but people with addictions (commonly referred to as *addicts*) share some characteristics. As mentioned, many use a substance or activity as a substitute for healthier coping strategies. People vary in their ability to manage their lives, and those who have trouble dealing with stress and painful emotions may be susceptible to addiction. For this

Table 10.2	Psychoactive Drugs and Their Potential for Substance Use Disorder and Addiction
Very high	Heroin
High	Nicotine, morphine
Moderate/high	Cocaine, pentobarbital
Moderate	Alcohol, ephedra, Rohypnol
Moderate/low	Caffeine, marijuana, MDMA (methylenedioxymethamphetamine), nitrous oxide
Low/very low	Ketamine, LSD (lysergic acid diethylamide), mescaline, psilocybin

SOURCE: Adapted from Gable, R. S. 2006. Acute toxicity of drugs versus regulatory status. In J. M. Fish (Ed.), *Drugs and Society: U.S. Public Policy*, pp. 149–162. Lanham, MD: Rowman & Littlefield.

Drug use in college has long been recognized as a significant health problem that affects many students. According to the most recent survey data from the National Survey on Drug Use and Health (NSDUH), almost 24% of young adults aged 18–25 reported using an illicit drug in the past 30 days, with marijuana the most commonly used drug (refer to Table 10.1). Other surveys show a spike in marijuana vaping by high school seniors and college students. Over 11% of students reported nonmedical use of prescription stimulants within the past year.

Drug use on college campuses has been examined extensively, and many experts believe that no single factor can explain the widespread cause of this phenomenon. Family history, peer pressure, depression, anxiety, low self-esteem, and the dynamics of college life (for example, the drive to compete and a distorted perception of drug use among peers) have been suggested as potential explanations for college-age drug use.

Excessive alcohol use often accompanies illicit drug use, and the risk of combining drugs and alcohol increases with the number of drinks a young adult consumes during a single session. In 2015, among the 17.3 million heavy drinkers aged 12 and over, 32.5 percent were also current illicit drug users. Persons who were not current alcohol users were less likely to have used illicit drugs in the past month.

The term *AOD* (alcohol and other drug) has been coined to refer to this type of substance use among college students. Further, AOD use and depression and/or anxiety are generally recognized as coexisting conditions that require a comprehensive approach to prevention and treatment. Despite the growing awareness among college counselors and other health professionals who work with college students, it is not entirely clear whether anxiety and depression precede the onset of alcohol and drug use or whether early precollege exposure to alcohol and drug use exacerbates more serious psychiatric disorders by the time a student enters college. A third line of research suggests that AOD use, depression, and anxiety share common causes such as genetic predisposition and family history.

However, one aspect of drug use among college students remains clear: AOD use has dramatic consequences for the educational, family, and community lives of students. Poor academic performance has been linked with AOD use. Further, driving while intoxicated remains one of the most dangerous outcomes associated with AOD use affecting families and communities.

Several AOD prevention programs are now under way at college campuses. Several federal laws have been enacted to provide resources and a legislative framework for addressing AOD use at schools. The 1989 Drug-Free Schools and Communities Act and the 1998 Higher Education Amendments are examples of concerted federal legislative efforts to encourage the development of educational policies for preventing alcohol and other drug use and providing assistance to college students at risk for these harmful behaviors.

Factors Associated with Trying Drugs   Who are the young people most likely to try drugs? They share the following characteristics:

• *Male.* Males are more likely than females to use almost all types of illicit drugs. According to the National Institute on Drug Abuse, fewer women use marijuana. Women tend to use smaller amounts of heroin and for less time, and they are less likely than men to inject it. National overdose deaths from prescription drugs, cocaine, and heroin are consistently higher in males than in females. However, females are just as likely as males to develop a substance use disorder.

• *Troubled childhood.* Teens are more likely to try drugs if they have had behavioral issues in childhood, such as aggression, have suffered sexual or physical abuse, used tobacco at a young age, or suffer from certain mental or emotional problems.

• *Thrill-seeker.* Impulsivity and a sense of invincibility is a factor in drug experimentation.

• *Dysfunctional family.* A chaotic home life with poor supervision, constant tension or arguments, or parental abuse increases the risk of teen drug use. Having parents who misuse drugs or alcohol increases the risk for teen drug and alcohol use.

• *Trouble at school.* Young people who are uninterested in school, or have problems at school, or have difficulty fitting in, are more likely to find a peer group that accepts drug use.

• *Poor.* Young people who live in disadvantaged areas are more likely to be around drugs at a young age.

• *Adolescents engaged in risky sexual behavior.* There is a relationship between drug use and risky sexual behavior, such as with adolescent girls who date boys two or more years older than themselves; they are more likely to use drugs.

Factors Associated with Not Using Drugs   As a group, nonusers also share some characteristics. Not surprisingly, people who perceive drug use as risky and who disapprove of it are less likely to use drugs. Drug use is also less common among people who have positive self-esteem and self-concept and who are assertive, independent thinkers able to resist peer pressure. People with self-control, social competence, optimism, academic achievement, and religiosity (hold religious beliefs and attend religious services) are less likely to use drugs.

Home environments are also influential: Young people who communicate openly with and feel supported by their parents are also less likely to use drugs.

RISKS ASSOCIATED WITH DRUG MISUSE

Tracking emergency department visits is one way to measure levels of drug misuse or abuse. Close to 600,000 visits were reported for 2016 (Table 10.3), and the number could be much higher—1.3 million, according to a *Consumer Reports* survey. The highest rate of emergency department visits was among those aged 15–24. The following are serious concerns:

- *Intoxication.* People who are intoxicated may act in uncharacteristic and unsafe ways because their physical and mental functioning are impaired. They are more likely to be injured from a variety of causes, to have unsafe sex, and to be involved in incidents of aggression and violence.

- *Unexpected side effects.* Psychoactive drugs have many physical and psychological effects that can range from nausea and constipation to paranoia, depression, and heart failure. Some drugs also carry the risk of fatal overdose.

- *Unknown drug constituents.* A drug may have been mixed with other drugs or substances to boost its effects. Illicit drugs can be contaminated or even poisonous.

Table 10.3	Estimated Drug-Related Emergency Department (ED) Visits: 2016

REASON FOR ED VISIT	NUMBER OF ED VISITS*
All opioid poisonings	197,970
Heroin poisonings	123,272
Methadone poisonings	3,434
Poisonings by other opioids	72,065
Cocaine poisonings	8,617
Methamphetamine poisonings	13,131
All drug poisonings	**577,794**

*Does not include persons who were hospitalized, died, or transferred to another facility. Visits with missing age and sex were also excluded.

SOURCE: Centers for Disease Control and Prevention. 2019. *Annual Surveillance Report of Drug-Related Risks and Outcomes—United States, 2019.* Centers for Disease Control and Prevention, U.S. Department of Health and Human Services (https://www.cdc.gov /drugoverdose/pdf/pubs/2019-cdc-drug-surveillance-report.pdf).

Ask Yourself

QUESTIONS FOR CRITICAL THINKING AND REFLECTION

Have you ever tried a psychoactive drug for fun? What were your reasons for trying it? Whom were you with, and what were the circumstances? What was your experience? What would you tell someone who was thinking about trying a drug?

- *Infection and injection drug use.* Heroin is the most commonly injected drug, but users can also inject cocaine, amphetamines, and other drugs. Many injection drug users (IDUs) share or reuse needles, syringes, and other injection supplies, which can become contaminated with the user's blood. Small amounts of blood can carry enough human immunodeficiency virus (HIV) and hepatitis C virus (HCV) to be infectious. According to the CDC, one in ten new diagnoses of HIV infection is due to injection drug use. Injection drug use also accounts for the majority of new HCV infections.

In states with legal syringe services programs (SSPs)—where IDUs can trade a used syringe for a new one—HIV and HCV rates have dropped an estimated 50%, and other health problems and costs associated with drug injection use have also decreased. Philadelphia is attempting to become the first U.S. city to approve the opening of a supervised injection facility (SIF), where IDUs can administer their own drugs using sterile needles under health care supervision.

Opponents of SSPs and SIFs argue that providing any medical support for addicts to inject drugs sends the message that illegal drug use is acceptable and worsens the nation's drug problem. However, studies have shown that well-implemented SSPs and SIFs do not increase the use of drugs; in fact, such programs have been found to help people stop or reduce drug use, overdoses, and infections.

- *Legal consequences.* Many psychoactive drugs are illegal, so possessing them can result in large fines and imprisonment. According to the FBI, the highest arrest counts for all types of crimes were for drug use violations (estimated at 1.7 million out of 10.3 million total arrests in 2018).

HOW DRUGS AFFECT THE BODY

Beyond a fairly predictable change in brain chemistry, the effects of a drug may vary depending on drug factors, user factors, and social factors.

Changes in Brain Chemistry

The quicker a drug reaches the brain, the more likely the user becomes dependent on it. Once a psychoactive drug reaches the brain, it interferes with the way neurons (nerve cells that communicate with other cells) send, receive, and process signals sent by **neurotransmitters**. Drugs like cocaine and amphetamines increase the amount of dopamine, a neurotransmitter thought to play a key role in the process of reinforcement—the brain's way of telling itself, "I feel good; do the same thing again." This is a reward pathway.

When a neuron releases a neurotransmitter, it travels across a gap, called a *synapse*, to signal another neuron. The signaling is controlled in part by removing the neurotransmitter molecules from the synapse by a process called reuptake. Some drugs, such as cocaine, inhibit the resorption of dopamine, thereby extending or intensifying their action (Figure 10.1).

Other drugs, like marijuana and heroin, can activate neurons because their chemical structure mimics that of a natural neurotransmitter in the body. For example, the body produces natural opioids, which include endorphins, as well as natural cannabinoids (named after the marijuana plant Cannabis sativa). These natural chemicals interact with specific receptors throughout the body and brain to regulate important body functioning—but the chemical similarity of the drugs allows them to attach onto and activate the same neurons. Although they mimic the brain's own chemicals, these drugs don't activate neurons in the same way as a natural neurotransmitter, and they lead to abnormal messages being sent through the network.

The duration of a drug's effect depends on many factors and may range from 5 minutes (crack cocaine) to 12 or more hours (LSD). As drugs circulate through the body, they are metabolized by the liver and eventually excreted by the kidneys in urine. Small amounts may also be eliminated in other ways, including in sweat, in breast milk, and via the lungs.

Physical Factors

Certain physical characteristics help determine how a person will respond to a drug. Body mass is one variable: The effects of a certain dose of a drug on a 150-pound person will exceed its effect on a 200-pound person. Other variables include general health and genetic factors. For example, some people have an inherited ability to rapidly metabolize a cough suppressant called dextromethorphan, which also has psychoactive properties. These people must take a higher-than-normal dose to get a given cough suppressant effect.

If a person's biochemical state is already altered by another drug, this too can make a difference. Some drugs intensify the effects of other drugs, as is the case with alcohol and sedatives. Some drugs block the effects of other drugs, such as when a tranquilizer is used to relieve anxiety caused by cocaine. Interactions between drugs, including many prescription and over-the-counter (OTC) medications, can be unpredictable and dangerous.

One physical condition that requires special precautions is pregnancy. It can be risky for a woman to use any drugs at all

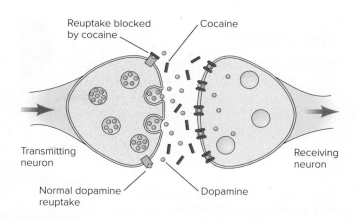

FIGURE 10.1 **Effect of cocaine on brain chemistry.** Under normal circumstances, the transmitting neuron controls the reuptake of dopamine at a synapse. Cocaine blocks the removal of dopamine from a synapse; the resulting buildup of dopamine causes continuous stimulation of the receiving neurons.

during pregnancy, including alcohol and common OTC products like cough medicine.

Psychological Factors

Sometimes a person's response to a drug is strongly influenced by the user's expectations of how the drug will affect them. With large doses, the drug's chemical properties seem to have the strongest effect on the user's response. But with small doses, psychological (and social) factors are often more important. If people believe that a given drug will affect them a certain way, they are more likely to experience those effects regardless of the drug's pharmacological properties. In one study, regular users of marijuana reported a moderate level of intoxication (**high**) after using a cigarette that smelled and tasted like marijuana but contained no THC, the active ingredient in marijuana. This is an example of the **placebo effect**—when a person receives an inert substance yet responds as if it were an active drug. In other studies, subjects who smoked low doses of real marijuana that they believed to be a placebo experienced no effects from the drug. Clearly the user's expectations had a greater effect than the drug itself.

Social Factors

The *setting* is the physical and social environment surrounding the drug use. If a person uses marijuana at home with trusted

---

TERMS

neurotransmitter A brain chemical that transmits nerve impulses.

high The subjectively pleasing effects of a drug, usually felt quite soon after the drug is taken.

placebo effect A response to an inert or innocuous substance given in place of an active drug.

friends and pleasant music, the effects are likely to differ from the effects if the same dose is taken in an austere experimental laboratory with an impassive research technician. Similarly, a dose of alcohol that produces mild euphoria and stimulation at a noisy, active cocktail party might induce sleepiness and slight depression when taken at home while alone.

GROUPS OF PSYCHOACTIVE DRUGS

The following sections and Figure 10.2 introduce six representative groups of psychoactive drugs: opioids, central nervous system (CNS) depressants, CNS stimulants, marijuana and other cannabis products, hallucinogens, and inhalants. Some of these drugs are classified according to how they affect the body. Others—the opioids and the cannabis products—are classified according to their chemical makeup.

Opioids

Opioids are natural or synthetic (laboratory-made) drugs that relieve pain, cause drowsiness, and induce **euphoria.** Natural opioid-like hormones released by the brain, called endorphins, can inhibit pain and induce euphoria. Opium, morphine, heroin, methadone, codeine, hydrocodone, oxycodone, meperidine, and fentanyl are opioids. When taken at prescribed doses, opioids have beneficial medical uses, including

> **QUICK STATS**
>
> **Opioids were responsible for almost 47,600 overdose deaths in 2017, compared to 40,000 killed in car accidents, 40,000 by guns, or more than 40,000 from breast cancer.**
>
> —Centers for Disease Control and Prevention, 2019

> **TERMS**
>
> **opioid** Any of several natural or synthetic drugs that relieve pain and cause drowsiness and/or euphoria; examples are opium, morphine, and heroin; also called a *narcotic.*
>
> **euphoria** An exaggerated feeling of well-being.
>
> **depressant, sedative-hypnotic** A drug that decreases nervous or muscular activity, causing drowsiness or sleep.
>
> **tranquilizer** A central nervous system (CNS) depressant that reduces tension and anxiety.
>
> **central nervous system (CNS)** The brain and spinal cord.

pain relief and cough suppression. Opioids tend to reduce anxiety and produce lethargy, apathy, and an inability to concentrate.

Although the euphoria associated with opioids is an important factor in their misuse, many people experience a feeling of uneasiness when they first use these drugs. Even so, the misuse of opioids often results in addiction. Tolerance can develop rapidly and be pronounced. Withdrawal symptoms include cramps, chills, sweating, nausea, tremors, irritability, and feelings of panic.

The opioid epidemic in the United States claims the lives of around 130 people each day. According to the CDC, between 1999 and 2017 there were 400,000 deaths from opioid-related overdoses.

The opioid epidemic has emerged in three waves. The first wave began in the 1990s with prescription opioids like oxycodone, hydrocodone, and methadone. Healthcare providers began overprescribing opioid pain relievers as pharmaceutical companies reassured them that patients would not become addicted. This led to widespread misuse, and by 2011 there were around 16,000 overdose deaths on pills annually (Figure 10.3).

The second wave began in 2010 as addicts shifted to heroin, a cheaper alternative to prescription pills. From 2010 to 2017, heroin deaths increased fivefold; in 2017, 15,000 people suffered fatal overdoses. The third wave surfaced with a rise in synthetic opioids like fentanyl and carfentanil. Fifty times stronger than heroin, fentanyl and other synthetic opioids caused more than 28,000 overdose deaths in 2017. Of the more than 67,000 drug overdose deaths in 2018, almost 70% involved a prescription or illicit opioid.

When taken as prescribed in tablet form, these drugs treat moderate to severe chronic pain and do not typically lead to misuse. When taken in large doses or combined with other drugs, oxycodone and hydrocodone can cause fatal respiratory depression.

In 2016, the Centers for Disease Control and Prevention announced a new effort to reduce the number of inappropriate prescriptions written for opioid painkillers.

Kratom Kratom, a plant in the coffee family, has both stimulant properties (like khat) and opioid-like properties. It has been used to aid in opioid withdrawal and to act as a substitute in opioid addiction. In February 2018, the FDA echoed the declaration of the Drug Enforcement Administration (DEA) five years earlier that there are no known medical uses of kratom, and little is known about its safety.

Central Nervous System Depressants

Central nervous system **depressants,** also known as **tranquilizers** or **sedative-hypnotics,** slow the **central nervous system (CNS).**

Category	Representative drugs	Street names	Appearance	Methods of use	Short-term effects
Opioids 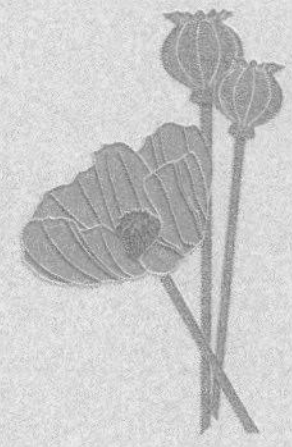	Heroin	Dope, H, junk, brown sugar, smack	White/dark brown powder; dark tar or coal-like substance	Injected, smoked, snorted	Relief of anxiety and pain; euphoria; lethargy, apathy, drowsiness, confusion, inability to concentrate; nausea, constipation, respiratory depression
	Opium	Big O, black stuff, hop	Dark brown or black chunks	Swallowed, smoked	
	Morphine	M, Miss Emma, monkey, white stuff	White crystals, liquid solution	Injected, swallowed, smoked	
	Oxycodone, codeine, hydrocodone	Oxy, O.C., killer, Captain Cody, schoolboy, vike	Tablets, powder made from crushing tablets	Swallowed, injected, snorted	
Central nervous system depressants 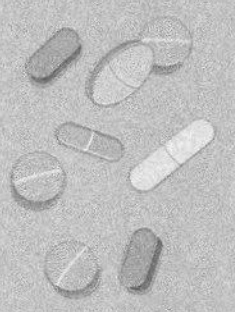	Barbiturates	Barbs, reds, red birds, yellows, yellow jackets	Colored capsules	Swallowed, injected	Reduced anxiety, mood changes, lowered inhibitions, impaired muscle coordination, reduced pulse rate, drowsiness, loss of consciousness, respiratory depression
	Benzodiazepines (e.g., Valium, Xanax, Rohypnol)	Candy, downers, tranks, roofies, forget-me pill	Tablets	Swallowed, injected	
	Methaqualone	Ludes, quad, quay	Tablets	Injected, swallowed	
	Gamma hydroxy butyrate (GHB)	G, Georgia home boy, grievous bodily harm	Clear liquid, white powder	Swallowed	
Central nervous system stimulants 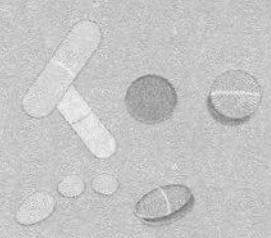	Amphetamine, methamphetamine	Bennies, speed, black beauties, uppers, chalk, crank, crystal, ice, meth	Tablets, capsules, white powder, clear crystals	Injected, swallowed, smoked, snorted	Increased and irregular heart rate, blood pressure, metabolism; increased mental alertness and energy; nervousness, insomnia, impulsive behavior; reduced appetite
	Cocaine, crack cocaine	Blow, C, candy, coke, flake, rock, toot, snow	White powder, beige pellets or rocks	Injected, smoked, snorted	
	Ritalin	JIF, MPH, R-ball, Skippy	Tablets	Injected, swallowed, snorted	
	Synthetic cathinones ("bath salts")	Bliss, Blue Silk, Flakka, Ivory Wave, Meow Meow, Vanilla Sky, White Lightning	Fine white, off-white, or slightly yellow-colored powder or crystals; can be tablets or capsules	Swallowed, smoked, vaporized, sniffed, snorted, and injected	Increased blood pressure, rapid heartbeat, panic attacks in some people
Marijuana and other cannabis products 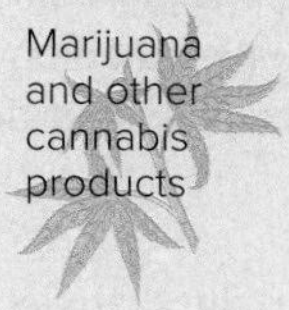	Marijuana	Dope, grass, joints, Mary Jane, reefer, skunk, weed, pot	Dried leaves and stems	Smoked, swallowed	Euphoria, slowed thinking and reaction time, confusion, anxiety, impaired balance and coordination, increased heart rate
	Hashish	Hash, hemp, boom, gangster	Dark, resin-like compound formed into rocks or blocks	Smoked, swallowed	
	K-2, Spice	Black Mamba, Bliss, Bombay Blue, Fake Weed, Genie, Spice, Zohai	Dried leaves	Smoked, teas	Increased blood pressure and heartbeat, paranoia, panic attacks
Hallucinogens 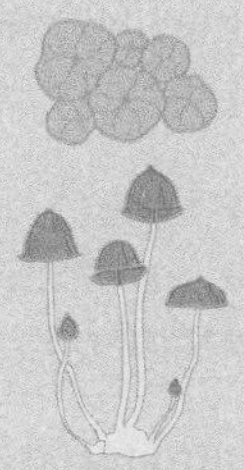	LSD	Acid, boomers, blotter, yellow sunshines	Blotter paper, liquid, gelatin tabs, pills	Swallowed, absorbed through mouth tissues	Altered states of perception and feeling; nausea; increased heart rate, blood pressure; delirium; impaired motor function; numbness, weakness
	Mescaline (peyote)	Buttons, cactus, mesc	Brown buttons, liquid	Swallowed, smoked	
	Psilocybin	Shrooms, magic mushrooms	Dried mushrooms	Swallowed	
	Ketamine	K, special K, cat valium, vitamin K	Clear liquid, white or beige powder	Injected, snorted, smoked	
	PCP	Angel dust, hog, love boat, peace pill	White to brown powder, tablets	Injected, swallowed, smoked, snorted	
	MDMA (Ecstasy)	X, peace, clarity, Adam, Molly	Tablets	Swallowed	
Inhalants 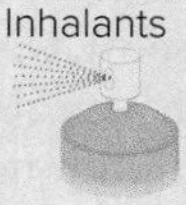	Solvents, aerosols, nitrites, anesthetics	Laughing gas, poppers, snappers, whippets	Household products, sprays, glues, paint thinner, petroleum products	Inhaled through nose or mouth	Stimulation, loss of inhibition, slurred speech, loss of motor coordination, loss of consciousness

FIGURE 10.2 **Commonly misused drugs and their effects.**

SOURCES: The Partnership to End Addiction. 2020. *Drug Guide* (http://www.drugfree.org/drug/); National Institute on Drug Abuse. 2020. *Commonly Abused Drugs Chart* (https://www.drugabuse.gov/drugs-abuse/commonly-abused-drugs-charts).

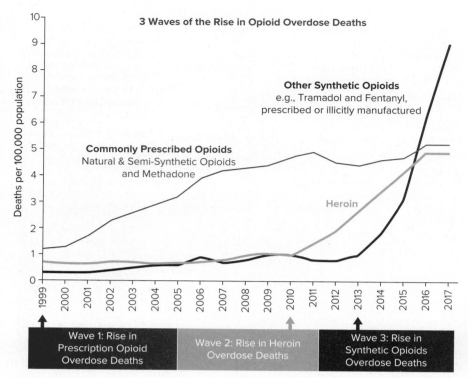

3 Waves of the Rise in Opioid Overdose Deaths

Commonly Prescribed Opioids
Natural & Semi-Synthetic Opioids
and Methadone

Other Synthetic Opioids
e.g., Tramadol and Fentanyl,
prescribed or illicitly manufactured

Heroin

Deaths per 100,000 population

Wave 1: Rise in Prescription Opioid Overdose Deaths

Wave 2: Rise in Heroin Overdose Deaths

Wave 3: Rise in Synthetic Opioids Overdose Deaths

FIGURE 10.3

SOURCE: Centers for Disease Control and Prevention. 2020. *Understanding the Epidemic* (https://www.cdc.gov/drugoverdose/epidemic/index.html)

They were mainly developed as antianxiety agents. The effects of these depressants can range from feeling relaxed with mild **sedation** to coma and death.

Types   CNS depressants include alcohol as well as **barbiturates** such as amobarbital, secobarbital, phenobarbital, pentobarbital, and butalbital. Barbiturates are used for the treatment of seizures and migraines; they are sometimes used in euthanasia and capital punishment. They had been on the market since the early 1900s, but in the 1950s the dangers of barbiturate dependence and overdose were recognized, and these drugs were eventually replaced by other antianxiety agents, known as the **benzodiazepines**. Benzodiazepines include alprazolam (Xanax), diazepam (Valium), chlordiazepoxide (Librium), triazalom (Halcion), clonazepam (Klonopin), midalzolam, and flunitrazepam (Rohypnol, also called "roofies"). Other CNS depressants include methaqualone

> **QUICK STATS**
>
> **Over 100 billion doses of oxycodone and hydrocodone were shipped nationwide in 2006–2014.**
>
> —*The Washington Post*, 2020

(Quaalude), ethchlorvynol (Placidyl), chloral hydrate, and gamma hydroxybutyrate (GHB). An additional class of sedative-hypnotics is called the "Z-drugs" and includes the sleeping pills known as Ambien (zolpidem), Lunesta (eszopiclone), and Sonata (zaleplon). These drugs act like benzodiazepines but do not belong to this group.

Effects   CNS depressants reduce anxiety and cause mood changes, impaired muscular coordination, slurring of speech, and drowsiness or sleep. Mental functioning is also affected, but the degree varies from person to person and also depends on the kind of task the person is trying to do. Most people become drowsy with small doses, although a few become more active.

Medical Uses   The CNS depressants listed above are used for their calming properties in combination with **anesthetics** before operations and other medical or dental procedures.

From Use to Misuse   People are usually introduced to CNS depressants either through a medical prescription or through drug-using peers. The use of Rohypnol and GHB (discussed in greater detail later in this chapter) is often associated with dance clubs and raves. The misuse of CNS depressants by a medical patient may begin with repeated use for insomnia and progress to dependence through increasingly larger doses at night, coupled with doses during stressful times of the day.

> **TERMS**
>
> **sedation**   The induction of a calm, relaxed, often sleepy state.
>
> **barbiturates**   CNS depressants used to treat seizures, headaches, and sometimes used in euthanasia.
>
> **benzodiazepines**   CNS depressants used for sleep and anxiety disorders.
>
> **anesthetic**   A drug that produces a loss of sensation with or without a loss of consciousness.

Most CNS depressants, including alcohol, can lead to addiction. Tolerance, sometimes for up to 15 times the usual dose, can develop with repeated use. CNS depressants can produce physical dependence even at ordinary prescribed doses. Withdrawal symptoms can be more severe than those accompanying opioid addiction and are similar to the DTs of alcoholism (see Chapter 11). They may begin as anxiety, shaking, and weakness but may turn into seizures and possibly cardiovascular collapse and death.

While intoxicated, people on depressants cannot function well. They are often confused and may be obstinate, irritable, or abusive. Long-term use of depressants, including alcohol, can lead to serious physical effects, including brain damage, with impaired ability to reason and make judgments.

Overdosing with CNS Depressants
Too much depression of the central nervous system slows respiration and may stop it entirely. CNS depressants are particularly dangerous in combination with another depressant, such as alcohol, or with opioids, which are respiratory depressants. People who combine depressants with alcohol, opioids, or both account for thousands of emergency department visits and hundreds of overdose deaths each year.

Club Drugs
Some people refer to club drugs as soft drugs because they see them as recreational—for the casual weekend user—rather than as addictive. But club drugs can lead to a substance use disorder and have many potential negative effects; they are particularly potent and unpredictable when mixed with alcohol. Substitute drugs are often sold in place of club drugs, putting users at risk for taking dangerous combinations of unknown drugs.

Rohypnol (flunitrazepam) is a sedative that is 10 times more potent than Valium. Its effects, which are magnified by alcohol, include reduced blood pressure, dizziness, confusion, gastrointestinal disturbances, and loss of consciousness. Users of Rohypnol may develop physical and psychological dependence on the drug. Rohypnol has never been approved for medical use by the U.S. Food and Drug Administration (FDA); along with some other club drugs such as GHB, it is used as a "date rape drug." Because they can be added to beverages surreptitiously, these drugs may be unknowingly consumed by intended rape victims. In addition to depressant effects, some drugs also cause *anterograde amnesia*—the loss of memory of things occurring while under the influence of the drug. Rohypnol can be fatal if combined with alcohol.

GHB (gamma hydroxybutyrate) can be produced in clear liquid, white powder, tablet, and capsule form. GHB, used to treat narcolepsy, is a CNS depressant that, when taken in large doses or in combination with alcohol or other depressants, can cause sedation, loss of consciousness, respiratory arrest, and death. GHB may cause prolonged and potentially life-threatening withdrawal symptoms. GHB is often produced clandestinely, resulting in widely varying degrees of purity; it has been responsible for many poisonings and deaths.

Central Nervous System Stimulants

Central nervous system **stimulants** speed up the activity of the nervous or muscular system. Under their influence, the heart rate accelerates, blood pressure rises, blood vessels constrict, the pupils and bronchial tubes dilate, and gastric and adrenal secretions increase. There is greater muscular tension and sometimes an increase in motor activity. Small doses usually make people feel more awake and alert, and less fatigued and bored. The most common CNS stimulants are cocaine, amphetamines, nicotine (see Chapter 12), ephedrine, and caffeine.

Cocaine
Usually derived from the leaves of coca shrubs that grow high in the Andes in South America, cocaine is a potent CNS stimulant. For centuries, natives of the Andes have chewed coca leaves both for pleasure and to increase their endurance. For a short time during the 19th century, some physicians were enthusiastic about the use of cocaine to cure alcoholism and addiction to the painkiller morphine. Enthusiasm waned after the drug's adverse side effects became apparent.

Cocaine quickly produces a feeling of euphoria, which makes it a popular recreational drug. Cocaine use surged in popularity during the early 1980s, when the drug's high price made it somewhat of a status drug. The introduction of crack cocaine during the 1980s made the drug available in smaller quantities and at lower prices to more people, a shift affecting poorer inner-city neighborhoods. Cocaine use peaked in 1985 with an estimated 3% of adult Americans reporting use.

METHODS OF USE Cocaine is usually snorted and absorbed through the nasal mucosa or injected intravenously, with fast, intense effects. Processing cocaine with baking soda and water yields the ready-to-smoke form of cocaine known as crack. Crack is typically used as small beads or pellets smokable in glass pipes.

EFFECTS The effects of cocaine are usually intense but short-lived. The euphoria lasts from 5 to 20 minutes and ends abruptly with irritability, anxiety, or slight depression. When cocaine is absorbed by either smoking or inhalation, it reaches the brain in about 10 seconds, and the effects are particularly intense. This is part of the appeal of smoking crack. The effects from IV injections occur almost as quickly—in about 20 seconds. Since the mucous membranes in the nose briefly slow absorption, the onset of effects from snorting

> **Rohypnol** (flunitrazepam) A sedative that is 10 times more potent than Valium; used as a "date rape drug."
>
> **GHB** (gamma hydroxybutyrate) A central nervous system depressant that can be produced in clear liquid, white powder, tablet, and capsule form.
>
> **stimulant** A drug that increases nervous or muscular activity.
>
> **TERMS**

takes 2–3 minutes. Heavy users may inject cocaine intravenously every 10–20 minutes to maintain the effects.

The larger the cocaine dose and the more rapidly it is absorbed into the bloodstream, the greater the immediate—and sometimes lethal—effects. Sudden death from cocaine is often the result of excessive CNS stimulation that causes convulsions and respiratory collapse, irregular heartbeat, extremely high blood pressure, blood clots, and possibly heart attack or stroke. Although rare, fatalities can occur in healthy young people; among people aged 18–59, cocaine users are seven times more likely than nonusers to have a heart attack. Chronic cocaine use produces inflammation of the nasal mucosa, which can lead to persistent bleeding and ulceration of the septum between the nostrils. The use of cocaine may also cause paranoia and aggressiveness.

When steady cocaine users stop taking the drug, they experience a sudden "crash" characterized by depression, agitation, and fatigue, followed by a period of withdrawal. Their depression can be relieved temporarily by taking more cocaine, reinforcing its continued use. A binge cocaine user may go for weeks or months without using any cocaine and then take large amounts repeatedly. Although they may not be physically dependent, a binge cocaine user who misses work or school and risks serious health consequences is clearly abusing the drug.

COCAINE USE DURING PREGNANCY A woman who uses cocaine during pregnancy is at higher risk for miscarriage, premature labor, and stillbirth. Her infant may be at increased risk for defects of the genitourinary tract, cardiovascular system, central nervous system, and extremities. Infants whose mothers use cocaine may also be born intoxicated, and effects continue into childhood. They are typically irritable and jittery and do not eat or sleep normally. Cocaine also passes into breast milk and can intoxicate a breastfeeding infant.

Amphetamines

Amphetamines (uppers) are a group of synthetic chemicals that are potent CNS stimulants. Some common drugs in this family are amphetamine (Benzedrine), dextroamphetamine (Dexedrine), and methamphetamine (Methedrine). Crystal methamphetamine (also called ice) is a smokable, high-potency form of methamphetamine, or meth. Crystal meth is easy to manufacture and cheaper than crack cocaine, and it produces a similar but longer-lasting euphoria. The use of crystal meth can quickly lead to addiction.

EFFECTS Small doses of amphetamines usually make people feel more alert. Amphetamines generally increase motor activity but do not measurably alter a normal, rested person's ability to perform tasks calling for challenging motor skills or complex thinking. When amphetamines improve performance,

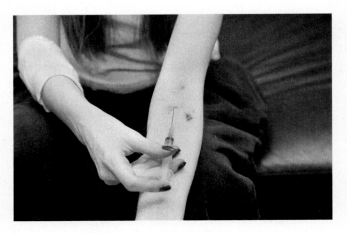

Heavy users may inject cocaine intravenously every 10–20 minutes to maintain the effects. Ttatty/Shutterstock

it is primarily by counteracting fatigue and boredom. In small doses, amphetamines increase heart rate and blood pressure and change sleep patterns.

Amphetamines are sometimes misused to curb appetite, but after a few weeks the user develops tolerance, and higher doses are necessary. When people stop taking the drug, their appetite usually returns, and they gain back the weight they lost unless they have made permanent changes in eating behavior.

MISUSE AND ADDICTION Much amphetamine misuse begins as an attempt to cope with a temporary situation. A student cramming for an exam or an exhausted long-haul truck driver can go a little longer by taking amphetamines, but the results can be disastrous. The likelihood of making bad judgments increases significantly. The stimulating effects may also wear off suddenly, and the user may precipitously feel exhausted or fall asleep ("crash").

Performance may deteriorate when students use drugs to study and then take tests in their normal, nondrug state. Users of antihistamines may also experience this problem. Repeated use of amphetamines can lead to severe disturbances in behavior, including a temporary state of paranoid **psychosis,** with delusions of persecution and episodes of unprovoked violence. If injected in large doses, amphetamines produce a feeling of intense pleasure, followed by sensations of vigor and euphoria that last for several hours. As these feelings wear off, they are replaced by feelings of irritability and vague uneasiness. Long-term use of amphetamines at high doses can cause paranoia, hallucinations, delusions, and incoherence.

Methamphetamine is more addictive than other forms of amphetamine. It also is more dangerous because it is more toxic and its effects last longer. In the short term, meth can cause rapid breathing, increased body temperature, insomnia, tremors, anxiety, and convulsions. Meth use has been linked to high-risk sexual behavior and increased rates of sexually transmitted infections, including HIV infection. In the long term, the effects of meth can include weight loss, severe acne, hallucinations, paranoia, violence, and psychosis.

> **psychosis** A severe mental disorder characterized by a distortion of reality; symptoms might include delusions or hallucinations. **TERMS**

Meth use may cause extensive tooth decay and tooth loss, a condition referred to as "meth mouth," but this may be due to poor hygiene associated with chronic meth use and severe drug dependence in general. Meth takes a toll on the user's heart and can cause heart attack and stroke. Methamphetamine users have signs of brain damage similar to those seen in Parkinson's disease patients. These symptoms can persist even after drug use ceases, causing impaired memory and motor coordination problems. Withdrawal from meth causes symptoms that may include muscle aches and tremors, profound fatigue, deep depression, despair, and apathy. Addiction to methamphetamine is associated with pronounced psychological cravings and obsessive drug-seeking behavior.

Women who use amphetamines during pregnancy risk premature birth, stillbirth, low birth weight, and early infant death. Babies born to amphetamine-using mothers have a higher incidence of cleft palate, cleft lip, and deformed limbs. They may also experience symptoms of withdrawal.

Stimulant ADHD Medications

A stimulant with amphetamine-like effects, Ritalin (methylphenidate) is used to treat attention-deficit/hyperactivity disorder (ADHD). Prescription stimulants such as Ritalin, Adderall, or Concerta in low dosages have a calming effect on people with ADHD, allowing greater attention and focus. When methylphenidate is injected or snorted, dependence and tolerance can result rapidly. Often misused by students to raise school performance and grades, studies have found that prescription stimulants do not enhance learning or thinking ability when taken by people who do not have ADHD. Taken in higher dosages, or by people who do not have ADHD, prescription stimulants can increase dopamine in a rapid and amplified manner (similar to methamphetamine), thereby disrupting normal communication between brain cells, producing euphoria and, as a result, increasing the risk of addiction.

Ephedrine

Although somewhat less potent than amphetamine, ephedrine produces stimulant effects. Ephedrine has been linked to heart arrhythmia, stroke, psychotic reactions, seizures, and some deaths, and it may be particularly dangerous at high doses or when combined with another stimulant such as caffeine. The FDA has banned the sale of ephedrine.

Caffeine

Caffeine is a very popular psychoactive drug and also one of the most ancient. It is found in coffee, tea, cocoa, soft drinks, headache remedies, and OTC preparations like NoDoz. In ordinary doses, caffeine produces greater alertness and a sense of well-being. It also decreases feelings of fatigue or boredom, so using caffeine may enable a person to keep at physically tiring or repetitive tasks longer. Such use is usually followed, however, by a sudden crash. Caffeine does not noticeably influence a person's ability to perform complex mental tasks unless fatigue, boredom, or other factors have already affected normal performance.

Caffeine mildly stimulates the heart and respiratory system, increases muscular tremor, and enhances gastric secretion. Higher doses may cause nervousness, anxiety, irritability, headache, disturbed sleep, and gastric irritation or peptic ulcers. In people with high blood pressure, caffeine can cause blood pressure to rise even further above normal; in people with type 2 diabetes, caffeine may cause glucose and insulin levels to rise after meals.

Drinks containing caffeine are rarely harmful for most people, but some tolerance develops, and withdrawal symptoms of irritability, headaches, and even mild depression occur. Thus although we don't usually think of caffeine as a dependence-producing drug, for some people it is. The *DSM-5* does not include caffeine in the substance use disorder category, but it does suggest further research on the impact of caffeine use. People can usually avoid problems by simply decreasing their daily intake of caffeine. If intake is decreased gradually, withdrawal symptoms can be reduced or avoided. About 80–90% of American adults consume caffeine regularly. The average daily intake is about 280 mg.

ENERGY "SHOTS" The popularity of small (1.5- to 3-ounce) energy drinks has increased dramatically in recent years. Because these products are sold as dietary supplements rather than food, the FDA does not regulate their caffeine content. Each two-ounce "shot" typically contains the same amount of caffeine (roughly 100 mg) as a regular-size cup of coffee. A growing body of scientific evidence shows that energy drinks can have serious health effects, particularly in children, teenagers, and young adults.

Marijuana and Other Cannabis Products

With 43.5 million users in 2018, marijuana is the most widely used federally illegal drug in the United States. This statistic will likely change as more states legalize both medical and recreational marijuana. At the time of this writing, 33 states and the District of Columbia (DC) have legalized medical marijuana, and 11 states and DC allow for recreational usage. Since the new laws took effect, general marijuana use among twelfth graders has remained steady, although the number of students vaping it has risen. More use has been reported among eighth and tenth graders, as well as college students. THC (tetrahydrocannabinol) is the main active ingredient in marijuana. Marijuana plants that grow wild often have less than 1% THC in their leaves. When selected strains are cultivated by separation of male and female plants (*sinsemilla*), the buds from the flowering tops may contain 10-20% THC or more. Hashish, a potent preparation made from the thick resin that exudes from the marijuana leaves, may contain up to 15% THC or more.

Short-Term Effects and Uses

At low doses, marijuana users typically experience euphoria, a heightening of subjective sensory experiences, a slowing down of the perception of passing time, and a relaxed attitude. These pleasant effects are the reason this drug is so widely used. With moderate doses, marijuana's effects become stronger, and the user can also expect to have impaired memory function, disturbed

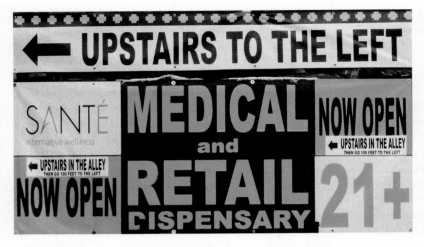

Some states permit the sale of both medical and recreational marijuana. The regulations typically differ for the two types of sales: In Colorado, for example, medical marijuana is taxed at a lower rate and is less expensive than recreational marijuana. KaraGrubis/iStock Editorial/Getty Images

thought patterns, lapses of attention, and feelings of **depersonalization,** in which the mind seems to be separated from the body.

At higher doses, marijuana's effects are determined mostly by the drug itself rather than by the user's expectations and setting. Very high doses produce feelings of depersonalization, marked sensory distortion, and changes in body image (such as a feeling that the body is very light). Inexperienced users sometimes think these sensations mean they are going crazy and become anxious or even panicky. Unexpected reactions are the leading reason for emergency department visits by users of marijuana or hashish. Consuming food or candy infused with marijuana can increase the risk of an unexpected reaction. Edibles take longer to digest and produce a high; people often overconsume edibles in a mistaken attempt to speed up the process. Additionally, THC dosage levels are difficult to measure and are often unknown in edible marijuana products.

Physiologically, marijuana increases heart rate and dilates certain blood vessels in the eyes, which creates the characteristic bloodshot eyes. The user may also feel less inclined toward physical exertion and may feel particularly hungry or thirsty. Because THC affects parts of the brain that control balance, coordination, and reaction time, marijuana use impairs driving performance. The combination of alcohol and marijuana is even more dangerous: Even a low dose of marijuana, when combined with alcohol, significantly impairs driving performance and increases crash risk.

The U.S. Supreme Court has held that state laws permitting medical marijuana use cannot supersede federal law.

---

depersonalization   A state in which a person loses the sense of his or her reality or perceives his or her body as unreal.

hallucinogen   Any of several drugs that alter perception, feelings, or thoughts; examples are LSD, mescaline, and PCP.

TERMS

Thus, anyone using marijuana can still be prosecuted under federal drug laws.

Research shows benefits for using cannabis to treat muscle spasms in multiple sclerosis and cancer-related pain that is not otherwise relieved by opioid medications. Two FDA-approved drugs containing THC, dronabinol and nabilone, are used to treat nausea caused by chemotherapy and increase appetite in patients with extreme weight loss caused by AIDS. The FDA has also approved a cannabidiol-based liquid medication for the treatment of two forms of severe childhood epilepsy. Additional research is focused on synthesizing compounds that target symptoms without the psychoactive effects of cannabinoids, standardizing doses, and conducting clinical trials on the efficacy of these cannabinoids that conform with procedures used with other drugs that are in development.

Long-Term Effects   The most probable long-term effect of smoking marijuana is respiratory damage, including impaired lung function and chronic bronchial irritation. Although no evidence links marijuana use to lung cancer, it may cause changes in lung tissue that promote cancer growth. Marijuana users may be at increased risk for emphysema and cancer of the head and neck, and among people with chronic conditions like cancer and AIDS, marijuana use is associated with increased risk of fatal lung infections. (These are key reasons why the National Academy of Medicine has recommended the development of alternative methods of delivering the potentially beneficial compounds in marijuana.) Heavy users may experience learning problems, as well as subtle impairments of attention and memory that may or may not be reversible following long-term abstinence. Long-term use may also affect sperm productivity and quality.

Studies show that marijuana use during pregnancy may affect the fetus's neural development. Children exposed to cannabis in-utero showed cognitive deficits, suggesting that maternal use of marijuana has interfered with the proper development of the brain. Babies born to mothers who used marijuana during pregnancy also had increased startles and tremors as well as difficulty adjusting to light. Their sleep patterns were altered, and they showed increased irritability. Moreover, THC rapidly enters breast milk and may impair an infant's early motor development. As children developed into adolescents, memory, impulsivity, and attention problems emerged. There is growing evidence that adolescent initiation of cannabis use is associated with the development of psychiatric disorders such as depression, anxiety, and psychosis.

Hallucinogens

As shown in Figure 10.2, **hallucinogens** are a group of drugs whose primary pharmacological effect is to alter the user's perceptions, feelings, and thoughts.

LSD LSD (lysergic acid diethylamide) is one of the most powerful psychoactive drugs. Tiny doses will produce noticeable effects in most people, such as an altered sense of time, visual disturbances, an improved sense of hearing, mood changes, and distortions in perception. Dilation of the pupils and slight dizziness, weakness, and nausea may also occur. With larger doses, users may experience a phenomenon known as **synesthesia**: feelings of depersonalization and other alterations in the perceived relationship between the self and external reality.

Many hallucinogens induce tolerance so quickly that after only one or two doses their effects decrease substantially. The user must then stop taking the drug for several days before his or her system can be receptive to it again. Most hallucinogens cause little drug-seeking behavior and no physical dependence or withdrawal symptoms; PCP (phencyclidine), however, is addictive.

The immediate effects of low doses of hallucinogens are determined largely by expectations and setting. Reports of many effects vary because they involve subjective and unusual dimensions of awareness—the **altered states of consciousness** for which these drugs are famous. For this reason, hallucinogens have acquired a certain aura not associated with other drugs. People have taken LSD in search of a religious or mystical experience or in the hope of exploring new worlds. During the 1960s some psychiatrists gave LSD to their patients to help them talk about their feelings. In the past several years, the FDA has allowed clinical trials for psilocybin-assisted therapy for depression and approved esketamine (Spravato) for severe depression in patients who do not respond to other treatments.

A severe panic reaction, which can be terrifying, can result from taking any dose of LSD. It is impossible to predict when a panic reaction will occur. Some LSD users report having had hundreds of pleasurable and ecstatic experiences before having a "bad trip." If the user is already in a serene mood and feels no anger or hostility and if he or she is in secure surroundings with trusted companions, a bad trip may be less likely, but a tranquil experience is not guaranteed.

Even after the drug's chemical effects have worn off, spontaneous flashbacks and other psychological disturbances can occur. **Flashbacks** in this context are perceptual distortions and bizarre thoughts that occur after the drug has been entirely eliminated from the body. Although they are relatively rare phenomena, flashbacks can be extremely distressing. They are often triggered by specific psychological cues associated with the drug-taking experience, such as certain mood states or even types of music.

MDMA MDMA (methylenedioxymethamphetamine), and variants called Ecstasy (MDMA with a stimulant such as caffeine added) and Molly (a powder that may be "purer" than Ecstasy, but which often contains synthetic cathinone, or bath salts, discussed later), may be classified as a hallucinogen or a stimulant, having both hallucinogenic and amphetamine-like properties. Tolerance to MDMA develops quickly, leading users to take the drug more frequently, use higher doses, or combine MDMA with other drugs to enhance the drug's effects. High doses can cause anxiety, delusions, and paranoia. Users may experience euphoria, increased energy, and a heightened sense of belonging. Using MDMA can produce dangerously high body temperature and potentially fatal dehydration with kidney failure; several cases have been reported of low total body salt concentrations (hyponatremia). Some users experience confusion, depression, anxiety, paranoia, muscle tension, involuntary teeth clenching, blurred vision, nausea, and seizures. Even low doses can affect concentration, judgment, and driving ability.

Other Hallucinogens Most other hallucinogens have the same general effects as LSD, but there are some variations. For example, a DMT (dimethyltryptamine) or ketamine high does not last as long as an LSD high.

PCP (phencyclidine) reduces and distorts sensory input, especially proprioception—the sensation of body position and movement—and creates a state of sensory deprivation. PCP was initially used as an anesthetic but was unsatisfactory because it caused agitation, confusion, and delirium (loss of contact with reality). Because it can be easily made, PCP is often available illegally and is sometimes used as an inexpensive replacement for other psychoactive drugs.

The effects of ketamine are similar to those of PCP—confusion, agitation, aggression, lack of coordination, and distorted perceptions of sight and sound that produce feelings of dissociation from the environment and self—but they tend to be less predictable. Tolerance to either drug can develop rapidly.

Mescaline, derived from the peyote cactus, is the ceremonial drug of the Native American Church. It causes effects similar to LSD, including altered perception and feeling; increased body temperature, heart rate, and blood pressure; weakness and trembling; and sleeplessness. Mescaline is expensive, so most street mescaline is diluted LSD or a mixture of other drugs. Hallucinogenic effects can be obtained from certain mushrooms (*Psilocybe mexicana*, or "magic mushrooms"), certain morning glory seeds, nutmeg, jimsonweed, and other botanical products; but unpleasant side effects, such as dizziness, have limited the popularity of these products.

TERMS

synesthesia A condition in which a stimulus evokes not only the sensation appropriate to it but also another sensation of a different character, such as when a color evokes a specific smell.

altered states of consciousness Profound changes in mood, thinking, and perception.

flashback A perceptual distortion or bizarre thought that recurs after the chemical effects of a drug have worn off.

Inhalants

Inhaling certain chemicals can produce effects ranging from heightened pleasure to delirium and death. Inhalants fall into several major groups:

- Volatile solvents, which are found in products such as paint thinner, glue, and gasoline
- Aerosols, which are sprays that contain propellants and solvents
- Nitrites, such as butyl nitrite and amyl nitrite
- Anesthetics, which include nitrous oxide (laughing gas)

Inhalant use tends to be highest among younger adolescents and declines with age. Inhalant use is difficult to control because inhalants are easy to obtain. They are present in a variety of seemingly harmless products, from dessert-topping sprays to underarm deodorants, that are both inexpensive and legal. Using the drugs also requires no illegal or suspicious paraphernalia. Inhalant users get high by sniffing, snorting, "bagging" (inhaling fumes from a plastic bag), or "huffing" (placing an inhalant-soaked rag in the mouth).

Although different in makeup, nearly all inhalants produce effects similar to those of anesthetics, which slow down body functions. Low doses may cause users to feel slightly stimulated; at higher doses, users may feel less inhibited and less in control. Sniffing high concentrations of the chemicals in solvents or aerosol sprays can cause loss of consciousness, heart failure, and death. High concentrations of any inhalant can also cause death from suffocation by displacing oxygen in the lungs and central nervous system. Deliberately inhaling from a bag or in a closed area greatly increases the chances of suffocation. Other possible effects of the excessive or long-term use of inhalants include damage to the nervous system, hearing loss, increased risk of cancer, and damage to the liver, kidneys, and bone marrow.

Prescription Drug Misuse

The National Institute on Drug Abuse describes prescription drug misuse as the use of a medication without a prescription, in a way other than as prescribed, or to feel euphoria. Over the past decade, misuse of prescription drugs has increased, and national surveys now show that prescription medications—such as those used to treat pain, ADHD, and anxiety—are being misused at a rate second only to marijuana,

Ask Yourself

QUESTIONS FOR CRITICAL THINKING AND REFLECTION

Do you know anyone who may be at risk for using inhalants? If so, would you try to intervene in some way? What would you tell a teenager to convince him or her to stop inhaling chemicals?

tobacco, and alcohol among Americans aged 12 and over. In 2017, over 17,000 people died from drug overdoses involving prescription opioids.

New Psychoactive Substances

In recent years, herbal or synthetic recreational drugs have become increasingly available. These drugs are part of a group called new psychoactive substances; they are intended to have pharmacological effects similar to those of illicit drugs while being chemically distinct from them and therefore either legal or impossible to detect in drug screening. The drugs fall into two main groups. One group is marketed as synthetic marijuana and sold as "herbal incense," or "herbal highs," with names such as Spice, K2, Genie, and Mr. Nice Guy. The other group is marketed as stimulants with properties like those of cocaine or amphetamine and sold as "bath salts" with names such as Zoom, Ivory Wave, and White Rush.

Spice and other synthetic mimics of THC are human-made chemicals that are either sprayed onto plant material for smoking or sold in liquid form for vaping devices. Their active ingredients are synthetic cannabinoids that act on brain cells to produce effects similar to those of THC, such as physical relaxation, but may also include psychotic effects like extreme anxiety, confusion, paranoia, and hallucinations. Misleadingly marketed as safe and natural, synthetic cannabinoids went through a period of initial popularity among teens and young adults. In 2011, 11.4% of high school seniors reported having used synthetic cannabinoids at least once during the year. Since then levels have dropped—by 2019 to about 3%.

The blends of ingredients vary widely, but these products typically contain more than a dozen different substances that give rise to a variety of drug combinations. Calls to poison control centers for exposure to synthetic cannabinoids typically involve symptoms like rapid heart rate, vomiting, violent behavior, and suicidal thoughts; these drugs can also raise blood pressure and cause liver damage and seizures. In 2018, hundreds of cases of severe bleeding and bruising in midwestern states were linked to synthetic cannabinoids contaminated with brodifacoum, a blood-thinning compound commonly used in rat poison.

"Bath salts," marketed as cocaine or methamphetamine substitutes, are widely available on the internet. They contain synthetic cathinones such as mephedrone, methylone, or methylenedioxypyrovalerone (MDPV). Similar in effect to MDMA (Ecstasy), these cathinones are synthetic but more powerful versions of the active ingredient found in the stimulant khat, a chewable leaf that is widely used in countries of the Middle East and Africa. The products are sold in small packets of salt-like crystals with warnings like "novelty only" and "not for human consumption." Bath salts, not to be confused with products like Epsom salts used for bathing, can be ingested by smoking, eating, injecting, or snorting. The effects of bath salts can be severe and include combative violent behavior, extreme agitation, confusion, hallucinations, hypertension, chest pain, and suicidal thoughts. Bath salts can be highly addictive; in 2018, researchers developed a vaccine that blunts the drug's effects on the brain, which could help recovering drug users who experience a relapse.

PREVENTING DRUG-RELATED PROBLEMS

New psychoactive drugs may present unexpected possibilities for therapy, social use, and misuse. Making honest and unbiased information about drugs available to everyone, however, may cut down on their misuse.

Although the use of some drugs, both legal and illegal, has declined dramatically since the 1970s, the use of others has increased. Efforts to address the problem include workplace drug testing, tougher law enforcement and prosecution, and treatment and education. These drugs enter the country on a massive scale from South America, Southeast Asia, and elsewhere, and are distributed through drug-smuggling organizations and street gangs.

Drugs, Society, and Families

The economic cost of drug misuse is staggering. Use and misuse of alcohol, nicotine, and illicit drugs and misuse of prescription drugs cost Americans more than $700 billion a year in increased health care costs, crime, and lost productivity. The cost of the opioid epidemic in 2018 alone—including taxpayer-funded services and the costs paid by individuals, families, employers, and private insurers—was $179.4 billion. But the costs are more than just financial—they are also paid in human pain and suffering.

It is a crime to possess certain drugs. Some crimes are committed in order to obtain drugs, and some crimes are committed because of the loss of control associated with drug use. The criminal justice system is inundated with people accused of crimes related to drug possession, sale, or use. The FBI reports that roughly 1.65 million arrests were made for drug violations in 2018, and over 1 million for driving under the influence. In 2019, almost half of federal inmates (73,660) were in prison because of drug offenses. The Bureau of Justice Statistics reports that about half of all state and federal prisoners—roughly 850,000 men and women—meet diagnostic criteria for drug abuse or addiction. Many assaults and murders are committed when people try to acquire or protect drug territories, settle disputes about drugs, or steal from dealers. Violence and gun use are common in neighborhoods where drug trafficking is prevalent. Addicts commit more robberies and burglaries than criminals not on drugs. People under the influence of drugs, especially alcohol, are more likely to commit violent crimes like rape and murder than are people who do not use drugs.

To what extent is drug misuse also a health care issue for society? In the United States, alcohol and prescription and illicit drug use leads to hundreds of thousands of emergency department admissions and nearly 90,000 deaths annually. Drug addicts who want to quit, especially among the urban poor, often have to wait months for acceptance into a residential care or other treatment program.

Children born to women who use drugs such as alcohol, tobacco, or cocaine may have long-term health problems. Drug misuse in families can become a vicious cycle. Children who observe adults using drugs may assume it is acceptable. Abuse, neglect, lack of opportunity, and unemployment become contributing factors to drug use, perpetuating the cycle (see the box "Drug Use and Race/Ethnicity: A Look at High School Students").

Legalizing Drugs

Pointing out that many social problems associated with drugs are related to prohibition (which failed for alcohol from 1920 to 1933) rather than to the effects of the drugs themselves, some people argue for drug legalization or decriminalization. Proposals range from making drugs such as marijuana and heroin available by prescription to allowing licensed dealers to sell some of these drugs to adults. Proponents argue that legalizing some currently illicit drugs—but putting controls on them similar to those used for alcohol, tobacco, and prescription drugs—could eliminate many problems. Some states have adopted policies that decriminalize possession of small amounts of marijuana—that is, possession for recreational use either is legal or is treated as a misdemeanor crime without significant penalty. Opponents of drug legalization argue that allowing easier access to drugs would expose many more people to possible addiction. Drugs would be cheaper and easier to obtain, and drug use would be more socially acceptable. Legalizing drugs could cause an increase in drug use among children and teenagers. Opponents point out that alcohol and tobacco—drugs that already are legal—are major causes of disease and death in our society.

Drug Testing

According to recent surveys, the majority of substance users hold full-time jobs. Drug use in the workplace not only creates health problems for individual users but also has a negative effect on productivity and on the safety of coworkers. Illicit drug use is highest among workers in the accommodations and food service industry and construction sectors, while heavy alcohol use is greatest among mining and construction workers. A

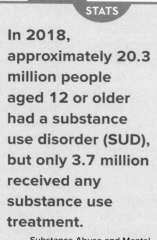

QUICK STATS

In 2018, approximately 20.3 million people aged 12 or older had a substance use disorder (SUD), but only 3.7 million received any substance use treatment.

—Substance Abuse and Mental Health Services Administration, 2018

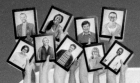

DIVERSITY MATTERS
Drug Use and Race/Ethnicity: A Look at High School Students

Surveys of the U.S. population find a variety of trends in drug use and misuse among racial and ethnic groups (see the accompanying table). In addition to these general trends, there are also trends relating to specific drugs.

According to the Monitoring the Future survey, African American high school students have for many years had significantly lower rates of illicit drug use compared to white students. The gap has narrowed in recent years, however, due to increased rates of marijuana use among black students and a leveling off of marijuana use among whites. African American high school students at all grade levels report higher usage of bath salts and lower usage of hallucinogens, synthetic cannabinoids, and lower prescription drug misuse. Among twelfth graders in 2018, heroin use was higher among black students (0.6%) than among whites (0.2%) and Hispanics (0.4%).

A similar rise in marijuana use has been seen among Hispanic students in recent years, with Hispanics reporting the highest levels of past-year marijuana use among students at grades 8, 10, and—until 2018—12. Among twelfth

Past Year for Illicit Drug Use for High School Seniors

Race/Ethnicity	Percentage
Non-Hispanic, Non-Latino white	39.5
Black or African American	38.8
Hispanic or Latino	37.2

SOURCE: Johnston, L. D., et al. 2019. *Demographic Subgroup Trends among Adolescents in the Use of Various Licit and Illicit Drugs, 1975–2018* (Monitoring the Future Occasional Paper No. 92). Ann Arbor, MI: Institute for Social Research, The University of Michigan.

graders, Hispanic students report the highest past-year use of synthetic marijuana, cocaine, crystal methamphetamines and sedatives. Overall, Hispanic students report the highest levels of illicit drug use in eighth grade, with the gap among groups narrowing by twelfth grade; the higher dropout rates among Hispanic students compared to whites and African Americans may contribute to this pattern.

White twelfth graders report the highest nonmedical use of several prescription drugs, including Oxycontin and Vicodin. In 2018, nonmedical use of Adderall among twelfth graders was

reported by 6.6% of white students, 1.6% of black students, and 3.6% of Hispanic students. Alcohol use was also highest among white students: the 30-day prevalence of alcohol use reported in 2018 among twelfth graders was 21.2% among blacks, 26.4% among Hispanics, and 38.0% among whites.

SOURCES: Center for Behavioral Health Statistics and Quality. 2019. 2018 *National Survey on Drug Use and Health: Detailed Tables.* SAMHSA, Rockville, MD. Schulenberg, J. E., et al. 2017. *Monitoring the Future National Survey Results on Drug Use, 1975–2018: Key Findings on Adolescent Drug Use.* Ann Arbor: Institute for Social Research, The University of Michigan.

2019 study found that those in the construction field were also the most likely to use cocaine and misuse opioids, and the second most likely to use marijuana.

Despite controversial aspects of drug testing in the workplace, a growing number of U.S. workers recognize the need for such screening. According to the Quest Diagnostics Drug Testing Index, overall drug use among U.S. workers has declined since the Drug-Free Workplace Act of 1988, although positive urine tests for marijuana increased 5% from 2017 to 2018; positive opioid tests, however, declined by 21% in the same period.

Treating Drug Addiction

In 2017, the Trump administration declared an opioid crisis and issued an executive order to establish a commission to combat the overdose deaths. Under the Affordable Care Act enacted under the Obama administration, all insurance sold on health insurance exchanges or provided by Medicaid to certain newly eligible adults must include services for treat-

ment of substance use disorders such as alcohol or drug addiction.

The 2016 United Nations General Assembly Special Session on Drugs put out recommendations, including the following: Eliminate stigma and discrimination toward people with substance use disorders; implement evidence-based prevention programs and treatment for addiction; engage scientific data and experts in policy making, public health, education, law enforcement, and health care; support drug-related research; and ensure that scheduled medications are available for therapeutic use.

Treating addiction as a public health issue instead of as a crime is also far less expensive. For example, a year of methadone treatment for a person with opioid use disorder costs on average $4700; a year of incarceration costs around $24,000 per person.

Despite changes to brain structure and function caused by addiction, which make relapse possible even after long periods of abstinence, effective treatment makes a drug-free life possible. Adequate time is essential. Most addicts need at least three months in treatment, and better outcomes occur with longer duration.

Treatment for addiction should assess for other mental disorders as well as infectious disease. Addiction is a mental disorder that often co-occurs with other mental illnesses, and drug-related behaviors put people at risk for diseases like HIV/AIDS, hepatitis B and C, and tuberculosis.

Medically assisted detoxification is the first, not the only stage of treatment. Behavioral therapies and counseling, often combined with appropriate medications, are crucial components of effective treatment.

Medication-Assisted Treatment

Medications are increasingly being used in addiction treatment to reduce the craving for the abused drug or to block its effects. Perhaps the best-known medication for drug use is methadone, a synthetic drug used as a substitute for heroin. Methadone prevents withdrawal reactions and reduces the craving for heroin. Its use enables heroin-addicted people to function normally in social and vocational activities, although they remain dependent on methadone. The drug buprenorphine, a partial opioid agonist, in combination with naloxone, approved for treatment of opioid addiction, reduces cravings and relapse but also leaves one dependent on buprenorphine. An opioid blocker called naltrexone in both oral and injection forms has also shown efficacy for the treatment of both opioid and alcohol use disorders. There is now a growing movement to intervene in emergency departments (EDs) with a brief course of either buprenorphine or naltrexone with coordination of outpatient addiction and primary care for follow-up. This reduces the risk for relapse and overdose immediately following discharge from the ED. Many other medications are under study; drugs used specifically in the treatment of alcohol and nicotine dependence are discussed in Chapters 11 and 12.

Medication therapy can appear efficacious and efficient and is therefore popular among patients and health care providers. However, the relapse rate remains high. Combining drug therapy with psychological and social services improves success rates, underscoring the importance of psychological factors in drug dependence.

Treatment Centers

Treatment centers offer a variety of short-term and long-term services, including hospitalization, detoxification, counseling, and other mental health services. The therapeutic community is a specific type of residential program run in a completely drug-free environment. Administered by recovering addicts, these centers use confrontation, strict discipline, and unrelenting peer pressure to attempt to resocialize the addicted individual with a different set of values. Halfway houses, which are transitional settings between a 24-hour-a-day program and independent living, are an important phase of treatment for some people. Strategies for evaluating programs are given in the box "Choosing a Drug Treatment Program."

Groups and Peer Counseling

Groups such as Alcoholics Anonymous (AA) and Narcotics Anonymous (NA) have helped many people. People receiving treatment in drug substitution programs or substance use treatment centers are often urged or required to join a mutual-help group as part of their recovery. Many of these groups follow a 12-step program. Group members' first step is to acknowledge that they have a problem over which they have no control. Peer support is a critical ingredient of these programs, and members usually meet at least once a week. As part of a 12-step program, each member is paired with a sponsor to call on for advice and guidance in working through the 12 steps and getting support if the temptation to relapse becomes overwhelming. With such support, thousands of substance-dependent people have been able to recover, remain abstinent, and reclaim their lives. Chapters of AA and NA meet on some college campuses; community-based chapters are listed in the phone book, in local newspapers, and online. Other organizations provide an alternative to the 12 steps such as LifeRing Secular Recovery, Rational Recovery, SMART Recovery, Women for Sobriety, and Refuge Recovery.

Many colleges also have peer counseling programs, in which students are trained to help other students who have drug problems. A peer counselor's role may be as limited as referring a student to a professional with expertise in substance dependence for an evaluation or as involved as helping arrange a leave of absence from school for participation in a drug treatment program. Most peer counseling programs are founded on principles of strict confidentiality. Peer counselors may also be able to help students who are concerned about a classmate or loved one with an apparent drug problem (see the box "If Someone You Know Has a Drug Problem . . ."). Information about peer counseling programs is usually available from the student health center.

Harm Reduction Strategies

Because many attempts at treatment are at first unsuccessful, some experts advocate the use of harm reduction strategies. The goal of harm reduction is to minimize the negative effects of drug use and misuse. A common example is the use of designated drivers to reduce alcohol-related motor vehicle crashes. Drug substitution programs such as methadone maintenance are another well-known form of harm reduction; although participants remain drug dependent, the negative consequences of their drug use are reduced. Additional examples of harm reduction strategies include the following:

- Syringe exchange programs, designed to reduce transmission of HIV and hepatitis C
- Safe injection facilities or sites where heroin users can go to inject heroin under medical supervision
- Provision of easy-to-use forms of naloxone, a drug that rapidly reverses opioid overdose, to family members and caregivers of heroin users; in 2014, the FDA approved a handheld naloxone autoinjector or nasal spray
- Free testing of street drugs for purity and potency to help users avoid unintentional toxicity or overdose

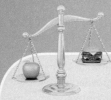

CRITICAL CONSUMER
Choosing a Drug Treatment Program

When evaluating different facilities or programs for drug treatment, consider the following issues:

• *What type of treatment or facility is most appropriate?* Intensive outpatient treatment is available through many community mental health centers, as well as through specialized drug treatment facilities. Such programs typically require several sessions per week, combining individual therapy, group counseling, and attendance at 12-step meetings. Residential, or inpatient, facilities may be associated with a medical facility such as a hospital, or they may be freestanding programs that focus solely on substance use treatment. Some residential treatment programs last longer or cost more per week than many health insurance plans will cover.

• *How will treatment be paid for?* Many health insurance plans limit residential treatment to a maximum number of weeks. They may also require that the insured first attempt an intensive outpatient treatment before they will approve coverage for a residential facility.

• *Is there likely to be a need for medical support?* Chronic abusers of alcohol or other CNS depressants may experience life-threatening seizures or other withdrawal symptoms during the first few days of detoxification. Malnutrition is common among substance abusers, and injection drug users may suffer from local infections and bloodborne diseases such as hepatitis or HIV infection. Medical problems such as these are best handled in an inpatient program with good medical support.

• *Is the treatment center or program certified and licensed? What type of oversight is in place? What is the level of professional training of the staff?* Is there a medical doctor on-site or making frequent visits? Are there trained nurses? Licensed psychologists or social workers? Many successful programs are staffed primarily by recovering alcohol or drug users. Those staff members should have training and certification as addiction specialists. Finally, is the facility listed under SAMHSA's National Review of State Alcohol and Drug Treatment Programs and Certification Standards for Substance Abuse Counselors and Prevention Professionals?

• *Does the program provide related services, such as family and job counseling and posttreatment follow-up?* These types of services are extremely important for the long-term success of drug use treatment.

• *Can a prospective client visit the facility and speak with the staff and clients?* A prospective client and his or her family should be allowed to visit any treatment center or program.

Codependency Many treatment programs also offer counseling for those who are close to drug abusers. Drug misuse takes a toll on friends and family members, and counseling can help people work through painful feelings of guilt and powerlessness. **Codependency,** in which a person close to the drug abuser is controlled by the addict's behavior, sometimes develops. Codependent people may come to believe that love, approval, and emotional and physical security are contingent on their taking care of the addicted person. People can become codependent naturally because they want to help when someone they love becomes dependent on a drug. They may assume that their good intentions will persuade the drug user to stop.

Codependent people often engage in *enabling* behaviors that remove or soften the effects of drug use on the user. The habit of enabling can inhibit a drug abuser's recovery because the person never has to experience the consequences of his or her behavior. Often the enabler is dependent, too—on the patterns of interaction in the relationship. People who need to take care of others often marry people who need to be taken care of. Children in these families often develop the same behavior pattern as one of their parents—either becoming helpless or becoming a caregiver. For this reason, many treatment programs involve the whole family.

Have you ever been an enabler in a relationship? You may have if you've ever done any of the following:

• Given someone countless chances to stop abusing drugs

• Made excuses or lied for someone to his or her friends, teachers, or employer

• Joined someone in drug use and blamed others for your behavior

• Lent money to someone to continue drug use

• Stayed up late waiting for or gone out searching for someone who uses drugs

• Felt embarrassed or angry about the actions of someone who uses drugs

• Ignored the drug use because the person got defensive when you brought it up

• Avoided confronting a friend or relative who was obviously intoxicated or high on a drug

> **codependency** A relationship in which a non-substance-abusing partner or family member is controlled by the abuser's behavior; codependent people frequently engage in enabling behaviors.
>
> **TERMS**

Changes in behavior and mood in someone you know may signal a growing dependence on drugs. Signs that a person's life is beginning to focus on drugs include the following:

- Sudden withdrawal or emotional distance

- Rebellious or unusually irritable behavior

- A loss of interest in usual activities or hobbies

- A decline in school performance

- A sudden change in the chosen group of friends

- Changes in sleeping or eating habits

- Frequent borrowing of money or stealing

- Secretive behavior about personal possessions, such as a backpack or the contents of a drawer

- Deterioration of physical appearance

If you believe a family member or friend has a drug problem, locate information about drug treatment resources available on campus or in your community. Communicate your concern, provide him or her with information about treatment options, and offer your support during treatment. If the person continues to deny having a problem, talk with an experienced counselor about setting up an intervention—a formal, structured confrontation designed to end denial by having family, friends, and other caring people present their concerns to the drug user. Participants in an intervention would indicate the ways in which the individual is hurting others as well as himself or herself. If your friend or family member agrees to treatment, encourage him or her to attend a support group such as Narcotics Anonymous or Alcoholics Anonymous.

And finally, examine your relationship with the abuser for signs of codependency. If necessary, get help for yourself; friends and family of drug users can often benefit from counseling.

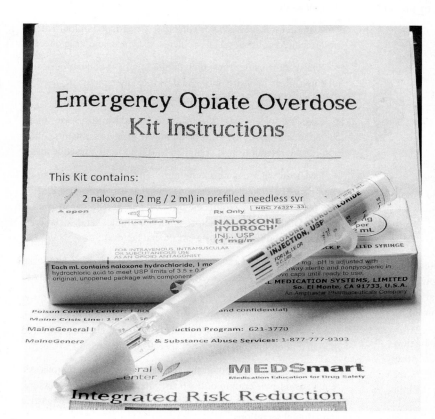

A naloxone kit is an example of a harm reduction strategy for people at risk of an opioid overdose. Portland Press Herald/Joe Phelan/Getty Images

If you come from a codependent family or see yourself developing codependency relationships or engaging in enabling behaviors, consider acting now to make changes in your patterns of interaction. Remember, you cannot cause or cure drug addiction in another person.

Preventing Drug Misuse

Obviously the best solution to drug misuse is prevention. Government attempts at controlling the drug problem have historically focused on stopping the production, importation, and distribution of illegal drugs. A national drug policy announced in 2010, however, redirects federal funding and efforts into stopping the demand for drugs. Developing persuasive antidrug educational programs may offer the best hope for solving the drug problem in the future. Indirect approaches to prevention involve building young people's self-esteem, improving their academic skills, and increasing their recreational opportunities. Direct approaches involve providing information about the adverse effects of drugs and teaching tactics that help students resist peer pressure to use drugs in various situations.

Do you have a substance abuse problem or a behavioral addiction? If so, how has it affected you? How has it affected others? Have you taken any steps to help yourself? Have friends or family offered help?

Developing strategies for resisting peer pressure is one of the more effective techniques.

Prevention efforts need to focus on the different motivations individuals have for using and misusing specific drugs at different ages. For example, grade-school children seem receptive to programs that involve their parents or well-known adults such as professional athletes. Adolescents in junior or senior high school are often more responsive to peer counselors. Many young adults tend to be influenced by efforts that focus on health education. For all ages, it is important to provide nondrug alternatives—such as recreational facilities, counseling, greater opportunities for leisure activities, and places to socialize—that speak to the individual's or group's specific reasons for using drugs. Reminding young people that most people, no matter what age, are *not* users of illegal drugs, do *not* smoke cigarettes, and do *not* get drunk frequently is a critical part of preventing substance misuse.

TIPS FOR TODAY AND THE FUTURE

RIGHT NOW YOU CAN:

- Assess your own relationship with any substances you consume or behaviors in which you frequently engage.
- Consider whether you or someone you know might benefit from drug counseling. Find out what types of services are available on campus or in your area.

IN THE FUTURE YOU CAN:

- Think about the drug-related attitudes of people you know. For example, talk to two older adults and two fellow students about their attitudes toward legalizing marijuana. What are the differences in their opinions, and how do they account for them?
- Analyze media portrayals of drug use. As you watch television shows and movies, note the way they depict drug use among people of different ages and backgrounds. How realistic are the portrayals, in your view? Think about the influence they have on you and your peers.

SUMMARY

- Addiction is a bio-psycho-social-spiritual process that is a chronic medical condition.

- Some common behaviors are potentially addictive, including gambling, shopping, sexual activity, internet use, eating, exercising, and working.

- Addictions, whether to a substance or an activity, are self-reinforcing. Addicts experience a strong compulsion for the substance or behavior and a loss of control over it; an escalating pattern of misuse with serious negative consequences may result.

- Addictions often persist despite adverse social, psychological, or medical consequences.

- Addiction involves taking a drug or engaging in a behavior compulsively, neglecting constructive activities because of it, and continuing to use or engage in it despite the adverse effects. Tolerance and withdrawal symptoms are often present.

- The development of addiction includes factors like genetics, heredity, age, gender, personality, lifestyle, social and physical environment, and the nature of the substance or behavior. People may use a substance or behavior as a means of alleviating stress or painful emotions.

- Drug misuse is use of a drug that is not consistent with medical or legal guidelines.

- Criteria for a substance use disorder are grouped in four categories: impaired control, social problems, risky use, and drug effects.

- Reasons for using drugs include the lure of the illicit, curiosity, rebellion, peer pressure, and the desire to alter mood or alleviate boredom, anxiety, depression, or other psychiatric symptoms.

- Risks associated with drug misuse include intoxication, unexpected side effects, ingestion of unknown drug constituents, injection-related infections and complications, and legal consequences.

- Psychoactive drugs affect the mind and body by altering brain chemistry. The effect of a drug depends on its properties and on how it's used (drug factors), the physical and psychological characteristics of the user (user factors), and the physical and social environment surrounding the drug use (social factors).

- Opioids relieve pain, cause drowsiness, and induce euphoria; they reduce anxiety and produce lethargy, apathy, and an inability to concentrate.

- CNS depressants slow down the overall activity of the central nervous system; they reduce anxiety and cause mood changes, impaired muscular coordination, slurring of speech, and drowsiness or sleep.

- CNS stimulants speed up the activity of the central nervous system, causing acceleration of the heart rate, a rise in blood pressure, dilation of the pupils and bronchial tubes, and an increase in gastric and adrenal secretions.

- Marijuana usually causes euphoria and a relaxed attitude at low doses; very high doses produce feelings of depersonalization and sensory distortion. Use during pregnancy may impair fetal growth.

- Hallucinogens alter perception, feelings, and thoughts and may cause an altered sense of time, visual disturbances, and mood changes.

- Inhalants are present in a variety of everyday products; they can cause delirium. Their use can lead to loss of consciousness, heart failure, suffocation, and death.

- Economic and social costs of drug misuse include the financial costs of law enforcement, treatment, and health care and the social costs of crime, violence, and family problems. Drug testing and drug legalization have been proposed to address some of the problems related to drug use.

- Approaches to treatment include medication, treatment centers, self-help groups, and peer counseling; many programs also offer counseling to family members.

FOR MORE INFORMATION

American Society of Addiction Medicine: Patient Resources. Provides information about treatment and support groups.

https://www.asam.org/Quality-Science/resource-links/patient-resources

Drug Enforcement Administration (DEA): Drug Facts Sheets. Provides basic facts about major drugs of abuse.

https://www.dea.gov/druginfo/factsheets.shtml

Generation Rx. Works to educate people about the risks of prescription medication misuse and abuse.

https://www.generationrx.org/

Go Ask Alice. A health question-and-answer resource produced by Columbia University; see "Alcohol & Other Drugs" in the Health Answers section.

http://goaskalice.columbia.edu

Higher Education Center for Alcohol and Drug Misuse Prevention and Recovery. Based at The Ohio State University, it promotes information and solutions to drug and alcohol abuse on college campuses.

http://hecaod.osu.edu/

National Center on Addiction and Substance Abuse. Provides information on addiction, including prevention and treatment.

http://www.centeronaddiction.org

National Council on Problem Gambling. Provides information and help for people with gambling problems and their families.

http://www.ncpgambling.org

National Drug Information, Treatment, and Referral Hotlines (SAMHSA: see below)

800-662-HELP

800-729-6686 (Spanish)

800-487-4889 (TDD for hearing impaired)

National Institute on Drug Abuse (NIDA). Develops and supports research on drug addiction prevention; provides background information on drugs of abuse.

http://www.drugabuse.gov

Net Addiction: FAQs. Provides background information on internet addiction disorder.

http://netaddiction.com

Partnership for Drug-Free Kids: Drug Guide. A comprehensive source of information on specific drugs.

http://www.drugfree.org/drug-guide

Substance Abuse and Mental Health Services Administration (SAMHSA). Provides statistics, information, and other resources related to substance abuse prevention and treatment.

http://www.samhsa.gov

The following additional organizations/websites provide support services:

Cocaine Anonymous (CA)

https://ca.org

Gamblers Anonymous (GA)

http://www.gamblersanonymous.org/ga/

Marijuana Anonymous (MA)

http://www.marijuana-anonymous.org

Narcotics Anonymous (NA)

http://www.na.org

Overeaters Anonymous (OA)

https://oa.org

Refuge Recovery

http://www.refugerecovery.org

Sex Addicts Anonymous (SAA)

https://saa-recovery.org

SMART® Recovery

http://www.smartrecovery.org

BEHAVIOR CHANGE STRATEGY
Changing Your Drug Habits

This behavior change strategy focuses on one of the most commonly used drugs—caffeine. If you are concerned about your use of a different drug or another type of addictive behavior, you can devise your own plan based on this one and on the steps outlined in Chapter 1.

Like many Americans, you may find yourself relying on coffee (or tea, chocolate, or cola) to get through a busy schedule. When you are studying for exams, for example, the forced physical inactivity and the need to concentrate even when fatigued may lead you to over use caffeine. But caffeine doesn't help unless you are already sleepy. And it does not relieve any underlying condition (you are just more tired when it wears off). How can you change this pattern?

Self-Monitor

Keep a log of how much caffeine you eat or drink. Be sure to include all forms, such as chocolate and OTC medications, as well as colas, tea, and coffee. Use Table 4.1 in Chapter 4 to convert the amounts you drink into an estimate expressed in milligrams of caffeine.

Self-Assess

At the end of the week, add up your daily totals and divide by 7 to get your daily average in milligrams. At more than 250 mg per day, you may be experiencing some adverse symptoms. If you are experiencing at least five of the following symptoms, you may want to cut down:

- Restlessness
- Nervousness
- Excitement
- Insomnia
- Flushed face
- Excessive sweating
- Gastrointestinal problems
- Muscle twitching
- Rambling thoughts and speech
- Irregular heartbeat
- Periods of inexhaustibility
- Excessive pacing or movement

Set Limits

Can you restrict your caffeine intake to a daily total, and stick to this contract? If so, set a cutoff point, such as the amount of caffeine in one cup of coffee. If you cannot stick to your limit, you may want to cut out caffeine altogether: Abstinence can be easier than moderation for some people. If you experience caffeine withdrawal symptoms (headache, fatigue), you may want to cut your intake more gradually.

Find Other Ways to Keep Up Your Energy

Get enough sleep or exercise more, rather than drowning the problem in coffee or tea. Remember that exercise raises your metabolic rate for hours afterward—a handy fact to exploit when you need to feel more awake and want to avoid an irritable caffeine jag. And if you've been compounding your fatigue by not eating properly, try filling up on complex carbohydrates such as whole-grain bread or crackers instead of candy bars.

SELECTED BIBLIOGRAPHY

American College Health Association. 2017. *American College Health Association–National College Health Assessment II: Reference Group Executive Summary Spring 2017.* Hanover, MD: American College Health Association.

American College Health Association. 2019. *American College Health Association–National College Health Assessment II: Reference Group Executive Summary Spring 2019.* Hanover, MD: American College Health Association (https://www.acha.org/NCHA/ACHA-NCHA_Data/Publications_and_Reports/NCHA/Data/Reports_ACHA-NCHAIIc.aspx).

American Psychiatric Association. 2013. *Diagnostic and Statistical Manual of Mental Disorders,* 5th ed. Washington, DC: American Psychiatric Publishing.

American Psychiatric Association. 2020. *Addictions* (https://www.apa.org/topics/addiction/).

American Psychiatric Association. 2016. Can you be addicted to the internet? *APA Blog* (https://www.psychiatry.org/news-room/apa-blogs/apa-blog/2016/07/can-you-be-addicted-to-the-internet).

Bagot, K. S., R. Milin, and Y. Kaminer. 2015. Adolescent initiation of cannabis use and early-onset psychosis. *Substance Abuse* 36(4): 524–533.

Bush, D. M., and R. N. Lipari. 2015. Substance use and substance use disorder by industry. *The CBHSQ Report.* Substance Abuse and Mental Health Services Administration (https://www.samhsa.gov/data/sites/default/files/report_1959/ShortReport-1959.html).

Caspi, A., et al. 2005. Moderation of the effect of adolescent-onset cannabis use on adult psychosis by a functional polymorphism in the catechol-o-methyltransferase gene: Longitudinal evidence of a gene × environment interaction. *Biological Psychiatry* 57: 1117–1127.

Centers for Disease Control and Prevention. 2019. *Annual Surveillance Report of Drug-Related Risks and Outcomes—United States, 2019.* Centers for Disease Control and Prevention, U.S. Department of Health and Human Services (https://www.cdc.gov/drugoverdose/pdf/pubs/2019-cdc-drug-surveillance-report.pdf).

Centers for Disease Control and Prevention. 2019. Syringe Services Programs (SSPs) Fact Sheet (https://www.cdc.gov/ssp/docs/SSP-FactSheet.pdf).

Centers for Disease Control and Prevention. 2020. *Opioid Overdose* (https://www.cdc.gov/drugoverdose/data/analysis.html).

Cidambi, I. 2017. Actual cost of drug abuse in U.S. tops $1 trillion annually. *Psychology Today* (https://www.psychologytoday.com/us/blog/sure-recovery/201708/actual-cost-drug-abuse-in-us-tops-1-trillion-annually).

Consumer Reports National Research Center. 2017. Consumer Reports National Research Center's nationally representative survey of 1,947 adults, conducted April 2017.

Cox, C., M. Rae, and B. Sawyer. 2018. A look at how the opioid crisis has affected people with employer coverage. *Peterson-Kaiser Health System Tracker* (https://www.healthsystemtracker.org/brief/a-look-at-how-the-opioid-crisis-has-affected-people-with-employer-coverage/#item-start).

Drug Enforcement Administration, U.S. Department of Justice. 2017. *Drugs of Abuse: A DEA Resource Guide, 2017 Edition* (https://www.dea.gov/sites/default/files/drug_of_abuse.pdf).

Federal Bureau of Prisons. 2018. *Inmate Statistics: Offenses* (https://www.bop.gov/about/statistics/statistics_inmate_offenses.jsp).

Garnier-Dykstra, L. M., et al. 2012. Nonmedical use of prescription stimulants during college: Four-year trends in exposure opportunity, use, motives, and sources. *Journal of American College Health* 60(3): 226–234.

Griffiths, M. D., et al. 2016. The evolution of addiction: A global perspective. *Addictive Behaviors* 53: 193–195.

Johnston, L. D., et al. 2019. Demographic subgroup trends among adolescents in the use of various licit and illicit drugs, 1975–2018 (Monitoring the Future Occasional Paper No. 92). Ann Arbor, MI: Institute for Social Research, The University of Michigan (http://monitoringthefuture.org/pubs/occpapers/mtf-occ92.pdf).

Johnston, L. D., et al. 2019. Monitoring the Future National Survey Results on Drug Use 1975-2018: Overview, Key Findings on Adolescent Drug Use. Ann Arbor: Institute for Social Research, University of Michigan (http://www.monitoringthefuture.org//pubs/monographs/mtf-overview2018.pdf).

Kraus, S. W., V. Voon, and M. N. Potenza. 2016. Should compulsive sexual behavior be considered an addiction? *Addiction* 111(12): 2097–2106.

Miech, R. A., et al. 2019. Monitoring the Future National Survey Results on Drug Use, 1975–2018: Volume I, Secondary School Students. Ann Arbor: Institute for Social Research, The University of Michigan (http://monitoringthefuture.org/pubs.html#monographs).

National Academies of Sciences, Engineering, and Medicine. 2017. *The Health Effects of Cannabis and Cannabinoids: The Current State of Evidence and Recommendations for Research*. Washington, DC: The National Academies Press.

National Council on Problem Gambling. 2016. *What Is Problem Gambling?* (http://www.ncpgambling.org/help-treatment/faq/).

National Institute on Drug Abuse. 2014. *Stimulant ADHD Medications* (https://www.drugabuse.gov/sites/default/files/drugfacts_stimulantadhd_1.pdf).

National Institute on Drug Abuse. 2018. *Misuse of Prescription Drugs* (https://www.drugabuse.gov/publications/research-reports/misuse-prescription-drugs/what-scope-prescription-drug-misuse).

National Institute on Drug Abuse. 2018. *The Science of Drug Abuse and Addiction: The Basics* (https://www.drugabuse.gov/publications/media-guide/science-drug-abuse-addiction-basics).

National Institute on Drug Abuse. 2018. *Synthetic Cannabinoids (K2/Spice)* (https://www.drugabuse.gov/publications/drugfacts/synthetic-cannabinoids-k2spice).

National Institute on Drug Abuse. 2019. Drug and Alcohol Use in College-Age Adults in 2018. (https://www.drugabuse.gov/related-topics/trends-statistics/infographics/drug-alcohol-use-in-college-age-adults-in-2018).

National Institute on Drug Abuse. 2020. *What can be done for a heroin overdose?* (https://www.drugabuse.gov/publications/research-reports/heroin/what-can-be-done-for-heroin-overdose).

National Institute on Drug Abuse. 2020. *Opioid Overdose Crisis* (https://www.drugabuse.gov/drugs-abuse/opioids/opioid-overdose-crisis).

National Institute on Drug Abuse. 2020. *Sex and Gender Differences in Substance Use.* (https://www.drugabuse.gov/publications/research-reports/substance-use-in-women/sex-gender-differences-in-substance-use).

Office of National Drug Control Policy. 2015. *National Drug Control Strategy* (https://obamawhitehouse.archives.gov/ondcp/policy-and-research/ndcs).

Quest Diagnostics. 2019. *Workforce Drug Testing Positivity Climbs to Highest Rate Since 2004, According to New Quest Diagnostics Analysis* (https://www.questdiagnostics.com/home/physicians/health-trends/drug-testing/).

The Recovery Village. 2020. *Pornography Facts and Statistics* (https://www.therecoveryvillage.com/process-addiction/porn-addiction/related/pornography-statistics/#gref).

Rich, S., S. Higham, and S. Horwitz. 2020. More than 100 billion pain pills saturated the nation over nine years. *The Washington Post*, 14 January (https://www.washingtonpost.com/investigations/more-than-100-billion-pain-pills-saturated-the-nation-over-nine-years/2020/01/14/fde320ba-db13-11e9-a688-303693fb4b0b_story.html).

Schulenberg, J. E., et al. 2017. *Monitoring the Future National Survey Results on Drug Use, 1975–2016: Volume 2, College Students and Adults Ages 19–55.* Ann Arbor: Institute for Social Research, The University of Michigan.

Schulenberg, J. E., et al. 2019. Monitoring the Future National Survey Results on Drug Use, 1975–2018: Volume II, College Students and Adults Ages 19–60. Ann Arbor: Institute for Social Research, The University of Michigan (http://monitoringthefuture.org/pubs.html#monographs).

Substance Abuse and Mental Health Services Administration. 2019. Key Substance Use and Mental Health Indicators in the United States: Results from the 2018 National Survey on Drug Use and Health (HHS Publication No. PEP19-5068, NSDUH Series H-54). Rockville, MD: Center for Behavioral Health Statistics and Quality, Substance Abuse and Mental Health Services Administration (https://www.samhsa.gov/data/).

Substance Abuse and Mental Health Services Administration. 2019. Results from the 2018 National Survey on Drug Use and Health: Detailed Tables. Rockville, MD: Center for Behavioral Health Statistics and Quality, Substance Abuse and Mental Health Services Administration (https://www.samhsa.gov/data/).

Swan, S. C., et al. 2016. Just a dare or unaware? Outcomes and motives of drugging ("drink spiking") among students at three college campuses. *Psychology of Violence,* May 23 (advance online publication).

United States Sentencing Commission. 2019. *Federal Offenders in Prison* (https://www.ussc.gov/research/quick-facts/federal-offenders-prison).

U.S. Department of Justice, Federal Bureau of Investigation. 2018. *Crime in the United States: Persons Arrested* (https://ucr.fbi.gov/crime-in-the-u.s/2018/crime-in-the-u.s.-2018/topic-pages/persons-arrested).

Volkow, N. D., and A. T. McLellan. 2016. Opioid abuse in chronic pain—misconceptions and mitigation strategies. *New England Journal of Medicine* 374: 1253–1263.

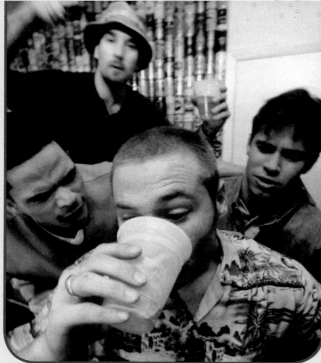

Chuck Savage/The Image Bank/Getty Images

CHAPTER 11

CHAPTER OBJECTIVES

- Understand how alcoholic beverages work in your body
- Describe the immediate and long-term health effects of drinking alcohol
- Understand what constitutes excessive use of alcohol
- Evaluate the role of alcohol in your life, and list strategies for using it responsibly

Alcohol: The Most Popular Drug

TEST YOUR KNOWLEDGE

1. "Moderate drinking" is having three or fewer drinks per day.
   True or False?

2. If a man and a woman of the same weight drink the same amount of alcohol, the woman will become intoxicated more quickly than the man.
   True or False?

3. Drinking too much alcohol in too short a time can cause death from alcohol poisoning.
   True or False?

4. Drinking coffee will help you sober up.
   True or False?

ANSWERS

1. **FALSE.** Moderate drinking is having no more than one drink per day for women and no more than two drinks per day for men.

2. **TRUE.** Women have a less active form of a stomach enzyme that breaks down alcohol. This causes them to become intoxicated more quickly and to a greater degree.

3. **TRUE.** Having a number of drinks over a period of several hours is likely to cause intoxication, followed by a hangover; chugging the same amount in an hour or less can be lethal.

4. **FALSE.** Once alcohol has been absorbed by the body, nothing speeds its metabolism.

Despite numerous prohibitions against it throughout history, alcohol has remained the most popular psychoactive drug in the Western world. Alcohol plays contradictory roles in human behavior. Used in moderation, alcohol can enhance social occasions by loosening inhibitions and creating pleasant feelings of relaxation. But alcohol can also be harmful. Like other drugs, alcohol produces physiological effects that can impair functioning in the short term and cause devastating damage in the long term. For some people, alcohol can become addictive, leading to a lifetime of recovery or to debilitation and death.

Some people choose to drink in moderation; some choose not to drink at all (in a 2018 survey, 49% of U.S. adults reported not drinking in the previous month). Still others realize too late that they've had too much. This chapter discusses the complexities of alcohol use and provides information that will help you make choices that are right for you. See Chapter 10 for a discussion of the terms *abuse, use,* and *misuse.* Here they are used somewhat interchangeably.

ALCOHOL AND THE BODY

You have probably noticed that alcohol affects people in different ways. One person may seem to get drunk after just a drink or two, while another appears to tolerate a great deal of alcohol without apparent effect. These differences make alcohol's effects on the body seem mysterious and account for many misconceptions about alcohol use.

Common Alcoholic Beverages

Technically speaking, there are many kinds of **alcohols,** which are organic compounds. In this book, however, the term *alcohol* refers only to ethyl alcohol (or ethanol). Several kinds of alcohol chemically resemble ethyl alcohol, such as methanol (wood alcohol) and isopropyl alcohol (rubbing alcohol), but these are highly toxic; if consumed, they can cause serious illness, blindness, and death.

There are several basic types of alcoholic beverages. Ethanol is the psychoactive ingredient in each of them:

• Beer is a mild intoxicant brewed from a mixture of grains. By volume, beer usually contains 3–6% alcohol.

• Ales and malt liquors, which also have grain bases and are similar to beer in their processing, typically contain 6–8% alcohol by volume.

• Wines are made by fermenting the juices of grapes or other fruits. During *fermentation,* sugars from the fruit react with yeast to create ethanol and other by-products. In table wines, the concentration of alcohol is about 9–14%. A more potent type of wine, *fortified wine,* is called this because extra alcohol is added during its production. Fortified wines—such as sherry, port, and Madeira—contain about 20% alcohol.

• Hard liquor—such as gin, whiskey, rum, tequila, vodka, and liqueur—is made by *distilling* brewed or fermented grains or other plant products. Hard liquors usually contain 35–50% alcohol but can be much stronger.

The concentration of alcohol in a beverage is indicated by its **proof value,** which amounts to two times the percentage concentration. For example, if a beverage is 100 proof, it contains 50% alcohol by volume. Two ounces of 100-proof whiskey contain 1 ounce of pure alcohol. The proof value of hard liquor can usually be found on the bottle's label.

"Standard Drinks" versus Actual Servings When discussing alcohol consumption, the term **one drink** (or *a standard drink*) refers to the amount of a beverage that typically contains about 0.6 ounces or 14 grams of alcohol. Figure 11.1 shows the amounts of popular beverages that are considered to be one standard drink, based on their alcohol content.

A typical serving of most alcoholic beverages is larger (sometimes significantly larger) than a single standard drink. This is particularly true of mixed drinks, which often include more than one type of hard liquor. Alcoholic beverages are usually sold in packages that contain multiple servings, as shown in Table 11.1.

Caloric Content Alcohol provides 7 calories per gram, and the alcohol in one drink (14–17 grams) supplies about 100–120 calories. Most alcoholic beverages also contain some carbohydrate; for example, one beer provides about 150 total calories. The "light" in light beer refers to calories; a light beer typically has close to the same alcohol content as a regular beer and about 100 calories. A 5-ounce glass of red wine has 100 calories; white wine has 96. A 3-ounce margarita supplies 157 calories, a 6-ounce cosmopolitan has 143 calories, and a 6-ounce rum and Coke contains about 180 calories.

Drinking alcoholic beverages significantly increases food and total energy intake. A recent meta-analysis on 12 studies suggests that adults do not compensate for alcohol energy by eating less, and a relatively modest alcohol dose may lead to an increase in food consumption.

Absorption

Have you ever had too much to drink? The rate at which your body absorbs alcohol will affect how quickly you feel drunk or how quickly your behavior is impaired. In fact, the speed at which your blood alcohol concentration rises has been linked to the degree of impairment, more than the concentration itself. Several factors determine the rate of absorption: how fast you drink, how fast your stomach empties its

---

alcohol   The intoxicating ingredient in fermented or distilled beverages; a colorless, pungent liquid.

TERMS

proof value   Two times the percentage of alcohol, by volume, in an alcoholic beverage; a "100-proof" beverage is 50% alcohol by volume.

one drink   The amount of a beverage that typically contains about 0.6 ounces of alcohol; also called a *standard drink.*

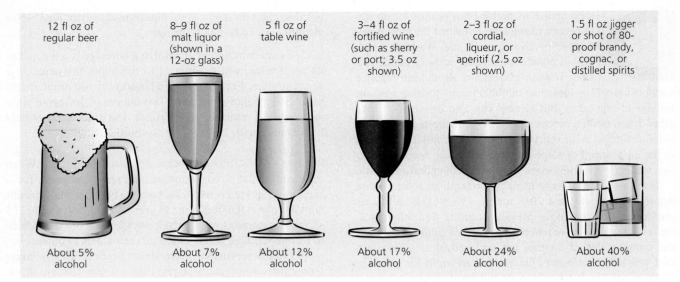

| 12 fl oz of regular beer | 8–9 fl oz of malt liquor (shown in a 12-oz glass) | 5 fl oz of table wine | 3–4 fl oz of fortified wine (such as sherry or port; 3.5 oz shown) | 2–3 fl oz of cordial, liqueur, or aperitif (2.5 oz shown) | 1.5 fl oz jigger or shot of 80-proof brandy, cognac, or distilled spirits |
| About 5% alcohol | About 7% alcohol | About 12% alcohol | About 17% alcohol | About 24% alcohol | About 40% alcohol |

FIGURE 11.1 One standard drink contains about 0.6 fluid ounces of alcohol. To determine the drink size of other beverages, use the National Institutes of Health drink size calculator (http://rethinkingdrinking.niaaa.nih.gov/Tools/Calculators/drink-size-calculator.aspx) or do your own calculation by dividing 0.6 by the percentage alcohol volume of the beverage, expressed as a decimal. For example, to calculate the size of a standard drink of beer labeled as having 5% alcohol content:

$$\frac{0.6}{0.05} = 12 \text{ oz.}$$

SOURCE: National Institute on Alcohol Abuse and Alcoholism. 2015. *Rethinking Drinking: Alcohol and Your Health* (NIH Publication No. 15-3770). Rockville, MD: National Institute on Alcohol Abuse and Alcoholism.

Table 11.1	Serving Sizes versus Standard Drinks of Common Alcoholic Beverages	
BEVERAGE	**SERVING/ CONTAINER SIZE**	**NUMBER OF STANDARD DRINKS**
Beer (5% alc/vol)	12 oz.	1*
	16 oz.	1.3
	22 oz.	2
	40 oz.	3.3
Malt liquor (7% alc/vol)	12 oz.	1.5
	16 oz.	2
	22 oz.	2.5
	40 oz.	4.5
Table wine (12% alc/vol)	750-mL (25 oz.) bottle	5
Hard liquor (80 proof) (40% alc/vol)	1 shot (1.5 oz. glass/50 ml bottle)	1
	1 mixed drink	1 or more
	Half pint (8 oz.) bottle	4.5
	1 pint (16 oz.) bottle	8.5
	1 fifth (25 oz.) bottle	17

*Approximate values. For different types of beer, wine, or malt liquor, the alcohol content can vary greatly.

SOURCE: National Institute on Alcohol Abuse and Alcoholism. 2019. *Rethinking Drinking: Alcohol and Your Health* (NIH Publication No. 15-3770). Rockville, MD: National Institute on Alcohol Abuse and Alcoholism (https://www.rethinkingdrinking.niaaa.nih.gov/How-much-is-too-much/What-counts-as-a-drink/How-Many-Drinks-Are-In-Common-Containers.aspx).

contents, and how much and what type of food and other drugs are in your system. Food in the stomach slows the rate of absorption.

The kind of alcohol (volume, concentration, and nature) also affects absorption. For example, the carbonation in a beverage like champagne increases the rate of alcohol absorption, as do artificial sweeteners (commonly used in drink mixers). You may be surprised to know that drinking highly concentrated alcoholic beverages such as hard liquor slows absorption. Gender and ethnicity also affect the rate of absorption.

How does alcohol get into the bloodstream? When a person drinks alcohol, a small amount is absorbed by the oral mucosa (the lining of the mouth). About 20% is absorbed in the stomach, and about 75% is absorbed through the upper part of the small intestine. Any remaining alcohol enters the bloodstream farther along the gastrointestinal (GI) tract. Once in the bloodstream, alcohol produces sensations of intoxication.

Metabolism and Excretion

Once alcohol has been absorbed, it is metabolized, meaning that the body transforms it into usable substances and waste. The usable parts are transformed into energy and fat reserves in the following way.

The circulatory system quickly transports alcohol throughout the body. Because alcohol easily moves through most biological membranes, it is rapidly distributed throughout most body tissues. Although a small amount of alcohol is metabolized in the stomach, most is metabolized in the liver. There, several enzymes convert the alcohol to acetaldehyde, then to acetate. Individuals vary slightly in the enzymes they have, and thus they may react differently to alcohol. (See the box "Metabolizing Alcohol: Our Bodies Work Differently.")

About 2–10% of ingested alcohol is not metabolized in the liver or other tissues but is excreted unchanged by the lungs,

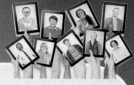
Do you and your friends react differently to alcohol? If so, your reactions may be affected by genetic differences in alcohol metabolism. **Metabolism** refers to the chemical transformation of alcohol and other substances in your body into energy and waste. Alcohol is metabolized mainly in the liver, where an enzyme, alcohol dehydrogenase, converts the alcohol into a toxic substance called acetaldehyde. Acetaldehyde causes many of alcohol's noxious effects. Ideally it is quickly broken down to a less active by-product, acetate, by another enzyme, acetaldehyde dehydrogenase (ALDH). Acetate can then separate into water and carbon dioxide and easily be eliminated. But people vary in the length of time it takes to break down the toxins in alcohol and in how efficiently they can process them. Some differences in metabolism are associated with ethnicity.

Some people, primarily those of Asian descent, inherit ineffective or inactive variations of that latter enzyme, acetaldehyde dehydrogenase. Others, including some people of African and Jewish descent, have forms of alcohol dehydrogenase that metabolize alcohol to acetaldehyde very quickly. Either way, toxic acetaldehyde builds up when these people drink alcohol. They experience a reaction called *flushing syndrome*. Their skin feels hot, their heart and respiration rates increase, and they may get a headache, vomit, or break out in hives. The severity of their reactions is affected by the inherited form of their alcohol-metabolizing enzymes. These adverse reactions to drinking makes some people so uncomfortable that they are unlikely to develop alcohol addiction.

The body's response to acetaldehyde is the basis for treating alcohol misuse with the drug disulfiram (Antabuse), which inhibits the action of acetaldehyde dehydrogenase. When a person taking disulfiram ingests alcohol, acetaldehyde levels increase rapidly, and he or she develops an intense flushing reaction along with weakness, nausea, vomiting, and other disagreeable symptoms.

How people behave in relation to alcohol is influenced in complex ways by a wide range of factors, including liver size, body mass, and social and cultural influences. But individual choices and behavior are also strongly influenced by specific genetic characteristics.

---

kidneys, and sweat glands. Excreted alcohol causes the telltale smell on a drinker's breath and is the basis of breath and urine analyses for alcohol levels. Although such analyses do not give precise measurements of alcohol concentrations in the blood, they provide a reasonable approximation if done correctly.

When alcohol enters the human brain, it affects neurotransmitters—the chemicals that carry messages between brain cells. Alcohol changes the ability of brain cells to receive these messages and disrupts networks within the brain that connect different brain regions. These changes are temporary, creating many of the immediate effects of drinking alcohol.

With chronic heavy use, however, alcohol's disruptive effects can become permanent, resulting in loss of brain function and changes in brain structure. Alcohol interferes with the production of new brain cells (neurogenesis) in unborn children, young children, adolescents, and young adults, whose brains continue to develop until about age 21. Alcohol may also negatively affect neurogenesis in mature adults.

Alcohol Intake and Blood Alcohol Concentration

Blood alcohol concentration (BAC) is the ratio of alcohol in a person's blood by weight, expressed as the percentage of alcohol measured in a deciliter of blood. BAC is affected by the amount of alcohol consumed in a given amount of time and by these individual factors:

- *Body weight.* In most cases, a smaller person develops a higher BAC than a larger person after drinking the same amount of alcohol (Figure 11.2). A smaller person has less overall body tissue into which alcohol can be distributed.

- *Percentage of body fat.* A person with a higher percentage of body fat will usually develop a higher BAC than a more muscular person of the same weight when they drink the same amount. Alcohol does not concentrate as much in fatty tissue as in muscle and most other tissues, in part because fat has fewer blood vessels.

- *Sex.* Women metabolize less alcohol in the stomach than men do because the stomach enzyme that breaks down alcohol before it enters the bloodstream is four times more active in men than in women. Hormonal fluctuations may also affect the rate of alcohol metabolism, making a woman more susceptible to high BACs at certain times during her menstrual cycle.

BAC also depends on the balance between the rate of alcohol absorption and the rate of alcohol metabolism. A man who weighs 150 pounds and has normal liver function metabolizes about 0.3 ounces of alcohol per hour, the equivalent of about half a 12-ounce bottle of beer or half a 5-ounce glass of wine.

The rate of alcohol metabolism varies among people and is determined largely by genetic factors and drinking behavior. Chronic drinking activates enzymes that metabolize alcohol in the liver, so people who drink frequently metabolize

---

metabolism The chemical transformation of food and other substances in the body into energy and wastes, first through breaking apart the components and then using them in other forms. **TERMS**

blood alcohol concentration (BAC) The amount of alcohol in the blood expressed as the percentage of alcohol in a deciliter of blood; used as a measure of intoxication.

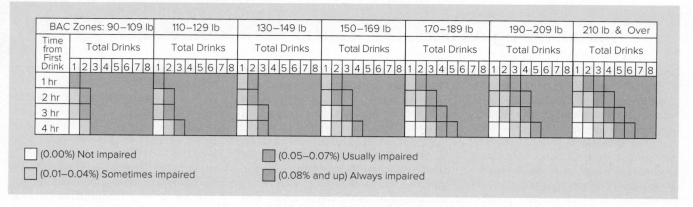

FIGURE 11.2 **Approximate blood alcohol concentration (BAC) and body weight.** This chart illustrates the BAC an average person of a given weight would reach after drinking the specified number of drinks in the time shown. The federal legal limit for BAC for drivers is 0.08%; for drivers under 21 years of age, many states have zero-tolerance laws that set BAC limits of 0.01% or 0.02%.

alcohol at a more rapid rate than nondrinkers. Other than that, nothing will sober you up faster than the time it takes for your sweat, urine, breath, and the enzyme alcohol dehydrogenase to eliminate the alcohol from your body. Although the rate of alcohol absorption can be slowed by factors like food, the metabolic rate *cannot* be influenced by exercise, breathing deeply, eating, drinking coffee, or taking other drugs. Whether a person is asleep or awake, the rate of alcohol metabolism is the same.

If a person absorbs slightly less alcohol each hour than can be metabolized in an hour, their BAC remains low. People can drink large amounts of alcohol this way over a long period of time without becoming noticeably intoxicated; however, they still run the risk of long-term health problems (described later in the chapter). If people drink more alcohol than they can metabolize (for example, two drinks within 30 minutes), the BAC will increase steadily, and they will become more and more intoxicated (see Figure 11.3). Drinking too much alcohol too quickly can be lethal: Think of a quantity of alcohol consumed over a period of two or three hours—enough to cause intoxication and a hangover the next day. Now imagine chugging that same amount in an hour or less.

ALCOHOL'S IMMEDIATE AND LONG-TERM EFFECTS

The effects of alcohol consumption on health depend on the person, the circumstances, and the amount of alcohol consumed.

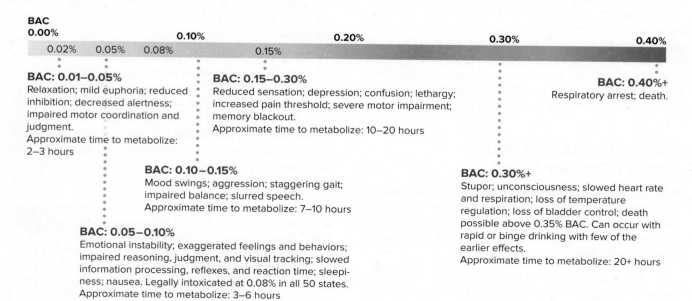

FIGURE 11.3 **Effects of blood alcohol concentration (BAC) at each stage of intoxication.**

Immediate Effects

The amount of alcohol in the blood is a primary factor determining the effects of alcohol. At low concentrations, alcohol tends to make people feel relaxed and jovial, but at higher concentrations, people are more likely to feel angry, sedated, or sleepy. In general, alcohol slows reactions, impairs coordination and judgment, and eventually, sedates to inactivity. The senses become less acute.

Low Concentrations of Alcohol

The effects of alcohol can first be felt at a BAC of 0.03–0.05%. These effects may include lightheadedness, relaxation, and a release of inhibitions. Most drinkers experience mild euphoria and become more sociable. When people drink in social settings, alcohol often seems to act as a stimulant, enhancing friendliness or confidence. This apparent stimulation occurs because alcohol depresses inhibitory centers in the brain.

Higher Concentrations of Alcohol

At higher concentrations, the pleasant effects tend to be replaced by more negative ones: interference with motor coordination, verbal performance, and intellectual functions. The drinker often becomes irritable and may be easily angered or given to crying.

When the BAC reaches 0.1%, most sensory and motor functioning is reduced, and many people become sleepy. Vision, smell, taste, and hearing become less acute. At 0.2%, most drinkers are completely unable to function, either physically or psychologically, because of the pronounced depression of the central nervous system, muscles, and other body systems. Coma usually occurs at a BAC of 0.35%, and any higher level can be fatal.

Small doses of alcohol may initially improve sexual functioning for people who are especially anxious or self-conscious, but higher doses often have negative effects, such as reduced erectile response. Effects of chronic heavy drinking include reducing testosterone levels and impairing sperm production.

Alcohol causes blood vessels near the skin to dilate, so drinkers often feel warm initially; their skin flushes, and they may sweat more. Flushing and sweating contribute to heat loss, however, so the internal body temperature falls. High doses of alcohol may impair the body's ability to regulate temperature, causing it to drop sharply, especially if the surrounding temperature is low. Drinking alcoholic beverages to keep warm in cold weather does not work and can even be dangerous.

Since alcohol is a sedative, it induces sleepiness. But its utility is short-lived because people quickly build up a tolerance to it. Moreover, large amounts of alcohol disturb normal sleep patterns. The sleep that follows drinking can be poor quality—and unrefreshing because the person awakens after fitful dreams, and often stays wakeful. Alcohol can also cause or worsen sleep apnea. (Sleep and sleep disorders are discussed in Chapter 4.)

Alcohol Hangover

Alcohol's effects wear off slowly, and anyone who has experienced a severe hangover knows they are not fun. The symptoms include headache, shakiness, nausea, diarrhea, fatigue, and impaired mental functioning.

Ask Yourself

QUESTIONS FOR CRITICAL THINKING AND REFLECTION

Have you ever had a hangover or watched someone else suffer through one? Did the experience affect your attitude about drinking? In what way?

But even after a person sobers up, at high BACs the resulting hangover can continue to leave the person impaired for several hours.

A hangover is probably caused by a combination of the toxic products of alcohol breakdown, dehydration, and hormonal effects. During a hangover, heart rate and blood pressure increase, making some individuals more vulnerable to heart attacks. Electroencephalography (brain wave measurement) shows slowing of brain waves for up to 16 hours after BAC drops to 0.0%. Studies of pilots, drivers, and skiers all indicate that coordination and cognition are impaired in a person with a hangover, increasing the risk of injury.

The best treatment for hangover is prevention. Nearly all men can expect a hangover if they drink more than five to six standard drinks; for women, the number is three to four drinks. Drinking less, drinking slowly, and eating food decrease the risk of hangover. If you ever suffer through a hangover, remember that your driving ability is impaired even after your BAC returns to 0.0%.

Alcohol Poisoning

Acute alcohol poisoning occurs much more frequently than most people realize, and all too often it causes death. Drinking large amounts of alcohol in a short time can rapidly raise the BAC into the lethal range. Alcohol, either alone or in combination with other drugs, is responsible for more toxic overdose deaths than any other drug.

Death from alcohol poisoning may be caused either by central nervous system (CNS) and respiratory depression or by inhaling fluid or vomit into the lungs. The amount of alcohol that renders a person unconscious is dangerously close to a fatal dose. Although passing out may prevent someone from drinking more, BAC can keep rising during unconsciousness because the body continues to absorb ingested alcohol into the bloodstream. Special care should be taken to ensure the safety of anyone who has been drinking heavily, especially if he or she passes out (see the box "Dealing with an Alcohol Emergency").

Using Alcohol with Other Drugs

Alcohol–drug combinations are a leading cause of drug-related deaths. Using alcohol while taking a medication that depresses the CNS increases the effects of both drugs, potentially leading to coma, respiratory depression, and death. Such drugs include barbiturates, Valium-like drugs, narcotics such as codeine, and over-the-counter antihistamines such as Benadryl. For people who consume three or more drinks per day, use of over-the-counter pain relievers like aspirin, ibuprofen, or acetaminophen increases the risk of stomach bleeding and liver damage. Some antacids, antibiotics, and diabetes medications can also interact dangerously with alcohol.

Many illegal drugs are especially dangerous when combined with alcohol. Life-threatening overdoses occur at much lower doses when heroin and other narcotics are combined with alcohol. When cocaine and alcohol are used together, they form a toxic substance in the liver called cocaethylene, which can produce effects that neither drug alone does.

A trend among young drinkers involves mixing alcoholic beverages with caffeinated ones, especially highly caffeinated energy drinks (see the box "Alcoholic Energy Drinks"). The safest strategy is to avoid combining alcohol with any other drug—prescription, over-the-counter, or illegal. If in doubt, ask your pharmacist or doctor before combining any drug with alcohol. Better, just don't do it.

Alcohol-Related Injuries and Violence

The combination of impaired judgment, weakened sensory perception, reduced inhibitions, impaired motor coordination, and increased aggressiveness and hostility that characterizes alcohol intoxication can be dangerous and deadly. Through homicide, suicide, automobile crashes, and other traumatic incidents, alcohol use is linked to about 90,000 deaths each year in the United States. The majority of people who attempt suicide have been drinking. Among successful suicides, alcohol use is common as well; an analysis of studies involving over 420,000 participants reveals that alcohol use disorder is an important predictor of suicide. Alcohol use more than triples the risk of fatal injuries during leisure activities such as swimming and boating. More than 50% of fatal falls and serious burns happen to people who have been drinking.

Alcohol and Aggression

Eighty percent of arrests happen for drug- and alcohol-related offenses (domestic violence, driving under the influence of alcohol, public drunkenness, and property and drug offenses). Alcohol use contributes to 40% of all murders, assaults, and rapes. It is frequently found in the bloodstream of victims as well as perpetrators. Some people become violent under alcohol's influence, and alcohol is an important component of gang life, maintaining the solidarity of the group, and contributing to gang violence. Doubly risky is the effect of alcohol on people predisposed to aggressive or impulsive behavior. In some cases these people may have an underlying psychiatric condition called *antisocial personality disorder*. Their destructive behaviors—repeated criminal acts, deceitfulness, impulsiveness, repeated fights or assaults, and disregard for the safety of others—gain momentum under the influence of alcohol. They are also more likely to become alcohol-dependent. However, all drinkers under the influence of alcohol are subject to unpredictable and injurious consequences.

Alcohol misuse can wreak havoc on home life. Marital discord and domestic violence often exist in the presence of excessive alcohol consumption. Heavy drinking by parents is associated with abuse of their children, typically emotional or psychological abuse. Links between parental drinking and

QUICK STATS

In 2018, **8.1%** of drivers aged 16–25 years reported driving under the influence of alcohol at least once in the past year, down from **19.9%** in 2000.

—Substance Abuse and Mental Health Services Administration, 2019

A popular trend is to mix alcohol with energy drinks or other caffeinated beverages. Slightly more than a third of young people consume these mixed drinks—among others, espresso martinis, rum and coke, vodka Red Bull®, and Jägerbombs. This practice is dangerous for many reasons.

For one, combining energy drinks with alcohol increases alcohol absorption, but caffeine does not speed alcohol metabolism. This means that people who consume more caffeine–alcohol drinks reach higher BAC levels, consume more drinks, and spend more time drinking than those who consume alcohol by itself. There is also a greater correlation with alcohol dependence when people consume caffeine with alcohol than when they consume alcohol alone.

Another striking problem with these mixed drinks is that consumers *perceive* themselves to be more alert than they actually are. They expect the caffeine (sometimes five times greater than in a cup of coffee) to counteract the negative effects of the alcohol, leading some drinkers to take risks they might not take with alcohol alone, such as driving a car. Along with impaired decision making, there is an increased risk for injury and aggression.

The myth that caffeine–alcohol drinks keep the drinker alert played a big role in a 2018 study about expectations. Some participants were led to believe that caffeine would offset negative effects of the alcohol. These participants showed more impairment in completing tasks than did the participants who did not expect the caffeine to help them remain sharp.

Some gender differences, however, emerged in a 2019 study on a predominantly female student sample: Up to a 0.13% blood alcohol level, the women overestimated the amount of alcohol in their blood as they drank more caffeine. In other words, caffeine did not increase their alertness, but instead their feelings of intoxication. Whatever the disparity between perception and actual levels of intoxication, making decisions after consuming any alcoholic beverages is often dangerous.

A growing body of evidence highlights the risks associated with energy drinks. These include risk-seeking behavior, such as substance abuse and aggression, mental health problems such as anxiety and stress, and physical problems such as increased blood pressure, obesity, kidney damage, fatigue, and stomachaches. According to SAMHSA, 1 in 10 emergency department visits of patients aged 12 and over in 2011 was related to highly caffeinated drinks. Nearly half the emergencies resulted from mixing the beverages with alcohol or other drugs.

In 2010, the FDA reported that premixed, commercial, caffeinated alcoholic beverages (CABs) are a public health concern and that adding caffeine to malt alcoholic beverages amounts to using an "unsafe food additive" that violates the Federal Food, Drug, and Cosmetic Act. Effectively, the FDA banned the sale of premixed drinks. Still, a general lack of regulation of energy drinks has led to vigorous marketing campaigns by CAB manufacturers, making unsubstantiated claims about the performance-enhancing properties of their product. It is important that individual consumers personally investigate what they are consuming.

SOURCES: Al-Shaar, L., et al. 2017. Health effects and public health concerns of energy drink consumption in the United States: A mini-review. *Frontiers in Public Health* 5 (https://doi.org/10.3389/fpubh.2017.00225); Marczinski, C. A., et al. 2018. Alcohol-induced impairment of balance is antagonized by energy drinks. *Alcoholism: Clinical and Experimental Research* 42(1): 144–152; Norberg, M. M., et al. 2019. Why are caffeinated alcoholic beverages especially risky? *Addictive Behaviors* 98 10.1016/j.addbeh.2019.106062; Roldán, M., et al. 2017. Red Bull® energy drink increases consumption of higher concentrations of alcohol. *Addiction Biology* (https://doi-org.laneproxy.stanford.edu/10.1111/adb.12560); Substance Abuse and Mental Health Services Administration. 2014. *The DAWN Report: 1 in 10 Energy Drink-Related Emergency Department Visits Results in Hospitalization*. Rockville, MD: Substance Abuse and Mental Health Services Administration (http://www.samhsa.gov/data/sites/default/files /spot124-energy-drinks-2014.pdf).

physical or sexual abuse are not found consistently, but when such mistreatment does take place, the damaging effect is often long-lasting and associated with alcohol misuse in the grown child.

Alcohol and Sexual Decision Making

Alcohol seriously impairs a person's ability to make wise decisions about sex. A recent survey of college students revealed that frequent binge drinkers were five times more likely to engage in unplanned sexual activity and five-and-a-half times more likely to have unprotected sex than non–binge drinkers. **Binge drinking** is a pattern of rapid, periodic drinking that brings a person's blood alcohol concentration up to 0.08% or higher, typically with five or more drinks for men, or four drinks for women, typically within about two hours. The difference between *bingeing* and *heavy drinking* is that heavy drinking involves bingeing on five or more days in the past month, according to the Substance Abuse and Mental Health Services Administration (SAMHSA).

Heavy drinkers are also more likely to have multiple sex partners and to engage in other forms of high-risk sexual behavior. Rates of sexually transmitted infections (including HIV) and unwanted pregnancy are higher among people who drink heavily than among people who drink moderately or not at all. People who binge-drink are at increased risk of rape and other forms of nonconsensual sex. The laws regarding sexual consent are clear: A person who is very drunk or passed out cannot consent to sex. Having sex with a person who is drunk or unconscious is rape.

binge drinking   Periodically drinking alcohol to the point of severe intoxication: about four drinks (for women) and five drinks (for men) consumed within a period of about two hours. **TERMS**

Drinking and Driving

Drunk driving remains a serious problem in the United States. In 2018, 10,511 Americans were killed in accidents involving alcohol-impaired drivers—close to one-third of all traffic fatalities for the year. Men are more likely than women to be driving drunk in fatal crashes. The National Highway Transportation Safety Administration reports that in 2018, 21% of men were drunk in these crashes, compared to 14% of women. Of all drivers involved in fatal crashes, those aged 21–24 had the highest percentage of BACs of 0.08% or higher.

People who drink are unable to drive safely because their judgment is impaired, their reaction time is slower, and their coordination is reduced. Some driving skills are affected at BACs of 0.02% and lower. At a BAC of 0.05%, visual perception, reaction time, and certain steering tasks are impaired. Any amount of alcohol impairs your ability to drive safely, and fatigue augments the effects of alcohol.

Can we predict which behaviors or traits factor into young adults' driving under the influence (DUI) of alcohol? Impulsivity—the tendency to act without thinking—is a predictor of DUI. However, the specific facets of impulsivity that predict DUI and how they vary with gender differences remain unclear. Men appear to exhibit higher sensation seeking and alcohol use than women. Women exhibit greater perception of risk and greater perseverance (staying focused on long, complex tasks). Men report more DUIs and have more of them. However, prevention strategies should be tailored to all sexes and should focus on personality traits associated with impulsivity, especially in women with sensation-seeking behaviors.

The *dose-response function* is the relationship between the amount of alcohol or drug consumed and the type and intensity of the resulting effect. Higher doses of alcohol are associated with a much greater probability of automobile crashes (Figure 11.4). A person driving with a BAC of 0.14% is over

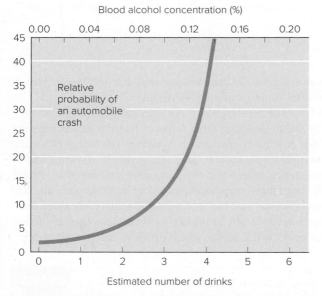

FIGURE 11.4   The dose-response relationship between BAC and automobile crashes.

Ask Yourself

QUESTIONS FOR CRITICAL THINKING AND REFLECTION

Have you ever witnessed or been involved in an alcohol emergency? Did you think the situation was urgent at the time? What were the circumstances surrounding the event? How did the people involved deal with it?

40 times more likely to be involved in a crash than someone with no alcohol in their blood. For those with a BAC above 0.14%, the risk of a fatal crash is estimated to be 380 times higher. The risks for young drivers are even greater, even at very low BACs. Younger drivers have less experience with both driving and alcohol, which results in significant impairment even with BACs as low as 0.02%.

In addition to increasing the risk of injury and death, driving while intoxicated can have serious legal consequences. Drunk driving is against the law. The legal limit for BAC is 0.08% in the United States, but alcohol impairs the user even at much lower BACs. Stiff penalties for drunk driving include fines, loss of license, confiscation of vehicle, and jail time. Under current zero-tolerance laws in many states, drivers under age 21 who have consumed *any* alcohol may have their licenses suspended. Increasingly, states are passing laws against having open containers of alcohol in a vehicle and are allowing stricter punishment for repeat offenders.

If you are out of your home and drinking, find alternative transportation or appoint a *designated driver* who doesn't drink and can provide safe transportation home. Although difficult in the face of social pressure, this is the critical moment to be fearless and stand against the pressure. It is reasonable to insist on not being driven by anyone who has been drinking. Ridesharing apps (such as Uber and Lyft) make it easy to get a ride if needed. Remember, you risk more than your own life when you drink and drive. Causing serious injury or death results in lifelong feelings of sadness and guilt for the driver and grief for friends and families of victims.

It's more difficult to protect yourself against someone else who drinks and drives. Learn to be alert to the erratic driving that signals an impaired driver.

The following behaviors typically indicate that someone is driving while drunk:

- Wide, abrupt, and illegal turns
- Straddling the center line or lane marker
- Driving against traffic
- Driving on the shoulder
- Weaving, swerving, or nearly striking objects or other vehicles
- Following too closely
- Erratic speed
- Driving with headlights off at night
- Driving with the windows down in very cold weather

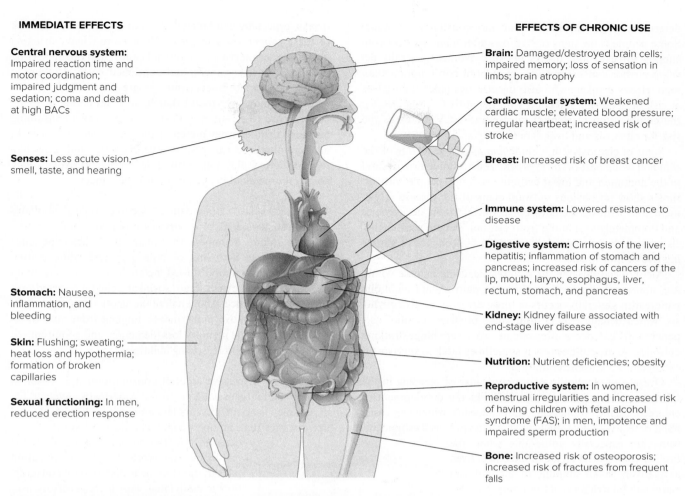

Central nervous system: Impaired reaction time and motor coordination; impaired judgment and sedation; coma and death at high BACs

Senses: Less acute vision, smell, taste, and hearing

Stomach: Nausea, inflammation, and bleeding

Skin: Flushing; sweating; heat loss and hypothermia; formation of broken capillaries

Sexual functioning: In men, reduced erection response

Brain: Damaged/destroyed brain cells; impaired memory; loss of sensation in limbs; brain atrophy

Cardiovascular system: Weakened cardiac muscle; elevated blood pressure; irregular heartbeat; increased risk of stroke

Breast: Increased risk of breast cancer

Immune system: Lowered resistance to disease

Digestive system: Cirrhosis of the liver; hepatitis; inflammation of stomach and pancreas; increased risk of cancers of the lip, mouth, larynx, esophagus, liver, rectum, stomach, and pancreas

Kidney: Kidney failure associated with end-stage liver disease

Nutrition: Nutrient deficiencies; obesity

Reproductive system: In women, menstrual irregularities and increased risk of having children with fetal alcohol syndrome (FAS); in men, impotence and impaired sperm production

Bone: Increased risk of osteoporosis; increased risk of fractures from frequent falls

FIGURE 11.5 **The immediate and long-term effects of alcohol misuse.**

If you see any of these signs in another driver, avoid that vehicle by pulling off the road or turning at the nearest intersection. Report the driver to the police.

Long-Term Effects of Chronic Misuse

Because alcohol is distributed throughout most of the body, it affects many organs and tissues (Figure 11.5). This section considers problems associated with chronic or habitually excessive use of alcohol, including damaged brain cells, impaired memory, possible loss of sensation in the limbs, and brain atrophy. Diseases of the digestive system include cirrhosis of the liver, hepatitis, inflamed stomach and pancreas, and increased risk of cancers throughout the GI tract. The cardiovascular system may show weakened heart muscle, elevated blood pressure, and increased risk of stroke. Drinking during pregnancy risks the health of both the mother and her developing fetus, discussed in more detail later in this chapter.

The Digestive System   Even in the short term, alcohol can alter the functioning of the liver, which is essential for digesting and absorbing fat. Within just a few days of heavy alcohol consumption, fat begins to accumulate in liver cells,

resulting in the development of "fatty liver." If drinking continues, inflammation of the liver can occur, resulting in alcoholic hepatitis, a frequent cause of hospitalization and death among alcoholics. Both fatty liver and alcoholic hepatitis are potentially reversible if the person stops drinking. With continued alcohol use, however, liver cells are progressively damaged and then destroyed.

Young men who consume alcohol (about two or more drinks regularly) show an increased risk of eventual severe liver disease, even up to 40 years later in life. Even those who drink less regularly show a trend toward later liver disease. Current guidelines for safe alcohol intake in men may have to be revised.

Destroyed liver cells are replaced by fibrous scar tissue, a condition known as **cirrhosis.** As cirrhosis develops, a drinker may gradually lose his or her capacity to tolerate alcohol because fewer and fewer healthy cells remain in the liver to metabolize it.

As with most health hazards, the risk of cirrhosis depends on an individual's susceptibility, which is largely genetically

cirrhosis   A disease in which the liver is severely damaged by alcohol, other toxins, or infection.

determined, and the amount of alcohol consumed over time. Some people show signs of cirrhosis after a few years of consuming three to four drinks per day. Women generally develop cirrhosis at lower levels of alcohol consumption than men. Heavy drinkers who also inject drugs place themselves at risk of acquiring infection with hepatitis C virus (HCV); the combination of alcohol misuse and HCV increases the risk for cirrhosis and liver cancer.

Signs of cirrhosis can include *jaundice* (a yellowing of the skin and white part of the eyes) and the accumulation of fluid in the abdomen and lower extremities. Some people with cirrhosis show no obvious outward signs of the disease. Treatment for cirrhosis includes correcting nutrient deficiencies and completely abstaining from alcohol. People with cirrhosis who continue to drink have only a 50% chance of surviving five or more years.

Alcohol can inflame the pancreas, causing nausea, vomiting, abnormal digestion, and severe pain. Acute alcoholic pancreatitis generally occurs in binge drinkers. Unlike cirrhosis, which usually occurs after years of heavy alcohol use, pancreatitis can occur after one or two severe binge-drinking episodes. Acute pancreatitis is sometimes fatal; in survivors it can become a chronic condition.

Overuse of alcohol is a common cause of bleeding in the GI tract. Cirrhosis frequently results in the development of enlarged, fragile esophageal and rectal veins, which can easily burst or tear with potentially fatal results. Enlarged esophageal veins are especially vulnerable when the drinker vomits after an alcoholic binge. Even a relatively small amount of alcohol can cause painful irritation of the stomach lining.

The Cardiovascular System The effects of alcohol on the cardiovascular system depend on the amount of alcohol consumed. Moderate doses of alcohol—one drink or less a day for women and one to two drinks a day for men—may reduce the risk of heart disease and heart attack in some people.

However, higher doses of alcohol harm the cardiovascular system. In some people, more than two drinks a day will elevate blood pressure, making stroke and heart attack more likely. Some alcoholics show a weakening of the heart muscle, a condition known as **cardiac myopathy.** Binge drinking can cause "holiday heart," characterized by serious abnormal heart rhythms, which usually appear within 24 hours of a binge episode.

Cancer In 2000, the U.S. Department of Health and Human Services added alcoholic beverages to its list of known human carcinogens. Chronic alcohol consumption is a clear risk factor for cancers of the mouth, throat, larynx, and esophagus (cancers also associated with use of tobacco, with which alcohol frequently acts as a cocarcinogen). Five or six daily

> **QUICK STATS**
>
> About **11%** of pregnant women drink alcohol, and **3%** engage in binge drinking.
> —Centers for Disease Control and Prevention, 2020

drinks, especially combined with smoking, increases the risk of these cancers by a factor of 50 or more. Heavy drinking also puts users at risk for colorectal cancer and the most common form of liver cancer; and continued heavy drinking in people with hepatitis accelerates progression to this cancer.

Studies have also found that light to moderate drinking can increase your risk. A 2015 study suggests that consuming even one drink per day increases the risk of breast cancer. In all alcohol-related cancers, however, genetics and other biological factors play important roles and help explain why some chronic alcohol abusers do not get cancer.

Brain Damage Brain damage due to chronic alcohol misuse is also tempered by a person's physiology and genetics. Imaging studies document that many alcoholics experience brain shrinkage with loss of both gray and white matter, reduced blood flow, and slowed metabolic rates in some brain regions. To some extent, brain shrinkage can be reversed over time with abstinence. About half of the alcoholics in the United States have cognitive impairments, ranging from mild to severe. These include memory loss, dementia, and compromised problem-solving and reasoning abilities.

Mortality Excessive alcohol consumption is a factor in several leading causes of death for Americans. Average life expectancy is about 15 years less among people with alcohol use disorder than among people who do not have the disorder. Early in the coronavirus (COVID-19) pandemic, the World Health Organization put out the statement that alcohol consumption is associated with a range of diseases and mental health disorders that can compromise the body's immune system. Therefore, people should minimize their alcohol consumption at any time, and particularly during the COVID-19 pandemic. About half the deaths caused by alcohol are due to chronic conditions such as cirrhosis and cancer; the other half are due to acute conditions or events such as car crashes, falls, and suicide. Because many deaths from acute conditions occur in youths and young adults, alcohol is responsible for 2.5 million years of potential life lost each year.

Alcohol Use during Pregnancy

During pregnancy, alcohol and its metabolic product acetaldehyde easily cross the placenta, harming the developing fetus. Damage to the fetus depends on the amount of alcohol the mother consumes and the stage of fetal development. Early in pregnancy, heavy drinking can cause spontaneous abortion or miscarriage. Alcohol in early pregnancy, during critical fetal development periods, can also cause a collection of birth defects known as *fetal alcohol syndrome (FAS)*, which was discussed in Chapter 9.

Because rapid brain development continues throughout pregnancy, the fetal brain stays vulnerable to alcohol use until birth. Although effects of drinking later in pregnancy do not

> **cardiac myopathy** Weakening of the heart muscle through disease.
> **TERMS**

typically cause the characteristic physical deformities of FAS, getting drunk just once during the final three months of pregnancy can damage a fetal brain.

FAS is a permanent, incurable condition that causes lifelong disability. CDC studies identify the number of FAS cases as ranging from two to nine infants for every 10,000 live births in the United States. About three times as many babies are born with **alcohol-related neurodevelopmental disorder (ARND).** Children with ARND appear physically normal but often have significant learning and behavioral disorders. As adults, they are more likely to develop substance use disorders and to have criminal records. ARND must be treated as early as possible to avoid long-term physiological as well as social consequences. Treatments include medical care, medication, behavior and education therapy, parent training, and other approaches such as biofeedback, yoga, and art therapy. The whole range of FAS and ARND is commonly called *fetal alcohol spectrum disorder (FASD).*

No one is sure exactly how much alcohol causes FASD. Like other untoward effects of alcohol, genetics and individual differences in metabolism, along with environmental factors such as diet, are thought to affect vulnerability. The American Academy of Pediatrics stresses that no amount of alcohol at any point during pregnancy is considered safe: Exposure to alcohol is "the leading preventable cause of birth defects and intellectual and neurodisabilities in children."

Women who are trying to conceive, or who are sexually active without using effective contraception, should abstain from alcohol to avoid inadvertently harming their fetus in the first few days or weeks of pregnancy, before they know they're expecting.

Any alcohol consumed by a nursing mother quickly enters her milk. What impact this consumption has on the child or on the mother's milk production is a matter of controversy. Dosage may again be the key issue. Many physicians advise nursing mothers to abstain from drinking alcohol because of the possibility that any amount may have negative effects on the baby's brain development.

Possible Health Benefits of Alcohol?

Researchers are changing their tune on the effects of moderate drinking. Previous studies showed that light to moderate drinking may improve heart health by raising blood levels of HDL (the beneficial form of cholesterol), by thinning the blood, and by reducing inflammation and the risk of dangerous blood clots, all of which can contribute to the risk of a heart attack.

Newer studies, however, cast doubt on such benefits. A 2017 meta-analysis of 45 studies found no benefit of moderate drinking in protecting against cardiovascular disease (CVD) to people 55 years or younger. For those over 55, studies that controlled for heart health also found no protective effects of alcohol. In fact, alcohol consumption in older people may be dangerous. The American Heart Association reported on new research among older adults showing that women who drank moderately had small reductions in heart function. "In spite of potential benefits of low alcohol intake," the researchers report, "our findings highlight the possible hazards to cardiac structure and function by increased amounts of alcohol consumption in the elderly, particularly among women."

The previous idea that moderate drinking could protect us against all causes of death in general now looks less likely, maybe a complete impossibility. This is also true for younger people: current research finds no evidence that drinking in one's twenties and thirties has any health benefits.

EXCESSIVE USE OF ALCOHOL

Excessive use of alcohol affects more than just the drinker. Friends, family members, coworkers, strangers that drinkers encounter on the road, and society as a whole pay the physical, emotional, and financial costs of the misuse of alcohol. As discussed in Chapter 10, the *DSM-5* is refocusing general understanding of excessive alcohol use. It diagnoses behavior based on a continuum of mild, moderate, and severe symptoms. In this case, behaviors are symptoms. Rather than using the terms *alcoholic* or *nonalcoholic,* the *DSM-5* prefers **alcohol use disorder.** Meeting two of the following criteria indicates an alcohol use disorder; two to three symptoms indicates a mild disorder, four to five a moderate disorder, and six or more a severe disorder.

To determine a person's place on the disorder spectrum, ask these questions:

1. Do you often consume alcohol in large amounts over a long period?
2. Do you find that your efforts to control your alcohol use are unsuccessful?
3. Do you spend excessive time using alcohol or recovering from its effects?
4. Do you have a strong desire or craving to use alcohol?
5. Does your persistent alcohol use cause a failure to fulfill obligations at work, school, or home?
6. Do you continue using alcohol despite recurrent social or interpersonal problems caused by its effects?
7. Have you reduced important social or recreational activities because of your alcohol use?
8. Do you persist in using alcohol in situations that are physically risky?
9. Do you continue using alcohol despite knowing that it can cause or worsen a recurrent physical or psychological problem?
10. Do you have a need for increased amounts of alcohol to achieve a desired effect (increased tolerance)?
11. Do you experience symptoms of withdrawal, such as greater amounts of any of the following: sweating, increased pulse rate, hand tremor, insomnia, nausea, and anxiety?

---

alcohol-related neurodevelopmental disorder (ARND) TERMS   Cognitive and behavioral problems seen in people whose mothers drank alcohol during pregnancy.

alcohol use disorder   Misuse of alcohol that leads to clinically significant impairment.

Statistics on Alcohol Use

The CDC estimates that about 60% of Americans aged 18 and over drink alcohol routinely or infrequently. Approximately 15% of Americans are former drinkers, and 25% are lifetime abstainers.

According to the 2018 National Survey on Drug Abuse and Health, 6% of Americans aged 12 or older were classified as heavy alcohol users. Excessive alcohol use is responsible for 88,000 deaths per year among Americans and is the third leading lifestyle-related cause of death.

Alcohol Use Disorder: From Mild to Severe

Alcohol misuse is recurrent alcohol use that has negative consequences, such as drinking in dangerous situations (before driving, for instance) or drinking patterns that result in academic, professional, interpersonal, or legal difficulties. The person who drinks only once a month, but then drives while intoxicated, is a dangerous alcohol user. One in four full-time college students have participated in alcohol misuse or experienced alcohol abuse or dependence in the past year. Nearly half of college student treatment admissions are for primary alcohol abuse.

Severe alcohol use disorder, or **alcoholism,** involves more extensive problems with alcohol use, usually involving physical tolerance and withdrawal.

How can you tell if you or someone you know has serious problems with alcohol? Look for the following warning signs:

- Drinking alone or secretively
- Using alcohol deliberately and repeatedly to perform or get through difficult situations
- Using alcohol as a way to "self-medicate" in order to dull strong emotions or negative feelings
- Feeling uncomfortable on certain occasions when alcohol is not available
- Escalating alcohol consumption beyond an already established drinking pattern
- Consuming alcohol heavily in risky situations, such as before driving
- Getting drunk regularly or more frequently than in the past
- Drinking in the morning

Binge Drinking

In 2018, 37% of Americans aged 18–25 reported that they engaged in binge drinking in the past month; 9% reported that they engaged in heavy drinking in the past month. Surprisingly, most binge drinkers are not alcohol dependent. If their judgment were not impaired, many would decide not to binge. Among Americans under age 21, most drinking occurs in the form of bingeing, and over 90% of the alcohol they drink is consumed while binge drinking. Over half the alcohol consumed by all adults in the United States is downed during binge drinking.

The price of binge drinking is huge, and everyone has to pay. Binge drinking caused more than half the 90,000 deaths and three-fourths of the estimated economic cost of excessive drinking—$249 billion—in 2010 (the latest available data). Students also often mention that they pay in other, nonmonetary ways when they binge-drink (see the box "Peer Pressure and College Binge Drinking"). Frequent binge drinkers are three to seven times more likely than non–binge drinkers to engage in unplanned or unprotected sex, drive after drinking, get hurt or injured, fall behind in schoolwork, or argue with friends.

Alcoholism (Severe Alcohol Use Disorder)

As mentioned earlier, alcoholism is usually characterized by tolerance to alcohol and withdrawal symptoms. Everyone who drinks—even if not suffering from an alcohol use disorder—develops tolerance after repeated alcohol use, whereas withdrawal symptoms suggest a severe disorder.

Patterns and Prevalence   Alcoholism occurs among people of all racial and ethnic groups and at all socioeconomic levels. The stereotype of the homeless, impoverished alcoholic accounts for less than 5% of all alcohol-dependent people and usually represents the final stage of a drinking career that began years earlier. Patterns of excessive alcohol use vary, including these four common variations:

1. Regular daily intake of large amounts
2. Regular heavy drinking limited to weekends
3. Long periods of sobriety interspersed with binges of daily heavy drinking lasting for weeks or months
4. Heavy drinking limited to periods of stress

Once established, alcoholism often exhibits a pattern of exacerbations and remissions. The person may stop drinking and abstain from alcohol for days or months after a frightening problem develops. After a period of abstinence, an alcoholic often attempts controlled drinking, which almost inevitably leads to an escalation in drinking and more problems. Alcoholism is not hopeless, however. Many misusers of alcohol achieve permanent abstinence.

Health Effects   Tolerance and withdrawal can have a serious impact on health. As described in Chapter 10, *tolerance* means that a drinker needs more alcohol to achieve intoxication or the desired effect, that the effects of continued use of the same amount of alcohol are diminished, or that the drinker can function adequately at doses or a BAC that would produce significant impairment in a casual user. Heavy users of alcohol may need to consume about 50% more than they

> **alcoholism**   A pathological use of alcohol or impairment in functioning due to alcohol; characterized by tolerance to alcohol and withdrawal symptoms.   **TERMS**

Peer Pressure and College Binge Drinking

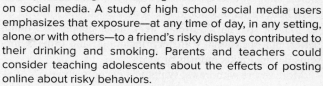

College drinking is pervasive. Approximately 55% of college students drink alcohol and, of those, 37% report having binged on alcohol; both rates are higher than those for similarly aged people not in college. Every year, more than 1800 college students aged 18–24 die from alcohol-related injuries. Another 600,000 sustain unintentional alcohol-related injuries; 700,000 are assaulted by other students who have been drinking; and close to 100,000 are victims of alcohol-related date rape or sexual assault.

These statistics have shocked many students, administrators, and parents into demanding changes in college attitudes and policies regarding alcohol. In response, the National Institute on Alcohol Abuse and Alcoholism (NIAAA) created task forces that bring together research and calls for action. Its reports focus on three levels of action:

1. Ultimately *each student* is accountable and must take responsibility for his or her own behavior. Programs that encourage and support the development of healthy attitudes toward alcohol are needed. These programs should target students at increased risk of developing alcohol problems: first-year students, Greek organization members, and athletes. Treatment should be readily available for problem drinkers.

2. The *student body as a whole* must work to discourage alcohol abuse. These efforts include promoting alcohol-free activities, reducing the availability of alcohol, and avoiding social and commercial promotion of alcohol on campus. The environment should be designed to accept students who choose to abstain and disapprove of students who drink to excess. Fraternities, sororities, eating clubs, and other campus organizations should be held accountable for inappropriate alcohol use, especially involving underage students, that takes place on their premises.

3. *Colleges and surrounding communities* must cooperate to discourage excessive drinking. College administrators, law enforcement, bar and liquor store owners, residents who live near campus, and the court system must all do their part to reduce the availability of cheap alcohol and to enforce existing laws. Those who enable students to drink irresponsibly must be held accountable.

Peer Pressure

The pressure to think and act along certain peer-prescribed guidelines plays a major role in drinking motivations. Late adolescence and early adulthood are times of life in which we are particularly susceptible to frequent alcohol abuse, risky behavior, and peer pressure. A study of young adult men examined direct versus indirect peer pressure. The researchers found that indirect pressure, as in the ideas contributing to our beliefs about alcohol, had more influence than direct pressure, such as offers or dares to drink at parties. The most common motivations of the young adult men were to get high and to forget their worries, rather than to fit in socially or make their social gatherings more fun. Thus, the authors of the study recommend targeting motives over peer pressure as a way to change behaviors.

A vehicle for peer-pressuring young people in particular is the display of drinking and smoking on social media. A study of high school social media users emphasizes that exposure—at any time of day, in any setting, alone or with others—to a friend's risky displays contributed to their drinking and smoking. Parents and teachers could consider teaching adolescents about the effects of posting online about risky behaviors.

Ten Ways to Decline a Drink

1. No thanks.
2. My religious beliefs or health condition prohibit me from drinking.
3. I have offered to be the designated driver.
4. I am an athlete or musician who cannot compromise my general performance.
5. I must do something tomorrow (e.g., work, an exam, a family function), and I won't be able to do it if I drink tonight.
6. I'm dancing (or DJing).
7. I already have a drink (whether alcoholic or not can be hard to tell).
8. I'm cutting calories.
9. I don't like the taste of alcohol.
10. The last time I drank I became violent.

What Schools Are Doing

Some schools have attempted to shift classes to Fridays and even Saturdays after they found that binge drinking increases when students don't have Friday classes. Increasingly, incoming students are required to take a three-hour online class about alcohol. And some campuses apply stricter punishment for underage drinking and public drunkenness, with the likelihood of suspension for repeat offenders.

Many colleges ban ads for alcoholic drinks in college newspapers and during broadcasts of college athletic events. Flyers, posters, and other promotions for cheap drinks, such as two-for-one specials, happy hours, all you can drink, and ladies' night, are banned on many campuses. In these college communities, bars and restaurants that cater to students are discouraged from offering patrons cheap alcohol.

SOURCES: Huang, G. C., et al. 2014. Peer influences: The impact of online and offline friendship networks on adolescent smoking and alcohol use. *Journal of Adolescent Health* 54(5): 508–514; Substance Abuse and Mental Health Services Administration. 2019. *Results from the 2018 National Survey on Drug Use and Health: Detailed Tables*. Rockville, MD: Center for Behavioral Health Statistics and Quality, Substance Abuse and Mental Health Services Administration; National Institute on Drug Abuse. 2015. *6 Tactful Tips for Resisting Peer Pressure to Use Drugs and Alcohol* (https://teens.drugabuse.gov/blog/post/6-tactful-tips-resisting-peer-pressure-to-use-drugs-and-alcohol); Studer, J., et al. 2014. Peer pressure and alcohol use in young men: A mediation analysis of drinking motives. *International Journal of Drug Policy* 25(4): 700–708.

originally needed in order to experience the same degree of intoxication.

When people with severe alcohol use disorder stop drinking or sharply decrease their intake, they experience *withdrawal*. Symptoms include trembling hands (shakes or jitters), a rapid pulse and accelerated breathing rate, insomnia, nightmares, anxiety, and GI upset. These symptoms usually begin 5–10 hours after alcohol intake is decreased and improve after four or five days. After a week most people feel much better; but occasionally anxiety, insomnia, and other symptoms persist for six months or more.

More severe withdrawal symptoms occur in about 5% of alcoholics. These include seizures (sometimes called "rum fits"), confusion, and **hallucinations** such as seeing visions or hearing voices. Still less common is **delirium tremens (the DTs)**, a medical emergency characterized by severe disorientation, confusion, epileptic-like seizures, and vivid hallucinations, often of vermin and small animals. The mortality rate from the DTs can be as high as 15%, especially in very debilitated people with preexisting medical illnesses.

Alcoholics face all the physical health risks associated with intoxication and chronic drinking described earlier in the chapter. Some damage is compounded by nutritional deficiencies that often accompany alcoholism. A mental problem associated with alcohol use is profound memory gaps (commonly known as blackouts), which the drinker sometimes tries to cover up by conscious or unconscious lying.

The specific health effects of alcoholism tend to vary from person to person. For example, one person may suffer from problems with memory and CNS defects and have no problems with liver or GI tract. Another person with a similar drinking and nutritional history may develop advanced liver disease but no memory gaps.

Social and Psychological Effects   Alcohol use causes more serious social and psychological problems than all other forms of drug abuse combined. For every person who is an alcoholic, another three or four people are directly affected. More than half of all adults have a family history of alcoholism or problem drinking, and more than 7 million children live in a household where at least one parent is dependent on or has abused alcohol.

People suffering from an alcohol use disorder frequently have mental disorders. They are much more likely to have clinical depression, panic disorder, schizophrenia, borderline personality disorder, or antisocial personality disorder. People with anxiety or panic attacks may try to use alcohol to lessen their anxiety, even though alcohol often intensifies these disorders. Alcohol use disorder often co-occurs with other substance abuse problems as well.

Causes of Alcoholism   The precise causes of severe alcohol use disorder are unknown, but many factors are probably involved. Studies of twins and adopted children clearly demonstrate the importance of genetics. If one of a pair of fraternal twins has severe alcohol use disorder, the other has about twice the normal risk of developing the disorder. For the identical twin of an alcoholic, the risk of alcoholism is about four times that of the general population. These risks persist even when the twins have little contact with each other or their biological parents. Similarly, adoption studies show an increased risk among children of alcoholics, even if they were adopted at birth into nondrinking families. Alcoholism in adoptive parents, by contrast, doesn't make their adopted children more or less likely to become alcoholic. Some studies suggest that as much as 50–60% of a person's risk for alcoholism is determined by genetic factors.

Not all children of alcoholics develop alcohol use disorder, however, and it is clear that other factors are involved. A person's risk of developing alcoholism may be increased by having certain personality disorders, having grown up in a violent or otherwise troubled household, and imitating the alcohol abuse of peers and other role models. People who begin drinking excessively in their teens are especially prone to binge drinking and alcoholism later in life. Common psychological features of individuals who misuse alcohol are denial ("I don't have a problem") and rationalization ("I drink because I need to socialize with my clients"). Certain social factors have also been linked with alcoholism, including urbanization, disappearance of the extended family, a general loosening of kinship ties, increased mobility, and changing values.

Treatment   Some alcoholics recover without professional help. How often this occurs is unknown, but it is estimated that as many as one-third stop drinking on their own or reduce their drinking enough to eliminate problems. Often these spontaneous recoveries are linked to an alcohol-related crisis, such as a blackout or an alcohol-related automobile crash, a health problem (especially one that can be made worse by alcohol use), or the threat of losing one's job. Not all alcoholics must hit bottom before they are motivated to stop. People vary markedly in what induces them to change their behavior.

Most alcoholics, however, require a treatment program of some kind in order to stop drinking. Many different kinds of programs exist. No single treatment works for everyone, so a person may have to try different programs before finding the right one.

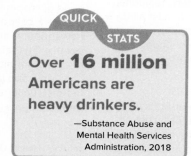

QUICK STATS

Over **16 million** Americans are heavy drinkers.

—Substance Abuse and Mental Health Services Administration, 2018

hallucination   A false perception that does not correspond to external reality, such as seeing visions or hearing voices that are not there.   TERMS

delirium tremens (the DTs)   A state of confusion brought on by the reduction of alcohol intake in an alcohol-dependent person; other symptoms are sweating, trembling, anxiety, hallucinations, and seizures.

Although treatment is not successful for all alcoholics, considerable optimism has replaced the older view that nothing can be done. Many alcoholics have patterns of drinking that fluctuate widely over time. These fluctuations indicate that their alcohol misuse is a response to environmental factors, such as life stressors or social pressures, and therefore may be influenced by treatment.

One of the oldest and best-known recovery programs is Alcoholics Anonymous (AA). In many communities, AA consists of self-help groups that meet several times each week and follow a 12-step program. Important steps for people in these programs include recognizing that they are "powerless over alcohol" and must seek help from a "higher power" to regain control of their lives. By verbalizing these steps, the alcoholic directly addresses the denial that is often prominent in alcoholism and other addictions. Many AA members have a sponsor of their choosing who is available by phone 24 hours a day for individual support and crisis intervention. AA convincingly shows the alcoholic that abstinence can be achieved and also provides a sober peer group of people who share the same identity—that of recovering alcoholics. Many AA members find that this method works best in combination with counseling and medical care.

Other recovery approaches are available. Some, like Rational Recovery and Women for Sobriety, deliberately avoid any emphasis on higher spiritual powers. A more controversial approach to problem drinking is offered by the group Moderation Management, which encourages people to manage their drinking behavior by limiting intake or abstaining.

Al-Anon and Alateen are companion programs to AA for families and friends of alcoholics. In Al-Anon, spouses and others explore how they **enable** the alcoholic to drink by denying, rationalizing, or covering up his or her drinking and how they can change this codependent behavior.

Employee assistance programs and school-based programs represent another approach to alcoholism treatment. These programs can deal directly with work and campus issues, which are often important sources of stress for the alcohol misuser. They encourage effective coping responses for internal and external stressors.

Inpatient hospital rehabilitation is useful for some alcoholics, especially if they have serious medical or mental problems or if life stressors threaten to overwhelm them. When patients return to the community, however, it is critical that there be some form of active, continuing, long-term treatment. Those who return to a spouse or family often need to address issues involving those significant others, and to establish new routines and shared recreational activities that do not involve drinking.

There are also several medical treatments for alcoholism. All of these work best in combination with counseling or other nonpharmacological programs:

- *Disulfiram* (Antabuse) inhibits the metabolic breakdown of acetaldehyde and causes patients to flush and feel ill when they drink, theoretically inhibiting impulse drinking. However, disulfiram is potentially dangerous if the user continues to drink.

- *Naltrexone* (ReVia, Depade) binds to a brain pleasure center that reduces the craving for alcohol and decreases its pleasant, reinforcing effects. When taken correctly, naltrexone usually does not make the user feel ill.

- *Injectable naltrexone* (Vivitrol) acts the same as oral naltrexone, but it is a single monthly shot administered by a health professional. Compliance with a monthly regimen may be better for some alcoholics.

- *Acamprosate* (Campral) helps people maintain abstinence after they have stopped drinking. It is unclear how acamprosate works, but it appears to act on brain pathways related to alcohol abuse.

A variety of other drugs to treat alcoholism are undergoing clinical trials—alone, in combination, or in combination with counseling therapies.

In people who misuse alcohol and have significant depression or anxiety, the use of antidepressant or antianxiety medication can improve both mental health and drinking behavior. In addition, drugs such as diazepam (Valium) are sometimes prescribed to replace alcohol during initial stages of withdrawal. Such chemical substitutes are usually useful for only a week or so because alcoholics are at particularly high risk for developing dependence on other drugs.

Alcohol treatment programs are successful in achieving an extended period of sobriety for about half of those who participate. Success rates of conventional treatment programs are about the same for men and women and for people from different racial and ethnic groups. Women, minorities, and the poor often face major economic and social barriers to receiving treatment. Most inpatient treatment programs are financially out of reach for people with low income or those without insurance coverage. AA remains the mainstay of treatment for most people and is often a component of even the most expensive treatment programs. Special AA groups exist in many communities for young people, women, gay men and lesbians, non–English speakers, and a variety of interest groups.

Gender and Ethnic Differences

People who misuse alcohol come from all socioeconomic levels and cultural groups, but notable differences appear in drinking patterns between men and women and among different racial and ethnic groups (Table 11.2).

Men Men are more likely than women to drink alcohol, to misuse alcohol, and to develop an alcohol use disorder. Among white American men, excessive drinking often begins in the teens or twenties and progresses gradually through the thirties until the man is clearly identifiable as an alcoholic by

enable Provide misguided support or the means that facilitates self-destructive behavior of another person with substance-abuse issues.

TERMS

Table 11.2 — Alcohol Use and Binge Alcohol Use by Sex and Race/Ethnicity in 2018, Aged 12 and Over

	PAST MONTH PREVALENCE (PERCENTAGE OF TOTAL POPULATION)	
	ALCOHOL USE	BINGE ALCOHOL USE
Gender		
Male	54.5	28.5
Female	47.9	20.7
Race and Ethnicity		
Not Hispanic or Latino	53.0	24.5
White	56.7	25.7
Black or African American	43.0	23.0
American Indian and Alaska Native	35.9	22.4
Native Hawaiian/Pacific Islander	35.4	24.4
Asian American	39.3	14.7
Two or more races	46.0	23.3
Hispanic or Latino	41.7	24.6
Total Population	**51.1**	**24.5**

SOURCE: Center for Behavioral Health Statistics and Quality. 2019. *2018 National Survey on Drug Use and Health: Detailed Tables*. SAMHSA, Rockville, MD.

the time he is in his late thirties or early forties. Other men may remain controlled drinkers until later in life, sometimes becoming alcoholic in association with retirement, the loss of friends and loved ones, boredom, illness, or psychological disorders.

Men account for the majority of alcohol-related deaths and injuries in the United States, the greatest proportion occurring in men age 35 and under. Most alcohol-related deaths and injuries among men result from motor vehicle crashes, falls, drowning, suicide, and homicide.

Various factors contribute to men's higher rates of alcohol use and abuse. The pressure of traditional or stereotypical gender roles and ideas regarding masculinity and drinking behavior may promote excessive alcohol consumption among men. Young men in particular are also more likely to engage in all types of risky health behaviors. Men drive more miles, drive more dangerously, and are more likely to drive while intoxicated. They tend to have greater access to firearms, contributing to their increased rates of suicide and homicide. Men may also be more likely than women to use alcohol to cope with stress and other life challenges.

Women Because of differences in body chemistry—for example, hormones and enzymes—women become intoxicated at lower doses of alcohol than men, and they tend to experience adverse physical effects of chronic drinking sooner and at lower levels of alcohol consumption. Their progression of drinking alcohol usually differs from men's: Women tend to become alcoholic at later ages and with fewer years of heavy drinking. It is not unusual for women in their forties or fifties to succumb to alcoholism after years of controlled drinking.

Rates of alcohol abuse and dependence among women have increased in the past decade. Alcoholic women develop cirrhosis and other medical complications more often and after a shorter period of heavier drinking than men, and have higher death rates—including deaths from cirrhosis—than male alcoholics. Some alcohol-related health issues are unique to women, including increased risk of breast cancer and menstrual disorders, and exposing a fetus to alcohol during pregnancy. Women are more vulnerable to the anticlotting effects of alcohol, which can raise the risk of bleeding strokes. Female alcoholics are less likely to seek early treatment for drinking problems, possibly because of the social stigma attached to problem drinking. Women from all walks of life and all racial and ethnic groups can develop alcohol problems, but those who have never married or are divorced are more likely to drink heavily than married or widowed women. Women who have multiple life roles, such as parent, worker, and spouse, are less vulnerable to alcohol problems than women who have fewer socially connecting roles.

African Americans As a group, African Americans use less alcohol than the average for American adults, but they face disproportionately high levels of alcohol-related birth defects, cirrhosis, cancer, hypertension, and other medical problems. In addition, African Americans are more likely than members of other racial or ethnic groups to be victims of alcohol-related homicides, criminal assaults, and injuries. African American women are more likely to abstain from alcohol use than white women, but among black women who drink there is a higher percentage of heavy drinkers. Urban black males commonly start drinking excessively and develop serious neurological illnesses at an earlier age than urban white males. They also have a higher rate of alcoholism-related suicide.

AA groups of predominantly African Americans are effective, perhaps because essential elements of AA—sharing common experiences, mutual acceptance of one another as human beings, and trusting a higher power—are already a part of many African American practices. Treatments that use the extended family and occupational training can also be effective.

Latinos Drinking patterns among Latinos vary significantly, depending on their specific cultural background and level of acculturation. Drunk driving and cirrhosis are the most common causes of alcohol-related death and injury among Hispanic men. Hispanic women are more likely to abstain from alcohol than white or black women, but those who drink are at special risk for problems. Treating the entire family as a unit is an important part of treatment because family pride, solidarity, and support are important aspects of Latino culture. Some Hispanics may do better if treatment efforts integrate spirituality, and traditional cultural values.

Asian Americans   As a group, Asian Americans have lower-than-average rates of alcohol misuse. However, acculturation may somewhat weaken the generally strong Asian taboos and community sanctions against alcohol use. Asian American men consume much more alcohol than do Asian American women (60% versus 39%). For many Asian Americans, though, the genetically based physiological aversion to alcohol remains a deterrent to misuse. Ethnic agencies, health care professionals, and ministers seem to be the most effective sources of treatment for members of this group, when needed. That alcohol may interact with hepatitis B virus is of special concern because Asian Americans have a higher prevalence of this hepatitis infection.

American Indians and Alaska Natives   As a group, American Indians and Alaska Natives have a relatively low rate of drinking overall (more abstainers) and a rate of binge drinking that is similar to the overall population rate. However, alcohol use disorder is significantly more prevalent among Native Americans than among other groups, as is the death rate from alcohol-related causes such as motor vehicle crashes. Socioeconomic disadvantage can be a barrier to adequate health care. Treatment may be more effective if it reflects tribal values.

Helping Someone with an Alcohol Problem

Helping a friend or relative with an alcohol problem requires skill and tact. Start by making sure you are not enabling someone to continue excessive use of alcohol. Enabling takes many forms, such as making excuses for the alcohol misuser—for example, saying "he has the flu" when it is really a hangover.

Another important step is open, honest labeling—"I think you have a problem with alcohol." Such explicit statements usually elicit emotional rebuttals and may endanger a relationship. However, you are not helping your friends by allowing them to deny their problems with alcohol or other drugs. Taking action shows that you care.

Even when problems are acknowledged, there is usually reluctance to get help—it takes hard work. You can't cure a friend's drinking problem, but you can guide him or her to

QUICK STATS

49% of American adults report not drinking alcohol in the past month.

—SAMHSA
2018 National Survey on Drug Use and Health

appropriate help. Your best role might be to obtain information about the available resources and persistently encourage their use. Consider making an appointment for your friend at the student health center and then go with him or her to the appointment. Most student health centers will be able to recommend local options for self-help groups and formal treatment; the counseling center is another excellent source for help. You can also check the phone book and the Internet for local chapters of AA and other groups (see For More Information at the end of the chapter). And don't underestimate the power of families to help. An honest phone call to your friend's parents could save a life if your friend is in serious trouble with alcohol.

DRINKING BEHAVIOR AND RESPONSIBILITY

Responsible use of alcohol means keeping your BAC low so that your behavior is always under your control. In addition to controlling your own drinking, you can promote responsible alcohol use in others.

Examine Your Drinking Behavior

When you want to drink responsibly, it's helpful to know, first of all, why you drink. The following are common reasons given by college students:

- "It lets me go along with my friends."
- "It makes me less self-conscious and more social."
- "It makes me less inhibited."
- "It relieves depression, anxiety, tension, or worries."
- "It enables me to experience a different state of consciousness."

If you drink alcohol, what are your reasons for doing so?

After examining your reasons for drinking, take a closer look at your drinking behavior. Is it moderate and responsible? Or do you overindulge and suffer negative consequences? The *CAGE* screening test can help you determine whether you, or someone close to you, may have a drinking problem. Answer yes or no to the following questions:

Have you ever felt you should . . .
   Cut down on your drinking?
Have people . . .
   Annoyed you by criticizing your drinking?
Have you ever felt bad or . . .
   Guilty about your drinking?
Have you ever had an . . .
   Eye-opener (a drink first thing in the morning to steady your nerves or get rid of a hangover)?

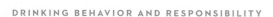

The Alcohol Use Disorders Identification Test (AUDIT) is a screening tool for problem drinking. It can also be used for self-assessment. For each question, choose the answer that best describes your behavior. Then total your scores.

Questions	POINTS					YOUR SCORE
	0	1	2	3	4	
1. How often do you have a drink containing alcohol?	Never	Monthly or less	2–4 times a month	2–3 times a week	4 or more times a week	_____
2. How many drinks containing alcohol do you have on a typical day when you are drinking?	1 or 2	3 or 4	5 or 6	7–9	10 or more	_____
3. How often do you have five or more drinks on one occasion?	Never	Less than monthly	Monthly	Weekly	Daily or almost daily	_____
4. How often during the past year have you found that you were not able to stop drinking once you had started?	Never	Less than monthly	Monthly	Weekly	Daily or almost daily	_____
5. How often during the past year have you failed to do what was normally expected because of drinking?	Never	Less than monthly	Monthly	Weekly	Daily or almost daily	_____
6. How often during the past year have you needed a first drink in the morning to get yourself going after a heavy drinking session?	Never	Less than monthly	Monthly	Weekly	Daily or almost daily	_____
7. How often during the past year have you had a feeling of guilt or remorse after drinking?	Never	Less than monthly	Monthly	Weekly	Daily or almost daily	_____
8. How often during the past year have you been unable to remember what happened the night before because you had been drinking?	Never	Less than monthly	Monthly	Weekly	Daily or almost daily	_____
9. Have you or has someone else been injured as a result of your drinking?	No		Yes, but not in the past year (2 points)	Yes, during the past year (4 points)		_____
10. Has a relative, friend, doctor, or other health worker been concerned about your drinking or suggested you cut down?	No		Yes, but not in the past year (2 points)	Yes, during the past year (4 points)		_____
					Total	_____

A total score of 8 or more indicates a strong likelihood of hazardous or harmful alcohol consumption. Even if you score below 8, if you are encountering drinking-related problems with your academic performance, job, relationships, health, or the law, you should consider seeking help.

SOURCE: Saunders, J. B., et al. 1993. Development of the Alcohol Use Disorders Identification Test (AUDIT): WHO Collaborative Project on Early Detection of Persons with Harmful Alcohol Consumption. Box 4, page 17.

One yes response suggests a possible alcohol problem; if you answered yes to more than one question, it is highly likely that a problem exists. For a more detailed evaluation of your drinking habits, complete the *AUDIT* questionnaire in the box "Do You Have a Problem with Alcohol?" If the results of either assessment test indicate a potential problem, get help right away.

Drink Moderately and Responsibly

Sometimes people lose control when they misjudge how much they drink. At other times, they set out deliberately to get drunk. Following are some strategies for keeping your drinking and your behavior under control.

• **Drink slowly.** Sip your drinks instead of gulping them. If you are actually thirsty, use nonalcoholic beverages to quench your thirst. Avoid drinks made with carbonated mixers, especially if you're thirsty; you'll be more likely to gulp them down.

• **Space your drinks.** Drink nonalcoholic drinks at parties, or alternate them with alcoholic drinks. Learn to refuse a round: "I've had enough for right now." Parties are easier for some people if they hold a glass of something nonalco-

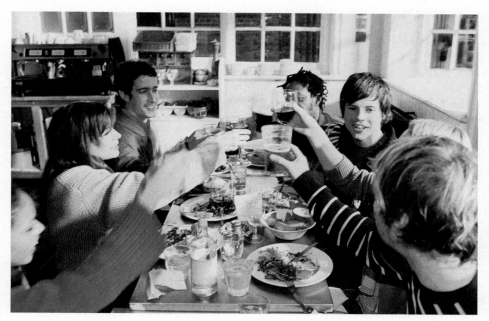

Eating food while you are drinking will slow the rate of alcohol absorption and lower your peak BAC.
Digital Vision/Getty Images

holic that has ice and a twist of lime floating in it so that it looks like an alcoholic drink.

• *Eat before and while drinking.* Avoid drinking on an empty stomach. Food in your stomach will not prevent alcohol from eventually being absorbed, but it will slow down the rate somewhat and lower the peak BAC. In restaurants, order your food before you order a drink. Try to have something to eat before you go to a party where alcohol will be served.

• *Know your limits and your drinks.* Review the BAC chart in Figure 11.2 or try one of the many apps or websites that provide estimates of BAC. You can learn how different BACs affect you by seeing how you respond to a set amount—say one or two drinks in an hour. (Try this experiment only in a safe setting and only if drinking is legal for you.) A good test is walking heel to toe in a straight line with your eyes closed or standing with your feet crossed and trying to touch your finger to your nose with your eyes closed.

Be aware that in different settings your performance, and especially your ability to judge your behavior, may change. At a given BAC, you will perform less well when surrounded by activity and boisterous companions than you will in a quiet test setting with just one or two other people. This impairment results partially because alcohol reduces your ability to perform when your brain is bombarded by multiple stimuli.

Promote Responsible Drinking

Although you cannot control the drinking behavior of others, you can promote responsible drinking.

Encourage Responsible Attitudes   Our society teaches us attitudes toward drinking that contribute to alcohol-related

problems. Many of us have difficulty expressing disapproval about someone who has had too much to drink, and we are amused by the antics of a funny drunk. We accept the alcohol industry's linkage of drinking with virility or sexuality (see the box "Alcohol Advertising"). And many people treat nondrinkers as nonconformists in social settings. Recognize that the choice to abstain is neither odd nor unusual. More than one-third of adults do not drink at all or drink only infrequently. Most people are capable of enjoying their leisure time without alcohol or drugs.

Be a Responsible Host   When you are the host, serve nonalcoholic beverages as well as alcohol. Have only enough alcohol on hand for each guest to have a moderate amount. Don't put out large kegs of beer because these invite people to overindulge. For parties hosted by a dorm, fraternity, or other campus group, don't allow guests to have unlimited drinks for a single admission fee because this also encourages binge drinking.

Always serve food along with alcohol, and stop serving alcohol an hour or more before people will leave. If possible, arrange carpools with designated nondrinking drivers in advance. Remind your guests who are under 21 about the zero-tolerance laws in many states—even a single drink can result in an illegal BAC. Insist that guests who drink too much take a rideshare or taxi, ride with someone else, or stay overnight rather than drive.

Plan social functions with no alcohol at all. Outdoor parties, hikes, and practically every other type of social occasion can be enjoyable without alcohol. If that doesn't seem possible to you, then examine your drinking patterns and attitudes toward alcohol. If you can't have fun without drinking, you may have a problem with alcohol.

Hold the Drinker Responsible   Anyone who consumes alcohol must take full responsibility for his or her behavior. Pardoning unacceptable behavior fosters the attitude that the behavior is caused by the drug. The drinker is thereby excused from responsibility and learns to expect minimal adverse consequences for bad behavior. The opposite approach—holding the individual fully accountable—is a more effective policy. For example, alcohol-impaired drivers who receive strict penalties have fewer subsequent rearrests than those who receive only mandatory treatment. Other people's drunkenness can impinge on your living or study environment. Speak up against this behavior—and insist on your rights.

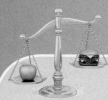

CRITICAL CONSUMER
Alcohol Advertising

Alcohol manufacturers spend $6 billion every year on advertising and promotions. They claim that the purpose is to persuade adults who already drink to choose a certain brand. But in reality, ads appeal far more broadly and subconsciously: They cleverly engage young people and children by clearly linking alcohol and good times.

Alcohol ads are common during sporting events and other shows popular with teenagers. Studies show that the more television adolescents watch, the more likely they are to take up drinking in their teens. New alcoholic drinks geared to the tastes of young people are heavily promoted. "Hard lemonade" and other drinks ("alcopops") have been described by teens as a way to get drunk without experiencing a bitter taste. Almost half of 14- to 18-year-olds report having tried them.

Alcohol manufacturers also reach out to young people at activities like concerts and sporting events. Product logos are heavily marketed through sales of T-shirts, hats, and other items. Many colleges allow alcohol manufacturers to advertise at campus events in exchange for sponsorship.

Many ads give the impression that drinking alcohol is a normal part of everyday life and good times. This message seems to work, as many young people believe that heavy drinking at parties is normal and fun. The use of famous musicians, athletes, or actors in commercials increases the appeal of alcohol by associating it with fame, wealth, sex, and popularity.

What ads don't show is the darker side of drinking. You never see hangovers, car crashes, slipping grades, or violence. Although some ads include a brief message such as "drink responsibly," the impact of such cautions is small compared to that of the image of happy, attractive young people having fun while drinking.

The next time you see an advertisement for alcohol, look critically and be aware of its effect on you.

Take Community Action Consider joining an action group such as Students Against Destructive Decisions (SADD). Through lesson plans, peer counseling, and the promotion of better communication between students and parents, SADD helps students avoid the dangers of drinking, drug use, impaired driving, and other destructive choices.

TIPS FOR TODAY AND THE FUTURE

The responsible use of alcohol means drinking in moderation or not at all.

RIGHT NOW YOU CAN:

- Consider whether there is a history of alcohol abuse or dependence in your family.
- Think about your current drinking habits. For example, count the number of parties you attended in the past month and how many drinks you had at each one.
- Take stock of the number of alcoholic beverages in your home. Does there always seem to be a lot on hand? Do you find yourself purchasing alcohol frequently? What do your purchasing habits say about your drinking?

IN THE FUTURE YOU CAN:

- Think about the next party you plan to attend. Decide how much you will drink at the party, and how you will get home afterward.
- Watch your friends' behavior at events where drinking is involved. Do any of them show signs of a drinking problem? If so, consider what you can do to help.

SUMMARY

- Although alcohol has long been a part of human celebrations, it is a psychoactive drug capable of causing addiction.

- After being absorbed into the bloodstream, alcohol is transported throughout the body. The liver metabolizes alcohol as blood circulates through it.

- If people drink more alcohol each hour than the body can metabolize, blood alcohol concentration (BAC) increases. The rate of alcohol metabolism depends on a variety of individual factors.

- Alcohol is a CNS depressant. At low doses, it tends to make people feel relaxed.

- At higher doses, alcohol interferes with motor and mental functioning; at very high doses, alcohol poisoning, coma, and death can occur. Effects may be increased if alcohol is combined with other drugs.

- Alcohol use increases the risk of injury and violence; drinking before driving is particularly dangerous, even at low doses.

- Chronic alcohol use has negative effects on the digestive and cardiovascular systems and increases cancer risk and overall mortality.

- Pregnant women who drink risk giving birth to children with a cluster of birth defects known as fetal alcohol syndrome (FAS). Even occasional drinking during pregnancy can cause brain injury in the fetus.

- Alcohol misuse involves drinking in dangerous situations or drinking to a degree that causes academic, professional, interpersonal, or legal difficulties.

- Alcoholism is characterized by more extensive problems with alcohol, usually involving tolerance and withdrawal.

- Binge drinking is a common form of misusing alcohol that negatively affects both drinkers and nondrinkers. For numerous reasons, college students may be especially prone to binge drinking.

- Physical consequences of alcoholism include the direct effects of tolerance and withdrawal, as well as all the problems associated with chronic drinking. Psychological problems associated with alcoholism include memory loss and additional mental disorders such as depression.

- Alcoholism treatment includes mutual support groups like AA, job- and school-based programs, inpatient hospital programs, and pharmacological treatments.

- Helping someone who misuses alcohol means not enabling them and finding useful information about available resources, e.g., treatment programs and support groups, and persistently encouraging their use.

- Strategies for controlling drinking include examining attitudes about drinking and drinking behavior, drinking slowly, spacing drinks, eating before and while drinking, and knowing one's limits.

- Strategies for promoting responsible drinking in others include encouraging responsible attitudes, being a responsible host, holding the drinker responsible for his or her actions, learning about prevention programs, and taking community action.

FOR MORE INFORMATION

Al-Anon Family Group Headquarters. Provides information and referrals to local Al-Anon and Alateen groups. The website includes a self-quiz to determine if you are affected by someone's drinking.

http://www.al-anon.alateen.org

Alcoholics Anonymous (AA) World Services. Provides general information about AA, literature about alcoholism, and information about AA meetings and related 12-step organizations.

http://www.aa.org

AlcoholScreening.Org. Provides information about alcohol and health, referrals for treatment and support groups, and a drinking self-assessment.

http://www.alcoholscreening.org

Alcohol Treatment Referral Hotline. Provides referrals to local intervention and treatment providers.

800-ALCOHOL

College Drinking: Changing the Culture. Created by the National Institute on Alcohol Abuse and Alcoholism (NIAAA), this site gives comprehensive research-based information on issues related to alcohol abuse and binge drinking among college students.

http://www.collegedrinkingprevention.gov

Mothers Against Drunk Driving (MADD). Supports efforts to develop solutions to the problems of drunk driving and underage drinking and provides news, information, and brochures about many topics, including a guide for giving a safe party.

http://www.madd.org

National Association for Children of Addiction (NACoA). Provides information and support for children of alcoholics.

http://www.nacoa.org

National Council on Alcoholism and Drug Dependence (NCADD). Provides information and counseling referrals. Website URLs depend on your state and local chapter.

800-NCA-CALL (24-hour Hope Line)

National Institute on Alcohol Abuse and Alcoholism (NIAAA). Provides booklets and other publications on a variety of alcohol-related topics, including fetal alcohol syndrome, alcoholism treatment, and alcohol use and minorities.

http://www.niaaa.nih.gov

Substance Abuse and Mental Health Services Administration. Provides statistics and information about alcohol abuse, including resources for people who want to help friends and family members overcome alcohol abuse problems.

http://www.samhsa.gov

See also the listings for Chapter 10.

SELECTED BIBLIOGRAPHY

Addolorato, G., et al. 2006. Baclofen: A new drug for the treatment of alcohol dependence. *International Journal of Clinical Practice* 60(8): 1003–1008.

American Heart Association. 2015. The downside to alcohol: Moderate drinking in later years may damage heart. *Heart Insight* (http://heartinsight.heart.org/Fall-2015/The-Downside-to-Alcohol/).

American Psychiatric Association. 2013. *Diagnostic and Statistical Manual of Mental Disorders,* 5th ed. *(DSM-5).* Washington, DC: American Psychiatric Publishing.

Anton, R. F., et al. 2006. Combined pharmacotherapies and behavioral interventions for alcohol dependence: The COMBINE study: A randomized controlled trial. *Journal of the American Medical Association* 295(17): 2003–2017.

Cao, Y., et al. 2015. Light to moderate intake of alcohol, drinking patterns, and risk of cancer: Results from two prospective US cohort studies. *British Medical Journal* 351: h4238.

Centers for Disease Control and Prevention. 2019. *Alcohol and Public Health: Fact Sheets—Binge Drinking* (http://www.cdc.gov/alcohol/fact-sheets/binge-drinking.htm).

Centers for Disease Control and Prevention. 2017. *Alcohol-Attributable Deaths Due to Excessive Alcohol Use* (https://chronicdata.cdc.gov/browse?category=alcohol-related+disease+impact).

Centers for Disease Control and Prevention. 2020. *Fetal Alcohol Spectrum Disorders (FASD)* (https://www.cdc.gov/ncbddd/fasd/index.html).

College Drinking Prevention. 2017. *A Snapshot of Annual High-Risk College Drinking Consequences* (http://www.collegedrinkingprevention.gov/StatsSummaries/snapshot.aspx).

Collins, G. B., et al. 2006. Drug adjuncts for treating alcohol dependence. *Cleveland Clinic Journal of Medicine* 73(7): 641–644.

Costello, R. M. 2006. Long-term mortality from alcoholism: A descriptive analysis. *Journal of Studies on Alcohol and Drugs* 67(5): 694–699.

Cunningham, J. K., T. A. Solomon, and M. L. Muramoto. 2016. Alcohol use among Native Americans compared to whites: Examining the veracity of the 'Native American elevated alcohol consumption' belief. *Drug and Alcohol Dependence* 160: 65–75.

Darvishi, N., et al. 2015. Alcohol-related risk of suicidal ideation, suicide attempt, and completed suicide: A meta-analysis. *PLOS ONE* e0126870.

Daube, M. 2015. Alcohol's evaporating health benefits. *British Medical Journal* 350: h407.

Dawson, D. A., et al. 2005. Recovery from DSM-IV alcohol dependence: United States, 2001–2002. *Addiction* 100(3): 281–292.

Gonçalves, A., et al. 2015. Relationship between alcohol consumption and cardiac structure and function in the elderly: The Atherosclerosis Risk in Communities Study. *Circulation: Cardiovascular Imaging* 8(6): e002846.

Gruenewald, P. J., and L. Remer. 2006. Changes in outlet densities affect violence rates. *Alcoholism: Clinical and Experimental Research* 30(7): 1184–1193.

Hagström, H., et al. 2018. Alcohol consumption in late adolescence is associated with an increased risk of severe liver disease later in life. *Journal of Hepatology* 68(3): 505–510.

Heilig, M., and M. Egli. 2006. Pharmacological treatment of alcohol dependence: Target symptoms and target mechanisms. *Pharmacology & Therapeutics* 111(3): 855–876.

Kane, J. C., et al. 2016. Differences in alcohol use patterns between adolescent Asian American ethnic groups: Representative estimates from the National Survey on Drug Use and Health 2002–2013. *Addictive Behaviors* 64: 154–158.

Klarich, D. S., Brasser, S. M., and M. Y. Hong. 2015. Moderate alcohol consumption and colorectal cancer risk. *Alcoholism: Clinical and Experimental Research* 398(8): 1280–1291.

Kwok, A., A. L. Aimee, and G. Paton. 2019. Effect of alcohol consumption on food energy intake: A systematic review and meta-analysis. *British Journal of Nutrition* 121(5): 481–495.

Lipari, R. N., and B. Jean-Francois. 2016. *A Day in the Life of College Students Aged 18 to 22: Substance Use Facts.* Rockville, MD: Center for Behavioral Health Statistics and Quality, Substance Abuse and Mental Health Services Administration.

Mallett, K. A., et al. 2013. An update of research examining college student alcohol-related consequences: New perspectives and implications for interventions. *Alcoholism: Clinical and Experimental Research* 37(5): 709–716.

Naimi, T. S. 2019. A fresh approach to the development of national alcohol guidelines. *Addiction* 114(4): 601–602.

National Center for Health Statistics. 2010. *National Hospital Ambulatory Medical Care Survey: 2007 Emergency Department Summary* (*National Health Statistics Reports* 26). Hyattsville, MD: National Center for Health Statistics.

National Highway Traffic Safety Administration. 2019. *Traffic Safety Facts. 2018 Fatal Motor Vehicle Crashes: Overview.* Washington, DC: National Highway Traffic Safety Administration, DOT HS. 812–826.

National Institute on Alcohol Abuse and Alcoholism. 2020. Alcohol Facts and Statistics (https://www.niaaa.nih.gov/publications/brochures-and-fact-sheets/alcohol-facts-and-statistics).

Navasa, J. F.,et al. 2019. Sex differences in the association between impulsivity and driving under the influence of alcohol in young adults: The specific role of sensation seeking. *Accident Analysis & Prevention* 124:174–179.

Painter, K. 2015. Alcohol good for your heart? Evidence is evaporating. *USA Today,* February 15 (http://www.usatoday.com/story/news/2015/02/15/alcohol-heart-cardiovascular-health/23109823/).

Parker-Pope, T. 2012. *America's drinking binge. New York Times,* January 11 (http://well.blogs.nytimes.com/2012/01/11/americas-drinking-binge).

Penn State. 2012. Early intervention may curb dangerous college drinking. *Science Daily* (http://www.sciencedaily.com/releases/2012/01/120130131204.htm).

Sacks, J., et al. 2015. 2010 national and state costs of excessive alcohol consumption. *American Journal of Preventive Medicine* 49(5): e73–e79.

Substance Abuse and Mental Health Services Administration. 2012. *Nearly Half of College Student Treatment Admissions Were for Primary Alcohol Abuse* (http://www.samhsa.gov/data/spotlight/Spotlight054College2012.pdf).

Substance Abuse and Mental Health Services Administration. 2015. *Behavioral Health Trends in the United States: Results from the 2014 National Survey on Drug Use and Health* (HHS Publication No. SMA 15-4927, NSDUH Series H-41). Rockville, MD: Substance Abuse and Mental Health Services Administration.

Substance Abuse and Mental Health Services Administration Center for Behavioral Health Statistics and Quality. 2019. *Results from the 2018 National Survey on Drug Use and Health* (https://www.samhsa.gov/data/sites/default/files/cbhsq-reports/NSDUHNationalFindingsReport2018/NSDUHNationalFindingsReport2018.pdf).

Svanberg, J., et al., eds. 2014. *Alcohol and the Adult Brain.* London: Taylor and Francis.

Torre, L. A., et al. 2016. Cancer statistics for Asian Americans, Native Hawaiians, and Pacific Islanders, 2016: Converging incidence in males and females. *CA: A Cancer Journal for Clinicians* 66(3): 182–202.

U.S. Department of Health and Human Services. 2007. *The Surgeon General's Call to Action to Prevent and Reduce Underage Drinking.* Washington, DC: Department of Health and Human Services, Office of the Surgeon General.

Vander Ven, T. 2011. *Getting Wasted: Why College Students Drink Too Much and Party So Hard.* New York: NYU Press.

Williams, J. F., and V. C. Smith, the Committee on Substance Abuse. 2015. Fetal alcohol spectrum disorders. *American Academy of Pediatrics* 136(5): e1395–e1406.

World Health Organization. 2020. Alcohol does not protect against COVID-19; access should be restricted during lockdown (http://www.euro.who.int/en/health-topics/disease-prevention/alcohol-use/news/news/2020/04/alcohol-does-not-protect-against-covid-19-access-should-be-restricted-during-lockdown).

Zhao, J., et al. 2017. Alcohol consumption and mortality from coronary heart disease: An updated meta-analysis of cohort studies. *Journal of Studies on Alcohol and Drugs* 78: 375–386.

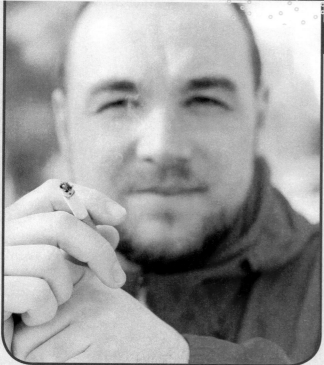

Fredrikke Wetherilt/Alamy Stock Photo

- Explain the demographic patterns related to tobacco use
- List the reasons why people use tobacco, including electronic cigarettes
- Explain the health hazards associated with tobacco use, whether smoked, chewed, or vaped
- Discuss the effects of smoking on nonsmokers
- List social and legislative actions that can be taken to combat smoking and vaping
- Explain strategies that help people stop using tobacco

CHAPTER **12**

Tobacco Use

TEST YOUR KNOWLEDGE

1. **"Light" or low-tar cigarettes are safer than regular cigarettes.**
   True or False?

2. **Which of the following substances are found in tobacco smoke?**
   a. Acetone (nail polish remover)
   b. Ammonia (cleaner)
   c. Hexamine (lighter fluid)
   d. Toluene (industrial solvent)

3. **Every day more than 3000 Americans start smoking.**
   True or False?

4. **Cigarette smoking increases the risk for which of the following conditions?**
   a. Facial wrinkling
   b. Miscarriage
   c. Impotence

5. **A person who quits smoking now will reduce his or her risk of lung cancer within 10 years.**
   True or False?

ANSWERS

1. **FALSE.** Smokers who choose "light" or low-tar cigarettes do not reduce tar intake or smoking-related disease risks, nor is there any evidence that switching to "light" cigarettes helps smokers quit.

2. **ALL FOUR.** Tobacco contains thousands of chemical substances, including many that are poisonous or linked to the development of cancer.

3. **TRUE.** Each day, nearly 3200 Americans under the age of 18 smoke their first cigarette.

4. **ALL THREE.** Cigarette smoking reduces the quality of life and is the leading preventable cause of death in the United States.

5. **TRUE.** The lung cancer rate of a former smoker is half that of a continuing smoker within 10 years of quitting.

Cigarette smoking is still the leading cause of preventable disease, disability, and death in the United States. Despite a significant drop in numbers of smokers since the 1960s, when the first U.S. Surgeon General's report came out, a sizeable 34 million adults in the United States still smoke. And there are close to 59 million people ages 12 and over who use any tobacco product. The 2020 Surgeon General's report discusses the continued diversification of the tobacco product landscape: Because of the increasing availability and use of products such as electronic cigarettes, efforts to raise awareness of devastation from tobacco-related disease and death need to be vigorously renewed. Vaping has become an insidious inducement for young people.

Estimates from the Centers for Disease Control and Prevention (CDC) show that more than 480,000 Americans—nonsmokers as well as smokers—die prematurely from tobacco-related causes every year (Figure 12.1). That's nearly *half a million* Americans who are dying from tobacco-related illnesses every year.

On average, smokers live about 10 years less than nonsmokers. But nonsmokers, especially the children of parents who smoke, also suffer the effects of tobacco smoke. Exposure to secondhand, also called environmental, tobacco smoke kills approximately 41,000 nonsmokers every year, including 400 infants.

This chapter discusses the reasons why people use tobacco, the negative impacts of smoking, and the measures being taken to stop this public health threat.

WHO USES TOBACCO?

Rates of tobacco use vary based on gender, age, race and ethnicity, and education level (Figure 12.2). According to the CDC National Health Interview Survey, 14% of Americans aged 18 and over were cigarette smokers in 2018. About 26% of men and 14% of women reported that they currently used any tobacco product. Adults with a twelfth-grade education or less were much more likely to smoke cigarettes than were those who went on to earn a college degree. Other groups with higher-than-average smoking rates include those who live below the poverty level, those without health insurance (or insured through Medicaid), those who have a physical disability or psychological disorder, those living in the Midwest or South, and LGBT people.

The number of people in the United States who smoke cigarettes (every day or some days) has been decreasing overall, however, with about a 66% decline since 1965. In fact, cigarette smoking is at an all-time low. The largest decrease has been in young adults (aged 18–24), with a 68% decrease from 2005 to 2018. Their use of e-cigarettes, however, increased to 8% of the young adult population.

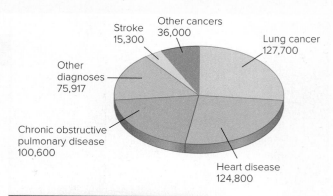

VITAL STATISTICS

FIGURE 12.1 **Estimated annual mortality among cigarette smokers directly attributable to smoking.**
Note: Data based on final death data from 2005 to 2009.

SOURCE: U.S. Department of Health and Human Services. 2014. *The Health Consequences of Smoking—50 Years of Progress: A Report of the Surgeon General.* Atlanta: U.S. Department of Health and Human Services, Centers for Disease Control and Prevention, National Center for Chronic Disease Prevention and Health Promotion, Office on Smoking and Health.

Young People and Alternative Tobacco Products

Young adults use fewer cigarettes and cigars but more e-cigarettes than other adults. Although cigarette smoking has declined over the past two decades, the number of "occasional" and "very light" smokers has increased, as has the use of alternative tobacco products. Occasional smoking is that which occurs some days but not every day, and very light smoking indicates five or fewer cigarettes per day.

Regulations passed in 2010 made it a federal crime to sell tobacco products to anyone under 18 years of age. Even so, minors smoke an estimated 800 million packs of cigarettes each year; more than half of these cigarettes are purchased at retail stores. According to the 2019 Monitoring the Future survey, among twelfth graders, 6% smoked cigarettes, 26% vaped nicotine, and 14% vaped marijuana in the past month. (See the discussion of e-cigarettes later in the chapter.)

College students, who make up 40% of young adults, often fit the "very light smoker" category, and most of those very light smokers use at least one type of alternative tobacco product. Advertisements may claim these products have lower health risks, but many pose considerable danger. These products also do not help very light smokers reduce their tobacco use.

Gender and Smoking

American men are currently more likely than women to use any tobacco product, including cigarettes and e-cigarettes, but women younger than age 23 are becoming

QUICK STATS

About **12.5%** of middle and **31%** of high school students used some type of tobacco product in 2019.

—Centers for Disease Control and Prevention, 2019

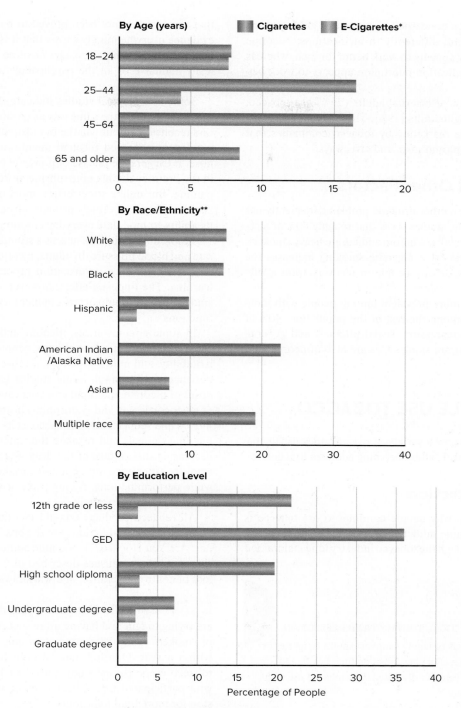

By Age (years) ◼ Cigarettes ◼ E-Cigarettes*

By Race/Ethnicity**

By Education Level

Percentage of People

FIGURE 12.2 Who is smoking and who is vaping? Among U.S. adults in 2018, almost 20% were currently using any tobacco product. However, smoking and vaping rates vary significantly by age, race/ethnicity, and education level.

*Missing e-cigarette bars indicate no data available

**Unless noted, all racial/ethnic groups are non-Hispanic; Hispanics can be of any race.

SOURCE: Centers for Disease Control and Prevention. 2019. Tobacco product use and cessation indicators among adults—United States, 2018. *Morbidity and Mortality Weekly Report* 68(45): 1013–1019.

smokers at a faster rate than any other population segment. When women decide to try to stop smoking, they are more likely than men to join a support group. Overall, though, women are less successful than men in quitting. Women report more severe withdrawal symptoms when they stop

smoking and are more likely than men to report cravings in response to social and behavioral cues associated with smoking.

For men, relapse to smoking is often associated with work or social pressure; women are more likely to relapse when sad or depressed or when concerned about weight gain. Women and men also respond differently to medications: Nicotine replacement therapy appears to work better for men, whereas the non-nicotine medication bupropion appears to work better for women.

More lesbian, gay, or bisexual adults (29%) use tobacco, compared with straight adults (19%). These higher rates may be due to aggressive marketing by tobacco companies that sponsor events, bar promotions, and giveaways.

Tobacco and Other Factors

Men and women with other drug-use problems frequently use tobacco. For example, studies show that roughly 80% of alcoholics and more than 90% of heroin addicts are heavy smokers. New research suggests that cigarette smoking increases the likelihood of relapse among people in recovery from a substance use disorder.

Smoking also is more prevalent among people with mental disorders than among the rest of the population: 40% of people with major depression, social phobias, and generalized anxiety disorder are smokers, as are 80% of people with schizophrenia.

WHY PEOPLE USE TOBACCO

People start smoking for a variety of reasons; they usually become long-term smokers after becoming addicted to nicotine.

Nicotine Addiction

The primary reason why people continue to use **tobacco** is that they have become addicted to a powerful **psychoactive drug: nicotine.** Although the tobacco industry long maintained

tobacco   The leaves of cultivated tobacco plants prepared for smoking, chewing, or use as snuff.   **TERMS**

psychoactive drug   A chemical substance that affects brain function and changes perception, mood, or consciousness.

nicotine   A toxic, addictive substance found in tobacco and responsible for many of the effects of tobacco.

tolerance   A need for increasingly more of a substance to achieve the desired effect or a diminished effect with continued use of the same amount of the substance.

that nicotine had not been proved to be addictive, scientific evidence overwhelmingly shows that it is highly addictive. In fact, many researchers consider nicotine to be the most physically addictive of all the psychoactive drugs, including cocaine and heroin.

Some neurological studies indicate that nicotine acts on the brain in much the same way as cocaine and heroin. Nicotine reaches the brain via the bloodstream seconds after it is inhaled or absorbed through membranes of the mouth or nose. It triggers the release of powerful chemical messengers in the brain, including epinephrine, norepinephrine, and dopamine. But unlike street drugs, most of which are used to achieve a high, nicotine's primary attraction seems to lie in its ability to modulate everyday emotions.

At low doses, nicotine acts as a stimulant, increasing heart rate and blood pressure. In adults, nicotine can enhance alertness, concentration, information processing, memory, and learning. The opposite effect, however, occurs in teens who smoke; they show impairment in memory and other cognitive functions.

In some circumstances, nicotine acts as a mild sedative. Most commonly, nicotine relieves symptoms such as anxiety, irritability, and mild depression in tobacco users who are experiencing withdrawal. Some studies have shown that high doses of nicotine and rapid smoking cause increases in levels of glucocorticoids and endorphins, hormones that moderate moods and reduce stress. Tobacco users are able to fine-tune nicotine's effects and regulate their moods by increasing or decreasing their intake of the drug. Studies have shown that smokers experience milder mood variation than nonsmokers while performing long, boring tasks or while watching emotional movies, for example.

All tobacco products contain nicotine, and using any of them can lead to addiction (see the box "Tobacco Use Disorder: Are You Hooked?"). Nicotine addiction fulfills the criteria for substance misuse described in Chapter 10, including loss of control, tolerance, and withdrawal.

Loss of Control   Within the past decade, more people are trying to quit and having more success. Still, the majority of smokers (94%) who attempt to quit start smoking again within a year. Quitting may be even harder for smokeless tobacco users: In one study, only 1 in 14 spit tobacco users who participated in a tobacco cessation clinic was able to stop for more than four hours.

Regular tobacco users live according to a rigid cycle of need and gratification. On average, they can go no more than 40 minutes between doses of nicotine; otherwise, they begin feeling edgy and irritable and have trouble concentrating. If ignored, nicotine cravings build until getting tobacco becomes a paramount concern, crowding out other thoughts. Tobacco users may plan their daily schedule around opportunities to satisfy their nicotine cravings; this loss of control and personal freedom can affect all the dimensions of wellness.

Tolerance and Withdrawal   Tobacco users build up **tolerance** to nicotine—a condition in which higher doses of

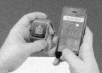

If you meet two of the following criteria within a one-year period, then you have a tobacco use disorder, according to the American Psychiatric Association's *Diagnostic and Statistical Manual of Mental Disorders*, 5th edition (*DSM-5*):

1. Smoke, vape, or chew more tobacco and for a longer time than you intended.
2. Have a persistent desire or are unsuccessful in your efforts to control your tobacco use.
3. Spend a lot of time trying to get or use tobacco.
4. Crave or strongly desire tobacco.
5. Continue to use tobacco even though it interferes with work, school, or home obligations.
6. Continue to use tobacco even though it exacerbates interpersonal problems (e.g., causes arguments with others about your tobacco use).
7. Give up important social, occupational, or recreational activities because of tobacco use.
8. Use tobacco in hazardous situations, such as smoking in bed.
9. Use tobacco even though you know you have a physical or psychological problem that probably comes from smoking.
10. Experience tolerance.
11. Experience withdrawal.

Tobacco users become adept at keeping a steady amount of nicotine circulating in the blood and going to the brain. In one experiment, smokers were given cigarettes that looked and tasted alike but varied in nicotine content. The subjects automatically adjusted their rate and depth of inhalation so that they absorbed their usual amount of nicotine. In other studies, heavy smokers were given nicotine without knowing it, and they cut down on their smoking without a conscious effort. Smokeless tobacco users and those who vape maintain blood nicotine levels as high as those of cigarette smokers.

nicotine are required to produce the same initial effect. Whereas one cigarette may make a beginning smoker nauseated and dizzy, a long-term smoker may have to chain-smoke a pack or more to experience the same effects. For most regular tobacco users, sudden abstinence from nicotine produces predictable **withdrawal** symptoms. These symptoms, which come on several hours after the last dose of nicotine, can include severe cravings, insomnia, confusion, tremors, difficulty concentrating, fatigue, muscle pains, headache, nausea, irritability, anger, and depression. Users experiencing withdrawal undergo measurable changes in brain waves, heart rate, and blood pressure, and they perform poorly on tasks requiring sustained attention. Although most of these symptoms of physical dependence pass in two or three days, the craving associated with addiction persists. Even years after quitting, many ex-smokers report intermittent, intense urges to smoke.

Social and Psychological Factors

Social and psychological forces combine with physiological addiction to maintain the tobacco habit. Many people, for example, have established patterns of smoking or vaping while doing something else—while talking, working, drinking, and so on. The spit tobacco pattern is also associated with certain situations—studying, drinking coffee, or play-

ing sports. These associations can make it more difficult for users to break their habits because the activities they associate with tobacco use continue to trigger urges. Such activities are called **secondary reinforcers;** they act together with physiological addiction to keep the user dependent on nicotine.

Genetic Factors

Genetics play an important role in some aspects of tobacco use. Inherited factors may be more important than social and environmental factors in smoking initiation and in the development of nicotine dependence.

For example, nicotine is broken down in the body, meaning it is metabolized, with the help of an enzyme called CYP2A6. Genetic differences can determine the activity level of this enzyme in the body. When people with slow CYP2A6 metabolism smoke tobacco, the nicotine remains in

withdrawal Symptoms such as irritability, anxiety, and insomnia that can be relieved by taking more of an addictive substance.

secondary reinforcers Stimuli that are not necessarily pleasurable in themselves but that are associated with other stimuli that are pleasurable.

TERMS

their blood longer than in people who have the gene for a faster-metabolizing form of the enzyme. The slow metabolizers are more likely to feel nausea or dizziness when they first use tobacco, are less likely to continue smoking if they try it, and find it easier to quit if they do become regular smokers.

Scientists have also shown that a gene called *DRD2* (associated with the brain chemical dopamine, which plays a key role in the pleasurable effects of nicotine) appears to influence the progression of smoking in adolescence. Among tenth graders who took one puff of a cigarette, those with one form of the gene were more than three times as likely as those with the other form to be regular smokers when they finished eleventh grade.

A couple of recent studies identified gene variants that increase the likelihood of developing a nicotine dependence (in people of both European and African descent) and of developing a preference for menthol-flavored cigarettes (in people of only African descent).

Why Start in the First Place?

In the United States, the legal age to purchase cigarettes is 18 in most states; 15 states and the District of Columbia have raised the legal age to 21. Despite this, nearly 90% of all adult smokers report that they started smoking before age 18. The average age for starting smokers and smokeless tobacco users is around 15. The earlier people begin smoking, the more likely they are to become heavy smokers—and to die of tobacco-related disease.

Not all young people are equally vulnerable to the lure of tobacco. Research suggests that the following characteristics are related to youth tobacco use:

- A parent, sibling, or peer who uses tobacco
- Lack of support or involvement from parents
- Lower socioeconomic status, including lower income or education
- Doing poorly in or dropping out of school
- Low self-image or self-esteem
- Positive attitudes about tobacco use
- Accessibility, availability, and price of tobacco products
- Tobacco advertising in stores, on TV, on the internet, in movies, or in print

Young people start using tobacco for a variety of reasons. Many young, white, male athletes, for example, begin using spit tobacco to emulate professional athletes. Young women commonly take up smoking because they think it will help them lose weight or stay thin. A third of e-cigarette users in grades 6 through 12 said they vape because of the available flavors. Most often, however, young people start using tobacco simply because their peers are already doing it; smoking or vaping gives them a way to fit in with a crowd.

Rationalizing the Dangers   Making the decision to smoke requires minimizing or denying both the health risks

and the tremendous costs—disability, emotional trauma, family stress, and financial expense involved in tobacco-related diseases such as cancer and emphysema. A sense of invincibility, characteristic of many young people, also contributes to the decision to use tobacco. They may persuade themselves they are too intelligent, too lucky, or too healthy to be vulnerable to tobacco's dangers.

Many teenagers believe they can stop smoking when they want to. In fact, adolescents are more vulnerable to nicotine than are older tobacco users. Compared with older smokers, adolescents become heavy smokers and develop dependence after fewer cigarettes. Nicotine addiction can start within a few days of smoking and after just a few cigarettes. Over half of teenagers who try cigarettes progress to daily use, and about half of those who ever smoke daily progress to nicotine dependence. One National Institute on Drug Abuse (NIDA) survey revealed that about 75% of smoking teens state they wish they had never started. Another survey revealed that only 5% of high school smokers predicted they would definitely be smoking in five years; in fact, close to 75% were smoking seven to nine years later.

Emulating Smoking in the Media   Television ads for cigarettes have been banned for 50 years; however, just a few years ago, e-cigarette company JUUL began advertising on social media sites. Then they launched a $10 million TV ad campaign. By September 2019, in light of the epidemic of lung illnesses and multiple deaths attributable to vaping, many media corporations responded. CBS, Viacom, WarnerMedia, and others promised to ban e-cigarette advertising on their channels.

Media portrayals of smoking are a key influence on young people. In fact, studies by the National Cancer Institute have concluded that a direct causal relationship exists between media portrayals of smoking and smoking initiation. This holds true for vaping, too. And a study conducted by researchers at the Dartmouth Medical School found that more than 50% of young people surveyed began smoking after watching repeated favorable portrayals of smoking in movies.

In general, the fictional portrayal of smoking or vaping in films and television does not reflect actual U.S. patterns of tobacco use. The prevalence of smoking among lead characters is three to four times that among comparable Americans. Films typically show smokers as white, male, well educated, successful, and attractive. In reality, smokers tend to be poor and to have less education (see Figure 12.2). Public campaigns to reduce images of smoking in movies have succeeded somewhat; smoking is shown less often in films and television shows now than even just a decade ago. The University of California at San Francisco (UCSF) supports a website (smokefreemovies.ucsf.edu) that ranks actors, directors, and movies by their use of tobacco. It also describes tobacco company sales tactics and supports an R rating for every film that depicts tobacco products.

Still, films remain a critical and highly successful form of advertising for the tobacco industry (see the box "Tobacco Advertising").

Advertising is a powerful influence. In 2018, tobacco companies spent over $9 billion marketing cigarettes and smokeless tobacco to U.S. viewers. A number of other nicotine-rich products are also entering the marketplace: electronic products such as e-cigarettes, e-cigars, and e-pipes. Most tobacco advertising portrays users as young, confident, popular, fit, and sexually attractive. Tobacco companies attract younger smokers through strategies like flavored tobacco products. Flavors such as fruit, herb, spice, alcohol, and candy are popular among young smokers. They are distinguishable from the smell and taste of tobacco, and researchers are working to identify the components of these flavors to more easily regulate them. Brazil and Canada have already banned most flavors.

Young people are a prime target of tobacco ads because nicotine addiction can lead to a lifetime of purchasing tobacco. The most heavily advertised cigarettes are the choice of 90% of teen smokers. In the 1980s and 1990s, for example, R.J. Reynolds Tobacco Company's promotion of the Camel brand recruited millions of new smokers—many of them teenagers or younger. In surveys, more than 90% of 6-year-olds recognized the Camel character ("Joe Camel"), who became as familiar to children as Mickey Mouse.

Cigarette ads don't target only children. Certain brands are designed to appeal primarily either to men or to women, or to a specific racial or ethnic group. Magazines that target African American audiences, for example, receive proportionately more revenues from cigarette ads than do other consumer magazines. Before being made illegal in 1998, billboards advertising tobacco products were placed in black communities four or five times more often than in primarily white communities.

The federal government began regulating tobacco advertising in 1967, requiring broadcasters to air antismoking messages along with cigarette advertisements. Within a few years, cigarette consumption dropped by 7%. Broadcast ads for cigarettes were banned in 1971.

In 1998, lawsuits brought against the tobacco industry by the attorneys general of 39 states achieved these limits or bans on the following marketing tools:

- Billboard and transit ads for tobacco products
- The use of cartoon characters in ads and on packaging
- Tobacco logos on T-shirts, hats, and other promotional items
- Brand-name sponsorship of sporting events
- Product placement in movies, TV shows, and concerts

The 2009 Family Smoking Prevention and Tobacco Control Act further allowed the Food and Drug Administration (FDA) to regulate all tobacco products, including the banning of vending machine sales and product sampling (except in adult-only facilities).

Regardless, the tobacco industry spends billions to promote its products. Much of this money is spent on print ads and coupons, but a great deal is also given to retailers to help offset ever-increasing taxes levied on tobacco products by states.

The industry's promotional efforts are most apparent in convenience stores, where tobacco products and promotions are prominently placed at checkout counters. Tobacco products are presented as a colorful and commonplace part of the retail environment—as acceptable as a candy bar or a carton of milk.

Many states, as well as the federal government, have filed lawsuits against the tobacco industry to reclaim money spent on tobacco-related health care. A 1998 agreement requires tobacco companies to pay states $206 billion over 25 years. For these and other reasons, tobacco consumption in the United States is declining among some groups. In response, the U.S. tobacco industry has increased its efforts to sell in foreign markets, especially in developing nations with few restrictions on tobacco advertising.

HEALTH HAZARDS

Tobacco adversely affects nearly every part of the body, including the brain, stomach, mouth, and reproductive organs.

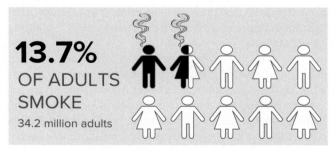

13.7%
OF ADULTS
SMOKE
34.2 million adults

Campaign for Tobacco-Free Kids, 2019 (https://www.tobaccofreekids.org/problem/toll-us).

Tobacco Smoke: A Toxic Mix

Tobacco smoke contains thousands of chemical substances, several hundred of which are known to be harmful to humans, including acetone (found in nail polish remover), ammonia, hexamine (lighter fluid), and toluene (industrial solvent). Smoke from a typical unfiltered cigarette contains about 5 billion particles per cubic millimeter—50,000 times as many as are found in an equal volume of smoggy urban air. These particles, when condensed, form a brown, sticky mass called **cigarette tar.**

cigarette tar A brown, sticky mass created when the chemical particles in tobacco smoke condense. **TERMS**

Carcinogens and Poisons When burned, cigarettes create more than 7000 chemicals. At least 69 of them are linked to cancer. Some, such as benzo(a)pyrene and urethane, are **carcinogens**—that is, they directly cause cancer. Other chemicals, such as formaldehyde, are **cocarcinogens;** they do not themselves cause cancer but combine with other chemicals to stimulate the growth of certain cancers, at least in laboratory animals. Other substances in tobacco cause health problems because they damage the lining of the respiratory tract or decrease the lungs' ability to fight off infection.

Tobacco also contains acutely poisonous substances, including arsenic and hydrogen cyanide. In addition to being an addictive psychoactive drug, nicotine is a poison that can be fatal in high doses. Many cases of nicotine poisoning occur each year in toddlers and infants who eat cigarette butts they find at home or on the playground. In addition, children and adults have been poisoned by swallowing, breathing, or absorbing e-cigarette liquid through their skin or eyes.

Cigarette smoke contains carbon monoxide, the deadly gas in automobile exhaust, in concentrations 400 times greater than is considered safe in industrial workplaces. Carbon monoxide displaces oxygen in red blood cells, depleting the body's supply of oxygen needed for extra work. Not surprisingly, smokers often complain of breathlessness when they exert themselves. Carbon monoxide also impairs visual acuity, especially at night.

Additives Tobacco manufacturers use additives to manipulate the taste and effect of cigarettes and other tobacco products. Additives account for roughly 10%, by weight, of a cigarette, and include flavoring agents, humectants (compounds that keep tobacco from drying out), and chemicals that enhance nicotine's addicting properties. Some additives and their uses are described below:

- *Sugars (such as licorice, cocoa, honey).* These additives mask the bitter taste of tobacco, allowing for deeper inhalation. Burning sugar produces acetaldehyde, which is an addictive carcinogen.

- *Other flavorings.* Theobromine and glycyrrhizin are flavorings that also act as bronchodilators, opening the lungs' airways and making it easier for nicotine to get into the bloodstream.

- *Ammonia.* The main purpose of this additive is to boost nicotine delivery. Ammonia reduces the acidity of tobacco smoke and releases nicotine in the form of a

---

Ask Yourself

QUESTIONS FOR CRITICAL THINKING AND REFLECTION
What has influenced your decision to try, continue, or quit smoking or vaping or using some other form of tobacco? Have you ever felt that images or messages in the media were encouraging you to use tobacco? How do you react to such messages?

base (alkaline) rather than a salt, which would bind to other acid components of smoke. As a free base, nicotine is more readily absorbed into the blood.

- *Potassium citrate, aluminum, and clay.* These additives make **sidestream smoke** (the uninhaled smoke from a burning cigarette) less obvious and objectionable. They are added to cigarette wrappers to convert particulate ash into an invisible gas with less irritating odor. These are intended to reduce social pressures from nonsmokers.

Nearly 600 chemicals, approved as safe when used as food additives, are used in manufacturing cigarettes. In 1994, U.S. cigarette manufacturers submitted a list of tobacco additives to the U.S. Department of Health and Human Services (HHS), which made the list public and accompanied it with the notice that "although these ingredients are regarded as safe when ingested in foods, some may form carcinogens when heated or burned."

Inhaling Tobacco Smoke All smokers absorb some gases, tar, and nicotine from cigarette smoke, but smokers who inhale cigarette smoke into their lungs bring most of these substances into their bodies and keep them there. In a year, a typical pack-a-day smoker takes in 50,000–70,000 puffs. Smoke from a cigarette, pipe, or cigar directly assaults the mouth, throat, and respiratory tract. The nose, which normally filters about 75% of foreign matter we breathe, is bypassed completely.

In a cigarette, the unburned tobacco itself acts as a filter. As a cigarette burns down, there is less and less filter. Thus more chemicals are absorbed into the body during the last third of a cigarette than during the first. A smoker can cut down on the absorption of harmful chemicals by not smoking cigarettes down to short butts. Any gains, of course, are offset by smoking more cigarettes, inhaling more deeply, or puffing more frequently.

"Reduced Harm" Cigarettes There is no such thing as a safe cigarette, and smoking behavior is a more important factor in tar and nicotine intake than the type of cigarette smoked. Smokers who switch to a low-nicotine or low-tar brand often compensate by smoking more cigarettes, inhaling more deeply, taking larger or more frequent puffs, or blocking ventilation holes with lips or fingers to offset the effects of filters.

QUICK STATS

More than 249 billion cigarettes were sold in the United States in 2017.

—Centers for Disease Control and Prevention, 2018

TERMS

carcinogen Any substance that causes cancer.

cocarcinogen A substance that works with a carcinogen to cause cancer.

sidestream smoke The uninhaled smoke from a burning cigarette.

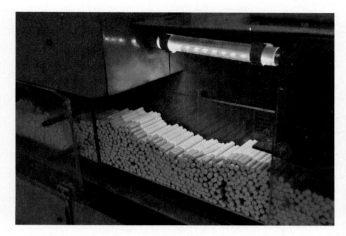

Cigarette making is an elaborate process involving industrial machinery and chemistry. Dozens of compounds may be added to tobacco to produce a specific brand of cigarette. CristiNistor/Getty Images

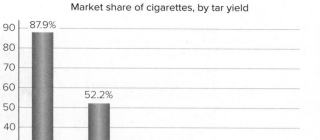

Market share of cigarettes, by tar yield

VITAL STATISTICS

FIGURE 12.3 **U.S. market share of cigarettes, by tar level: 2016.**

SOURCE: Federal Trade Commission. 2019. *Federal Trade Commission Cigarette Report for 2017.* Washington, DC: Federal Trade Commission.

Studies have found that people who smoke "light" cigarettes inhale up to eight times as much tar and nicotine as printed on the label. Studies also show that smokers of light cigarettes are less likely to quit than smokers of regular cigarettes, probably due to the misperception that light cigarettes are safer. Use of light and low-tar cigarettes does not reduce the risk of smoking-related illnesses.

In June 2010, federal regulations prohibited cigarette manufacturers from labeling their products with descriptors such as "light," "mild," or "low"—terms that have effectively convinced many consumers that such cigarettes are safer alternatives to higher-tar cigarettes. Manufacturers that want to apply such labels have to receive special permission from the U.S. Food and Drug Administration (FDA). To sidestep labeling regulations, some cigarette companies shifted to color-coded packaging in order to distinguish different types of cigarettes. For example, Camel Lights are now called Camel Blues, and Marlboro Ultralights are now Marlboro Silver. Despite the availability of lower-tar cigarettes, consumers heavily favor higher-tar products. As shown in Figure 12.3, less than 17% of the market goes to cigarettes with a tar level of 9 mg or less.

Menthol Cigarettes Concerns have also been raised about menthol cigarettes. Menthol is a bronchodilator; as mentioned earlier, bronchodilators open the lungs' airways and make it easier for nicotine to enter the bloodstream. About 70% of black smokers smoke these cigarettes, as compared to 30% of white smokers. Studies have found that African Americans absorb more nicotine than other groups and metabolize it more slowly; they also have lower rates of successful quitting. The anesthetizing effect of menthol, which may allow smokers to inhale more deeply and hold smoke in their lungs for a longer period, may be partly responsible for these differences. Research is needed to determine if the effects of menthol and differences in smoking behavior can help explain the higher rates of smoking-related diseases among African Americans.

The Immediate Effects of Smoking

The beginning smoker often has symptoms of mild nicotine poisoning, including the following:

- Dizziness
- Faintness
- Rapid pulse
- Cold, clammy skin
- Nausea
- Vomiting
- Diarrhea

The seasoned smoker occasionally suffers these effects of nicotine poisoning, particularly after quitting and then returning to a previous level of consumption. The effects of nicotine on smokers vary, largely depending on the size of the nicotine dose and how much tolerance the smoker has built up through previous smoking. Nicotine can either excite or tranquilize the nervous system, depending on dosage.

Nicotine has many other immediate effects (see Figure 12.4). It stimulates the part of the brain called the **cerebral cortex.** It also stimulates the adrenal glands to release adrenaline, which accelerates heart rate, elevates blood pressure, and restricts blood flow to the heart. Nicotine inhibits the formation of urine and constricts blood vessels, especially in the skin. Higher blood pressure, faster heart rate, and constricted blood vessels require the heart to pump more blood. In healthy people, the heart can usually meet this demand; but in people whose coronary arteries are damaged, the heart muscle may be strained.

cerebral cortex The outer region of the brain, which controls complex behavior and mental activity. **TERMS**

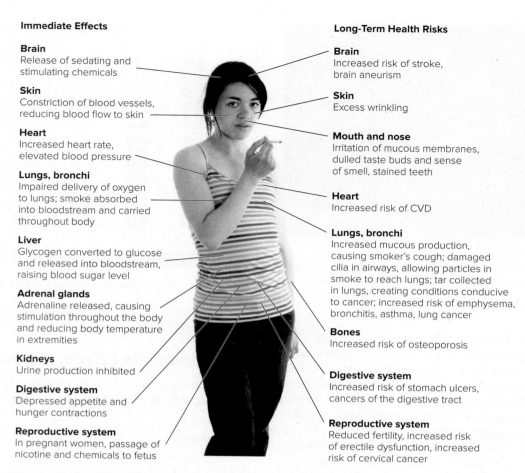

Immediate Effects

Brain
Release of sedating and stimulating chemicals

Skin
Constriction of blood vessels, reducing blood flow to skin

Heart
Increased heart rate, elevated blood pressure

Lungs, bronchi
Impaired delivery of oxygen to lungs; smoke absorbed into bloodstream and carried throughout body

Liver
Glycogen converted to glucose and released into bloodstream, raising blood sugar level

Adrenal glands
Adrenaline released, causing stimulation throughout the body and reducing body temperature in extremities

Kidneys
Urine production inhibited

Digestive system
Depressed appetite and hunger contractions

Reproductive system
In pregnant women, passage of nicotine and chemicals to fetus

Long-Term Health Risks

Brain
Increased risk of stroke, brain aneurism

Skin
Excess wrinkling

Mouth and nose
Irritation of mucous membranes, dulled taste buds and sense of smell, stained teeth

Heart
Increased risk of CVD

Lungs, bronchi
Increased mucous production, causing smoker's cough; damaged cilia in airways, allowing particles in smoke to reach lungs; tar collected in lungs, creating conditions conducive to cancer; increased risk of emphysema, bronchitis, asthma, lung cancer

Bones
Increased risk of osteoporosis

Digestive system
Increased risk of stomach ulcers, cancers of the digestive tract

Reproductive system
Reduced fertility, increased risk of erectile dysfunction, increased risk of cervical cancer

FIGURE 12.4   Tobacco use: Immediate effects and long-term health risks.

Tim Large - Youth Social Issues/Alamy Stock Photo

Smoking depresses hunger sensations and dulls the taste buds. Smokers who quit often notice that food tastes much better. Smoking is not useful for weight loss, however. Smoking for decades may lessen or prevent age-associated weight gain for some smokers, but for people under age 30, smoking is not associated with weight loss.

The Long-Term Effects of Smoking

Smoking is linked to many deadly and disabling diseases (refer to Figure 12.4). Research indicates that the total amount of tobacco smoke inhaled is a key factor contributing to disease. People who begin smoking at early ages run a greater risk of disease than nonsmokers.

As more research is done, even more diseases associated with smoking are being discovered. The costliest ones—to society as well as to the individual—are cardiovascular disease, cancer, and respiratory diseases.

Cardiovascular Disease   Cardiovascular disease is the most widespread cause of death for cigarette smokers, not lung cancer. **Coronary heart disease (CHD),** a form of cardiovascular disease, often results when the arteries that supply the heart muscle with blood develop **atherosclerosis.** In atherosclerosis, fatty deposits called **plaques** form on the inner walls of arteries, causing them to narrow and stiffen. Smoking and exposure to environmental tobacco smoke (ETS) accelerate the rate of plaque accumulation in the coronary arteries—50% for smokers, 25% for ex-smokers, and 20% for people regularly exposed to ETS. The crushing chest pain of **angina pectoris,** a primary symptom of CHD, results when the heart muscle, or *myocardium,* does not get enough oxygen. Sometimes a plaque forms at a narrow point in a main coronary artery. If the plaque completely blocks the flow of

coronary heart disease (CHD)   Cardiovascular **TERMS** disease caused by hardening of the arteries that supply oxygen to the heart muscle; also called *coronary artery disease.*

atherosclerosis   Cardiovascular disease caused by the deposit of fatty substances (called *plaque*) in the walls of the arteries.

plaque   A deposit on the inner wall of blood vessels; blood can coagulate around plaque and form a clot.

angina pectoris   Chest pain due to coronary heart disease.

blood to a portion of the heart, that portion may die. This type of heart attack is called a **myocardial infarction.**

CHD can also interfere with the heart's electrical activity, resulting in disturbances of the normal heartbeat rhythm. Sudden and unexpected death is a common result of CHD, particularly among smokers. (See Chapter 16 for a more extensive discussion of cardiovascular disease.)

Smokers have a death rate from CHD that is 70% higher than that of nonsmokers. Deaths from CHD associated with cigarette smoking are most common in people aged 40–50. (In contrast, deaths from lung cancer caused by smoking are most likely to occur in 60- to 70-year-olds.) Among people *under* age 40, smokers are five times more likely than nonsmokers to have a heart attack. Cigar and pipe smokers run a lower risk than cigarette smokers.

Smoking reduces the amount of "good" cholesterol (high-density lipoprotein, or HDL) in the blood, thereby promoting plaque formation in artery walls. Smoking may also increase tension in heart muscle walls, speeding up the rate of muscular contraction and accelerating the heart rate. The workload of the heart thus increases, as does its need for oxygen and other nutrients. Carbon monoxide produced by cigarette smoking combines with hemoglobin in the red blood cells, displacing oxygen and thus providing less oxygen to the heart. One study showed that the additional blood supply available to the heart during stress was 21% less in smokers than in nonsmokers. This reduced blood flow is an early indicator of future heart attacks or strokes.

The risks of CHD decrease rapidly when a person stops smoking. This is particularly true for younger smokers, whose coronary arteries have not yet been damaged extensively.

Cigarette smoking has been linked to other cardiovascular diseases, including the following:

• *Stroke.* A sudden interference with the circulation of blood in a part of the brain, resulting in the destruction of brain cells.

• *Aortic aneurysm.* A bulge in the aorta caused by a weakening in its walls.

• *Pulmonary heart disease.* A disorder of the right side of the heart, caused by changes in the blood vessels of the lungs.

Lung Cancer and Other Cancers   About 30% of all cancer deaths are caused by smoking. Cigarette smoking is the primary cause of lung cancer and is responsible for 87% of lung cancer deaths. Research has identified the precise mechanism: Benzo(a)pyrene, a chemical in tobacco smoke, causes genetic mutations in lung cells that are identical to those found in many patients with lung cancer. Those who smoke two or more packs of cigarettes a day have lung cancer death rates 12–25 times greater than those of nonsmokers. The dramatic rise in lung cancer rates among women in the past

40 years clearly parallels the increase in smoking in this group; lung cancer now exceeds breast cancer as the leading cause of cancer deaths among women. The risk of developing lung cancer increases with the number of cigarettes smoked each day and the number of years of smoking. The younger you are when you start smoking, and the longer you continue, the greater your risk of developing a smoking-related cancer. But as Figure 12.5 shows, the younger a smoker is when he or she stops smoking, the lower the risk of ultimately dying from lung cancer. Evidence suggests that after 1 year without smoking, the risk of lung cancer decreases substantially. After 10 years, the risk of lung cancer among ex-smokers is half that of active smokers.

Although cigar and pipe smokers have a higher risk of lung cancer than nonsmokers do, their risk is lower than that for cigarette smokers. Smoking filter-tipped cigarettes slightly reduces health hazards unless the smoker compensates by smoking more, as is often the case.

Research has also linked smoking to cancers of the trachea, mouth, pharynx, esophagus, larynx, pancreas, bladder,

myocardial infarction   A heart attack caused by the complete blockage of a main coronary artery.   TERMS

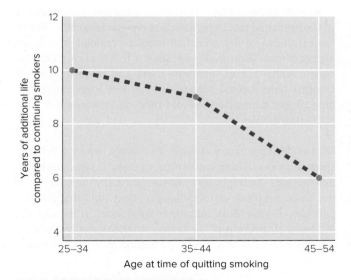

VITAL STATISTICS

FIGURE 12.5   Increased life expectancy. Data show that quitting smoking at younger ages substantially reduces the risk of death from smoking-related causes: Quitting at age 25–34 adds 10 more years, and at age 45–54 adds 6 years.

SOURCE: WHO. 2020. Tobacco Free Initiative (https://www.who.int/tobacco/quitting/benefits/en/).

kidney, breast, cervix, stomach, liver, colon, and skin. For more information about cancer, see Chapter 17.

Chronic Obstructive Pulmonary Disease The stresses smoking places on the lungs can permanently damage lung function and lead to *chronic obstructive pulmonary disease* (*COPD*), also known as chronic obstructive lung disease or chronic lower respiratory disease. COPD is a disorder that consists of several diseases, including emphysema and chronic bronchitis. It is caused by the overtaxing of smokers' lungs, which need to work harder to respond to the constant exposure to chemicals and irritants. COPD was the fourth leading cause of death in the United States in 2016.

For most Americans, cigarette smoking is a primary cause of COPD, whereas in poorer countries COPD often develops from exposure to the fumes of burning fuels used for heating and cooking. In the U.S., cigarette smokers are up to 18 times more likely than nonsmokers to die from emphysema and chronic bronchitis. (Pipe and cigar smokers have a smaller risk.) In a study of 605 people with COPD, 62% used tobacco.

EMPHYSEMA Smoking is the primary cause of **emphysema,** a disabling condition in which the air sacs in the walls of the lungs lose their elasticity and are gradually destroyed. The lungs' ability to take in oxygen and expel carbon dioxide is impaired. A person with emphysema is often breathless, gasps for air, and has the feeling of drowning. The heart must pump harder and may become enlarged. People with emphysema often die from a damaged heart. There is no known way to reverse this disease. In its advanced stage, emphysema leaves the victim bedridden and severely disabled.

CHRONIC BRONCHITIS Persistent, recurrent inflammation of the bronchial tubes characterizes **chronic bronchitis.** When the cell lining of the bronchial tubes is irritated, it secretes excess mucus. Bronchial congestion is followed by a chronic cough, which makes breathing more and more difficult. If smokers have chronic bronchitis, they face a greater risk of lung cancer, no matter how old they are or how many cigarettes they smoke.

Other Respiratory Damage Even when a smoker shows no signs of lung impairment or disease, cigarette smoking damages the respiratory system. Normally the cells lining the bronchial tubes secrete *mucus,* a sticky fluid that collects particles of soot, dust, and other substances in inhaled air. Mucus is cleared out of the lungs into the throat by the continuous motion of *cilia,* which are hairlike structures that pro-

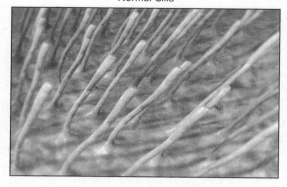

Normal Cilia

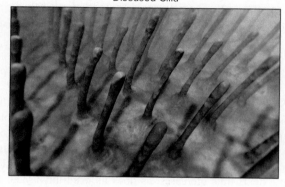

Diseased Cilia

Smoking causes damage to the lungs, bronchial tubes, their cilia, and the mouth. MedicalRF.com/Corbis

trude from the inner surface of the bronchial tubes. If the cilia are destroyed or impaired, or if inhaled air contains more pollutants than the system can remove, the protection provided by cilia is lost.

Cigarette smoke first slows and then stops the action of the cilia. Eventually it destroys them, leaving delicate membranes exposed to injury from substances inhaled in cigarette smoke or air pollution. Special cells called *macrophages* (a type of white blood cell) also work to remove foreign particles from the respiratory tract by engulfing them. Smoking appears to make macrophages work less efficiently. This respiratory interference often leads rapidly to conditions known as *smoker's throat* and *smoker's cough,* as well as to shortness of breath. Even smokers of high school age show impaired respiratory function compared with nonsmokers of the same age. Other respiratory effects of smoking include a worsening of allergy and asthma symptoms and an increase in smokers' susceptibility to colds.

Although cigarette smoking can cause many respiratory disorders and diseases, the damage is not always permanent. Once a person stops smoking, steady improvement in overall lung function usually takes place. Chronic coughing subsides, mucus production returns to normal, and breathing becomes easier. The likelihood of lung disease drops sharply. People of all ages, even those who have been smoking for decades, enjoy improved health after they stop smoking.

> **emphysema** A disease characterized by a loss **TERMS** of lung tissue elasticity and destruction of the air sacs, impairing the lungs' ability to take in oxygen and expel carbon dioxide.
>
> **chronic bronchitis** Recurrent, persistent inflammation of the bronchial tubes.

Additional Health, Cosmetic, and Economic Concerns

- **Ulcers.** People who smoke are more likely to develop and die from peptic ulcers (especially stomach ulcers) because smoking impairs the body's healing ability. Smoking also increases the risk of gastroesophageal reflux, which causes heartburn and can raise the risk of esophageal cancer.

- **Thinning of the brain's cortex.** Long-term cigarette smoking appears to hasten the thinning of the brain's cortex, which could lead to cognitive deterioration.

- **Erectile dysfunction.** Smoking affects blood flow and is an independent risk factor for erectile dysfunction (ED). In one recent study, smokers were twice as likely as nonsmokers to experience ED.

- **Reproductive health problems.** Smoking is linked to reduced fertility. A study of 18-year-old male smokers found that they had a significantly higher proportion of abnormally shaped sperm and sperm with genetic defects than nonsmokers. In women, smoking can contribute to menstrual disorders, early menopause, and pregnancy complications.

- **Dental diseases.** Smokers are at increased risk for tooth decay and gum diseases, with symptoms appearing by the mid-twenties.

- **Diminished senses.** Smoking dulls the senses of taste and smell. Over time it increases the risk of hearing loss and of macular degeneration and cataracts (serious eye conditions that can result in blindness).

- **Injuries.** Smokers have higher rates of motor vehicle crashes, fire-related injuries, and back pain.

- **Cosmetic concerns.** Smoking can cause premature skin wrinkling, premature baldness, stained teeth, discolored fingers, and a persistent tobacco odor in clothes and hair.

- **Economic costs.** In 2019, the average per-pack price of cigarettes was $6.96. A pack-a-day habit can exceed $3600 per year. It costs cigarette companies only about 6 cents to make a pack of cigarettes.

In addition, smoking contributes to osteoporosis, increases the risk of complications from diabetes, and accelerates the course of multiple sclerosis.

Cumulative Effects The cumulative effects of tobacco use fall into two general categories. The first is reduced life expectancy. A male who takes up smoking before age 15 and continues to smoke is only half as likely to live to age 75 as a male who never smokes. Females who have similar smoking habits also have a reduced life expectancy.

The second category involves quality of life. Smokers become disabled at younger ages than nonsmokers and have more years of illness. A national health survey started in 1964 shows that smokers spend one-third more time away from their jobs because of illness than nonsmokers. Female smokers spend 17% more days sick in bed than female nonsmokers. Lost workdays due to smoking cost businesses and workers who smoke billions of dollars every year.

Gender Differences in Health Hazards Although overall risks of tobacco-related illness are similar for women and men, sex appears to make a difference in some diseases. Women, for example, are more at risk for smoking-related blood clots and strokes, and the risk is even greater for women using oral contraceptives. Among men and women with the same smoking history, the odds for developing three major types of cancer, including lung cancer, are 1.2–1.7 times higher in women. More American women die each year from lung cancer than from breast cancer. Women may also have a greater biological vulnerability to lung cancer, and a greater risk than men for coronary heart disease.

Men who smoke carry a greater risk of dying from bronchitis and emphysema and from cancer of the trachea, lung, and bronchus. They also increase their risk of erectile dysfunction and infertility due to reduced sperm density and motility. Women who smoke have higher rates of osteoporosis (a bone-thinning disease that can lead to fractures), thyroid-related diseases, and depression.

> QUICK STATS
> **Smoking costs the United States $170 billion in direct medical care each year.**
> —Centers for Disease Control and Prevention, 2019

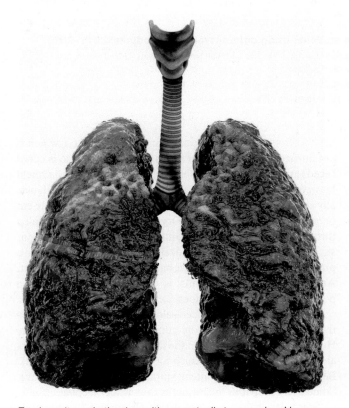

Tar deposits and other impurities eventually turn smokers' lungs black. Pavel Chagochkin/Shutterstock

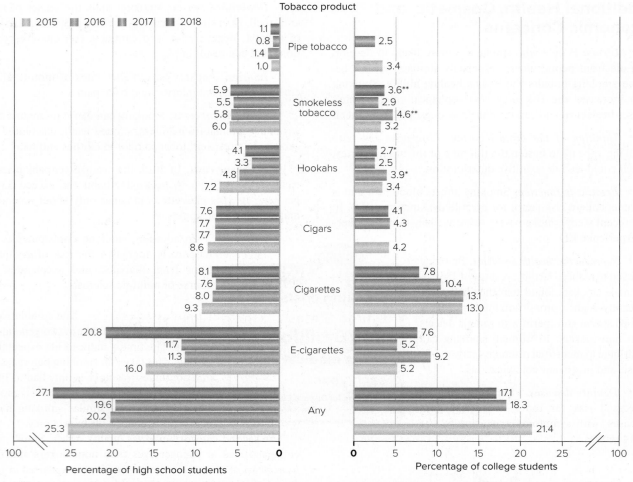

FIGURE 12.6 **Estimated percentages of high school and college students using different tobacco products, 2015–2018.**

SOURCE: Centers for Disease Control and Prevention. 2019. Vital Signs: Tobacco Product Use Among Middle and High School Students–United States, 2011–2018. *Morbidity and Mortality Weekly Report* 68(6): 157–164 (https://www.cdc.gov/mmwr/volumes/68/wr/mm6806e1.htm?s_cid=mm6806e1_w#T1_down).

*Data from American College Health Association-National College Health Assessments, 2016 and 2018. (80% participants 18–24 years.)

**Schulenberg, J. E., et al. 2017. Monitoring the Future national survey results on drug use, 1975–2018; Volume II, College students and adults ages 19-55. Ann Arbor, MI: Institute for Social Research, The University of Michigan.

Women who smoke also have risks associated with reproduction and the reproductive organs. Smoking is associated with greater menstrual bleeding, greater duration of painful menstrual cramps, and more variability in menstrual cycle length. Smokers have a more difficult time becoming pregnant, and they reach menopause on average a year or two earlier than nonsmokers. When women smokers become pregnant, they face increased chances of miscarriage or placental disorders that lead to bleeding and premature delivery; rates of ectopic pregnancy, preeclampsia, and stillbirth are also higher among women who smoke. In addition, smoking is a risk factor for cervical cancer.

Risks Associated with Other Forms of Tobacco Use

Many smokers have switched from cigarettes to other forms of tobacco, such as spit tobacco, cigars, pipes, clove cigarettes, bidis, hookahs, and e-cigarettes (see Figure 12.6). These alternatives, however, can be just as harmful.

Smokeless (Spit) Tobacco Smokeless tobacco, which is not burned, comes in several forms. Chewing tobacco is cured (aged) and sold in pouches. Often flavored, it is chewed or held between the cheek and gums to release the nicotine. Snuff, usually sold in small tins, is cured tobacco that has been finely cut or processed into a powder. Dry, powdered snuff is inhaled through the nose; powdered snuff also comes in lozenges or strips that are sucked on. Smokeless tobacco increases saliva production, and the resulting tobacco juice is usually spat out. Another product, called snus, is moist snuff contained in a pouch (like a teabag) and does not require spitting.

The nicotine in spit tobacco–along with flavorings and additives–is absorbed through the gums and lining of the mouth. Holding an average-size dip in the mouth for 30 minutes delivers about the same amount of nicotine as two or three cigarettes. Because of its nicotine content, spit tobacco is highly addictive. Some users keep it in their mouths even while sleeping.

Smokeless tobacco is not a safe alternative to cigarettes. Gums and lips become dried and irritated and may bleed. White or red patches may appear inside the mouth; this condition, known as *leukoplakia,* can lead to oral cancer. About 25% of regular smokeless tobacco users have *gingivitis* (inflammation), tooth loss, and recession of the gums and bone loss around the teeth, especially where the tobacco is typically placed. The senses of taste and smell are usually dulled. In addition, other people are repelled by wads of tobacco in the mouth, stained teeth, bad breath, and frequent spitting.

One of the most serious effects of smokeless tobacco is an increased risk of oral cancer—cancers of the lip, tongue, cheek, throat, gums, roof and floor of the mouth, and larynx. Smokeless tobacco contains at least 28 chemicals known to cause cancer, and long-term snuff use may increase the risk of oral cancer by as much as 50 times. Surgery to treat oral cancer is often disfiguring and may involve removing parts of the face, tongue, cheek, or lip. Using smokeless tobacco can also cause heart and gum disease.

Smokeless tobacco produces blood levels of nicotine similar to those in cigarette smokers. Other chemicals in smokeless tobacco are believed to pose risks to developing fetuses.

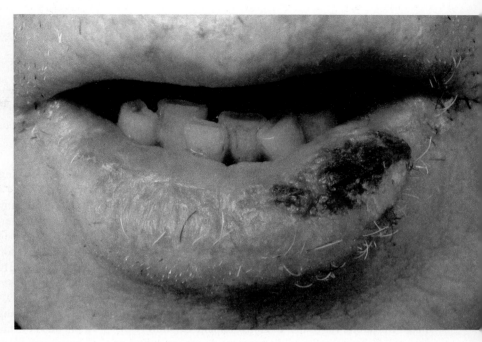

Cigar smokers have 27 times the risk of oral cancer compared to nonsmokers. BSIP/UIG/Getty Images

Cigars and Pipes
Cigars are most popular among African American males aged 18–44, but women are also smoking cigars in record numbers. In government surveys, 7.6% of American high school students reported having smoked at least one cigar in the previous month. Fewer than 1% of Americans, mostly males who smoke cigarettes, are pipe smokers.

Because cigar and pipe smoke is more alkaline than cigarette smoke, users of cigars and pipes do not need to inhale in order to ingest nicotine; instead they absorb nicotine through the gums and lining of the mouth. Cigars contain more tobacco than cigarettes and so contain more nicotine and produce more tar when smoked. Large cigars may contain as much tobacco as a whole pack of cigarettes and may take one or two hours to smoke.

The health risks of cigars depend on the number of cigars smoked and whether the smoker inhales. Because most cigar and pipe users do not inhale, they have a lower risk of cancer and cardiovascular and respiratory diseases than cigarette smokers. However, their risks are substantially higher than those of nonsmokers. For example, compared to nonsmokers, people who smoke one or two cigars per day without inhaling have six times the risk of cancer of the larynx. The risks are much higher for cigar smokers who inhale: They have 27 times the risk of oral cancer and 53 times the risk of cancer of the larynx compared to nonsmokers, and their risk of heart and lung diseases approaches that of cigarette smokers. Smoking a cigar immediately impairs the ability of blood vessels to dilate, reducing the amount of oxygen delivered to tissues, including the heart muscle, especially during stress. Pipe and cigar smoking are also risk factors for pancreatic cancer, which is almost always fatal.

The recent rise in cigar use among teens also raises concerns because nicotine addiction almost always develops in the teen or young adult years. More research is needed to determine if cigar use by teens will develop into nicotine addiction.

Hookah
The practice of puffing flavored tobacco through a water pipe—a **hookah**—has grown in the United States, particularly among college students. The smoker inhales through a hose, drawing air over a piece of burning charcoal, heating the tobacco, and producing smoke that travels through the body of the pipe, an urn filled with water, and the hose.

Many people assume that hookahs provide a safer way of using tobacco. One study showed that over a quarter of college students believed hookahs did not contain tobacco, and over a third believed that hookahs did not contain nicotine. However, research has found hookah smoke contains many harmful chemicals, including 10 times more carbon monoxide than the smoke from a single cigarette. One hour of hookah smoking involves 200 puffs, whereas an average cigarette involves 20 puffs. The volume of smoke inhaled during a typical hookah session is about 90,000 milliliters (ml), compared with 500–600 ml inhaled when smoking a cigarette. Smoke from both tobacco and nontobacco hookah products contains toxic compounds that increase the risk for smoking-related cancers, heart disease, and lung disease. Depending on which toxic compound is measured, a single hookah session is the equivalent of smoking between 1 and 50 cigarettes.

> **hookah** A pipe used for smoking specially flavored tobacco (e.g., apple, mint, cherry); sometimes called a water pipe or *shisha*.
>
> **TERMS**

E-Cigarettes Electronic cigarettes, also known as e-cigarettes or e-cigs, are battery-powered devices that look like traditional cigarettes, pens, or even USB flash drives. They use a changeable cartridge containing a liquid form of nicotine, flavorings, and other chemicals; cartridges can also contain tetrahydrocannabinol (THC) or cannabinoid (CBD) oils. When the user "smokes" or "vapes" an e-cig by sucking the filtered end, the battery heats the chemicals to create an inhalable vapor.

Because they deliver nicotine in aerosol form instead of smoke, e-cigs have been advertised as a safe alternative to traditional cigarettes, despite exposing users to nicotine and other toxic chemicals. E-cigarettes get hot enough to produce carcinogens and other toxic chemicals like formaldehyde, found in traditional cigarettes, or diethylene glycol, a toxic chemical in antifreeze.

E-cigarettes also produce nanoparticles, which have been linked to inflammation leading to asthma, stroke, and heart disease. One study found that vaping may make antibiotic-resistant bacteria even harder to kill. Another recent study linked e-cigarette flavorants to an irreversible respiratory disease called bronchiolitis obliterans, or "popcorn lung," in which the airways become inflamed and scarred, resulting in a permanent cough and shortness of breath. A recent study found that even nicotine-free e-cigarette solutions contain chemicals that damage lung cells.

No evidence submitted to the FDA supports the claim that e-cigarettes can be used as a smoking cessation product like nicotine gums and patches. Instead, sleek advertisements, appealing flavors, and a perception of safety have made e-cigarettes extremely popular among teenagers and first-time smokers.

The vaping trends of young people were declared an epidemic by the Surgeon General in 2018. From 2017 to 2018, rates climbed to over 20% of high school students and almost 5% of middle school students. By 2019, e-cigarette rates among high-schoolers spiked to 27.5%. Most young e-cigarette users cited appealing flavors as the primary reason of use. As more young people become addicted to nicotine, they are also vaping more often. The adverse effects of nicotine on brain development in adolescents and young adults is of particular concern. Studies have linked nicotine use in teenagers and young adults to long-term cognition and attention problems and to an increased risk for mood disorders. Furthermore, early nicotine exposure increases the chance of nicotine dependence later in life and the likelihood of using other dependence-producing substances.

According to the Monitoring the Future Study, vaping also increased among college students from 2017 to 2018;

Ask Yourself

QUESTIONS FOR CRITICAL THINKING AND REFLECTION

Do you know anyone who has suffered from an illness related to tobacco use? If so, what problems did that person face? What was the outcome? Did the experience have any effect on your views about using tobacco?

nicotine vaping rose from 6% to 16% and marijuana vaping from 5% to 11%. These were among the greatest one-year increases for any substance monitored since the survey was first administered in 1975.

In response to the outbreak of vaping-related lung disease, the CDC recommends that people not use vaping products containing THC, nor purchase any type of vaping products, including those containing nicotine, from informal sources like friends, family, or at in-person or online dealers. They should also not add any substances to e-cigarette products that are not intended by the manufacturer. In 2019, 2300 people across 49 states were sickened and 47 died from e-cigarette-associated lung injury.

THE EFFECTS OF SMOKING ON THE NONSMOKER

Tens of thousands of nonsmokers die each year because of exposure to secondhand smoke, and the latest research points to similar devastating effects from thirdhand smoke. The medical and societal costs of tobacco use are enormous.

Environmental Tobacco Smoke

The U.S. Environmental Protection Agency (EPA) has designated **environmental tobacco smoke (ETS)**—more commonly called *secondhand smoke* and *thirdhand smoke*—a Class A carcinogen. The National Toxicology Program classifies ETS as a "known human carcinogen." These designations put ETS in the same category as notorious cancer-causing agents like asbestos. The Surgeon General has concluded that for some people there is no safe level of exposure to ETS; even brief exposure can cause serious harm.

Environmental tobacco smoke consists of mainstream smoke and sidestream smoke. Smoke exhaled by smokers is referred to as **mainstream smoke.** Sidestream smoke enters the atmosphere from the burning end of a cigarette, cigar, or pipe. Nearly 85% of the smoke in a room where someone is smoking comes from sidestream smoke. Sidestream smoke is not filtered through either a cigarette filter or a smoker's lungs. It has twice as much tar and nicotine, three times as much benzo(a)pyrene, almost three times as much carbon monoxide, and three times as much ammonia as mainstream smoke.

In rooms where people are smoking, levels of carbon monoxide can exceed those permitted by federal air quality

environmental tobacco smoke (ETS) Smoke **TERMS** that enters the atmosphere from the burning end of a cigarette, cigar, or pipe, as well as smoke that is exhaled by smokers; also called *secondhand smoke.*

mainstream smoke Smoke that is inhaled by a smoker and then exhaled into the atmosphere.

Given the health risks of exposure to ETS, try these strategies to keep the air around you safe:

- **Speak up tactfully.** Smokers may not know the dangers they are causing or may not know it bothers you.

- **Display reminders.** Put up signs asking smokers to refrain in your home, work area, and car.

- **Don't allow smoking in your home or room.** Get rid of ashtrays and ask smokers to light up outside.

- **Open a window.** If you cannot avoid being in a room with a smoker, at least try to provide some ventilation.

- **Sit in the nonsmoking section in restaurants and other public areas.** Complain to the manager if none exists.

- **Fight for a smoke-free work environment.** Join with your coworkers to either eliminate all smoking indoors or confine it to certain areas.

- **Make sure schools and day care sites are tobacco-free.** Teach children to stay away from secondhand smoke.

- **Discuss quitting strategies.** Social pressure is a major factor in many former smokers' decisions to quit. Help the smokers in your life by sharing quitting strategies with them.

standards for outside air. In a typical home with the windows closed, it takes about six hours for 95% of the airborne cigarette smoke particles to clear. The carcinogens in the secondhand smoke from a single cigar exceed those of three cigarettes, and cigar smoke contains up to 30 times more carbon monoxide. E-cigarettes produce secondhand aerosol. While it contains fewer toxins than cigarette smoke, the Surgeon General has concluded that e-cigarette aerosol is not harmless; it may expose bystanders to nicotine, heavy metals, ultrafine particulates, volatile organic compounds, and other toxins.

The CDC estimates that 58 million nonsmoking Americans (including 15 million children) are exposed to some level of ETS every year.

Thirdhand Smoke   A further complicating factor is *thirdhand smoke*, the toxic residues and chemicals that linger on indoor surfaces, curtains, and furniture, and in dust. Although it may seem like only a stale smell, thirdhand smoke contains the chemicals of secondhand smoke from tobacco: gases and particulate matter, including carcinogens and heavy metals such as arsenic, lead, and cyanide. Highly toxic particulates like nicotine can cling to walls and ceilings; gases can be absorbed into dust, fabrics, and upholstery. These toxic mixes can then recombine to form harmful compounds that remain at high levels long after smoking has stopped.

The transition from secondhand to thirdhand smoke is gradual, so the distinct chronic effects of each are not yet clear. The predicted health damage caused by thirdhand smoke ranges from 5% to 60% of total harm, much of which may currently be attributed to secondhand smoke. We do know that nicotine in thirdhand smoke forms carcinogens that are then inhaled, absorbed, or ingested, increasing the risk of respiratory illnesses and other tobacco-related health problems. Young children who crawl and put objects in their mouths are more likely to come in contact with contaminated surfaces and are therefore the most vulnerable to thirdhand

smoke's harmful effects. Homes of former smokers remained polluted with thirdhand smoke for months after residents quit smoking. Nicotine could be measured in the bodies of nonsmokers who moved into homes that had been smoked in, cleaned, and left empty several months.

ETS Effects   Nonsmokers subjected to ETS frequently develop coughs, headaches, nasal discomfort, and eye irritation. Other symptoms range from breathlessness to sinus problems. People with allergies tend to suffer the most (see the box "Avoiding ETS").

ETS causes an estimated 7300 lung cancer deaths and 34,000 deaths from heart disease each year in people who do not smoke. Exposure to ETS is also associated with a 20% increase in the progression of atherosclerosis and raises the risk of developing heart disease and stroke by up to 30%. ETS aggravates asthma and increases the risk for breast and cervical cancers. For an individual, greater and longer exposure to ETS may be associated with greater risk, although as with many chronic conditions, multiple risk factors are involved.

Scientists have been able to measure changes that contribute to lung tissue damage and potential tumor promotion in the bloodstreams of healthy young people who spend just three hours in a smoke-filled room. After just 30 minutes of exposure to ETS, the function in the coronary arteries of healthy nonsmokers is reduced to the same level as that of smokers. And nonsmokers can still be affected by the harmful effects of ETS hours after they have left a smoky environment. Carbon monoxide, for example, lingers in the bloodstream five hours after exposure.

Infants, Children, and ETS   Infants and children are perhaps the group most vulnerable to the harmful effects of ETS. Recent studies have shown that infants exposed to smoke from more than 21 cigarettes a day are more than *23 times* more likely to die of sudden infant death syndrome (SIDS) than are babies not exposed to ETS. The National

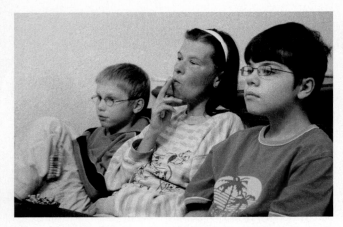

Millions of American infants and children are regularly exposed to environmental tobacco smoke. Kuttig - People/Alamy Stock Photo

Ask Yourself

QUESTIONS FOR CRITICAL THINKING AND REFLECTION

What antismoking ordinances are in effect in your community? Does your school prohibit smoking on campus? Do you think these rules have been effective in reducing smoking or exposure to ETS? Do you support such regulations? Why or why not?

Cancer Institute recently estimated that ETS causes up to 18,600 cases of low birth weight each year. Children under age 5 whose primary caregiver smokes 10 or more cigarettes per day have measurable blood levels of nicotine and tobacco carcinogens. Chemicals in tobacco smoke also show up in breast milk, and breastfeeding may pass more chemicals to the infant of a smoking mother than the infant receives through direct exposure to ETS.

ETS triggers bronchitis, pneumonia, and other respiratory infections in infants and toddlers up to age 18 months, resulting in as many as 15,000 hospitalizations each year.

Older children suffer, too. ETS is a risk factor for asthma and aggravates symptoms in children who already have asthma. ETS is also linked to reduced lung function and fluid buildup in the middle ear, a contributing factor in middle-ear infections, a leading reason for childhood surgery. Children and teens exposed to ETS score lower on tests of reading and reasoning. Later in life, people exposed to ETS as children are at increased risk for lung cancer, emphysema, and chronic bronchitis.

Smoking and Pregnancy

Smoking almost doubles a pregnant woman's chance of having a miscarriage, and it significantly increases her risk of ectopic pregnancy. Maternal smoking causes approximately 1000 infant deaths in the United States each year, primarily due to premature delivery and smoking-related problems with the placenta. Maternal smoking is a major factor in low birth weight, which puts newborns at high risk for infections and other serious problems. If a nonsmoking mother is regularly exposed to ETS, her infant is also at greater risk for low birth weight. Recent studies have also shown that babies whose mothers smoked during pregnancy have higher rates of colic, clubfoot, cleft lip and palate, and impaired lung function; they may also have other genetic damage.

Babies born to mothers who smoke more than two packs a day perform poorly on developmental tests in the first hours after birth, compared to babies of nonsmoking mothers.

Later in life, obesity, hyperactivity, short attention span, and lower scores on spelling and reading tests all occur more frequently in children whose mothers smoked during pregnancy than in those born to nonsmoking mothers. Prenatal tobacco exposure has also been associated with behavioral problems in children, including immaturity, emotional instability, physical aggression, and hyperactivity. Other research shows that teenagers whose mothers smoked during pregnancy have lower scores on tests of general intelligence and poorer performance on tasks requiring auditory memory than do children who were not exposed to cigarette smoke before birth. Males born to smoking mothers have higher rates of adolescent and adult criminal activity, suggesting that maternal smoking may cause brain damage that increases the risk of criminal behavior. Nevertheless, 1 in 14 pregnant women smoked during pregnancy in 2016.

According to the CDC, e-cigarettes are not safe to use during pregnancy. Nicotine can damage a developing baby's brain and lungs, and certain flavorants found in e-cigarettes may also cause harm.

The Cost of Tobacco Use to Society

The annual health care expenditures related to smoking total nearly $170 billion, and the annual cost of lost productivity is about $156 billion. These costs far exceed the tax revenues that states collect on the sale of tobacco products, even though the average cigarette tax was $2.14 per pack in 2019 (including federal taxes) and is rising in some states.

WHAT CAN BE DONE TO COMBAT SMOKING?

There are many ways to act against this public health threat.

Action at the Local Level

Since the 1980s, local government agencies—such as city councils, school boards, and county boards of commissioners—have been passing ordinances designed to discourage smoking in public places. Thousands of local ordinances across the nation now restrict or ban smoking in restaurants, stores, workplaces, and even public outdoor areas. In 2019, nearly 82% of Americans lived in municipalities that restrict or ban smoking in public buildings, workplaces, restaurants, and bars. Hundreds of colleges and universities now have totally smoke-free campuses or prohibit smoking in residential buildings. As local nonsmoking laws proliferate, evidence mounts that environmental restrictions are effective in encouraging smokers to quit.

Action at the State and Federal Levels

State legislatures have passed many tough new anti-tobacco laws. As of 2019, comprehensive smoke-free air laws were in effect in 28 states, the District of Columbia, Puerto Rico, and the U.S. Virgin Islands. These laws prohibit smoking in almost all public areas, as well as in workplaces, restaurants, and bars. But do these bans do more than prevent smoking at certain venues? The answer is yes!

Researchers looked for decreased birth weights and increased prevalence of asthma in young children, which would show evidence for exposure to smoke. They found no such evidence. The workplace bans seemed to be changing behaviors and culture at large. Not only were people smoking less, but they were also exposing coworkers and children at home less. Smoke-free legislation has contributed to a decline in heart disease morbidity and respiratory symptoms; a decrease in acute coronary events; and a decrease in rates of hospital admissions or deaths for cardiac events, other heart diseases, cerebrovascular accidents, and respiratory disease.

Additionally, studies have shown that smoking bans help increase tobacco cessation and reduce tobacco use among adults and youth. After 47 deaths linked to e-cigarettes, cities and some states are starting to ban them. The Trump administration responded to the epidemic of deaths by vowing to ban flavored e-cigarettes but was persuaded by political advisers and lobbyists to abandon the effort.

Do cigarette tax increases affect smoker behavior? Evidence says yes: smokers smoke less when prices go up. But tobacco consumers also find ways around the price increases. Low-income smokers, especially, continue to smoke as much or more because they buy cartons of cigarettes, which are less expensive than individual packs. Other money-saving strategies include buying a cheaper brand, using discounts and coupons, finding a cheaper vendor, rolling their own cigarettes, and sharing fewer cigarettes with others. In addition to consumers' compensating for tax increases, tobacco companies also grant discounts to cigarette retailers to reduce the cost of the cigarettes.

One way to mitigate these countermeasures is to increase taxes on all tobacco products, including cigarettes, cigars, pipe tobacco, and roll-your-own tobacco, as is done by the Children's Health Insurance Program Reauthorization Act of 2009.

California has one of the most aggressive—and successful—tobacco control programs, combining taxes on cigarettes, graphic advertisements, and bans on smoking in bars and

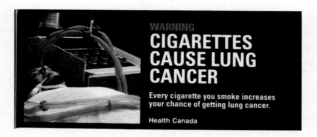

Canada's graphic cigarette labels have greatly helped reduce smoking rates. Staff/Getty Images News/Getty Images

restaurants. California now has the second-lowest rate of smoking (11%) in the U.S. Utah, with a smoking rate of 9%, is the first (and only) state to meet the *Healthy People 2010* target. Kentucky and West Virginia have the highest rates: 25% and 26%, respectively.

FDA Regulation of Tobacco

Tobacco products—all of which are ingested, contain psychoactive drugs, and include many of the same additives used in food products—have historically not been regulated by the FDA. But that changed in 2009 when Congress gave the FDA broad regulatory powers over the production, marketing, and sale of cigarettes. In 2016, this authority was extended to all tobacco products, including e-cigarettes, cigars, and hookah and pipe tobacco, banning their sale to minors and requiring identification for purchase.

As of 2018, the FDA has the authority to do the following:

• Set nicotine standards. Although the FDA is not empowered to ban nicotine outright (Congress retains that power), the agency can dictate how much nicotine is included in tobacco products. In 2017, the FDA proposed a new regulatory effort to decrease the level of nicotine in tobacco products in order to make them less addictive. In late 2019, however, the proposal to reduce nicotine was dropped.

• Enforce tougher rules on the marketing and sales of tobacco products, especially to minors. For example, the FDA can ban tobacco brands from sponsoring sports and entertainment events.

• Make it more difficult for minors to purchase tobacco by requiring retailers to display such products behind the counter in stores. The agency also has the authority to strengthen enforcement and raise penalties to discourage the sale of tobacco products to minors.

• Ban the use of terms such as "light," "mild," or "low" in product advertising and packaging.

• Require bigger, more informative health warnings on tobacco products. The warnings mark the first change in more than 25 years and significantly advance communicating the dangers of smoking. For instance, larger graphic warnings in Canada have been attributed to an estimated 12–20%

reduction in smoking rates between 2000 and 2009. Similar reductions in smoking rates could emerge in the United States once graphic warning labels like those in Canada are implemented.

• Require manufacturers to provide detailed disclosure of their products' ingredients. The disclosures must include nicotine levels, specific additives used, and harmful components in the products' smoke.

• Create a content standard that tobacco products must meet. If needed, the FDA can require manufacturers to modify products to meet the standard.

• Eliminate or control levels of the thousands of chemical additives used to make tobacco more appealing and addictive, and ban all cigarette flavorings, including menthol.

• Regulate so-called reduced harm products. In order to market or sell a product as being less harmful than others, the manufacturer must provide proof of the claim and receive special FDA permission.

• Establish a minimum age of 21 for the purchase of tobacco products.

• Prohibit manufacturers from giving away free samples of cigarettes and restrict the giving away of smokeless products.

• Fund regulatory activity through a user fee on tobacco products, to be collected from manufacturers.

• Protect states' ability to pass other tobacco control laws.

• Regulate electronic cigarette products with the same restrictions as other tobacco products.

The FDA has been criticized for the slow regulation of e-cigarettes and other vaping products. Vaping devices and e-liquids that were on the market before 2016, when the FDA was given authority over tobacco products, do not have explicit FDA authorization. Companies had until May 2020 to retroactively apply for authority, at which point the FDA could remove products or ingredients they found unsafe.

International Action

Many countries are following the United States' lead in restricting smoking. Smoking is now banned on many international air flights, as well as in many restaurants and hotels and on public transportation in some countries. The World Health Organization has taken the lead in international anti-tobacco efforts by sponsoring the Framework Convention on Tobacco Control. Another international activity is the annual commemoration of World No Tobacco Day (May 31), on which smokers are encouraged to stop smoking for one day. (This is similar

to the American Cancer Society's Great American Smokeout, held each November.) The smoker who successfully takes the first step of quitting for a day may be encouraged enough to follow through on the commitment and become a permanent nonsmoker. With more than 1 billion smokers worldwide, addressing the global impact of tobacco use requires a massive coordinated effort.

Action in the Private Sector

The number of smoke-free restaurants has increased dramatically in recent years, and the vast majority of the nation's shopping malls now prohibit smoking. Efforts at the local, state, national, and international levels represent progress, but health activists warn that tobacco industry influence remains strong. The tobacco industry contributes heavily to sympathetic legislative officeholders and candidates. In 1998 alone, it spent almost $73 million on federal lobbying. Since then, the annual amount has dropped to about $20 million per year, but the total is more than $500 million. Many states have relatively weak antismoking laws that are backed by the tobacco industry and include clauses that prevent the passage of stricter local ordinances. During the 2018 election cycle, the industry gave $2.4 million directly to federal candidates.

Individual Action

Nonsmokers have the right not only to breathe clean air but also to take action to help solve one of society's most serious public health threats. Here are just some of the many ways in which individuals can help support tobacco prevention and stop-smoking efforts.

• When a smoker violates a no-smoking designation, complain.

• If your favorite restaurant or shop doesn't have a non-smoking policy, ask the manager to adopt one.

• If you see children buying tobacco, report this illegal activity to the facility manager or the police.

• Learn more about addiction and tobacco cessation so that you can better support the tobacco users you know.

> **QUICK STATS**
>
> If smoking among U.S. youth continues at the current rate, **5.6 million** of today's Americans younger than 18 will die early from a smoking-related illness.
> —Centers for Disease Control and Prevention, 2019

Ask Yourself

QUESTIONS FOR CRITICAL THINKING AND REFLECTION

What are your views on the government's role in regulating tobacco products? Is current regulation enough, or should the government go further in controlling the production and marketing of these products? What events or experiences have shaped your views on this issue?

- Vote for candidates who support anti-tobacco measures; contact local, state, and national representatives to express your views.
- Cancel your subscriptions to magazines that carry tobacco advertising; send a letter to the publisher explaining your decision.
- Voice your opinion about other positive representations of tobacco use. (A recent study found that more than two-thirds of children's animated feature films have featured tobacco or alcohol use with no clear message that such practices were unhealthy.)
- Volunteer with the American Lung Association, the American Cancer Society, or the American Heart Association.

HOW A TOBACCO USER CAN QUIT

Giving up tobacco is a long-term, intricate process. Heavy smokers who say they simply stopped "cold turkey" don't tell of the struggle and mental processes that contributed to their final conquest over this powerful addiction.

Research shows that tobacco users move through predictable stages—from being uninterested in stopping, to thinking about change, to making a serious effort to stop, to finally maintaining abstinence. But most attempt to quit several times before they finally succeed. Relapse is a normal part of the process.

Benefits of Quitting

Giving up tobacco provides immediate health benefits to people of all ages (Table 12.1). People who quit smoking find that food tastes better. Their sense of smell is sharper. Circulation improves, heart rate and blood pressure drop, and lung function and heart efficiency increase. Ex-smokers can breathe more easily, their coughing stops, and their capacity for exercise improves. Many ex-smokers report feeling more energetic and alert. They experience fewer headaches. Even their complexions may improve.

Quitting also has a positive effect on long-term disease risk. From the first day without tobacco, ex-smokers begin to decrease their risk of cancer of the lung, larynx, mouth, pancreas, bladder, cervix, and other organs. Risk of heart attack, stroke, and other cardiovascular diseases drops quickly, too.

The younger people are when they stop smoking, the more pronounced the health improvements. And these improvements gradually but invariably increase as the period of nonsmoking lengthens. It's never too late to quit, though. According to a Surgeon General's report, people who quit smoking, regardless of age, live longer than people who continue to smoke. Even smokers who have already developed chronic bronchitis or emphysema may show some improvement when they quit.

Table 12.1	Benefits of Quitting Smoking

Within 20 minutes of your last cigarette:
- Blood pressure drops to normal
- Pulse rate drops to normal
- Temperature of hands and feet increases to normal
- You stop polluting the air

8 hours:
- Carbon monoxide level in blood drops to normal
- Oxygen level in blood increases to normal

24 hours:
- Chance of heart attack decreases

48 hours:
- Nerve endings start regrowing
- Ability to smell and taste is enhanced

2–3 months:
- Circulation improves
- Walking becomes easier
- Lung function increases up to 30%

1–9 months:
- Coughing, sinus congestion, fatigue, and shortness of breath all decrease

1 year:
- Heart disease death rate is half that of a smoker

5 years:
- Stroke risk drops nearly to the risk for nonsmokers

10 years:
- Lung cancer death rate drops to 50% of that of continuing smokers
- Incidence of other cancers (mouth, throat, larynx, esophagus, bladder, kidney, and pancreas) decreases
- Risk of ulcer decreases

15 years:
- Risk of lung cancer is about 25% of that of continuing smokers
- Risks of heart disease and death are close to those of nonsmokers

SOURCES: American Cancer Society. 2018. *Benefits of Quitting Smoking Over Time* (https://www.cancer.org/healthy/stay-away-from-tobacco/benefits-of-quitting-smoking-over-time.html); U.S. National Library of Medicine. 2017. *Benefits of Quitting Tobacco* (https://www.nlm.nih.gov /medlineplus/ency/article/007532.htm).

Options for Quitting

More than two-thirds of adult tobacco users want to quit, and the majority will make an attempt this year. What are their options? No single method works for everyone, but each works for some people some of the time. In June 2000, the U.S. Public Health Service issued guidelines for medical professionals on how to help their patients quit smoking, emphasizing the benefits of both behavioral and pharmacological interventions. In 2008, the agency updated those guidelines and urged all physicians to provide antismoking intervention and treatment to all their patients who use tobacco. In essence, the health service set a goal of

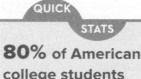

QUICK STATS

80% of American college students report that they have never smoked a cigarette.
—American College Health Association, 2019

The U.S. Public Health Service suggests a "5 Rs" strategy to enhance motivation to quit. If you are a smoker or are trying to help one, think about these areas of concern and see if they help develop a desire and readiness to make a real attempt at quitting.

• **Relevance.** Think about the personal relevance of quitting tobacco use. What would be the effects on your family and friends? How would your daily life improve? What is the most important way that quitting would change your life?

• **Risks.** Immediate risks include shortness of breath, infertility, and impotence, and long-term risks include cancer, heart disease, and respiratory problems. Remember, smoking is harmful both to you and to anyone you expose to your smoke.

• **Rewards.** The list of the rewards of quitting is almost endless, including improving immediate and long-term health, saving money, and feeling better about yourself. You can also stop worrying about quitting and set a good example for others.

• **Roadblocks.** What are the potential obstacles to quitting? Are you worried about withdrawal symptoms, weight gain, or lack of support? How can you overcome these barriers?

• **Repetition.** Revisit your reasons for quitting and strengthen your resolve until you are ready to prepare a plan. Most people make several attempts to quit before they succeed. Relapsing does not mean that you will never succeed.

---

helping every American smoker to quit—not just those who ask their doctors for help.

Behavior Change Choosing to quit requires developing a strategy for success (see the box "Strategies to Quit Smoking"). Some people quit cold turkey, whereas others taper off slowly. Over-the-counter and prescription products help many people. Support from others and regular exercise are behavioral factors that have been shown to increase the chances that a smoker will stop smoking permanently. Support can come from friends and family and/or formal group programs sponsored by organizations such as the American Cancer Society and the American Lung Association, or by a college health center or community hospital. Programs that combine group support with nicotine replacement therapy have rates of continued abstention as high as 35% after one year.

Most smokers in the process of quitting experience both physical and psychological effects of nicotine withdrawal, and exercise can help with both. For many smokers, tobacco use is associated with certain times and places—following a meal, for example. Resolving to walk after dinner instead of lighting up provides a distraction from cravings and eliminates the cues that trigger a desire to smoke. In addition, many people worry about weight gain associated with quitting. Although most ex-smokers do gain a few pounds, at least temporarily, incorporating exercise into a new tobacco-free routine lays the foundation for healthy weight management. The health risks of adding a few pounds are minimal compared to the risks of continued smoking. It's estimated that a smoker would have to gain 75–100 pounds to equal the health risks of smoking a pack a day.

Telephone Quitlines The use of free telephone quitlines are emerging as a popular and effective way to get help to stop smoking. Quitlines are staffed by trained counselors who help each caller plan a personal quitting strategy, usually including a combination of nicotine replacement therapy, changes in daily habits, and emotional support. Counselors provide printed materials that match the smoker's needs and schedule phone counseling sessions for key days after a smoker quits. Smokers can arrange for sessions to fit their schedule, and some quitlines may provide stop-smoking medications at reduced prices. Almost all smokers make more than one attempt to stop before they succeed in quitting for good; quitline counselors can help smokers understand what leads to relapse, review their reasons for wanting to quit, and make a better plan for the next attempt. The goal is for smokers to find a support system and techniques that work for them.

HHS has a national toll-free number, 1-800-QUITNOW (1-800-784-8669), to serve as a single access point for smokers seeking information and assistance in quitting. Callers are routed to their state's smoking cessation quitline or, in states that have not established quitlines, to one maintained by the National Cancer Institute.

As with any significant change in health-related behavior, giving up tobacco requires planning, sustained effort, and support. It is an ongoing process, not a one-time event. The "Kicking the Tobacco Habit" box at the end of the chapter describes the steps that successful quitters follow.

Smoking Cessation Products Each year millions of Americans visit their doctors in the hope of finding a drug that can help them stop smoking. Although pharmacological options are limited, the few available drugs have proved successful.

CHANTIX (VARENICLINE) The newest smoking cessation drug, marketed under the name Chantix, works in two ways: It reduces nicotine cravings, easing the withdrawal process, and it blocks the pleasant effects of nicotine. The drug acts on neurotransmitter receptors in the brain.

Six clinical trials, which included more than 3600 long-term, chronic smokers, demonstrated that Chantix is an effective smoking cessation aid. In one of the studies, nearly 25% of Chantix users stopped smoking for a full year. Results varied with the dosage and duration of treatment.

Unlike most smoking cessation products currently on the market, Chantix is not a nicotine replacement. For this reason, smokers may be advised to continue smoking for the first few days of treatment to avoid withdrawal and to allow the drug to build up in their bodies. The approved course of treatment is 12 weeks, but the duration and recommended dosage depend on several factors, including the smoker's general health and the length and severity of his or her nicotine addiction.

Side effects reported with Chantix include nausea, headaches, vomiting, sleep disruptions, and changes in taste perception. People with kidney problems or who take certain medications should not take Chantix, and it is not recommended for women who are pregnant or nursing. Further, the FDA has been investigating reports of the drug causing adverse reactions, such as behavioral changes, agitation, depression, suicidal thoughts, and attempted suicide. Anyone taking Chantix should immediately notify his or her doctor of any sudden change in mood or behavior.

ZYBAN (BUPROPION) Bupropion is an antidepressant (prescribed under the name Wellbutrin) as well as a smoking cessation aid (prescribed under the name Zyban). As a smoking cessation aid, bupropion eases the symptoms of nicotine withdrawal and reduces the urge to smoke. Like Chantix, it acts on neurotransmitter receptors in the brain.

Bupropion is not a nicotine replacement, so the user may need to continue smoking for the first few days of treatment. A nicotine replacement product, such as a patch or gum, may be recommended to further ease withdrawal symptoms after the user stops smoking.

Bupropion users have reported an array of side effects, but they are rare. Side effects may be reduced by changing the dosage, taking the medicine at a different time of day, or taking it with or without food. Bupropion is not recommended for people with specific physical conditions or who take certain drugs. Zyban and Wellbutrin should not be taken together.

NICOTINE REPLACEMENT PRODUCTS The most widely used smoking cessation products replace the nicotine that the user would normally get from tobacco. The user continues to get nicotine, so withdrawal symptoms and cravings are reduced. Although still harmful, nicotine replacement products provide a cleaner form of nicotine without the thousands of poisons and tars produced by burning tobacco. Less of the product is used over time as the need for nicotine decreases.

Nicotine replacement products come in several forms, including patches, gum, lozenges, nasal sprays, and inhalers. They are available in a variety of strengths and can be worked into many different smoking cessation strategies. Most are available without a prescription.

The nicotine patch is popular because it can be applied and forgotten until it needs to be removed or changed, usually every 16 or 24 hours. Placed on the upper arm or torso, it releases a steady stream of nicotine, which is absorbed through the skin. The main side effects are skin irritation and redness. Nicotine gum and nicotine lozenges have the advantage of allowing the smoker to use them whenever he or she craves nicotine. Side effects of nicotine gum include mouth sores and headaches; nicotine lozenges can cause nausea and heartburn. Nicotine nasal sprays and inhalers are available only by prescription.

Although all these products have proved to be effective in helping users stop smoking, experts recommend them only as one part of a complete smoking cessation program. Such a program should include regular professional counseling and physician monitoring.

TIPS FOR TODAY AND THE FUTURE

For most smokers, quitting is one of the hardest things they'll ever do.

RIGHT NOW YOU CAN:
- If you smoke, throw away the pack and lighter.
- If you smoke, think about the next time you'll want a cigarette, such as while talking on the phone this afternoon or relaxing after dinner tonight. Visualize yourself enjoying this activity without smoking.
- If you use tobacco, go outside for a short walk or a stretch to limber up. Breathe deeply. Tell a friend you've just decided to quit.

IN THE FUTURE YOU CAN:
- Resolve to talk to someone you know who uses tobacco, offering support and assistance if the person is interested in quitting.
- Resolve to quit smoking. Research your options for quitting and choose the one you think will work best for you.
- Recruit a friend or family member to help you quit smoking. Arrange to talk to this person whenever you feel the urge to smoke.

SUMMARY

- Smoking is the largest preventable cause of premature disease and death in the United States. Nevertheless, millions of Americans use tobacco.

- Regular tobacco use causes physical dependence on nicotine, characterized by loss of control, tolerance, and withdrawal. Habits can become associated with tobacco use and trigger the urge for a cigarette.

- People who begin smoking are usually imitating others or responding to seductive advertising. Smoking is associated with low education level and the use of other drugs.

- Tobacco smoke is made up of thousands of chemicals, including some that are carcinogenic or toxic or that damage the respiratory system.

- Nicotine acts on the nervous system as a stimulant or a depressant. It can cause blood pressure and heart rate to increase, straining the heart.

BEHAVIOR CHANGE STRATEGY
Kicking the Tobacco Habit

Congratulations! You've decided to quit smoking. You likely already know that your first day without cigarettes may be difficult. Here are six steps you can take to handle your "quit day" and be confident about being able to stay quit.

1. Make a Quit Plan

Having a quit plan helps you stay focused, confident, and motivated to quit. No single approach to quitting works for everyone. If you don't know what quit method might be right for you, visit the Quit Smoking Methods Explorer (http://smokefree.gov/explore-quit-methods) to learn more. As part of your plan, identify your reasons for quitting: for example, to be healthier, save money, smell better, relieve the worrying of your loved ones.

2. Set a Quit Date

Choose a date within the next two weeks. This will give you enough time to prepare:

- Start to get rid of smoking reminders—e.g., wash your clothes, clean your car, get rid of matches and ashtrays.
- Identify your smoking triggers. Triggers are the people, places, things, and situations that set off your urge to smoke. Some are emotional, such as feeling stressed or down; others are habitual, such as talking on the phone or drinking alcohol; still others are social, such as going to a bar or a party. Being aware of your triggers will help you avoid them or think of strategies for defusing them.
- Consider how you will fight the inevitable cravings—for example, think of ways to keep your hands and mouth busy; find new ways to relieve stress or improve your mood.

3. Stay Busy on Your Quit Day

Being busy will help you keep your mind off smoking and distract you from cravings. Try some of these activities:

- Go out for walks. Notice details about your neighborhood.
- Chew gum or hard candy.
- Keep your hands busy with a pen or toothpick.
- Drink lots of water.
- Relax with deep breathing.
- Go to a movie.
- Spend time with nonsmoking friends and family.
- Go to dinner at your favorite smoke-free restaurant.

4. Avoid Smoking Triggers

On your quit day, try to avoid all your triggers.

- Throw away all your cigarettes, lighters, and ash trays if you haven't already.
- Avoid caffeine, which can make you feel jittery. Try drinking water instead.

- Spend time with nonsmokers.
- Go to places where smoking isn't allowed.
- Get plenty of rest and eat healthy foods. Being tired can trigger you to smoke.
- Change your routine to avoid the things you associate with smoking.

5. Stay Positive

Quitting smoking is difficult. It happens one minute . . . one hour . . . one day at a time. Try not to think of quitting as forever. Pay attention to *today,* and the time will add up. Your quit day might not be perfect; what matters is that you don't smoke—not even one puff. Reward yourself for being smoke-free for 24 hours. You deserve it.

6. Ask for Help

You don't need to rely on willpower alone to be smoke-free. Tell your family and friends when your quit day is. Ask them for support on quit day and in the first few days and weeks after. Let them know exactly how they can support you. Don't assume they'll know. Be honest about your needs. If using nicotine replacement therapy is part of your plan, be sure to start using it first thing in the morning. Finally, Smokefree.gov has many tools to help you, including a text message program, apps to help you track cravings and monitor your progress, online chats with a cessation counselor, and a Facebook page.

SOURCES: Smokefree.gov. n.d. Build Your Quit Plan (http://smokefree.gov/build-your-quit-plan); Smokefree.gov. n.d. *Quit Day: 5 Steps* (http://smokefree.gov /steps-on-quit-day).

- Cardiovascular disease is the most widespread cause of death for cigarette smokers. Cigarette smoking is the primary cause of lung cancer and is linked to many other cancers and respiratory diseases.

- Cigarette smoking is linked to ulcers, impotence, reproductive health problems, dental diseases, and other conditions. Tobacco use leads to lower life expectancy and to a diminished quality of life.

- The use of smokeless tobacco leads to nicotine addiction and is linked to a variety of cancers of the head and neck.

- Cigars, pipes, clove cigarettes, bidis, hookahs, and e-cigarettes are not safe alternatives to cigarettes. Using them results in lung, lip, larynx, and pancreatic cancers, COPD, and emphysema, among other conditions.

- Environmental tobacco smoke (ETS) contains high concentrations of toxic chemicals and can cause headaches, eye and nasal irritation, and sinus problems. Long-term exposure to ETS causes cancer and heart disease. Both secondhand and thirdhand smoke contribute to these devastating effects.

- Infants and young children take in more pollutants than adults do; children whose parents smoke are especially susceptible to respiratory diseases.

- Smoking during pregnancy increases the risk of miscarriage, stillbirth, congenital abnormalities, premature birth, and low birth weight. SIDS, behavior problems, and long-term impairments in development are also risks to infants and children of mothers who smoke during pregnancy.

- The overall cost of tobacco use to society includes the cost of both medical care and lost worker productivity.

- Individuals and groups have many options for acting against tobacco use. Nonsmokers can use social pressure and legislative channels to assert their rights to breathe clean air.

- Giving up smoking is a difficult and long-term process. Although most ex-smokers quit on their own, some smokers benefit from stop-smoking programs, over-the-counter and prescription medications, and support groups.

FOR MORE INFORMATION

Action on Smoking and Health (ASH). Provides statistics, news briefs, and other information.

http://ash.org

American Cancer Society (ACS). Provides information about the dangers of tobacco, as well as tools for prevention and cessation for both smokers and users of smokeless tobacco; sponsors the annual Great American Smokeout.

http://www.cancer.org

American Lung Association. Provides information about lung diseases, tobacco control, and environmental health.

http://www.lungusa.org

CDC's Tobacco Information and Prevention Source (TIPS). Provides research results, educational materials, and tips on how to quit smoking; website includes special sections for kids and teens.

http://www.cdc.gov/tobacco

Center for Responsive Politics (CRP). A nonprofit, nonpartisan research group based in Washington, DC, that tracks the effects of money and lobbying on elections and public policy, including spending and lobbying by the tobacco industry.

http://www.opensecrets.org

Environmental Protection Agency Indoor Air Quality/ETS. Provides information and links about secondhand smoke.

https://www.epa.gov/indoor-air-quality-iaq/secondhand-smoke -and-smoke-free-homes

Nicotine Anonymous. A 12-step program for tobacco users.

http://www.nicotine-anonymous.org

Smokefree.gov. Provides step-by-step strategies for quitting as well as expert support via telephone or instant messaging.

http://www.smokefree.gov

Tobacco BBS. A resource center on tobacco and smoking issues that includes news and information, assistance for smokers who want to quit, and links to related sites.

http://www.tobacco.org

World Health Organization Tobacco Free Initiative. Promotes the goal of a tobacco-free world.

http://www.who.int/tobacco/en

World No Tobacco Day (WNTD). Provides information about the annual worldwide event to encourage people to quit smoking; includes general information about tobacco use and testimonials of ex-smokers.

https://www.who.int/tobacco/wntd/en/

See also the listings for Chapters 10, 16, and 17.

SELECTED BIBLIOGRAPHY

Allen, J. G., et al. 2016. Flavoring chemicals in e-cigarettes: Diacetyl, 2, 3-pentanedione, and acetoin in a sample of 51 products, including fruit-, candy-, and cocktail-flavored e-cigarettes. *Environmental Health Perspectives* 124(6) (http://ehp.niehs.nih.gov/15-10185/).

American Cancer Society. 2019. *Cancer Facts and Figures, 2019.* Atlanta, GA: American Cancer Society.

American College Health Association. 2019. *American College Health Association–National College Health Assessment IIc: Reference Group Executive Summary Spring 2019.* Hanover, MD: American College Health Association.

American Lung Association. 2019. *Smokefree Air Laws* (http://www.lung.org/policy-advocacy/tobacco/smokefree-environments/smokefree-air -laws.html).

American Lung Association. 2019. *What's in a Cigarette?* (https://www.lung.org/stop-smoking/smoking-facts/whats-in-a-cigarette.html)

American Nonsmokers' Rights Foundation. 2020. *Overview List –Number of Smokefree and Other Tobacco-Related Laws* (http://no-smoke.org /wp-content/uploads/pdf/mediaordlist.pdf).

Andrews, M. 2019. Cigarettes can't be advertised on TV. Should Juul ads be permitted? National Public Radio (https://www.npr.org/sections/health -shots/2019/08/20/752553108/cigarettes-cant-be-advertised-on-tv-should -juul-ads-be-permitted).

Armstrong, D., and Bloomberg. 2019. Slashing cigarette nicotine levels no longer on FDA's agenda. *Fortune* (https://fortune.com/2019/11/20/fda -nicotine-plan-cigarettes-no-longer-on-agenda/).

Booker, B. 2019. TV broadcasters to stop taking e-cigarette ads. National Public Radio (https://www.npr.org/sections/health-shots/2019/09/19 /762410165/tv-broadcasters-to-stop-taking-e-cigarette-ads).

Campaign for Tobacco-Free Kids. 2020. *State Cigarette Excise Tax Rates and Rankings.* Washington, DC: Campaign for Tobacco-Free Kids.

Campaign for Tobacco-Free Kids. 2018. *Tobacco Company Political Action Committee (PAC) Contributions to Federal Candidates* (https://www .tobaccofreekids.org/what_we_do/federal_issues/campaign_contributions).

Center for Responsive Politics. 2019. *Tobacco: Industry Profile: Summary,* 2019 (https://www.opensecrets.org/lobby/indusclient.php?id=A02).

Center for Responsive Politics. 2019. *Tobacco: Opensecrets* (https://www .opensecrets.org/industries/lobbying.php?cycle=2018&ind=A02).

Centers for Disease Control and Prevention. 2018. *Lesbian, Gay, Bisexual, and Transgender Persons and Tobacco Use* (https://www.cdc.gov/tobacco /disparities/lgbt/index.htm).

Centers for Disease Control and Prevention. 2018. *Smoking & Tobacco Use: Tobacco-Related Mortality* (https://www.cdc.gov/tobacco/data_statistics /fact_sheets/health_effects/tobacco_related_mortality/index.htm#cigs).

Centers for Disease Control and Prevention. 2019. Current cigarette smoking among adults–United States, 2018. *MMWR* 68(45): 1013–1019.

Centers for Disease Control and Prevention. 2019. *Economic Trends in Tobacco* (https://www.cdc.gov/tobacco/data_statistics/fact_sheets/economics /econ_facts/index.htm).

Centers for Disease Control and Prevention. 2019. *Smoking & Tobacco Use* (https://www.cdc.gov/tobacco/data_statistics/fact_sheets/index.htm).

Centers for Disease Control and Prevention. 2019. *Smoking & Tobacco Use: Youth and Tobacco Use* (https://www.cdc.gov/tobacco/data_statistics /fact_sheets/youth_data/tobacco_use/index.htm).

Centers for Disease Control and Prevention. 2019. *State Tobacco Activities Tracking and Evaluation (STATE) System* (http://www.cdc.gov /STATESystem).

Centers for Disease Control and Prevention. 2020. *Outbreak of Lung Injury Associated with the Use of E-Cigarette, or Vaping, Products* (https://www.cdc.gov/tobacco/basic_information/e-cigarettes/severe-lung-disease.html).

Centers for Disease Control and Prevention. 2020. *Smoking & Tobacco Use: Secondhand Smoke* (https://www.cdc.gov/tobacco/basic_information/secondhand_smoke/index.htm).

Choi, K., and R. G. Boyle. 2018. Changes in cigarette expenditure minimising strategies before and after a cigarette tax increase. *Tobacco Control* 27(1): 99-104.

Creamer, M. R., et al. 2016. College students' perceptions and knowledge of hookah use. *Drug and Alcohol Dependence* 168: 191-195.

Creamer, M. R., et al. 2019. Tobacco product use and cessation indicators among adults — United States, 2018. *MMWR* 68:1013-1019.

Dean, M. 2007. *Empty Cribs: The Impact of Smoking on Child Health.* New York: Arts & Sciences Publishing.

Division of Reproductive Health, National Center for Chronic Disease Prevention and Health Promotion. 2019. *Tobacco Use and Pregnancy* (http://www.cdc.gov/reproductivehealth/TobaccoUsePregnancy/index.htm).

Drake, P., A. K. Driscoll, and T. J. Mathews. 2018. Cigarette smoking during pregnancy: United States, 2016. *NCHS Data Brief* 305. Hyattsville, MD: National Center for Health Statistics (https://www.cdc.gov/nchs/products/databriefs/db305.htm).

Ducharme, J. 2019. As the number of vaping-related deaths climbs, these states have implemented e-cigarette bans. *Time* (https://time.com/5685936/state-vaping-bans/).

Federal Trade Commission. 2019. *Federal Trade Commission Cigarette Report for 2017.* Washington, DC: Federal Trade Commission.

Food and Drug Administration. 2019. *How FDA Is Regulating E-Cigarettes* (https://www.fda.gov/news-events/fda-voices/how-fda-regulating-e-cigarettes).

Jha, P., et al. 2013. 21st century hazards of smoking and benefits of cessation in the United States. *New England Journal of Medicine* 368: 341-350.

Johnston, L. D., et al. 2017. *Monitoring the Future National Results on Adolescent Drug Use 1975-2017: Overview of Key Findings.* Ann Arbor: Institute for Social Research, University of Michigan.

Kaplan, R. M. 2020. Cancer deaths, smoking, and Rodney Dangerfield. *Health Affairs* (https://www.healthaffairs.org/do/10.1377/hblog20200417.775123/full/).

Karama, S., et al. 2015. Cigarette smoking and thinning of the brain's cortex. *Molecular Psychiatry* 20: 778-785.

Karni, A., M. Haberman, and S. Kaplan. 2019. Trump retreats from flavor ban for e-cigarettes. *The New York Times*, 17 November (https://www.nytimes.com/2019/11/17/health/trump-vaping-ban.html).

Kochanek K. D., et al. 2017. Mortality in the United States, 2016. *NCHS Data Brief* 293. Hyattsville, MD: National Center for Health Statistics.

Krüsemann, E. J. Z., et al. 2018. Identification of flavour additives in tobacco products to develop a flavour library. *Tobacco Control* 27(1): 105-111.

Li, X., A. Loukas, and C. L. Perry. 2018. Very light smoking and alternative tobacco use among college students. *Addictive Behaviors* 81: 22-25.

Matt, G., et al. 2017. When smokers quit: Exposure to nicotine and carcinogens persists from thirdhand smoke pollution. *Tobacco Control* 26(5): 548-556.

Maxwell, J. C. 2016. *The Maxwell Report: Year End & Fourth Quarter 2015 Cigarette Industry.* Richmond, VA: John C. Maxwell, Jr.

McDaniel, P. A., and R. E. Malone. 2009. Creating the "desired mindset": Philip Morris's efforts to improve its corporate image among women. *Women & Health* [published online], October 21.

McGeary, K. A., et al. 2017. *Impact of Comprehensive Smoking Bans on the Health of Infants and Children.* Working Paper 23995. Cambridge, MA: National Bureau of Economic Research.

National Institute on Drug Abuse. 2018. *Cigarette Smoking Increases the Likelihood of Drug Use Relapse* (https://www.drugabuse.gov/news-events/nida-notes/2018/05/cigarette-smoking-increases-likelihood-drug-use-relapse).

NIH/National Institute on Deafness and Other Communication Disorders. 2019. Genetic Vulnerability to Menthol Cigarette Use: Unexpected Sensory Variant Exclusive to African-Americans (https://www.nidcd.nih.gov/news/2019/researchers-find-genetic-vulnerability-menthol-cigarette-use).

Perrone, M. 2014. Senators warn of carcinogen risk with e-cigarettes. *Associated Press, SFGate,* May 8.

Rosenberry, Z. R., W. B. Pickworth, and B. Koszowski. 2018. Large cigars: Smoking topography and toxicant exposure. *Nicotine & Tobacco Research* 20(2): 183-191.

RTI International. 2017. Gene that influences nicotine dependence identified: Discovery creates the possibility for new research in addiction treatment. *ScienceDaily,* 10 October (https://www.sciencedaily.com/releases/2017/10/171010124112.htm).

SAMHSA Center for Behavioral Health Statistics and Quality. 2019. *Results from the 2018 National Survey on Drug Use and Health* (https://www.samhsa.gov/data/sites/default/files/cbhsq-reports/NSDUHDetailedTabs2018R2/NSDUHDetailedTabs2018.pdf).

SAMHSA Newsroom. 2017. Report Shows That 8.7 Million Americans Used Smokeless Tobacco in the Past Month (https://www.samhsa.gov/data/sites/default/files/cbhsq-reports/NSDUHFFR2017/NSDUHFFR2017.pdf).

Schaeffer, K. 2019. Before recent outbreak, vaping was on the rise in U.S., especially among young people. *Pew Research Center* (https://www.pewresearch.org/fact-tank/2019/09/26/vaping-survey-data-roundup/).

Schulenberg, J. E., et al. 2017. *Monitoring the Future National Survey Results on Drug Use, 1975-2016; Volumne II, College Students and Adults Ages 19-55.* Ann Arbor: Institute for Social Research, The University of Michigan.

Schulenberg, J. E., et al. 2019. *Monitoring the Future National Survey Results on Drug Use, 1975-2018; Volume II, College Students and Adults Ages 19-60.* Ann Arbor: Institute for Social Research, The University of Michigan.

Schweitzer, K. S., et al. 2015. Endothelial disruptive pro-inflammatory effects of nicotine and e-cigarette vapor exposures. *American Journal of Physiology-Lung Cellular and Molecular Physiology.* DOI: 10.1152/ajplung.00411.2014.

Sleiman, M., et al. 2010. Formation of carcinogens indoors by surface-mediated reactions of nicotine with nitrous acid, leading to potential thirdhand smoke hazards. *Proceedings of the National Academy of Sciences* 107(15): 6576-6581.

Titus-Ernstoff, L., et al. 2008. Longitudinal study of viewing smoking in movies and initiation of smoking by children. *Pediatrics* 121(1): 15-21.

U.S. Department of Health and Human Services. 2014. *The Health Consequences of Smoking—50 Years of Progress: A Report of the Surgeon General.* Atlanta, GA: HHS, Centers for Disease Control and Prevention, National Center for Chronic Disease Prevention and Health Promotion, Office on Smoking and Health.

U.S. Department of Health and Human Services. 2016. *E-Cigarette Use Among Youth and Young Adults. A Report of the Surgeon General.* Atlanta, GA: HHS, Centers for Disease Control and Prevention, National Center for Chronic Disease Prevention and Health Promotion, Office on Smoking and Health.

U.S. Department of Health and Human Services. 2020. *Smoking Cessation: A Report of the Surgeon General.* Atlanta, GA: HHS, Centers for Disease Control and Prevention, National Center for Chronic Disease Prevention and Health Promotion, Office on Smoking and Health.

U.S. Food and Drug Administration Center for Tobacco Products. 2019. *Vaporizers, E-Cigarettes, and other Electronic Nicotine Delivery Systems (ENDS).* (https://www.fda.gov/tobacco-products/products-ingredients-components/vaporizers-e-cigarettes-and-other-electronic-nicotine-delivery-systems-ends).

U.S. Surgeon General. 2006. *The Health Consequences of Involuntary Exposure to Tobacco Smoke* (http://www.surgeongeneral.gov/library/secondhandsmoke/report/).

Zhang, J., et al. 2014. Comparison of clinical features between non-smokers with COPD and smokers with COPD: A retrospective observational study. *International Journal of Chronic Obstructive Pulmonary Disease* 9: 57-63.

- List the components of a healthy diet
- Explain how to make informed choices about foods
- Put together a personal nutrition plan

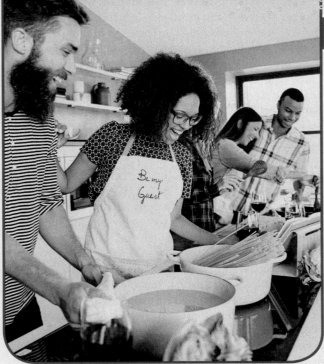
Flamingo Images/Shutterstock

CHAPTER **13**

Nutrition Basics

TEST YOUR KNOWLEDGE

1. It is recommended that adults consume only one serving of fruits and one of vegetables every day.
   True or False?

2. How many french fries are considered to be one half-cup serving?
   a. 10
   b. 15
   c. 25

3. Candy is the leading source of added sugars in the American diet.
   True or False?

4. Which of the following is not likely to be a whole grain?
   a. Brown rice
   b. Wheat flour
   c. Popcorn

5. Which of the following are important food safety principles?
   a. Use or freeze fresh meats within 1 day of purchase.
   b. Cook hamburgers to at least 160°F.
   c. If a food looks and smells fine, it is safe.
   d. If you are a young child or an older person, you should not drink unpasteurized juices or unpasteurized milk.

ANSWERS

1. **FALSE.** The recommendation for someone consuming 2000 calories daily is 2½ cups (3-5 servings) of vegetables and 2 cups (2-4 servings) of fruit.

2. **A.** Many people underestimate the size of the portions they eat, leading them to exceed their recommended daily intakes for total energy and fat.

3. **FALSE.** Regular (nondiet) sodas are the leading source of sugar, with an average of 55 gallons consumed per person per year. Each 12-ounce soda supplies about 10 teaspoons of sugar, or nearly 10% of the calories in a 2000-calorie diet.

4. **B.** Unless labeled as whole wheat, wheat flour is processed to remove the bran and the germ and is not a whole grain.

5. **B AND D.** Use or freeze fresh meats within 3–5 days and fresh poultry, fish, and ground meat within 1–2 days; cook hamburgers to at least 160°F. Even if a food looks and smells fine, it may not be safe. If you are a young child or an older person, or pregnant, you should not drink unpasteurized (raw) juices or unpasteurized milk.

iane, a college nutrition instructor, gave her students a challenging assignment: "Write about a time when you changed something in your life because of something you learned in nutrition class." She was impressed with her students' responses—and with one student's in particular.

Hannah reported having gone to her parents' house for dinner the evening following a class lecture on sodium. Hannah first observed her father with his leg propped up on a chair because of a swollen ankle. She watched him take one of his blood pressure pills with a glass of wine. At dinner, before even tasting his rice, vegetables, and fish, he proceeded to salt everything. She wondered whether his swollen ankle and high blood pressure were related and possibly the result of his oversalting.

Hannah suggested to her father that he not salt his food for one month to see what would happen. He agreed. After just two weeks, his ankle returned to its normal size, and his blood pressure dropped enough that he wondered whether he still needed to take his medication. Outcomes such as this are just one reason why Diane loves being a nutrition instructor.

This chapter examines the role of personal dietary choices and the basic principles of **nutrition**. It introduces the six classes of essential nutrients and explains their roles in health and disease. It also provides guidelines for designing a healthy diet plan. The chapter emphasizes the importance of making a personal commitment to eating right, engaging in physical activity, and staying educated about public health policies, current food systems, and global nutrition trends.

COMPONENTS OF A HEALTHY DIET

If you're like most people, you think about your diet in terms of the foods you like to eat. More important for your health, though, are the nutrients contained in those foods. Your body requires proteins, fats, carbohydrates, vitamins, minerals, and water—about 45 **essential nutrients.** In this context, the word *essential* means that you must get these substances from food because your body is unable to manufacture them or make an adequate amount to meet your physiological needs. The six classes of nutrients, along with their functions and major sources, are listed in Table 13.1. The body needs some essential nutrients in relatively large amounts; these **macronutrients** include protein, fat, carbohydrate, and water. **Micronutrients,** such as vitamins and minerals, are required in much smaller amounts. This section reviews the functions, sources, and recommendations for each class of nutrients; in the next section, we'll focus on the guidelines for patterns of food choices that can help you meet these nutrient goals.

Choosing foods that provide the nutrients you need while limiting the substances linked to disease should be an important part of your daily life. Your dietary needs change as you

TERMS

nutrition   The science of food and dietary supplements, and how the body uses them in health and disease.

essential nutrients   Dietary components the body must get from foods or supplements because it cannot manufacture them to meet its needs.

macronutrient   An important nutrient required by the body in relatively large amounts.

micronutrient   An important nutrient required by the body in minute amounts.

Table 13.1	The Six Major Classes of Dietary Components	
NUTRIENT	**FUNCTION**	**MAJOR SOURCES**
Proteins	Form important parts of muscles, bone, blood, enzymes, some hormones, and cell membranes, which are essential for growth and repair of tissue; regulate water and acid–base balance; help maintain a healthy immune system; used for energy supply in case of excess protein intake or insufficient energy intake	Meat (e.g., beef, pork, fish, poultry), eggs, milk, milk products, legumes, quinoa, and nuts
Carbohydrates	Provide main source of energy for cells in all body parts including the brain, nervous system, blood, and muscles at rest and during exercise	Grains in form of breads and cereals, fruits, vegetables, milk, and natural and added sugars
Fats	Supply energy; insulate, support, and cushion organs; provide medium for absorption of fat-soluble vitamins; contribute in the regulation of function of various genes (gene expression)	Animal foods, grains, nuts, seeds, fish, and vegetables
Vitamins	Promote specific chemical reactions within cells, and influence the regulation of gene expression	Abundant in fruits, vegetables, grains, liver, and dairy products; found either naturally or through food fortification
Minerals	Help regulate body functions; aid in growth and maintenance of body tissues; act as catalysts for release of energy	Found in most food groups naturally; fortified foods may contain minerals (e.g., calcium in some juices)
Water	Provides medium for chemical reactions; transports chemicals; regulates temperature; removes waste products	Beverages including water and juices, fresh fruits and vegetables, and cooked semisolid foods

go through different life stages, guided by your current energy needs, daily nutrient requirements, locally available foods, foods you choose to eat, and your health condition. When you are actively involved in sports, for example, your energy needs will be higher than when you are inactive, even if your age and body size remain the same. Similarly, energy needs for lactating mothers are higher than those for nonlactating mothers with similar body size and physical activity levels.

Most nutrients become available to the body through the process of **digestion,** in which the foods we eat are broken down into compounds the gastrointestinal tract can absorb and that the body processes further and uses for normal body functions (Figure 13.1). An adequate diet must provide enough essential nutrients and energy to support and regulate various vital body functions.

Energy

The amount of energy in foods is expressed as **kilocalories (kcal)**. One kilocalorie represents the amount of heat required to raise the temperature of 1 liter of water by 1°C. An average person needs about 2000 kilocalories per day to meet his or her energy needs. Although technically inaccurate, people usually refer to kilocalories as *calories*. This chapter uses the term *calorie* when discussing the energy unit, and food labels do as well. What's the difference between "energy" and "calorie?" **Energy** is the capacity to do work. Calories are used to measure energy. The energy in food is chemical energy, which the body converts to mechanical, electrical, or heat energy.

Of the six broad classes of essential nutrients, three supply energy:

- Fat = 9 calories per gram
- Protein = 4 calories per gram
- Carbohydrate = 4 calories per gram

Alcohol, though not an essential component of our diet, also supplies energy, providing 7 calories per gram. (One gram equals a little less than 0.04 ounce.) Certain calories consumed in excess of your energy needs may be converted into fat that is then stored in the body.

Just meeting energy needs is not enough. Our bodies also need an adequate amount of the essential nutrients to function properly. Many Americans consume sufficient or excess calories but not enough essential nutrients. Nearly all foods contain combinations of nutrients, although foods are sometimes classified according to their predominant nutrient; for example, pastas are considered carbohydrate foods even though they also contain other nutrients.

Nutrient density is an important concept related to food energy. Nutrient-dense foods are high in essential nutrients but relatively low in calories. Think of your daily calorie intake as a budget: You need to spend your calories wisely on nutrient-dense foods to obtain all essential nutrients while staying within your budget.

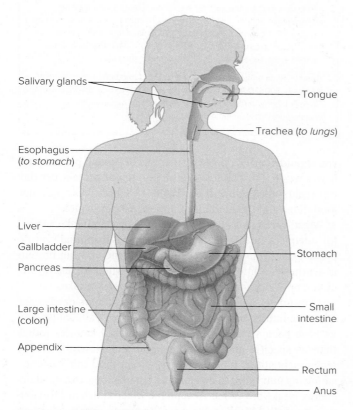

Salivary glands
Tongue
Trachea (*to lungs*)
Esophagus (*to stomach*)
Liver
Gallbladder
Pancreas
Stomach
Large intestine (colon)
Small intestine
Appendix
Rectum
Anus

FIGURE 13.1 The digestive system. Food is partially broken down by being chewed and mixed with saliva in the mouth. After traveling to the stomach via the esophagus, food is broken down further by stomach acids and other secretions. As food moves through the digestive tract, it is mixed by muscular contractions to facilitate further digestion and absorption. Most absorption of nutrients occurs via the lining of the small intestine. The large intestine reabsorbs excess water; the remaining solid wastes are collected in the rectum and excreted through the anus.

TERMS

digestion The process of breaking down foods into compounds the gastrointestinal tract can absorb and the body can use.

kilocalorie (kcal) A measure of energy content in food; 1 kilocalorie represents the amount of heat needed to raise the temperature of 1 liter of water 1°C; commonly referred to as a *calorie*.

energy The capacity to do work, measured by calories. We get energy from certain nutrients in food.

nutrient density The ratio of a food's essential nutrients to its calories.

Proteins—The Basis of Body Structure

Proteins form important parts of the body's main structural components: muscles and bones. Proteins also form important parts of blood, enzymes, some hormones, and cell membranes. When consumed, proteins also provide energy (4 calories per gram) for the body.

Amino Acids   The building blocks of proteins are called **amino acids.** Twenty common amino acids are found in food proteins. Nine of these amino acids are essential (sometimes called indispensable). As long as foods supply certain nutrients, the body can produce the other 11 amino acids.

Complete and Incomplete Proteins   Individual protein sources are considered *complete* if they supply all the essential amino acids in adequate amounts and *incomplete* if they do not. Meat, fish, poultry, eggs, milk, cheese, and soy provide complete proteins. Incomplete proteins, which come from other plant sources such as nuts and legumes (dried beans and peas), are good sources of most essential amino acids but are usually low in one or more.

Certain combinations of vegetable proteins, such as grains and legumes (peanut butter on whole wheat bread) allow each vegetable protein to make up for the amino acids missing in the other protein. The combination yields a complete protein. Many traditional food pairings, such as beans and rice or corn and beans, have emerged as dietary staples because together they provide complementary proteins.

About two-thirds of the protein in the typical American diet comes from animal sources (meat and dairy products); therefore, the American diet is rich in essential amino acids. It was once believed that vegetarians had to complement their proteins at each meal to receive the benefit of a complete protein. It is now known that proteins consumed throughout the course of the day can complement each other as part of a pool of amino acids that the body can draw from to produce the necessary proteins in the body. Vegetarians should include a variety of vegetable protein sources in their diets to make sure they get enough of all the essential amino acids. (Healthy plant-based diets are discussed later in the chapter.)

Recommended Protein Intake   The Food and Nutrition Board of the National Academy of Medicine has established goals to help ensure adequate intake of protein as well as the other macronutrients (Table 13.2). For protein, adequate daily intake for adults is 0.8 gram per kilogram (0.36 gram per pound) of body weight. So, if you weigh 140 pounds,

---

TERMS

protein   An essential nutrient that forms important parts of the body's main structures (muscles and bones) as well as blood, enzymes, hormones, and cell membranes; also provides energy.

amino acid   One of the building blocks of proteins; 20 common amino acids are found in foods.

| Table 13.2 | Goals for Protein, Fat, and Carbohydrate Intake |

	DAILY ADEQUATE INTAKE DISTRIBUTION (GRAMS)*		ACCEPTABLE MACRONUTRIENT DISTRIBUTION RANGE (PERCENTAGE OF TOTAL DAILY CALORIES)
	MEN	WOMEN	
Protein**	56	46	10–35
Fat (total)			20–35
Linoleic acid	17	12	
Alpha-linolenic acid	1.6	1.1	
Carbohydrate	130	130	45–65

*To meet daily energy needs, you must consume more than the minimally adequate amounts of the energy-providing nutrients listed here, which alone supply only 800–900 calories. Use the AMDRs to set overall daily goals.

**Protein-intake goals can be calculated more specifically by multiplying your body weight in pounds by 0.36.

NOTE: Individuals can allocate total daily energy intake among the three classes of macronutrients to suit individual preferences. To translate percentage goals into daily-intake goals expressed in calories and grams, multiply the appropriate percentages by your total daily energy intake and then divide the results by the corresponding calories per gram. For example, a fat limit of 35% applied to a 2200-calorie diet would be calculated as follows: 0.35 × 2200 = 770 calories of total fat; 770 ÷ 9 calories per gram = 86 grams of total fat.

SOURCE: Recommendations from Food and Nutrition Board, Institute of Medicine. 2005. *Dietary Reference Intakes for Energy, Carbohydrate, Fiber, Fat, Fatty Acids, Cholesterol, Protein, and Amino Acids.* Washington, DC: National Academies Press.

---

you should consume at least 50 grams of protein per day, and if you weigh 180 pounds, then 65 grams of protein per day represents adequate intake. Table 13.3 lists some popular food items and the amount of protein each provides.

Most Americans meet or exceed the protein intake needed for adequate nutrition. If you consume substantially more protein than your body needs, the extra energy from protein is synthesized into fat for storage or burned for energy requirements, depending on your overall energy intake.

Consuming some protein above the amount needed for adequate nutrition is not harmful; suggested daily intake limits have been set as a proportion of overall calories rather than as specific amounts. The Food and Nutrition Board recommendations for how much protein (and other energy-supplying nutrients) to consume as a percentage of total daily energy intake are called Acceptable Macronutrient Distribution Ranges (AMDRs); the AMDRs aim to ensure adequate intake of essential nutrients and also reduce the risk of chronic diseases. The AMDR for protein for adults aged 19 years and over is 10–35% of total daily calorie intake (see Table 13.2): For someone consuming a 2000-calorie diet, this percentage range corresponds to a suggested daily intake of between 50 and 175 grams per day. Healthy protein-rich food choices are described in detail later in the chapter.

Table 13.3 — Protein Content of Common Food Items

ITEM	PROTEIN (GRAMS)*
3 ounces lean meat, poultry, or fish	20–27
¼ block (3 ounces) tofu	7
1 cup cooked beans (black, white, pinto)	15–17
1 cup yogurt	8–13
1 ounce cheese (cheddar, Swiss)	6–8
½–1 cup cereals	1–6
1 egg cooked	6
1 cup ricotta cheese	28
1 cup milk	8
1 ounce nuts	2–6

*For the specific protein content of a food, check the food label or the searchable USDA food composition database (https://ndb.nal.usda.gov/ndb/search).

SOURCE: U.S. Department of Agriculture, Agricultural Research Service, Food Data Central (https://fdc.nal.usda.gov/) accessed March 2, 2020.

Fat—Another Essential Nutrient

At 9 calories per gram, fats, also known as *lipids,* are the most concentrated source of energy. The fats stored in your body represent usable energy, help insulate your body, and support and cushion your organs. Fats in the diet help your body to absorb fat-soluble vitamins, and they add important flavor and texture to foods. Fats are the major fuel for the body during rest and light activity.

Two fats, linoleic acid and alpha-linolenic acid, are essential fatty acids and necessary components of the diet. They are used to make compounds that are key regulators of body functions such as the maintenance of blood pressure and the progress of a healthy pregnancy.

Types and Sources of Fats Called *triglycerides,* most fats in foods are fairly similar in their basic composition, generally including a molecule of glycerol (an alcohol) with three fatty acid chains attached to it. Animal fat, for example, is made primarily of triglycerides.

Within a triglyceride, differences in the fatty acid structure result in different types of fats. Depending on this structure, a fat may be saturated or unsaturated, monounsaturated or polyunsaturated, depending on how many double bonds exist in the structure of the fatty acid chains. The essential fatty acids linoleic acid and alpha-linolenic acid are both polyunsaturated (they have two or more double bonds). Different types of fatty acids have different characteristics and therefore varied effects on health, as discussed in the box "Fats and Health."

Food fats are usually composed of both saturated and unsaturated fatty acids. The dominant type of fatty acid determines the fat's characteristics. Food fats containing large amounts of saturated fatty acids or trans fatty acids are usually solid at room temperature; they are generally found naturally in animal products or in products containing hydrogenated oils. The leading sources of saturated fat in the American diet are red meats (hamburger, steak, roasts), whole milk, cheese, hot dogs, and lunch meats. Palm and coconut oils, also known as "tropical oils," although derived from plants, are also highly saturated and are solid or semisolid at room temperature. Most monounsaturated and polyunsaturated fatty acids in foods usually come from plant sources and are liquid at room temperature. Olive, canola, safflower, and peanut oils contain mostly monounsaturated fatty acids. Soybean, corn, and cottonseed oils contain mostly polyunsaturated fatty acids. (See Table 13.4.)

Hydrogenation and Trans Fats When unsaturated vegetable oils undergo the chemical process known as **hydrogenation,** the result is a more solid fat from a liquid oil. The mixture contains both saturated and unsaturated fatty acids. Hydrogenation also changes some unsaturated fatty acids into **trans fatty acids**—unsaturated fatty acids that raise your risk of heart disease.

Food manufacturers use hydrogenation to increase the stability of an oil so that it can be reused for deep frying, to improve the texture of certain foods (to make pie crusts flakier, for example), and to extend the shelf life of foods made with oil. In general, the more solid a hydrogenated oil is, the more saturated or trans fats it contains. For example, hard stick margarines typically contain more saturated and trans fats than do soft tub or squeeze margarines. In some studies, trans fats are associated with an increase in **low-density lipoprotein (LDL) cholesterol,** or "bad" cholesterol, and a lowering of **high-density lipoprotein (HDL) cholesterol,** or "good" cholesterol, resulting in a double-negative effect on heart health.

Consuming trans fats appears to increase the risk for both cardiovascular disease and type 2 diabetes. As aware-

TERMS

hydrogenation A chemical process by which hydrogen atoms are added to molecules of unsaturated fats, increasing the degree of saturation and turning liquid oils into solid fats. Hydrogenation produces a mixture of saturated fatty acids, and *cis* (standard) and *trans* forms of unsaturated fatty acids.

trans fatty acid A type of unsaturated fatty acid produced during the process of hydrogenation; trans fats have an atypical shape that affects their chemical activity. Trans fats are associated with an increase in LDL cholesterol and a lowering of HDL cholesterol, attributes associated with risk of heart disease.

cholesterol A waxy substance in the blood and cells, needed for synthesis of cell membranes, vitamin D, and hormones.

low-density lipoprotein (LDL) cholesterol Blood fat that transports cholesterol to organs and tissues; excess amounts result in the accumulation of deposits in artery walls, causing hardening of the arteries and potentially cardiovascular disease.

high-density lipoprotein (HDL) cholesterol Blood fat that helps transport cholesterol out of the arteries, thereby protecting against cardiovascular disease.

Table 13.4	Types of Fatty Acids

TYPE OF FATTY ACID	FOUND IN*
Saturated	• Animal fats (especially fatty meats and poultry fat and skin) • Butter, cheese, and other high-fat dairy products • Palm and coconut oils
Trans	• Some frozen pizza • Some types of popcorn • Deep-fried fast foods • Stick margarines, shortening • Packaged cookies and crackers • Processed snacks and sweets
Monounsaturated	• Olive, canola, and safflower oils • Avocados, olives • Peanut butter (without added fat) • Many nuts, including almonds, cashews, pecans, and pistachios
Polyunsaturated—omega-3[†]	• Fatty fish, including salmon, white albacore tuna, mackerel, anchovies, and sardines • Compared to fish, lesser amounts are found in canola and soybean oils; tofu; walnuts; flaxseeds; and dark green leafy vegetables
Polyunsaturated—omega-6[†]	• Corn, soybean, and cottonseed oils (often used in margarine, mayonnaise, and salad dressings)

*Food fats contain a combination of types of fatty acids in various proportions. For example, canola oil is composed mainly of monounsaturated fatty acids (62%) but also contains polyunsaturated (32%) and saturated (6%) fatty acids.

[†]The essential fatty acids are polyunsaturated: Linoleic acid is an omega-6 fatty acid and alpha-linolenic acid is an omega-3 fatty acid.

ness of these health risks has grown, cities and states have banned the use of trans fats in restaurants and food prepared for retail sale, and food manufacturers have reduced the amount of trans fats they use. The Food and Drug Administration (FDA) required that food manufacturers stop using trans fats by June 2018, although some foods produced prior to the ban can be distributed through 2021.

Small amounts of trans fats occur naturally in animal fat, particularly beef, lamb, and dairy products, but the majority of trans fats in the American diet are artificial and come from partially hydrogenated oils. Many baked and fried foods are prepared with hydrogenated vegetable oils, which means they can be relatively high in saturated and trans fatty acids. The leading sources of trans fats in the American diet are fried fast foods such as french fries and fried chicken (typically fried in vegetable shortening rather than oil), baked and snack foods, and stick margarine.

Recommended Fat Intake   It takes only 3–4 teaspoons (15–20 grams) of vegetable oil per day incorporated into your diet to supply essential fats. To meet the body's demand for essential fats, adult men need about 17 grams per day of linoleic acid and 1.6 grams per day of alpha-linolenic acid; adult women need 12 grams of linoleic acid and 1.1 grams of alpha-linolenic acid. Most Americans consume sufficient amounts of the essential fats; limiting unhealthy fats is a much greater health concern.

Limits for total fat, saturated fat, and trans fat intake have been set by several government and research organizations. As with protein, a limited range of fat consumption is associated with good health. The AMDR for total fat is 20–35% of total daily calories. AMDRs have also been set for omega-6 fatty acids (5–10% of total calories) and omega-3 fatty acids (0.6–1.2% of total calories) as part of total daily fat intake. However, these are more difficult for consumers to monitor.

The latest federal guidelines place greater emphasis on choosing healthy unsaturated fats in place of saturated and trans fats. It is also important to avoid highly processed reduced-fat foods that substitute refined carbohydrates and added sugars for fats. Information about the types of fats present in a food can be found on the food label or, for unlabeled products, in nutrition guides and online. It is important to check ingredient labels for partially hydrogenated oils: As long as a product has no more than half a gram of trans fats, the label may claim zero. (See for more Information at the end of the chapter.)

Look at your choices in the overall context of your diet. For example, peanut butter eaten on whole-wheat bread and served with a banana, carrot sticks, and a glass of reduced-fat milk makes a nutritious lunch. In comparison, peanut butter on high-fat crackers with potato chips, cookies, and whole milk is a less healthy combination.

Carbohydrates—An Important Source of Energy

Carbohydrates are needed in the diet primarily to supply energy for body cells. Some cells, such as those in the brain, in (parts of)

carbohydrate   An essential nutrient, required for energy for cells; sugars, starches, and dietary fiber are all carbohydrates. **TERMS**

Fats are a major source of energy and help us absorb vitamins and minerals. Polyunsaturated and monounsaturated fats are healthy, we know that. Trans fats are clearly unhealthy. But what about the in-betweens . . . the saturated fats?

Artificial Trans Fats: Heading for the Exit

Health experts and public health recommendations agree on the dangers of artificial trans fats because of their double-negative effect on heart health—raising LDL and lowering HDL. Consuming trans fats appears to increase the risk of both cardiovascular disease and type 2 diabetes. As awareness of these health risks grew, cities and states banned the use of trans fats in restaurants and foods prepared for retail sales, and food manufacturers reduced the amount of trans fats in processed foods. According to the U.S. Food and Drug Administration (FDA), trans fat consumption declined by almost 80% between 2003 and 2012.

In 2015, the FDA removed partially hydrogenated oils (the primary source of artificial trans fats) from the category of food additives "generally regarded as safe" for use in human foods. This change will substantially lower trans fat consumption in the United States and is expected to reduce the incidence of coronary heart disease and prevent thousands of fatal heart attacks each year.

Until trans fats are eliminated from processed foods, consumers can check for them by examining the ingredient list of a food for "partially hydrogenated oil" or "vegetable shortening." In addition, if a food contains 0.5 g or more of trans fats, the amount will be listed on the Nutrition Facts label.

Saturated Fats: Mixed Evidence?

Many studies have examined the effects of dietary-fat intake on blood cholesterol levels and the risk of heart disease. Although a handful of recent studies have challenged the link between heart disease and saturated fats, long-standing advice has been to limit them. A meta-analysis of 21 studies concluded that not enough evidence supports the link to heart disease. But the analysis did favor replacing saturated fats with unsaturated ones because they may reduce the risk of heart disease. Reduce your fats from red meats, whole milk, cheese, coconut oil, and many bought and processed baked goods and choose instead fats from nuts, avocados, and vegetable oils. Another two studies reinforced this replacement idea, also warning against substituting refined, processed carbs for saturated fats, which only increases our risk.

The greater consensus stands by the advice to lower saturated-fat intake and aim for a dietary pattern that achieves only 5-6% of total calories from saturated fat, especially for people with risk factors for heart disease. This recommendation comes from the 2020 Dietary Guidelines Advisory Committee, American Heart Association, and American College of Cardiology.

Research on the health effects of saturated fats is ongoing. For example, do saturated fats in beef, butter, milk, and chocolate all have the same effect on heart disease risk? And what are the health effects of shifts in the intake of particular fats within the overall context of the diet? Also, dietary fat—and the foods that contain it—affect health in other ways besides heart disease risk. Diets high in saturated fat such as in rich fatty red meats are associated with an increased risk of certain forms of cancer, especially colon cancer.

Type Over Total, Pattern Over Individual

Both the latest federal dietary guidelines and changes to food labels reflect a greater emphasis on the types of fats consumed rather than the total. Overall fat intake is important, especially if the fats are in foods with few other nutrients. On average, Americans' intake of total fats is within the AMDR, but saturated-fat intake is over the recommended levels.

To find good sources of polyunsaturated fats, look for omega-3 fatty acids in fatty fish such as salmon and sardines, and in walnuts, flaxseeds, and canola or unhydrogenated soybean oil. Look for the other main type of polyunsaturated fat, omega-6 fatty acids, in vegetable oils such as safflower, soybean, sunflower, walnut, and corn oils.

But aren't dietary patterns more important for health than a focus on a single nutrient? Yes. The fats in your diet are found in foods that contain other nutrients, and the foods you consume are in the pattern of your overall diet. Increased body weight, aging, and gender are more important for predicting negative health events than is eating one kind of dietary fat rather than another.

SOURCES: Dietary Guidelines Advisory Committee. 2020. *Scientific Report of the 2020 Dietary Guidelines Advisory Committee: Advisory Report to the Secretary of Agriculture and the Secretary of Health and Human Services.* U.S. Department of Agriculture, Agricultural Research Service, Washington, DC; U.S. Food and Drug Administration. 2015. *Final Determination Regarding Partially Hydrogenated Oils (Removing Trans Fat)* (https://www.fda.gov/Food/IngredientsPackagingLabeling /FoodAdditivesIngredients/ucm449162.htm Harvard Health Publishing. 2019. The Truth about fats: The good, the bad, and the in-between. (https://www.health.harvard.edu/staying-healthy/the-truth-about-fats-bad -and-good); American Heart Association. *Saturated Fat* (https://www.heart .org/en/healthy-living/healthy-eating/eat-smart/fats/saturated-fats).

the nervous system, and in blood, prefer the carbohydrate glucose for fuel. During high-intensity exercise, muscles also use energy from carbohydrates as their primary fuel source. Eating the equivalent of just three or four slices of bread supplies the body's daily minimum need for carbohydrates.

When we don't eat enough carbohydrates to satisfy the energy needs of the brain and red blood cells, our bodies synthesize fuel from fats and proteins. In situations of extreme deprivation, when the diet lacks a sufficient amount of both carbohydrates and proteins, the body turns to its own organs and tissues, breaking down proteins in muscles, the heart, kidneys, and other vital organs to supply carbohydrate needs.

Simple and Complex Carbohydrates Carbohydrates are classified into two groups: simple and complex. *Simple carbohydrates* include single sugar molecules (monosaccharides) and double sugar molecules (disaccharides). The monosaccharides are glucose, fructose, and galactose. Glucose is the most common sugar and is used by both animals and plants for energy. Fructose is a very sweet sugar that is found in fruits, and galactose is the sugar in milk. The disaccharides are pairs of single sugars; they include sucrose or table sugar (fructose + glucose), maltose or malt sugar (glucose + glucose), and lactose or milk sugar (galactose + glucose). Simple carbohydrates add sweetness to foods; they are found naturally in fruits and milk and are added to soft drinks, fruit drinks, candy, sweet desserts, and a variety of other processed foods. As described below, diets high in added sugars are linked to obesity.

---

glucose A simple sugar that is the body's basic fuel.

TERMS

glycogen A starch stored in the liver and muscles.

whole grain The entire edible portion of a grain (such as wheat, rice, or oats), consisting of the germ, endosperm, and bran; processing removes parts of the grain, often leaving just the endosperm.

Complex carbohydrates include starches and most types of dietary fiber. Starches are found in a variety of plants, especially grains (wheat, rye, rice, oats, barley, and millet), legumes (dry beans, peas, and lentils), and tubers (potatoes and yams). Most other vegetables contain a mixture of complex and simple carbohydrates. Fiber, discussed in the next section, is found in grains, fruits, and vegetables.

During digestion, your body breaks down carbohydrates into simple sugar molecules, such as **glucose,** for absorption. Once glucose is in the bloodstream, the pancreas releases the hormone insulin, which allows cells to take up glucose and use it for energy. The liver and muscles take up glucose to provide carbohydrate storage in the form of a starch called **glycogen.** Some people have problems controlling their blood glucose levels, a disorder called *diabetes mellitus* (Chapter 15).

Refined versus Whole Grains Complex carbohydrates from grains can be further divided into processed (refined) carbohydrates and whole grains (unrefined carbohydrates). Before they are processed, all grains are **whole grains,** consisting of an inner layer, the germ; a middle layer, the endosperm; and an outer layer, the bran (Figure 13.2). During processing, the germ and bran are often removed, leaving just the starchy endosperm. The refinement of whole grains transforms whole-wheat flour into white flour, brown rice into white rice, and so on.

Processed grains usually retain all the calories of their unrefined counterparts, but they tend to be much lower in fiber, vitamins, minerals, and other beneficial compounds—in other words, they are less nutrient dense. Processed grain products may be enriched or fortified with vitamins and minerals, but not all the nutrients lost in processing are replaced.

Whole grains tend to take longer to chew and digest than refined ones; they also enter the bloodstream more slowly. This slower digestive pace tends to make people feel full sooner and for a longer period. Also, a slower rise in blood glucose levels following the consumption of unrefined complex carbohydrates may help in the management of diabetes. Whole grains are also high in dietary fiber and so have all the benefits of fiber (discussed later).

FIGURE 13.2 **The parts of a whole grain kernel.** Lynx/Iconotec.com/Glowimages

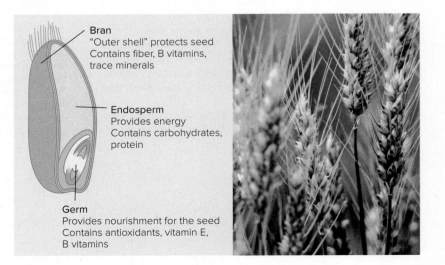

Bran
"Outer shell" protects seed
Contains fiber, B vitamins, trace minerals

Endosperm
Provides energy
Contains carbohydrates, protein

Germ
Provides nourishment for the seed
Contains antioxidants, vitamin E, B vitamins

Because whole-grain foods offer so many health benefits, federal dietary guidelines recommend six or more servings of grain products every day, with at least half of those servings from whole grains. Currently, however, Americans average less than one serving of whole grains per day.

What Are Whole Grains?

The first step in increasing your intake of whole grains is to correctly identify them. The following are whole grains:

Whole wheat	Whole-grain corn
Whole rye	Popcorn
Whole oats	Brown rice
Oatmeal	Whole-grain barley

More unusual choices include bulgur (cracked wheat), millet, kasha (roasted buckwheat kernels), quinoa, wheat and rye berries, amaranth, wild rice, graham flour, whole-grain kamut, whole-grain spelt, and whole-grain triticale.

Wheat flour, unbleached flour, enriched flour, and degerminated corn meal are not whole grains. Wheat germ and wheat bran are also not whole grains, but they are the constituents of wheat typically left out when wheat is processed and so are healthier choices than regular wheat flour, which typically contains just the grain's endosperm.

Checking Packages for Whole Grains

To find packaged foods—such as bread or pasta—that are rich in whole grains, read the list of ingredients and check for special health claims related to whole grains. The *first* item on the list of ingredients should be one of the whole grains in the preceding list. Product names and food color can be misleading. *When in doubt, always check the list of ingredients and make sure "whole" is the first word on the list.* The word "enriched" means that it is white flour to which some of the nutrients that were removed in the milling process have been added back.

The U.S. Food and Drug Administration (FDA) allows manufacturers to include special health claims for foods that contain 51% or more whole-grain ingredients. Such products may display a statement such as the following on their packaging:

"Rich in whole grain."
"Made with 100% whole grain."
"Diets rich in whole-grain foods may help reduce the risk of heart disease and certain cancers."

However, many whole-grain products do not carry such claims. This is one more reason to check the ingredient list to make sure you're buying a product made from one or more whole grains.

Consumption of whole grains has been linked to a reduced risk of heart disease, diabetes, obesity, and cancer and plays an important role in gastrointestinal health and body weight management. For all these reasons, whole grains are recommended over those that have been processed. This does not mean that you should never eat processed carbohydrates such as white bread or white rice—simply that whole-wheat bread, brown rice, and other whole grains are healthier choices. See the box "Choosing More Whole-Grain Foods" for tips on increasing your intake of whole grains.

Added Sugars Food manufacturers or individuals sometimes add sugars to foods. The term *added sugars* refers to white sugar, brown sugar, high-fructose corn syrup, and other sweeteners added to processed foods. Naturally occurring sugars in fruit and milk are not considered added sugars. Foods high in added sugar tend to be higher in calories and lower in essential nutrients and fiber, thus providing "empty calories." High intake of added sugars from foods and sugar-sweetened beverages is associated with dental caries (cavities), excess body weight, and increased risk of type 2 diabetes, and it may also increase risk for hypertension, stroke, and heart disease.

Added sugars currently contribute about 250–300 calories in the typical daily American diet, representing about 13–17% of total energy intake. A limit of 10% is suggested by the U.S. Department of Agriculture (USDA) and other organizations;

even lower intakes may meet all nutrient needs at a given level of calorie intake. Major sources of added sugar in the U.S. diet are sugar-sweetened beverages, snacks, and sweets. Added sugars now appear on food labels as manufacturers adopt the new Nutrition Facts food-labeling format.

The sugars in your diet should be those that occur naturally, coming mainly from whole fruits, which are excellent sources of vitamins and minerals, and from low-fat milk and other dairy products, which are high in protein and calcium. Dietary patterns low in added sugars are described in detail later in the chapter.

Recommended Carbohydrate Intake On average, Americans consume 200–300 grams of carbohydrate per day—well above the 130 grams needed to meet the body's requirement for essential carbohydrate. The AMDR for carbohydrates is 45–65% of total daily calories. That's about 225–325 grams of carbohydrate for someone who consumes 2000 calories per day. The focus should be on consuming a variety of foods rich in complex carbohydrates, especially whole grains.

Athletes can especially benefit from high-carbohydrate diets (60–70% of total daily calories), which can increase the amount of carbohydrates stored in their muscles and therefore provide more fuel for use during endurance events or long workouts. Carbohydrates consumed during prolonged athletic events (e.g., low-sugar sports beverages and gels) provide fluid, electrolytes, and glucose to help fuel muscles and can extend the availability of glycogen stored in muscles. You should be aware, however, that overconsumption of carbohydrates often leads to underconsumption of other nutrients.

Fiber—A Closer Look

Dietary fiber is the term given to nondigestible carbohydrates naturally present in plants such as whole grains, fruits, legumes, and vegetables. Instead of being digested, fiber helps move waste through the intestinal tract and provides bulk for feces in the large intestine, which in turn facilitates elimination. In the large intestine, bacteria break down some types of fiber into acids and gases, which explains why consuming too much fiber can lead to intestinal gas. Even though humans don't digest fiber, we need it for good health.

Types of Fiber   There are two types of fiber: soluble and insoluble. Both types are important for health. **Soluble (viscous) fiber** such as that found in oat bran or legumes can delay stomach emptying, slow the movement of glucose into the blood after eating, and reduce absorption of cholesterol. Soluble fiber dissolves or swells in water (like oatmeal that gets soft). In contrast, **insoluble fiber** does not dissolve in water. It increases fecal bulk and helps prevent constipation, hemorrhoids, and other digestive disorders. We can find insoluble fiber in all plants, and especially in wheat bran, or psyllium seed.

The Food and Nutrition Board gives three other descriptions of fiber:

- **Dietary fiber** refers to the nondigestible carbohydrates (and the noncarbohydrate substance *lignin*) that are naturally present in plants such as grains, fruits, legumes, and vegetables.

- **Functional fiber** refers to nondigestible carbohydrates that have been either isolated from natural sources or synthesized in a laboratory and then added to a food product or dietary supplement.

---

dietary fiber   Nondigestible carbohydrates and lignin that are intact in plants.

TERMS

soluble (viscous) fiber   Fiber that dissolves in water or is broken down by bacteria in the large intestine.

insoluble fiber   Fiber that does not dissolve in water and is not broken down by bacteria in the large intestine.

functional fiber   Nondigestible carbohydrates either isolated from natural sources or synthesized; these may be added to foods and dietary supplements.

total fiber   The total amount of dietary fiber and functional fiber in the diet.

vitamins   Carbon-containing substances needed in small amounts to help promote and regulate chemical reactions and processes in the body.

- **Total fiber** refers to the sum of dietary and functional fiber in your diet.

A high-fiber diet can help reduce the risk of type 2 diabetes, heart disease, and cancer, as well as improve gastrointestinal health and aid in the management of metabolic syndrome and body weight. Many studies have linked high-fiber diets with a reduced risk of colon and rectal cancer. Other studies have suggested that it is the total dietary pattern—one rich in fruits, vegetables, and whole grains—that may be responsible for this reduction in risk (see Chapter 17). A high-fiber diet has also been linked to healthier gut bacteria, which may improve immunity and reduce the risk of obesity.

Sources of Fiber   All plant foods contain some dietary fiber. Fruits, legumes, oats (especially oat bran), and barley all contain the viscous types of fiber that help lower blood glucose and cholesterol levels. Wheat (especially wheat bran), other grains and cereals, and vegetables are good sources of cellulose and other fibers that help prevent constipation. Psyllium, which is often added to cereals or used in fiber supplements and laxatives, improves intestinal health and also helps control glucose and cholesterol levels. The processing of packaged foods can remove fiber, so it is important to rely on fresh fruits and vegetables and foods made from whole grains as your main sources of fiber. Ideally, fiber should come from foods, not supplements.

Recommended Fiber Intake   To reduce the risk of chronic disease and maintain intestinal health, the Food and Nutrition Board recommends a daily fiber intake of 38 grams for adult men and 25 grams for adult women. Americans generally consume about half this amount.

Vitamins—Organic Micronutrients

Vitamins are organic (carbon-containing) substances required in small amounts to regulate various processes within living cells (Table 13.5). Humans need 13 vitamins; of these, 4 are fat-soluble (A, D, E, and K), and 9 are water-soluble (C, and the B vitamins thiamin, riboflavin, niacin, vitamin B-6, folate, vitamin B-12, biotin, and pantothenic acid).

Solubility affects how a vitamin is absorbed, transported, and stored in the body. The water-soluble vitamins are absorbed directly into the bloodstream, where they travel freely; excess

---

Ask Yourself

?

QUESTIONS FOR CRITICAL THINKING AND REFLECTION

Experts say that two of the most important factors in a healthy diet are eating the "right" kinds of carbohydrates and eating the "right" kinds of fats. Based on what you've read so far in this chapter, which are the "right" carbohydrates and fats? How would you say your own diet stacks up when it comes to carbohydrates and fats?

Table 13.5 — Facts about Vitamins

VITAMIN AND RECOMMENDED INTAKES*	IMPORTANT DIETARY SOURCES	MAJOR FUNCTIONS	SIGNS OF PROLONGED DEFICIENCY	TOXIC EFFECTS OF MEGADOSES
Fat-soluble				
Vitamin A Men: 900 µg Women: 700 µg	Liver, milk, butter, cheese, fortified margarine, carrots, spinach, orange and deep green vegetables and fruits	Immune function and maintenance of vision; skin; and linings of the nose, mouth, and digestive and urinary tracts	Night blindness, scaling skin, increased susceptibility to infection, loss of appetite, anemia, kidney stones	Liver damage, miscarriage, birth defects, headache, vomiting, diarrhea, vertigo, double vision, bone abnormalities
Vitamin D Men: 15 µg Women: 15 µg	Fortified milk and margarine, fish oils, butter, egg yolks; sunlight on skin also produces vitamin D	Development and maintenance of bones and teeth, promotion of calcium absorption	Rickets (bone deformities) in children; bone softening, loss, and fractures in adults	Kidney damage, calcium deposits in soft tissues, depression, death
Vitamin E Men: 15 mg Women: 15 mg	Vegetable oils, whole grains, nuts and seeds, green leafy vegetables, asparagus, peaches	Protection and maintenance of cellular membranes	Red blood cell breakage and anemia, weakness, neurological problems, muscle cramps	Relatively nontoxic, but may cause excess bleeding or formation of blood clots
Vitamin K Men: 120 µg Women: 90 µg	Green leafy vegetables; smaller amounts widespread in other foods	Production of factors essential for blood clotting and bone metabolism	Hemorrhaging	None reported
Water-soluble				
Biotin Men: 30 µg Women: 30 µg	Cereals, yeast, egg yolks, soy flour, liver; widespread in foods	Synthesis of fats, glycogen, and amino acids	Rash, nausea, vomiting, weight loss, depression, fatigue, hair loss	None reported
Folate Men: 400 µg Women: 400 µg	Green leafy vegetables, yeast, oranges, whole grains, legumes, liver	Amino acid metabolism, synthesis of RNA and DNA, new cell synthesis	Anemia, weakness, fatigue, irritability, shortness of breath, swollen tongue	Masking of vitamin B-12 deficiency
Niacin Men: 16 mg Women: 14 mg	Eggs, poultry, fish, milk, whole grains, nuts, enriched breads and cereals, meats, legumes	Conversion of carbohydrates, fats, and proteins into usable forms of energy	Pellagra (symptoms include diarrhea, dermatitis, inflammation of mucous membranes, dementia)	Flushing of the skin, nausea, vomiting, diarrhea, liver dysfunction, glucose intolerance
Pantothenic acid Men: 5 mg Women: 5 mg	Animal foods, whole grains, broccoli, potatoes; widespread in foods	Metabolism of fats, carbohydrates, and proteins	Fatigue, numbness and tingling of hands and feet, gastrointestinal disturbances	None reported
Riboflavin Men: 1.3 mg Women: 1.1 mg	Dairy products, enriched breads and cereals, lean meats, poultry, fish, green vegetables	Energy metabolism; maintenance of skin, mucous membranes, and nervous system structures	Cracks at corners of mouth, sore throat, skin rash, hypersensitivity to light, purple tongue	None reported
Thiamin Men: 1.2 mg Women: 1.1 mg	Whole-grain and enriched breads and cereals, organ meats, lean pork, nuts, legumes	Conversion of carbohydrates into usable forms of energy, maintenance of appetite and nervous system function	Beriberi (symptoms include muscle wasting, mental confusion, anorexia, enlarged heart, nerve changes)	None reported
Vitamin B-6 Men: 1.3 mg Women: 1.3 mg	Eggs, poultry, fish, whole grains, nuts, soybeans, liver, kidney, pork	Metabolism of amino acids and glycogen	Anemia, convulsions, cracks at corners of mouth, dermatitis, nausea, confusion	Neurological abnormalities and damage
Vitamin B-12 Men: 2.4 µg Women: 2.4 µg	Meat, fish, poultry, fortified cereals	Synthesis of blood cells, other metabolic reactions	Anemia, fatigue, nervous system damage, sore tongue	None reported
Vitamin C Men: 90 mg Women: 75 mg	Peppers, broccoli, spinach, brussels sprouts, citrus fruits, strawberries, tomatoes, potatoes, cabbage, other fruits and vegetables	Maintenance and repair of connective tissue, bones, teeth, and cartilage; promotion of healing; absorption of iron	Scurvy, anemia, reduced resistance to infection, loosened teeth, joint pain, poor wound healing, hair loss, poor iron absorption	Urinary stones in some people, acid stomach from ingesting supplements in pill form, nausea, diarrhea, headache, fatigue

*Recommended intakes for adults aged 19–30; to calculate your personal Dietary Reference Intakes (DRIs) based on age, sex, and other factors, visit the Interactive DRI website (https://www.nal.usda.gov/fnic/dri-calculator/).

SOURCES: The following reports may be accessed via www.nap.edu: *Dietary Reference Intakes for Thiamin, Riboflavin, Niacin, Vitamin B6, Folate, Vitamin B12, Pantothenic Acid, Biotin and Choline* (1998); *Dietary Reference Intakes for Vitamin C, Vitamin E, Selenium, and Carotenoids* (2000); *Dietary Reference Intakes for Vitamin A, Vitamin K, Arsenic, Boron, Chromium, Copper, Iodine, Iron, Manganese, Molybdenum, Nickel, Silicon, Vanadium, and Zinc* (2001); and *Dietary Reference Intakes for Calcium and Vitamin D* (2011); Ross, A. C., et al., eds. 2014. *Modern Nutrition in Health and Disease*, 11th ed. Baltimore, MD: Lippincott Williams & Wilkins.

water-soluble vitamins are detected and removed by the kidneys and excreted in urine. However, extended use of large doses of water-soluble vitamins can cause toxicities and may interfere with some medications. Fat-soluble vitamins require a more complex absorptive process. They are usually carried in the blood by special lipoproteins or other carrier proteins and are stored in the liver and in fat tissues rather than excreted.

Functions of Vitamins   Many vitamins help chemical reactions take place. They provide no energy to the body directly but help release the energy stored in carbohydrates, proteins, and fats. Other vitamins are critical in the production of red blood cells and the maintenance of the nervous, skeletal, and immune systems. Some vitamins act as **antioxidants,** which help preserve the health of cells.

Sources of Vitamins   The human body does not manufacture most of the vitamins it requires and must obtain them from foods. Vitamins are abundant in fruits, vegetables, and grains. In addition, many processed foods, such as flour and breakfast cereals, contain added vitamins. There are a few vitamins made in the body: When exposed to sunlight, the skin makes vitamin D. Intestinal bacteria make vitamin K. Nonetheless, we still need additional vitamin D and vitamin K from foods. Table 13.5 lists good food sources of vitamins.

Vitamin Deficiencies   If your diet lacks a particular vitamin, characteristic symptoms of deficiency can develop (see Table 13.5). Physicians have known about some common deficiency-related ailments for generations. For example, *scurvy* is a potentially fatal illness caused by a long-term lack of vitamin C. Children who do not get enough vitamin D can develop *rickets,* which can lead to disabling bone deformations. Low intake of folate during the early weeks of pregnancy increases a woman's risk of giving birth to a baby with a neural tube defect (a congenital malformation of the central nervous system). Vitamin A deficiency may cause blindness, and anemia can develop in people whose diet lacks vitamin B-12, folate, or B-6. Although the data are not conclusive, low levels of folate and vitamins B-6 and B-12 have been linked to an increased risk of heart disease and stroke. Plant foods are not a source of B-12. Vegetarians and especially vegans must rely on fortified cereals or supplements for B-12.

In addition to vitamin D, studies show that vitamins C, A, and K as well as several B vitamins play a role in bone health.

While vitamin-deficiency diseases are common in rural areas of developing countries, they are relatively rare in the United States because vitamins are readily available from our fortified food supply. Still, many Americans consume lower-than-recommended amounts of several vitamins. Supplementation is discussed in detail later in this chapter.

Vitamin Excesses   Extra vitamins in the diet can also be harmful, especially when taken as supplements for an extended period of time. For example, although vitamin A plays an important role in bone growth, too much of it can trigger bone loss and increase the risk of fracture. Megadoses of fat-soluble vitamins are particularly dangerous because the excess is stored in the body rather than excreted, increasing the risk of toxicity. Even when vitamins are not taken in excess, relying on supplements for an adequate intake of vitamins can be a problem because many health benefits from other, nonvitamin ingredients in foods are likely to be missed. Later, this chapter discusses specific recommendations for vitamin intake and when a vitamin supplement is advisable. For now, keep in mind that it's best to get most of your vitamins from foods rather than supplements.

Keeping the Nutrient Value in Food   Vitamins and minerals can be lost or destroyed during the storage and cooking of foods. To retain nutrients, eat vegetables as soon as possible after purchasing. Raw fruits and vegetables should be stored in the refrigerator in covered containers or plastic bags to minimize moisture loss. Freeze foods that won't be eaten within a few days. Frozen and canned vegetables are usually as high in nutrients as fresh vegetables because nutrients are locked in when produce is frozen or canned. To reduce nutrient losses during food preparation, minimize the amount of water used and the total cooking time. Baking, steaming, broiling, grilling, and microwaving are all good methods of preparing vegetables.

Minerals—Inorganic Micronutrients

Minerals are inorganic (non-carbon-containing) elements you need in relatively small amounts to help regulate body functions, aid in the growth and maintenance of body tissues, and help release energy (Table 13.6). There are about 17 essential minerals. The major minerals, which the body needs in amounts exceeding 100 milligrams per day, include calcium, phosphorus, magnesium, sodium, potassium, and chloride. The essential trace minerals, which you need in minute amounts, include copper, fluoride, iodide, iron, selenium, and zinc.

Characteristic symptoms develop if an essential mineral is consumed in a quantity too large or too small for good health. For example, approximately 90% of Americans consume the mineral sodium in excess as part of dietary salt. More than 70% of sodium in the diet comes from processed foods and restaurant meals. High sodium consumption can raise blood pressure, and as blood pressure increases, the risk for heart disease and stroke does as well. Blood pressure begins to decrease within weeks of lowering sodium intake; therefore,

TERMS

antioxidant   A substance that can reduce the breakdown of food or body constituents by free radicals; the actions of antioxidants include binding oxygen, donating electrons to free radicals, and repairing damage to molecules.

minerals   Inorganic compounds needed in relatively small amounts for regulation, growth, and maintenance of body tissues and functions.

reducing dietary salt has become an important public health initiative.

The minerals commonly lacking in the American diet are iron, calcium, potassium, and magnesium. Iron-deficiency **anemia** is a problem in some age groups, but particularly among menstruating women and among women who have had multiple pregnancies. Poor calcium and vitamin D intakes during childhood contribute to a risk of future **osteoporosis,** especially in women. The box "Eating for Healthy Bones" has tips for building and maintaining bone density; also see Chapter 23 for more information about osteoporosis. Low fluoride intake contributes to dental caries; low iodine increases the risk of goiter. Public health fortification programs have minimized deficiencies in geographic areas where fortification (fluoridated water and iodized salt) is common practice.

Table 13.6 Facts about Selected Minerals

MINERAL AND RECOMMENDED INTAKES*	IMPORTANT DIETARY SOURCES	MAJOR FUNCTIONS	SIGNS OF PROLONGED DEFICIENCY	TOXIC EFFECTS OF MEGADOSES
Calcium Men: 1000 mg Women: 1000 mg	Milk and milk products, tofu, fortified orange juice and bread, green leafy vegetables, bones in fish	Formation of bones and teeth, control of nerve impulses, muscle contraction, blood clotting	Stunted growth in children, bone mineral loss in adults, urinary stones	Kidney stones, calcium deposits in soft tissues, inhibition of mineral absorption, constipation
Fluoride Men: 4 mg Women: 3 mg	Fluoridated water, tea, marine fish eaten with bones	Maintenance of tooth and bone structure	Higher frequency of tooth decay	Increased bone density, mottling of teeth, impaired kidney function
Iodine Men: 150 µg Women: 150 µg	Iodized salt, seafood, processed foods	Essential part of thyroid hormones, regulation of body metabolism	Goiter (enlarged thyroid), cretinism (birth defect)	Depression of thyroid activity, hyperthyroidism in susceptible people
Iron Men: 8 mg Women: 18 mg	Meat and poultry, fortified grain products, dark green vegetables, dried fruit	Component of hemoglobin, myoglobin, and enzymes	Iron-deficiency anemia, weakness, impaired immune function, gastrointestinal distress	Nausea, diarrhea, liver and kidney damage, joint pains, sterility, disruption of cardiac function, death
Magnesium Men: 400 mg Women: 310 mg	Widespread in foods and water (except soft water); especially found in grains, legumes, nuts, seeds, green vegetables, milk	Transmission of nerve impulses, energy transfer, activation of many enzymes	Neurological disturbances, cardiovascular problems, kidney disorders, nausea, growth failure in children	Nausea, vomiting, diarrhea, central nervous system depression, coma; death in people with impaired kidney function
Phosphorus Men: 700 mg Women: 700 mg	Present in nearly all foods, especially milk, cereal, peas, eggs, meat	Bone growth and maintenance, energy transfer in cells	Impaired growth, weakness, kidney disorders, cardiorespiratory and nervous system dysfunction	Drop in blood calcium levels, calcium deposits in soft tissues, bone loss
Potassium Men: 4700 mg Women: 4700 mg	Meats, milk, fruits, vegetables, grains, legumes	Nerve function, body water balance	Muscular weakness, nausea, drowsiness, paralysis, confusion, disruption of cardiac rhythm	Cardiac arrest
Selenium Men: 55 µg Women: 55 µg	Seafood, meat, eggs, whole grains	Defense against oxidative stress, regulation of thyroid hormone action	Muscle pain and weakness, heart disorders	Hair and nail loss, nausea and vomiting, weakness, irritability
Sodium Men: 1500 mg Women: 1500 mg	Salt, soy sauce, salted foods, tomato juice	Body water balance, acid–base balance, nerve function	Muscle weakness, loss of appetite, nausea, vomiting; deficiency is rarely seen	Edema (excess fluid buildup), hypertension in sensitive people
Zinc Men: 11 mg Women: 8 mg	Whole grains, meat, eggs, liver, seafood (especially oysters)	Synthesis of proteins, RNA, and DNA; wound healing; immune response; ability to taste	Growth failure, loss of appetite, impaired taste acuity, skin rash, impaired immune function, poor wound healing	Vomiting, impaired immune function, decline in blood HDL levels, impaired copper absorption

*Recommended intakes for adults aged 19–30; to calculate your personal DRIs based on age, sex, and other factors, visit the Interactive DRI website (https://www.nal.usda.gov/fnic/dri-calculator/).

SOURCES: The following reports may be accessed via www.nap.edu: *Dietary Reference Intakes for Calcium, Phosphorous, Magnesium, Vitamin D, and Fluoride* (1997); *Dietary Reference Intakes for Vitamin A, Vitamin K, Arsenic, Boron, Chromium, Copper, Iodine, Iron, Manganese, Molybdenum, Nickel, Silicon, Vanadium, and Zinc* (2001); *Dietary Reference Intakes for Water, Potassium, Sodium, Chloride, and Sulfate* (2005); and *Dietary Reference Intakes for Calcium and Vitamin D* (2011). Ross, A. C., et al., eds. 2014. *Modern Nutrition in Health and Disease,* 11th ed. Baltimore, MD: Lippincott Williams & Wilkins.

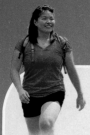

TAKE CHARGE
Eating for Healthy Bones

Osteoporosis is a condition in which the bones become dangerously thin and fragile over time. An estimated 10 million Americans over age 50 have osteoporosis, and another 34 million are at risk. Women account for about 80% of osteoporosis cases. Most of our adult bone mass is built by age 18 in girls and age 20 in boys. After bone density peaks between ages 25 and 35, bone mass is lost slowly over time and then at an increasing rate after menopause. To prevent osteoporosis, the best strategy is to build as much bone as possible during your youth and do everything you can to maintain it as you age. Up to 50% of bone loss is determined by controllable lifestyle factors such as resistance training and diet. Key nutrients for bone health include the following:

• **Calcium.** Getting enough calcium is important throughout life to build and maintain bone mass. Milk, yogurt, and calcium-fortified orange juice, bread, and cereals are all good sources.

• **Vitamin D.** Vitamin D is necessary for bones to absorb calcium. The National Academy of Medicine recommends a daily intake of 600 IU (15 mg) of vitamin D for most adults and 800 IU (20 mg) of vitamin D for men and women over the age of 70 years. Vitamin D can be obtained from foods and is manufactured by the skin when exposed to sunlight. Candidates for vitamin D supplements include people who don't eat many foods rich in vitamin D; those who don't expose their faces, arms, and hands to the sun (without sunscreen) for 5–15 minutes a few times each week; and people who live north of an imaginary line roughly between Boston and the Oregon–California border (where the sun is weaker).

• **Vitamin K.** Vitamin K promotes the synthesis of proteins that help keep bones strong. Broccoli and leafy green vegetables are rich in vitamin K.

• **Other nutrients.** Other nutrients that may play an important role in bone health include vitamin C, vitamin A, magnesium, potassium, phosphorus, fluoride, manganese, zinc, copper, and boron.

Several dietary substances may have a *negative* effect on bone health, especially if consumed in excess. These include alcohol, sodium, caffeine, and retinol (a form of vitamin A). Drinking lots of soda, which often replaces milk in the diet, has been shown to increase the risk of bone fractures in teenage girls.

The effect of protein intake on bone mass depends on other nutrients. Protein helps build bone as long as calcium and vitamin D intake are adequate. But if intake of calcium and vitamin D is low, high protein intake can lead to bone loss.

Weight-bearing aerobic exercise helps maintain bone mass throughout life, and strength training improves bone density, muscle mass, strength, and balance. Drinking alcohol only in moderation, refraining from smoking, and managing depression and stress are also important for maintaining strong bones. For people who develop osteoporosis, a variety of medications are available to treat the condition.

SOURCES: Movassagh, E. Z., and H. Vatanparast, 2017. Current evidence on the association of dietary patterns and bone health: A scoping review. *Advances in Nutrition* 8(1), 2017, 1–16; Institute of Medicine of the National Academies. 2011. *Dietary Reference Intakes for calcium and vitamin D.*

Water—Vital but Underappreciated

Water is the major component in both foods and the human body: We are composed of about 50–60% water. Our need for other nutrients, in terms of weight, is much less than our need for water. We can live up to 50 days without food but only a few days without water.

Water is distributed among lean and other tissues and in blood and other body fluids. Water is used in the digestion and absorption of food and is the medium in which most chemical reactions take place within the body. Some water-based fluids, like blood, transport substances around the body, whereas other fluids serve as lubricants or cushions. Water also helps regulate body temperature.

Water is part of most foods, particularly liquids, fruits, and vegetables. The foods and beverages you consume provide 80–90% of your daily water intake; the remainder is generated through metabolism. You lose water each day in urine, feces, and sweat and through evaporation from your lungs.

Most people can maintain a healthy water balance by consuming beverages at meals and drinking fluids when thirsty. The Food and Nutrition Board has set levels of adequate water intake to maintain hydration. Under these guidelines, men need about 3.7 total liters of water daily, with 3.0 liters (about 13 cups) coming from beverages; women need 2.7 total liters, with 2.2 liters (about 9 cups) coming from beverages. All fluids, including those containing caffeine, can count toward your total daily fluid intake. If you exercise vigorously or live in a hot climate, you need to consume additional fluids to maintain a balance between water consumed and water lost. Severe dehydration causes weakness and can lead to death.

> **QUICK STATS**
>
> Osteoporosis is more common in women; in people ages 65 and over with low bone mass, it occurs in about 25% of women and 5% of men.
>
> —Centers for Disease Control and Prevention, 2019

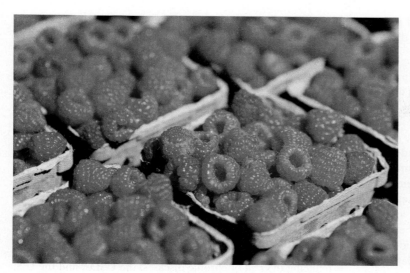

Berries are rich in antioxidants, vitamins, and dietary fiber. Nash Photos/ Photographer's Choice/Getty Images

Other Substances in Food

There are many other substances in food that are not essential nutrients but may influence health.

Antioxidants   When the body uses oxygen or breaks down certain fats or proteins as a normal part of metabolism, it gives rise to substances called **free radicals.** Environmental factors such as cigarette smoke, exhaust fumes, radiation, excessive sunlight, certain drugs, and stress can increase free radical production. A free radical is a chemically unstable molecule that reacts with fats, proteins, and DNA, damaging cell membranes and mutating genes. Free radicals have been implicated in aging, cancer, cardiovascular disease, and other degenerative diseases like arthritis.

Antioxidants found in foods can help protect the body from damage by free radicals in several ways. Some prevent or reduce the formation of free radicals; others remove free radicals from the body; still others repair some types of free radical damage after it occurs. Some antioxidants, such as vitamin C, vitamin E, and selenium, are also essential nutrients. Others—such as the carotenoids found in yellow, orange, and deep green vegetables—are not. Some of the top antioxidant-containing foods and beverages include berries, walnuts, artichokes, green tea, pecans, cloves, grape juice, dark chocolate, sour cherries, and red wine. Also high in antioxidants are brussels sprouts, kale, cauliflower, and pomegranates.

Phytochemicals   Antioxidants fall into the broader category of **phytochemicals,** which are substances found in plant foods that may help prevent chronic disease. Researchers have identified and studied hundreds of compounds found in foods and how they affect our health, and many findings are promising. For example, certain substances found in soy foods may help lower cholesterol levels. Sulforaphane, a compound isolated from broccoli and other **cruciferous vegetables,** may render some carcinogenic compounds harmless. Allyl sulfides, a group of chemicals found in garlic and onions, appear to boost the activity of immune cells and lower total cholesterol concentrations. Carotenoids found in green vegetables may help preserve eyesight with age. Phytochemicals found in whole grains are associated with a reduced risk of cardiovascular disease, diabetes, and cancer. Currently, research on phytochemicals extends the role of nutrition to the prevention and treatment of many chronic diseases.

If you want to increase your intake of phytochemicals, eat a variety of fruits, vegetables, and unprocessed grains rather than relying on supplements. Like many vitamins and minerals, isolated phytochemicals may be harmful if taken in high doses. Another reason to get your phytochemicals from foods is that their health benefits could be the result of many chemical substances from whole foods working in combination. Eating more fruits and vegetables is a smart alternative to less healthy foods. In contrast, people who rely more on supplements may take them and eat large portions of unhealthy foods, erroneously thinking that this can create a net positive health benefit. The role of phytochemicals in disease prevention is discussed further in Chapter 17.

NUTRITIONAL GUIDELINES: PLANNING YOUR DIET

Scientific and government groups have created a variety of tools to help people design healthy diets:

• **Dietary Reference Intakes (DRIs).** Standards for nutrient intake designed to prevent nutritional deficiencies and reduce the risk of chronic diseases

free radical   An electron-seeking compound that **TERMS** can react with fats, proteins, and DNA, damaging cell membranes and mutating genes in its search for electrons; produced through chemical reactions in the body and by exposure to environmental factors such as sunlight and tobacco smoke.

phytochemical   A naturally occurring substance found in plant foods that may help prevent and treat chronic diseases like cancer and heart disease; *phyto* means "plant."

cruciferous vegetables   Vegetables of the cabbage family, including cabbage, broccoli, brussels sprouts, kale, and cauliflower; the flower petals of these plants form the shape of a cross, hence the name.

Dietary Reference Intakes (DRIs)   An umbrella term for four types of nutrient standards designed to prevent nutritional deficiencies and reduce the risk of chronic diseases. Estimated Average Requirement (EAR) is the amount estimated to meet the nutrient needs of half the individuals in a population group; Adequate Intake (AI) and Recommended Dietary Allowance (RDA) are levels of intake considered adequate to prevent nutrient deficiencies and reduce the risk of chronic disease for most individuals in a population group; and Tolerable Upper Intake Level (UL) is the maximum daily intake that is unlikely to cause health problems.

- *Dietary Guidelines for Americans.* Established to promote health and reduce the risk of major chronic diseases through diet and physical activity

- **MyPlate.** Provides a food guidance system to help people apply the *Dietary Guidelines for Americans* to their own diets

Dietary Reference Intakes (DRIs)

The Food and Nutrition Board of the National Academy of Medicine establishes dietary standards, or recommended intake levels, for Americans of all ages. The current set of standards, the Dietary Reference Intakes (DRIs), was introduced in 1997. The DRIs are reviewed frequently and are updated as new nutrition-related information becomes available. The DRIs have a broad focus, being based on research that looks not just at the prevention of nutrient deficiencies but also at the role of nutrients in promoting health and preventing chronic diseases such as cancer, osteoporosis, and heart disease.

The DRIs include a set of four reference values used as standards for both recommended intakes and maximum safe intakes. The recommended intake of each nutrient is expressed as either a *Recommended Dietary Allowance (RDA)* or an *Adequate Intake (AI).* An AI is set when there is not enough information available to set an RDA value; regardless of the type of standard used, however, the DRI represents the best available estimate of intake for optimal health.

Used primarily in nutrition policy and research, the *Estimated Average Requirement (EAR)* is the average daily nutrient intake level estimated to meet the requirement of half the healthy individuals in a given gender and life stage. The *Tolerable Upper Intake Level (UL)* is the maximum daily intake that is unlikely to cause health problems in a healthy person. For example, the RDA for calcium for an 18-year-old female is 1300 mg per day; the UL is 3000 mg per day.

Because of lack of data, ULs have not been set for all nutrients. The absence of ULs does not mean that people can tolerate chronic intakes of these vitamins and minerals above recommended levels. Like all chemical agents, nutrients can produce adverse effects if intakes are excessive. There is no established benefit from consuming nutrients at levels above the RDA or AI.

The DRIs for many nutrients are found in Tables 13.2, 13.5, and 13.6. For a personalized DRI report for all nutrients,

appropriate for your sex and life stage, visit the Interactive DRI website (https://www.nal.usda.gov/fnic/dri-calculator/).

Because the DRIs are too cumbersome to use as a basis for food labels, the FDA uses another set of dietary standards, the **Daily Values.** The Daily Values are based on several different sets of guidelines and include standards for fat, cholesterol, carbohydrate, dietary fiber, and selected vitamins and minerals. The Daily Values represent appropriate intake levels for a 2000-calorie diet. The Daily Value percentage on a food label shows how well that food contributes to your recommended daily intake, assuming you follow a 2000-calorie-per-day diet. Food labels are described in detail later in this chapter.

Dietary Guidelines for Americans

To provide general guidance for choosing a healthy diet and reducing the risk of chronic diseases, the USDA and the U.S. Department of Health and Human Services issue the *Dietary Guidelines for Americans,* revising them every five years. The information in the *Dietary Guidelines* is used in developing federal food, nutrition, and health policies and programs and also serves as the basis for federal nutrition education materials.

The *Dietary Guidelines* are designed to help Americans make healthy and informed food choices. The main objectives of the 2020–2025 *Dietary Guidelines* are projected to encourage healthy eating patterns and regular physical activity among Americans, over 70% of whom are overweight or obese and yet at the same time undernourished in several key nutrients. The guidelines focus on the total diet and offer practical tips for how people can make *shifts* in their diet to integrate healthier choices. And they include findings on the broader environmental and societal aspects of the American diet—that is, the "food environment."

Earlier versions of the *Dietary Guidelines* focused more on individual dietary components such as food groups and nutrients. However, people do not eat individual nutrients or single foods but rather foods in combination, to form an overall **eating pattern** that has cumulative effects on health. The more recent *Dietary Guidelines* point out the large discrepancy between the recommendations and the actual American diet, which includes too much added sugar, solid fat, refined grain, and sodium and not enough vegetables, fruits, high-fiber whole grains, low-fat milk and milk products, and seafood.

Recommended eating patterns and their food and nutrient characteristics are based on the growing body of research that has examined the relationship between overall eating patterns, health, and risk of chronic disease. Following these guidelines promotes health and reduces the risk of diseases such as heart disease, cancer, diabetes, stroke, osteoporosis, and obesity.

The *2020-2025 Dietary Guidelines,* to be released at the end of 2020, also feature a whole lifespan approach. Previously, the guidelines focused on children aged 2 and over. The new guidelines will emphasize how diet during early life stages promotes health and prevents chronic disease throughout childhood and into adulthood. This means we take into account good nutrition for babies and children under 24 months, as well as for mothers who are pregnant and breastfeeding.

TERMS

Dietary Guidelines for Americans National nutritional recommendations issued jointly by the U.S. Department of Agriculture and the U.S. Department of Health and Human Services every five years; designed to promote health and reduce the risk of chronic diseases.

MyPlate The USDA food guidance system designed to help Americans make healthy food choices.

Daily Values A simplified version of the RDAs used on food labels; also included are values for nutrients with no RDA per se.

eating pattern The result of choices on multiple eating occasions over time, both at home and away from home.

Each of the guidelines is supported by an extensive review of scientific and medical evidence.

General Recommendations

The major themes expected to influence the *2020–2025 Dietary Guidelines* include the following;

1. **Approach food choices from a full lifespan perspective.** Special nutrition considerations exist at each life stage: for the fetus during pregnancy and birth, the baby through to age 24 months, and the child, adolescent, and adult. Improvements in recommended dietary patterns at each stage influence health food choices at each subsequent life stage.

2. **Focus on dietary patterns.** Emphasize healthy foods and combinations of foods that contribute to a dietary pattern, because individual nutrients have a synergistic and interactive effect on overall health, wellness, and risk of disease.

3. **Shift to healthier food and beverage choices.** Choose more vegetables, fruits, legumes, whole grains, low- or nonfat dairy, lean meat and poultry, seafood, nuts, and unsaturated vegetable oils.

4. **Limit calories from red and processed meats, sugar-sweetened foods and beverages, and refined grains.** Consume an eating pattern low in added sugars, saturated fats, and sodium. Cut back on foods and beverages higher in these components to amounts that fit within healthy eating patterns. If alcohol is consumed, drink only one alcoholic beverage.

5. **Support healthy eating patterns for all.** More than 37 million people in the U.S., including 6 million children, live with food insecurity. The disproportionate lack of access to healthy and affordable foods that affects low-income, black, and Hispanic households has become even more apparent during the COVID-19 pandemic. Everyone has a role in supporting healthy eating in our homes and communities, and reaching out especially to those people who are isolated and marginalized.

The *Dietary Guidelines* acknowledge the challenges that make it difficult for Americans to reach their food and fitness goals. The *Guidelines* argue that all segments of our society, from families to food producers and restaurants to policymakers, have a responsibility in supporting healthy choices. The *Dietary Guidelines* emphasize that a healthy eating pattern is not a rigid prescription, but rather an adaptable framework in which individuals can enjoy foods that meet their personal, cultural, and traditional preferences and fit within their budget and lifestyle. Adopting a healthy eating pattern and engaging in regular physical activity will go a long way toward improving health and reducing the risk of chronic disease in every life stage.

QUICK STATS

More than **70%** of Americans consume too much added sugars and saturated fats; **89%** have intakes that are too high for sodium.

—U.S. Department of Health and Human Services and U.S. Department of Agriculture, 2018b

Building Healthy Eating Patterns

A healthy eating pattern is one that meets nutrient needs while not exceeding calorie requirements and while staying within limits for dietary components that are typically overconsumed. The *Dietary Guidelines* highlight three healthy eating patterns:

- **Healthy U.S.-Style Pattern.** Based on the types and proportions of foods Americans typically consume, but in nutrient-dense forms and appropriate amounts.

- **Healthy Vegetarian Pattern.** Includes more legumes, processed soy products, nuts and seeds, and whole grains; it contains no meat, poultry, or seafood but is close to the Healthy U.S.-Style Pattern in amounts of all other food groups. Dairy and eggs are still included because the majority of vegetarians eat them; however, the plan can be vegan with plant-based substitutions.

- **Healthy Mediterranean-Style Pattern.** Reflecting a dietary pattern associated with many cultures bordering the Mediterranean Sea, which includes more fruit and seafood and less dairy than the Healthy U.S.-Style Pattern. The Mediterranean diet has been associated with positive health outcomes such as lower rates of heart disease and lower total mortality.

All three patterns are based on amounts of food from different food groups (and subgroups) according to overall energy intake. They share an emphasis on whole fruits, vegetables, whole grains, beans and peas, fat-free and low-fat milk and milk products, and healthy oils; they include less red meat and more seafood than the typical American diet. Healthy dietary patterns include oils, but they limit the amount of energy that people should consume from solid fats.

A fundamental principle of all healthy dietary patterns is that people should eat nutrient-dense foods—foods with little or no solid fats, added sugars, and added refined starches—so that they can obtain all the needed nutrients without exceeding their daily energy requirements. In addition, people should strive to get their nutrients from foods rather than from dietary supplements, although supplements or fortification may be helpful for certain populations.

Following a healthy pattern allows you to meet all the DRIs for essential nutrients and stay within the AMDRs established by the Food and Nutrition Board for nutrients that supply energy. Table 13.7 compares the three patterns for a 2000-calorie diet. See the Nutrition Resources section at the end of the chapter for a more detailed breakdown of the recommendations for the three healthy dietary patterns.

Although the greatest emphasis of the *Dietary Guidelines* is on consuming an overall healthy eating pattern, specific recommendations have been set for dietary components of particular public health concern. A summer 2020 report from the Dietary Guidelines Advisory Committee previewed some specific suggestions from the 2020-2025 publication. After

Table 13.7   USDA Healthy Food Patterns at the 2000-Calorie Level

FOOD GROUP	HEALTHY U.S.-STYLE PATTERN	HEALTHY VEGETARIAN PATTERN	HEALTHY MEDITERRANEAN-STYLE PATTERN
Vegetables	**2½ c-eq/day**	**2½ c-eq/day**	**2½ c-eq/day**
Dark green	1½ c-eq/wk	1½ c-eq/wk	1½ c-eq/wk
Red and orange	5½ c-eq/wk	5½ c-eq/wk	5½ c-eq/wk
Legumes (beans and peas)	1½ c-eq/wk	3 c-eq/wk*	1½ c-eq/wk
Starchy	5 c-eq/wk	5 c-eq/wk	5 c-eq/wk
Other	4 c-eq/wk	4 c-eq/wk	4 c-eq/wk
Fruit	**2 c-eq/day**	**2 c-eq/day**	**2½ c-eq/day**
Grains	**6 oz-eq/day**	**6½ oz-eq/day**	**6 oz-eq/day**
Whole grains	3 oz-eq/day	3½ oz-eq/day	3 oz-eq/day
Refined grains	3 oz-eq/day	3 oz-eq/day	3 oz-eq/day
Dairy	**3 c-eq/day**	**3 c-eq/day**	**2 c-eq/day**
Protein Foods	**5½ oz-eq/day**	**3½ oz-eq/day**	**6½ oz-eq/day**
Seafood	8 oz-eq/wk	N/A	15 oz-eq/wk
Meat, poultry, eggs	26 oz-eq/wk	3 oz-eq/wk (eggs)	26 oz-eq/wk
Nuts, seeds, soy products	5 oz-eq/wk	15 oz-eq/wk	5 oz-eq/wk
Oils	**27 g/day**	**27 g/day**	**27 g/day**
Limit on calories for other uses (% of total calories)**	270 cal/day (14%)	290 cal/day (15%)	260 cal/day (13%)

*For the Vegetarian Pattern, half of total legume intake counts as vegetables and half as protein foods.

**If all food choices to meet food group recommendations are in nutrient-dense forms, a small number of calories remain within the overall calorie limit of the pattern (i.e., limit on calories for other uses). Calories up to the specified limit can be used to consume added sugars, added refined starches, solid fats, or alcohol, or to eat more than the recommended amount of food in a food group.

NOTE: c-eq = cup-equivalent, the amount of a food or beverage product that is considered equal to 1 cup from the vegetables, fruits, or dairy food groups; oz-eq = ounce-equivalent, the amount of a food product that is considered equal to 1 ounce from the grain or protein food groups; N/A = not applicable.

SOURCE: U.S Department of Health and Human Services and U.S. Department of Agriculture. 2015. *2015–2020 Dietary Guidelines for Americans,* 8th ed. (http://health.gov/dietaryguidelines/2015/guidelines/).

completing a scientific review, the committee recommends these actions for staying within calorie limits while sticking to a dietary pattern that has healthy amounts of vegetables, fruits, legumes, whole grains, nuts and seeds, with some vegetable oils, low-fat dairy, lean meat and poultry, and fatty fish.

FATS Replace saturated fats with unsaturated fats, particularly polyunsaturated fat. Reducing saturated fats lowers the incidence of cardiovascular disease in adults and LDL cholesterol in all adults and some children, especially boys.

BEVERAGES Hydrate with water and drinks that don't have sugars added. Sugar-sweetened beverages, not including coffee and tea with added sugar, account for approximately one-third of all drinks that young children consume. They account for 50% of the beverages consumed by adolescents, and 60% of those consumed by adults. These beverages provide energy but contribute very little toward meeting nutrient and food group recommendations; rather, they increase overweight and obesity.

Alcohol has no confirmed health benefits: The Committee concluded that no evidence exists to relax current guidelines; in fact, the evidence points to tightening them for men. Both men and women who drink should consume just one drink per day on days when alcohol is consumed.

SUGAR Consume less than 6% of energy from added sugars. This proportion is lower than the 10% recommended in the *2015-2020 Dietary Guidelines for Americans.* Nearly 70 percent

of added sugars intake comes from 5 food categories: sweetened beverages, desserts and sweet snacks, coffee and tea (with their additions), candy and sugars, and breakfast cereals and bars.

In addition, all Americans should strive to meet the federal physical activity guidelines (described in detail in Chapter 14) and aim to achieve and maintain a healthy body weight.

Making Shifts to Align with Healthy Eating Patterns Every food choice is an opportunity to move toward a healthy eating pattern. Making small positive dietary changes over time can cumulatively make a big difference and support your efforts at maintaining a healthy body weight, meeting nutrient needs, and reducing your risk for chronic disease. See the box "Positive Changes to Improve Your Diet" for some strategies to get you started.

People have many options for incorporating the recommendations of the *Dietary Guidelines* into healthy eating patterns that (1) meet nutrient needs; (2) stay within calorie limits; (3) accommodate cultural, ethnic, traditional, and personal preferences; and (4) take into account food cost and availability. For tips on eating healthfully in a variety of ethnic restaurants, see the box "Ethnic Foods."

Supporting Healthy Eating Patterns Making healthy choices can be challenging, but ultimately each person makes decisions about what, where, when, and how much to eat. Individuals are more likely to shift their eating patterns toward

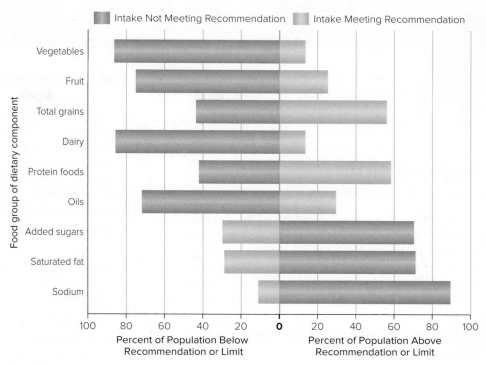

FIGURE 13.3 Dietary intakes compared to recommendations.
The bars show the percentages of the U.S. population aged 1 year and over who are below, at, or above each dietary goal or limit. The center (0) line is the goal or limit. For most people, meaning those represented by the red sections of the bars, shifting toward the center line will improve eating patterns. For example, over 80% of people do not eat enough vegetables—they fall below the recommendation. Within the area of the graph demonstrating our consumption of foods we should limit—added sugars, saturated fat, and sodium—the red bars show that over 80% of people exceed the recommended limit for sodium intake.

SOURCES: What We Eat in America, NHANES 2007–2010 for average intakes by age-sex group. Healthy U.S.-Style Food Patterns, which vary based on age, sex, and activity level, for recommended intakes and limits (see National Cancer Institute. Usual Dietary Intakes: Food Intakes, U.S. Population, 2007–10. *Epidemiology and Genomics Research Program* website; https://epi.grants.cancer.gov/diet/usualintakes).

the guidelines if we make a collaborative effort across all segments of society. By doing so, we create a culture in which healthy lifestyle choices at home, school, work, and everywhere else are easy, accessible, affordable, and normative.

Are healthy food options available and affordable at your school and worksite? How far is it from your home to the nearest place to purchase fruits and vegetables? How many food advertisements are you exposed to daily, and what are they for? Factors such as these can have an enormous influence on individual behavior—both positive and negative—sometimes without our awareness. If the environment supports public health guidelines, individuals are more likely to reach fitness, nutritional, health, and body weight goals. Although societal policies can promote health at all stages of the life cycle, managing health, chronic diseases, body weight, and physical activity still remains a personal responsibility (see Figure 13.4).

Planning and Budgeting for Healthy Eating Students often complain that they cannot afford fruits and vegetables. But many also spend hundreds of dollars on unnecessary supplements, eating out, and fast foods. Buying groceries and eating at home is cheaper and gives you more control over the ingredients added to your food.

Before heading out to the store:

- Plan for a couple of meals and write down the necessary ingredients.
- Create a grocery list so that you do not spontaneously pick up prepackaged food, frozen meals, and desserts.
- Shop on a full stomach so that the chips and cookies do not tempt you.

At the store:

- Buy foods that take more prep work but save money—choose fresh fruits and vegetables instead of precut, bagged, and canned produce; make your own guacamole, bean dips, and salad dressings.
- Stock up on organic black beans, low-fat refried beans, whole-grain pasta, and other staples when they go on sale; buy in bulk.
- Alternate meats with other sources of protein (e.g., quinoa, nuts, tofu, and cottage cheese).

USDA's MyPlate

To help consumers put the *Dietary Guidelines for Americans* into practice, the USDA issues the food-guidance system called MyPlate. MyPlate provides a simple graphic showing how to use the five food groups to build a healthy plate at each meal (Figure 13.5). If you need to make changes in your dietary pattern, use MyPlate to build a healthy eating style by focusing on variety, amount of food consumed, and nutrition. Follow the recommendations in the *Dietary Guidelines* to limit saturated fat, added sugars, and sodium. Start with small changes; they will add up over time.

You can get a personalized version of MyPlate recommendations by visiting ChooseMyPlate.gov. Using the daily food plan feature, you can determine the amount of each food group you need daily based on your calorie allowance. Your plan is personalized based on your age, gender, weight,

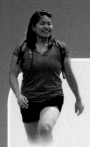

TAKE CHARGE
Positive Changes to Improve Your Diet

Remember to focus on nutrient-dense options for the majority of your food choices: Use your calorie budget wisely. The tips here focus on the types of changes and swaps needed for the majority of Americans to move toward the dietary pattern recommended in the *Dietary Guidelines*.

Vegetables: Eat More

- Increase the vegetable content of mixed dishes while decreasing the amounts of other food components that you may overconsume—for example, cut the meat or cheese in half and double the vegetables in a soup, stew, or casserole.
- Always choose a green salad or a vegetable as a side dish.
- Incorporate vegetables into most meals and snacks.
- Replace foods high in calories, saturated fat, or sodium, such as some meats, poultry, cheeses, and snack foods, with vegetables.

Fruits: Increase Fruit Intake, Especially Whole Fruits

- Choose more fruits as snacks, in salads, as side dishes, and as desserts in place of foods with added sugars such as cookies, pies, cakes, and ice cream.

Grains: Swap Processed for Whole Grains

- Shift from refined to whole-grain versions of commonly eaten foods—from white to 100% whole-wheat breads, white to whole-grain pasta, and white to brown rice (see the section on whole grains earlier in the chapter for more information on using food labels to identify whole grains).
- Cut back on refined-grain desserts and sweet snacks that are high in added sugars, solid fats, or both. Choose smaller portions and eat them less often. For healthy swaps, try plain popcorn instead of buttered and bread instead of a croissant or biscuit, for example.

Dairy: Increase Intake

- Drink fat-free or low-fat milk (or soy beverage) with meals, choose yogurt as a snack, or use yogurt as an ingredient in salad dressings, spreads, and other prepared dishes.
- Favor milk and yogurt for additional dairy servings; cheese has more sodium and saturated fat and less potassium, vitamin A, and vitamin D than milk and yogurt.

Protein: Add Variety and Make More Plant-Based Choices

- Increase low-mercury seafood intake if yours is low: Try seafood as the protein choice in meals twice per week in place of meat, poultry, or eggs—for example, a tuna sandwich or a salmon steak.
- Use legumes or nuts and seeds in mixed dishes instead of some meat or poultry—for example, bean chili instead of a mixed-meat dish or almonds instead of ham on a main-dish salad.

Oils: Choose Healthier Fats

- Use oils rather than solid fats in food preparation where possible—for example, vegetable oil in place of butter, stick margarine, shortening, lard, or coconut oils when cooking.
- Increase intake of foods that naturally contain oils, such as seafood and nuts, in place of some meat and poultry.
- Choose options for salad dressings and spreads made with oils instead of solid fats.

Saturated Fats: Reduce to Less Than 10% of Calories per Day

- Substitute foods high in unsaturated fats for foods high in saturated fats; for example, use oils rather than solid fats for food preparation.
- Read food labels to identify the types of fats in prepared foods; compare and choose lower-fat forms of foods and beverages that contain solid fats (e.g., fat-free milk instead of 2% or whole).
- Adjust proportions of ingredients in mixed dishes to increase vegetables, whole grains, lean meat, and lower-fat cheeses in place of some of the fatty meat or regular cheeses.
- Consume foods higher in solid fats less often and in smaller portions.

Added Sugars: Reduce as Much as Possible

- Choose beverages with no added sugars, such as water, in place of sugar-sweetened beverages.
- Reduce portion sizes of sugar-sweetened beverages, and choose them less often.
- Limit servings and decrease portion sizes of grain-based and dairy desserts and sweet snacks.
- Choose unsweetened or no-sugar-added versions of canned fruit, fruit sauces, and yogurt.

Sodium: Lower Intake

- Read food labels to compare sodium content, choosing products with less sodium.
- Choose fresh, plain frozen, or no-salt-added canned vegetables and fresh protein sources rather than processed meat and poultry.
- Eat at home more often; cooking from scratch allows you to control the sodium content.
- Limit sauces, mixes, and "instant" flavoring packs that come with rice and noodles; use your own flavorings based on herbs and spices rather than salt.

Physical Activity: Do More!

- Increase weekly physical activity; target transportation and leisure activities.
- Reduce sedentary time; take frequent breaks during sedentary activities.

SOURCE: U.S. Department of Health and Human Services and U.S. Department of Agriculture. 2015. *2015–2020 Dietary Guidelines for Americans,* 8th ed. (http://health.gov/dietaryguidelines/2015/guidelines/).

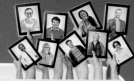

No single ethnic diet clearly surpasses all others in providing people with healthful foods. However, every diet has advantages and disadvantages and, within each cuisine, some foods are better choices. The dietary guidance described in this chapter can be applied to any ethnic cuisine. For additional guidance, refer to the table below.

	Choose More Often	Choose Less Often
Chinese	Dishes that are zheng (steamed), jum (poached), chu (boiled), kao (roasted), shu (barbecued), or lightly stir-fried Hoisin sauce, oyster sauce, wine sauce, plum sauce, velvet sauce, or hot mustard Fresh fish and seafood, skinless chicken, tofu Mixed vegetables, Chinese greens Steamed rice, steamed spring rolls, soft noodles	Fried wontons or egg rolls Crab rangoon Crispy (Peking) duck or chicken Sweet-and-sour dishes made with breaded and deep-fried meat, poultry, or fish Fried rice Fried or crispy noodles
French	Dishes prepared au vapeur (steamed), en brochette (skewered and broiled), or grillé (grilled) Fresh fish, shrimp, scallops, or mussels or skinless chicken, without sauces Clear soups	Dishes prepared à la crème (in cream sauce), au gratin or gratinée (baked with cream and cheese), or en croûte (in pastry crust) Drawn butter, hollandaise sauce, and remoulade (mayonnaise-based sauce)
Greek	Dishes that are stewed, broiled, or grilled, including shish kebabs (souvlaki) Dolmas (grape leaves) stuffed with rice Tzatziki (yogurt, cucumbers, and garlic) Tabouli (bulgur-based salad) Pita bread, especially whole wheat	Moussaka, saganaki (fried cheese) Vegetable pies such as spanakopita and tyropita Dolmas stuffed with ground meat Deep-fried falafel (chickpea patties) Gyros stuffed with ground meat Baklava
Indian	Dishes prepared masala (curry), tandoori (roasted in a clay oven), or tikke (pan roasted); kebabs Raita (yogurt and cucumber salad) and other yogurt-based dishes and sauces Dal (lentils), pullao or pilau (basmati rice) Chapati (baked bread)	Ghee (clarified butter) Korma (meat in cream sauce) Samosas, pakoras (fried dishes) Molee and other coconut milk–based dishes Poori, bhatura, or paratha (fried breads) Mango lassi
Italian	Pasta primavera or pasta, polenta, risotto, or gnocchi with marinara, red or white wine, white or red clam, or light mushroom sauce Dishes that are grilled or prepared cacciatore (tomato-based sauce), marsala (broth and wine sauce), or piccata (lemon sauce) Cioppino (seafood stew) Vegetable soup, minestrone or fagioli (beans)	Antipasto (cheese, smoked meats) Dishes that are prepared alfredo, frito (fried), crema (creamed), alla panna (with cream), or carbonara Veal scaloppini Chicken, veal, or eggplant parmigiana Italian sausage, salami, and prosciutto Buttered garlic bread Cannoli
Japanese	Dishes prepared nabemono (boiled), shabu-shabu (in boiling broth), mushimono (steamed), nimono (simmered), yaki (broiled), or yakimono (grilled) Sushi or domburi (mixed rice dish) Steamed rice or soba (buckwheat), udon (wheat), or rice noodles	Tempura (battered and fried) Agemono (deep fried) Katsu (fried pork cutlet) Sukiyaki Fried tofu
Mexican	Soft corn or wheat tortillas Burritos, fajitas, enchiladas, soft tacos, and tamales filled with beans, vegetables, or lean meats Refried beans, nonfat or low-fat; rice and beans, brown rice Ceviche (fish marinated in lime juice) Salsa, enchilada sauce, and picante sauce Gazpacho, menudo, or black bean soup Fruit or flan for dessert	Crispy, fried tortillas Dishes that are fried, such as chile rellenos, chimichangas, flautas, and tostadas Nachos and cheese, chili con queso, and other dishes made with cheese or cheese sauce Sour cream and extra cheese Refried beans made with lard Fried ice cream
Thai	Dishes that are barbecued, sautéed, broiled, boiled, steamed, braised, or marinated Sâté (skewered and grilled meats) Fish sauce, basil sauce, chili or hot sauces, lime sauce or juice Bean thread noodles, Thai salad	Coconut milk soup Peanut sauce or dishes topped with nuts Mee-krob (crispy noodles) Red, green, and yellow curries, which typically contain coconut milk

SOURCES: National Heart, Lung, and Blood Institute. 2014. *Aim for a Healthy Weight: Maintaining a Healthy Weight on the Go: A Pocket Guide.* NIH Publication No. 14-7415.; Duyff, R. L. 2012. *The American Dietetic Association Complete Food and Nutrition Guide*, 4th ed. Hoboken, NJ: Wiley.

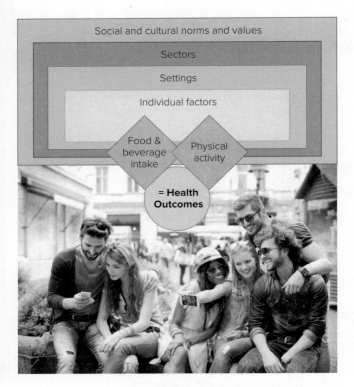

FIGURE 13.4 **A Social-Ecological Model (SEM) for food and physical activity decisions.** The model shows that various factors influence food and beverage intake, physical activity patterns, and ultimately health outcomes.
Social and cultural norms and values, including traditions, religion, lifestyle, body image, and priorities
Sectors, including government, education, health care, and transportation systems; public health and community organizations; and business and industries related to agriculture, food and beverage, entertainment, marketing, and media
Settings, such as home, school, worksite, and food retail
Individual factors, such as age, sex, socioeconomic status, race/ethnicity, knowledge and skills, and food preferences
SOURCE: U.S. Department of Health and Human Services and U.S. Department of Agriculture. 2015. *2015–2020 Dietary Guidelines for Americans,* 8th ed. (http://health.gov/dietaryguidelines/2015/guidelines/chapter-3 /social -ecological-model/), accessed March 2018. svetikd/Getty Images

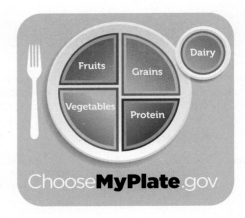

FIGURE 13.5 **MyPlate.** The USDA's MyPlate is designed as a simple graphic to help Americans apply the *Dietary Guidelines* to their own diets.
SOURCE: U.S. Department of Agriculture, www.choosemyplate.gov.

level for your eating plan, monitor your body weight and adjust calorie intake and physical activity based on changes in weight over time.

The *Dietary Guidelines* recommend that adults who are obese or overweight shift their eating and physical-activity behaviors to prevent additional weight gain and/or promote weight loss. Weight management is discussed in Chapter 15.

Most people underestimate not only the number of calories they consume but also the size of their portions. See the box "Judging Portion Sizes" for strategies to improve the accuracy of your estimates. MyPlate doesn't use number of portions as the basis of recommendations; instead, amounts are listed in terms of cup-equivalents and ounce-equivalents. These units of measurement allow for the alignment of servings of foods that differ—those that are concentrated versus those that are more airy or contain more water. For example, ½ cup of blueberries and ¼ cup of raisins both count as ½ cup-equivalent of fruit.

Next, let's take a brief look at each food group.

height, and level of physical activity. MyPlate is available in Spanish, and it offers special recommendations for dieters, preschoolers aged 2–5, children aged 6–11, and pregnant and breastfeeding women.

Energy Intake and Portion Sizes To build a healthy eating style, your food group goals should be based on an appropriate level of energy intake. Table 13.8 provides ranges for calorie intake for weight maintenance. Everyone is different, however, and the number of calories you need will vary depending on multiple factors. If your weight is stable, your current energy intake is in balance with calories expended; you can set a more personal calorie goal by carefully tracking your food intake for several days to determine your current calorie intake. Once you select a calorie

Fruits: Focus on Whole Fruits People who eat more vegetables and fruits as part of an overall healthy diet are likely to have a reduced risk of some chronic diseases. Fruits are rich in carbohydrates, dietary fiber, and many vitamins, especially vitamin C. A 2000-calorie diet should include 2 cups of fruit daily. Each of the following counts as 1 cup-equivalent from the fruit group:

- 1 cup fresh, canned, or frozen fruit
- 1 cup fruit juice (100% juice)
- 1 small whole fruit
- ½ cup dried fruit

Choose whole fruits often; they are higher in fiber and often lower in energy than fruit juices. Fruit *juices* typically

Table 13.8	Estimated Daily Calorie Needs		
AGE (YEARS)	SEDENTARY*	MODERATELY ACTIVE**	ACTIVE***
Females**			
16–18	1800	2000	2400
19–25	2000	2200	2400
26–30	1800	2000	2400
31–50	1800	2000	2200
51–60	1600	1800	2200
61 & up	1600	1800	2000
Males			
16–18	2400	2800	3200
19–20	2600	2800	3000
21–25	2400	2800	3000
26–35	2400	2600	3000
36–40	2400	2600	2800
41–45	2200	2600	2800
46–55	2200	2400	2800
56–60	2200	2400	2600
61–65	2000	2400	2600
66–75	2000	2200	2600
76 & up	2000	2200	2400

*Sedentary means a lifestyle that includes only the physical activity of independent living.

**Moderately active means a lifestyle that includes physical activity equivalent to walking about 1.5–3 miles per day at 3–4 miles per hour, in addition to the activities of independent living.

***Active means a lifestyle that includes physical activity equivalent to walking more than 3 miles per day at 3–4 miles per hour, in addition to the activities of independent living.

****Estimates for females do not include women who are pregnant or breastfeeding.

SOURCES: U.S. Department of Health and Human Services and U.S. Department of Agriculture. 2015. *2015–2020 Dietary Guidelines for Americans*, 8th ed. (http://health.gov/dietaryguidelines/2015 /guidelines/); Food and Nutrition Board, Institute of Medicine. 2002. *Dietary Reference Intakes for Energy, Carbohydrate, Fiber, Fat, Fatty Acids, Cholesterol, Protein, and Amino Acids.* Washington, DC: National Academies Press.

contain more nutrients and less added sugar than fruit *drinks*. When buying canned fruits, choose those packed in 100% fruit juice or water rather than in syrup.

Vegetables: Vary Your Veggies   Together, fruits and vegetables should make up half your plate. Vegetables contain carbohydrates, dietary fiber, carotenoids, vitamin C, folate, potassium, and other nutrients. They are naturally low in calories and fat and contain no cholesterol. A 2000-calorie diet should include 2½ cups of vegetables daily. Each of the following counts as 1 cup-equivalent from the vegetable group:

- 1 cup raw or cooked vegetables
- 2 cups raw leafy salad greens
- 1 cup vegetable juice

Because vegetables vary in the nutrients they provide, eat a variety to obtain maximum nutrition. MyPlate recommends weekly servings from the five subgroups within the vegetables group (see Table 13.7). Eat vegetables from several subgroups each day.

- Dark green vegetables (e.g., broccoli, bok choy, romaine lettuce, spinach, collards, kale)
- Red and orange vegetables (e.g., tomatoes, carrots, sweet potatoes, red peppers, winter squash)
- Beans and peas (e.g., split and black-eyed peas; lentils; soybeans; black, kidney, navy, pinto, and white beans)
- Starchy vegetables (e.g., corn, potatoes, green peas)
- Other vegetables (e.g., artichokes, asparagus, beets, cauliflower, green beans, head lettuce, onions, mushrooms, zucchini)

Grains: Make Half Your Grains Whole Grains   Foods from this group are usually low in fat and rich in complex carbohydrates, dietary fiber (if grains are unrefined), and vitamins and minerals, including thiamin, riboflavin, iron, niacin, folic acid (if enriched or fortified), and zinc. A 2000-calorie diet should include 6 ounce-equivalents each day, with half of those servings from whole grains. The following items count as 1 ounce-equivalent:

- 1 slice of bread
- 1 small (2½-inch diameter) muffin
- 1 cup ready-to-eat cereal flakes
- ½ cup cooked cereal, rice, grains, or pasta
- 1 6-inch tortilla

Choose foods that are typically made with little fat or sugar (bread, rice, pasta) over those that are high in fat and sugar (croissants, chips, cookies).

Protein Foods: Vary Your Protein Routine   This group includes meat, poultry, fish, dried beans and peas, eggs, nuts and seeds, and processed soy foods. These foods provide protein, niacin, iron, vitamin B-6, zinc, and thiamin. The animal foods in this group also provide vitamin B-12. A 2000-calorie diet should include 5½ ounce-equivalents daily. Each of the following counts as 1 ounce-equivalent:

- 1 ounce cooked lean meat, poultry, or fish
- ¼ cup cooked dried beans (legumes) or tofu
- 1 egg
- 1 tablespoon peanut butter
- ½ ounce nuts or seeds

Choose a variety of lean meats and skinless poultry, select a variety of protein foods, and watch serving sizes carefully. Choose at least one serving of plant proteins, such as black beans, lentils, or tofu, every day, and include at least 8 ounces of cooked seafood per week. Vegetarian options in the protein foods group include beans and peas, processed soy products, and nuts and seeds.

Studies have shown that most people under-estimate the size of their food portions, in many cases by as much as 50%. If you need to retrain your eye, try using measuring cups and spoons and an inexpensive kitchen scale when you eat at home. With a little practice, you'll learn the difference between 3 and 8 ounces of chicken or meat and what a half-cup of rice really looks like. For quick estimates, use the following equivalents:

- 1 teaspoon margarine = the tip of your thumb

- 1 ounce cheese = your thumb, four dice stacked together, or an ice cube

- 3 ounces chicken or meat = a deck of cards

- 1 cup pasta = a small fist or a tennis ball

- ½ cup rice or cooked vegetables = an ice cream scoop or one-third of a can of soda

- 2 tablespoons peanut butter = a Ping-Pong ball or a large marshmallow

- 1 medium potato = a computer mouse

- 2-ounce muffin or roll = a plum or a large egg

- 2-ounce bagel = a hockey puck or a yo-yo

- 1 medium fruit (apple or orange) = a baseball

- ¼ cup nuts = a golf ball

- small cookie or cracker = a poker chip

Dairy: Move to Low-Fat and Fat-Free Dairy   This group includes milk and milk products, such as yogurt and cheeses that retain their calcium, as well as calcium-fortified soy milk. Foods from this group are high in protein, carbohydrate, calcium, potassium, riboflavin, and vitamin D (if fortified). Dairy choices should be fat-free or low-fat as much as possible to reduce energy intake. A 2000-calorie diet should include 3 cups of milk or the equivalent daily. Each of the following counts as 1 cup-equivalent:

- 1 cup milk

- 1 cup yogurt

- ½ cup ricotta cheese

- 1½ ounces natural cheese

- 2 ounces processed cheese

Cottage cheese is lower in calcium than most other cheeses; ½ cup is equivalent to ¼ cup milk. Ice cream is also lower in calcium and higher in sugar and fat than many other dairy products; one scoop counts as ⅓ cup milk.

Oils   Included in this category are oils and fats that are liquid at room temperature; they come mostly from plant and fish sources. Also included are soft margarines, soft vegetable oil table spreads, mayonnaise, and some salad dressings that have no trans fats. Oils are major sources of vitamin E and unsaturated fatty acids, including essential fatty acids, but

they are *not a food group*. A 2000-calorie diet should include 6 teaspoons (27 g) of oils per day. A 1-teaspoon serving is the equivalent of the following:

- 1 teaspoon vegetable oil or soft margarine

- 1 tablespoon mayonnaise-type salad dressing

Foods that are mostly oils include nuts, olives, avocados, and some fish. The following portions include about 1 teaspoon of oil: 8 large olives, ⅙ medium avocado, ½ tablespoon peanut butter, and ⅓ ounce roasted nuts. Food labels can help you identify the types and amounts of fat in various foods.

Solid Fats and Added Sugars   If you choose nutrient-dense foods from all food groups, you will have a small proportion of your daily calorie budget left to "spend" on additional food choices. For those wanting to maintain weight, these calories may be used to increase the amount of food from a food group, to consume foods that contain solid fats or added sugars, or to consume alcohol. People who are trying to lose weight and improve their health should limit solid fats and added sugars as much as possible. The average American consumes nearly 800 calories daily from solid fats and added sugars—far higher than the recommended limits.

For an evaluation of your diet, complete the activity in the box "Your Diet versus MyPlate Recommendations."

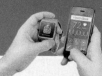
1. **Keep a food record.** To evaluate your daily diet, begin by keeping a record of everything you eat on a typical day. To help with your analysis, break down each food item into its component parts and note your portion sizes. For example, you might list a turkey sandwich as 2 slices of sourdough bread, 3 ounces of turkey, 1 tomato, 1 tablespoon of mayonnaise, and so on.

2. **Compare your servings to the recommendations of MyPlate.** Complete the following chart to compare your daily diet to the USDA Food Intake Patterns and MyPlate. See Figures 1–3 in the Nutrition Resources section at the end of the chapter for the recommended amount for your calorie level. It may be difficult to track values for added sugars, and especially for oils and fats, but be as accurate as you can. Check food labels for information about fat and sugar. (*Note:* For a more complete and accurate analysis of your diet, keep food records for three days and then average the results.) ChooseMyPlate.gov has additional guidelines for counting discretionary calories.

Food Group	Recommended Daily Amounts for Your Energy Intake	Your Actual Daily Intake (Amounts)	Serving Sizes and Equivalents
Grains (total)			1 ounce-equivalent = 1 slice of bread; 1 small muffin; 1 cup ready-to-eat cereal flakes; or ½ cup cooked cereal, rice, grains, or pasta
Whole grains			
Processed grains			
Vegetables (total)			1 cup or equivalent = 1 cup raw or cooked vegetables; 2 cups raw leafy salad greens; or 1 cup vegetable juice
Dark green*			
Red/orange*			
Legumes*			
Starchy*			
Other*			
Fruits			1 cup or equivalent = 1 cup fresh, canned, or frozen fruit; 1 cup fruit juice; 1 small whole fruit; or ½ cup dried fruit
Dairy			1 cup or equivalent = 1 cup milk or yogurt; 1½ oz natural cheese; or 2 oz processed cheese
Protein foods			1 ounce-equivalent = 1 oz lean meat, poultry, or fish; ¼ cup cooked dry beans or tofu; 1 egg; 1 tablespoon peanut butter; or ½ oz nuts or seeds
Seafood*			
Meat, poultry, eggs*			
Nuts, seeds, soy products*			
Oils			1 teaspoon or equivalent = 1 teaspoon vegetable oil or 1 tablespoon mayonnaise-type salad dressing
Solid fats & added sugars			

*Calculate daily intake from the weekly amounts shown in Figures 1–3 in the Nutrition Resources section at the end of the chapter.

3. **Further evaluate your food choices within the groups.** Based on the data you collected and what you learned in this chapter, what were the especially healthy choices you made (e.g., whole grains and citrus fruits), and what were your less healthy choices? Identify and list foods in the latter category because these are areas where you can make changes to improve your diet. In particular, you may want to limit your intake of the following: processed, sweetened grains; high-fat meats and poultry skin; deep-fried fast foods; full-fat dairy products; regular sodas, sweetened teas, and fruit drinks; alcoholic beverages; and other foods that provide primarily sugar and solid fats and few other nutrients.

4. **Make healthy changes.** Bring your diet in line with MyPlate by adding servings from food groups for which you fall short of the recommendations. To maintain a healthy weight, you may need to balance these additions by making reductions in other areas—by eliminating some of the fats, sweets, and alcohol you consume; by cutting extra servings from food groups for which your intake is more than adequate; or by making healthier choices within the food groups. Make a list of foods to add and a list of foods to eliminate, and post your lists in a prominent location.

For a more detailed and customized analysis of your current diet, including intakes of specific nutrients, many smartphone apps are available to help you track your diet.

Physical Activity The *Dietary Guidelines for Americans* and MyPlate strongly encourage all Americans to be physically active as much as possible. Daily physical activity improves health, reduces the risk of chronic diseases, and helps people manage body weight. The MyPlate recommendation for adults is 2½ hours of moderate physical activity or 1¼ hours of vigorous physical activity per week, equivalent to the 150 minutes of moderate activity or 75 minutes of vigorous activity recommended in the *2008 Physical Activity Guidelines for Americans*.

See Figure 13.6 for a summary of the MyPlate recommendations for a 2000-calorie diet. The Nutrition Resources section at the end of the chapter includes detailed food group amounts for other calorie levels and for all three healthy eating patterns featured in the *Dietary Guidelines*.

DASH Eating Plan

Other food-group plans have been proposed by a variety of experts and organizations, some to address the needs of special populations. One well-studied eating plan is called Dietary Approaches to Stop Hypertension (DASH). It was developed to help people control high blood pressure, and it is tailored with special attention to sodium, potassium, and other nutrients that affect blood pressure. Figure 4 in the Nutrition Resources section at the end of the chapter provides a more detailed look at the DASH Eating Plan.

Choosing a Plant-Based Diet

People following a plant-based diet choose a diet with one basic difference from the diets described previously—they restrict or exclude foods of animal origin (meat, poultry, fish, eggs, and milk) and instead choose more plant-based foods. Commonly referred to as vegetarian, plant-based diets are lower in total fat, saturated fat, cholesterol, and animal protein and higher in complex carbohydrates, dietary fiber, magnesium, folate, vitamins C and E, carotenoids, and phytochemicals. **Vegetarians** generally have a lower body mass index than nonvegetarians and have diet patterns associated with lower mortality rates and lower rates of heart disease, obesity, hypertension, and type 2 diabetes. Many people adopt a vegetarian diet for health reasons, whereas others do so out of concern for the environment, for financial reasons, or for reasons related to ethics or religion. Since meat, dairy, and eggs are the only food sources for vitamin B-12 and for highly bioavailable iron, vegetarians must rely on fortified cereals and supplements.

Types of Plant-Based Diets There are various vegetarian styles. The wider the variety of foods eaten, the easier it is to meet nutritional needs.

- *Vegans* eat only plant foods.
- *Lacto-vegetarians* eat plant foods and dairy products.
- *Lacto-ovo-vegetarians* eat plant foods, dairy products, and eggs.

Others can be categorized as partial vegetarians, semi-vegetarians, or pesco-vegetarians. The latter—also called

> **vegetarian** Someone who follows a diet that restricts or eliminates foods of animal origin. **TERMS**

Food Group Amounts for 2000 Calories a Day

Fruits	Vegetables	Grains	Protein	Dairy
2 cups	**2½ cups**	**6 ounces**	**5½ ounces**	**3 cups**
Focus on whole fruits	**Vary your veggies**	**Make half your grains whole grains**	**Vary your protein routine**	**Move to low-fat or fat-free milk or yogurt**
Focus on whole fruits that are fresh, frozen, canned, or dried.	Choose a variety of colorful fresh, frozen, and canned vegetables—make sure to include dark green, red, and orange choices.	Find whole-grain foods by reading the Nutrition Facts label and ingredients list.	Mix up your protein foods to include seafood, beans and peas, unsalted nuts and seeds, soy products, eggs, and lean meats and poultry.	Choose fat-free milk, yogurt, and soy beverages (soy milk) to cut back on your saturated fat.

Limit **Drink and eat less sodium, saturated fat, and added sugars. Limit:**
- Sodium to **2300 milligrams** a day.
- Saturated fat to **22 grams** a day (less than 10% of total daily calories).
- Added sugars to **50 grams** a day (less than 10% of total daily calories).
- If alcohol is consumed, it should be consumed in moderation—up to one drink per day for women and up to two drinks per day for men—and only by adults of legal drinking age.

Activity **Be active your way:**
Adults:
- Be physically active at least **2½ hours** per week.

FIGURE 13.6 **MyPlate food group amounts and recommendations for a 2000-calorie diet.**

SOURCE: MyPlate.gov. 2016. *MyPlate Daily Checklist for 2,000 Calories* (http://www.choosemyplate.gov/resources/MyPlatePlan/MyPlatePlan_2000cals_Age14plus).

pescatarians or pescetarians—have diets that are mainly plant-based but also include fish and other seafood. Partial vegetarians generally eat plant foods, dairy products, eggs, and usually a small selection of poultry, fish, and other seafood. Many other people choose vegetarian meals frequently but are not strictly vegetarians. A quarter of Americans make dietary choices to limit their meat intake. Including some animal protein (such as dairy products) in a vegetarian diet makes planning easier, but it is not necessary.

Health professionals now recommend plant-based diets as a primary method in the prevention and treatment of chronic diseases. A plant-based diet need not be fully vegetarian. Instead, it can contain more whole foods consisting of fruits, vegetables, legumes, whole grains, nuts, seeds, and herbs. You may have heard of the trend "meatless Mondays" as one option to encourage more people to move toward a more plant-based eating pattern.

A Plant-Based Food Plan Figure 2 in the Nutrition Resources section at the end of the chapter outlines the USDA's Healthy Vegetarian diet plan for a 2000-calorie diet. Adapting MyPlate for vegetarians requires only a few key modifications: For the meat and beans group, vegetarians can focus on the nonmeat choices of dry beans, nuts, seeds, eggs, and soy foods like tofu. Vegans and other vegetarians who do not consume any dairy products must find other rich sources of calcium. Fruits, vegetables, and whole grains are healthy choices for people following all types of vegetarian diets.

People following a more plant-based diet may choose to include meat alternatives—foods that approximate the taste and texture of meat but are made from vegetarian ingredients such as soy, gluten, or legumes. Many new plant-based products mimic beef patties, sausages, chicken strips, and similar animal foods. Recently developed products like the Impossible Burger and the Beyond Burger are promoted as especially meat-like and are even created to "bleed" like beef. As with any processed food, consider the overall nutritional profile of meat alternatives you select.

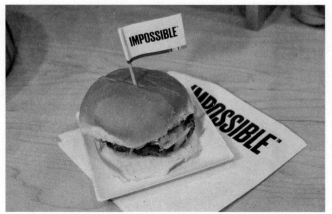

John D. Ivanko/Alamy Stock Photo

Unlike most animal proteins, most plant proteins do not contain all the necessary amino acids for good health. Thus, a healthy vegetarian diet must emphasize a wide variety of plant foods in order to include all the necessary amino acids. Choosing minimally processed and unrefined foods will maximize nutrient value and provide ample dietary fiber. Daily consumption of a variety of plant foods in amounts that meet total energy needs can provide all needed nutrients, except vitamin B-12 and possibly calcium, iron, zinc, and vitamin D. Strategies for obtaining nutrients of concern include the following:

- *Vitamin B-12* occurs naturally only in animal foods. If dairy products and eggs are limited or avoided, B-12 can be obtained from fortified foods such as ready-to-eat cereals, soy beverages, meat substitutes, and special yeast products or from supplements.

- *Vitamin D* can be obtained by spending 5–15 minutes a day in the sun (without sunscreen), from vitamin D–fortified products like ready-to-eat cereals, fortified orange juice, and soy or rice milk, or by taking a supplement.

- *Calcium* is found in legumes; tofu processed with calcium; dark green leafy vegetables; nuts; tortillas made from lime-processed corn; and fortified orange juice, soy milk, bread, and other foods.

- *Iron* can be obtained from whole grains, fortified bread and breakfast cereals, dried fruits, green leafy vegetables, nuts and seeds, legumes, and soy foods. The iron in plant foods is more difficult for the body to absorb than is the iron from animal sources; consuming a good source of vitamin C with most meals is helpful because vitamin C improves iron absorption.

- *Zinc* is found in whole grains, nuts, legumes, and soy foods.

If you're a vegetarian, or just trying to follow a more plant-based diet, remember that it's especially important to eat as wide a variety of foods as possible to ensure that all your nutritional needs are satisfied. Consulting with a registered dietitian nutritionist (RDN) will make meal planning easier. Vegetarian diets for children, teens, and pregnant and lactating women warrant professional guidance.

Dietary Challenges for Various Population Groups

The *Dietary Guidelines for Americans* and MyPlate can help nearly anyone create a healthy diet. However, some population groups face special dietary challenges.

Children and Teenagers How can we encourage young people to eat healthy foods? Perhaps the best thing a parent

Eating Strategies for College Students

All the Time

• Eat a colorful, varied, and plant-based diet. The more colorful your diet is, the more varied and rich in fruits and vegetables it will be. Fruits and vegetables are typically inexpensive, delicious, and nutrient-dense.

• Don't skip meals, especially breakfast. You'll have more energy in the morning and be less likely to grab an unhealthy snack later on. Skipping meals leads to poorer food choices throughout the day.

• Choose healthy snacks—fruits, vegetables, whole grains, and cereals.

• Drink nonfat milk, water, mineral water, or 100% fruit juice more often than soft drinks or sweetened beverages.

• Pay attention to portion sizes. Enjoy your food, but eat less.

• Plan to eat meals with friends and family members who choose healthy foods and can provide support and inspiration.

• Combine physical activity with healthy eating.

• Choose plant-based (meatless) meals more often. Ask about vegetarian options when eating out or consider cooking your own meat-free burgers, tacos, or "meat" balls and spaghetti.

Eating in the Dining Hall

• Choose a meal plan that includes breakfast.

• Decide what you want to eat before you get in line, and stick to your choices.

• Build your meals around whole grains and vegetables. Ask for small servings of meat and high-fat main dishes.

• Choose leaner poultry, fish, or bean dishes without added sugar or high sodium rather than high-fat meats and fried entrees.

• Ask that gravies and sauces be served on the side; limit your intake.

• Choose broth-based or vegetable soups, not cream soups.

• At the salad bar, load up on leafy greens, beans, and fresh vegetables. Avoid mayonnaise-coated salads, bacon, croutons, and high-fat dressings. Put dressing on the side, and dip your fork into it rather than pouring it over the salad.

• Choose fruit for dessert rather than baked goods.

• Skip the soda machine and opt for water or low-fat dairy for your beverage choices.

Eating in Fast-Food Restaurants

• Most fast-food chains can provide a brochure with the nutritional content of their menu items. Ask for it, or check the restaurant's website for nutritional information. Order small single burgers with no cheese instead of double burgers with many toppings. If possible, get them broiled instead of fried.

• Ask for items to be prepared without mayonnaise, tartar sauce, sour cream, or other high-fat sauces. Ketchup, mustard, and fat-free mayonnaise or sour cream are better choices and are available at many fast-food restaurants.

• Choose whole-grain bread for burgers and sandwiches.

• Choose chicken items made from chicken breast, not processed chicken.

• Order vegetable pizzas without extra cheese.

• Try a salad or fruit as a side item. If you can't resist french fries or onion rings, get the smallest size.

• For food truck meals, use the same strategies suggested for fast-food restaurants: Choose lean proteins and ask for condiments on the side. If your favorite food truck doesn't have healthy options, ask that they be added to the menu.

Eating on the Run

• When you need to eat in a hurry, carry healthy foods in your backpack or a small insulated lunch sack (with a frozen gel pack to keep fresh food from spoiling). Also carry a refillable water bottle.

• Carry items that are small and convenient but nutritious, such as fresh fruits or vegetables, whole-wheat buns or muffins, snack-size cereal boxes, and water.

• When buying beverages from vending machines, choose water or 100% fruit juice. When buying snacks, choose whole-grain crackers, pretzels, nuts or seeds, baked chips, low-fat popcorn, or low-fat granola bars.

---

can do for younger children is to provide them with a variety of nutrient-dense food options. Allowing children to help prepare meals is another good way to increase food variety and develop a child's interest in eating well. Many children and teenagers enjoy eating at fast-food restaurants, but they should be encouraged to select the healthiest choices from fast-food menus and to balance the day's diet with low-fat, nutrient-rich foods.

College Students Convenient foods are not always the healthiest choices. Students who eat in buffet-style dining halls can easily overeat, and the foods offered are not necessarily high in nutrients or low in fat, sodium, and added sugars. The same is true of meals at fast-food restaurants. See the box "Eating Strategies for College Students" for tips on making healthy eating convenient and affordable.

Pregnant and Breastfeeding Women   Good nutrition is essential to a healthy pregnancy. Before conception, nutrition counseling can help a woman establish a balanced eating plan and healthy body weight for pregnancy. During pregnancy and while breastfeeding, women have special nutritional needs and are often advised to take nutrient supplements (discussed in more detail later in this chapter and in Chapter 9).

Older Adults   Nutrient needs do not change much as people age, but because older adults tend to become less active, they don't need as much energy intake to maintain body weight. At the same time, older adults absorb some nutrients less efficiently (e.g., vitamin B-12) because of age-related changes in the digestive tract. For these reasons, older adults should focus on eating nutrient-dense foods. Foods fortified with vitamin B-12 and/or B-12 supplements are recommended for people over age 50, and calcium and vitamin D supplements may be recommended for older adults to reduce bone loss and lower the risk of osteoporosis. Antioxidants from fruits and vegetables are important in older adults to reduce age-related changes in vision, immunity, and cognitive functioning. Because constipation is a common problem for older adults, eating high-fiber foods and drinking enough fluids are important goals.

Athletes   Key dietary concerns for athletes are meeting their increased energy requirements and drinking enough fluids during practice and throughout the day to remain fully hydrated. Endurance athletes and athletes in heavy training may also benefit from increasing the amount of carbohydrates in the diet to 60–70% of total daily energy intake; this increase should take the form of complex, rather than simple, carbohydrates. Athletes who need to maintain a low body weight—such as skaters, gymnasts, and wrestlers—must avoid unhealthy eating patterns, which can lead to eating disorders. Eating for exercise is discussed in more detail in Chapter 14; see Chapter 15 for information about eating disorders.

People with Special Health Concerns   People with diabetes benefit from a well-balanced diet that is low in simple sugars and high in complex carbohydrates. People with high blood pressure need to control their weight and limit their sodium consumption. If you have a health concern that requires a special diet, discuss your situation with a physician or registered dietitian nutritionist.

A PERSONAL PLAN: MAKING INFORMED CHOICES ABOUT FOOD

Understanding the basics of good nutrition should get you started on creating a healthy diet that works for you. But eating for health involves other skills, as well. For example, it's helpful to be able to interpret the labels on food products and dietary supplement labels. Everyone who handles and pre-

pares food should know how to avoid foodborne illnesses and environmental contaminants. In addition to understanding the nutritional content of foods, you can be an even smarter consumer if you know about other food contents, such as additives, and the various ways foods can be processed before going to market. The sections that follow address these issues.

Reading Food Labels

All processed foods regulated by either the FDA or the USDA include standardized nutrition information on their labels. Every food label shows serving sizes and the amounts of fat, saturated fat, trans fat, cholesterol, sodium, total carbohydrate, dietary fiber, total sugars, added sugars, and protein in each serving. To make informed choices about food, learn to read and *understand* food labels (see the box "Using Food Labels").

Food label regulations also require that foods meet strict definitions if their packaging includes terms such as *light, low-fat,* or *high-fiber* (Table 13.9). Health claims such as "good source of dietary fiber" or "low in saturated fat" on packages are also regulated and can be signals that a product can be wisely included in your diet. Overall, the food label is an important tool to help you choose a healthy dietary pattern.

Fresh meat, poultry, fish, fruits, and vegetables are not required to have food labels, and many of these products are not packaged. You can find information about the nutrient content of these items from basic nutrition books, registered dietitian nutritionist, nutrient analysis computer software, the internet, and the companies that produce or distribute these foods. Supermarkets may also have large posters or pamphlets listing the nutrient contents of these foods.

Calorie Labeling: Restaurants and Vending Machines

In 2014, the FDA issued new regulations requiring that calorie information be available on restaurant menus and vending machines; these new rules were required as part of the 2010 Affordable Care Act. As of May 2018, calorie information is required on menus and menu boards in chain restaurants and

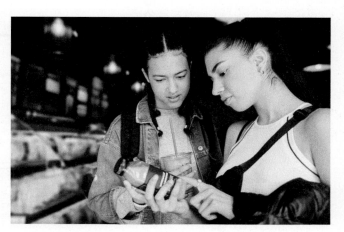

We Are/Getty Images

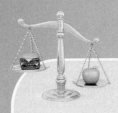

CRITICAL CONSUMER
Using Food Labels

The Nutrition Facts panel on a food label is designed to help consumers make food choices based on the nutrients that are most important to good health. In addition to listing nutrient content by weight, the label puts the information in the context of a daily diet of 2000 calories, with the understanding that your calorie needs may be higher or lower depending on your age, gender, height, weight, and physical activity level.

Food labels contain uniform serving sizes. This means that if you look at different brands of salad dressing, for example, you can compare calories and fat content based on the serving amount. Food label serving sizes, however, may be larger or smaller than MyPlate serving-size equivalents.

The Nutrition Facts label had been in use without major changes since the 1990s. Based on research into how consumers use food labels as well as changes to the nutrients of most concern to Americans, the FDA announced changes to the look and content of the label in 2016. Some new features include:

- Adding added sugars, vitamin D, and potassium to all labels; Vitamins A and C will no longer be required because deficiencies in these vitamins are rare today
- Removing the listing for "Calories from Fat" because research shows the type of fat is more important than the amount
- Revising Daily Values for certain nutrients to reflect the latest recommendations
- Updating serving-size labeling for certain packages to be more realistic and to reflect amounts typically eaten at one time
- Refreshing the design to highlight calorie content and serving size and to make other parts of the label easier to read

The new Nutrition Facts label is required on all foods by January 1, 2021. Many manufacturers have already started to adopt the new label on their products.

SOURCE: U.S. Food and Drug Administration. 2020. *Changes to the Nutrition Facts Label.* (https://www.fda.gov/Food/GuidanceRegulation/Guidance DocumentsRegulatoryInformation/LabelingNutrition/ucm385663.htm).

Previous Label

1. Serving size and calories: Based on the amount of food expected to be eaten at one time.

2. Daily Values: Generally based on a 2,000-calorie diet, Daily Value percentages tell you whether the nutrients in a serving contribute much to your total daily diet.

5% or less is low
20% or more is high

3. Limit these nutrients: Look for foods low in saturated fat, trans fat, and sodium.

4. Get enough of these nutrients: Look for foods high in dietary fiber, vitamin A, vitamin C, calcium, and iron.

Footnote: This section shows recommended daily intake for two levels of calorie consumption and values for dietary calculations.

Nutrition Facts

Serving Size 1-1/2 cup (208g)
Servings per container 2

Amount per Serving

Calories 240 Calories from Fat 36

	% Daily Value*
Total Fat 4g	**5%**
Saturated Fat 1.5g	**8%**
Trans Fat 0g	
Cholesterol 5mg	**2%**
Sodium 430mg	**19%**
Total Carbohydrate 46g	**17%**
Dietary Fiber 7g	**25%**
Sugars 4g	
Protein 11g	
Vitamin A	10%
Vitamin C	2%
Calcium	20%
Iron	35%

*Percent Daily Values are based on a 2,000 calorie diet. Your daily values may be higher or lower depending on your calorie needs:

		Calories	2,000	2,500
Total Fat	Less than		65g	80g
Sat Fat	Less than		20g	25g
Cholesterol	Less than		300mg	300mg
Sodium	Less than		2,400mg	2,400mg
Total Carbohydrate			300g	375g
Dietary Fiber			25g	30g

Ingredients: Bulgur Wheat, Sauce (Water, Half and Half [Milk, Cream], Parmesan Cheese [Pasteurized Skim Milk, Cultures, Salt, Enzymes], Cheddar Cheese [Pasteurized Milk, Cultures, Salt, Enzymes], Olive Oil, Spice, Butter, Sugar, Xanthan Gum), Lentils, Corn, Green Beans, Red Beans, Potatoes.

Contains: Wheat and Milk

New Label

1. Servings sizes and calories: Information larger and bolder; some serving sizes have been updated to reflect what people actually eat or drink. "Calories from Fat" has been removed because research shows the type of fat consumed is more important than the amount.

2. Daily Values: Updated based on new scientific evidence; still based on 2,000-calorie diet.

3. Nutrients to look for: Look for new information on added sugars, vitamin D, and potassium. Overall, choose foods low in added sugars, saturated and trans fats, and sodium; choose foods high in fiber, vitamin D, calcium, iron, and potassium. Actual amounts of each nutrient will be listed.

Nutrition Facts

2 servings per container
Serving size 1 1/2 cup (208g)

Amount per serving
Calories   240

	% Daily Value*
Total Fat 4g	**5%**
Saturated Fat 1.5g	**8%**
Trans Fat 0g	
Cholesterol 5mg	**2%**
Sodium 430mg	**19%**
Total Carbohydrate 46g	**17%**
Dietary Fiber 7g	**25%**
Total Sugars 4g	
Includes 2g Added Sugars	**4%**
Protein 11g	
Vitamin D 2mcg	10%
Calcium 260mg	20%
Iron 6mg	35%
Potassium 240mg	6%

*The % Daily Value (DV) tells you how much a nutrient in a serving of food contributes to a daily diet. 2,000 calories a day is used for general nutrition advice.

Ingredients: Bulgur Wheat, Sauce (Water, Half and Half [Milk, Cream], Parmesan Cheese [Pasteurized Skim Milk, Cultures, Salt, Enzymes], Cheddar Cheese [Pasteurized Milk, Cultures, Salt, Enzymes], Olive Oil, Spice, Butter, Sugar, Xanthan Gum), Lentils, Corn, Green Beans, Red Beans, Potatoes.

Contains: Wheat and Milk

All Food Packages

Ingredient list: Specifies each ingredient in a food by its common or usual name in descending order by weight; potential allergens must be declared at least once on a food label, in the ingredient list and/or immediately after it.

Table 13.9 — Food Package Nutrient Claims

TERM	DEFINITION
Healthy*	A food that is low in total fat, is low in saturated fat; has no more than 360–480 mg sodium and 60 mg cholesterol; and provides 10% or more of the Daily Value for vitamin A, vitamin C, protein, calcium, iron, or dietary fiber
Light or lite	33% fewer calories or 50% less fat than a similar product
Reduced or fewer	At least 25% less of a nutrient than a similar product; can be applied to fat ("reduced fat"), saturated fat, cholesterol, sodium, and calories
Extra or added	10% or more of the Daily Value per serving when compared to a similar product
Good source	10–19% of the Daily Value for a particular nutrient per serving
High, rich in, or excellent source of	20% or more of the Daily Value for a particular nutrient per serving
Low calorie	40 calories or less per serving
High fiber	5 grams or more of fiber per serving
Good source of fiber	2.5–4.9 grams of fiber per serving
Fat-free	Less than 0.5 gram of fat per serving
Low-fat	3 grams or less of fat per serving
Saturated- or trans-fat-free	Less than 0.5 gram of saturated fat and 0.5 gram of trans fatty acids per serving
Low saturated fat	1 gram or less of saturated fat per serving and no more than 15% of total calories
Low sodium	140 mg or less of sodium per serving
Very low sodium	35 mg or less of sodium per serving
Lean	Cooked seafood, meat, or poultry with less than 10 grams of fat, 4.5 grams or less of saturated fat, and less than 95 mg of cholesterol per serving
Extra lean	Cooked seafood, meat, or poultry with less than 5 grams of fat, 2 grams of saturated fat, and 95 mg of cholesterol per serving

*In mid-2016, the FDA began the process of redefining the "healthy" nutrient content claim.

NOTE: The FDA has not yet defined nutrient claims relating to carbohydrates, so foods labeled low- or reduced-carbohydrate do not conform to any approved standard.

SOURCE: U.S. Food and Drug Administration. 2018. *FDA Nutrient Content Claims* (http://www.fda.gov/Food/LabelingNutrition/ucm2006880.htm). Accessed March 4, 2020.

similar retail food establishments (those with 20 or more locations). In addition, chain restaurants are also required to provide more detailed nutrition information on their menu items—on posters, tray liners, signs, handouts, or other similar locations—so look for it!

Calorie labels are also now required for vending machine operators who own or operate 20 or more machines. Calories will be shown on a sign or digital display near the food items or selection button. To disclose calories on food items in vending machines, vendors can rely on front-of-pack labeling. Use the information as you consider your options and monitor your calorie intake.

Dietary Supplements

National food guidance encourages people to meet their nutritional needs with a nutritionally balanced diet of whole foods rather than with vitamin and mineral supplements. Although dietary supplements are sold over the counter, they are not necessarily proven effective or safe, especially when consumed over a long period of time. Some vitamins and minerals are dangerous when taken in excess. Large doses of particular nutrients can also cause health problems by affecting the absorption of certain vitamins or minerals or interacting with medications. For this reason, it is prudent to talk to your doctor, pharmacist, or a registered dietitian nutritionist before taking any high-dosage supplement.

People Who Benefit from Supplements In establishing the DRIs, the Food and Nutrition Board recommended supplements of particular nutrients for specific groups:

- Women who are capable of getting pregnant should get 400 µg per day of folic acid (the synthetic form of the vitamin folate) from fortified foods and supplements in addition to folate from a varied diet. This level of folate can reduce the risk of neural tube defects in a developing fetus. Enriched breads, flours, cornmeal, rice, noodles, and other grain products are fortified with folic acid. Folate is found naturally in leafy green vegetables, legumes, oranges, and strawberries.

- As noted earlier, people over age 50 should eat foods fortified with vitamin B-12, take a B-12 supplement, or combine the two to meet the RDA of 2.4 µg daily. Up to 30% of people over age 50 may have trouble absorbing protein-bound B-12 in foods.

- Because of the oxidative stress caused by smoking, smokers should get 35 mg more vitamin C per day than the RDA set for their age and sex. Supplements aren't usually necessary, however, because this extra vitamin C can easily be found in foods. For example, an 8-ounce glass of orange juice has about 100 mg of vitamin C.

Supplements may be recommended in other cases. Women with heavy menstrual flows, for example, may need extra iron. Older adults, people with dark skin, and people exposed to little sunlight may need extra vitamin D. Other people may benefit from supplementation based on their physical condition, the medicines they take, or their dietary habits.

Before deciding whether to take a vitamin or mineral supplement, consider whether you already eat a fortified breakfast cereal every day. Many breakfast cereals contain almost as many nutrients as a multivitamin pill. If you elect to take a supplement, choose one that contains 50–100% of the Daily Values for vitamins and minerals. Avoid supplements containing large doses at levels exceeding the tolerable upper intake level (UL).

Reading Supplement Labels

Dietary supplements include vitamins, minerals, amino acids, herbs, carotenoids, enzymes, and other compounds. They are available as tablets, capsules, liquids, and powders. Although dietary supplements are often thought to be safe and sometimes labeled "natural," they can contain powerful bioactive chemicals that have the potential for harm. About one-quarter of all pharmaceutical drugs are derived from botanical sources—morphine from poppies and digoxin from foxglove, for example. And as described earlier, even essential vitamins and minerals can have toxic effects if consumed in excess.

In the United States, dietary supplements are not legally considered drugs and are not regulated the same way drugs are. Before a drug is approved by the FDA and put on the market, it must undergo clinical studies to determine safety, effectiveness, side effects and risks, possible interactions with other substances, and appropriate dosages. The FDA does not authorize or test dietary supplements, and supplement manufacturers are not required to demonstrate either safety or effectiveness prior to marketing. Although dosage guidelines exist for some of the compounds in dietary supplements, dosages for many are not well established, and purity can vary widely.

There are also key differences in how drugs and supplements are manufactured. FDA-approved medications are standardized for potency, and quality control and proof of purity are required. Dietary supplement manufacture is not as closely regulated, and there is no guarantee that a product even contains a given ingredient, let alone in the appropriate amount. The potency of herbal supplements tends to vary widely due to differences in growing and harvesting conditions, preparation methods, and storage. Some manufacturers attempt to standardize their products by isolating the compounds believed to be responsible for an herb's action. However, potency is often still highly variable and several compounds may be responsible for an herb's effect. In addition, herbs can be contaminated or misidentified at any stage

from harvest to packaging. (See Chapter 21 for more about herbal remedies.) The FDA has recalled several products due to the presence of dangerous contaminants, including heavy metals and pharmaceutical drugs.

To provide consumers with more reliable and consistent information about supplements, the FDA requires supplements to have labels similar to those found on foods (see the box "Using Dietary Supplement Labels" for more information). Label statements and claims about supplements are also regulated.

Most importantly, remember that dietary supplements are not a substitute for a healthy diet. Supplements do not provide all the benefits of whole foods. Be sure to inform your health care provider about all dietary and herbal supplements you take, and remember that supplements should also not be used as a replacement for medical treatment for serious illnesses.

Protecting Yourself against Foodborne Illness

The CDC estimates that approximately 48 million illnesses, 128,000 hospitalizations, and 3000 deaths occur each year in the United States due to foodborne illnesses. Symptoms include diarrhea, vomiting, fever, pain, headache, and weakness. Although the effects of foodborne illnesses are usually not serious, some groups, such as children, pregnant women, individuals with immune deficits, and older adults, are more at risk for severe complications such as rheumatic diseases, seizures, blood poisoning, hemolytic uremic syndrome, and death.

Causes of Foodborne Illnesses

Most cases of foodborne illness are caused by 31 known **pathogens**—disease-causing microorganisms. Food can be contaminated with pathogens through improper handling, and pathogens can grow if food is prepared or stored improperly. According to the CDC, 8 pathogens contribute to the vast majority of illnesses, hospitalizations, and deaths related to foodborne illnesses:

- *Salmonella*—most often found in eggs, on vegetables, and on poultry
- *Norovirus*—most often found in salad ingredients and shellfish
- *Campylobacter jejuni*—most often found in meat and poultry
- *Toxoplasma*—most often found in meat
- *Escherichia coli (E. coli)* O157:H7—most often found in meat and water
- *Listeria monocytogenes*—most often found in lunch meats, sausages, and hot dogs
- *Clostridium perfringens*—most often found in meat and gravy
- *Staphylococcus aureus*—most often resulting from improper hand washing leading to food contamination

pathogen A microorganism that causes disease. **TERMS**

Since 1999, specific types of information have been required on the labels of dietary supplements. In addition to basic information about the product, labels include a "Supplement Facts" panel, modeled after the "Nutrition Facts" panel used on food labels (see the label illustrated in this box). Under the Dietary Supplement Health and Education Act (DSHEA) and food labeling laws, supplement labels can make three types of health-related claims:

- **Nutrient content claims,** such as "high in calcium," "excellent source of vitamin C," or "high potency." The claims "high in" and "excellent source of" mean the same as they do on food labels. A "high-potency" single-ingredient supplement must contain 100% of that nutrient's Daily Value; a "high-potency" multi-ingredient product must contain 100% or more of the Daily Value of at least two-thirds of the nutrients present for which Daily Values have been established.

- **Health claims,** if they have been authorized by the FDA or another authoritative scientific body. The association between adequate calcium intake and lower risk of osteoporosis is an example of an approved health claim. Since 2003, the FDA has also allowed so-called qualified health claims for situations in which there is emerging but as yet inconclusive evidence for a particular claim. These claims must include qualifying language such as "scientific evidence suggests but does not prove [the claim]."

- **Structure–function claims,** such as "antioxidants maintain cellular integrity" or "this product enhances energy levels." Because these claims are not reviewed by the FDA, they must carry a disclaimer (see the sample label).

Tips for Choosing and Using Dietary Supplements

- Check with your physician before taking a supplement. Many are not meant for children, older adults, women who are pregnant or breastfeeding, people with chronic illnesses or upcoming surgery, or people taking prescription or over-the-counter medications. When you visit your doctor, bring a list of all dietary supplements you are taking. Do not take megadoses (more than double the DRI levels) without your doctor's approval.

- Choose brands made by nationally known food and drug manufacturers or house brands from large retail chains. Due to their size and visibility, such sources are likely to have high manufacturing standards.

- Look for the "USP" (United States Pharmacopeial Convention) verification mark on the label, indicating that the product meets minimum safety and purity standards developed under the USP Dietary Supplement Verification Program. The USP mark means that the product (1) contains the listed ingredients, (2) has the declared amount and strength of ingredients, (3) will dissolve effectively, (4) has been screened for harmful contaminants, and (5) has been manufactured using safe, sanitary, and well-controlled procedures. The National Nutritional Foods Association (NNFA) has a self-regulatory testing program for its members; other associations and laboratories, including ConsumerLab.com, also test and rate dietary supplements.

Courtesy of The United States Pharmacopeial Convention. Registered trademark of The United States Pharmacopeial Convention.

- Follow the label's cautions, directions for use, and dosage.

- If you experience side effects, stop using the product and contact your physician. Report any serious reactions to the FDA's MedWatch monitoring program (800-FDA-1088 or online at http://www.fda.gov/Safety/MedWatch/default.htm).

For More Information about Dietary Supplements

NIH Office of Dietary Supplements (http://ods.od.nih.gov)
FDA (http://www.fda.gov/food/dietarysupplements)
USDA (http://fnic.nal.usda.gov/dietary-supplements)

Statement of identity and net quantity

MOOD ENHANCER
DIETARY SUPPLEMENT

60 capsules

Structure-function claim

Specially formulated to enhance your mood, maintain healthy energy levels, and help you deal with daily stresses.

Directions for use and storage

DIRECTIONS FOR USE: Take one capsule twice daily with a meal.

Keep out of reach of children. Store in a cool, dry place, tightly closed. Color variation is normal in this product.

Warnings may appear on some labels

WARNING: FOR ADULTS ONLY. Do not exceed the recommended dosage. Do not use if you are pregnant, lactating, or taking prescription antidepressant or anti-anxiety medication. Do not use with alcohol. Do not use if you have allergies to the ragweed family. Limit exposure to the sun as St. John's wort may cause increased sensitivity to light. Discontinue use in the event of a rash.

PHENYLKETONURICS:
CONTAINS PHENYLALANINE.

Disclaimer accompanying structure-function claim

*This statement has not been evaluated by the Food and Drug Administration. This product is not intended to diagnose, treat, cure, or prevent any disease.

Supplement Facts
Serving Size 1 capsule

Amount per capsule	% Daily Value*
Vitamin B₆ (as pyroxidine hydrochloride) 2.0 mg	100%
Folic acid 200 mcg	50%
Vitamin B₁₂ (as cyanocobalamin) 6 mcg	100%
St. John's wort aerial parts extract 300 mg (*Hypericum perforatum*)	†
Kava root extract 250 mg (*Piper methysticum*)	†
Siberian ginseng root extract 200 mg (*Eleutherococcus senticosus*)	†
Phenylalanine (as L-phenylalanine hydrochloride) 100 mg	†

*Percent Daily Values are based on a 2000 calorie diet.
†Daily Value not established.

Other ingredients: Rice flour, gelatin, water.

Standardization levels: St. John's wort: 0.3% hypericin; kava: 30% kavalactones; Siberian ginseng: 1% eleutherosides.

Made by JKS Herbal Supplements, P.O. Box 2000, San Francisco, CA 94444.

Serving size

Source and amount of ingredients with established Daily Values

Name, source, and amount of ingredients without established Daily Values

Standardization levels may appear on some labels

Address to write to for more product information

Salmonella is the leading cause of foodborne hospitalizations. Other causes of foodborne illness include the bacteria *Clostridium perfringens, Vibrio vulnificus,* and *Yersinia enterocolytica;* the hepatitis A virus; the parasites *Trichinella spiralis* (found in pork and wild game), *Anisakis* (found in raw fish), *Giardia lamblia, Cyclospora cayetanensis,* and tapeworms; and certain molds.

Preventing and Treating Foodborne Illnesses Because every teaspoon of the soil that our food grows in contains about 2 billion bacteria (only some of them pathogenic), we are always exposed to the possibility of a foodborne illness. You can't tell by taste, smell, or sight whether a food is contaminated. Raw foods are the most common source of foodborne illnesses. Examples include raw meat and poultry that may have become contaminated during slaughter, and produce such as spinach, lettuce, tomatoes, sprouts, and melons that become contaminated with *Salmonella, Shigella,* or *E. coli* during growing, harvesting, processing, storing, shipping, or final preparation. One in 10,000 eggs may be contaminated with *Salmonella* inside the eggshell.

Although foodborne illness outbreaks associated with food-processing plants make headlines, most cases of illness trace back to poor food handling in the home or in restaurants. Food safety experts encourage people to follow four basic food safety principles:

- *Clean* hands, food contact surfaces, and vegetables and fruits.
- *Separate* raw, cooked, and ready-to-eat foods while shopping, storing, and preparing foods.
- *Cook* foods to a safe temperature.
- *Chill* (refrigerate) perishable foods promptly.

If you think you may be having a bout of foodborne illness, drink plenty of fluids to prevent dehydration and consult a physician. For more details on handling food safely, see the box "Safe Food Handling."

Although pathogens are usually destroyed during cooking, the U.S. government has taken steps to bring down levels of contamination by improving national surveillance and testing. Careful food handling greatly reduces the risk of foodborne illness. Raw meat and poultry products are now

sold with safe handling and safe cooking instructions, and all packaged, unpasteurized fresh fruit and vegetable juices carry warnings about potential contamination. In 2011, the Food Safety Modernization Act (FSMA) was signed into law to reform the food safety system in the United States and further ensure the safety of the U.S. food supply. The FSMA allows the FDA to focus more on preventing food safety problems than on reacting to problems after they occur.

Environmental Contaminants

In addition to pathogens, environmental contaminants are also present in the food-growing environment. They include various minerals, antibiotics, hormones, pesticides, industrial chemicals known as **PCBs (polychlorinated biphenyls),** metals such as methyl mercury, and naturally occurring substances such as cyanogenic glycosides (found in lima beans and the pits of some fruits) and certain molds. Their effects depend on many factors, including concentration, length of exposure, and the age and health status of the person involved. Regulations attempt to keep our exposure to contaminants at safe levels, but monitoring is difficult, and many substances (such as pesticides) persist in the environment long after being banned from use.

Organic Foods

Some people who are concerned about pesticides and other environmental contaminants choose foods that are **organic.** To be certified as organic by the USDA, foods must meet strict production, processing, handling, and labeling criteria. Organic crops must meet limits on pesticide residues. For meat, milk, eggs, and other animal products to be certified organic, animals must be given organic feed and access to the outdoors and may not be given antibiotics or growth hormones. The use of genetic engineering, ionizing radiation, and sewage sludge is prohibited. Products can be labeled "100% organic" if they contain all organic ingredients and "organic" if they contain at least 95% organic ingredients; all such products may carry the USDA organic seal. A product with at least 70% organic ingredients can be labeled "made with organic ingredients" but cannot use the USDA seal.

Although organic foods may be contaminated with pesticides used on neighboring lands or on foods transported in the same train or truck, they tend to have lower levels of pesticide residues than conventionally grown crops. Some experts recommend that consumers who want to buy organic produce spend their money on those fruits and vegetables that have the highest levels of pesticide residue when grown conventionally (the "dirty dozen"): apples, bell peppers, celery, cherries, imported grapes, nectarines, peaches, pears, potatoes, red raspberries, spinach, and strawberries.

TERMS

polychlorinated biphenyl (PCB) An industrial chemical linked to certain cancers; banned worldwide in 1977 but persistent in the environment.

organic A designation applied to foods grown and produced according to strict guidelines limiting the use of pesticides, nonorganic ingredients, hormones, antibiotics, irradiation, genetic engineering, and other practices.

- Thoroughly wash your hands with warm, soapy water for 20 seconds before and after handling food, especially raw meat, fish, shellfish, poultry, or eggs.

- Don't buy food in containers that leak, bulge, or are severely dented. Refrigerated foods should be cold, and frozen foods should be solid when you buy them.

- Refrigerate perishable items as soon as possible after purchase. Use or freeze fresh meats within 3–5 days and fresh poultry, fish, and ground meat within 1–2 days.

- Store raw meat, poultry, fish, and shellfish in containers in the refrigerator so that the juices don't drip onto other foods. Keep these items away from other foods, surfaces, utensils, or serving dishes to prevent cross-contamination.

- Thaw frozen food in the refrigerator or in the microwave oven, not on the kitchen counter. Cook foods immediately after thawing.

- Make sure counters, cutting boards, dishes, utensils, and other equipment are cleaned thoroughly with hot, soapy water before and after use. Wash dishcloths frequently.

- If possible, use separate cutting boards for meat, poultry, and seafood and for foods that will be eaten raw. Replace cutting boards once they become worn or develop hard-to-clean grooves.

- Thoroughly rinse and scrub fruits and vegetables with a brush, if possible, or peel off the skin.

- Cook foods thoroughly, especially beef, poultry, fish, pork, wild game, and eggs; cooking kills most microorganisms. Use a food thermometer to ensure that foods are cooked to a safe temperature. Hamburgers should be cooked to at least 160°F. Turn or stir microwaved food to make sure it is heated evenly throughout. When eating out, order hamburger cooked well-done and make sure foods are served piping hot.

- Keep hot foods hot (140°F or above) and cold foods cold (40°F or below). Harmful bacteria can grow rapidly between these two temperatures. Refrigerate foods within two hours of purchase or preparation, and within one hour if the air temperature is above 90°F. Refrigerate foods at or below 40°F and freeze at or below 0°F. Use refrigerated leftovers within 3–4 days.

- Don't eat raw animal products, including raw eggs in homemade hollandaise sauce or eggnog. Use only pasteurized milk and juice, and look for pasteurized eggs, which are now available in some states.

- Cook eggs until they're firm, and fully cook foods containing eggs. Store eggs in the cooler parts of the refrigerator, not in the door, and use them within 3–5 weeks.

- Avoid raw sprouts. Even sprouts grown under clean conditions in the home can be risky because bacteria may be present in the seeds. Cook sprouts before eating them.

- Read the food label and package information, and follow safety instructions such as "Keep Refrigerated" and the "Safe Handling Instructions."

- According to the USDA, "When in doubt, throw it out." Even if a food looks and smells fine, it may not be safe. If you aren't sure that a food has been prepared, served, and stored safely, don't eat it.

Additional precautions are recommended for people at particularly high risk for foodborne illness—pregnant women, very young children, older people, and people with weakened immune systems or certain chronic illnesses. If you are a member of one of these groups, don't eat or drink any of the following products: unpasteurized juices; raw sprouts; unpasteurized (raw) milk and products made from unpasteurized milk; raw or undercooked meat, poultry, eggs, fish, or shellfish; and soft cheeses such as feta, Brie, Camembert, or blue-veined cheeses. To protect against *Listeria,* avoid ready-to-eat foods such as hot dogs, luncheon meats, and cold cuts unless they are reheated until they are steaming hot.

Experts also recommend buying organic beef, poultry, eggs, dairy products, and baby food. Fruits and vegetables that carry little pesticide residue whether grown conventionally or organically include asparagus, avocados, bananas, broccoli, cauliflower, corn, kiwi, mangoes, onions, papaya, pineapples, and peas. All foods are subject to strict pesticide limits; the debate about the health effects of small amounts of residue is ongoing.

Organic farming is better for the environment. Benefits include sustainable farming practices, preservation of biodiversity, healthier soil, protection of water supplies, reduced use of fossil fuels, improved animal welfare, protection of ecosystems, and safer conditions for farmworkers. Buying organic food, buying locally grown foods, and participating in a community garden are ways to support food production that benefits and sustains the environment.

Guidelines for Fish Consumption

A specific area of concern has been mercury contamination in fish. Overall, fish and shellfish are healthy sources of protein, omega-3 fats, and other nutrients. Prudent choices can minimize the risk of any possible negative health effects. High mercury concentrations are most likely to be found in predator fish—large fish that eat smaller fish. Mercury can cause brain damage in fetuses and young children.

According to 2019 FDA and Environmental Protection Agency (EPA) guidelines, women who are or may become pregnant and nursing mothers should follow these guidelines to minimize their exposure to mercury:

- Do not eat shark, swordfish, king mackerel, marlin, orange roughy, bigeye tuna, or tilefish (from the Gulf of Mexico).
- Eat 2–3 servings (8–12 ounces) a week of a variety of fish and shellfish that are lower in mercury, such as shrimp, canned light tuna, salmon, pollock, and catfish. Limit consumption of albacore tuna to 1 serving (4 ounces) per week.
- Check advisories about the safety of recreationally caught fish from local lakes, rivers, and coastal areas; if no information is available, limit consumption to 4 ounces per week.

The same FDA/EPA guidelines apply to children, although they should consume smaller servings.

Additives in Food

According to the FDA's "Everything Added to Food in the United States (EAFUS)" database, approximately 3000 substances are intentionally added to foods to maintain or improve nutritional quality, maintain freshness, help in processing or preparation, or alter taste or appearance. The most widely used food additives are sugar, salt, and corn syrup; these three plus citric acid, baking soda, vegetable colors, mustard, and pepper account for 98% by weight of all food additives used in the United States.

Some additives may be of concern for certain people, either because they are consumed in large quantities or because they cause some type of reaction. Additives having potential health concerns include nitrates and nitrites, used in processed meats and associated with the synthesis of cancer-causing agents in the stomach; BHA (butylated hydroxyanisole) and BHT (butylated hydroxytoluene), used to maintain freshness and possibly associated with an increased risk of some cancers; and sulfites, used to keep vegetables from turning brown and associated with severe reactions in sensitive people.

Food additives pose no significant health hazard to most people because the levels used are well below any that could produce toxic effects. To avoid potential problems, eat a variety of foods in moderation. If you are sensitive to an additive, check food labels when you shop and ask questions when you eat out.

Functional Foods

The American diet contains numerous *functional foods*. This phrase generally refers to foods containing components that may provide positive health benefits. Two of the earliest functional foods introduced in the United States were iodized salt and milk fortified with vitamins A and D. More recently, manufacturers began fortifying breads and grains with folic acid to reduce the incidence of neural tube defects. Some foods are made functional by the addition of an ingredient with proven health-promoting or disease-preventing components. To be considered functional, a food must be able to claim a health benefit beyond what you would normally get consuming the food in nonfortified form. Some examples of functional foods are calcium-fortified orange juice; margarine enriched with sterols or stanols to lower the risk of heart disease; and soy milk enriched with calcium, vitamin D, yogurt with probiotics, and plant-based milks with vitamin B-12 for vegetarians.

Food Biotechnology

Food biotechnology techniques, such as crossbreeding, have been used by farmers for thousands of years to improve productivity and develop desirable qualities in animals and crops. Modern biotechnology tools, such as genetic engineering and cloning, allow for more precise, productive, and efficient development of crops and livestock. Internationally, 26 countries planted more than 191 million hectares of biotech crops. The top five countries with the largest area of biotech crops planted are the United States, Brazil, Argentina, Canada, and India, totaling about 91% of global biotech. Seventy percent of countries have adopted biotech crops to address problems of hunger, malnutrition, and climate change. In the United States, biotechnology is used in about 94% of the current soybean crops, 98% of cotton, and 90% of corn crops. The USDA, FDA, and EPA are the three federal agencies in charge of the regulatory oversight of biotechnology.

Irradiation   **Food irradiation** is the treatment of foods with gamma rays, X-rays, or high-voltage electrons to kill potentially harmful pathogens, including bacteria, parasites, insects, and fungi that cause foodborne illness. Irradiation also reduces spoilage and extends a product's shelf life. For example, irradiated strawberries stay unspoiled in the refrigerator up to 3 weeks, versus only 3–5 days for untreated berries. The government permits the irradiation of certain foods, including wheat and flour, white potatoes, pork, herbs and spices, fruits and vegetables, raw poultry, red meat, and certain leafy green vegetables.

Even though irradiation has been generally endorsed by agencies such as the World Health Organization (WHO), the CDC, and the American Medical Association (AMA), few irradiated foods are currently on the market due to consumer resistance and skepticism. Studies indicate that when consumers are given information about the process of irradiation and the benefits of irradiated foods, most want to purchase them. All primary irradiated foods (meat, vegetables, and so on) are labeled with the flowerlike Radura symbol and a brief

food irradiation The treatment of foods with gamma rays, X-rays, or high-voltage electrons to kill potentially harmful pathogens and increase shelf life.

TERMS

information label; spices and foods that are merely ingredients do not have to be so labeled.

Genetically Modified (GM) Foods   Genetic engineering involves altering the characteristics of a plant, animal, or microorganism by adding, rearranging, or replacing genes in its DNA; the result is a **genetically modified organism (GMO).** New DNA may come from related species or from entirely different types of organisms. Many GM crops are already grown in the United States. For example, some soybean crops in the United States have been genetically modified to be resistant to some herbicides used to kill weeds, and some GM corn crops carry genes for herbicide resistance or pest resistance. Products made with GMOs include juice, soda, nuts, tuna, frozen pizza, spaghetti sauce, canola oil, chips, salad dressings, and soup.

The potential benefits of GM foods cited by supporters include improved yields overall and in difficult growing conditions, increased disease resistance, improved nutritional content, lower prices, and less pesticide use. Critics of biotechnology argue that unexpected harmful effects may occur: Gene manipulation could elevate levels of naturally occurring toxins or allergens, permanently change the gene pool, reduce biodiversity, and produce pesticide-resistant insects. Experience has shown that GM products are difficult to keep separate from non-GM products. Animal escapes, cross-pollination, and contamination during processing are just a few ways in which GMOs could potentially appear unexpectedly in the food supply or the environment.

Labeling of GM Foods   Surveys indicate that most Americans want to know if their food contains ingredients from GMOs. The FDA does not require special labeling for foods from genetically modified or cloned food sources. Under current rules, the FDA requires special labeling only when a food's composition is changed significantly or when a known allergen such as a peanut gene is introduced into a food. The only foods guaranteed not to contain GM ingredients are those certified as organic.

Food Allergies and Food Intolerances

For some people, consuming a particular food causes symptoms such as itchiness, swollen lips, or abdominal pain. Adverse reactions like these may be due to a food allergy or a food intolerance, and symptoms may range from annoying to a severe and life-threatening reaction called anaphylaxis. If you've had an adverse reaction to a food, it's important to determine whether your symptoms are due to an allergy or an intolerance so that you can take appropriate action.

Food Allergies   A true **food allergy** is a reaction of the body's immune system to a food or food ingredient, usually a protein. The immune system perceives the reaction-provoking substance, or allergen, as foreign and acts to destroy it. This

immune reaction can occur within minutes of ingesting the food, resulting in symptoms that affect the skin (hives), gastrointestinal tract (cramps or diarrhea), respiratory tract (asthma), or mouth (swelling of the lips or tongue). The most severe response is a systemic reaction called *anaphylaxis,* which involves a potentially life-threatening drop in blood pressure and narrowing of airways blocking normal breathing. Repeated exposure to the allergen may result in more severe symptoms.

Food allergies affect 8% of infants and children and almost 11% of adults in the United States. Although numerous food allergens have been identified, just eight foods account for more than 90% of the food allergies in the United States: cow's milk, eggs, peanuts, tree nuts (walnuts, cashews, and so on), soy, wheat, fish, and shellfish. Food labels are now required to state the presence of the eight most common allergens in plain language in the ingredient list. Individuals with food allergies, especially those prone to anaphylaxis, must diligently avoid trigger foods. This involves carefully reading food labels and asking questions about ingredients when eating out. People at risk are usually advised to carry medications to treat anaphylaxis, such as injectable epinephrine. Refer to Chapter 18 for more about allergies.

Food Intolerances   Many people who believe they have food allergies may actually suffer from a much more common source of adverse food reactions—a **food intolerance.** In the case of a food intolerance, the problem usually lies with metabolism rather than with the immune system. Typically the body cannot adequately digest a food or food component, often because of some type of chemical deficiency; in other cases, the body reacts to a particular compound in a food. Lactose intolerance is a fairly common food intolerance.

A more serious condition may be intolerance of gluten, a protein component of some grains. In recent decades, the prevalence of celiac disease has risen in Western populations.

genetically modified organism (GMO)   A plant, **TERMS** animal, or microorganism in which genes have been added, rearranged, or replaced through genetic engineering.

food allergy   An adverse reaction to a food or food ingredient in which the immune system perceives a particular substance (allergen) as foreign and acts to destroy it.

food intolerance   An adverse reaction to a food or food ingredient that doesn't involve the immune system; intolerances are often due to a problem with metabolism.

Currently, almost 1% of Americans have a problem that causes the body to attack the small intestine when gluten is ingested and can lead to other debilitating medical problems. An additional 18 million people, or about 6% of the population, is believed to have gluten sensitivity, a less severe problem with the protein in wheat, barley, and rye and other foods that gives elasticity to dough and stability to the shape of baked goods.

Sulfite, a common food additive, can produce severe asthmatic reactions in sensitive individuals. Food intolerances have also been attributed to MSG and the sweetener aspartame.

Food intolerance reactions often produce symptoms similar to those of food allergies, such as diarrhea or cramps, but reactions are typically localized and not life-threatening. Many people with food intolerances can consume small amounts of the food that affects them; exceptions are gluten and sulfite, which must be avoided by sensitive individuals. Through trial and error, most people with food intolerances can adjust their intake of the trigger food to an appropriate level.

If you suspect that you have a food allergy or intolerance, a good first step is to keep a food diary. Note everything you eat or drink, any symptoms you develop, and how long after eating the symptoms appear. Then make an appointment with your physician to go over your diary and determine if any additional tests are needed.

TIPS FOR TODAY AND THE FUTURE

Opportunities to improve your diet present themselves every day, and small changes add up.

RIGHT NOW YOU CAN:
- Substitute a healthy snack for an unhealthy one.
- Drink a glass of water and put a reusable water bottle in your backpack for tomorrow.
- Plan to make healthy selections when you eat out, such as steamed vegetables instead of french fries, or salmon instead of steak.

IN THE FUTURE YOU CAN:
- Visit the MyPlate website at ChooseMyPlate.gov and use the online tools to create a personalized nutrition plan and begin tracking your eating habits.
- Learn to cook healthier meals. Hundreds of free websites and low-cost cookbooks provide recipes for healthy dishes.

SUMMARY

- To function at its best, the human body requires about 45 essential nutrients in certain relative proportions. People get these nutrients from foods; the body cannot synthesize most of them.

- Proteins, made up of amino acids, form muscles and bones and help make up blood, enzymes, hormones, and cell membranes. Foods from animal sources provide complete proteins; plants provide incomplete proteins and must be combined in order to attain the right balance of amino acids, especially if no or limited animal protein is in the diet. Protein intake should be 10–35% of total daily energy intake.

- Fats, a concentrated source of energy, also help to insulate the body and cushion the organs; 3–4 teaspoons of vegetable oil per day supplies the essential fats. Dietary fat intake should be 20–35% of total daily energy intake. In general, you can still eat high-fat foods, but avoid trans fats and limit the size of your portions and balance your intake with low-fat foods.

- Carbohydrates supply energy to the brain and other parts of the nervous system as well as to red blood cells. The body needs about 130 grams of carbohydrates a day, but more is recommended. Carbohydrates should make up 45–65% of total daily energy intake.

- Fiber includes nondigestible carbohydrates provided mainly by plants. A high-fiber diet can help people manage diabetes and high cholesterol levels and improve intestinal health.

- The 13 vitamins needed in the diet are organic substances that regulate various processes within living cells and promote specific chemical reactions. Deficiencies or excesses can cause serious illnesses and even death.

- The approximately 17 minerals needed in the diet are inorganic substances that regulate body functions, aid in the growth and maintenance of body tissues, and help in the release of energy from foods.

- Water helps digest and absorb food, transport substances around the body, and regulate body temperature.

- Foods contain other substances such as phytochemicals, which may not be essential nutrients but may help reduce chronic disease risk.

- Dietary Reference Intakes (DRIs) are standards for nutrient intake designed to prevent nutritional deficiencies and reduce the risk of chronic diseases.

- The *Dietary Guidelines for Americans* are designed to help people make healthy and informed food choices. Following the guidelines promotes health and reduces the risk of chronic disease. The *2020–2025 Dietary Guidelines,* to be released at the end of 2020, continue a focus on healthy eating patterns that start from the earliest life stages (in the womb) through adulthood.

- Choosing the right amount of foods from each food group in MyPlate every day ensures that you get enough necessary nutrients without overconsuming calories.

- A plant-based diet can meet human nutritional needs but must be planned carefully to prevent potential micronutrient deficiencies, especially of vitamin B-12 and readily bioavailable iron.

- Almost all foods have labels that show how much fat, cholesterol, protein, fiber, and sodium they contain. Serving sizes are standard-

Improving Your Diet by Choosing Healthy Beverages

After reading this chapter and completing the dietary assessment, you can probably identify several ways to improve your diet. As an example here, we focus on choosing healthy beverages to increase intake of nutrients and decrease intake of empty calories from added sugars and fat. This model can be applied to any change you want to make to your diet.

Gather Data and Establish a Baseline

Begin by tracking your beverage consumption in a journal. Write down the types and amounts of beverages you drink, including water. Also note where you were at the time and whether you got the beverage there or brought it with you. At the same time, investigate your options. Find out what other beverages you can easily find during your daily routine. This information will help you put together a successful plan for change.

Analyze Your Data and Set Goals

Evaluate your beverage consumption by dividing your typical daily consumption between healthy and less healthy choices. Use the following guide as a basis, and add other beverages to the lists as needed:

Choose More Often	Servings Daily	Choose Less Often	Servings Daily
Water: plain, mineral, sparkling		Regular soda	
Low-fat or fat-free milk		Whole milk	
Fruit juice (100%)		Fruit beverages made with little fruit juice	
Unsweetened or noncaloric sweetened herbal tea		Sugar-sweetened beverages such as iced tea and sports drinks	
Others		Others	

How many beverages do you consume daily from each category? What would be a healthy and realistic goal for change? For example, if your beverage consumption is currently evenly divided between the "choose more often" and "choose less often" categories (four from each list), you might set a final goal for your behavior change program of increasing your healthy choices by two (to six from the "more often" list and two from the "less often" list).

Develop a Plan for Change

Once you've set your goal, you need to develop strategies that will help you choose healthy beverages more often. Consider the following possibilities:

- Keep healthy beverages on hand. If you live in a dorm, rent a small refrigerator or keep water in a reusable bottle and other healthy choices in the dorm kitchen's refrigerator.
- Plan ahead, and carry a reusable bottle with water or 100% juice in your backpack every day.
- Check food labels on beverages for serving sizes, energy content, and nutrients; compare products to find the healthiest choices; and watch your serving sizes. Use this information to make your "choose more often" list longer and more specific.
- If you eat out frequently, examine all the beverages available at the places you typically eat your meals. You'll probably find that plain water or other healthy choices are available.

You may also need to make changes in your routine to decrease the likelihood that you'll make unhealthy choices. For example, your journal might reveal that you always buy a soda after class when you pass a particular vending machine. If this is the case, try another route that bypasses the machine. Guard against impulse buying by carrying water or a healthy snack with you every day.

To complete your plan, try some of the other behavior change strategies described in Chapter 1: Develop and sign a contract, set up a system of rewards, involve other people in your program, and develop strategies for challenging situations. Once your plan is complete, take action. Keep track of your progress by continuing to monitor and evaluate your beverage consumption.

ized, and health claims are regulated carefully. Dietary supplements also have uniform labels that provide supplement facts.

- Food additives, environmental containments, and foodborne illnesses from *Salmonella, E. coli, Norovirus,* and other microorganisms can pose threats to health. Other dietary issues of concern to some people include food irradiation, genetic modification of foods, and food allergies and intolerances.

FOR MORE INFORMATION

Academy of Nutrition and Dietetics (formerly the American Dietetic Association). Provides a variety of nutrition-related educational materials.

http://www.eatright.org

American Diabetes Association. An organization with the aim of leading the fight against the deadly consequences of diabetes and fighting for those affected by diabetes.

http://www.diabetes.org

The Dietary Guidelines. The official site for the *Dietary Guidelines for Americans, 2015.*

http://health.gov/dietaryguidelines/2015/guidelines/

FDA Center for Food Safety and Applied Nutrition. Offers information about topics such as food labeling, food additives, dietary supplements, and foodborne illness.

http://www.fda.gov/food

Food Safety Hotlines. Provide information on safe purchase, handling, cooking, and storage of food.

888-SAFEFOOD (FDA)

800-535-4555 (USDA)

Foodsafety.gov. Provides access to government resources relating to food safety and nutrition.

http://www.foodsafety.gov

Fruit and Veggies: More Matters. A nonprofit organization designed to increase consumption of fruits and vegetables to five or more servings a day to improve the health of Americans.

http://www.fruitsandveggiesmorematters.org

Harvard School of Public Health: The Nutrition Source. Provides recent key research findings, an overview of the Healthy Eating Plate, and suggestions for building a healthful diet.

http://www.hsph.harvard.edu/nutritionsource

Mayo Clinic: Nutrition Basics. Medical, nutrition, and health information and tools for healthy living.

http://www.mayoclinic.org/healthy-lifestyle/nutrition-and
-healthy-eating/basics/nutrition-basics/hlv-20049477

MyPlate. Provides personalized dietary plans and interactive food and activity tracking tools.

http://www.ChooseMyPlate.gov

National Academies' Food and Nutrition Board. Provides information about the Dietary Reference Intakes and related guidelines.

http://www.nap.edu/read/11537/chapter/1

Nutrition.gov. A USDA-sponsored website that provides reliable information to help consumers make healthy eating choices.

http://www.nutrition.gov

USDA Center for Nutrition Policy and Promotion. Established in 1994 to improve the nutrition and well-being of Americans. Includes information about the *Dietary Guidelines* and MyPlate.

http://www.choosemyplate.gov/

USDA Food and Nutrition Information Center. Provides a variety of materials and extensive links relating to the *Dietary Guidelines,* food labels, MyPlate, and many other topics.

https://fnic.nal.usda.gov

See also the resources listed in Chapters 14–17 and 23.

SELECTED BIBLIOGRAPHY

Academy of Nutrition and Dietetics. 2016. Position of the Academy of Nutrition and Dietetics: Vegetarian diets. *Journal of the Academy of Nutrition and Dietetics* 116: 1970-1980.

Afshin, A., et al. 2017. The prospective impact of food pricing on improving dietary consumption: A systematic review and meta-analysis. *PLoS One* 12(3): e0172277.

Ahluwalia, N., et al. 2016. Usual nutrient intakes of US infants and toddlers generally meet or exceed Dietary Reference Intakes: Findings from NHANES 2009–2012. *American Journal of Clinical Nutrition* 104(4): 1167–1174.

American Heart Association. 2017. *Diet and Lifestyle Recommendations* (https://www.heart.org/en/healthy-living/healthy-eating/eat-smart/nutrition-basics/aha-diet-and-lifestyle-recommendations).

American Heart Association. 2017. *The Facts on Fat* (https://www.heart.org/en/healthy-living/healthy-eating/eat-smart/fats/the-facts-on-fats).

American Heart Association. 2020. *How Does Plant-Forward (Plant-Based) Eating Benefit Your Health?* (https://www.heart.org/en/healthy-living/healthy-eating/eat-smart/nutrition-basics/how-does-plant-forward-eating-benefit-your-health).

American Heart Association. 2017. *Fish and Omega-3 Fatty Acids* (https://www.heart.org/en/healthy-living/healthy-eating/eat-smart/fats/fish-and-omega-3-fatty-acids).

American Heart Association. 2020. *Saturated Fats* (https://www.heart.org/en/healthy-living/healthy-eating/eat-smart/fats/saturated-fats).

American Heart Association. 2016. *The Greatness of Whole Grains.* (http://www.heart.org/HEARTORG/HealthyLiving/HealthyEating/HealthyDietGoals/The-Greatness-of-Whole-Grains_UCM_455739_Article.jsp#.WpRRxIPwYdU).

Bellavia, A., F. Stilling, and A. Wolk. 2016. High red meat intake and all-cause cardiovascular and cancer mortality: Is the risk modified by fruit and vegetable intake? *American Journal of Clinical Nutrition* 104(4): 1137–1143.

Billingsley, H. E., S. Carbone, and C. J. Lavie. 2018. Dietary fats and chronic noncommunicable diseases. *Nutrients* 10(10): 1385. DOI: 10.3390/nu10101385.

Centers for Disease Control and Prevention. 2015. *CDC and the Food Safety Modernization Act* (https://www.cdc.gov/foodsafety/fsma/index.html).

Centers for Disease Control and Prevention. 2015. *Percentage of Adults Aged 65 and Over with Osteoporosis or Low Bone Mass at the Femur, Neck or Lumbar Spine: United States, 2005–2010* (http://www.cdc.gov/nchs/data/hestat/osteoporsis/osteoporosis2005_2010.pdf).

Centers for Disease Control and Prevention. 2017. *Incidence and Trends of Infections with Pathogens Transmitted Commonly Through Food and the Effect of Increasing Use of Culture-Independent Diagnostic Tests on Surveillance—Foodborne Diseases Active Surveillance Network, 10 U.S. Sites, 2013–2016. 2017. MMWR* 66(15); 397–403. (https://www.cdc.gov/mmwr/volumes/66/wr/mm6615a1.htm)

Centers for Disease Control and Prevention. 2017. *Sodium: The Facts* (http://www.cdc.gov/salt/pdfs/Sodium_Fact_Sheet.pdf).

Centers for Disease Control and Prevention. 2018. *Burden of Foodborne Illness: Findings* (https://www.cdc.gov/foodborneburden/2011-foodborne-estimates.html).

Centers for Disease Control and Prevention. 2018. *Estimates of Foodborne Illness in the United States* (https://www.cdc.gov/foodborneburden/index.html).

Centers for Disease Control and Prevention. 2019. CDC Genomics and Precision Health. *Does Osteoporosis Run in Your Family?* (http://www.cdc.gov/features/osteoporosis/).

Centers for Disease Control and Prevention. 2019. *Foodborne Germs and Illnesses* (http://www.cdc.gov/foodsafety/foodborne-germs.html).

Centers for Disease Control and Prevention. 2020. *CDC Healthy Schools: Food Allergies.* (https://www.cdc.gov/healthyschools/foodallergies/index.htm).

Centers for Disease Control and Prevention. 2020. *Patient Stories: Was It Something I Ate?* (https://www.cdc.gov/foodsafety/patient-stories.html).

Centers for Disease Control and Prevention. 2020. Overweight & Obesity. *Adult Obesity Facts: Obesity Is a Common, Serious and Costly Disease* (https://www.cdc.gov/obesity/data/adult.html).

Centers for Disease Control and Prevention. 2020. Overweight & Obesity. *Childhood Obesity Facts: Prevalence of Childhood Obesity in the United States* (https://www.cdc.gov/obesity/data/childhood.html).

Chowdhury, R., et al. 2014. Association of dietary, circulating, and supplement fatty acids with coronary risk: A systematic review and meta-analysis. *Annals of Internal Medicine* 160(6): 398–406.

Coleman-Jensen, A., M. P. Rabbitt, C. A. Gregory, and A. Singh. 2017. *Household Food Security in the United States in 2016*, ERR-237, U.S. Department of Agriculture, Economic Research Service.

Council for Responsible Nutrition. *Dietary Supplements—Safe, Regulated and Beneficial* (https://www.crnusa.org/resources/dietary-supplements-safe-beneficial-and-regulated).

Dahl, W. J., and M. L. Steward. 2015. Position of the Academy of Nutrition and Dietetics: Health implications of dietary fiber. *Journal of the Academy of Nutrition and Dietetics* 115(11): 1861–1870.

Dietary Guidelines Advisory Committee. 2020. *Scientific Report of the 2020 Dietary Guidelines Advisory Committee: Advisory Report to the Secretary of Agriculture and the Secretary of Healthand Human Services.* U.S. Department of Agriculture, Agricultural Research Service, Washington, DC.

Edwards, B. J. 2015. Anticancer effects of vitamin D. *Physicians Education Resource* (https://www.gotoper.com/publications/ajho/2015/2015oct/anticancer-effects-of-vitamin-d).

Environmental Protection Agency. 2019. EPA-FDA advice about eating fish and shellfish. July 17. (https://www.epa.gov/fish-tech/epa-fda-advice-about-eating-fish-and-shellfish).

FAO, IFAD, UNICEF, WFP, and WHO. 2019. *The State of Food Security and Nutrition in the World 2019.* Safeguarding against economic slowdowns and downturns. (https://www.wfp.org/publications/2019-state-food-security-and-nutrition-world-sofi-safeguarding-against-economic).

Food and Nutrition Board, Institute of Medicine. 2005. *Dietary Reference Intakes for Energy, Carbohydrate, Fiber, Fat, Fatty Acids, Cholesterol, Protein, and Amino Acids.* Washington, DC: National Academies Press.

Food and Nutrition Board, Institute of Medicine. 2005. *Dietary Reference Intakes for Water, Potassium, Sodium, Chloride, and Sulfate.* Washington, DC: National Academies Press.

Food and Nutrition Board, Institute of Medicine. 2011. *Dietary Reference Intakes for Calcium and Vitamin D.* Washington, DC: National Academies Press.

Grosse, Charlene C. S. J., et al. 2020. The role of a plant-based diet in the pathogenesis, etiology and management of the inflammatory bowel diseases. *Expert Review of Gastroenterology & Hepatology.* DOI: 10.1080/17474124.2020.1733413.

Gupta, R. S., et al. 2019. Prevalence of food allergies among U.S. adults. *JAMA Open Network.* 2019 Jan;2(1): e185630.

Harvard Health Publishing. 2020, January 29. The right plant-based diet for you. (https://www.health.harvard.edu/staying-healthy/the-right-plant-based-diet-for-you).

Harvard Medical School. 2019. *The Truth about Fats: The Good, the Bad, and the In-Between* (https://www.health.harvard.edu/staying-healthy/the-truth-about-fats-bad-and-good).

Harvard School of Public Health, Department of Nutrition. 2020. *The Nutrition Source* (http://www.hsph.harvard.edu/nutritionsource).

Hedrick, V. E., et al. 2017. Dietary quality changes in response to a sugar-sweetened beverage-reduction intervention: Results from the Talking Health randomized controlled clinical trial. *American Journal of Clinical Nutrition.* DOI:10.3945/ajcn.116.144543

Hever, J. 2016. Plant-based diets: A physician's guide. *Permanente Journal* 20(3): 93–101.

Hever, J., and R. J. Cronise. 2017. Plant-based nutrition for healthcare professionals: Implementing diet as a primary modality in the prevention and treatment of chronic disease. *Journal of Geriatric Cardiology* 14(5): 355–368.

Hooper, L., et al. 2015. Reduction in saturated fat intake for cardiovascular disease. *Cochrane Database of Systematic Reviews* 6:CD011737.

The Hunger Project. 2020. *Know Your World: Facts about Hunger and Poverty* (http://www.thp.org/knowledge-center/know-your-world-facts-about-hunger-poverty/).

Insel, P., et al. 2021. *Nutrition,* 7th ed. Burlington, MA: Jones & Bartlett Learning.

ISAAA. 2018. Brief 54: Global Status of Commercialized Biotech/GM Crops: 2018. (http://www.isaaa.org/resources/publications/briefs/54/default.asp).

Islam, M. A., et al. 2019. Trans fatty acids and lipid profile: A serious risk factor to cardiovascular disease, cancer and diabetes. *Diabetes & Metabolic Syndrome* 13(2):1643–1647.

Jackson, S. L., et al. 2016. Prevalence of excess sodium intake in the United States—NHANES, 2009–2012. *MMWR* 64(52): 1393–1397.

Jeon, S-M., and E-A. Shin. 2018. Exploring vitamin D metabolism and function in cancer. *Experimental & Molecular Medicine* 50: 20 (https://www.nature.com/articles/s12276-018-0038-9).

Jesri, M., W. Y. Lou, and M. R. L'Abbé. 2016. 2015 Dietary Guidelines for Americans is associated with a more nutrient-dense diet and lower risk of obesity. *American Journal of Clinical Nutrition* 104(5): 1378–1392.

Johnson, R., et al. 2009. Dietary sugars intake and cardiovascular health: A scientific statement from the American Heart Association. *Circulation* 120: 1011-1020.

Kirwan, J. P., et al. 2016. A whole-grain diet reduces cardiovascular risk factors in overweight and obese adults: A randomized controlled trial. *Journal of Nutrition* 146(11): 2244–2251.

Li, W., et al. 2016. Dietary phytochemical and cancer chemoprevention: A perspective on oxidative stress, inflammation, and epigenetics. *Chemical Research in Toxicology* 29(12): 2071–2095.

Lebwohl, B., J. F. Ludvigsson, and P. H. Green. 2015. Celiac disease and non-celiac gluten sensitivity. *BMJ* 351: h4347. DOI: 10.1136/bmj.h4347.

Micha, R., et al. 2017. Association between dietary factors and mortality from heart disease, stroke, and type 2 diabetes in the United States. *Journal of the American Medical Association* 317(9): 912–924.

National Academy of Sciences. 2020. *Genetically Engineered Crops: Experience and Prospects* (http://nas-sites.org/ge-crops).

National Institutes of Health. 2020. Osteoporosis and Related Bone Diseases. National Resource Center. *Bone Basics* (https://www.bones.nih.gov/health-info/bone/bone-basics).

National Osteoporosis Foundation. 2020. *Food and Your Bones—Osteoporosis Nutrition Guidelines* (https://www.nof.org/patients/treatment/nutrition/).

National Osteoporosis Foundation. 2020. *What Is Osteoporosis and What Causes It?* (https://www.nof.org/patients/what-is-osteoporosis/).

Nettleton, J. A. et al. 2017. Saturated fat consumption and risk of coronary heart disease and ischemic stroke: A scientific update. *Annals of Nutrition & Metabolism* 70(1): 26–33.

Niaz, K., E. Zaplatic E, and J. Spoor J. 2018. Extensive use of monosodium glutamate: A threat to public health? *EXCLI Journal* 2018;17: 273-278.

Nowak, V., J. Du, and R. Charrondière. 2016. Assessment of the nutritional composition of quinoa (*Chenopodium quinoa* Willd.) *Food Chemistry* 193:47–54.

Orlich, M. J., et al. 2015. Vegetarian dietary patterns and the risk of colorectal cancers. *JAMA Internal Medicine* 175(5): 767–776.

Park S, et al. 2013. Prevalence of sugar-sweetened beverage intake among adults—23 states and the District of Columbia. *MMWR* 2016(65): 169–174.

Physicians Committee for Responsible Medicine. 2020. *Plant-Based Diets.* (https://www.pcrm.org/good-nutrition/plant-based-diets).

Rodriguez, L. A., et al. 2016. Added sugar intake and metabolic syndrome in U.S. adolescents. *Public Health Nutrition* 19(13): 2424–2434.

Rosinger, A., et al. 2017. Sugar-sweetened beverage consumption among U.S. adults, 2011–2014. *National Center for Health Statistics Data Brief* No. 270.

Ross, S. M. 2015. Cardiovascular disease mortality: The deleterious effects of excess dietary sugar intake. *Holistic Nursing Practice* 29(1): 53–57.

Sacks, F. M., et al. 2017. Dietary fats and cardiovascular disease: A presidential advisory from the American Heart Association. *Circulation* 135. DOI: 10.1161/CIR.0000000000000510.

Sirsikar, S., and A. Sirsikar. 2015. Prevention and management of postmenopausal osteoporosis. *International Journal of Innovative and Applied Research* 3(6): 5–26.

Sonnenburg, E. D., et al. 2016. Diet-induced extinctions in the gut microbiota compound over generations. *Nature* 529(7585): 212–215.

Strate, L. L., et al. 2017. Western dietary pattern increases, whereas prudent dietary pattern decreases, risk of incident diverticulitis in a prospective cohort study. *Gastroenterology* S0016-5085(17)30006-9.

U.S. Department of Agriculture. 2015. Choose MyPlate.gov Nutrients and Health Benefits. *Why Is It Important to Eat Grains, Especially Whole Grains?* (https://www.choosemyplate.gov/eathealthy/grains/grains-nutrients -health).

U.S. Department of Agriculture. 2018. *Household Food Security in the United States in 2018,* Economic Research Report No. ERR-270. (https://www .ers.usda.gov/webdocs/publications/94849/err-270.pdf?v=963.1).

U.S. Department of Agriculture, 2020. *Biotechnology.* (https://www.usda.gov /topics/biotechnology).

U.S. Department of Agriculture. 2020. *ChooseMyPlate* (http://www .choosemyplate.gov).

U.S. Department of Agriculture, Agricultural Research Service, *Food Data Central*. 2020. (https://fdc.nal.usda.gov/).

U.S. Department of Agriculture, Agriculture Research Service. 2019. *What We Eat in America.* (https://www.ars.usda.gov/northeast-area/beltsville -md-bhnrc/beltsville-human-nutrition-research-center/food-surveys -research-group/docs/wweianhanes-overview).

U.S. Department of Agriculture, Economic Research Service. 2019. *Biotechnology* (https://www.ers.usda.gov/topics/farm-practices-management /biotechnology).

U.S. Department of Agriculture and Centers for Disease Control and Prevention. 2020. *What We Eat in America* (https://www.cdc.gov/nchs/nhanes /wweia.htm).

U.S. Department of Health and Human Services and U.S. Department of Agriculture. 2020. *2015–2020 Dietary Guidelines for Americans*, 8th ed. (http://health.gov/dietaryguidelines/2015/guidelines/).

U.S. Department of Health and Human Services and U.S. Department of Agriculture. 2020. *Scientific Report of the 2015 Dietary Guidelines Advisory Committee,* Figure D1.33 (http://www.health.gov/dietaryguidelines /2015-scientific-report).

U.S. Department of Health and Human Services and U.S. Food and Drug Administration. *Substances Added to Food* (formerly EAFUS). (https:// www.fda.gov/food/food-additives-petitions/substances-added-food-formerly -eafus).

U.S. Food and Drug Administration. Trans *Fats* (https://www.fda.gov/food /food-additives-petitions/trans-fat).

U.S. Environmental Protection Agency. 2020. *Choose Fish and Shellfish Wisely.* (https://www.epa.gov/choose-fish-and-shellfish-wisely).

U.S. Food and Drug Administration. 2018. *Use of the Term Healthy on Food Labeling* (https://www.fda.gov/food/food-labeling-nutrition/use-term -healthy-food-labeling).

U.S. Food and Drug Administration. 2018. *Food Allergies: What You Need to Know* (https://www.fda.gov/Food/ResourcesForYou/Consumers/ucm079311 .htm).

U.S. Food and Drug Administration. 2019. *Advice About Eating Fish.* (https:// www.fda.gov/food/consumers/advice-about-eating-fish).

U.S. Food and Drug Administration. 2019. *Calories on the Menu.* (https:// www.fda.gov/food/nutrition-education-resources-materials/calories -menu).

U.S. Food and Drug Administration. 2019. Vending Machine Labeling Requirements. Final Rule Information. (https://www.fda.gov/food/food -labeling-nutrition/vending-machine-labeling-requirements).

van den Heuvel, E. G. H. M., and J. M. J. M. Steijns. 2018. Dairy products and bone health: How strong is the scientific evidence? *Nutrition Research Reviews* 31(2):164–178. DOI: 10.1017/S095442241800001X

Vos, M. B., et al. 2017. Added sugars and cardiovascular risk in children: A scientific statement from the American Heart Association. *Circulation* 135(19): e1017–e1034.

Wang, D. D., et al. 2017. Association of specific dietary fats with total and cause-specific mortality. *JAMA Internal Medicine* 176(8): 1134–1145.

Wang, X., et al. 2014. Fruit and vegetable consumption and mortality from all causes, cardiovascular disease, and cancer: Systematic review and dose-response meta-analysis of prospective cohort studies. *BMJ* 349: g4490.

Watowicz, R. P., et al. 2015. Energy contribution of beverages in US children by age, weight, and consumer status. *Childhood Obesity* 11(4): 475–483.

Whelton, P. K., et al. 2017. ACC/AHA/AAPA/ABC/ACPM/AGS/APhA/ ASH/ASPC/NMA/PCNA guideline for the prevention, detection, evaluation, and management of high blood pressure in adults: A report of the American College of Cardiology/American Heart Association Task Force on Clinical Practice Guidelines. *Journal of the American College of Cardiology* 71:e127–248.

World Health Organization. 2020. Global Health Observatory (GHO) data. *Child Malnutrition* (https://www.who.int/gho/child-malnutrition/en/).

World Health Organization. 2020. *Global Strategy on Diet, Physical Activity, and Health: Child Overweight and Obesity* (http://www.who.int /dietphysicalactivity/childhood/en/).

Wu, J. H. Y., R. Micha, and D. Mozaffarian. 2019. Dietary fats and cardiometabolic disease: Mechanisms and effects on risk factor and outcomes. *Nature Reviews Cardiology* 16(10):581-601.

Wu, L., and D. Sun. 2017. Adherence to Mediterranean diet and risk of developing cognitive disorders: An updated systematic review and meta-analysis of prospective cohort studies. *Scientific Reports* 7: 41317. DOI:10.1038/srep41317.

Yang, W. S., et al. 2019. Association between plasma N-6 polyunsaturated fatty acid levels and the risk of cardiovascular disease in a community-based cohort study. *Scientific Reports* 9(1):19298. DOI: 10.1038/s41598 -019-55686-7.

Zhang, P., et al. 2019. Dietary fats in relation to total and cause-specific mortality in a prospective cohort of 521120 individuals with 16 years of follow-up. *Circulation Research* 124(5):757–768. DOI: 10.1161/ CIRCRESAHA.118.314038.

Zong, G., et al. 2016. Intake of individual saturated fatty acids and risk of coronary heart disease in US men and women: Two prospective longitudinal cohort studies. *BMJ* 355: i5796. DOI:10.1136/bmj.i5796.

Healthy US-Style Food Patterns

Calorie level of pattern	1600	1800	2000	2200	2400	2600	2800	3000
Food Group	**Daily amount** of food from each group (vegetable and protein foods subgroup amounts are per week)							
Vegetables	**2 c-eq**	**2.5 c-eq**	**2.5 c-eq**	**3 c-eq**	**3 c-eq**	**3.5 c-eq**	**3.5 c-eq**	**4 c-eq**
Dark green veg	1.5 c/wk	1.5 c/wk	1.5 c/wk	2 c/wk	2 c/wk	2.5 c/wk	2.5 c/wk	2.5 c/wk
Red/orange veg	4 c/wk	5.5 c/wk	5.5 c/wk	6 c/wk	6 c/wk	7 c/wk	7 c/wk	7.5 c/wk
Legumes (beans, peas)	1 c/wk	1.5 c/wk	1.5 c/wk	2 c/wk	2 c/wk	2.5 c/wk	2.5 c/wk	3 c/wk
Starchy veg	4 c/wk	5 c/wk	5 c/wk	6 c/wk	6 c/wk	7 c/wk	7 c/wk	8 c/wk
Other veg	3.5 c/wk	4 c/wk	4 c/wk	5 c/wk	5 c/wk	5.5 c/wk	5.5 c/wk	7 c/wk
Fruits	**1.5 c-eq**	**1.5 c-eq**	**2 c-eq**	**2 c-eq**	**2 c-eq**	**2 c-eq**	**2.5 c-eq**	**2.5 c-eq**
Grains	**5 oz-eq**	**6 oz-eq**	**6 oz-eq**	**7 oz-eq**	**8 oz-eq**	**9 oz-eq**	**10 oz-eq**	**10 oz-eq**
Whole grains	3 oz-eq	3 oz-eq	3 oz-eq	3.5 oz-eq	4 oz-eq	4.5 oz-eq	5 oz-eq	5 oz-eq
Refined grains	2 oz-eq	3 oz-eq	3 oz-eq	3.5 oz-eq	4 oz-eq	4.5 oz-eq	5 oz-eq	5 oz-eq
Dairy	**3 c-eq**	**3 c-eq**	**3 c-eq**	**3 c-eq**	**3 c-eq**	**3 c-eq**	**3 c-eq**	**3 c-eq**
Protein foods	**5 oz-eq**	**5 oz-eq**	**5.5 oz-eq**	**6 oz-eq**	**6.5 oz-eq**	**6.5 oz-eq**	**7 oz-eq**	**7 oz-eq**
Seafood	8 oz-eq/wk	8 oz-eq/wk	8 oz-eq/wk	9 oz-eq/wk	10 oz-eq/wk	10 oz-eq/wk	10 oz-eq/wk	10 oz-eq/wk
Meat, poultry, eggs	23 oz-eq/wk	23 oz-eq/wk	26 oz-eq/wk	28 oz-eq/wk	31 oz-eq/wk	31 oz-eq/wk	33 oz-eq/wk	33 oz-eq/wk
Nuts, seeds, soy	4 oz-eq/wk	4 oz-eq/wk	5 oz-eq/wk	5 oz-eq/wk	5 oz-eq/wk	5 oz-eq/wk	6 oz-eq/wk	6 oz-eq/wk
Oils	**22 g**	**24 g**	**27 g**	**29 g**	**31 g**	**34 g**	**36 g**	**44 g**
Limit on calories for other uses (calories and % of calories)*	**130 cal (8%)**	**170 cal (9%)**	**270 cal (14%)**	**280 cal (13%)**	**350 cal (15%)**	**380 cal (15%)**	**400 cal (14%)**	**470 cal (16%)**

Food group amounts shown in cup equivalents (c-eq) or ounce equivalents (oz-eq). Oils are shown in grams (g).
Quantity equivalents for each food group are:
- Grains, 1 ounce equivalent is: ½ cup cooked rice, pasta, or cooked cereal; 1 ounce dry pasta or rice; 1 slice bread; 1 cup ready-to-eat cereal flakes.
- Fruits and vegetables, 1 cup equivalent is: 1 cup raw or cooked fruit or vegetable, 1 cup fruit or vegetable juice, 2 cups leafy salad greens.
- Protein Foods, 1 ounce equivalent is: 1 ounce lean meat, poultry, or seafood; 1 egg; ¼ cup cooked beans or tofu; 1 Tbsp peanut butter; ½ ounce nuts/seeds.
- Dairy, 1 cup equivalent is: 1 cup milk or yogurt, 1½ ounces natural cheese such as cheddar cheese or 2 ounces of processed cheese.

*All foods are assumed to be in nutrient-dense forms, lean or low-fat, and prepared without added fats, sugars, refined starches, or salt. If all food choices to meet food group recommendations are in nutrient-dense forms, a small number of calories remain within the overall calorie limit of the pattern. Calories up to the specified limit can be used for added sugars, added refined starches, solid fats, alcohol, or to eat more than the recommended amount of food in a food group. The overall eating pattern also should not exceed the limits of less than 10% of calories from added sugars and less than 10% of calories from saturated fats. At most calorie levels, amounts that can be accommodated are less than these limits. For adults of legal drinking age who choose to drink alcohol, a limit of up to one drink per day for women and up to two drinks per day for men within limits on calories for other uses applies; and calories from protein, carbohydrate, and total fats should be within the Acceptable Macronutrient Distribution Ranges (AMDRs).

FIGURE 1   **Healthy U.S.-Style Food Patterns.**

SOURCE: U.S. Department of Health and Human Services and U.S. Department of Agriculture. *2015–2020 Dietary Guidelines for Americans.* 8th Edition. December 2015. Available at http://health.gov/dietaryguidelines/2015/guidelines.

Healthy Vegetarian Patterns

Calorie level of pattern	1600	1800	2000	2200	2400	2600	2800	3000
Food Group	Daily amount[a] of food from each group (vegetable and protein foods subgroup amounts are per week)							
Vegetables	2 c-eq	2.5 c-eq	2.5 c-eq	3 c-eq	3 c-eq	3.5 c-eq	3.5 c-eq	4 c-eq
Dark green veg	1.5 c/wk	1.5 c/wk	1.5 c/wk	2 c/wk	2 c/wk	2.5 c/wk	2.5 c/wk	2.5 c/wk
Red/orange veg	4 c/wk	5.5 c/wk	5.5 c/wk	6 c/wk	6 c/wk	7 c/wk	7 c/wk	7.5 c/wk
Legumes (beans, peas)	1 c/wk	1.5 c/wk	1.5 c/wk	2 c/wk	2 c/wk	2.5 c/wk	2.5 c/wk	3 c/wk
Starchy veg	4 c/wk	5 c/wk	5 c/wk	6 c/wk	6 c/wk	7 c/wk	7 c/wk	8 c/wk
Other veg	3.5 c/wk	4 c/wk	4 c/wk	5 c/wk	5 c/wk	5.5 c/wk	5.5 c/wk	7 c/wk
Fruits	1.5 c-eq	1.5 c-eq	2 c-eq	2 c-eq	2 c-eq	2 c-eq	2.5 c-eq	2.5 c-eq
Grains	5.5 oz-eq	6.5 oz-eq	6.5 oz-eq	7.5 oz-eq	8.5 oz-eq	9.5 oz-eq	10.5 oz-eq	10.5 oz-eq
Whole grains	3 oz-eq	3.5 oz-eq	3.5 oz-eq	4 oz-eq	4.5 oz-eq	5 oz-eq	5.5 oz-eq	5.5 oz-eq
Refined grains	2.5 oz-eq	3 oz-eq	3 oz-eq	3.5 oz-eq	4 oz-eq	4.5 oz-eq	5 oz-eq	5 oz-eq
Dairy	3 c-eq	3 c-eq	3 c-eq	3 c-eq	3 c-eq	3 c-eq	3 c-eq	3 c-eq
Protein foods	2.5 oz-eq	3 oz-eq	3.5 oz-eq	3.5 oz-eq	4 oz-eq	4.5 oz-eq	5 oz-eq	5.5 oz-eq
Eggs	3 oz-eq/wk	3 oz-eq/wk	3 oz-eq/wk	3 oz-eq/wk	3 oz-eq/wk	3 oz-eq/wk	4 oz-eq/wk	4 oz-eq/wk
Legumes (beans, peas)[b]	4 oz-eq/wk	6 oz-eq/wk	6 oz-eq/wk	6 oz-eq/wk	8 oz-eq/wk	9 oz-eq/wk	10 oz-eq/wk	11 oz-eq/wk
Tofu/processed soy	6 oz-eq/wk	6 oz-eq/wk	8 oz-eq/wk	8 oz-eq/wk	9 oz-eq/wk	10 oz-eq/wk	11 oz-eq/wk	12 oz-eq/wk
Nuts and seeds	5 oz-eq/wk	6 oz-eq/wk	7 oz-eq/wk	7 oz-eq/wk	8 oz-eq/wk	9 oz-eq/wk	10 oz-eq/wk	12 oz-eq/wk
Oils	22 g	24 g	27 g	29 g	31 g	34 g	36 g	44 g
Limit on calories for other uses (calories and % of calories)[c]	180 cal (11%)	190 cal (11%)	290 cal (15%)	330 cal (15%)	390 cal (16%)	390 cal (15%)	400 cal (14%)	440 cal (15%)

[a]Food group amounts shown in cup equivalents (c-eq) or ounce equivalents (oz-eq). Oils are shown in grams (g). Quantity equivalents for each food group are:
  • Grains, 1 ounce equivalent is: ½ cup cooked rice, pasta, or cooked cereal; 1 ounce dry pasta or rice; 1 slice bread; 1 cup ready-to-eat cereal flakes.
  • Fruits and vegetables, 1 cup equivalent is: 1 cup raw or cooked fruit or vegetable, 1 cup fruit or vegetable juice, 2 cups leafy salad greens.
  • Protein Foods, 1 ounce equivalent is: 1 ounce lean meat, poultry, or seafood; 1 egg; ¼ cup cooked beans or tofu; 1 tbsp peanut butter; ½ ounce nuts/seeds.
  • Dairy, 1 cup equivalent is: 1 cup milk or yogurt, 1½ ounces natural cheese (e.g. cheddar cheese) or 2 ounces of processed cheese.

[b]About half of total beans and peas are shown as vegetables, in cup eqs, and half as protein foods, in ounce eqs. Total beans and peas in cup eq is amount in vegetables plus the amount in protein foods/4:

	1600	1800	2000	2200	2400	2600	2800	3000
Total beans/peas	2 c-eq/wk	3 c-eq/wk	3 c-eq/wk	3.5 c-eq/wk	4 c-eq/wk	5 c-eq/wk	5 c-eq/wk	6 c-eq/wk

[c]All foods are assumed to be in nutrient-dense forms, lean or low-fat, and prepared without added fats, sugars, refined starches, or salt. If all food choices to meet food group recommendations are in nutrient-dense forms, a small number of calories remain within the overall calorie limit of the pattern. Calories up to the specified limit can be used for added sugars, added refined starches, solid fats, alcohol, or to eat more than the recommended amount of food in a food group. The overall eating pattern also should not exceed the limits of less than 10% of calories from added sugars and less than 10% of calories from saturated fats. At most calorie levels, amounts that can be accommodated are less than these limits. For adults of legal drinking age who choose to drink alcohol, a limit of up to one drink per day for women and up to two drinks per day for men within limits on calories for other uses applies; and calories from protein, carbohydrate, and total fats should be within the Acceptable Macronutrient Distribution Ranges (AMDRs).

FIGURE 2 Healthy Vegetarian Food Patterns.

source: U.S. Department of Health and Human Services and U.S. Department of Agriculture. *2015–2020 Dietary Guidelines for Americans.* 8th Edition. December 2015. Available at http://health.gov/dietaryguidelines/2015/guidelines.

Healthy Mediterranean-Style Patterns

Calorie level of pattern	1600	1800	2000	2200	2400	2600	2800	3000
Food Group	**Daily amount** of food from each group (vegetable and protein foods subgroup amounts are per week)							
Vegetables	**2 c-eq**	**2.5 c-eq**	**2.5 c-eq**	**3 c-eq**	**3 c-eq**	**3.5 c-eq**	**3.5 c-eq**	**4 c-eq**
Dark green veg	1.5 c/wk	1.5 c/wk	1.5 c/wk	2 c/wk	2 c/wk	2.5 c/wk	2.5 c/wk	2.5 c/wk
Red/orange veg	4 c/wk	5.5 c/wk	5.5 c/wk	6 c/wk	6 c/wk	7 c/wk	7 c/wk	7.5 c/wk
Legumes (beans, peas)	1 c/wk	1.5 c/wk	1.5 c/wk	2 c/wk	2 c/wk	2.5 c/wk	2.5 c/wk	3 c/wk
Starchy veg	4 c/wk	5 c/wk	5 c/wk	6 c/wk	6 c/wk	7 c/wk	7 c/wk	8 c/wk
Other veg	3.5 c/wk	4 c/wk	4 c/wk	5 c/wk	5 c/wk	5.5 c/wk	5.5 c/wk	7 c/wk
Fruits	**2 c-eq**	**2 c-eq**	**2.5 c-eq**	**2.5 c-eq**	**2.5 c-eq**	**2.5 c-eq**	**3 c-eq**	**3 c-eq**
Grains	**5 oz-eq**	**6 oz-eq**	**6 oz-eq**	**7 oz-eq**	**8 oz-eq**	**9 oz-eq**	**10 oz-eq**	**10 oz-eq**
Whole grains	3 oz-eq	3 oz-eq	3 oz-eq	3.5 oz-eq	4 oz-eq	4.5 oz-eq	5 oz-eq	5 oz-eq
Refined grains	2 oz-eq	3 oz-eq	3 oz-eq	3.5 oz-eq	4 oz-eq	4.5 oz-eq	5 oz-eq	5 oz-eq
Dairy	**2 c-eq**	**2 c-eq**	**2 c-eq**	**2 c-eq**	**2.5 c-eq**	**2.5 c-eq**	**2.5 c-eq**	**2.5 c-eq**
Protein foods	**5.5 oz-eq**	**6 oz-eq**	**6.5 oz-eq**	**7 oz-eq**	**7.5 oz-eq**	**7.5 oz-eq**	**8 oz-eq**	**8 oz-eq**
Seafood	11 oz-eq/wk	15 oz-eq/wk	15 oz-eq/wk	16 oz-eq/wk	16 oz-eq/wk	17 oz-eq/wk	17 oz-eq/wk	17 oz-eq/wk
Meat, poultry, eggs	23 oz-eq/wk	23 oz-eq/wk	26 oz-eq/wk	28 oz-eq/wk	31 oz-eq/wk	31 oz-eq/wk	33 oz-eq/wk	33 oz-eq/wk
Nut, seeds, soy	4 oz-eq/wk	4 oz-eq/wk	5 oz-eq/wk	5 oz-eq/wk	5 oz-eq/wk	5 oz-eq/wk	6 oz-eq/wk	6 oz-eq/wk
Oils	**22 g**	**24 g**	**27 g**	**29 g**	**31 g**	**34 g**	**36 g**	**44 g**
Limit on calories for other uses (calories and % of calories)*	**140 cal (9%)**	**160 cal (9%)**	**260 cal (13%)**	**270 cal (12%)**	**300 cal (13%)**	**330 cal (13%)**	**350 cal (13%)**	**430 cal (14%)**

Food group amounts shown in cup equivalents (c-eq) or ounce equivalents (oz-eq). Oils are shown in grams (g).
Quantity equivalents for each food group are:
- Grains, 1 ounce equivalent is: ½ cup cooked rice, pasta, or cooked cereal; 1 ounce dry pasta or rice; 1 slice bread; 1 cup ready-to-eat cereal flakes.
- Fruits and vegetables, 1 cup equivalent is: 1 cup raw or cooked fruit or vegetable, 1 cup fruit or vegetable juice, 2 cups leafy salad greens.
- Protein Foods, 1 ounce equivalent is: 1 ounce lean meat, poultry, or seafood; 1 egg; ¼ cup cooked beans or tofu; 1 Tbsp peanut butter; ½ ounce nuts/seeds.
- Dairy, 1 cup equivalent is: 1 cup milk or yogurt, 1½ ounces natural cheese such as cheddar cheese or 2 ounces of processed cheese.

*All foods are assumed to be in nutrient-dense forms, lean or low-fat, and prepared without added fats, sugars, refined starches, or salt. If all food choices to meet food group recommendations are in nutrient-dense forms, a small number of calories remain within the overall calorie limit of the pattern. Calories up to the specified limit can be used for added sugars, added refined starches, solid fats, alcohol, or to eat more than the recommended amount of food in a food group. The overall eating pattern also should not exceed the limits of less than 10% of calories from added sugars and less than 10% of calories from saturated fats. At most calorie levels, amounts that can be accommodated are less than these limits. For adults of legal drinking age who choose to drink alcohol, a limit of up to one drink per day for women and up to two drinks per day for men within limits on calories for other uses applies; and calories from protein, carbohydrate, and total fats should be within the Acceptable Macronutrient Distribution Ranges (AMDRs).

FIGURE 3 Healthy Mediterranean-Style Patterns.

SOURCE: U.S. Department of Health and Human Services and U.S. Department of Agriculture. *2015–2020 Dietary Guidelines for Americans.* 8th Edition. December 2015. Available at http://health.gov/dietaryguidelines/2015/guidelines.

Nutrition Resources

FOLLOWING THE DASH EATING PLAN
for 1,800 to 2,000 calories per day

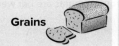

Grains
6–8 Servings per day

Sources of fiber and magnesium

Serving Size
1 slice bread
1 oz dry cereal
½ cup cooked rice, pasta, or cereal

Examples
Oatmeal, grits, brown rice, unsalted pretzels and popcorn, whole grain cereal, whole wheat bread, rolls, pasta, English muffin, pita bread, bagel

Vegetables
4–5 Servings per day

Sources of potassium, magnesium, and fiber

Serving Size
1 cup raw leafy vegetables
½ cup cut-up raw or cooked vegetable
½ cup vegetable juice

Examples
Broccoli, carrots, collards, green beans, green peas, kale, lima beans, potatoes, spinach, squash, sweet potatoes, tomatoes

Fruits
4–5 Servings per day

Sources of potassium, magnesium, and fiber

Serving Size
1 medium fruit
¼ cup dried fruit (unsweetened)
½ cup fresh, frozen, or canned fruit, or fruit juice

Examples
Apples, apricots, bananas, dates, grapes, oranges, grapefruit, grapefruit juice, mangoes, melons, peaches, pineapples, raisins, strawberries, tangerines

Dairy
2–3 Servings per day

Sources of calcium and protein

Serving Size
1 cup milk
1 cup yogurt
1½ oz cheese

Examples
Fat-free (skim) or low-fat (1%) milk or buttermilk; fat-free, low-fat, or reduced-fat cheese; fat-free or low-fat regular or frozen yogurt; fortified soy beverage; lactose-free products

Lean meats, fish, poultry, and eggs
6 servings or less per day

Sources of protein and magnesium

Serving Size
1 oz cooked meats, fish, or poultry
1 egg

Examples
Chicken or turkey without skin; salmon, tuna, trout; lean cuts of beef, pork, and lamb

Fats and oils
2–3 Servings per day

Sources of energy and vitamin E

Serving Size
1 tsp soft margarine
1 tsp vegetable oil
1 tbsp mayonnaise
2 tbsp salad dressing

Examples
Soft margarine, vegetable oil (such as canola, corn, olive, or safflower), low-fat mayonnaise, light salad dressing

Nuts, seeds and legumes
4–5 Servings per week

Sources of energy magnesium, protein, and fiber

Serving Size
⅓ cup or **1½ oz** nuts (unsalted)
2 tbsp peanut butter
2 tbsp or **½ oz** seeds
½ cup cooked legumes (dry beans and peas)

Examples
Almonds, hazelnuts, mixed nuts, peanuts, walnuts, sunflower seeds, peanut butter, kidney beans, lentils, split peas

Sweets and Added sugars
5 Servings or less per week

Sweets should be low in fat

Serving Size
1 tbsp sugar
1 tbsp jelly or jam
½ cup sorbet, gelatin
1 cup lemonade

Examples
Fruit-flavored gelatin, fruit punch, hard candy, jelly, maple syrup, sorbet and ices, sugar

FIGURE 4 The DASH Eating Plan.

SOURCE: National Institutes of Health, National Heart, Lung, and Blood Institute. 2020. Following the DASH Eating Plan for 1800-2000 Calories per Day. https://www.nhlbi.nih.gov/health-topics/all-publications-and-resources/whats-your-plate-1800–2000-caloriesday

Design Elements: Assess Yourself icon: Aleksey Boldin/Alamy Stock Photo; Diversity Matters icon: Rawpixel Ltd/Getty Images; Wellness on Campus icon: Rawpixel Ltd/Getty Images; Take Charge icon: VisualCommunications/Getty Images; Critical Consumer icon: pagadesign/Getty Images.

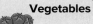

CHAPTER 14

CHAPTER OBJECTIVES

- Describe the benefits of exercise
- Define physical fitness
- Explain the components of an active lifestyle
- Put together a personalized exercise program
- Explain strategies for staying on track with an exercise program

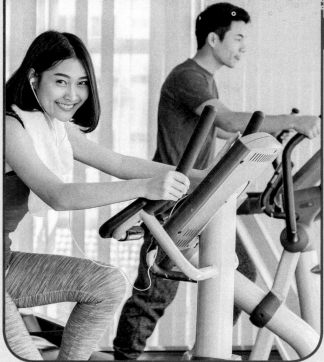

Manop_Phimsit/Shutterstock

Exercise for Health and Fitness

TEST YOUR KNOWLEDGE

1. To improve your health, you must exercise vigorously for at least 30 minutes straight, five or more days per week.
   True or False?

2. Which of the following is (are) considered a form of cardiorespiratory endurance exercise?
   a. Walking
   b. Swimming
   c. Step aerobics

3. Developing strength in the trunk muscles is the most important way to prevent low-back pain.
   True or False?

4. The terms *physical activity* and *exercise* mean the same thing.
   True or False?

ANSWERS

1. **FALSE.** For substantial health benefits, adults should do at least 150 minutes (2.5 hours) a week of moderate-intensity aerobic physical activity, or 75 minutes (1 hour and 15 minutes) a week of vigorous-intensity aerobic physical activity, or an equivalent combination of moderate- and vigorous-intensity aerobic activities. The activity can be done in short bouts—10-minute sessions, for example—spread out over the week.

2. **ALL THREE.** You can develop cardiorespiratory endurance through activities that involve continuous, rhythmic movements of large muscle groups, such as the legs. Many kinds of activities count as cardiorespiratory endurance exercise.

3. **FALSE.** Although muscular strength is an important factor in low-back health, muscular endurance in the trunk and hips, along with good posture, is most important for preventing low-back pain.

4. **FALSE.** Physical activity is any body movement carried out by the skeletal muscles that requires energy. Exercise is planned, structured, repetitive movement performed specifically to improve or maintain physical fitness. Increase your physical activity—in addition to your structured exercise program.

Your body is a wonderful moving machine made to work best when it is physically active. It readily adapts to practically any level of activity and exercise: The more you ask of your body, the stronger and more fit it becomes. The opposite is also true. Left unchallenged, bones lose their density, joints stiffen, muscles weaken, and the body's energy systems degenerate. To be truly healthy, human beings must be active.

This chapter gives you the basic information you need to put together a physical fitness program that will work for you. If approached correctly, physical activity and exercise can contribute immeasurably to overall wellness, add fun and joy to life, and provide the foundation for a lifetime of fitness.

THE BENEFITS OF EXERCISE

The human body is adaptable. The greater the demands, the more it adjusts and the more fit it becomes. Over time, immediate, short-term adjustments translate into long-term changes and improvements (Figure 14.1).

Reduced Risk of Premature Death

Physically active people have a reduced risk of dying prematurely from all causes; the most active people experience the greatest health benefits (Figure 14.2).

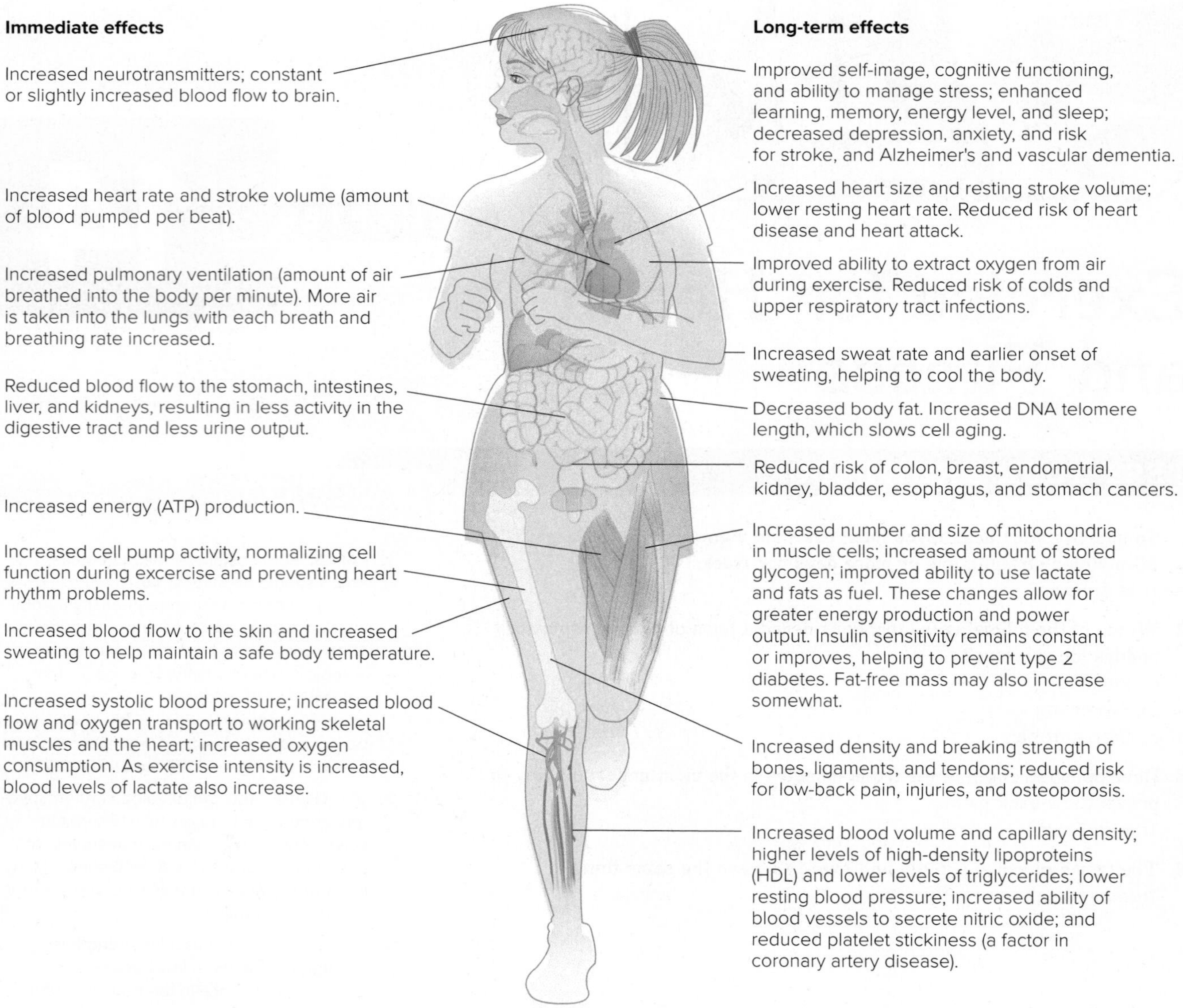

Immediate effects

Increased neurotransmitters; constant or slightly increased blood flow to brain.

Increased heart rate and stroke volume (amount of blood pumped per beat).

Increased pulmonary ventilation (amount of air breathed into the body per minute). More air is taken into the lungs with each breath and breathing rate increased.

Reduced blood flow to the stomach, intestines, liver, and kidneys, resulting in less activity in the digestive tract and less urine output.

Increased energy (ATP) production.

Increased cell pump activity, normalizing cell function during excercise and preventing heart rhythm problems.

Increased blood flow to the skin and increased sweating to help maintain a safe body temperature.

Increased systolic blood pressure; increased blood flow and oxygen transport to working skeletal muscles and the heart; increased oxygen consumption. As exercise intensity is increased, blood levels of lactate also increase.

Long-term effects

Improved self-image, cognitive functioning, and ability to manage stress; enhanced learning, memory, energy level, and sleep; decreased depression, anxiety, and risk for stroke, and Alzheimer's and vascular dementia.

Increased heart size and resting stroke volume; lower resting heart rate. Reduced risk of heart disease and heart attack.

Improved ability to extract oxygen from air during exercise. Reduced risk of colds and upper respiratory tract infections.

Increased sweat rate and earlier onset of sweating, helping to cool the body.

Decreased body fat. Increased DNA telomere length, which slows cell aging.

Reduced risk of colon, breast, endometrial, kidney, bladder, esophagus, and stomach cancers.

Increased number and size of mitochondria in muscle cells; increased amount of stored glycogen; improved ability to use lactate and fats as fuel. These changes allow for greater energy production and power output. Insulin sensitivity remains constant or improves, helping to prevent type 2 diabetes. Fat-free mass may also increase somewhat.

Increased density and breaking strength of bones, ligaments, and tendons; reduced risk for low-back pain, injuries, and osteoporosis.

Increased blood volume and capillary density; higher levels of high-density lipoproteins (HDL) and lower levels of triglycerides; lower resting blood pressure; increased ability of blood vessels to secrete nitric oxide; and reduced platelet stickiness (a factor in coronary artery disease).

FIGURE 14.1   Immediate and long-term effects of regular cardiorespiratory endurance exercise. When endurance exercise is performed regularly, short-term changes in the body develop into more permanent adaptations; these include improved ability to exercise, reduced risk of many chronic diseases, and improved psychological and emotional well-being.

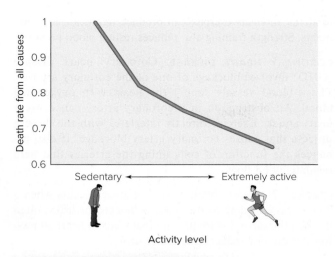

FIGURE 14.2 **Exercise promotes longevity.** The risk of death each year from all causes decreases with increased amounts and intensities of weekly physical activity.

SOURCES: Adapted from a composite of 12 studies involving over 200,000 men and women. Wen, M., et al. 2014. Physical activity and mortality among middle-aged and older adults in the United States. *Journal Physical Activity & Health* 11: 303–312; Physical Activity Guidelines Advisory Committee. *Physical Activity Guidelines Advisory Committee Report, 2008*. Washington, DC: 2008. U.S. Department of Health and Human Services; Schnohr, P., et al. 2015. Dose of jogging and long-term mortality: The Copenhagen City Heart Study. *Journal of the American College of Cardiology* 65(5): 411–419.

Improved Cardiorespiratory Functioning

Every time you take a breath, oxygen enters your lungs and is picked up by red blood cells and transported to your heart. From there, the heart pumps oxygenated blood throughout the body to organs and tissues that use it. During exercise, the cardiorespiratory system (heart, lungs, and circulatory system) must work harder to meet the body's increased demand for oxygen. Regular cardiorespiratory endurance exercise improves the functioning of the heart and the ability of the cardiorespiratory system to carry oxygen to body tissues. Exercise directly affects the health of your arteries, keeping them from stiffening or clogging with plaque and reducing the risk of cardiovascular disease. Exercise also improves sexual function and general vitality.

More Efficient Metabolism and Improved Cell Health

Endurance exercise improves metabolism—the process that converts food to energy and builds tissue. This process involves oxygen, nutrients, hormones, and enzymes. A physically fit person's body can more efficiently use energy from carbohydrates and fats and better regulate hormones. Exercise may also protect cells from damage from free radicals, which are destructive chemicals produced normally during metabolism (see Chapter 13), and from inflammation caused by obesity, high blood pressure or cholesterol, nicotine, and overeating. Training activates antioxidants that prevent free radical damage and

maintain cell health. Regular physical activity and exercise prevent the deterioration of telomeres, which form the protective ends of chromosomes that are vital for cell health and repair.

Improved Body Composition

Healthy body composition means that the body has a high proportion of fat-free mass and a relatively small proportion of fat. Too much body fat, particularly abdominal fat, is linked to a variety of health problems, including heart disease, high blood pressure, cancer, and diabetes. Healthy body composition can be difficult to achieve and maintain because a diet that contains enough essential nutrients can be relatively high in calories, especially for someone who is sedentary. Excess calories can be stored in the body as fat.

Exercise can improve body composition in several ways. Endurance exercise increases daily calorie expenditure. It can also slightly raise *metabolic rate,* the rate at which the body burns calories, for several hours after an exercise session. Strength training increases muscle mass, tipping the body composition ratio toward fat-free mass and away from fat. It can also help with losing fat because metabolic rate is directly proportional to fat-free mass: The more muscle mass, the higher the metabolic rate.

Physical activity reduces the risk of death regardless of its effect on body composition. Greater levels of activity and physical fitness are associated with lower death rates, no matter your weight, although this effect is especially true for people who are overweight or obese. A 2015 literature review concluded that death rates from all causes are lower in fit people and that "being fat and fit is better than unfat and unfit" (Figure 14.3).

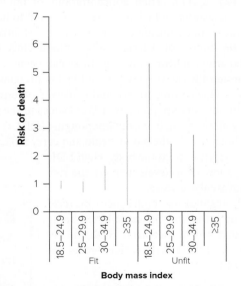

FIGURE 14.3 **Relationship among fitness, body mass index, and risk of death from all causes in men and women.**

SOURCE: Yerrakalva, D., et al. 2015. The associations of "fatness," "fitness," and physical activity with all-cause mortality in older adults: a systematic review. *Obesity* 23(10): 1944–1956.

A study of 1.3 million Swedish men, however, found that men who were overweight as young men had a higher risk of premature death, regardless of fitness. Physical activity does not eliminate the health risks associated with overweight, but it reduces its effects.

Disease Prevention and Management

Regular physical activity and exercise lower your risk of many chronic, disabling diseases.

Cardiovascular Disease   A sedentary lifestyle is one of six major risk factors for cardiovascular disease (CVD), including heart attack and stroke. The other major risk factors are smoking, abnormal blood fats, high blood pressure, diabetes, and obesity. Most of these risk factors are linked by a group of symptoms called the *metabolic syndrome*. These symptoms include insulin resistance, high blood pressure, abnormal blood fats, abdominal fat deposits, type 2 diabetes, blood clotting abnormalities, and blood vessel inflammation. Sedentary people have CVD death rates significantly higher than those of fit individuals. Physical inactivity increases the risk of CVD by as much as 240%. (See Chapter 16 for an in-depth discussion of cardiovascular disease and its risk factors.)

The benefits of physical activity begin at moderate levels of exercise and increase as the amount and intensity of activity rise. Exercise positively affects the risk factors for CVD, including cholesterol levels, insulin resistance, and blood pressure. Exercise also directly interferes with the disease process itself, lowering the risk of heart disease and stroke.

BLOOD FAT LEVELS   High concentrations of lipids (fats), such as cholesterol and triglycerides, are linked to heart disease because they contribute to the formation of fatty deposits on the linings of arteries. When blood clots block a narrowed artery, a heart attack or stroke can occur.

Cholesterol is carried in the blood by lipoproteins, which are classified according to size and density. Cholesterol carried by low-density lipoproteins (LDLs) sticks to the walls of coronary arteries. High-density lipoproteins (HDLs) pick up excess cholesterol in the bloodstream and carry it back to the liver for excretion from the body. High LDL levels and low HDL levels increase the risk of cardiovascular disease.

Cardiorespiratory endurance exercise and strength training influence blood lipids in a positive way by increasing HDL and decreasing LDL and triglycerides—reducing the risk of CVD.

HIGH BLOOD PRESSURE   Regular cardiorespiratory endurance exercise tends to reduce high blood pressure (hypertension), a contributing factor in diseases such as coronary heart disease, stroke, heart failure, kidney failure, sexual dysfunction, and blindness. Intense exercise works best, but even moderate-intensity exercise can produce significant improvements. Strength training also reduces resting blood pressure.

CORONARY HEART DISEASE   Coronary heart disease (CHD) involves blockage of one of the coronary arteries. These blood vessels supply the heart with oxygenated blood. An obstruction in a coronary artery can cause a heart attack. Exercise directly interferes with the disease process that causes coronary artery blockage. It also enhances the function of cells lining the arteries that help regulate blood flow.

STROKE   The most common kind of stroke occurs when a blood vessel leading to the brain is blocked or leaks, often through the same disease process that leads to heart attacks. Regular exercise reduces the risk of stroke.

Cancer   Studies have shown a relationship between increased physical activity and a reduced risk of cancer. Specifically, a new analysis of data from studies of 1.44 million subjects concludes that higher levels of leisure-time physical activity were associated with lower risks for 13 of 26 types of cancer, including kidney, colon, head and neck, bladder, rectal, and liver cancer. Most of these associations applied whether the participants were overweight/obese or had a history of smoking. Exercise may decrease the risk of colon cancer by speeding the movement of food through the gastrointestinal tract (quickly eliminating potential carcinogens), lowering blood-insulin levels, enhancing immune function, and reducing blood fats. Physical activity during high school and college years may be important for preventing breast cancer later in life.

Osteoporosis   A special benefit of exercise, especially for women, is protection against osteoporosis, a disease that results in loss of bone density and poor bone strength. Weight-bearing exercise, which includes almost everything except swimming, helps build bone during childhood and the teens and twenties. Older people with denser bones can better endure the bone loss that occurs with aging. Strength training and impact exercises such as jumping rope help maintain bone and muscle health throughout life. With stronger bones and muscles and better balance, fit people are less likely to experience debilitating falls and bone fractures. Along with exercise, a well-balanced diet containing adequate calcium and vitamin D and normal hormone function are also essential for strong bones. (One caution: Too much exercise can depress levels of estrogen, leading to bone loss, even in young women. Estrogen helps maintain bone density.)

Type 2 Diabetes   People with diabetes are prone to heart disease, blindness, and severe problems of the nervous and circulatory systems. Exercise prevents type

2 diabetes, the most common form of the disease. Exercise burns excess sugar and makes cells more sensitive to insulin. When people have a condition called *insulin resistance*, the body produces insulin but fails to use it effectively. Instead of the insulin enabling their cells to absorb and burn excess calories, insulin-resistant people store the excess calories as fat. Exercise helps keep body fat at healthy levels, which is important because obesity is a key risk factor for type 2 diabetes. For people with diabetes, physical activity and exercise are important for treatment. See Chapter 15 for more about diabetes.

Improved Psychological and Emotional Wellness

Physically active people enjoy many social, psychological, and emotional benefits, including:

- **Reduced anxiety.** Exercise reduces symptoms of anxiety, such as worry and self-doubt, both in people who are anxious most of the time and in people who become anxious in response to a particular experience. Exercise is associated with a lower risk for panic attacks, generalized anxiety disorder, and social anxiety disorder.

- **Reduced depression and improved mood.** Exercise relieves feelings of sadness and hopelessness and can be as effective as psychotherapy in treating mild to moderate cases of depression. Exercise improves mood and increases feelings of well-being in both depressed and nondepressed people.

- **Improved sleep.** Regular physical activity and exercise help people fall asleep more easily; they also improve sleep quality.

- **Reduced stress.** Exercise reduces the body's overall response to all forms of stressors and helps people deal more effectively with stress.

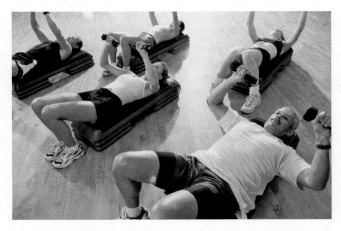

Because exercise improves workers' quality of work and mental and physical abilities, many large companies provide on-site fitness facilities or gym memberships as employee benefits. Purestock/SuperStock

- **Enhanced self-esteem, self-confidence, and self-efficacy.** Exercise can boost self-esteem and self-confidence by providing opportunities for people to succeed and excel. Exercise also improves body image. Sticking with an exercise program increases people's belief in their ability to be active, boosting self-efficacy.

- **Enhanced creativity and intellectual functioning.** In studies of people of all ages, physically active people score higher than sedentary people on tests of creativity and mental function. Exercise improves alertness and memory in the short term. Over time, exercise helps maintain reaction time, short-term memory, and nonverbal reasoning skills and enhances brain metabolism.

- **Improved work productivity.** Studies show that workers' quality of work, time management abilities, and mental and interpersonal performance are better on days they exercise.

- **Increased opportunities for social interaction.** Exercise provides many chances for people to have positive interactions with other people.

Improved Immune Function

Exercise can have either positive or negative effects on the immune system—the physiological processes that protect us from disease. Moderate endurance exercise boosts immune function, whereas excessive training depresses it. Physically fit people get fewer colds and upper respiratory tract infections than people who are not fit. The immune system and ways to strengthen it are discussed further in Chapter 18.

Prevention of Injuries and Low-Back Pain

Increased muscle strength and endurance provide protection against injury because they help people maintain spinal stability, good posture, and body mechanics when performing everyday activities such as walking, lifting, and carrying. Good muscle endurance in the abdomen, hips, lower back, and legs supports the back in proper alignment and helps prevent low-back pain, which afflicts over 85% of Americans in their lives.

Improved Wellness for Life

Although people differ in the maximum levels of fitness they can achieve through exercise, the wellness benefits of exercise are available to everyone. Exercising regularly may be the most important thing you can do now to improve the quality of your life. All the benefits of exercise continue to accrue but gain new importance as the resilience of youth wanes. Exercising can help you live a longer and healthier life.

WHAT IS PHYSICAL FITNESS?

Physical fitness is a set of physical attributes that allow the body to respond or adapt to the demands and stress of physical effort—to perform moderate to vigorous levels of physical activity without becoming overly tired. A person's level of fitness depends on physiological factors, such as the heart's ability to pump blood and the energy-generating capacity of the cells. These factors depend on genetics—a person's inborn potential for physical fitness—and on behavior—getting enough physical activity to stress the body and cause long-term physiological changes.

Some components of fitness are related to specific activities or sports, whereas others relate to general health. **Health-related fitness** includes these components::

- Cardiorespiratory endurance
- Muscular strength
- Muscular endurance
- Flexibility
- Body composition

Health-related fitness helps you withstand physical challenges and protects you from diseases.

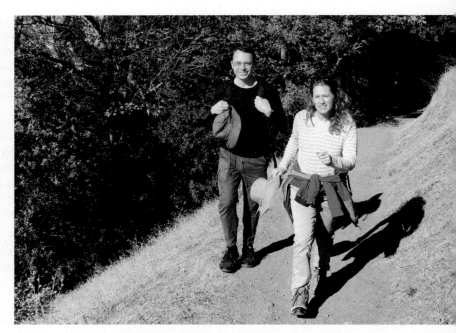

Cardiorespiratory endurance is a critical component of a fitness plan and, in this case, a mountaintop marriage proposal. Claire Insel

Cardiorespiratory Endurance

Cardiorespiratory endurance is the ability to perform prolonged, large-muscle, dynamic exercise at moderate to high intensity. It depends on factors such as the lungs' ability to deliver oxygen to the bloodstream, the heart's capacity to pump blood, the ability of the nervous system and blood vessels to regulate blood flow, and the cells' ability to use oxygen and process fuels for exercise.

When cardiorespiratory fitness is low, the heart has to work hard during normal daily activities and may not work hard enough to sustain high-intensity physical activity in an emergency. Poor cardiorespiratory fitness is linked with heart disease, diabetes, colon cancer, stroke, depression, anxiety, and premature death from all causes.

Regular **cardiorespiratory endurance training,** however, conditions the heart and metabolism. Endurance training makes the heart stronger and improves the function of the entire cardiorespiratory system. As cardiorespiratory fitness improves, related physical functions also improve:

- The heart pumps more blood per heartbeat.
- Resting heart rate slows and resting blood pressure decreases.
- Blood volume increases.
- Blood supply to tissues improves.
- The body can cool itself better.
- Metabolic health improves, which helps the body process fuels and regulate cell function.

A healthy heart can better withstand the strains of daily life, the stress of occasional emergencies, and the wear and tear of time.

Endurance training also improves the function of the body's chemical systems, particularly in the muscles and liver, enhancing the body's ability to use energy from food and to do more exercise with less effort.

You can develop cardiorespiratory endurance through activities that involve continuous, rhythmic movements of large muscle groups, such as the legs. Such activities include walking, jogging, cycling, and group aerobics.

Muscular Strength

Muscular strength is the amount of force a muscle can produce with a single maximum effort. It depends on factors such as the size of muscle cells and the ability of nerves to activate muscle cells. Strong muscles are important for everyday activities, such as climbing stairs, as well as for emergencies. Strong muscles help keep the skeleton in proper alignment, preventing back and leg pain and providing the support necessary for good posture. Recreational activities also require

---

physical fitness   The body's ability to respond or **TERMS** adapt to the demands and stress of physical effort.

health-related fitness   Physical capabilities that contribute to health, including cardiorespiratory endurance, muscular strength, muscular endurance, flexibility, and body composition.

cardiorespiratory endurance   The ability of the body to perform prolonged, large-muscle, dynamic exercise at moderate to high levels of intensity.

cardiorespiratory endurance training   Exercise intended to improve cardiorespiratory endurance.

muscular strength   The amount of force a muscle can produce with a single maximum effort.

muscular strength: Strong people can hit a tennis ball harder, kick a soccer ball farther, and ride a bicycle uphill more easily.

Muscle tissue is an important element of overall body composition. Greater muscle mass makes possible a higher rate of metabolism and faster energy use, which help people to maintain a healthy body weight.

Maintaining strength and muscle mass is vital for healthy aging. Older people lose muscle cells (a condition called *sarcopenia*), and many of the remaining muscle cells become nonfunctional because they lose their attachment to the nervous system. Strength training helps maintain muscle mass, function, and balance in older people, which greatly enhances their quality of life and prevents injuries. Strength training promotes cardiovascular health, reduces the risk of osteoporosis (bone loss), and prevents premature death from all causes.

Muscular strength can be developed by training with weights or by using the weight of the body for resistance during calisthenic exercises such as push-ups and curl-ups.

Muscular Endurance

Muscular endurance is the ability to resist fatigue and sustain a level of muscle tension—that is, to hold a muscle contraction for a long time or to contract a muscle repeatedly. For example, you need good muscle endurance to hold your spine in a neutral position when you sit in class or drive a car. Muscular endurance depends on factors such as the size of muscle cells, the ability of muscles to store fuel, the content of mitochondria (cell energy centers), and the blood supply to muscles.

Muscular endurance is important for good posture and for injury prevention. For example, if abdominal and back muscles cannot hold the spine correctly, the chances of low-back pain and back injury are increased. Good muscular endurance in the trunk muscles is more important than muscular strength for preventing back pain. Muscular endurance helps people cope with the physical demands of everyday life and enhances performance in sports and work.

Stressing the muscles with a greater load (weight) than they are accustomed to develops muscle endurance and muscular strength. How much strength or endurance develops depends on the type and amount of stress applied.

Flexibility

Flexibility is the ability of joints to move through their full range of motion. It depends on joint structure, the length and elasticity of connective tissue, and nervous system activity. Flexible, pain-free joints are important for good health and well-being. Inactivity causes the joints to become stiffer with age. Stiffness often causes older people to assume unnatural body postures that can stress joints and muscles. Stretching exercises can help ensure a healthy range of motion for all major joints.

Body Composition

Body composition refers to the proportion of fat and **fat-free mass** (muscle, bone, and water) in the body. Healthy body composition involves a high proportion of fat-free mass and an acceptably low level of body fat, adjusted for age and sex. The best way to lose fat is through a lifestyle that includes a sensible diet and exercise. The best way to add muscle mass is through resistance training such as weight training. (Chapter 15 discusses body composition in detail.)

Skill-Related Components of Fitness

In addition to the five health-related components of physical fitness, the ability to perform a particular sport or activity may depend on **skill-related fitness** components such as:

- *Speed.* The ability to perform a movement quickly.
- *Power.* The ability to exert force rapidly, based on strength and speed.
- *Agility.* The ability to change the body's position quickly and accurately.
- *Balance.* The ability to maintain equilibrium while either moving or stationary.
- *Coordination.* The ability to perform motor tasks accurately and smoothly using body movements and the senses.
- *Reaction time.* The ability to respond quickly to a stimulus.

Skill-related fitness is sport specific and is best developed through practice. For example, playing basketball best develops the speed, coordination, and agility needed to play basketball. Playing a sport can be fun, can help build fitness, and may contribute to other areas of wellness.

COMPONENTS OF AN ACTIVE LIFESTYLE

Despite the many benefits of an active lifestyle, levels of physical activity and exercise remain low for all populations of Americans. In 2018, the Centers for Disease Control and Prevention (CDC) reported the following statistics about the proportion of adult Americans who meet the CDC recommendations for aerobic and muscle-strengthening exercise:

- Over 23% of U.S. adults met both aerobic and muscle-strengthening guidelines, compared with 16% in 2006. More people living in metropolitan areas complied with the guidelines than people living in less populated areas.

> **TERMS**
>
> **muscular endurance** The ability of a muscle or group of muscles to remain contracted or to contract repeatedly for a long period of time.
>
> **flexibility** The joints' ability to move through their full range of motion.
>
> **body composition** The proportion of fat and fat-free mass (muscle, bone, and water) in the body.
>
> **fat-free mass** The nonfat components of the human body, consisting of skeletal muscle, bone, and water.
>
> **skill-related fitness** Physical abilities that contribute to performance in a sport or activity, including speed, power, agility, balance, coordination, and reaction time.

- Over 53% of adults met the aerobics recommendation, but only 28% met the muscle-strengthening guidelines.

- People with higher levels of education were more active than people with lower educational attainment, younger people were more active than older people, and men were more active than women.

- Other studies found that 12% of Americans report exercising vigorously for more than 20 minutes, three times per week. However, electronic measurements of people involved in normal daily activity showed that the actual proportion is closer to 3%.

Most surveys show large gaps in exercise habits of Americans based on ethnicity, socioeconomic status, and education level. Regardless of statistics, however, evidence is growing that becoming more physically active may be the single most important lifestyle change for promoting health and well-being.

Levels of Physical Activity

Physical activity is any body movement carried out by the skeletal muscles that requires energy. Different types of physical activity can be arranged on a continuum based on the amount of energy they require. Quick, easy movements such as standing up or walking down a hallway require little energy or effort. More intense, sustained activities such as cycling five miles or running in a race require considerably more.

Exercise refers to a subset of physical activity—planned, structured, repetitive movement of the body intended specifically to improve or maintain physical fitness. To develop fitness, a person must perform enough physical activity to stress the body and cause long-term physiological changes.

Moderate-intensity physical activity is essential to health and confers wide-ranging health benefits, but more intense exercise is necessary to improve physical fitness. This important distinction between physical activity and exercise is a key concept in understanding the guidelines discussed in this chapter.

Increasing Physical Activity and Exercise

In 2011, the American College of Sports Medicine (ACSM) released the newest version of its exercise guidelines for healthy adults, which were largely based on the landmark 2008 report from the U.S. Department of Health and Human Services, *Physical Activity Guidelines for Americans.* These reports stress the importance of regular physical activity for health, wellness, and the prevention of chronic diseases and premature death.

The current guidelines include the following key recommendations for adults:

- For substantial health benefits, adults should do at least 150 minutes (2.5 hours) a week of moderate-intensity exercise, or 75 minutes (1 hour and 15 minutes) a week of vigorous-intensity aerobic exercise or an equivalent combination of moderate- and vigorous-intensity aerobic exercise. Exercise should preferably be spread throughout the week.

- For additional and more extensive health benefits, adults should increase their aerobic exercise to 300 minutes (5 hours) a week of moderate-intensity activity, or 150 minutes (2.5 hours) a week of vigorous-intensity activity, or an equivalent combination of moderate- and vigorous-intensity activity. Adults can enjoy additional health benefits by engaging in physical activity beyond this amount.

- Adults should also do muscle-strengthening exercises that are moderate or high intensity and involve all major muscle groups on two or more days a week; these activities provide additional health benefits.

- Everyone should avoid inactivity. Adults, teenagers, and children should spend less time in front of a television or computer screen because it decreases metabolic health and contributes to a sedentary lifestyle and increases the risk of obesity.

The reports state that physical activity benefits people of all ages and of all racial and ethnic groups, including people with disabilities. The benefits of activity outweigh the dangers.

These levels of exercise promote health and wellness by lowering the risk of high blood pressure, stroke, heart disease, type 2 diabetes, colon cancer, and osteoporosis and by reducing feelings of mild to moderate depression and anxiety. What's the difference between moderate- and vigorous-intensity physical activity? *2008 Physical Activity Guidelines for Americans* defines moderate-intensity exercise as activity that causes a noticeable increase in heart rate, such as brisk walking. Vigorous-intensity exercise is activity that causes rapid breathing and a substantial increase in heart rate, such as jogging. Figure 14.4 shows examples of moderate activities. Brisk walking, dancing, swimming, cycling, and yard work can all help you meet the physical activity recommendations. You can burn the same

TERMS

physical activity Any body movement carried out by the skeletal muscles that requires energy.

exercise Planned, structured, repetitive movement of the body intended to improve or maintain physical fitness.

Ask Yourself

QUESTIONS FOR CRITICAL THINKING AND REFLECTION

When you think about exercise, do you think of only one or two of the five components of health-related fitness, such as muscular strength or body composition? If so, where do you think your ideas come from? What role do the media play in shaping your ideas about fitness?

Common Activities	Duration (min.)	
Washing and waxing a car	45–60	**Less Vigorous, More Time**
Washing windows or floors	45–60	
Gardening	30–45	
Wheeling self in wheelchair	30–40	
Pushing a stroller 1½ miles	30	
Raking leaves	30	
Walking 2 miles	30 (15 min/mile)	
Shoveling snow	15	
Stairwalking	15	

Sporting Activities		
Playing volleyball	45–60	
Playing touch football	45	
Walking 1¾ miles	35 (20 min/mile)	
Basketball (shooting baskets)	30	
Bicycling 5 miles	30	
Dancing fast (social)	30	
Water aerobics	30	
Swimming laps	20	
Basketball (playing game)	15–20	
Bicycling 4 miles	15	**More Vigorous, Less Time**
Jumping rope	15	
Running 1½ miles	15 (10 min/mile)	

FIGURE 14.4   Examples of moderate amounts of physical activity.

NOTE: Each example uses about 150 calories.

SOURCE: National Heart, Lung, and Blood Institute. n.d. *Guide to Physical Activity* (https://www.nhlbi.nih.gov/health/educational/lose_wt/phy_act.htm).

number of calories by doing a moderate-intensity exercise for a longer time or higher-intensity activity for a shorter time. For more examples of moderate and vigorous activities, see Table 14.1. Table 14.2 summarizes the physical activity recommendations for promoting general health, fitness, and weight management.

The daily total of physical activity can be accumulated in multiple bouts of 10 or more minutes—for example, two 10-minute bike rides to and from class and a brisk 10-minute walk to the store. In this lifestyle approach to physical activity, people can choose activities they find enjoyable and that fit into their daily routine. Everyday tasks at school, work, and home can be structured to contribute to the daily activity total (see the box "Making Time for Physical Activity"). If all sedentary Americans were to increase their lifestyle exercise to 150 minutes per week, the benefit to public health and individual well-being would be enormous.

Managing Weight with Physical Activity   Because over two-thirds of Americans are overweight, the U.S. Department of Health and Human Services also published physical activity guidelines focusing on weight management. These guidelines recognize that to prevent weight gain, lose weight, or maintain weight loss, 150 minutes per week of exercise may not be enough. Instead they recommend up to 90 minutes of exercise per day.

Exercising to Improve Physical Fitness   As mentioned earlier, moderate-intensity exercise confers significant health and wellness benefits, especially for those who are sedentary and become moderately active. However, people can obtain even greater health and wellness benefits by increasing the duration and intensity of exercise. With increased activity, they will see more improvements in quality of life and greater reductions in disease and mortality risk.

More vigorous activity—as in a structured, systematic exercise program—is also needed to improve physical fitness; moderate exercise alone is not enough. Physical fitness requires more intense movement that poses a substantially greater challenge to the body.

Reducing Sedentary Time

Regardless of whether we meet physical activity goals, too much sedentary time—sitting too much—is detrimental to health. Sedentary time is associated with increased risk of disease and death independent of activity level. The risk of negative outcomes from sedentary time was lower among people with higher levels of exercise.

Table 14.1	Examples of Moderate- and Vigorous-Intensity Exercise
MODERATE-INTENSITY PHYSICAL ACTIVITY (moderate effort, noticeable increase in heart rate)	**VIGOROUS-INTENSITY PHYSICAL ACTIVITY** (large effort, significant increase in heart rate and breathing)
Speedwalking or moderate bicycling	Hiking
	Jogging, running, or sprinting
Raking leaves, doing yardwork	Indoor cycling (e.g., spinning)
Vacuuming, household cleaning	Surfing
Doubles tennis	Singles tennis
Active play, running after a toddler, dancing	Soccer, basketball, flag football
Light manual labor, home repairs and improvements	Intense manual labor, shoveling snow/dirt
Load-bearing activities involving less than 45 pounds	Load-bearing activities involving 45 pounds or more

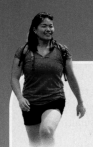

"Too little time" is a common excuse for not being physically active. Learning to manage your time successfully is crucial if you are to maintain a wellness lifestyle. Begin by keeping a record of how you spend your time. List each type of activity and the total time you engaged in it—for example, sleeping, 7 hours; eating, 1.5 hours; studying, 3 hours; and so on. Prioritize your activities according to how important they are to you, from essential to somewhat important to not important.

Change your daily schedule by subtracting time from other activities to make time for physical activity. Look carefully at your leisure-time activities and your methods of transportation—these are areas where it is easy to build in physical activity. For example, you may reduce the total time you spend playing computer games to make time for an after-dinner bike ride or a walk with a friend. You may watch 10 fewer minutes of television in the morning to change your 5-minute drive to class into a 15-minute walk.

Here are just a few ways to incorporate more physical activity into your daily routine:

- Take the stairs instead of the elevator or escalator.

- Walk to the mailbox, post office, store, bank, or library.

- Do at least one chore every day that requires physical activity: Wash the windows or your car, clean your room or house, mow the lawn, or rake the leaves.

- Take study or work breaks to avoid sitting for over 30 minutes at a time. Get up and walk around the library, your office, or your home or dorm; go up and down a flight of stairs.

- When you take public transportation, get off one stop early and walk to your destination.

- Take the dog for a walk every day.

- If weather or neighborhood safety rule out walking outside, look for alternative locations—an indoor track, an enclosed shopping mall, or even a long hallway.

- Seize every opportunity to get up and walk around. Move more and sit less.

How does excessive sedentary time affect health? Although not understood, sedentary time is associated with poor metabolic functioning, including unhealthy levels of blood glucose, insulin, and blood fats, and a large waist circumference. A study that looked at the impact of increased sedentary time in moderately active individuals found that sitting for over 30 or 60 minutes at a time resulted in elevated glucose and insulin levels. Sedentary time also

Table 14.2	Physical Activity and Exercise Recommendations for Promoting General Health, Fitness, and Weight Management
GOAL	**RECOMMENDATION**
General health	Perform moderate-intensity aerobic exercise for at least 150 minutes per week or 75 minutes of vigorous-intensity exercise per week. Also, be more active in your daily life: Walk instead of driving, take the stairs instead of the elevator, and watch less television.
Increased health and fitness benefits	Exercise at a moderate intensity for 300 minutes per week or at a vigorous intensity for 150 minutes per week.
Achieve or maintain weight loss	Exercise at a moderate intensity for 60–90 minutes per day on most days of the week.
Muscle strength and endurance	Perform one or more sets of resistance exercises that work the major muscle groups for 8–12 repetitions (10–15 reps with a lighter weight for older adults) on 2 or 3 nonconsecutive days per week. Examples include weight training and exercises that use body weight as resistance (such as core-stabilizing exercises, pull-ups, push-ups, lunges, and squats).
Flexibility	Perform range-of-motion (stretching) exercises at least 2 days per week. Hold each stretch for 10–30 seconds.
Neuromuscular training	Older people should do balance training 2 or 3 days per week. Examples include yoga, tai chi, and balance exercises (standing on one foot, step-ups, and walking lunges). These exercises are also beneficial for young and middle-aged adults.

SOURCES: Garber, C. E., et al. 2011. Quantity and quality of exercise for developing and maintaining cardiorespiratory, musculoskeletal, and neuromotor fitness in apparently healthy adults: Guidance for prescribing exercise. *Medicine & Science in Sports & Exercise* 43(7): 1334–1359; American Heart Association. 2015. *American Heart Association Recommendations for Physical Activity in Adults and Kids* (https://www.heart.org/en/healthy-living/fitness /fitness-basics/aha-recs-for-physical-activity-in-adults).

Regular exercise provides huge wellness benefits, but it does not cancel out all the negative effects of too much sitting during the day. Advances in technology promote sedentary behavior: We can now work or study at a desk, watch TV or play video games in our leisure time, order take-out and delivery for meals, and shop and bank online. To avoid the negative health effects of too little daily activity, try some of the following strategies:

• Stand up and/or walk when you are at work or making personal phone calls.

• Take the stairs whenever and wherever you can; walk up and down escalators instead of riding them.

• At work, walk to a coworker's desk rather than emailing or calling, take the long route to the restroom, and take a walk break whenever you take a coffee or snack break. Drink plenty of water so that you must take frequent restroom breaks.

• Set reminders to get up and move: Use commercial breaks while watching TV to remind yourself to move or stretch. At work or while using a digital device, set the clock function on your computer or phone to remind you to get up at least every hour. Moving every 20 or 30 minutes is even better.

• Engage in active chores and leisure activities.

• Track your sedentary time to get a baseline, and then continue monitoring to note any improvements. You can also use a step counter to track your general activity level and movement patterns.

Ask Yourself

QUESTIONS FOR CRITICAL THINKING AND REFLECTION

Does your current lifestyle include enough exercise—150 minutes of moderate-intensity activity a week—to support health and wellness? Do you go beyond this level to include enough vigorous activity and exercise to build physical fitness? What changes could you make in your lifestyle to start developing physical fitness?

affects blood fats and inflammation. All these factors can contribute to the development of type 2 diabetes, metabolic syndrome, heart disease, and cancer.

What does this mean for an individual? Studies have found that average American adults spend more than half their waking day in sedentary activities, such as using a computer, studying, or watching television. Fortunately, evidence so far suggests that frequent breaks from sedentary time—2 minutes every 20 or 30 minutes, for example—protect against some impacts of sedentary time. So, take frequent breaks when you are engaged in sedentary activities, whether at work or school or during leisure time. Try the strategies suggested in the box "Move More, Sit Less" and invent your own.

DESIGNING YOUR EXERCISE PROGRAM

The best exercise program has two primary characteristics: It promotes your health and fun for you to do. Exercise can provide some of the most pleasurable moments of your day, once you make it a habit. A little thought and planning will help you achieve these goals.

Figure 14.5 shows a physical activity pyramid. The wide section at the bottom of the pyramid shows activities you should engage in more frequently throughout the day: walking, climbing stairs, doing yard work, and sweeping the floor. From there, work up to meeting the goal of 150 minutes of moderate-intensity exercise per week. Be active whenever you can. If weight management is a concern for you, begin by achieving the goal of 150 minutes per week and then gradually increase your activity level to 300 minutes per week while reducing caloric intake, especially from added sugars and other empty calories (see Chapter 13).

For even greater benefits, look to the next two levels of the pyramid, which illustrate parts of a formal exercise program. They take up less of your time than the activities on the lower two levels of the pyramid, but they will develop all the health-related components of physical fitness. Regardless of your pattern of physical activity and formal exercise, you should limit your overall sedentary time (the tip of the pyramid) and take frequent active breaks.

New research shows that high-intensity interval training—repetitions of high-intensity exercise followed by rest—builds fitness rapidly in less time than traditional aerobic training (see the box "Interval Training: Pros and Cons"). The remaining sections of this chapter will show you how to develop a personalized exercise program. For a summary of the health and fitness benefits of different levels of physical activity, see Figure 14.6.

First Steps

Are you thinking about starting a formal exercise program? A little planning can help make it a success.

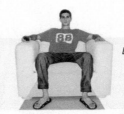
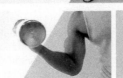

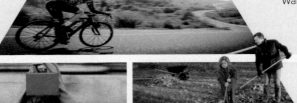

Sedentary Activities
Watching television, surfing the internet, talking on the telephone

Limit your sedentary activities

Strength Training
2–3 nonconsecutive days per week (all major muscle groups)
Biceps curls, push-ups, abdominal curls, bench press, calf raises

Flexibility Training
At least 2–3 days per week, ideally 5–7 days per week (all major joints)
Calf stretch, side lunge, step stretch, hurdler stretch

Cardiorespiratory Endurance Exercise
3–5 days per week (20–60 minutes)

Walking, jogging, bicycling, swimming, aerobic dancing, in-line skating, cross-country skiing, dancing, basketball

Moderate-Intensity Physical Activity
150 minutes per week; for weight loss or prevention of weight regain 60–90 minutes per day

Walking to the store or bank, climbing stairs, working in your yard, walking your dog, cleaning your room

FIGURE 14.5 **Physical activity pyramid.** Make activities at the base of the pyramid part of your everyday life; limit the amount of time you spend in the sedentary activities listed at the top. George Doyle/Stockbyte/Getty Images; Ryan McVay/Photodisc/Getty Images; Seth Foley/McGraw Hill; Rattanasak Khuentana/Shutterstock; Doug Menuez/Forrester Images/Photodisc/Getty Images; UpperCut Images/Alamy Stock Photo

	Lifestyle physical activity	**Moderate exercise program**	**Vigorous exercise program**
Description	Moderate physical activity (150 minutes per week; muscle-strengthening exercises 2 or more days per week)	Cardiorespiratory endurance exercise (20–60 minutes, 3–5 days per week); strength training (2–3 nonconsecutive days per week); and stretching exercises (2 or more days per week)	Cardiorespiratory endurance exercise (20–60 minutes, 3–5 days per week); interval training; strength training (3–4 nonconsecutive days per week); and stretching exercises (5–7 days per week)
Sample activities or program	*One of the following:* • Walking to and from work, 15 minutes each way • Cycling to and from class, 10 minutes each way • Yard work for 30 minutes • Dancing (fast) for 30 minutes • Playing basketball for 20 minutes	• Jogging for 30 minutes, 3 days per week • Weight training, 1 set of 8 exercises, 2 days per week • Stretching exercises, 3 days per week	• Running for 45 minutes, 3 days per week • Intervals: running 400 m at high effort, 4 sets, 2 days per week • Weight training, 3 sets of 10 exercises, 3 days per week • Stretching exercises, 6 days per week
Health and fitness benefits	Better blood cholesterol levels, reduced body fat, better control of blood pressure, improved metabolic health, and enhanced glucose metabolism; improved quality of life; reduced risk of some chronic diseases. Greater amounts of activity can help prevent weight gain and promote weight loss.	All the benefits of lifestyle physical activity, plus improved physical fitness (increased cardiorespiratory endurance, muscular strength and endurance, and flexibility) and even greater improvements in health and quality of life and reductions in chronic disease risk.	All the benefits of lifestyle physical activity and a moderate exercise program, with greater increases in fitness and somewhat greater reductions in chronic disease risk. Participating in a vigorous exercise program may increase risk of injury and overtraining.

FIGURE 14.6 **Health and fitness benefits of different amounts of physical activity and exercise.** Rubberball Productions/Photodisc/Getty Images; Tyler Stableford/Brand X Pictures/SuperStock; Thinkstock Images/Stockbyte/Getty Images

Few exercise techniques are more effective at improving fitness rapidly than *high-intensity interval training (HIIT)*—a series of very brief, high-intensity exercise sessions interspersed with short rest periods or low-intensity exercise. The four components of interval training are distance, repetition, intensity, and rest, defined as follows:

- *Distance* refers to either the distance or the time of the exercise interval.

- *Repetition* is the number of times the exercise is repeated.

- *Intensity* is the speed at which the exercise is performed.

- *Rest* is the time spent recovering between exercises.

Canadian researchers found that six sessions of high-intensity interval training (HIIT) on a stationary bike increased muscle oxidative capacity by almost 50%, muscle glycogen by 20%, and cycle endurance capacity by 100%. The subjects made these amazing improvements by exercising only 15 minutes in two weeks. Each workout consisted of 4–7 repetitions of high-intensity exercise (each repetition consisted of 30 seconds at near-maximum effort) on a stationary bike. Follow-up studies showed that practicing HIIT three times per week for six weeks improved endurance and aerobic capacity just as well as training five times per week for 60 minutes for six weeks. These studies (and more than 60 others) showed the value of high-intensity training for building aerobic capacity and endurance.

You can use interval training in your favorite aerobic exercises. In fact, the type of exercise you select is not important as long as you exercise at a high intensity. HIIT training can even be used to help develop sports skills. For example, a runner might do 4–7 repetitions of 200-meter sprints at near-maximum effort. A tennis player might practice volleys against a wall as fast as possible for 4–8 repetitions lasting 30 seconds

each. A swimmer might swim 4–8 repetitions of 50 meters at 100% effort. It is important to rest 3–5 minutes between repetitions, regardless of the type of exercise being performed.

If you add HIIT to your exercise program, do not practice interval training more than 3 days per week. Intervals are exhausting and easily lead to injury. Let your body tell you how many days you can tolerate. If you become overly tired after doing interval training 3 days per week, cut back to 2 days. If you feel good, try increasing the intensity or number of intervals (but not the number of days per week) and see what happens. As with any kind of exercise program, begin HIIT training slowly and progress conservatively. Although the Canadian studies showed that HIIT training produced substantial fitness improvements by themselves, it is best to integrate HIIT into a total exercise program.

High-intensity interval training appears to be safe and effective in the short term, but there are concerns about the long-term safety and effectiveness of this type of training, so consider the following issues:

- Maximal-intensity training could be dangerous for some people. A physician might be reluctant to give certain patients the green light for this type of exercise.

- Always warm up with several minutes of low-intensity exercise before practicing HIIT. Maximal-intensity exercise without a warm-up can cause cardiac arrhythmias (abnormal heart rhythms) even in healthy people.

- High-intensity interval training might trigger overuse injuries in unfit people. For this reason, it is essential to start gradually, especially for someone at a low level of fitness. Exercise at submaximal intensities for at least four to six weeks before starting HIIT. Cut back on interval training or rest if you feel overly fatigued or develop overly sore joints or muscles.

Medical Clearance   Previously inactive men over 40 and women over 50 should get a medical examination before beginning an exercise program. Diabetes, asthma, heart disease, and extreme obesity are conditions that may call for a modified program. If you have an increased risk of heart disease because of smoking, high blood pressure, or obesity, get a physical checkup, including an **electrocardiogram (ECG or EKG),** before beginning an exercise program.

Basic Principles of Physical Training   To put together an effective exercise program, you should first understand the basic principles of physical training.

SPECIFICITY   To develop a fitness component, you must perform exercises that are specifically designed for that component. This is the principle of **specificity.** Weight training, for example, develops muscular strength but is less effective for developing flexibility or cardiorespiratory endurance. Specificity also applies to the skill-related fitness components and to

the different parts of the body. A well-rounded exercise program includes exercises geared to each component of fitness, to different parts of the body, and to specific activities or sports.

PROGRESSIVE OVERLOAD   Your body adapts to the demands of exercise by improving its functioning. When the amount of exercise, or overload, is increased progressively, fitness continues to improve. This training principle is called **progressive overload.** Too little exercise has no effect on

---

electrocardiogram (ECG or EKG)   A recording **TERMS** of the changes in electrical activity of the heart.

specificity   The training principle that the body adapts to the particular type and amount of stress placed on it.

progressive overload   The training principle that placing increasing amounts of stress (in the form of exercise) on the body causes adaptations that improve fitness.

Ask Yourself

QUESTIONS FOR CRITICAL THINKING AND REFLECTION

Which benefits of exercise are most important and why? For example, is there a history of heart disease or diabetes in your family? Have you thought about how regular exercise could reduce your risks for specific diseases?

fitness; too much may cause injury. The appropriate amount depends on your current level of fitness, your genetic capacity to adapt to exercise, your fitness goals, and the fitness components being developed.

The overload needed to maintain or improve a particular level of fitness is determined in six dimensions, represented by the acronym FITT-VP, which stands for frequency, intensity, time, type, volume, and progression.

Frequency—how often a person exercises

Intensity—how hard or how fast a person exercises

Time—how long (duration) a period of exercise lasts

Type—mode of activity

Volume—how much (frequency × intensity × time) a person exercises

Progression—how a program advances over time

• *Frequency.* Optimum exercise frequency, expressed in number of days per week, varies with individual fitness goals. The time required to recover from exercise is important but highly dependent on factors such as training experience, age, and intensity of training. For example, 24 hours of rest between highly intense workouts involving heavy weights or track sprints is not enough recovery time for safe and effective training. Intense workouts need to be spaced out during the week to allow for sufficient recovery time. But, you can exercise every day if your program consists of moderate-intensity walking or cycling.

• *Intensity.* Fitness benefits occur when people exercise harder than their normal level. The appropriate exercise intensity varies with each fitness component. To develop cardiorespiratory endurance, for example, you must raise your heart rate above normal; you might do that by walking, swimming, or cycling faster. To develop muscular strength, you must lift a heavier weight than normal. To develop flexibility, you must stretch muscles beyond their normal length.

• *Time.* Benefits occur when you exercise for an extended period. The greater the intensity of exercise, the less time needed to obtain fitness benefits. High-intensity exercise poses a greater risk of injury than low-intensity exercise, so if you are a nonathletic adult, it's best to first emphasize low- to moderate-intensity activity of longer duration. To build muscular strength, muscular endurance, and flexibility, similar time is advisable, but training for these health components is more commonly organized in terms of a specific number of *repetitions* of a particular exercise.

• *Type.* The type of exercise varies with each fitness component and with your personal fitness goals. The frequency, intensity, and time of the exercise will be different for each type of activity.

• *Volume.* Volume is the product of frequency, intensity, and time (i.e., the FIT of exercise programming). Increasing volume is the best way to improve fitness. Excessive volume, however, can lead to injury and overtraining. Activity trackers can help you gauge and monitor your progress. They can also help quantify your program in total energy expenditure in terms of calories (calories per session, week, month, and/or year) and MET-minutes (exercise intensity in METs times minutes of exercise). A **MET** measures the *metabolic* cost of an exercise. One MET represents the body's resting metabolic rate—that is, the energy or calorie requirement of the body at rest. Exercise intensity is expressed in multiples of resting metabolic rate. For example, an exercise intensity of 2 METs is twice the resting metabolic rate.

• *Progression.* Fitness levels off as the body adapts to exercise training, so you need to gradually increase overload over time to improve fitness. How quickly you adapt to training depends not only on your genes but also on the effort you put into your training program. To avoid injury, progress slowly by increasing the volume of exercise; for example, add 5 minutes to your jogging workout or add 10 pounds for a weight training exercise. Don't increase frequency, intensity, and time all at once. With each increase, make sure you can maintain your program before moving forward.

REST AND RECUPERATION Fitness gains occur following exercise as the body adapts to the stress of training. Adequate rest is as important to this process as training. Overtraining—an imbalance between training and recovery—leads to injury, illness, and excessive fatigue.

REVERSIBILITY The body adjusts to lower levels of physical activity as it adjusts to higher levels—this is the principle of **reversibility.** When you stop exercising, you can lose up to 50% of fitness improvements within two months. Try to exercise consistently, and don't quit if you miss a few workouts. If you must temporarily curtail your training, you can maintain your fitness improvements by keeping the intensity of your workouts constant while reducing their frequency or duration.

INDIVIDUAL DIFFERENCES There are large individual differences among people in their ability to improve fitness, achieve a desirable body composition, and perform and learn sports skills. Studies show that some people on a diet and exercise program improve fitness by 50%, whereas others on the same program improve by only 2–3%. It is more difficult for those whose bodies don't respond as well to exercise to make changes in fitness or body fat levels. More than 800 genes are associated with endurance performance, and 100 of those determine individual differences in exercise capacity. However, regardless of heredity, physical training improves fitness. Elite athletes start out with a genetic advantage. But everyone has the capacity to improve fitness and reap the health benefits of exercise.

Selecting Activities   If you have been inactive, begin by gradually increasing the amount of moderate-intensity exercise in your life (the bottom of the activity pyramid shown in Figure 14.5). Once your body adjusts to your new level of activity, you can choose additional activities for your exercise program.

Be sure the activities you choose contribute to your overall wellness and make sense for you. Are you competitive? If so, try racquetball, basketball, or squash. Do you prefer to exercise alone? Then consider cross-country skiing, hiking, or road running. Have you been sedentary? A walking program may be a good place to start. If you think you may have trouble sticking with an exercise program, find a structured activity that you can do with a friend, a personal trainer, or a group.

Be realistic about the constraints presented by some sports, such as accessibility, expense, and time. For example, if you have to travel for hours to get to a ski area, skiing may not be a good choice for your regular exercise program. And if you've never played tennis, it will probably take some time to reach a reasonable skill level; you may be better off with a program of walking or jogging to get good workouts as you're improving your tennis game.

Cardiorespiratory Endurance Exercise

Exercises that condition your heart and lungs and improve your metabolism should play a central role in your fitness program.

Frequency   The optimal workout schedule for endurance training is 3–5 days per week. Beginners should start with 3 days and work up to 5 days. Training more than 5 days a week often leads to injury for recreational athletes. Although you get health benefits from exercising vigorously only 1 or 2 days per week, you risk injury because your body never gets a chance to adapt fully to regular exercise training.

Intensity   The most misunderstood aspect of conditioning, even among experienced athletes, is exercise intensity. Intensity is the crucial factor in attaining a significant training effect—that is, in increasing the body's cardiorespiratory capacity. A primary purpose of endurance training is to increase **maximal oxygen consumption** ($\dot{V}O_{2max}$).

$\dot{V}O_{2max}$ represents the cells' maximum ability to use oxygen and is considered the best measure of cardiorespiratory capacity. Intensity of training is the crucial factor in improving $\dot{V}O_{2max}$.

One of the easiest ways to determine exactly how intensely you should work involves measuring your heart rate. It is not necessary or desirable to exercise at your maximum heart rate—the fastest heart rate possible before exhaustion sets in—to improve your cardiorespiratory capacity. Beneficial effects occur at lower heart rates with a much lower risk of injury. Your **target heart rate zone** is the range of rates within which you should exercise to obtain cardiorespiratory benefits. To determine the intensity at which you should exercise, see the box "Determine Your Target Heart Rate" and Figure 14.7.

After you begin your fitness program, you may improve quickly because the body adapts readily to new exercises. The rate of improvement may slow after the first month or so. The more fit you become, the harder you will have to work to improve. By monitoring your heart rate, you will always know if you are working hard enough to improve, not hard enough, or too hard. For most people, a fitness program involves attaining an acceptable level of fitness and then maintaining that level. There is no need to keep working indefinitely to improve; doing so only increases the chance of injury. After you have reached the level you want, you can maintain fitness by exercising at the same intensity 3–5 days per week.

If you have been sedentary, start by exercising at the lower end of your target heart rate range (65% of maximum heart rate) for at least 4–6 weeks. Exercising closer to the top of the range can cause fast and significant gains in maximal oxygen consumption, but you may increase your risk of injury and overtraining. You *can* achieve significant health benefits by exercising at the bottom of your target range, so don't feel pressure to exercise at an unnecessarily intense level. If you exercise at a lower intensity, you can increase the duration or frequency of training to obtain as much benefit to your health, as long as you are above the 65% training threshold. For people with a very low initial level of fitness, a lower training intensity of 55–64% of maximum heart rate may be sufficient to achieve improvements in maximal oxygen consumption, especially at the start of an exercise program. Intensities of 70–85% of maximum heart rate are appropriate for average individuals.

As your program progresses and your fitness improves, you will need to jog, cycle, or walk faster in order to reach your target heart rate zone. To monitor your heart rate during exercise, count your pulse while you're still moving or

maximal oxygen consumption ($\dot{V}O_{2max}$)   The **TERMS** body's maximum ability to transport and use oxygen.

target heart rate zone   The range of heart rates that should be reached and maintained during cardiorespiratory endurance exercise to obtain benefits.

TAKE CHARGE
Determine Your Target Heart Rate

One of the best ways to monitor the intensity of cardiorespiratory endurance exercise is to measure your heart rate. It isn't necessary to exercise at your maximum heart rate to improve maximal oxygen consumption. Fitness adaptations occur at lower heart rates with a much lower risk of injury.

According to the American College of Sports Medicine, your target heart rate zone—rates at which you should exercise to experience cardiorespiratory benefits—is between 65% and 90% of your maximum heart rate. To calculate your target heart rate zone, follow these steps:

1. Estimate your maximum heart rate (MHR) by subtracting your age from 220, or have it measured precisely by undergoing an exercise stress test in a doctor's office, hospital, or sports medicine lab. (*Note:* The formula to estimate MHR carries an error of about ±10–15 beats per minute [bpm] and can be very inaccurate for some people, particularly older adults and young children.)

2. Multiply your MHR by 65% and 90% to calculate your target heart rate zone. Very unfit people should use 55% of MHR for their training threshold.

For example, a 19-year-old would calculate her target heart rate zone:

MHR = 220 − 19 = 201
65% training intensity = 0.65 × 201 = 131 bpm
90% training intensity = 0.90 × 201 = 181 bpm

To gain fitness benefits, the young woman in our example would have to exercise at an intensity that raises her heart rate to between 131 and 181 bpm.

An alternative method for calculating target heart rate range uses heart rate reserve, the difference between maximum heart rate and resting heart rate. With this method, target heart rate is equal to resting heart rate plus between 50% (40% for very unfit people) and 85% of heart rate reserve. Although some people (particularly those with very low levels of fitness) will obtain more accurate results using this more complex method, both methods provide reasonable estimates of an appropriate target heart rate zone.

immediately after you stop exercising. Count beats for 15 seconds and then multiply that number by 4 to see if your heart rate is in your target zone. Table 14.3 shows target heart rate ranges and 15-second counts based on the maximum heart rate formula.

Heart rate monitors are useful if close tracking of heart rate is important in your program. They offer several advantages:

- They are accurate, and they reduce the risk of mistakes when checking your own pulse.

- They are easy to use, although a sophisticated, multifunction monitor may take some time to master.

- They do the monitoring for you, so you don't have to worry about checking your own pulse.

- Heart rate can be integrated into workout information provided by smartphone apps such as Cyclemeter, Strava, Spotify, and Garmin Connect.

- The Apple Watch 5 can perform a one-lead electrocardiogram during recovery from exercise

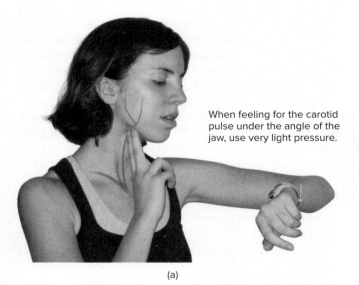

When feeling for the carotid pulse under the angle of the jaw, use very light pressure.

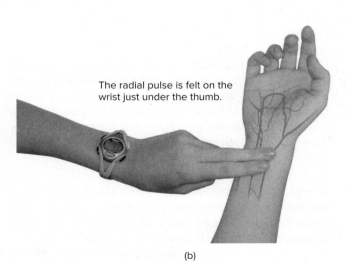

The radial pulse is felt on the wrist just under the thumb.

(a)

(b)

FIGURE 14.7   Checking your pulse. The pulse can be taken at the carotid artery in the neck (a) or at the radial artery in the wrist (b).
Courtesy of Robin Mouat

Table 14.3	Target Heart Rate Range and 15-Second Counts	
AGE (YEARS)	TARGET HEART RATE RANGE (bpm)*	15-SECOND COUNT (beats)
20–24	127–180	32–45
25–29	124–176	31–44
30–34	121–171	30–43
35–39	118–167	30–42
40–44	114–162	29–41
45–49	111–158	28–40
50–54	108–153	27–38
55–59	105–149	26–37
60–64	101–144	25–36
65+	97–140	24–35

*Target heart rates lower than those shown here are appropriate for individuals with a very low initial level of fitness. Ranges are based on the following formula: target heart rate = 0.65 to 0.90 of maximum heart rate, assuming maximum heart rate = 220 − age.

Table 14.4	Approximate MET and Caloric Costs of Selected Activities for a 154-Pound Person	
ACTIVITY	METS	CALORIC EXPENDITURE (kilocalories/min)
Rest	1	1.2
Light housework	2–4	2.4–4.8
Bowling	2–4	2.5–5
Walking	2–7	2.5–8.5
Archery	3–4	3.7–5
Dancing	3–7	3.7–8.5
Hiking	3–7	3.7–8.5
Horseback riding	3–8	3.7–10
Cycling	3–8	3.7–10
Basketball (recreational)	3–9	3.7–11
Swimming	4–8	5–10
Tennis	4–9	5–11
Fishing (fly, stream)	5–6	6–7.5
In-line skating	5–8	6–10
Skiing (downhill)	5–8	6–10
Rock climbing	5–10	6–12
Scuba diving	5–10	6–12
Skiing (cross-country)	6–12	7.5–15
Jogging	8–12	10–15

NOTE: Intensity varies greatly with effort, skill, and motivation.

SOURCE: Adapted from American College of Sports Medicine. 2013. *ACSM's Guidelines for Exercise Testing and Prescription*, 9th ed. Philadelphia, PA: Wolters Kluwer/Lippincott Williams & Wilkins Health.

When shopping for a heart rate monitor, do your homework. Quality, reliability, and warranties vary. Ask personal trainers for recommendations, and look for product reviews in consumer magazines or online.

Another way scientists describe fitness is in terms of the capacity to increase metabolism (energy usage level) above rest. METs are used to describe exercise intensities for occupational activities and exercise programs. Exercise intensities of less than 3–4 METs are considered low. Household chores and most industrial jobs fall into this category. Exercise at these intensities does not improve fitness for most people, but it will improve fitness for people with low physical capacities. Activities that increase metabolism by 6–8 METs are classified as moderate-intensity exercises and are suitable for most people beginning an exercise program. Vigorous exercise increases metabolic rate by over 10 METs. Fast running or cycling, as well as intense play in sports like racquetball, can place people in this category. Table 14.4 lists the MET ratings for various activities.

METs are only an approximation of exercise intensity. Skill, body weight, body fat, and environment affect the accuracy of METs. As a practical matter, however, these limitations can be disregarded. METs are a good way to express exercise intensity because this system is easy for people to remember and apply.

Time (Duration) A total time of 20–60 minutes per workout is recommended for cardiorespiratory endurance training. Exercise can be done in a single session or several sessions lasting 10 or more minutes. The total duration of exercise depends on its intensity. To improve cardiorespiratory endurance during a moderate-intensity activity such as walking or slow swimming, exercise for 45–60 minutes. For high-intensity exercise performed at the top of your target heart rate zone, a duration of 20 minutes is suffi-

cient. Start with less vigorous activities and gradually increase intensity.

Type The best exercises for developing cardiorespiratory endurance stress much of the body's muscle mass for a prolonged period. These include walking, jogging, running, swimming, bicycling, and aerobic dance. Many popular sports and recreational activities, such as racquetball, tennis, basketball, and soccer, are also good if the skill level and intensity of the game are sufficient to provide a vigorous workout.

Volume of Activity Exercise volume for cardiorespiratory endurance can be estimated using several measures; each of the following is approximately equivalent:

- 150 minutes per week of moderate-intensity activity
- Calories: 1000 calories per week in moderate-intensity exercise
- MET-minutes: 500 to 1000 MET-min per week
- Steps: 5400 to 7900 steps or more per day; for accuracy, combine step counts with recommended time (duration) of exercise.

Progression The rate of progression depends on your goals, fitness, health, age, and adaptation to training. For general health, most benefits occur at moderate training intensities for about 150 minutes per week. Higher levels of fitness require more intense training programs. Increasing intensity is most important for increasing fitness, while increasing time and frequency can promote a healthy body composition by increasing overall energy expenditure with moderate-intensity activity.

Highly motivated people will put up with the high levels of discomfort that accompany intense training programs. Less motivated people often stop exercising if the program is too intense or uncomfortable. Fitness determines your capacity to improve. Untrained people can make rapid gains, whereas highly fit people improve more slowly. Genetics also determine how fast you will improve. People vary in their response to identical training programs. Finally, health and age influence your adaptability and capacity for training progression.

The Warm-Up and Cool-Down Warm up before exercise and cool down afterward. Warming up enhances your performance and decreases your chances of injury. Your muscles work better when their temperature is elevated slightly above resting level. Warming up helps your body progress gradually from rest to exercise. Blood needs to be redirected to active muscles, and your heart needs time to adapt to the increased demands of exercise. A warm-up bathes joints with lubricating fluid, which helps protect joint surfaces from wear and tear.

A warm-up session should include low-intensity movements similar to those in the activity that will follow. For example, hit forehands and backhands before a tennis game or jog slowly for 400 meters before progressing to an 8-minute mile. A warm-up might include low-intensity whole-body exercises such as walking lunges, jumping jacks, or arm circles. Don't do static stretching exercises during the warm-up because they can temporarily decrease muscle strength and power. Do static stretching at the end of your workout, when your body temperature is elevated and you are no longer concerned with muscle performance. Stretching is discussed in detail later in this chapter.

Cooling down after exercise is important to restore the body's circulation to its normal resting condition. When you are at rest, a relatively small percentage of your total blood volume is directed to muscles, but during exercise, as much as 90% of the heart's output is directed to them. During recovery from exercise, continuing to exercise at a low level is im-

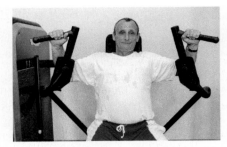

Pavel L Photo and Video/Shutterstock

portant to provide a smooth transition to the resting state. Cooling down helps regulate the return of blood to your heart. After exercising, avoid taking a hot shower until you have cooled down.

Exercises for Muscular Strength and Endurance

Any program designed to promote health should include exercises that develop muscular strength and endurance. Your ability to maintain correct posture and move efficiently depends in part on muscle fitness. Strengthening exercises also increase muscle tone, which improves the body's appearance.

Types of Strength-Training Exercises Muscular strength and endurance can be developed in many ways, from weight training to calisthenics. Common exercises such as curl-ups, push-ups, pull-ups, and unweighted squats maintain the muscular strength of most people if they practice them several times a week. To condition and tone your whole body, choose exercises that work the major muscles of the shoulders, chest, back, arms, abdomen, and legs.

To increase muscular strength and endurance, you must do **resistance exercise**—exercises in which your muscles must exert force against significant resistance. Resistance can be provided by weights, exercise machines, your own body weight, or even objects such as rocks.

Isometric (static) exercises involve applying force without movement, such as when you contract your abdominal muscles. This type of exercise is valuable for toning and strengthening muscles. Isometrics can be practiced anywhere and do not require any equipment. For maximum strength gains, hold an isometric contraction maximally for 6 seconds, and do 3–10 repetitions. Don't hold your breath: Doing so can restrict blood flow to your heart and brain. Within a few weeks, you will notice the effect of this exercise. Isometrics are particularly useful when recovering from an injury.

Isotonic (dynamic) exercises involve applying force with movement, as in weight training exercises such as the bench press. These types of exercises are the most popular for increasing muscle strength and seem to be most valuable for developing strength that can be transferred to other forms of physical activity. They include exercises using barbells, dumbbells, kettlebells, weight machines, and body weight (as in push-ups or pull-ups).

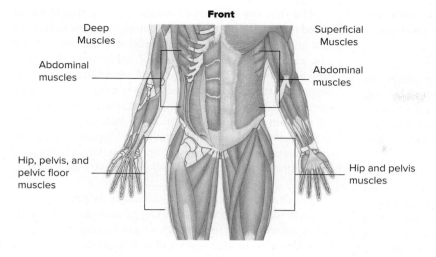

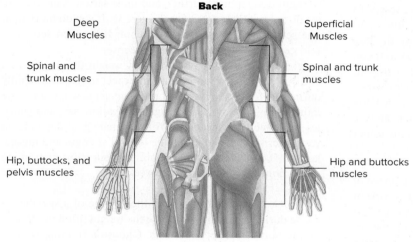

FIGURE 14.8 **Major core muscles.**

SOURCE: Fahey, T. D., P. M. Insel, C. E. Insel, and W. T. Roth. 2017. *Fit and Well: Core Concepts and Labs in Physical Fitness and Wellness,* 13th ed. New York: McGraw Hill. Copyright © 2019 The McGraw Hill Companies, Inc.

Core Training The core muscles include those in the abdomen, pelvic floor, sides of the trunk, back, buttocks, hips, and pelvis (Figure 14.8). They stabilize the midsection when you sit, stand, reach, walk, jump, twist, squat, throw, or bend. During any dynamic movement, the core muscles and active muscles work together. Some shorten to cause movement, whereas others contract and hold to provide stability, lengthen to brake the movement, or send signals to the brain about the movements and positions of the muscles, joints, and bones. When specific core muscles are weak or tired, the nervous system steps in and uses other muscles. This substitution causes abnormal stress on the joints, decreases power, and increases the risk of injury.

For over 100 years, traditional core training included dynamic exercises such as sit-ups, back extensions, and twists. However, since 2000, scientists have confirmed that spinal stability and stiffness are more important for health and performance than core movement strength. Isometric core exercises like side bridges build core stiffness, which strengthens core muscles and improves their endurance, reduces low back pain, and boosts sports performance. Greater core stiffness transfers strength and speed to the limbs, increases the load-bearing capacity of the spine, and protects the internal organs during sports movements. Studies directed by Stuart McGill from the University of Waterloo in Canada showed that isometric exercises for the core resulted in greater core stiffness than did whole-body dynamic exercises that activated core muscles. His studies on core stiffness are changing the way we train for sports.

The best exercises for low-back health are whole-body exercises that force the core muscles to stabilize the spine in many different directions. Exercises that focus on the core muscles include the lunge, side bridges, stir-the-pot, and bird dogs. These exercises are generally safe for beginning exercisers and, with physician approval, people with back pain.

Sex Differences in Muscular Strength
Within a given genetic population, men are generally stronger than women because their bodies are typically larger overall and a larger proportion of their total body mass is made up of muscle. But when strength is expressed per unit of muscle tissue, men are only 1–2% stronger than women in the upper body and about equal to women in the lower body. Individual muscle cells are larger in men, but the functioning of the cells is the same in both sexes.

Three factors that help explain the strength disparities between men and women are testosterone levels, skeletal size, and nerve-conduction velocity. Testosterone promotes the growth of muscle tissue in both males and females, but testosterone levels are about 6–10 times higher in men than in women, so men develop larger muscles. Also, men are usually bigger than women, which gives them more leverage. Nerve-conduction velocity in the brain and central nervous system is about 4% faster in men than women, which provides a slight advantage in muscle activation speed.

Most women will not develop large muscles from strength training. Resistance exercise helps women reduce their overall body fat levels and reduce fat in the midsection. Losing muscle over time is a much greater health concern for women than small gains in muscle weight in response to strength training, especially because any gains in muscle weight are typically more than balanced with loss of fat weight. Men and women lose muscle mass and power as they age, but because men start out with more muscle when they are young and don't lose power as quickly as women, older women often have greater impairment of muscle function than older men. This disparity may partially explain the higher incidence of life-threatening falls in older women.

Choosing Equipment Many people prefer weight machines to free-weights because they are safe, convenient, and easy to use. You set the resistance, sit down at the machine, and work. Free-weights require more care, balance, and coordination to use, but they strengthen your body in ways that are more adaptable to real life.

Choosing Exercises A complete weight training program works all the major muscle groups: neck, upper back, shoulders, arms, chest, core, thighs, buttocks, and calves. Different exercises work different muscles, so it usually takes about 8–10 exercises to get a complete workout for general fitness. For example, you can do bench presses to develop the chest, shoulders, and upper arms; pull-ups to work the biceps and upper back; squats to develop the legs and buttocks; toe raises to work the calves; and so on. If you are also training for a particular sport, include exercises to strengthen the muscles important for optimal performance and those that are most likely to be injured. Whole-body functional exercises, such as **kettlebell** swings and snatches, work many large muscle groups in the lower and upper body.

Frequency For general fitness, the American College of Sports Medicine (ACSM) recommends a strength workout frequency of at least 2 nonconsecutive days per week. This schedule allows your muscles one or more days of rest between workouts to avoid soreness and injury. If you enjoy weight training and would like to train more often, try working different muscle groups on alternate days.

Intensity and Time The amount of weight (resistance) you lift in weight training exercises is equivalent to intensity in cardiorespiratory endurance training, and the number of repetitions of each exercise is equivalent to time. To improve fitness, you must do enough repetitions of each exercise to temporarily fatigue your muscles. The number of repetitions needed to cause fatigue depends on the resistance: The heavier the weight, the fewer repetitions to reach fatigue. A heavy weight and a low number of repetitions (1–5) build strength, whereas a light weight and a high number of repetitions (10–25) build endurance. For a general fitness program to build both strength and endurance, try to do 8–12 repetitions of each exercise. For people over 50 years of age, 10–15 repetitions of each exercise using a lighter weight is recommended.

kettlebell A large iron ball with a handle attached **TERMS** varying in weight from about 5 pounds to more than 100 pounds; usually used to perform high-speed resistance exercises.

The first few sessions of weight training should be devoted to learning the exercises. To start, choose a weight you can move easily through 8–12 repetitions. Add weight when you can do over 12 repetitions of an exercise. If adding weight means you can do only 7 or 8 repetitions before your muscles fatigue, stay with that weight until you can again complete 12 repetitions. If you can do only 4–6 repetitions after adding weight, or if you can't maintain good form, you've added too much and should take some off. As a general guideline, try increases of approximately a half-pound of additional weight for each 10 pounds you are currently lifting.

For developing strength and endurance for general fitness, a single set (a group of repetitions) of each exercise is sufficient, provided you use enough weight to fatigue your muscles. Doing more than one set of each exercise may increase strength development further, and most serious weight trainers do at least three sets of each exercise. If you do more than one set of an exercise, rest long enough between sets (1–5 minutes) to allow your muscles to recover.

You should warm up before every weight training session and cool down afterward. You can expect to improve rapidly during the first 6–10 weeks of training; gains will then come more slowly. Factors such as age, motivation, sex, and genetics will affect your progress. Your ultimate goal depends on you. After you have achieved the level of strength and muscularity that you want, you can maintain your gains by training 2 or 3 nonconsecutive days per week.

Volume For weight training, the volume of a specific exercise during a workout would be the weight lifted multiplied by the number of reps and sets. Choose a training volume that promotes progress and that you will do consistently. Change the components occasionally—that is, increase the weight on some days and the sets and reps on other days. Changing the training volume prevents the body from adapting to exercise stress and results in more consistent improvements in fitness.

Progression Training intensity is the most important factor promoting improvements in strength and power. You will progress rapidly when you begin training, but progress slows as you become more fit. Set fitness goals and progress systematically by adding weight or sets as you gain strength and power; see the section "Getting Started and Staying on Track" for specific recommendations for adjusting training intensity in response to fitness improvements. After achieving your goal, maintain strength by training one to three times per week.

A Caution about Supplements No nutritional supplement or drug will change a weak person into a strong person. Those changes require regular training that stresses the body and causes physiological adaptations. Supplements or drugs that promise quick, large gains in strength rarely work and are often dangerous, expensive, or illegal. Over-the-counter supplements are not regulated carefully,

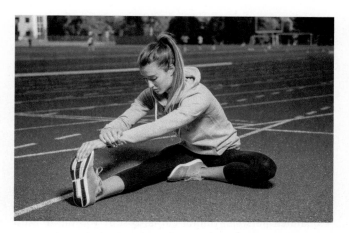

When performed regularly, stretching exercises help maintain or improve the range of motion in joints. Brian Caissie/fStop/Getty Images

and their long-term effects have not been studied systematically. Performance-enhancing drugs such as **anabolic steroids** and growth hormone have potentially dangerous side effects.

Flexibility Exercises

Flexibility, or stretching, exercises are important for maintaining the normal range of motion in the major joints of the body. Some exercises, such as running, can decrease flexibility because they require only a partial range of motion. Like a good weight training program, a good stretching program includes exercises for all the major muscle groups and joints of the body: neck, shoulders, back, hips, thighs, hamstrings, and calves. In tandem with core training, flexibility training is important for preventing low-back injuries and maintaining low-back health.

Proper Stretching Technique   Timing determines the best stretching technique: Do static stretching after a workout and dynamic or active stretching before a workout. *Static stretching* involves extending to a certain position and then holding it. *Dynamic stretching* is done by actively moving through the joints' ranges of motion. *Ballistic stretching* (known as "bouncing") is dangerous and counterproductive. The safest and most convenient technique for increasing flexibility may be active static stretching with a passive assist. For example, you might do a seated stretch of your calf muscles by contracting the muscles on the top of your shin and by grabbing your feet and pulling them toward you.

Frequency   Do stretching exercises at least 2 or 3 days per week (but 5–7 days is optimal). If you stretch during your cool-down after cardiorespiratory endurance exercise or strength training, you may develop more flexibility because your muscles are warmer then and can be stretched farther.

Intensity, Time, Volume, and Progression   Do stretching exercises statically. Stretch to the point of mild

discomfort, hold the position for 10–30 seconds, rest for 30–60 seconds, and then repeat, trying to stretch a bit farther. Stretch each muscle group for a total of 60 seconds. Older adults might benefit more from holding a stretch for 30–60 seconds.

Increase your intensity gradually. Improved flexibility takes many months to develop. There are large individual differences in joint flexibility. Don't feel you have to compete with others during stretching workouts. Progressively build flexibility, striving for a normal but not an excessive range of motion. Extremely flexible joints lose stability.

Training in Specific Skills

The final component in your fitness program is learning the skills required for the sports or activities in which you participate. By taking the time and effort to acquire competence, you can achieve a sense of mastery and add a new physical skill to your repertoire.

The first step in learning a new skill is getting help. Sports like tennis, golf, and skiing require mastery of basic movements and techniques, so instruction from a qualified teacher or coach can save you hours of frustration and increase your enjoyment. Skill is also important in conditioning activities such as jogging, swimming, and cycling. Even if you learned a sport as a child, additional instruction now can help you refine your technique, get over stumbling blocks, and relearn skills that you may have learned incorrectly.

Putting It All Together

Now that you know the basic components of a fitness program, you can put them all together in a program that works for you. Remember to include:

• *Cardiorespiratory endurance exercise.* Do at least 150 minutes of moderate-intensity aerobic exercise or 75 minutes of vigorous-intensity exercise per week (or a combination).

• *Muscular strength and endurance.* Work the major muscle groups (one or more sets of 8–10 exercises) at least 2–3 nonconsecutive days a week.

• *Flexibility exercise.* Do stretches at least 2 or 3 days a week and ideally 5–7 days a week, preferably after exercise when your muscles are warm.

• *Skill training.* Incorporate some or all of your aerobic or strengthening exercises into an enjoyable sport or physical activity.

See Figure 14.9 for a summary of the FITT-VP principle for the health-related components of fitness.

anabolic steroids   Synthetic male hormones used to increase muscle size and strength.   TERMS

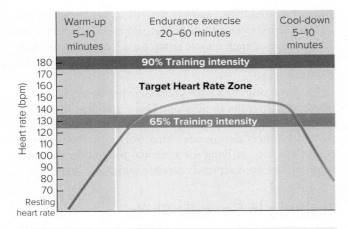

Frequency: 3–5 days per week

Intensity: 55/65–90% of maximum heart rate, 40/50–85% of heart rate reserve plus resting heart rate, or an RPE rating of about 4–8 (lower intensities—55–64% of maximum heart rate and 40–49% of heart rate reserve—apply to people who are quite unfit; for average individuals, intensities of 70–85% of maximum heart rate are appropriate)

Time (duration): 20–60 minutes (one session or multiple sessions lasting 10 or more minutes)

Type of activity: Cardiorespiratory endurance exercises, such as walking, jogging, biking, swimming, cross-country skiing, and rope skipping

Volume of activity: Equivalent to 150 minutes or 1,000 or more calories per week of moderate-intensity activity, consistent with individual fitness status and goals

Progression: Gradually increase volume (frequency, intensity, and/or time) over time, as appropriate for goals, fitness status, age, and adaptability

FIGURE 14.9 The FITT+VP principle for a cardiorespiratory endurance program. Longer-duration exercise at lower intensities can often be as beneficial for promoting health as shorter-duration, high-intensity exercise.

GETTING STARTED AND STAYING ON TRACK

Once a program fulfills your basic fitness needs and suits your personal tastes, adhering to a few basic principles will help you improve quickly, have fun, and minimize the risk of injury. These principles include buying equipment, eating and drinking properly, and managing your program so it becomes an integral part of your life.

Selecting Instructors, Equipment, and Facilities

Once you've chosen the activities for your program, you may need to look for the appropriate information, instruction, and equipment or find an appropriate facility.

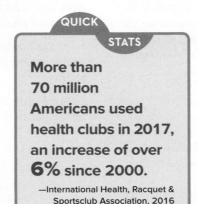

QUICK STATS

More than 70 million Americans used health clubs in 2017, an increase of over 6% since 2000.

—International Health, Racquet & Sportsclub Association, 2016

Finding Help and Advice One of the best places to get help is an exercise class, where an expert instructor can teach you the basics of training and answer your questions. A qualified personal trainer can also start you on an exercise program or a new form of training. Make sure that your instructor or trainer has proper qualifications, such as a college degree in exercise physiology, kinesiology, or physical education and certification by the American College of Sports Medicine, National Strength and Conditioning Association, International Sports Science Association, or another professional organization. Don't seek a person for advice simply because he or she looks fit. You can further your knowledge by reading articles by experts in fitness magazines such as *Fitness Rx for Men* and *Fitness Rx for Women*.

Many apps and websites provide fitness programs, including ongoing support and feedback via email. Many of these sites charge fees, so review the sites, decide which ones seem most appropriate, and go through a free trial period before subscribing. Also remember to consider the reliability of the information at fitness apps and websites, especially those that also advertise or sell products. A few popular sites are listed in the For More Information section at the end of the chapter.

Selecting Equipment Good equipment will enhance your enjoyment and decrease your risk of injury. Appropriate safety equipment, such as pads and helmets for skateboarding, is particularly important. If you shop around, you can often find bargains through mail-order companies and discount or used equipment stores.

Before you invest in a new piece of equipment, investigate it. Try it out at a local gym to make sure that you'll use it regularly. Make sure you have space to use and store it at home. Ask the experts (coaches, physical educators, and sports instructors) for their opinions. Also, educate yourself and become a lifelong student of physical activity and sport.

Footwear is an important piece of equipment for almost any activity; see the box "What to Wear" for shopping strategies.

Choosing a Fitness Center Are you thinking of joining a health club or fitness center? Choose one that has the right programs and equipment available at the times you will use them. You should feel comfortable with the classes and activities available;

Clothing

Modern exercise clothing is attractive, comfortable, and functional. Shorts made of elastic material, such as spandex, hug the body, supplying support. If you prefer, you can wear running shorts and a T-shirt. The main requirement for workout clothes is that they let you move easily but are not so loose that they get caught in the exercise machines or on fences when running outside. Don't wear street clothes when exercising because they can interfere with movement, and sweat, oil, and dirt can ruin them. If you run or cycle on the street, wear bright-colored clothing so that motorists can see you, and cyclists should wear a helmet to prevent head injury in case of an accident.

Specifics for Women and Men

- *For women.* Wear a good sports bra whenever you exercise. Breast support is important when running, playing volleyball, or weight training, The breasts can be injured if barbells press too firmly against them when you are weight-training or if they aren't properly supported when you run. A good sports bra should support the breasts in all directions, contain minimal elastic material, absorb moisture freely, and be easily laundered. Seams, hooks, and catches should not irritate the skin. You might buy a bra with an underwire for added support and a pocket in which to insert padding if you do exercises that could cause injury.

- *For men.* Wear a protective cup and jockstrap when participating in contact sports, such as football, baseball, cricket, hockey, wrestling, and karate. These protections can help guard against male infertility.

Footwear

Footwear is perhaps the most important item of equipment for almost any activity. Shoes protect and support your feet and improve traction. When you jump or run, you place as much as six times more force on your feet than when you stand still. Shoes can help cushion against the stress this additional force places on your lower legs, preventing injuries. Some athletic shoes are also designed to help prevent ankle roll-over, another common source of injury.

When choosing athletic shoes, first consider the activity you've chosen for your exercise program. Shoes appropriate for different activities have different characteristics. Foot type is another important consideration. If your feet roll inward excessively, you may need additional stability features on the inner side of the shoe to counteract this movement. If your feet roll outward excessively, you may need highly flexible and cushioned shoes that promote foot motion. Most women will get a better fit if they choose shoes specially designed for women's feet rather than downsized versions of men's shoes.

Barefoot Shoes or Minimalist Footwear

Two-thirds of runners experience an injury every year. Humans have evolved to run, so some scientists blame running shoes for the high injury rate. Most runners strike heel first when using heavily padded running shoes. Barefoot runners strike the

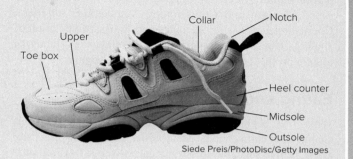

Siede Preis/PhotoDisc/Getty Images

ground with their forefoot (at least they're supposed to), which better uses the shock absorbing capacity of the skeleton. Some researchers speculated that using "minimalist" footwear allows people to run more naturally, which should cut down on the injury rate. Other research suggests that traditional running shoes provide a physiological advantage that makes running easier. We need more research to determine whether barefoot running is safe and viable or just the latest running fad.

Successful Shopping

For successful shoe shopping, remember the following strategies:

- Shop late in the day or, ideally, following a workout. Your foot size increases during the day and after exercise.

- Wear socks like those you plan to wear during exercise.

- Try on both shoes and wear them around for 10 minutes or more. Try walking on an uncarpeted surface. Approximate the movements of your activity: walk, jog, run, jump, and so on.

- Check the fit and style carefully:

  - Is the toe box roomy enough? Your toes will spread out when your foot hits the ground or you push off. There should be at least one thumb's width of space from the longest toe to the end of the toe box.

  - Do the shoes have enough cushioning? Do your feet feel supported when you bounce up and down? Try bouncing on your toes and on your heels.

  - Do your heels fit snugly in the shoe? Do they stay put when you walk, or do they slide up?

  - Are the arches of your feet on top of the shoes' arch supports?

  - Do the shoes feel stable when you twist and turn on the balls of your feet? Try twisting from side to side while standing on one foot.

  - Do you feel any pressure points?

- If you exercise at dawn or dusk, choose shoes with reflective sections for added visibility and safety.

- Replace athletic shoes about every three months or 300–500 miles of jogging or walking.

the age, fitness level, and dress of others in the club; and the music played in classes. The facility and equipment should be clean and well maintained, including the showers and lockers. The staff should be well trained and helpful.

Also make sure the facility is certified. Look for the displayed names American College of Sports Medicine, National Strength and Conditioning Association, American Council on Exercise, or Aerobics and Fitness Association of America. These trade associations have established standards to help protect consumer health, safety, and rights.

Eating and Drinking for Exercise

When they begin a fitness program, most people need not change their eating habits. Many athletes and other physically active people succumb to buying aggressively advertised vitamins, minerals, and protein supplements, but usually a well-balanced diet contains all the energy and nutrients needed to sustain an exercise program (see Chapter 13).

A balanced diet is also the key to improving body composition when you exercise more. One promise of a fitness program is a decrease in body fat and an increase in muscle mass. As a general rule, if you consume more calories than you expend through metabolism and exercise, fat increases. However, the control of body fat is determined by the amount and kind of calories you consume. Reduce your intake of added sugars and trans fats, and be physically active.

One of the most important principles to follow when exercising is to keep your body well hydrated by drinking enough fluids. Your body depends on water to sustain many chemical reactions and to maintain correct body temperature. Sweating during exercise depletes the body's water supply and can lead to dehydration if fluids are not replaced. Serious dehydration can cause reduced blood volume, accelerated heart rate, elevated body temperature, muscle cramps, heat stroke, and other serious problems.

Drinking fluids before and during exercise is important to prevent dehydration and enhance performance. Thirst receptors in the brain make you want to drink fluids, but during heavy or prolonged exercise or exercise in hot weather, thirst alone isn't a good indication of how much fluid you need to drink. Drink at least 16 ounces of fluid two to four hours before exercise and then drink enough during exercise to prevent significant fluid loss in sweat. Don't drink more than one quart per hour during exercise. After exercise, let thirst be your guide to your fluid needs. You can also check your weight before and after an exercise session; any weight loss is due to fluid loss that needs to be replaced.

Carry fluids when you exercise so that you can replace your fluids when they're depleted. For exercise sessions lasting less than 60–90 minutes, cool water is an excellent fluid replacement. For longer workouts, the ACSM recommends sports drinks that contain water and small amounts of electrolytes (sodium, potassium, and magnesium) and simple carbohydrates (sugar, usually in the form of sucrose or glucose). After your workout, replace any lost fluids. Nonfat or low-fat milk, for those who can tolerate dairy products, are excellent

postexercise fluid replacement beverages because they promote long-term hydration. Milk is digested more slowly than water or sports beverages and also contains electrolytes.

Managing Your Fitness Program

How can you tell when you're in shape? When do you stop improving and start maintaining? How can you stay motivated? For your program to become an integral part of your life, these questions are key.

Starting Slowly, Getting in Shape Gradually As Table 14.5 shows, an exercise program can be divided into three stages:

- *Initial stage.* The body adjusts to the new type and level of activity.
- *Improvement stage.* Fitness increases.
- *Maintenance stage.* The targeted level of fitness is sustained over the long term.

When beginning a program, start slowly to give your body time to adapt to the stress of exercise. Choose activities carefully according to your fitness status.

Exercising Consistently Consistency is the key to getting into shape without injury. Steady fitness improvement comes when you overload your body consistently. The best

| Table 14.5 | Sample Progression for a Walking and Running Program |

STAGE/WEEK	FREQUENCY (days/week)	INTENSITY* (beats/ minute)	TIME (duration in minutes)
Initial stage			
1	3	120–130	15–20
2	3	120–130	20–25
3	4	130–145	20–25
4	4	130–145	25–30
Improvement stage			
5–7	3–4	145–160	25–30
8–10	3–4	145–160	30–35
11–13	3–4	150–165	30–35
14–16	4–5	150–165	30–35
17–20	4–5	160–180	35–40
21–24	4–5	160–180	35–40
Maintenance stage			
25+	3–5	160–180	20–60

*The target heart rates shown here are based on calculations for a healthy 20-year-old. The program progresses from an initial target heart rate of 50% to a maintenance range of 70–90% of maximum heart rate.

SOURCE: Adapted from American College of Sports Medicine. 2018. *ACSM's Guidelines for Exercise Testing and Prescription,* 10th ed. Philadelphia, PA: Wolters.

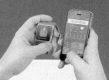

You can obtain a general rating of your cardiorespiratory fitness by taking the 1.5-mile run–walk test. Don't attempt this test unless you have completed at least 6 weeks of some conditioning activity. Also, if you are over age 35 or have questions about your health, check with your physician before taking this test.

You'll need a stopwatch, clock, or watch with a second hand and a running track or course that is flat and provides measurements of up to 1.5 miles. Pace yourself during the test to avoid going too fast at the start and becoming fatigued before you finish. Allow yourself a day or two to recover from a practice run before taking the test.

Warm up before taking the test with some walking, easy jogging, and stretching exercises. The idea is to cover the distance as fast as possible at a pace that is comfortable for you. You can run or walk the entire distance or use some combination of running and walking. Monitor your pace, or have someone call out your time at various intervals to help you determine whether your pace is correct.

When you have completed the test, refer to the table for your cardiorespiratory fitness rating. Cool down by walking or jogging slowly for about 5 minutes.

Standards for the 1.5-Mile Run–Walk Test (Minutes: Seconds)

	Superior	Excellent	Good	Fair	Poor	Very Poor
Women						
Age: 18–29	11:00 or less	11:01–12:59	13:00–14:29	14:30–15:59	16:00–17:29	17:30 or more
30–39	11:45 or less	11:46–13:29	13:30–15:29	15:30–16:29	16:30–18:29	18:30 or more
40–49	12:45 or less	12:46–14:29	14:30–16:29	16:30–18:29	18:30–19:29	19:30 or more
50–59	14:15 or less	14:16–16:29	16:30–18:29	18:30–19:29	19:30–20:29	20:30 or more
60 and over	16:29 or less	16:30–17:29	17:30–19:29	19:30–20:29	20:30–20:59	21:00 or more
Men						
Age: 18–29	9:15 or less	9:16–10:29	10:30–11:59	12:00–12:59	13:00–14:14	14:15 or more
30–39	9:45 or less	9:46–10:59	11:00–12:29	12:30–13:44	13:45–14:59	15:00 or more
40–49	10:00 or less	10:01–11:59	12:00–12:59	13:00–14:29	14:30–15:59	16:00 or more
50–59	10:45 or less	10:46–12:59	13:00–14:29	14:30–15:59	16:00–17:59	18:00 or more
60 and over	11:15 or less	11:16–13:59	14:00–15:59	16:00–17:59	18:00–20:59	21:00 or more

SOURCE: Adapted from *The Aerobics Program for Total Well Being* by Kenneth H. Cooper, M.D., M.P.H. Bantam Books, 1982.

way to ensure consistency is to record the details of your workouts in a journal: how far you ran, how much weight you lifted, and so on. This record will help you evaluate your progress and plan workout sessions intelligently. Don't increase your exercise volume by over 5–10% per week.

Table 14.5 shows how the overload is increased gradually over time in a sample walking–running program. Regardless of the activity chosen, an exercise program must begin slowly and progress gradually. Once you achieve the desired level of fitness, you can maintain it by exercising 3–5 days a week.

Assessing Your Fitness When are you in shape? It depends. One person may be out of shape running a mile in 5 minutes, but another may be in shape running a mile in 12

minutes. Your ultimate level of fitness depends on your goals, your program, and your natural ability. The important thing is to set goals that make sense for you. To assess your own approximate level of cardiorespiratory endurance, take the test in the box "The 1.5-Mile Run–Walk Test."

Preventing and Managing Athletic Injuries Although they are annoying, most injuries are neither serious nor permanent. If an injury is not cared for properly, however, it can escalate into a chronic problem. If you learn how to deal with injuries, they won't derail your fitness program (Table 14.6).

Some injuries require medical attention. See a physician right away if you suffer a head or eye injury, a possible

Table 14.6   Care of Common Exercise Injuries and Discomforts

INJURY	SYMPTOMS	TREATMENT
Blister	Accumulation of fluid in one spot under the skin	Don't pop or drain it unless it interferes too much with your daily activities. If it does pop, clean the area with antiseptic and cover with a bandage. Do not remove the skin covering the blister.
Bruise (contusion)	Pain, swelling, and discoloration	R-I-C-E: rest, ice, compression, elevation.
Fracture and/or dislocation	Pain, swelling, tenderness, loss of function, and deformity	Seek medical attention, immobilize the affected area, and apply cold.
Joint sprain	Pain, tenderness, swelling, discoloration, and loss of function	R-I-C-E. Apply heat when swelling has disappeared. Stretch and strengthen affected area.
Muscle cramp	Painful, spasmodic muscle contractions	Gently stretch for 15–30 seconds at a time and/or massage the cramped area. Drink fluids and increase dietary salt intake if exercising in hot weather.
Muscle soreness or stiffness	Pain and tenderness in the affected muscle	Stretch the affected muscle gently; exercise at a low intensity; apply heat. Nonsteroidal anti-inflammatory drugs, such as ibuprofen, help some people.
Muscle strain	Pain, tenderness, swelling, and loss of strength in the affected muscle	R-I-C-E. Apply heat when swelling has disappeared. Stretch and strengthen the affected area.
Plantar fasciitis	Pain and tenderness in the connective tissue on the bottom of the foot	Apply ice, take nonsteroidal anti-inflammatory drugs, and stretch. Wear night splints when sleeping.
Shin splint	Pain and tenderness on the front of the lower leg; sometimes also pain in the calf muscle	Rest. Apply ice or heat to the affected area several times a day and before exercise; wrap with tape for support. Stretch and strengthen muscles in the lower legs. Purchase good-quality footwear and run on soft surfaces.
Side stitch	Pain on the side of the abdomen	Stretch the arm on the affected side as high as possible; if that doesn't help, try bending forward while tightening the abdominal muscles.
Tendinitis	Pain, swelling, and tenderness of the affected area	R-I-C-E. Apply heat when swelling has disappeared. Stretch and strengthen the affected area.

SOURCE: Fahey, T. D., et al. 2019. *Fit & Well: Core Concepts and Labs in Physical Fitness and Wellness*, 13th ed. New York: McGraw Hill. Copyright © 2019 The McGraw Hill Companies, Inc.

ligament injury, a broken bone, or an internal disorder such as chest pain, fainting, or intolerance to heat. Also seek medical attention for apparently minor injuries that do not get better within a reasonable amount of time.

For minor cuts and scrapes, stop the bleeding and clean the wound with soap and water. Treat soft tissue injuries (muscles and joints) with the R-I-C-E principle:

Rest: Stop using the injured tissue when you experience pain, protect it from further injury, and avoid any activity that causes pain.

Ice: Ice reduces bleeding, but it also decreases inflammation, new blood vessel formation, and release of tissue growth factors. Ice decreases pain and spasm following an injury, but it might delay healing and eventual return to the playing field, so use it only during the early phases of injury rehabilitation. Apply ice to the injured tissue to reduce swelling and alleviate pain. Apply ice immediately for 10–20 minutes, and repeat every few hours until the swelling disappears.

Compression: Wrap the injured area with an elastic or compression bandage between icings. If the area throbs or changes color, the bandage may be wrapped too tightly. Do not sleep with the bandage on.

Elevation: Raise the injured area above heart level to decrease the blood supply and reduce swelling.

After 36–48 hours, if the swelling has disappeared, apply heat to relieve pain, relax muscles, and reduce stiffness. Immerse the affected area in warm water or apply warm compresses, a hot water bottle, or a heating pad.

After a minor athletic injury, gradually reintroduce the stress of the activity until you can return to full intensity. Before returning to full exercise participation, you should have a full range of motion in your joints; normal strength and balance; no injury compensation movements, such as limping; and little or no pain.

To prevent injuries, follow six basic guidelines:

1. Stay in condition: Haphazard exercise programs invite injury.

2. Warm up thoroughly before exercising.

3. Use proper body mechanics when lifting objects or executing sports skills.

4. Don't exercise when you're ill or overtrained (experiencing extreme fatigue due to overexercising).

5. Use the proper equipment.

6. Don't return to your normal exercise program until athletic injuries have healed.

You can minimize the risk of injury by following safety guidelines, respecting signals from your body that something may be wrong, and treating injuries promptly.

Use special caution in heat or humidity (over 80°F and over 60% humidity): Exercise slowly, rest frequently in the shade, wear clothing that breathes, and drink plenty of fluids. Slow down or stop if you feel uncomfortable. During hot weather, exercise in the early morning or evening when temperatures are lowest.

Staying with Your Program Once you have attained your desired level of fitness, you can maintain it by exercising regularly at a consistent intensity, 3–5 days a week. You must work at the intensity that brought you to your desired fitness level. If you don't, your body will become less fit because less is expected of it. If you exercise at the same intensity over a long period, your fitness will level out and can be maintained easily.

Adapt your program to changes in environment or schedule. Don't use wet weather or a new job as an excuse to give up your fitness program. If you walk in the summer, dress appropriately and walk in the winter. (Exercise is usually safe even in very cold temperatures if you dress warmly in layers and don't stay out too long.) If you can't go out because of darkness or an unsafe neighborhood, walk in a local shopping mall or on campus or join a gym and walk on a treadmill.

What if you run out of steam? Although good health is an important *reason* to exercise, it's a poor *motivator*. You'll find specific suggestions for staying with your program in the Behavior Change Strategy box at the end of the chapter.

TIPS FOR TODAY AND THE FUTURE

Physical activity and exercise offer benefits in nearly every area of wellness. Even a low to moderate level of activity provides valuable health benefits.

RIGHT NOW YOU CAN:
- Go outside and take a brisk 15-minute walk.
- Look at your calendar for the rest of the week and write in some physical activity—such as walking, running, or playing Frisbee—on as many days as you can. Schedule the activity for a specific time and stick to it.
- Call a friend and invite him or her to plan a regular exercise program with you.

IN THE FUTURE YOU CAN:
- Schedule a session with a qualified personal trainer who can evaluate your fitness level and help you set personalized fitness goals.
- Create seasonal workout programs for the summer, spring, fall, and winter. Develop programs varied but consistent with your overall fitness goals.

---

cross-training Participating in two or more activities to develop a variety of fitness components.

TERMS

Cross-training can add variety to your workouts. Cross-training emphasizes whole-body, high-intensity training using exercises such as deadlifts, cleans, squats, presses, jerks, kettlebell exercises, snatches, plyometrics, sled pulls, and weight carrying. Cross-trainers learn to handle their body weight by practicing gymnastics, pull-ups, dips, kettlebell swings and snatches, rope climbing, push-ups, Olympic lifts, handstands, pirouettes, flips, and splits. They also do aerobics such as running, cycling, rope skipping, and rowing, but the emphasis is on speed and intensity. Cross-training programs, such as CrossFit, attempt to develop well-rounded fitness by including exercises that build cardiovascular and respiratory endurance, stamina, strength, flexibility, power, speed, coordination, agility, balance, and accuracy. Explore many exercise options. Consider competitive sports at the recreational level, or find out how you can participate in an activity you've never done before. Try new activities, especially ones that you will be able to do for the rest of your life.

SUMMARY

- Exercise improves the functioning of the heart and the ability of the cardiorespiratory system to carry oxygen to the body's tissues. It also increases metabolic efficiency and improves body composition.

- Exercise lowers the risk of cardiovascular disease by improving blood fat levels, reducing high blood pressure, and interfering with the disease process that causes coronary artery blockage.

- Exercise reduces the risk of cancer, osteoporosis, and diabetes. It improves immune function and psychological health and helps prevent injuries and low-back pain.

- The five components of physical fitness most important to health are cardiorespiratory endurance, muscular strength, muscular endurance, flexibility, and body composition.

- Most people should accumulate at least 150 minutes of moderate-intensity or 75 minutes of vigorous-intensity exercise each week. Longer-duration or more vigorous activity produces additional health and fitness benefits.

- Cardiorespiratory endurance exercises stress a large portion of the body's muscle mass. Endurance exercise should be performed 3–5 days per week for 20–60 minutes per day. Intensity can be evaluated by measuring the heart rate.

- Warming up before exercising and cooling down afterward improve your performance and decrease your chances of injury.

- Exercises that develop muscular strength and endurance involve exerting force against a significant resistance. A strength-training program for general fitness typically involves one or more sets of 8–12 repetitions of 8–10 exercises performed on at least 2 nonconsecutive days per week.

- A good stretching program includes exercises for the major muscle groups and joints of the body. Do active, static stretches at least 2–3 days per week. Hold each stretch for 10–30 seconds and do 2–4 repetitions. Stretch when muscles are warm.

- Individuals should choose instructors, equipment, and facilities carefully to enhance enjoyment and prevent injuries.

- A well-balanced diet contains all the energy and nutrients needed to sustain a fitness program. When exercising, remember to drink enough fluids.

- Rest, ice, compression, and elevation (R-I-C-E) are treatments for minor muscle and joint injuries.

- People can maintain a desired level of fitness by exercising 3–5 days a week at a consistent intensity.

- Strategies for maintaining an exercise program over the long term include having meaningful goals, varying the program, and trying new activities.

FOR MORE INFORMATION

American College of Sports Medicine (ACSM). The principal professional organization for sports medicine and exercise science. Provides brochures, publications, and audio- and videotapes.

http://www.acsm.org

American Council on Exercise (ACE). Promotes exercise and fitness; the website features fact sheets on many consumer topics, including choosing shoes, cross-training, and steroids.

http://www.acefitness.org

Backfitpro. This site provides excellent information on preventing back pain and promoting core fitness. The site is maintained by Stuart McGill, a biomechanist and professor emeritus from University of Waterloo in Canada.

http://www.backfitpro.com/

CDC Physical Activity Information. Provides information about the benefits of physical activity and suggestions for incorporating moderate physical activity into daily life.

http://www.cdc.gov/physicalactivity/

Disabled Sports USA. Provides sports and recreation services to people with physical or mobility disorders.

http://www.disabledsportsusa.org

International Health, Racquet, & Sportsclub Association (IHRSA): Health Clubs. Provides guidelines for choosing a health or fitness facility and links to clubs that belong to IHRSA.

http://www.ihrsa.org

International Sports Sciences Association (ISSA). Trains and certifies personal trainers.

www.issaonline.com

Dan John. An excellent website for people serious about improving strength and fitness, written by a world-class athlete and coach in track and field and Highland games.

http://danjohn.net

MedlinePlus: Exercise and Physical Fitness. Provides links to news and reliable information about fitness and exercise from government agencies and professional associations.

https://medlineplus.gov/fitnessandexercise.html

President's Council on Physical Fitness and Sports (PCPFS). Provides information about PCPFS programs and publications, including fitness guides and fact sheets.

http://www.fitness.gov

http://www.presidentschallenge.org

Robert Wood Johnson Foundation. Promotes the health and health care of Americans through research and distribution of information on healthy lifestyles; publishes an annual report on the status of the national obesity problem.

http://www.rwjf.org

Shape America. A professional organization dedicated to promoting quality health and physical education programs.

https://www.shapeamerica.org

StrongFirst. A school of strength, directed by kettlebell master Pavel Tsatsouline, that teaches men and women how to reach high levels of strength and fitness without interfering with work, school, family, or sport. The program offers clinics and web-based information.

http://www.strongfirst.com

SELECTED BIBLIOGRAPHY

Aengevaeren, V. L., et al. 2017. Relationship between lifelong exercise volume and coronary atherosclerosis in athletes. *Circulation* 136(2): 136–148.

American College of Sports Medicine. 2013. Exercise and fluid replacement. *ACSM's Health & Fitness Journal* 17(4): 3.

American College of Sports Medicine. 2018. *ACSM's Guidelines for Exercise Testing and Prescription,* 10th ed. Philadelphia, PA: Wolters Kluwer.

American College of Sports Medicine. 2019. *ACSM's Health/Fitness Facility Standards and Guidelines,* 5th ed. Champaign, IL: Human Kinetics.

Arem, H., et al. 2015. Leisure time physical activity and mortality: A detailed pooled analysis of the dose-response relationship. *JAMA Internal Medicine* 175(6): 959–967.

Bajer, B., et al. 2015. Exercise associated hormonal signals as powerful determinants of an effective fat mass loss. *Endocrine Regulations* 49(3): 151–163.

Bangsbo, J., et al. 2019. Copenhagen consensus statement 2019: Physical activity and ageing. *British Journal of Sports Medicine.* 53: 856–858.

Biswas, A., et al. 2015. Sedentary time and its association with risk for disease incidence, mortality, and hospitalization in adults: A systematic review and meta-analysis. *Annals of Internal Medicine* 162: 123–132.

Blair-Kennedy, A., et al. 2018. Fitness or fatness. Which is more important? *Journal of the American Medical Association* 319(3): 231–232.

Centers for Disease Control and Prevention. 2013. Adult participation in aerobic and muscle-strengthening physical activities—United States, 2011. *MMWR* 62(17): 326–330.

Centers for Disease Control and Prevention. 2020. *Physical Activity Basics* (http://www.cdc.gov/physicalactivity/basics).

Centers for Disease Control and Prevention. 2019. *2018 National Health Interview Survey.* National Center for Health Statistics (https://www.cdc.gov/nchs/nhis/releases/released201905.htm#7A).

Chou, C. H., et al. 2019. High-intensity interval training enhances mitochondrial bioenergetics of platelets in patients with heart failure. *International Journal of Cardiology* 274: 214–220.

Dankel, S. J., et al. 2016. Does the fat-but-fit paradigm hold true for all-cause mortality when considering the duration of overweight/obesity? Analyzing the WATCH (Weight, Activity and Time Contributes to Health) paradigm. *Preventive Medicine* 83: 37–40.

Dorneles, G. P., et al. 2016. High intensity interval exercise decreases IL-8 and enhances the immunomodulatory cytokine interleukin-10 in lean and overweight-obese individuals. *Cytokine* 77: 1–9.

Fahey, T. D., et al. 2019. *Fit & Well: Core Concepts and Labs in Physical Fitness and Wellness*, 13th ed. New York: McGraw Hill.

Gaesser, G., and S. Blair. 2019. The health risks of obesity have been exaggerated. *Medicine & Science in Sports & Exercise.* 51(1):218-221.

Garber, C. E., et al. 2011. Quantity and quality of exercise for developing and maintaining cardiorespiratory, musculoskeletal, and neuromotor fitness in apparently healthy adults: Guidance for prescribing exercise. *Medicine & Science in Sports & Exercise* 43(7): 1334–1359.

Hogstrom, G., et al. 2015. Aerobic fitness in late adolescence and the risk of early death: A prospective cohort study of 1.3 million Swedish men. *International Journal of Epidemiology.* DOI: 10.1093/ije/dyv321.

Hussain, N., et al. 2018. Impact of cardiorespiratory fitness on frequency of atrial fibrillation, stroke, and all-cause mortality. *American Journal of Cardiology* 121: 41–49.

International Health, Racquet & Sportsclub Association. 2018. *Latest Data Shows U.S. Health Club Industry Serves 70.2 Million* (https://www.ihrsa.org/about/media-center/press-releases/latest-data-shows-u-s-health-club-industry-serves-70-2-million/).

Kennedy, A. B., et al. 2018. Fitness or fatness: Which is more important? *Journal of the American Medical Association* 319(3): 231-232.

Kim, Y., et al. 2018. The combination of cardiorespiratory fitness and muscle strength, and mortality risk. *European Journal of Epidemiology* 33(10): 953-964.

King, A.C., K. E. Powell, and W. E. Kraus. 2019. The U.S. Physical Activities Guidelines Advisory Committee report—introduction. *Medicine & Science in Sports & Exercise* 51(6): 1203–1205.

Klos, L. A., et al. 2015. Losing weight on reality TV: A content analysis of the weight loss behaviors and practices portrayed on *The Biggest Loser*. *Journal of Health Communication* 20(6): 639–646.

Koch, L. G., and S. L. Britton. 2018. Theoretical and biological evaluation of the link between low exercise capacity and disease risk. *Cold Spring Harbor Perspective Medicine* 8(1): a029868.

Kochanek, K. D. 2017. Mortality in the United States. *NCHS Data Brief*, No. 293.

Kyu, H. H., et al. 2016. Physical activity and risk of breast cancer, colon cancer, diabetes, ischemic heart disease, and ischemic stroke events: Systematic review and dose-response meta-analysis for the Global Burden of Disease Study 2013. *BMJ.* DOI: 10.1136/bmj.i3857.

Landi, F., et al. 2018. Impact of habitual physical activity and type of exercise on physical performance across ages in community living people. *PLoS ONE* 13(1): e0191820.

Lavie, C. J., et al. 2019. Sedentary behavior, exercise, and cardiovascular health. *Circulation Research* 124(5): 799-815.

Lee, B. C. Y., and S. M. McGill. 2015. Effect of long-term isometric training on core/torso stiffness. *Journal of Strength & Conditioning Research* 29(6): 1515-1526.

Lee, D. C., et al. 2017. Running as a key lifestyle medicine for longevity. *Progress in Cardiovascular Diseases* 60(1): 45-55.

Loprinzi, P. D., E. Frith, and M. K. Edwards. 2018. Resistance exercise and episodic memory function: A systematic review. *Clinical Physiology Functional Imaging* DOI: 10.1111/cpf.12507.

Lyden, K., et al. 2015. Discrete features of sedentary behaviors impact cardiometabolic risk factors. *Medicine & Science in Sports & Exercise* 47(5): 1079-1086.

Maughan, R. J., et al. 2016. A randomized trial to assess the potential of different beverages to affect hydration status: Development of a beverage hydration index. *American Journal of Clinical Nutrition* 103: 717-723.

McDermott, B. P., et al. 2017. National Athletic Trainer's Association position statement: Fluid replacement for the physically active. *Journal of Athletic Training* 52(9): 877-895.

McGill, S. M., et al. 2012. Kettlebell swing, snatch, and bottoms-up carry: Back and hip muscle activation, motion, and low back loads. *Journal of Strength & Conditioning Research* 26: 16-27.

McGill, S. M., et al. 2013. Low back loads while walking and carrying: Comparing the load carried in one hand or in both hands. *Ergonomics* 56(2): 293-302.

Moore, S. C., et al. 2016. Association of leisure-time physical activity with risk of 26 types of cancer in 1.44 million adults. *JAMA Internal Medicine.* DOI: 10.1001/jamainternmed.2016.1548.

Muntaner-Mas, A., et al. 2019. A systematic review of fitness apps and their potential clinical and sports utility for objective and remote assessment of cardiorespiratory fitness. *Sports Medicine* 49(4): 587-600.

O'Donovan, G., et al. 2017. Association of "weekend warrior" and other leisure time physical activity patterns with risks for all-cause, cardiovascular disease, and cancer mortality. *JAMA Internal Medicine* 177(3): 335-342.

Pedersen, B. K. 2019. Which type of exercise keeps you young? *Current Opinion in Clinical Nutrition & Metabolic Care.* 22(2): 167-173.

Physical Activity Guidelines Advisory Committee. 2008. *Physical Activity Guidelines Advisory Committee Report, 2008.* Washington, DC: U.S. Department of Health and Human Services.

Rivera-Torres, S., et al. 2019. Adherence to exercise programs in older adults: Informative report. *Gerontology and Geriatric Medicine* 5:1-10.

Ross, R.E., et al. 2019. High-intensity aerobic exercise acutely increases brain-derived neurotrophic factor. *Medicine & Science in Sports & Exercise* 51(8):1698-1709.

Schnohr, P., et al. 2013. Longevity in male and female joggers: The Copenhagen City Heart Study. *American Journal of Epidemiology* 177(7): 683-689.

Shiroma, E. J., et al. 2017. Strength training and the risk of type 2 diabetes and cardiovascular disease. *Medicine & Science in Sports & Exercise* 49(1): 40-46.

Song, J., et al. 2017. Do inactive older adults who increase physical activity experience less disability: Evidence from the osteoarthritis initiative. *Journal of Clinical Rheumatology* 23(1): 26-32.

Stephens, J., et al. 2015. Young adults, technology, and weight loss: A focus group study. *Journal of Obesity* 2015: 379769.

Stubbs, B., et al. 2016. Exercise improves cardiorespiratory fitness in people with depression: A meta-analysis of randomized control trials. *Journal of Affective Disorders* 190: 249-253.

Swain, D. P. 2013. *ACSM's Resource Manual for Guidelines for Exercise Testing and Prescription,* 7th ed. Philadelphia, PA: Lippincott Williams and Wilkins.

U.S. Department of Health and Human Services. 2020. *Healthy People 2020.* Washington, DC: U.S. Department of Health and Human Services (http://www.healthypeople.gov).

U.S. Department of Health and Human Services. 2018. *Physical Activity Guidelines for Americans,* 2nd ed. Washington, DC: U.S. Department of Health and Human Services.

U.S. Department of Health and Human Services and U.S. Department of Agriculture. 2015. *2015-2020 Dietary Guidelines for Americans,* 8th ed.

Viana, R. B., et al. 2019. Is interval training the magic bullet for fat loss? A systematic review and meta-analysis comparing moderate-intensity continuous training with high-intensity interval training (HIIT). *British Journal of Sports Medicine* 53(10):655-664.

Vollaard, N. B., et al. 2017. Effect of number of sprints in an SIT session on changes in $\dot{V}O_{2max}$: A meta-analysis. *Medicine & Science in Sports & Exercise.* 49(6): 1147-1156.

Williams, B. M., and R. R. Kraemer. 2015. Comparison of cardiorespiratory and metabolic responses in kettlebell high-intensity interval training versus sprint interval cycling. *Journal of Strength & Conditioning Research* 29(12): 3317-3325.

Young, D. R., et al. 2016. Sedentary behavior and cardiovascular morbidity and mortality. A science advisory from the American Heart Association. *Circulation* 134(13): e262-e279.

BEHAVIOR CHANGE STRATEGY
Planning a Personal Exercise Program

Although most people recognize the importance of incorporating exercise into their lives, many find it difficult to do. No single strategy will work for everyone, but the general steps outlined here should help you create an exercise program that fits your goals, preferences, and lifestyle. A carefully designed contract and program plan can help you convert your vague wishes into a detailed plan of action. And the strategies for program compliance outlined here and in Chapter 1 can help you enjoy and stick with your program for the rest of your life.

Step 1: Set Goals

Setting specific goals to accomplish by exercising is an important first step in a successful fitness program because it establishes the direction you want to take. Your goals might be specifically related to health, such as lowering your blood pressure and risk of heart disease, or they might relate to other aspects of your life, such as improving your tennis game or the fit of your clothes. If you can decide why you're starting to exercise, it can help you keep going. Make sure your goals meet the SMART criteria described in Chapter 1.

Think carefully about your reasons for incorporating exercise into your life, and then fill in the Fitness Goals portion of the Personal Fitness Contract.

Step 2: Select Activities

As discussed in the chapter, the success of your fitness program depends on the consistency of your involvement. Select activities that encourage your commitment: The right program will be its own incentive to continue, but poor activity choices provide obstacles and can turn exercise into a chore.

When choosing activities for your fitness program, consider the following:

- Is this activity fun? Will it hold my interest over time?

- Will this activity help me reach the goals I have set?

- Will my current fitness and skill level enable me to participate fully in this activity?

- Can I easily fit this activity into my daily schedule? Are there any special requirements (e.g., facilities, partners, equipment) that I must plan for?

- Can I afford any special costs required for equipment or facilities?

- If I have special exercise needs due to a particular health problem, does this activity conform to those exercise needs? Will it enhance my ability to cope with my specific health problem?

Using these guidelines listed, select a number of sports and activities. Fill in the Program Plan portion of the Personal Fitness Contract, including the fitness components your choices will develop and the frequency, intensity, and time standard you intend to meet for each activity. Does your program meet the criteria of a complete fitness program discussed in the chapter?

Step 3: Make a Commitment

Complete your Personal Fitness Contract by signing it and having it witnessed by someone who can help make you accountable for your progress. By completing a contract, you make a firm commitment and will be more likely to follow through until you meet your goals.

Step 4: Begin and Maintain Your Program

Start slowly and increase your intensity and duration gradually to allow your body time to adjust. Be realistic and patient—meeting your goals will take time. The important first step is to break your established pattern of inactivity. The following guidelines may help you start and stick with your program:

- *Set aside regular periods for exercise.* Choose times that fit in best with your schedule, and stick to them. Allow an adequate amount of time for warm-up, cool-down, and a shower.

- *Take advantage of any opportunity for exercise that presents itself.* For example, walk to class or take stairs instead of an elevator.

- *Do what you can to make your program fun and avoid boredom.* Do stretching exercises or jumping jacks to music, or watch the evening news while riding your stationary bicycle.

- *Exercise with a group that shares your goals and general level of competence.* The social side of exercise is an important motivator for many people.

- *Vary the program.* Change your activities periodically. Alter your route or distance if biking or jogging. Change racquetball partners, or find a new volleyball court.

- *Establish mini-goals or a point system, and work rewards into your program.* Until you reach your main goals, a series of small rewards will help you stick with your program. Rewards should be things you enjoy that are easily obtainable.

- *Focus on the positive.* Concentrate on the improvements you get from your program, and how good you feel during and after exercise. Visualize what it will be like to reach your goals, and keep these images in your mind as an incentive to stick to your program.

- *Revisit and revise.* If your program turns out to be unrealistic, revise it. Expect to make many adjustments in your program along the way.

- *Expect fluctuation and lapses.* On some days your progress will be excellent, but on others you'll barely be able to drag yourself through your scheduled activities. Don't let lapses discourage you or make you feel guilty. Instead make a renewed commitment to your exercise program.

- **Plan ahead for difficult situations.** Think about what circumstances might make it tough to keep up with your fitness routine, and develop strategies for sticking with your program. For example, devise a plan for your program during vacation, travel, bad weather, and so on.
- **Renew your attitude.** If you notice you're slacking off, try to list the negative thoughts and behaviors that are causing you to lose interest. Devise a strategy to reduce negative thoughts and behaviors. Make changes in your program plan and reward system to help renew your enthusiasm and commitment.

Step 5: Record and Assess Your Progress

Keeping a record that notes the daily results of your program will help remind you of your ongoing commitment to your program and give you a sense of accomplishment. It can also help you identify problems. Create daily and weekly program logs that you can use to track your progress, or use one of the many available apps for exercise tracking. Record the activity frequency, intensity, time, and type. Post or check your log frequently to remind you of your activity schedule and to provide incentive for improvement.

SOURCE: Adapted from Kusinitz, I., and M. Fine. 1995. *Your Guide to Getting Fit,* 3rd ed. Mountain View, CA: Mayfield.

Personal Fitness Contract

I, _____ , am contracting with myself to follow an exercise program to work at the following goals. I will begin my program on _____ .

Fitness Goals

1. _____   4. _____
2. _____   5. _____
3. _____   6. _____

Program Plan

Activities	Components (Check ✔)					Frequency (Check ✔)							Intensity	Time
	CRE	MS	ME	F	BC	M	Tu	W	Th	F	Sa	Su		
1.														
2.														
3.														
4.														
5.														

Note: You should conduct activities for achieving CRE goals at your target heart rate.

I agree to maintain a record of my activity, assess my progress periodically, and, if necessary, revise my goals.

Signed _____   Date _____

Witness _____

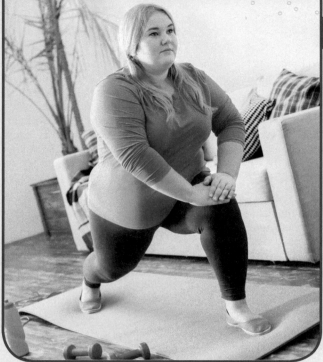
Viktoriia Hnatiuk/Getty Images

- Discuss methods for assessing body weight and body composition
- Explain the effects of body fat on wellness
- Explain factors that contribute to excess body fat
- Describe lifestyle factors associated with successful weight management
- Name and describe approaches to overcoming a weight problem
- Explain the relationship between body image and eating disorders and the associated health risks

CHAPTER 15

Weight Management

TEST YOUR KNOWLEDGE

1. **About what percentage of American adults are overweight?**
   a. 15%
   b. 35%
   c. 70%

2. **Genetic factors explain most cases of obesity.**
   True or False?

3. **The consumption of low-calorie sweeteners has helped Americans control their weight.**
   True or False?

4. **Which of the following is the most significant risk factor for type 2 diabetes (the most common type of diabetes)?**
   a. Smoking
   b. Low-fiber diet
   c. Overweight or obesity

5. **Approximately how many American girls and women have an eating disorder?**
   a. <1%
   b. 6–8%
   c. 10–15%

ANSWERS

1. **C.** About 70% of American adults are overweight, including almost 40% who are obese.

2. **FALSE.** Genetic factors may increase an individual's tendency to gain weight, but lifestyle is the key contributing factor.

3. **FALSE.** Ever since the introduction of low-calorie sweeteners, both total calorie and sugar intake have increased, as has the proportion of Americans who are overweight.

4. **C.** All are risk factors for diabetes, but overweight or obesity is the most significant. It is estimated that 90% of cases of type 2 diabetes could be prevented if people adopted healthy lifestyle behaviors.

5. **B.** About 6–8% currently. In the United States, about 20% of females and 14% of males will experience an eating disorder in their lifetime.

A chieving and maintaining a healthy body weight is a public health priority and a serious challenge for many Americans. According to standards developed by the National Institutes of Health (NIH), the prevalence of obesity among Americans is over 42% in adults (Figure 15.1). Of children and adolescents aged 2–19, about 18.5% are obese. Of adult men, almost 32% are obese, and of adult women, over 41% are obese. As millions struggle to lose weight, others fall into dangerous eating patterns such as binge eating or self-starvation.

This chapter explores body composition and the problems associated with excess body fat. It also explores factors that contribute to the development of overweight and suggests strategies for reaching and maintaining a healthy weight. Finally, it looks at body image and the development and treatment of eating disorders.

EVALUATING BODY WEIGHT AND BODY COMPOSITION

There are different methods for measuring and evaluating the health risks associated with body weight and body composition. First, let's look at the concept of body composition in more detail.

Body Composition

The human body can be divided into fat-free mass and body fat. Fat-free mass is composed of all the body's nonfat tissues: bone, water, muscle, connective tissue, organ tissues, and teeth.

A certain amount of body fat is necessary for the body to function. Fat is incorporated into the nerves, brain, heart, lungs, liver, mammary glands, and other body organs and tissues. It is the main source of stored energy in the body. It also cushions body organs and helps regulate body temperature. This **essential fat** makes up about 3–5% of total body weight in men and about 8–12% in women. The percentage is higher in women due to such factors as fat deposits in the breasts and uterus.

Most of the fat in the body is stored in fat cells, or **adipose tissue,** located under the skin (**subcutaneous fat**) and around major organs (**visceral fat** or *intra-abdominal fat*). People have a genetically determined number of fat cells, but these cells can increase or decrease in size depending on how much fat is being stored. The amount of stored fat depends on several factors, including age, sex, metabolism, diet, and activity level. The primary source of stored body fat comes from excess calories consumed in the diet—that is, calories consumed in excess of calories expended in metabolism, physical activity, and exercise. These factors are discussed in detail in the next section.

When looking at body composition, one important consideration is the proportion of the body's total weight that is

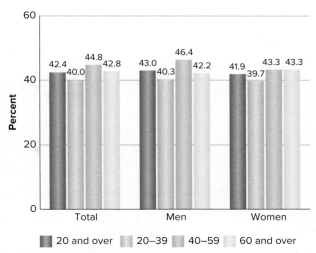

FIGURE 15.1 Prevalence of obesity and severe obesity among adults: United States, 2017–2018.

SOURCE: Hales, C. M., et al. 2020. NCHS Data Brief No. 360. Hyattsville, MD: National Center for Health Statistics.

fat—the **percent body fat.** For example, two women of the same height and weight may differ widely in percent body fat. If one has 19% body fat and the other 34% body fat, only the second woman's body composition will be considered unhealthy. A higher-than-healthy proportion of body fat is called overfat. Assessment methods based on body weight alone are less accurate than those based on body fat, but they are commonly used because body weight is easier to measure than body fat.

Defining Healthy Weight, Overweight, and Obesity

Many people struggle with body dissatisfaction and are concerned about their weight. But how do you decide if you are at a healthy weight? How thin is too thin, and at what point does being overweight present a health risk?

Overweight is defined as total body weight above the recommended range for good health, as determined by large-scale

---

essential fat Fat incorporated in various tissues of the body; critical for normal body functioning. **TERMS**

adipose tissue Connective tissue in which fat is stored.

subcutaneous fat Fat located under the skin.

visceral fat Fat located around major organs; also called *intra-abdominal fat.*

percent body fat The percentage of total body weight that is composed of fat.

overweight Body weight above the recommended range for good health.

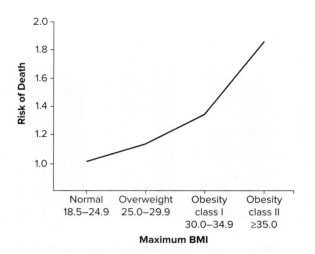

FIGURE 15.2 Weight history and all-cause mortality. Researchers followed more than 200,000 adults for 16 years and examined the relationship between an individual's maximum BMI over the period and subsequent mortality. A maximum BMI above the normal category was associated with an excess risk of death that increased with increasing BMI.

SOURCE: Yu, E., et al. 2017. Weight history and all-cause and cause-specific mortality in three prospective cohort studies. *Annals of Internal Medicine* 166(9): 613–620.

population surveys. **Obesity** is a more serious degree of overweight that carries multiple health risks, including a shorter life span (Figure 15.2). Both terms are used to identify weight ranges that are associated with increased likelihood of certain health problems.

Several methods can be used to measure and evaluate body weight and percent body fat. These assessments can give you information about the health risks associated with your current body weight and body composition. They can also help you establish reasonable goals and set a starting point for current and future decisions about weight loss and weight gain. We explore three methods used to determine how your current weight might be affecting your health. These methods are body composition, body mass index (BMI), and body fat distribution.

Estimating Body Composition

Methods for determining percent body fat provide only an estimate of the amount of body fat (or adipose tissue) and the amount of lean body mass (or lean tissue) you have. The margin of error for these methods can range from 3% to more than 20%. Margin of error means that, for example, if your

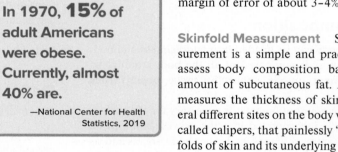

QUICK STATS

In 1970, **15%** of adult Americans were obese. Currently, almost **40%** are.

—National Center for Health Statistics, 2019

skinfold measurements were taken accurately and estimate that you have 20% body fat, the actual value could be as low as 17% or as high as 23% body fat. Because the value actually represents a range, these results should not be the only ones used to assess your health status.

As a reference, on average, women have about 10–12% more body fat than men. A healthy body fat range for men is considered to be about 12–20%, and for women, about 20–30%. Men with more than 25% body fat are considered obese, as are women with more than 33% body fat. Keep in mind that no matter which method of body composition analysis is used, the measurements should be performed by someone with appropriate training to ensure accuracy.

Bioelectrical Impedance Analysis (BIA) In this method, a person stands barefoot on a machine that resembles a scale, uses a handheld machine, or lies down with spot electrodes attached at various points on the body that are also connected to a bioelectrical machine. A very low level of electrical current is sent between electrodes through the body. Percent body fat is calculated from the measurements of resistance to the current. One disadvantage to this method is that, for the most accurate results, the person being tested must have followed the suggested guidelines for food and fluid intake, as well as restrictions on exercise prior to the test. BIA can estimate your body fat within a margin of error of about 3–4%.

Skinfold Measurement Skinfold measurement is a simple and practical way to assess body composition based on the amount of subcutaneous fat. A technician measures the thickness of skinfolds at several different sites on the body with a device, called calipers, that painlessly "pinches" the folds of skin and its underlying fat. The measurements are used in formulas that calculate body fat percentages. The accuracy of this method is highly dependent on

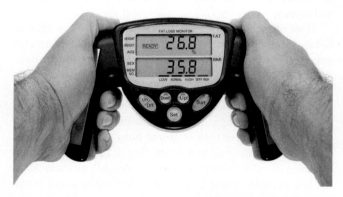

Bioelectrical impedance analysis calculates percent body fat by measuring resistance to a low level of electrical current. Lebazele/E+/Getty Images

> **obesity** Severe overweight, characterized by an excessive accumulation of body fat; may also be defined in terms of some measure of total body weight.
>
> TERMS

the expertise of the practitioner. When performed by a skilled technician, this method can estimate body fat within a 3–4% margin of error.

Scanning Procedures   High-tech scanning procedures are very accurate means of assessing body composition, but the costs are much higher compared to other methods. These procedures include computed tomography (CT), magnetic resonance imaging (MRI), dual-energy X-ray absorptiometry (DEXA), and dual-photon absorptiometry. Other procedures include near infrared reactance (Futrex 1100) and total body electrical conductivity (TOBEC). Considered to be very accurate, these techniques are generally offered only at medical or research facilities.

Body Mass Index

Body mass index (BMI) is a measure of body weight that is useful for estimating a person's weight status and for classifying the health risks of body weight if more sophisticated methods aren't available. BMI is based on the concept that weight should be proportional to height. Easy to calculate and rate, BMI is a fairly accurate measure of the health risks related to body weight for most average (nonathletic) people (see Table 15.1). BMI is correlated with body fat, but it does not directly measure body fat.

Calculating Your BMI   BMI is calculated by dividing your body weight (expressed in kilograms or pounds) by the square of your height (expressed in meters or inches). You can look up your BMI in the chart in Figure 15.3, or you can use the following formula to calculate it more precisely:

$$BMI = \frac{\text{weight in kg}}{(\text{height in meters})^2}$$

or $\frac{\text{weight in pounds}}{(\text{height in inches})^2} \times 703 \text{ (conversion factor)}$

Body weight status is categorized as underweight, healthy weight, overweight, or obese, compared with what is considered healthy for a given height. Under standards issued by the National Institutes of Health and adopted by the Dietary Guidelines for Americans, a BMI between 18.5 and 24.9 is considered healthy, a BMI of 25 or above is classified as overweight, and a BMI of 30 or above is classified as obese. A person with a BMI below 18.5 is classified as underweight, although low BMI values may be healthy in some cases if they are not the result of smoking, an eating disorder, or an underlying disease. A BMI of 17.5 or less is sometimes used as a diagnostic criterion for the eating disorder anorexia nervosa. For a more accurate assessment of health status, BMI is often combined with waist measurement (see Table 15.1);

body mass index (BMI)   A measure of relative body weight that takes height into account and is highly correlated with more direct measures of body fat; calculated by dividing total body weight (in kilograms) by the square of height (in meters).   **TERMS**

VITAL STATISTICS

| Table 15.1 | Body Mass Index (BMI) Classification and Disease Risk | | | |

| CLASSIFICATION | BMI (KG/M²) | OBESITY CLASS | DISEASE RISK RELATIVE TO NORMAL WEIGHT AND WAIST CIRCUMFERENCE[A] | |
			MEN ≤ 40 IN. (102 CM) WOMEN ≤ 35 IN. (88 CM)	>40 IN. (102 CM) >35 IN. (88 CM)
Underweight[b]	<18.5		—	—
Normal[c]	18.5–24.9		—	—
Overweight	25.0–29.9		Increased	High
Obese	30.0–34.9	I	High	Very high
	35.0–39.9	II	Very high	Very high
Extreme obesity	≥40.0	III	Extremely high	Extremely high

[a]Disease risk for type 2 diabetes, hypertension, and cardiovascular disease. The waist circumference cutoff points for increased risk are 40 inches (102 cm) for men and 35 inches (88 cm) for women.

[b]Research suggests that a low BMI can be healthy in some cases, as long as it is not the result of smoking, an eating disorder, or an underlying disease process. A BMI of 17.5 or less is sometimes used as a diagnostic criterion for the eating disorder anorexia nervosa.

[c]Increased waist circumference can also be a marker for increased risk, even in people of normal weight.

SOURCES: Adapted from National Heart, Lung, and Blood Institute. n.d. *Aim for a Healthy Weight: Classification of Overweight and Obesity by BMI, Waist Circumference, and Associated Disease Risks* (https://www.nhlbi.nih.gov/health/educational/lose_wt/BMI/bmi_dis.htm); U.S. Department of Health and Human Services, Centers for Disease Control and Prevention. *About BMI for Adults* (http://www.cdc.gov/healthyweight/assessing/bmi/adult_bmi/index.html#Athlete) 2020; Accessed March 26, 2020 National Heart, Lung, and Blood Institute. *Assessing Your Weight and Health Risk* (http://www.nhlbi.nih.gov/health/public/heart/obesity/lose_wt/risk.htm) Accessed March 26, 2020.

Category	<18.5 Underweight		18.5–24.9 Normal						25–29.9 Overweight					30–34.9 Obesity (Class I)					35–39.9 Obesity (Class II)					≥40 Extreme obesity
BMI	17	18	19	20	21	22	23	24	25	26	27	28	29	30	31	32	33	34	35	36	37	38	39	40
Height												Body Weight (pounds)												
4' 10"	81	86	91	96	101	105	110	115	120	124	129	134	139	144	148	153	158	163	168	172	177	182	187	192
4' 11"	84	89	94	99	104	109	114	119	124	129	134	139	144	149	154	159	163	168	173	178	183	188	193	198
5'	87	92	97	102	108	113	118	123	128	133	138	143	149	154	159	164	169	174	179	184	190	195	200	205
5' 1"	90	95	101	106	111	117	122	127	132	138	143	148	154	159	164	169	175	180	185	191	196	201	207	212
5' 2"	93	98	104	109	115	120	126	131	137	142	148	153	159	164	170	175	181	186	191	197	202	208	213	219
5' 3"	96	102	107	113	119	124	130	136	141	147	153	158	164	169	175	181	186	192	198	203	209	215	220	226
5' 4"	99	105	111	117	122	128	134	140	146	152	157	163	169	175	181	187	192	198	204	210	216	222	227	233
5' 5"	102	108	114	120	126	132	138	144	150	156	162	168	174	180	186	192	198	204	210	216	222	229	235	241
5' 6"	105	112	118	124	130	136	143	149	155	161	167	174	180	186	192	198	205	211	217	223	229	235	242	248
5' 7"	109	115	121	128	134	141	147	153	160	166	173	179	185	192	198	204	211	217	224	230	236	242	249	256
5' 8"	112	118	125	132	138	145	151	158	165	171	178	184	191	197	204	211	217	224	230	237	244	250	257	263
5' 9"	115	122	129	136	142	149	156	163	169	176	183	190	197	203	210	217	224	230	237	244	251	258	264	271
5' 10"	119	126	133	139	146	153	160	167	174	181	188	195	202	209	216	223	230	237	244	251	258	265	272	279
5' 11"	122	129	136	143	151	158	165	172	179	187	194	201	208	215	222	230	237	244	251	258	265	273	280	287
6'	125	133	140	148	155	162	170	177	184	192	199	207	214	221	229	236	243	251	258	266	273	280	288	295
6' 1"	129	137	144	152	159	167	174	182	190	197	205	212	220	228	235	243	250	258	265	273	281	288	296	303
6' 2"	132	140	148	156	164	171	179	187	195	203	210	218	226	234	242	249	257	265	273	281	288	296	304	312
6' 3"	136	144	152	160	168	176	184	192	200	208	216	224	232	240	248	256	264	272	280	288	296	304	312	320
6' 4"	140	148	156	164	173	181	189	197	206	214	222	230	238	247	255	263	271	280	288	296	304	312	321	329

FIGURE 15.3 Body mass index (BMI). To determine your BMI, find your height in the left column. Move across the appropriate row until you find the weight closest to your own. The number at the top of the column is the BMI at that height and weight.

SOURCES: U.S. Department of Health and Human Services and U.S. Department of Agriculture. 2015. *2015–2020 Dietary Guidelines for Americans*, 8th ed. (http://health.gov/dietaryguidelines/2015/guidelines). Accessed March 26, 2020.

as described in the next section, waist measurement provides an assessment of body fat distribution.

Limitations of BMI BMI is a valuable tool for assessing weight status, but it is not intended to determine body composition or track changes in body weight in relation to gains in muscle mass and loss of fat because BMI does not distinguish between fat weight and fat-free weight. It can also be inaccurate for some groups, including people shorter than 5 feet tall, muscular athletes, and older adults with little muscle mass due to inactivity or an underlying disease.

Body Fat Distribution

How is fat distributed throughout the body? The location of fat on your body is an important indicator of health, and it affects your risk for various diseases.

Two of the simplest methods for measuring body fat distribution are waist circumference measurement and waist-to-hip ratio calculation. In the first method, waist circumference is measured using a tape measure placed around your abdomen at the top of your hip bone. A waist circumference of greater than 40 inches (102 cm) for men or greater than 35 in (88 cm) for women is associated with an increased risk for chronic disease for most adults. In the second method, a mathematic formula (waist circumference divided by hip circumference) is used to find your waist-to-hip ratio. A waist-to-hip ratio above 0.94 for young men and above 0.82 for young women is associated with an increased risk of heart disease

and diabetes. More research is needed to determine the precise degree of risk associated with specific values for these two assessments of body fat distribution.

Men and postmenopausal women tend to store fat in the upper regions of their bodies, particularly in the abdominal area, as visceral fat. People with this *android* pattern of fat distribution are called apple shaped. Premenopausal women usually store fat in the hips, buttocks, and thighs, as subcutaneous fat. People with this *gynoid* pattern are called pear shaped.

Abdominal obesity increases the risk of high blood pressure, diabetes, early-onset heart disease, stroke, certain types of cancer, and mortality. This risk is independent of a person's BMI. Even people who have a BMI in the normal range may be at risk for diabetes, high blood pressure, and cardiovascular disease (CVD) if they have a large waist circumference, particularly if they have additional risk factors, such as high blood pressure. For example, a man with a BMI of 27 and a waist circumference above 40 inches is at greater risk for health problems than another man who has a BMI of 27 but has a smaller waist and no other risk factors. Abdominal obesity (as measured by waist circumference) is a primary component of metabolic syndrome and a forewarning of diabetes and heart disease.

Why is visceral fat more harmful than subcutaneous fat? The reason for the increased risk associated with abdominal obesity is that visceral fat is more easily mobilized and sent into the bloodstream, increasing disease-related blood fat levels. Visceral fat contains many biologically active substances such as inflammatory chemicals and growth factors, which can adhere to the lining of blood vessels, cause insulin resistance, and negatively affect cardiovascular health. Subcutaneous fat tends to be soft and flabby (whereas visceral fat is hard) and is not metabolically active the way visceral fat is.

What Is the Right Weight for You?

There are limits to the changes you can make to body weight and body shape, both of which are influenced by heredity. The changes that can and should be made are lifestyle changes, as described throughout this chapter.

To answer the question of what you should weigh, assess your health and body composition status and let your lifestyle be your guide. As described in Chapter 13, the *Dietary Guidelines for Americans 2015–2020* recommends that adults who are obese or overweight and have additional CVD risk factors should change their eating and physical activity behaviors to prevent additional weight gain and to promote weight loss. Instead of focusing on a particular weight, focus on living a lifestyle that includes following a healthy dietary pattern, getting plenty of exercise, thinking positively, and learning to cope with stress. Then let the pounds fall where they may. For many people, the result will be close to recommended weight ranges. For some, their weight will be somewhat higher than societal standards—but right for them. By letting a healthy lifestyle determine your weight, you can avoid developing unhealthy patterns of eating and a negative body image. Later in the chapter, we'll take a closer look at lifestyle recommendations for healthy weight management.

BODY FAT AND WELLNESS

The amount and distribution of fat in the body—both too much and too little—can have profound effects on health. Obesity doubles mortality rates and can reduce life expectancy by 10–20 years. In fact, if the current trends in overweight and obesity (and their related health problems) continue, some experts predict that the average American's life expectancy will soon decline by five years. However, very low levels of body fat can also be a threat to wellness. In this section, we explore both ends of the spectrum.

Compared with those of healthy weight, obese people have an increased risk of death from all causes. Obesity is associated with a number of chronic conditions such as diabetes, CVD, many kinds of cancer, impaired immune function, gallbladder and kidney diseases, skin problems, erectile dysfunction, sleep and breathing disorders, back pain, arthritis, and other bone and joint disorders. Obesity is also associated with complications of pregnancy, menstrual irregularities, urine leakage (stress incontinence), increased surgical risk, and psychological disorders and problems (such as depression, low self-esteem, and body dissatisfaction). Research has found that worldwide almost 3 million people die each year as a result of being overweight or obese.

In addition, studies show a decrease in the quality of life (measured by such things as self-image, bullying, bodily pain, quality of food intake, physical activity, and screen time) in overweight and obese children and adolescents compared to those of normal weight. It is also important to realize that small weight losses—5–10% of total body weight—can lead to significant health improvements. Current research finds that modest weight loss can increase quality of life for many individuals.

There is debate over the health risks for people who are overweight but not obese (BMI of 25–29), particularly for people who are overweight and physically active. These risks depend in part on an individual's overall health and other risk factors, such as high blood pressure, unhealthy cholesterol levels, body fat distribution, tobacco use, and level of physical activity.

Diabetes

According to the American Diabetes Association, more than 34 million Americans have one of the two major types of **diabetes mellitus,** a disease that disrupts normal metabolism. An estimated 1.5 million Americans are diagnosed with diabetes every year, and an estimated 88 million people 18 and older are believed to have prediabetes.

Obese people are more than three times as likely as nonobese people to develop type 2 diabetes, and the incidence of this disease among Americans has increased dramatically as the rate of obesity has climbed.

Diabetes involves a disruption in the process of metabolism. In normal metabolism, the pancreas secretes insulin, which stimulates cells to take up blood sugar (glucose) to produce energy (Figure 15.4). In diabetes, this process is disrupted, causing a buildup of glucose in the bloodstream. Diabetes is associated with kidney failure; nerve damage; circulation problems and amputations; retinal damage and blindness; and increased rates of heart attack, stroke, and hypertension. Diabetes is currently the seventh leading cause of death in the United States.

Types of Diabetes   About 1.6 million Americans have a form known as type 1 diabetes, a disease that usually begins in childhood or adolescence and is not related to obesity. The remaining people with diabetes have type 2 diabetes, a disease that is strongly associated with excess body fat. In type 1 diabetes, the body's immune system, triggered by a viral infection or some other environmental factor, destroys the insulin-producing cells in the pancreas. Little or no insulin is produced, so daily doses of insulin are required. In type 2 diabetes, the pancreas doesn't produce enough insulin, or

---

diabetes mellitus   A disease that disrupts normal metabolism, interfering with cells' ability to take in glucose for energy production.   **TERMS**

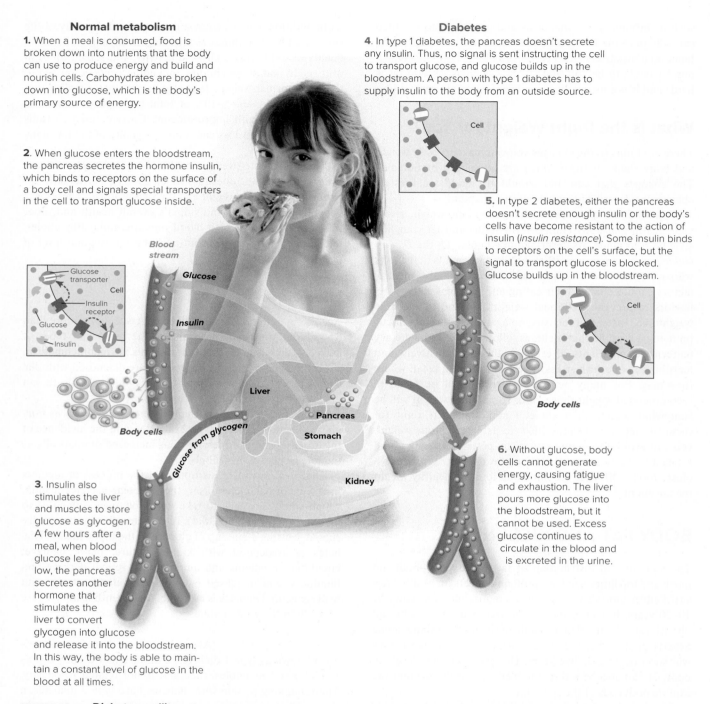

Normal metabolism

1. When a meal is consumed, food is broken down into nutrients that the body can use to produce energy and build and nourish cells. Carbohydrates are broken down into glucose, which is the body's primary source of energy.

2. When glucose enters the bloodstream, the pancreas secretes the hormone insulin, which binds to receptors on the surface of a body cell and signals special transporters in the cell to transport glucose inside.

Blood stream

Glucose transporter
Cell
Insulin receptor
Glucose
Insulin

Glucose

Insulin

Body cells

3. Insulin also stimulates the liver and muscles to store glucose as glycogen. A few hours after a meal, when blood glucose levels are low, the pancreas secretes another hormone that stimulates the liver to convert glycogen into glucose and release it into the bloodstream. In this way, the body is able to maintain a constant level of glucose in the blood at all times.

Glucose from glycogen

Liver

Pancreas

Stomach

Kidney

Diabetes

4. In type 1 diabetes, the pancreas doesn't secrete any insulin. Thus, no signal is sent instructing the cell to transport glucose, and glucose builds up in the bloodstream. A person with type 1 diabetes has to supply insulin to the body from an outside source.

Cell

5. In type 2 diabetes, either the pancreas doesn't secrete enough insulin or the body's cells have become resistant to the action of insulin (*insulin resistance*). Some insulin binds to receptors on the cell's surface, but the signal to transport glucose is blocked. Glucose builds up in the bloodstream.

Cell

Body cells

6. Without glucose, body cells cannot generate energy, causing fatigue and exhaustion. The liver pours more glucose into the bloodstream, but it cannot be used. Excess glucose continues to circulate in the blood and is excreted in the urine.

FIGURE 15.4 **Diabetes mellitus.** During digestion, carbohydrates are broken down in the small intestine into glucose, a simple sugar that enters the bloodstream. The presence of glucose signals the pancreas to release insulin, a hormone that helps cells take up glucose; once inside a cell, glucose can be converted to energy. In diabetes, this process is disrupted, resulting in a buildup of glucose in the bloodstream. webphotographeer/Getty Images

body cells are resistant to insulin (called *insulin resistance*), or both. About 25% of type 2 diabetics are unaware of their condition. About one-third of people with type 2 diabetes must take insulin; others may take medications that increase insulin production or stimulate the cells to take up glucose.

A third type of diabetes, called *gestational diabetes,* occurs in about 7% of women during pregnancy. The condition usually resolves after pregnancy, but about half of women who experience it eventually develop type 2 diabetes. *Prediabetes* is a condition in which blood sugar levels are higher than normal but not high enough for a diagnosis of full-blown diabetes. Nearly 85% of American adults with prediabetes don't even know they have it, and most will develop type 2 diabetes unless they adopt preventive lifestyle measures.

Warning Signs and Risk Factors   In the early stages, diabetes has no symptoms; possible warning signs include the following:

- Frequent urination
- Extreme hunger or thirst
- Unexplained weight loss
- Extreme fatigue
- Blurred vision
- Frequent infections
- Slow wound healing
- Tingling or numbness in the hands or feet
- Generalized dry skin and itching with no rash

The major risk factors for diabetes are age, obesity, physical inactivity, a family history of diabetes, and lifestyle. Race and ethnicity also play a role, with Native Americans, Alaska Natives, African Americans, and Hispanics having higher rates than Asian Americans and white Americans. Excess body fat reduces cell sensitivity to insulin, and insulin resistance is almost always a precursor of type 2 diabetes. More than 90% of people with type 2 diabetes are overweight or obese.

Screening involves a blood test to check glucose levels after either a period of fasting or the administration of a set dose of glucose. A fasting glucose level of 126 mg/dl or higher indicates diabetes; a level of 100–125 mg/dl indicates prediabetes. If you are concerned about your risk for diabetes, talk with your physician about being tested.

Prevention and Treatment   It is estimated that 90% of cases of type 2 diabetes could be prevented if people adopted healthy lifestyle behaviors. More than 40% of adults with type 2 diabetes are physically inactive, getting less than 10 minutes per week of physical activity. A moderate diet to control body fat and modest weight loss are also as important as exercise. Even a small amount of weight loss can be beneficial. For people with prediabetes, lifestyle measures are more effective than medication for delaying or preventing the development of diabetes. Exercise (endurance and/or strength training) makes cells more sensitive to insulin and helps stabilize blood glucose levels; it also helps keep body fat at healthy levels. Regular exercise and a healthy diet are often sufficient to control type 2 diabetes. There is no cure for diabetes, but it can be successfully managed by keeping blood sugar levels within safe limits through diet, exercise, and, if necessary, medication.

Heart Disease and Other Chronic Conditions

Obesity is one of the six major controllable risk factors for heart disease. Excess body fat is strongly associated with hypertension, unhealthy cholesterol and triglyceride levels, and impaired heart function. Many overweight and obese people—especially those who are sedentary and eat a poor diet—also suffer from a group of symptoms called *metabolic syndrome*. Symptoms include insulin resistance, high blood pressure, high blood glucose, unhealthy cholesterol levels, chronic inflammation, and abdominal fat. Metabolic syndrome increases the risk of heart disease, more so in men than in women (see Chapter 16 for more about metabolic syndrome).

Obesity is also a risk factor for certain types of cancer, including colon and rectal, breast, prostate, and ovarian cancer (see Chapter 17).

Problems Associated with Very Low Levels of Body Fat

Health experts have generally viewed very low levels of body fat—less than 8–12% for women and 3–5% for men—as a threat to wellness. Extreme leanness has been linked with reproductive, circulatory, and immune system disorders. Extremely lean people may experience muscle wasting and fatigue. They are also more likely to suffer from dangerous eating disorders.

In physically active women and girls, particularly those involved in sports where weight and appearance are important (ballet, gymnastics, skating, and distance running, for example), a condition called the **female athlete triad** may develop (Figure 15.5). The triad consists of three interrelated disorders: abnormal eating patterns (and excessive exercising), followed by **amenorrhea** (absence of menstruation), followed by

> **TERMS**
>
> **female athlete triad**   A condition consisting of three interrelated disorders: abnormal eating patterns (and excessive exercising) followed by lack of menstrual periods (amenorrhea) and decreased bone density (premature osteoporosis).
>
> **amenorrhea**   The absence of menstruation.

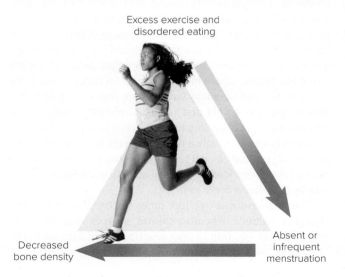

Excess exercise and disordered eating

Decreased bone density

Absent or infrequent menstruation

FIGURE 15.5   Female athlete triad. Some girls and women striving for unrealistic thinness develop a condition called the female athlete triad. Disordered eating combined with intense exercise can suppress the hormones that control the menstrual cycle, and absence of menstrual periods can lead to osteoporosis. *Alan Bailey/ Rubberball Productions/Getty Images*

decreased bone density (premature osteoporosis). Prolonged amenorrhea can cause bone density to erode to a point that a woman in her twenties will have the bone density of a woman in her sixties. Left untreated, the triad can lead to decreased physical performance, increased incidence of bone fractures, disturbances of heart rhythm and metabolism, and even death.

HOW DID I GET TO BE MY WEIGHT?

People vary in their ability to gain or lose weight. We all know someone who can eat large amounts of food without gaining weight while others will skip meals and never lose weight. Experts have developed theories and models that attempt to explain these individual variations. For decades we have heard that the best way to lose weight is through "energy balance" or "calories in, calories out." Drink a soda? Just jog off the calories. Exercise for an hour? Reward yourself with an ice cream sundae! But if the formula is so simple and easy to follow, why are so many of us obese or overweight and suffering a host of weight-related conditions?

In this section, we present several models that address factors complicating weight loss and maintenance, including the role of metabolism and hormonal responses to certain foods. Some factors are within our control, such as diet and exercise; genetic and environmental factors are not.

Energy Balance Model

Energy balance is the relationship between the amount of energy (calories) taken into the body through food and drink (energy in), and the amount of calories expended through metabolic and physical activity (energy out). If you burn the same amount of energy as you take in (a *neutral* energy balance), your weight can remain constant. The energy balance equation for many Americans today is tipped toward the energy-in side— a *positive energy balance* that promotes weight gain. This means that many people take in more calories than they expend. Even a very small positive energy balance can, over time, lead to significant gains in weight and fat. The opposite condition is a *negative energy balance*, which occurs when energy intake is less than energy use. To create a negative energy balance, the "calories in, calories out" model suggests you can burn more energy by increasing your level of physical activity and take in less energy by consuming fewer calories.

This model doesn't reflect other factors that may influence the balance. Specific calorie sources may promote weight gain in addition to their contribution of calories to the "energy in" side of the equation. For example, a portion of

> **energy balance**   A condition that occurs when energy intake equals energy expenditure; the key to achieving and maintaining a healthy body weight.   **TERMS**

unsalted nuts and a candy bar may have the same number of calories, but because the body absorbs fewer calories from nuts than from other foods, nuts do not cause much weight gain.

Carbohydrate-Insulin Model

In the carbohydrate-insulin model, the primary cause of obesity is overeating refined carbohydrates, which trigger an insulin response. When we eat processed food and other sugars that elevate insulin levels, the calories get trapped inside fat cells. Consequently, fewer calories remain available in the bloodstream, which makes us feel hungry and contributes to overeating. Insulin stimulates fat tissues to absorb glucose and also decreases the release of fatty acids from fat cells; it inhibits production of ketones in the liver and promotes fat and glycogen deposition. To put it simply: The problem is not overeating, but eating the wrong kind of calories, which expands fat tissue.

Multi-Factor Model

A third model puts less responsibility on your daily choices than the first two models. While it recognizes that fat accumulation does indeed depend on how much energy is consumed versus expended, the model suggests that obesity is a multifaceted problem that also includes genetic, metabolic, hormonal, psychological, cultural, and socioeconomic factors.

Genetic Factors   Scientists have so far identified more than 50 genes associated with obesity. Genes influence body size and shape, body fat distribution, and metabolic rate. Genetic factors also affect the ease with which weight is gained as a result of overeating and where on the body extra weight is added.

The *set-point theory* suggests that our bodies are designed to maintain a healthy and generally stable weight within a narrow range, or at a "set point," despite the variability in energy intake and expenditure. This theory is based on the idea that the rate at which our body burns calories adjusts according to the amount of food that we eat. Can we change our set point? It appears that when we maintain changes in our activity level and in our diets over a long period of time, our set point does change. Therefore, the set-point theory does not imply that we cannot maintain weight loss. However, physiological factors may make it easier to maintain a higher rather than a lower set point.

Fat Cells   The amount of fat (adipose tissue) the body can store is a function of the number and size of fat (adipose) cells, which is influenced by both genetic and lifestyle factors. Some people are born with an above-average number of fat cells and thus have the potential for storing more energy as body fat. Overeating at critical times, such as in childhood, can cause the body to create more fat cells. If a person loses weight, fat cell content is depleted, but the number of fat cells may not decrease. Fat tissue is not a passive form of energy storage; rather, fat cells send out chemical signals in order to be replenished. These signals affect multiple organs and systems, including those controlling appetite, metabolism, and immunity.

Metabolism　Metabolism is the sum of all the vital processes by which food energy and nutrients are made available to and used by the body. The largest component of metabolism, **resting metabolic rate (RMR)**, is the energy required to maintain vital body functions while the body is at rest, including respiration, heart rate, body temperature, and blood pressure. Resting metabolism (RMR) accounts for about 65–70% of daily energy expenditure. The energy required to digest food accounts for up to an additional 10% of daily energy expenditure. The remaining 20–30% is expended during physical activity.

Genetics affects metabolic rate. Men, who have a higher proportion of muscle mass than women, have a higher RMR because muscle tissue is more metabolically active than fat, requiring more energy to support its activities. A higher RMR means that a person burns more calories while at rest and can therefore take in more calories without gaining weight. Some individuals inherit a higher or lower RMR than others; RMR may vary by as much as 25% among same-weight individuals.

A number of factors reduce metabolic rate, making weight management challenging. Low-calorie intake and weight loss reduce RMR. When energy intake declines and weight is lost, the body responds by trying to conserve energy, reducing both RMR and the energy required to perform physical tasks. In essence, the body "defends" the original starting weight. Consider two people of the same size and activity level who both currently weigh 150 pounds, but one of whom used to weigh 170 pounds; the individual who lost weight will need to consume fewer calories to maintain the 150-pound weight than the person who had always been at that weight. This physiological response of the body points to the importance of preventing weight gain in the first place.

Exercise can have a modest positive effect on RMR. As described in Chapters 3 and 4, exercise temporarily raises RMR, and resistance training can increase muscle mass, which in turn boosts metabolism. In one recent study, a regular resistance training program increased RMR by an average of 5% in healthy adults. While relatively small, this degree of increase in RMR can still be helpful over the long term in maintaining a healthy weight. Resistance training may also protect against age-related declines in RMR.

Hormones　Hormones play a role in the accumulation of body fat, especially for women. Hormonal changes at puberty, during pregnancy, and at menopause contribute to the amount and location of fat accumulation. For example,

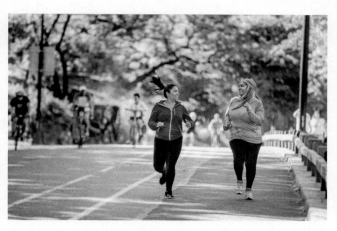

Regular physical activity is a key lifestyle strategy for weight loss and maintenance. LeoPatrizi/E+/Getty Images

during puberty, hormones cause the development of secondary sex characteristics such as larger breasts, wider hips, and added fat under the skin. This addition of body fat at puberty is normal and healthy.

In addition to insulin, two other hormones thought to be linked to obesity are leptin and ghrelin. Secreted by the body's fat cells, leptin is carried to the brain, where it appears to let the brain know how big or small the body's fat stores are. With this information, the brain can regulate appetite and metabolic rate accordingly. Leptin levels are higher in people who are obese, but obesity may cause the body to be less responsive to leptin's signals. Low-calorie diets may reduce leptin and cause an increase in appetite.

The hormone ghrelin, released by the stomach, is responsible for increasing appetite. Ghrelin levels go up before eating and down for approximately 3 hours after a meal. Together with leptin, ghrelin also has a role in regulating body weight. Adequate sleep and a diet high in whole grains and protein lower ghrelin levels.

Researchers hope to use leptin, ghrelin, and other hormones to develop treatments for obesity based on appetite control. As most of us will admit, however, feelings of hunger may often not be the primary reason we overeat.

Gut Microbiota　The human intestine houses millions of bacteria that form the intestinal flora (gut flora). These bacteria help digest the foods you eat, and they produce some vitamins, such as vitamin K. Studies show that lean people differ from overweight people in the composition of their intestinal flora,

QUICK STATS

Only 23% of U.S. adults meet the guidelines for both aerobic and muscle-strengthening activity.

—Centers for Disease Control and Prevention, 2019

TERMS

resting metabolic rate (RMR)　The energy required (in calories) to maintain vital body functions while the body is at rest, including respiration, heart rate, body temperature, and blood pressure.

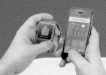

ASSESS YOURSELF
What Triggers Your Eating?

Hunger isn't the only reason people eat. Efforts to maintain a healthy body weight can be sabotaged by other factors, such as emotions, environment, and patterns of thinking. The following quiz is designed to provide you with a score for five factors that describe many people's eating habits. This information will put you in a better position to manage your eating behavior and control your weight. Circle the number that indicates to what degree each situation is likely to make you start eating.

Social

	VERY UNLIKELY									VERY LIKELY
1. Arguing or having a conflict with someone	1	2	3	4	5	6	7	8	9	10
2. Being with others when they are eating	1	2	3	4	5	6	7	8	9	10
3. Being urged to eat by someone else	1	2	3	4	5	6	7	8	9	10
4. Feeling inadequate around others	1	2	3	4	5	6	7	8	9	10

Emotional

5. Feeling bad, such as being anxious or depressed	1	2	3	4	5	6	7	8	9	10
6. Feeling good, happy, or relaxed	1	2	3	4	5	6	7	8	9	10
7. Feeling bored or having time on my hands	1	2	3	4	5	6	7	8	9	10
8. Feeling stressed or excited	1	2	3	4	5	6	7	8	9	10

Situational

9. Seeing an advertisement for food or eating	1	2	3	4	5	6	7	8	9	10
10. Passing by a bakery, cookie shop, or other enticement to eat	1	2	3	4	5	6	7	8	9	10
11. Being involved in a party, celebration, or special occasion	1	2	3	4	5	6	7	8	9	10
12. Eating out	1	2	3	4	5	6	7	8	9	10

Thinking

13. Making excuses to myself about why it's OK to eat	1	2	3	4	5	6	7	8	9	10
14. Berating myself for being fat or unable to control my eating	1	2	3	4	5	6	7	8	9	10
15. Worrying about others or about difficulties I'm having	1	2	3	4	5	6	7	8	9	10
16. Thinking about how things should or shouldn't be	1	2	3	4	5	6	7	8	9	10

Physiological

17. Experiencing pain or physical discomfort	1	2	3	4	5	6	7	8	9	10
18. Experiencing trembling, headache, or light-headedness associated with not eating or too much caffeine	1	2	3	4	5	6	7	8	9	10
19. Experiencing fatigue or feeling overtired	1	2	3	4	5	6	7	8	9	10
20. Experiencing hunger pangs or urges to eat, even though I've eaten recently	1	2	3	4	5	6	7	8	9	10

suggesting that intestinal flora may be involved in the development of obesity. Diets high in processed foods have been linked to less diverse intestinal microbiota. Such diets have also been linked to a higher proportion of bacteria types associated with increased energy absorption and hormonal changes that increase appetite—both factors that can contribute to obesity.

Psychology, Culture, and Behavior Many people have learned to use food as a means of coping with stress and

> **binge eating**   A pattern of eating in which normal food consumption is interrupted by episodes of high consumption.
>
> **TERMS**

negative emotions. Eating can provide a powerful distraction from difficult feelings—loneliness, anger, boredom, anxiety, shame, sadness, inadequacy. It can be used to combat low moods, low energy levels, and low self-esteem. (See the box "Assess Yourself: What Triggers Your Eating?") When eating becomes the primary means of regulating emotions, **binge eating** or other unhealthy eating patterns can develop.

A recent study shows a link between the misperception of weight and the condition of obesity. Teens who thought they weighed more or less than they actually did were more likely to engage in unhealthy eating behaviors, such as skipping meals. They were also more sedentary than those who accurately perceived their weight. Those who perceived themselves as obese or who were actually obese were the least likely to

Scoring

Total your scores for each category, and enter them below. Then rank the scores by marking the highest score 1, next highest score 2, and so on. Focus on the highest-ranked categories first, but any score above 24 is high and indicates that you need to work on that category.

Category	Total Score	Rank Order
Social (items 1–4)	_____	_____
Emotional (items 5–8)	_____	_____
Situational (items 9–12)	_____	_____
Thinking (items 13–16)	_____	_____
Physiological (items 17–20)	_____	_____

What Your Score Means

Social A high score here means you are very susceptible to the influence of others. Work on better ways to communicate more assertively, handle conflict, and manage anger. Challenge your beliefs about the need to be polite and the obligations you feel you must fulfill.

Emotional A high score here means you need to develop effective ways to cope with emotions. Work on developing skills in stress management, time management, and communication. Practicing positive but realistic self-talk can help you handle small daily upsets.

Situational A high score here means you are especially susceptible to external influences. Try to avoid external cues and respond differently to those you cannot avoid. Control your environment by changing the way you buy, store, cook, and serve food. Anticipate potential problems, and have a plan for handling them.

Thinking A high score here means that the way you think—how you talk to yourself, the beliefs you hold, your memories, and your expectations—has a powerful influence on your eating habits. Try to be less self-critical, less perfectionistic, and more flexible in your ideas about the way things ought to be. Recognize when you're making excuses or rationalizations that allow you to eat.

Physiological A high score here means that the way you eat, what you eat, or medications you are taking may be affecting your eating behavior. You may be eating to reduce physical arousal or deal with physical discomfort. Try eating three meals a day, supplemented with regular snacks if needed. Avoid too much caffeine. If any medication you're taking produces adverse physical reactions, switch to an alternative, if possible. If your medications may be affecting your hormone levels, discuss possible alternatives with your physician.

SOURCE: Adapted from Nash, Joyce D. "What Triggers Your Eating?" In *The New Maximize Your Body Potential*. Boulder, CO: Bull Publishing, 1997. Reprinted by permission.

exercise 60 minutes a day. One in four teens suffer from this misperception.

Obesity is strongly associated with socioeconomic status. The prevalence of obesity goes down as family income level goes up, especially among women and children. These differences may reflect greater access to unprocessed and low-calorie foods, to information about nutrition, and to physical activity among upper-income women. Upper-income women also may have acquired greater sensitivity and concern for a slim physical appearance. In contrast, the prevalence of obesity in some ethnic groups may reflect a greater acceptance of larger body types and different cultural values related to food choices in those groups. (See the box "Overweight and Obesity among U.S. Ethnic Populations.")

In some families and cultures, food is used as a symbol of love and caring. It is an integral part of social gatherings and celebrations. In such cases, it may be difficult to change established eating patterns because they are linked to cultural and family values.

Sleep In addition to diet and exercise habits, sleep is another health behavior that impacts weight management. Short sleep duration and sleep debt are associated with increased BMI and abdominal obesity, and researchers are still investigating how they might be linked. One possibility is that lack of sleep may affect hormone levels, appetite regulation, and metabolism. Short sleep duration is also associated with increased snacking and overall energy intake. Another factor is

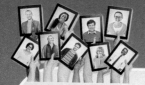

DIVERSITY MATTERS
Overweight and Obesity among U.S. Ethnic Populations

The prevalence of overweight and obesity is growing among all population groups in the United States. However, rates and trends vary by race and ethnicity and by other population characteristics:

- Certain groups, including African Americans, Latinos, and American Indians and Alaska Natives, have higher-than-average rates of obesity. Asian Americans have a low rate of obesity.

- The longer a foreign-born person lives in the United States, the more likely she or he is to become obese. BMI among immigrants begins to climb after about 10 years of U.S. residence, and after 15 years, it approaches the national average. This convergence may result from factors such as the availability of calorie-dense foods, less physical activity, and less time to prepare traditional meals.

- Cultural factors that influence dietary and exercise behaviors appear to play a role in the development of obesity. There are also cultural differences in acceptance of larger body size and in body image perception. For example, one study found that African Americans were more likely to think they were thinner than they really were, and whites were more likely to think they were fatter than they really were.

- The health consequences of obesity affect racial and ethnic populations in different ways. At a given level of BMI, Hispanics are significantly more likely to have type 2 diabetes than are non-Hispanic whites. Obesity in African

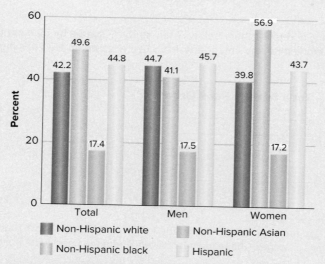

Prevalence of Obesity Among Adults: United States, 2017–2018

SOURCE: Hales, C. M., et al. 2020. NCHS Data Brief No. 360. National Health and Nutrition Examination Survey, 2017–2018 (https://www.cdc.gov/nchs/products/databriefs/db360.htm#fig1).

Americans is associated with increased risk of developing hypertension at a younger age and in a more severe form.

- For people of Asian descent, waist circumference is a better indicator of relative disease risk than BMI, and disease risk goes up at a lower level of BMI than for individuals of other groups. For Asian populations, World Health Organization (WHO) guidelines have a lower BMI cutoff for defining overweight (BMI $\geq$ 23 kg/m^2, compared to the general suggested cutoff of $\geq$ 25 kg/m^2); the same lower cutoff is recommended for diabetes screening by the American Diabetes Association.

- The prevalence of obesity differs among racial and ethnic groups in the United States in children as young as age

4 years. Obesity is twice as common in young American Indian/Native Alaskan children as it is in white and Asian American children, and obesity prevalence is higher in Hispanic and black children than it is in whites and Asian Americans. However, in some studies that controlled for family income, low socioeconomic status was a stronger predictor of obesity in children than was race/ethnicity.

- Fast-food restaurants are more prevalent in low-income areas compared with middle- to higher-income areas, and in areas with higher concentrations of racial/ethnic minority groups in comparison with whites. Higher BMIs may be associated with living in areas with increased exposure to fast food, although there is some debate about this hypothesis.

SOURCES: National Center for Health Statistics. 2016. *Health, United States, 2015: With Special Feature on Racial and Ethnic Health Disparities.* Hyattsville, MD: National Center for Health Statistics; Takeno, K., et al. 2016. Relationship between insulin sensitivity and metabolic abnormalities in Japanese men with BMI of 23–25 kg/m^2. *Journal of Clinical Endocrinology and Metabolism* 101(10): 3676-3684; Isasi, C. R., et al. 2015. Is acculturation related to obesity in Hispanic/Latino adults? Results from the Hispanic community health study/study of Latinos. *Journal of Obesity.* DOI: 10.1155/2015/186276; Rogers, R., et al. 2015. The relationship between childhood obesity, low socioeconomic status, and race/ethnicity. *Childhood Obesity* 11(6): 691–695; Mehta, N. K., et al. 2015. Obesity among U.S.- and foreign-born blacks by region of birth. *American Journal of Preventive Medicine* 49(2): 269–273.

Ask Yourself

QUESTIONS FOR CRITICAL THINKING AND REFLECTION

Is anyone in your family overweight? If so, can you identify factors that may contribute to this weight problem, such as heredity, eating patterns, or psychosocial factors? Has the person tried to address the problem? How is the issue handled in your family? Do family members help the situation or make it worse?

that use of multimedia devices may contribute to sleep deprivation and increase both energy intake and sedentary time. Getting adequate sleep is critical for overall wellness.

Food Marketing and Public Policy   The environment in which many Americans live and work can be "obesogenic"—meaning it encourages overconsumption of calories and discourages physical activity. This combination promotes weight gain rather than weight maintenance or loss. Food marketing and pricing, food production and distribution systems, and national agricultural policies all impact individual food choices.

The food industry promotes the sale of high-calorie processed foods at every turn. For example, vending machines offer mainly chocolate bars and unhealthy snacks, airlines offer complimentary soft drinks, and restaurants provide all-you-can-eat fried food buffets. Children are especially vulnerable to marketing that pushes ultra-processed foods high in sugar, salt, fat, and additives. Because they have a stronger preference for sweets than adults do, children are targeted from a young age and encouraged to make unhealthy choices.

Many experts observe that U.S. agricultural policy encourages farmers to produce corn and its by-product, high fructose corn syrup, at the expense of fruits and vegetables. As a result, over the past 30 years, the price of fruits and vegetables has risen much faster than the prices of other consumer goods, while the price of sugar, sweets, and carbonated drinks declined. Issues of price and availability of healthy food can have a profound effect on food choices. Low-income neighborhoods often have only fast-food venues offering high-calorie, highly processed foods.

Public policies can also have a positive influence. For example, the updated food labels and new regulations requiring chain restaurants and vending machine operators to post calorie information should help consumers make more informed choices. Other public health responses recommended by experts to support positive lifestyle choices for weight management include the following:

- Change food pricing to promote healthful options. For example, tax sugary beverages and offer incentives to farmers and food manufacturers to produce and market affordable healthy choices and smaller portion sizes.
- Limit advertising of unhealthy foods targeting children.
- Fund strategies to promote physical activity by creating more walkable communities, parks, and recreational facilities.

Rather than leaving all discussion to policy makers, public health experts are encouraging people to mobilize grassroots campaigns against the way food is currently distributed and marketed. Look around your community, school, and workplace: What aspects of the environment make it easier or more difficult to make healthy choices? What foods are available for purchase—and where and at what cost? Does the community environment and transportation system support walking or cycling, or is driving the only practical way to get around?

ADOPTING A HEALTHY LIFESTYLE FOR SUCCESSFUL WEIGHT MANAGEMENT

Are most weight problems lifestyle problems? Despite the growing prevalence of obesity in children and adolescents, many young adults get away with very unhealthy eating and exercise habits and don't develop a weight problem. But as the rapid growth of adolescence slows and school, family, and career obligations increase, maintaining a healthy weight becomes a greater challenge (see the box "The Freshman 15: Fact or Myth?"). Slow weight gain—just one or two pounds per year—is a major cause of overweight and obesity, so weight management is important for everyone, not just for people who are currently overweight. As you learned in the discussion of metabolism, it is easier to maintain a given weight than to maintain the same weight after weight loss, so avoiding slow weight gain is a critical goal for wellness.

A good time to develop a lifestyle for successful weight management is during your teens and early adulthood, when many behavior patterns form. Once established, it is important that you maintain healthy behaviors throughout life, including eating habits, level of physical activity, ability to think positively and manage your emotions effectively, and coping strategies you use to deal with the stresses and challenges in your life.

Dietary Patterns and Eating Habits

In contrast to *dieting,* which may involve some form of food restriction, a *diet* or *dietary pattern* refers to your daily food choices over the long term. Everyone has a diet, but not everyone is dieting. You need to develop a way of eating that you enjoy and that enables you to maintain a healthy body composition. Use the healthy dietary patterns recommended by the Dietary Guidelines for Americans, MyPlate, or the DASH Eating Plan as the basis for a healthy diet (see Chapter 13). For weight management, pay special attention to total calories, especially sugars, portion sizes, energy and nutrient density, and eating habits.

Total Calories   MyPlate suggests approximate daily energy needs based on gender, age, and activity level. However, individual energy balance may be a more important consideration for weight management than total calories consumed (refer back to Figure 15.6). Also, because of individual variations in RMR and other factors, your energy needs may differ from those estimated by MyPlate.

To maintain your current weight, the calories you eat must equal the number you burn, based on your personal energy balance. To lose weight, you must reduce your energy intake and/or increase the number of calories you burn; to gain weight, the reverse is true. If you choose to

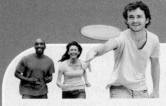

The Freshman 15: Fact or Myth?

According to popular belief, college students typically gain 15 pounds in their first year at school—the infamous "freshman 15." Is this the fate of all college students, or is it a myth that adds stress for body-conscious young adults?

In reality, the truth lies somewhere between these two scenarios. Many college freshmen gain weight, but usually not 15 pounds. More than 60% of college students gain an average of 7.5 pounds during their freshman year. Freshman men tend to gain more weight than women.

The reasons most often responsible for the weight gain include stress and a changed environment and lifestyle—newfound food independence, different eating habits, and social comparisons that come with the influence of roommates and friends. Another part of the transition from high school to university life is a drop in physical activity. Leaving high school has been associated with a decline both in moderate-vigorous physical activity and in diet quality. The unhealthy snacks widely available to college students, especially during times of higher stress such as the end of the semester, may also contribute.

Even small weight increases can pose a health risk or contribute to lower self-esteem. Changes in body composition—specifically, increased body fat—can become a troublesome pattern for students. Although men gain more weight than women, their weight gain involves less fat and more lean mass than women's weight gain. Even if they don't have a spike in weight during their first year, college-educated individuals tend to experience a moderate but steady weight gain during and after college.

More important, whether the weight gain is 5 pounds, 15 pounds, or even more, freshman weight gain is avoidable! In addition to the healthy eating strategies for college students described in Chapter 13, follow these tips and guidelines for avoiding freshman weight gain:

- Listen to your hunger cues, eating when you are hungry (and not for emotional reasons) and stopping when you are satisfied.

- Before you snack, ask yourself if you are really hungry or if you are eating out of stress, boredom, or anxiety.

- Watch portion sizes, and avoid second and third servings; many people underestimate portion sizes by up to 25%.

- Make healthy choices in the dining hall—if you are not sure what to eat, you can find a registered dietitian nutritionist (RDN) in the campus health center who will advise you.

- Avoid getting "too hungry"; don't go longer than 3–4 hours without eating.

- Plan ahead so that you have healthy snacks handy.

- Don't skip breakfast, and avoid late-night eating.

- Try not to drink your calories—limit high-calorie smoothies, coffee drinks, and alcoholic beverages.

SOURCES: Vadeboncoeur, C., N. Townsend, and C. Foster. 2015. A meta-analysis of weight gain in first year university students: Is freshman 15 a myth? *BMC Obesity* 2: 22; Eatright.org. 2019. 8 Ways to Beat the Freshman 15 (https://www.eatright.org/health/weight-loss/eating-out/8-ways-to-beat-the-freshman-15); Hootman, K. C., K. A. Guertin, and P. A. Cassano. 2018. Stress and psychological constructs related to eating behavior are associated with anthropometry and body composition in young adults. *Appetite* 125: 287–294; Winpenny, E. M., et al. 2020. Changes in physical activity, diet, and body weight across the education and employment transitions of early adulthood: A systematic review and meta-analysis. *Obesity Reviews* 21(4): e12962.

---

track calories, keep in mind that most people underestimate their energy intake and that energy needs change as body weight changes.

If weight loss is your goal, increase your physical activity and include strength and endurance training to build muscle mass and aerobic-type exercises to burn calories (see Chapter 14); this physical activity should be combined with moderate calorie reduction targeting added sugars, refined carbohydrates and other processed foods, and solid fats. A focus on calorie sources can be just as important as total energy intake for successful weight loss.

Maintaining weight loss may be more difficult than losing the weight. To maintain weight loss, you will need to maintain some degree of the calorie restriction you used to lose the weight (recall that RMR drops in response to calorie restriction and weight loss). Therefore, you need to adopt a practical level of food intake that provides all the essential nutrients and that you can live with over the long term.

Portion Sizes   Overconsumption of total calories is often tied closely to portion sizes. Many Americans are unaware that the portions of packaged foods and of foods served at restaurants have increased in size, and most of us significantly underestimate the amount of food we eat (Figure 15.6). Portion size is associated with body weight, so limiting portion sizes is critical for maintaining a healthy body weight. For many people, concentrating on portion sizes is easier than counting calories.

Quality of Food Choices: Energy (Calorie) Density and Nutrient Density   For successful weight management, be aware of both the number and the sources of calories you consume. Experts recommend that you pay attention to foods that are nutrient dense—that is, foods that are relatively low in calories but high in nutrients. For example, fresh fruits and vegetables and unprocessed whole-grain foods are low in calories and high in nutrients. Fresh

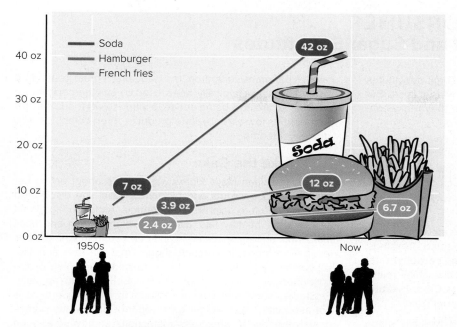

FIGURE 15.6 The new (ab)normal. Portion sizes have been growing. So have we. The average restaurant meal today is more than four times larger than in the 1950s. Adults today are, on average, 26 pounds heavier. To become healthier eaters, there are things we can do for ourselves and our community. Order the smaller meals on the menu, split a meal with a friend, or eat half and take the rest home. Ask the managers at favorite restaurants to offer smaller meals.

SOURCES: Centers for Disease Control and Prevention; for more information, visit http://MakingHealthEasier.org/TimeToScaleBack.

fruits contain fewer calories and more fiber than fruit juices. As you increase your consumption of foods high in nutrient density, you will want to decrease foods in your diet that are high in *energy density*. Energy density refers to the number of calories per ounce or gram of weight in a food. Ice cream, potato chips, croissants, crackers, and cakes and cookies are examples of foods high in energy density; in general, diets high in energy density are associated with higher rates of obesity. Foods that are low in energy density have more volume and bulk—that is, they are relatively heavy but have few calories, often due to high water and fiber content (Table 15.2). For example, for the same 100 calories, you could eat 21 baby carrots or 4 pretzel twists; you are more likely to feel full after eating the serving of carrots because it weighs 10 times as much as the serving of pretzels (10 ounces versus 1 ounce). Consuming foods low in energy density may reduce hunger and energy intake. When you do choose foods high in energy density, choose those with healthy fats, such as nuts, olives, and avocados; these foods have healthier overall nutrient profiles and usually aren't linked to weight gain.

Strategies for increasing the nutrient density of your diet while at the same time lowering its energy density include the following:

- Eat whole fruits with breakfast and for dessert.
- Add extra vegetables to sandwiches, casseroles, stir-fry dishes, pizza, pasta dishes, and fajitas.

- Start meals with a bowl of broth-based soup; include a green salad or fruit salad.
- Snack on fresh fruits and vegetables rather than crackers, chips, or other processed snack foods.
- Limit serving sizes of energy-dense foods such as butter, mayonnaise, cheese, fatty meats, croissants, and other sources of solid fats.
- Pay special attention to your beverage choices—many sweetened drinks are low in nutrients and high in calories from added sugar; for example, a can of regular soda may have more than 35 grams of added sugar but no other nutrients, while the same amount of low-fat milk has no added sugars and is rich in many essential nutrients.
- Limit processed foods, especially those high in added sugars and refined carbohydrates; these are usually energy dense, nutrient poor, and also high on the glycemic index, which may increase rather than reduce your appetite.

Processed foods labeled "fat-free" or "reduced fat" may be high in calories as well as high-glycemic-index refined carbohydrates; such products may also contain sugar and fat substitutes (see the box "Evaluating Fat and Sugar Substitutes"). Stick to the calorie and food pattern recommendations offered by the Dietary Guidelines for Americans, MyPlate, or the DASH Eating Plan (see Chapter 13).

Eating Habits Equally important to weight management is the habit of eating regular meals daily, including breakfast

Table 15.2	Examples of Foods Low in Energy Density	
FOOD	AMOUNT	CALORIES
Carrot, raw	1 medium	25
Popcorn, air popped	2 cups	62
Apple	1 medium	72
Vegetable soup	1 cup	72
Plain oatmeal	½ cup	80
Fresh blueberries	1 cup	80
Corn on the cob (plain)	1 ear	80
Cantaloupe	½ melon	95
Light (fat-free) yogurt with fruit	6 oz.	100
Unsweetened applesauce	1 cup	100
Pear	1 medium	100
Sweet potato, baked	1 medium	120

CRITICAL CONSUMER
Evaluating Fat and Sugar Substitutes

Foods made with fat and sugar substitutes are often promoted for weight loss. But what are fat and sugar substitutes? And can they really contribute to weight management?

Fat Substitutes

A variety of substances are used to replace fats in processed foods and other products. Some contribute calories, protein, fiber, or other nutrients; others do not. Fat replacers fall into three general categories:

- **Carbohydrate-based fat replacers.** These are often found in dairy and meat products, baked goods, salad dressings, and many other prepared foods. Adding carbohydrate-based fat replacers in these foods can successfully mimic the texture and taste of similar full-fat products. Carbohydrate-based fat replacers contribute 0–4 calories per gram.

- **Protein-based fat replacers.** These are typically made from milk, egg whites, soy, or whey; trade names include Simplesse, Dairy-lo, and Supro. They are used in cheese, sour cream, mayonnaise, margarine spreads, frozen desserts, salad dressings, and baked goods. Protein-based fat replacers typically contribute 1–4 calories per gram.

- **Fat-based fat replacers.** Some of these compounds are not absorbed well by the body and so provide fewer calories per gram (5 calories compared with the standard 9 for fats); others are impossible for the body to digest and so contribute no calories at all. Olestra, marketed under the trade name Olean and used in fried snack foods, is an example of the latter type of compound.

Nonnutritive Sweeteners and Sugar Alcohols

Sugar substitutes are often referred to as nonnutritive sweeteners because they provide only a few or no calories or essential nutrients. The U.S. Food and Drug Administration (FDA) has considered the following sweeteners safe for consumption: acesulfame-K (Sunett, Sweet One), advantame, aspartame (NutraSweet, Equal, Sugar Twin), Luo Han Guo fruit extracts (SGFE, Nectresse), saccharin (Sweet' N Low), steviol glycosides (Stevia, Truvia), sucralose (Splenda), and neotame. They are used in beverages, desserts, baked goods, yogurt, chewing gum, and products such as toothpaste, mouthwash, and cough syrup. Compared to table sugar, these high-intensity sweeteners are hundreds to thousands of times sweeter.

Sugar alcohols are made by altering the chemical form of sugars extracted from fruits and other plant sources; the best known of these is sorbitol. Sugar alcohols provide 0.2–2.5 calories per gram, compared to 4 calories per gram in standard sugar. They have typically been used to sweeten sugar-free candies but are now being added to many sweet foods that are promoted as low-carbohydrate products, often combined with other sweeteners.

Nuts Take the Cake

College freshman Maya Flores was worried about eating her favorite snack—walnuts and pistachios—until she discovered that it is difficult to gain weight from nuts. Although high in fat and calories, healthy fats, along with high protein and fiber, make nuts a filling snack and can keep you from eating other, less healthy foods. Researchers suggest that nuts have appetite-suppressing effects due to the increased production of the hormones peptide YY or cholecystokin. Both regulate appetite.

Studies show that consuming nuts in modest portions is not associated with weight gain, regardless of study participants' other dietary choices or restrictions; some studies even report that consuming nuts helps people to lose weight. One study of 65 overweight or obese people compared a low-calorie diet supplemented with almonds to a low-calorie diet supplemented with complex carbs. At the end of 24 weeks, those on the almond diet had a 62% greater reduction in weight and BMI, 50% greater reduction in waist circumference, and 56% greater reduction in fat mass.

Nut consumption has been connected with longevity and lower risk for heart disease, type 2 diabetes, metabolic syndrome, and certain cancers. Nuts are high in protein and fiber, nutrients such as magnesium, selenium, potassium, vitamins (E, K, and B-6), omega-3s, and antioxidants. Nuts are rich in unsaturated fats associated with heart health and disease prevention.

For the healthiest snack, choose nuts that are plain and unsalted.

Fat and Sugar Substitutes in Weight Management

Whether fat and sugar substitutes help you achieve and maintain a healthy weight depends on your overall eating and activity habits. The increase in the availability of fat-free and sugar-free foods in the United States has *not* been associated with a drop in calorie consumption. Reduced-fat foods often contain extra sugar to improve the taste and texture lost when fat is removed, so such foods may be as high or even higher in total calories than their fattier counterparts.

Finally, many of the foods containing fat and sugar substitutes are low-nutrient snack foods. Fruits, vegetables, and whole grains are healthier snack choices.

and snacks. Eating whole, unprocessed foods that are nutrient dense can help to fuel healthy metabolism, maintain muscle mass, and prevent between-meal hunger that often leads to unhealthy snacking. Intermittent fasting as an approach to weight loss has been tried for many years. Intermittent fasting aims to sync with a person's circadian rhythm and also extend their nighttime fasting period. Longer hours of nighttime fasting reduces evening eating, which is associated with a higher risk of obesity and diabetes. This extra fasting works to metabolic advantage as well as calorie reduction. The proposed longer-term benefits include weight loss, reduced blood pressure, lower inflammatory markers, reduced cancer risk, slower aging, and diabetes prevention.

In addition to establishing a regular pattern of eating, set some rules to govern your food choices. Balance your meals with whole grains, lean protein, fiber-rich fruits and vegetables, low-fat dairy, and moderate amounts of healthy fats. Rules for breakfast might be these, for example: Choose a high-fiber cereal that is low in added sugar with low-fat milk on most days; save pancakes and waffles for special occasions unless they are whole grain. Pay attention to portion sizes. Eating just enough, but not too much, helps to curb cravings and reduces chances of overeating.

Labeling some foods off-limits generally sets up a rule to be broken. A more sensible principle is "everything in moderation." A good goal is to eat in moderation; no foods need to be entirely off-limits, though some should be eaten judiciously.

Physical Activity and Exercise

Regular physical activity is another important lifestyle factor in weight management (see Chapter 14). It provides disease prevention benefits. It helps us sleep better, feel better, and perform daily tasks more easily. Physical activity and exercise burn calories and keep the metabolism geared to using food for energy instead of storing it as fat. Exercise has a positive effect on metabolism. When people exercise, they increase the number of calories their bodies burn at rest (resting metabolic rate). They also increase their muscle mass, which is associated with a higher metabolic rate. The exercise itself also burns calories, raising total energy expenditure. The higher the energy expenditure, the more the person can eat without gaining weight. So one of the most important reasons for exercising regularly is that it helps to maintain or increase your lean body mass and your metabolic rate. In contrast, energy restriction alone will cause a loss in lean body mass and a decrease in metabolic rate. Regular physical activity also improves cardiovascular and respiratory health, enhances mood, results in a higher quality of sleep, increases self-esteem, and gives us a sense of accomplishment. All these changes enhance our ability to engage in long-term healthful lifestyle behaviors.

The sooner you establish good habits, the better. The key to success is making exercise an integral part of the lifestyle you can enjoy now and in the future.

Thinking and Emotions

The way you think about yourself influences, and is influenced by, how you feel and how you act. In fact, research on people who struggle with their weight indicates that many of these individuals suffer from low self-esteem and the negative emotions that accompany it. Often people with low self-esteem mentally compare the actual self to an internally held picture of an "ideal self," an image based on perfectionistic goals and beliefs about how they and others should be. The more these two pictures differ, the larger the negative impact on self-esteem and the more likely the presence of negative emotions.

Besides the internal picture of ourselves, we all carry on an internal dialogue about events happening to us and around us. This *self-talk* can be self-deprecating or positively motivating, depending on our beliefs and attitudes (see Chapter 3). Having realistic beliefs and goals and practicing positive self-talk and problem solving support a healthy lifestyle.

Coping Strategies

Appropriate coping strategies help you deal with the stresses of life. They are also an important lifestyle factor in weight management. Many people use eating as a way to cope; others may cope by turning to drugs, alcohol, smoking, or gambling. Those who overeat might use food to alleviate loneliness or to serve as a pickup for fatigue, as an antidote to boredom, or as a distraction from problems. Some people even overeat to punish themselves for real or imagined transgressions.

Those who recognize that they are misusing food in such ways can analyze their eating habits with fresh eyes. They can consciously attempt to find new coping strategies and begin to use food appropriately—to fuel life's activities, to foster growth, and to bring pleasure, but *not* as a way to manage stress.

APPROACHES TO OVERCOMING A WEIGHT PROBLEM

Americans spend approximately $60 billion on weight loss efforts every year, including diet plans, diet products, and health club memberships. If you are overweight, you may already be creating a plan to lose weight and keep it off. You have many options (see the box "Lifestyle Strategies for Successful Weight Management").

Doing It Yourself

If you need to lose weight, focus on adopting the healthy lifestyle described throughout this book. The right weight for you will evolve naturally, and you won't have to diet. Combine modest cuts in energy intake with exercise, and avoid very-low-calorie diets.

Set Reasonable Goals   According to the Centers for Disease Control and Prevention, people who lose weight gradually (1–2 pounds weekly) and steadily are more successful at keeping weight off. Even modest weight loss improves blood sugar, cholesterol, and blood pressure levels. A reasonable weight loss for someone who is obese is 5–10% of body weight over six months. For example, for someone who weighs 200 pounds, a 5% weight loss equals 10 pounds, or reducing weight to 190 pounds. The person in this example may still be in the "overweight" or "obese" range, but this degree of weight loss can reduce the chronic disease risks related to obesity. Modest weight loss can also be easier to maintain. American Heart Association guidelines state that even smaller weight loss, in the 3–5% range, is beneficial if maintained. Relatively modest

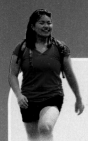

TAKE CHARGE
Lifestyle Strategies for Successful Weight Management

Food Choices

• Focus on making good choices from each food group, eating a variety of foods, and balancing your food intake with your energy expenditure.

• Select foods with high nutrient density, avoiding foods low in nutrient density.

• Limit calories in the form of sugar-sweetened beverages such as soda, fruit drinks, sports drinks, alcohol, and specialty coffees and teas.

• For very tempting high-calorie foods, try eating small amounts under controlled conditions. Go out for a scoop of ice cream, for example, rather than buying half a gallon for your freezer.

Planning and Serving

• Periodically monitor your calorie intake and compare this to your calorie expenditure—noting where your energy balance is. Do you need to exercise more? Eat less?

• Consume the majority of your calories during the day, not in the evening.

• Pay special attention to portion sizes. Use measuring cups and spoons and a food scale until you become familiar with appropriate portions.

• When you eat, just eat. Don't do anything else, such as reading, using the computer, or watching television.

• Eat slowly and stop eating when you are satisfied. It takes time for your brain to get the message that your stomach is full. Take small bites, chew thoroughly, and enjoy your food.

Special Occasions

• When you eat out, choose a restaurant where you can make healthy food choices. If portion sizes are large, share with a friend, or take half your food home for a later meal.

• Focus on the occasion and the people, not the food.

• If you cook a large meal for friends, send leftovers home with your guests or freeze them for later.

Physical Activity and Stress Management

• Engage in at least 150 minutes of moderate-intensity aerobic activity each week and muscle-strengthening activities on two or more days a week.

• Limit sedentary and screen time; get up and move around frequently while engaged in sedentary tasks.

• Try to get 8 hours of sleep a night.

• Develop techniques for handling stress that don't involve food. (See Chapter 2 for more about stress management.)

• Develop strategies for coping with nonhunger cues to eat, such as boredom, sleepiness, or anxiety. Try calling a friend, taking a shower, or going for a short walk.

• Tell family members and friends that you're changing your eating and exercise habits. Ask them to be supportive.

---

weight loss—and the lifestyle change used to achieve and maintain it—is likely to improve blood pressure as well as to improve blood lipids (reduce total and LDL cholesterol, lower triglycerides, and raise HDL cholesterol) and improve glucose levels and the risk for diabetes and heart disease.

Don't try to lose weight more rapidly than 0.5–2.0 pounds per week, which will require a negative energy balance of at least 250–1000 calories per day. Rapid weight loss not only relies on dramatic and unsustainable strategies like dehydration and extreme food restrictions, but it can also result in immediate and longer-term health problems, such as decreased bone formation.

Ask Yourself

QUESTIONS FOR CRITICAL THINKING AND REFLECTION

Have you ever used food as an escape when you were stressed out or distraught? Were you aware of what you were doing at the time? How can you avoid using food as a coping mechanism in the future?

A pound of body fat represents 3500 calories, meaning a negative energy balance of that amount over time should result in a loss of 1 pound of body weight. Although that may be true at the start of a diet, as described earlier in the chapter, because of physiological changes, as you reduce energy intake and lose weight, a greater negative calorie balance is needed to compensate for reductions in metabolism. In general, a low-calorie diet should provide at least 1200–1500 calories per day. The National Institutes of Health has a body weight planning tool that provides individual energy intake estimates for reaching a goal weight within a specific time period and to maintain it afterward (https://www.niddk.nih.gov/health-information/weight-management/body-weight-planner). Your individual energy balance may differ, but the tool can provide a starting point for planning, as well as a reality check on your goals.

Most low-calorie diets cause a rapid loss of body water at first. When this phase passes, weight loss declines. As a result, dieters are often misled into believing that their efforts are not working. They then give up, not realizing that smaller, mostly fat, losses later in the diet are actually better than the initial larger, mostly fluid losses.

Develop a Plan For many people, maintaining weight loss is a bigger challenge than losing weight. Most weight lost during a period of dieting is regained because the new diet and exercise routines require a new lifestyle. When you are planning a weight management program, it is extremely important to include strategies that you can maintain over the long term, both for food choices and for physical activity. Weight management is a lifelong project. A registered dietitian nutritionist (RDN) can recommend an appropriate plan. For more tips, refer to the Behavior Change Strategy section at the end of the chapter.

Diet Books, Websites, and Social Media Programs

Many people who try to lose weight by themselves fall prey to one or more of the hundreds of diet books, websites, and social media programs on the market. Although some contain useful advice and motivational tips, most make empty promises. Accept weight loss programs that advocate a balanced approach to diet plus exercise and sound nutritional advice, but reject any book that does the following:

- Advocates an unbalanced way of eating, such as a high-carbohydrate-only diet or a very-low-carbohydrate, high-protein diet, or that promotes a single food, such as cabbage or grapefruit

- Claims to be based on a "scientific breakthrough" or to have the "secret to success"

- Uses gimmicks, such as matching eating to blood type, hyping insulin resistance as the single cause of obesity, or combining foods in special ways to achieve weight loss

- Promises quick weight loss or severely limits food choices

Many diets can cause weight loss in the short term; however, the real difficulty is finding a safe and healthy pattern of food choices and physical activity that results in long-term maintenance of a healthy body weight and reduced risk of chronic disease (see the box "Are All Calories and Dietary Patterns Equal for Weight Loss?")

Dietary Supplements and Diet Aids

The number of dietary supplements and other weight loss aids on the market has also increased in recent years. Promoted in advertisements, magazines, direct mail, infomercials, blogs, websites, and social media, these products typically promise a quick and easy path to weight loss. Most of these products are marketed as dietary supplements and so are subject to fewer regulations than over-the-counter (OTC) medications. According to the Federal Trade Commission, more than half of advertisements for weight loss products make representations that are likely to be false. And although the FTC will order companies to stop making baseless and bogus product claims when monitors become aware of them, consumers are urged to critically evaluate any product that sounds too good to be true.

The following sections describe some commonly marketed OTC products for weight loss.

Formula Drinks and Food Bars Canned diet drinks, powders used to make shakes, and diet food bars and snacks are designed to achieve weight loss by substituting for some or all of a person's daily food intake. However, most people find it difficult to use these products for an extended period. Use of such products sometimes results in rapid short-term weight loss, but the weight is typically regained because users don't learn to change their eating and lifestyle behaviors.

Herbal Supplements Most herbal weight loss products work by increasing urination (causing water loss); by stimulating the central nervous system (causing body activities to speed up or metabolism to increase); or by affecting levels of brain chemicals (causing appetite suppression). As described in Chapter 13, herbs are marketed as dietary supplements, so little information is available about effectiveness, proper dosage, drug interactions, or side effects. In addition, labels may not accurately reflect the ingredients and dosages present, and safe manufacturing practices are not guaranteed.

Some of the more popular herbal stimulants on the market today are described in Table 15.3.

Other Supplements Fiber is another common ingredient in OTC diet aids, promoted for appetite control. Many diet aids contain only 3 or fewer grams of fiber, which does not contribute much toward the recommended daily intake of 25–38 grams. Other popular dietary supplements include chitosan, chromium picolinate, conjugated linoleic acid, glucomannan, carnitine, green tea extract, pyruvate, garcinia cambogia, caffeine, calcium, vitamin D, and a number of products labeled "fat absorbers," "fat blockers," and "starch blockers." The efficacy and safety of common ingredients in weight loss dietary supplements is reviewed on the Office of Dietary Supplements for Weight Loss web page (https://ods.od.nih.gov/factsheets/WeightLoss-Consumer/). Research has found most of these products to be ineffective, and many have adverse side effects.

Weight Loss Programs

Weight loss programs come in a variety of types, including noncommercial support organizations, commercial programs, websites, and clinical programs. According to the NIH, safe and effective weight loss programs should include the following:

- Healthy eating plans that reduce calories but do not exclude specific foods or food groups

- Tips on ways to increase moderate-intensity physical activity

- Information about how to get enough sleep, manage stress, and understand the pluses and minuses of weight loss medication

CRITICAL CONSUMER
Are All Calories and Dietary Patterns Equal for Weight Loss?

Many popular diets are promoted as the weight loss answer for all, but researchers continue to investigate the complex web of factors that influence the success or failure of efforts to lose weight and maintain that loss over time. Most researchers agree that total calorie intake is important, but preliminary evidence suggests some specific foods and eating patterns may help improve the odds for people trying to manage their weight.

Dietary Composition: Balance of Protein, Carbohydrates, and Fats

Scientists are investigating whether particular patterns of macronutrient intake (e.g., higher protein, lower fat, or lower carbohydrate) are better for weight loss, for weight loss maintenance, and for improving health markers such as blood fat levels. How might macronutrient balance impact weight management? Two possible areas of influence are appetite and resting metabolic rate (RMR).

Eating foods high in protein tends to make people feel fuller than eating foods high in fat or carbohydrate. This increase in satiety may help people refrain from overeating, thereby managing overall energy intake. Foods high in simple sugars and refined carbohydrates may cause an increase in appetite due to swings in the level of insulin.

A key challenge for weight loss maintenance is the drop in RMR that follows weight loss. In some small, short-term studies, researchers compared the impact on RMR following weight loss associated with low-fat, low-glycemic-index, and low-carbohydrate dietary patterns. On average, the low-carbohydrate dietary pattern showed the smallest reduction in RMR. However, additional studies are needed to confirm the findings and determine their importance over a longer time period. An additional challenge is that extreme shifts in macronutrient balance are difficult for people to maintain over time.

Researchers studying the impact of dietary composition over the long term have not found significant differences. A study comparing weight loss among adults assigned to one of four reduced-calorie diets differing in percentages of protein, carbohydrate, and fat found that weight loss at two years was similar for all four diets (about nine pounds). Weight loss was strongly associated with attendance at group sessions. Other studies have also found little difference in weight loss among popular reduced-calorie diets; most resulted in modest weight loss and reduced heart disease risk factors. The more closely people adhered to each diet, the more weight they lost. The American Heart Association notes that many dietary patterns can produce weight loss, and their latest guidelines list more than 15 dietary approaches that can lead to weight loss if calories are reduced.

An interesting finding of multiple weight loss and weight-maintenance studies is that different people seem to respond differently to different diets. So, for example, on a diet with a given balance of protein, carbohydrates, and fats, some people experience much greater weight loss than others. Similarly, changes in RMR after weight loss on different diets also vary. These findings point to individual differences in the factors affecting weight management—genetics, metabolism, hormones, intestinal flora. Thus, there is no single best diet for everyone. Researchers are looking to identify methods of matching people to an approach likely to be effective, but in the meantime, people can experiment with different dietary patterns to see what works best for them.

- Interaction and feedback from specialists to help you stick with healthier eating and physical activity

- A plan to monitor your own progress—keeping food journals and activity records

- Tips on healthy habits that also keep your cultural needs in mind, such as lower-fat versions of your favorite foods

- Slow and steady weight loss; depending on your starting weight, experts recommend losing weight at a rate of 0.5–2.0 pounds per week

- A recommendation for medical evaluation and care if you have health problems, are taking medication, or are planning to follow a special formula diet that requires monitoring by a doctor

- A plan to keep the weight off after you have lost it

QUICK STATS

A 16-ounce whole-milk latte has **265 calories;** beverages can have a significant impact on calorie intake.

—CDC, "Rethink Your Drink," 2020

Noncommercial Weight Loss Programs Noncommercial programs such as TOPS (Take Off Pounds Sensibly) and Overeaters Anonymous (OA) mainly provide group support. They do not advocate any particular diet but do recommend seeking professional advice for creating an individualized plan.

Like Alcoholics Anonymous, OA is a 12-step program with a spiritual orientation that promotes abstinence from compulsive overeating. These types of programs are generally free. Your physician or an RDN can also provide information and support for weight loss.

Commercial Weight Loss Programs Commercial weight loss programs typically provide group support, nutrition education, physical activity recommendations, and behavior modification advice. Some also make available packaged foods to assist in following dietary advice.

Quality Food Choices in Healthy Dietary Patterns

There is little evidence that dietary macronutrient composition affects the amount and duration of weight loss. What is clear is that the typical American dietary pattern—high in sugary beverages, refined carbohydrates, red meat, and solid fats—is associated with obesity. For weight loss, choose high-quality calorie sources in a healthier dietary pattern; refer back to the patterns and food choices recommended in Chapter 13. Remember that there is more to foods than just energy! Focus on diet quality by consuming high-quality calorie sources, whatever dietary composition you choose. Nutrient-dense foods can help with both weight management and chronic disease prevention:

- **Choose often:** unprocessed whole grains; a variety of vegetables from different MyPlate subgroups (e.g., don't overconsume potatoes, which have a high glycemic index); whole fruits; beans, fish, nuts, seeds, and other healthy protein sources; and plant oils.

- **Limit:** sugar-sweetened beverages, refined grains and sweets, red and processed meats, and solid fats (replace with plant oils and not with processed grains).

To reduce calorie intake, start by cutting empty calories from sugar-sweetened beverages and the processed foods that many Americans typically overeat. For some people, reducing sugar may be more effective than focusing on fats.

Weight Loss Maintenance: Clues from the National Weight Control Registry

Important lessons can be drawn from the National Weight Control Registry—an ongoing study of people who have lost significant amounts of weight and kept it off. The average participant in the registry has lost 71 pounds and kept the weight off for more than five years. Nearly all participants use a combination of diet and exercise to manage their weight. Common strategies include eating breakfast, self-monitoring weight and food intake, and getting regular exercise of about one hour per day. The most common dietary pattern used by registry participants was low-fat/high-carbohydrate. Greater weight regain in this group of individuals comes as a result of decreases in physical activity, having less dietary restraint, less individual monitoring of body weight, and increases in percentage of energy intake from fat. This study illustrates that to lose weight and keep it off, you must decrease daily calorie intake and/or increase daily physical activity—and continue to do so over your lifetime. Make sure your diet contains high-quality, nutrient-dense foods and that it is a pattern that you can maintain over the long term.

SOURCES: Hall, K. D., et al. 2016. Energy expenditure and body composition changes after an isocaloric ketogenic diet in overweight and obese men. *American Journal of Clinical Nutrition* 104(2): 324–333; Ebeling, C. B., et al. 2012. Effects of dietary composition on energy expenditure during weight-loss maintenance. *Journal of the American Medical Association* 307(24): 2627–2634; M. D. Jensen, et al. 2014. AHA/ACC/TOC guideline for the management of overweight and obesity in adults: A report of the American College of Cardiology/American Heart Association Task Force on Practice Guidelines and the Obesity Society. *Circulation* 129(25 Suppl. 2): S102–S138; Thomas, J. G., et al. 2014. Weight-loss maintenance for 10 years in the National Weight Control Registry. *American Journal of Preventive Medicine* 46(1): 17–23; U.S. Department of Health and Human Services and U.S. Department of Agriculture. 2015. *2015–2020 Dietary Guidelines for Americans,* 8th ed. (http://health.gov/dietaryguidelines/2015/guidelines); Seid H., M. Rosenbaum. 2019. Low carbohydrate and low-fat diets: What we don't know and why we should know it. *Nutrients* 11(11): 2749. Nutrition.gov. Interested in losing weight? (https://www.nutrition.gov/weight-management/strategies-success/interested-losing-weight), Accessed March 28, 2020.

In addition to the features of a safe and effective program outlined earlier, commercial weight loss programs should provide information about all fees and costs, including those of supplements and prepackaged foods, as well as data on risks and expected outcomes of participating in the program. They should also have a registered dietitian on staff along with qualified counselors and health professionals.

Weight Watchers is one of the best-known commercial weight loss programs. This program utilizes a point budget system considered by many as an easy tool for a person whose goal is to lose weight over time and to maintain the weight loss.

A strong commitment and a plan for maintenance are especially important because only about 10–15% of program participants maintain their weight loss—the rest gain back all or more than they had lost. Important predictors of weight loss and maintenance of weight loss in commercial programs include daily self-monitoring; an increased intake of vegetables, fruit, and low-fat dairy products; decreased intake of sweets; regular exercise; and adequate water consumption. Whereas regular exercise predicts maintaining weight loss, frequent television viewing predicts weight gain.

Ask Yourself

QUESTIONS FOR CRITICAL THINKING AND REFLECTION

Why do you think people continue to buy into fad diets and weight loss gimmicks, even though they are constantly reminded that the key to weight management is lifestyle change? Have you ever tried a fad diet or weight loss supplement? If so, what were your reasons for trying it? What were the results?

Table 15.3	Safety and Effectiveness of Common Over-the-Counter Weight Loss Pills		
INGREDIENT	PROPOSED MECHANISM OF ACTION	EVIDENCE OF EFFICACY	REPORTED ADVERSE EFFECTS
Alli (OTC form of orlistat)	Decreases absorption of dietary fat	Possible modest benefit; less effective than prescription strength form (Xenical)	Loose stools, gas with oily spotting, more frequent and hard to control bowel movements; reduced absorption of some nutrients; rare cases of liver damage
Bitter orange (synephrine)	Increased energy expenditure, mild appetite suppressant	Possible effect on resting metabolic rate; inconclusive effects on weight loss	Chest pain, anxiety, increased blood pressure and heart rate
Caffeine (as added caffeine or from guarana, kola nut, yerba mate, or other herbs)	Stimulates central nervous system, increases fat oxidation	Possible modest effect on body weight or decreased weight gain over time	Nervousness, jitteriness, vomiting, and tachycardia
Chitosan	Binds dietary fat in the digestive tract	Minimal effect on body weight	Bloating, flatulence, indigestion, constipation, nausea, heartburn
Chromium	Increases lean muscle mass; promotes fat loss; reduced hunger and fat cravings	Minimal effect on body weight and body fat	Headache, watery stools, constipation, weakness, vertigo, nausea, vomiting, hives
Conjugated linoleic acid	Promotes reduction in fat cells	Minimal effect on body weight and body fat	Abdominal pain, constipation, diarrhea, indigestion, and (possibly) adverse effects on blood lipid levels
Green tea extract	Increases energy expenditure and fat use, reduces fat absorption	Possible modest effect on body weight	Abdominal pain, constipation, nausea, increased blood pressure, liver damage
Guar gum	Acts as bulking agent in the gut, increases feelings of fullness	No effect on body weight	Abdominal pain, flatulence, diarrhea, nausea, cramps
Hoodia	Suppresses appetite, reduces food intake	Limited research, but no apparent effect on energy intake or body weight	Headache, dizziness, nausea, and vomiting
Pyruate	Increases fat burning and energy expenditure	Possible minimal effect on body weight and body fat	Diarrhea, gas, bloating, and (possibly) decreased "good" cholesterol (HDL).
Raspberry ketone	Alters fat metabolism	Insufficient research to draw firm conclusions	None known

SOURCE: Adapted from National Institutes of Health, Office of Dietary Supplements. 2020. *Dietary Supplements for Weight Loss: Fact Sheet for Health Professionals*, (http://ods.od.nih.gov/factsheets/WeightLoss-HealthProfessional).

Online and App-Based Weight Loss Programs Online diet websites and app-based weight loss programs have millions of subscribers worldwide. Most weight loss websites and apps combine self-help with group support through chat rooms, bulletin boards, and e-newsletters. Many sites offer online or in-app self-assessment for diet and physical activity habits as well as a meal plan; some provide access to a staff professional for individualized help.

Research suggests that this type of program provides an alternative to in-person diet counseling and can achieve weight loss for some people. Studies found that people who logged onto internet programs more frequently tended to lose more weight; regular online contact proved most successful for weight loss. The criteria used to evaluate commercial programs can also be applied to internet-based programs. In addition, good programs offer member-to-member support, motivational health coaching, and access to staff professionals.

Clinical Weight Loss Programs Medically supervised clinical programs are usually located in a hospital or other medical setting. Designed to help those who are severely obese, these programs typically involve a closely monitored, very-low-calorie diet. The cost of a clinical program is usually high, but insurance may cover part of the fee for those with obesity-related health problems.

Prescription Drugs

For a medicine to cause weight loss, it must help the user reduce energy consumption, increase energy expenditure, and/or interfere with energy absorption. The medications most often prescribed for weight loss are appetite suppressants that reduce feelings of hunger or increase feelings of fullness. Appetite suppressants usually work by increasing levels of catecholamine or serotonin—two brain chemicals that affect mood and appetite. Although some medications are approved only for short-term use, most experts agree that medications must be safe to use over the long term in order to be effective for treatment of obesity.

Appetite suppressants approved for long-term use include Belviq (lorcaserin), Qsymia (phentermine and topiramate extended-release), Contrave (bupropion and naltrexone), and Saxenda (liraglutide). All have potential side effects: Reported side effects include sleeplessness, nervousness, and euphoria, as well as increases in blood pressure and heart rate. Headaches, constipation or diarrhea, dry mouth, and insomnia are other side effects. If you are taking a prescription medication, discuss any concerns about side effects with your physician.

The other prescription medication approved for long-term use is Xenical (orlistat). This medication works differently: It is a lipid inhibitor that blocks fat absorption in the intestines. Orlistat prevents about 30% of the fat in food from being digested. Similar to the fat substitute olestra, orlistat reduces the absorption of fat-soluble vitamins and antioxidants. Therefore, taking a vitamin supplement is highly recommended for people taking orlistat. Side effects include diarrhea, cramping, and other gastrointestinal problems if users do not follow a low-fat diet. Alli is an FDA-approved, lower-dose version of orlistat that is sold over the counter.

Prescription medications work best in conjunction with behavior modification. Studies have generally found that appetite suppressants produce modest weight loss above the loss expected with nondrug obesity treatments. Researchers have found that people taking a prescription medication were two to three times more likely to have at least 5% weight loss than people taking a placebo. Individuals respond very differently, however, and some experience more weight loss than others. Unfortunately, weight loss tends to level off or reverse after four to six months on a medication, and many people regain the weight they've lost when they stop taking the medication.

Prescription weight loss drugs are not for people who want to lose only a few pounds. The latest federal guidelines advise people to try lifestyle modification for at least six months before trying drug therapy. Prescription drugs are recommended only in certain cases: for people who have been unable to lose weight with nondrug options and who have a BMI over 30 (or over 27 if two or more additional risk factors such as diabetes and high blood pressure are present). For severely obese people who have been unable to lose weight by other methods, prescription drugs may provide a good option.

Surgery

The National Health and Nutrition Examination Survey (NHANES) estimates almost 8% (1 in 13) of adult Americans aged 20 years and over have a BMI greater than 40, qualifying them as extremely or "morbidly" obese.

The number of severely obese people has nearly doubled in the past two decades. Extreme obesity is a serious medical condition that is often complicated by other health problems such as diabetes, heart disease, arthritis, and sleep disorders. Surgical intervention may be necessary as a treatment of last resort. According to the NIH, weight loss (bariatric) surgery is recommended for patients with a BMI greater than 40, or greater than 35 with obesity-related illnesses.

Due to the increasing prevalence of severe obesity, surgical treatment of obesity is growing worldwide. Obesity-related health conditions, as well as risk of premature death, generally improve after surgical weight loss. However, as with any surgery, gastric surgery is not without risks, including death. In the short term, the risks of gastric bypass surgery can include excessive bleeding, infection, reaction to anesthesia, blood clots, breathing problems, and leaks in the gastrointestinal system. Long-term complications can include bowel obstruction, diarrhea, nausea, vomiting, gallstones, and malnutrition. Bariatric surgery modifies the gastrointestinal tract by changing either the size of the stomach or how the intestine drains, thereby reducing food intake. Three common surgeries are the Roux-en-Y gastric bypass, the vertical sleeve gastrectomy, and the adjustable gastric banding procedure.

The *Roux-en-Y gastric bypass* surgery separates the stomach into two pouches. The smaller pouch is attached to the small intestine, and the larger one is bypassed. The procedure restricts food intake and reduces calorie absorption.

The *vertical sleeve gastrectomy* surgery removes approximately 80–85% of the stomach, leaving a new, smaller stomach shaped like a banana or garden hose. Like the bypass surgery, the procedure restricts food intake and causes the person to feel full after eating a small amount of food.

In the adjustable gastric banding procedure, commonly called the *Lap-Band,* an adjustable band is placed around the stomach to create a smaller stomach pouch. The band, which is filled with saline solution and can be tightened or loosened by adding or removing saline, ties off a portion of the stomach, restricting food intake. Results from the Lap-Band procedure may not be as significant as results from bypass surgery, in which part of the digestive system is rerouted. However, the Lap-Band procedure is often considered safer because it is less invasive, and patients generally have fewer complications. In mildly to moderately obese (BMI of 30–35) adults, gastric banding surgery has been found to be more effective in reducing weight and improving quality of life than nonsurgical methods. Over the course of a year, weight loss from surgery generally ranges between 40% and 70% of total body weight. Life behaviors and eating patterns can be changed permanently with adequate follow-up and sustained motivation.

Another procedure, *liposuction*, removes localized fat deposits beneath the skin. This cosmetic procedure does not improve health the way weight loss does and involves considerable pain and discomfort.

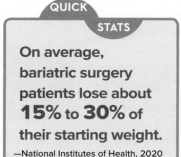

QUICK STATS

On average, bariatric surgery patients lose about **15%** to **30%** of their starting weight.
—National Institutes of Health, 2020

BODY IMAGE AND EATING DISORDERS

The collective picture of the body as seen through the mind's eye, **body image** consists of perceptions, images, thoughts, attitudes, and emotions. A negative body image is characterized by dissatisfaction with the body in general or some part of the body in particular. Most Americans, including those who are not overweight, are unhappy with their body weight or with some aspect of their appearance. People may be dissatisfied with their bodies for a variety of reasons, including sociocultural factors. For example, the ideal female body size in Western society has become progressively thinner, whereas actual female body size continues to increase, along with the frequency of unhealthy attitudes and behaviors surrounding food and body weight.

Losing weight or getting cosmetic surgery does not necessarily improve body image. In fact, improvements in body image may occur in the absence of changes in weight or appearance. Many experts now believe that body image issues must be dealt with as part of treating obesity and eating disorders. Developing a positive body image is an important aspect of psychological wellness and an important component of successful weight management.

Severe Body Image Problems

Poor body image can cause significant psychological distress. A person can become preoccupied with a perceived defect in appearance, thereby damaging self-esteem and interfering with relationships. Adolescents and adults who have a negative body image are more likely to diet restrictively, eat compulsively, or develop some other form of disordered eating.

When a person's dissatisfaction with his or her own body image becomes extreme, the condition is called *body dysmorphic disorder* (*BDD*). Although many people are dissatisfied with some part of their body or their appearance, these concerns usually do not constantly occupy their thoughts. Individuals with BDD are constantly preoccupied and upset about body imperfections, such as thinking their nose is too big or that their hair is never right. They cannot seem to stop checking or obsessing about their appearance, often focusing on perceived flaws that are not obvious to others. Low self-esteem is common in people with body dysmorphia. Individuals with BDD may spend hours every day thinking about their flaws and looking at themselves in mirrors, so that their preoccupation can interrupt daily activities, such as work and socializing. Some people with BDD may seek repeated cosmetic surgeries. BDD affects about 2% of Americans, males and

females in equal numbers. It usually begins before age 18 but can begin in adulthood, and it occurs in people with other mental health disorders such as major depression and anxiety.

This condition is related to obsessive-compulsive disorder and can lead to depression, social phobia, and suicide if left untreated. An individual with BDD needs to get professional evaluation and treatment. Medication and therapy can help people with BDD.

In some cases, body image may bear little resemblance to fact. People suffering from the eating disorder anorexia nervosa typically have a severely distorted body image—they believe themselves to be fat even when they have become emaciated. Distorted body image is also a hallmark of *muscle dysmorphia*, a disorder experienced by some bodybuilders and other active people who see themselves as small and out of shape despite being very muscular. Those who suffer from muscle dysmorphia may let obsessive exercise—particularly muscle-building exercise—interfere with their work and relationships. They may also use steroids and other potentially dangerous muscle-building drugs.

Eating Disorders

Problems with body weight and weight control are not limited to excessive body fat. A growing number of people, especially adolescent girls and young women, experience **eating disorders**—psychological disorders characterized by severe disturbances in body image, eating patterns, and eating-related behaviors. The main categories of eating disorders include anorexia nervosa, bulimia nervosa, binge-eating disorder, and other specified feeding or eating disorder (OSFED). During their lifetimes, one in seven males and one in five females will suffer from an eating disorder. Many more people have abnormal eating habits and attitudes about food that disrupt their lives, even though these habits do not meet the criteria for a major eating disorder.

Many factors are involved in the development of an eating disorder. Although widely differing explanations have been proposed, individuals with eating disorders share one central feature: a dissatisfaction with body image and body weight. Such dissatisfaction is created by distorted thinking, including

> **body image** The mental representation a person holds about his or her body at any given time, consisting of perceptions, images, thoughts, attitudes, and emotions about the body.
>
> **TERMS**
>
> **eating disorder** A serious disturbance in eating patterns or eating-related behavior, characterized by a negative body image and concerns about body weight or body fat.

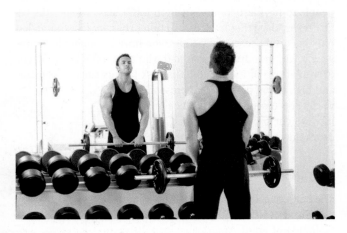

Exercise is a healthy practice, but people with muscle dysmorphia sometimes exercise compulsively, building their lives around their workouts. Compulsive exercise can lead to injuries and problems with work and relationships. Antonio Balaguer Soler/123RF

perfectionistic beliefs, unreasonable demands for self-control, and excessive self-criticism. Dissatisfaction with body weight can lead to dysfunctional attitudes about eating, such as fear of fat and preoccupation with food, and problematic eating behaviors, including excessive dieting, constant calorie counting, and checking body weight frequently.

Heredity and how genes interact with the environment appear to play an important role in the development of eating disorders. But as with other conditions, only the tendency to develop an eating disorder is explained by heredity; the expression of this tendency is affected by other factors. The home environment is one factor: Families in which there is hostility, abuse, or lack of cohesion provide fertile ground for the development of an eating disorder. A rigid or overprotective parent can also increase the risk. Cultural messages, as well as family, friends, and peers, shape attitudes toward the self and others. Comparing yourself negatively with others can damage self-esteem and increase vulnerability. Young people who see themselves as lacking control over their lives are also at high risk for eating disorders. About 90% of eating disorders begin during adolescence. Cases of eating disorders have increased among children as young as 6 years old, especially girls. It is reported that 40–60% of elementary school girls (aged 6–12) are concerned about their weight or about being too fat.

Certain turning points in life, such as leaving home for college, can trigger an eating disorder. Of a group of women surveyed on a college campus, 91% had attempted to control their weight through dieting, whereas 22% dieted "often" or "always." How a person copes with stress can influence risk, particularly in individuals who have few stress management skills. An eating disorder may become a means of coping: The abnormal eating behavior reduces anxiety by producing numbness and alleviating emotional pain. Restrictive dieting is another possible trigger for the development of eating disorders.

Anorexia Nervosa   A person with **anorexia nervosa** does not eat enough food to maintain a reasonable body weight. An estimated 0.5–3.7% of women suffer from anorexia nervosa in their lifetimes, and slightly less than 1% of female adolescents have anorexia. Anorexia typically develops during puberty and the late teenage years, with an average age of onset of about 19 years.

CHARACTERISTICS OF ANOREXIA NERVOSA   People with anorexia have an intense fear of gaining weight or becoming fat. Their body image is so distorted that even when emaciated they think they are fat. People with anorexia may engage in compulsive behaviors or rituals that help keep them from eating, though some may also binge and **purge.** A purge occurs when a person uses vomiting, laxatives, excessive exercise, restrictive dieting, enemas, diuretics, or diet pills to compensate for food that she or he has eaten and that the person fears will produce weight gain. Some people also use vigorous and prolonged exercise to reduce body weight as a way to purge. Although they may express a great interest in food, even taking over the cooking responsibilities for the rest of the family, their own diet becomes more and more restricted. People with anorexia nervosa often hide or hoard food without eating it.

People with anorexia are typically introverted, emotionally reserved, and socially insecure. They are often model children who rarely complain and are eager to please others and win their approval. Although school performance is typically above average, they are often critical of themselves and not satisfied with their accomplishments. For people with anorexia nervosa, their entire sense of self-esteem may be tied up in their evaluation of their body shape and weight.

HEALTH RISKS OF ANOREXIA NERVOSA   Because of extreme weight loss, females with anorexia often stop menstruating, become intolerant of cold, and develop low blood pressure and heart rate. They develop dry skin that is often covered by fine body hair like that of a newborn. Their hands and feet may swell and take on a blue tinge.

Anorexia nervosa has been linked to a variety of medical complications, including disorders of the cardiovascular, gastrointestinal, endocrine, and skeletal systems. When body fat is virtually gone and muscles are severely wasted, the body turns to its own organs in a desperate search for protein. Death can occur from heart failure caused by electrolyte imbalances. About 1 in 10 women with anorexia dies of starvation, cardiac arrest, or other medical complications—the highest death rate for any psychiatric disorder. Between 33% and 50% of patients with anorexia nervosa have a comorbid mood disorder such as depression. About half the fatalities related to anorexia are suicides.

Bulimia Nervosa   A person suffering from **bulimia nervosa** engages in recurrent episodes of binge eating followed by purging. Bulimia is often difficult to recognize because sufferers conceal their eating habits and usually maintain a normal weight, although they may experience weight fluctuations of 10–15 pounds. Although bulimia usually

---

TERMS

anorexia nervosa   An eating disorder characterized by a refusal to maintain body weight at a minimally healthy level and an intense fear of gaining weight or becoming fat; self-starvation.

purge   The use of vomiting, laxatives, excessive exercise, restrictive dieting, enemas, diuretics, or diet pills to compensate for food that has been eaten and that the person fears will produce weight gain.

bulimia nervosa   An eating disorder characterized by recurrent episodes of binge eating and purging—overeating and then using compensatory behaviors such as vomiting, laxatives, and excessive exercise to prevent weight gain.

begins in adolescence or young adulthood, it has begun to emerge at increasingly younger (11-12 years) and older (40-60 years) ages; the average age of onset is about 20 years.

CHARACTERISTICS OF BULIMIA NERVOSA During a binge, a bulimic person may rapidly consume thousands of calories. This is followed by an attempt to get rid of the food by purging, usually by vomiting or using laxatives or diuretics. During a binge, bulimics feel as though they have lost control and cannot stop or limit how much they eat. Some binge and purge only occasionally; others do so many times every day.

People with bulimia may appear to eat normally, but they are rarely comfortable around food. Binges usually occur in secret and can become nightmarish—uncontrollably raiding the kitchen for food, going from one grocery store to another to buy food, or stealing food. During the binge, food acts as an anesthetic, blocking out feelings. Afterward, bulimics feel physically drained and emotionally spent. They usually feel deeply ashamed and disgusted with both themselves and their behavior and terrified that they will gain weight from the binge.

Major life changes such as leaving for college, getting married, having a baby, or losing a job can trigger a binge-purge cycle. At such times, stress is high and the person may have no good outlet for emotional conflict or tension. As with anorexia nervosa, bulimia sufferers are often insecure and depend on others for approval and self-esteem. They may hide difficult emotions such as anger and disappointment from themselves and others. Binge eating and purging become a way of dealing with feelings.

HEALTH RISKS OF BULIMIA NERVOSA The binge-purge cycle of bulimia places a tremendous strain on the body and can have serious health effects. Contact with vomited stomach acids erodes tooth enamel. Bulimic people often develop tooth decay because they binge on foods that are high in simple sugars. Repeated vomiting or the use of laxatives, in combination with deficient calorie intake, can damage the liver and kidneys and cause cardiac arrhythmia. Chronic hoarseness and esophageal tearing with bleeding may also result from vomiting. More rarely, binge eating can lead to rupture of the stomach. Although many bulimic women maintain healthy weight, even a small weight loss can cause menstrual problems. Bulimia is associated with increased depression, excessive preoccupation with food and body image, and sometimes cognitive dysfunction.

Binge-Eating Disorder

Binge-eating disorder affects almost 1% of American adults and is almost twice as common in women as in men. It is characterized by uncontrollable eating, usually followed by feelings of guilt and shame about weight gain. Common eating patterns are eating more rapidly than normal, eating until uncomfortably full, eating when not hungry, and preferring to eat alone. Binge eaters may eat large amounts of food throughout the day, with no planned mealtimes. Many people with binge-eating disorder mistakenly see rigid dieting as the only solution to their problem. However, rigid dieting usually causes feelings of deprivation and a return to overeating.

Compulsive overeaters rarely eat because of hunger. Instead food is used as a means of coping with stress, conflict, and other difficult emotions or to provide solace and entertainment. People who do not have the resources to deal effectively with stress may be more vulnerable to binge-eating disorder. Inappropriate overeating often begins during childhood. In some families, eating may be used as an activity to fill otherwise empty time. Parents may reward children with food for good behavior or withhold food as a means of punishment, thereby creating distorted feelings about the experience of eating.

Binge eaters are almost always obese, so they face all the health risks associated with obesity. In addition, binge eaters may have higher rates of depression and anxiety. To overcome binge eating, a person must learn to put food and eating into proper perspective and develop other ways of coping with stress and painful emotions.

Other Patterns of Disordered Eating Eating habits and body image run along a continuum from healthy to seriously disordered. Where an individual falls along that continuum can change depending on life stresses, illnesses, and many other factors. People who have feeding or eating disorders that can cause significant distress or impairment, but who do not meet the criteria for another feeding or eating disorder, may be classified as having **other specified feeding or eating disorders (OSFED),** according to the American Psychiatric Association's *Diagnostic and Statistical Manual of Mental Disorders*. OSFED is the most commonly diagnosed eating disorder in adults and adolescents. Examples include atypical anorexia nervosa, a condition in which weight is not below normal; bulimia nervosa with limited duration, a condition with less frequent bulimic episodes; purging disorder, a condition without binge eating; and night eating syndrome, in which the individual engages in excessive nighttime food consumption. OSFED is present in approximately 30% of people who seek treatment for an eating disorder. OSFED is a serious mental illness, and affected people often have extremely disturbed eating habits, body image distortion, and intense fear of gaining weight.

Avoidant restrictive food intake disorder (ARFID) is a new DSM-5 diagnosis that was previously referred to as selective eating disorder. ARFID is similar to anorexia—both conditions involve severe limitations of amount and types of foods consumed—but individuals with ARFID do not have the same fears about body weight and shape as those with anorexia nervosa.

Individuals with *orthorexia* are so obsessed with healthy eating that it actually is damaging to their own health and well-being. Although not diagnosed with a DSM disorder,

> **TERMS**
>
> **binge-eating disorder** An eating disorder characterized by episodes of binge eating and a lack of control over eating behavior in general.
>
> **other specified feeding or eating disorders (OSFED)** A feeding or eating disorder that causes significant distress or impairment but does not meet the criteria for another feeding or eating disorder.

Secrecy and denial are two hallmarks of eating disorders, so it can be hard to know if someone has anorexia or bulimia. Signs that someone may have anorexia include sudden weight loss, excessive dieting or exercise, guilt or preoccupation with food or eating, frequent weighing, fear of becoming fat despite being thin, social withdrawal, and wearing baggy or layered clothes to conceal weight loss. Signs that someone may have bulimia include excessive eating without weight gain; secretiveness about food (stealing, hiding, or hoarding food); self-induced vomiting (bathroom visits during or after a meal); swollen glands or puffy face; erosion of tooth enamel; and use of laxatives, diuretics, or diet pills to control weight.

If you decide to approach a friend with your concerns, here are some tips to follow:

• Find out about treatment resources in your community (see the For More Information section for suggestions). You may want to consult a professional at your school clinic or counseling center about the best way to approach the situation.

• Arrange to speak with your friend in a private place, and allow enough time to talk.

• Express your concerns, with specific observations of your friend's behavior. Expect him or her to deny or minimize the problem and possibly to become angry with you. Stay calm and nonjudgmental, and continue to express your concern.

• Avoid giving simplistic advice about eating habits. Listen if your friend wants to talk, and offer your support and understanding. Give your friend the information you found about where he or she can get help, and offer to go along.

• If the situation is an emergency—if your friend has fainted, for example—call 911 for help immediately.

• If you are upset about the situation, consider talking to someone yourself. The professionals at the clinic or counseling center are there to help you. Remember, you are not to blame for another person's eating disorder.

---

people with orthorexia are compulsive about checking ingredient lists and nutritional labels and exhibit an inability to eat anything not on their narrow list of foods that they have deemed "pure" or "acceptable."

How do you know if you have disordered eating habits? When thoughts about food and weight dominate your life, you have a problem. If you're convinced that your worth as a person hinges on how you look and how much you weigh, it's time to get help. Other danger signs include frequent feelings of guilt after a meal or snack, any use of vomiting or laxatives after meals, or overexercising or severely restricting your food intake to compensate for what you've already eaten. Individuals who experience these issues, or who are concerned about eating and exercise habits, or about thoughts and emotions concerning food, physical activity, and body image, should address the situation with a health care provider.

If you suspect you have an eating problem, don't go it alone or delay getting help because disordered eating habits can develop into a full-blown eating disorder. Check with your student health or counseling center. If you are concerned about the eating habits of a family member or friend, refer to the suggestions in the box "If Someone You Know Has an Eating Disorder . . ."

Treating Eating Disorders The treatment of eating disorders must address both problematic eating behaviors and the misuse of food to manage stress and emotions. In many cases, anorexia nervosa treatment first involves averting a medical crisis by restoring adequate body weight; then the psychological aspects of the disorder can be addressed. The treatment of bulimia nervosa or binge-eating disorder involves first stabilizing the eating patterns, then identifying and changing the patterns of thinking that led to disordered eating, and then improving coping skills. Concurrent problems, such as depression, anxiety, and other mental disorders may be present and must also be addressed.

Treatment of eating disorders usually involves a combination of psychotherapy and medical management. The therapy may be done individually or in a group; sessions involving the entire family may be recommended. A support or self-help group can be a useful adjunct to such treatment. Medical professionals, including physicians, dentists, gynecologists, and RDNs, can evaluate and manage the physical damage caused by the disorder. If a patient is severely depressed or emaciated, hospitalization may be necessary.

Positive Body Image: Finding Balance

Knowing when you've reached the limits of healthy change—and learning to accept those limits—is crucial for overall wellness. Women in particular tend to measure self-worth in terms of their appearance. When they don't measure up to an unrealistic cultural ideal, they see themselves as

Ask Yourself

QUESTIONS FOR CRITICAL THINKING AND REFLECTION

Do you know someone you suspect may suffer from an eating disorder? Have you ever experienced disordered eating patterns yourself? If so, can you identify the reasons for them?

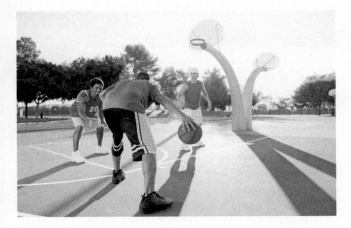

A balanced, realistic attitude toward weight management is part of overall wellness. Many healthy people do not fit society's image of ideal body size and shape. Dave and Les Jacobs/Blend Images LLC

defective, and their self-esteem falls. The result can be negative body image, disordered eating, or even a diagnosable eating disorder.

People who view their bodies positively tend to be more intuitive eaters, relying on internal hunger and fullness cues to regulate what and how much they eat. They think more about how their bodies feel and function than how they appear to others. Many healthy people do not fit society's image of ideal body size and shape. To minimize your risk of developing a body image problem, keep the following strategies in mind:

• Focus on healthy habits and good physical health.

• Put concerns about physical appearance in perspective. Your worth as a human being does not depend on how you look.

• Practice body acceptance. You can influence your body size and type through lifestyle to some degree, but the fact is that some people are genetically designed to be bigger or heavier than others.

• Find things to appreciate in yourself besides an idealized body image. People who can learn to value other aspects of themselves are more accepting of the physical changes that occur naturally with age.

• View eating as a morally neutral activity—eating dessert isn't "bad" and doesn't make you a bad person.

• See the beauty and fitness industries for what they are. Realize that their goal is to prompt you to feel dissatisfaction with yourself so that you will buy their products.

Weight management needs to take place in a positive and realistic atmosphere. For an obese person, losing as few as 10 pounds can reduce blood pressure and improve mood. The hazards of excessive dieting and being overly concerned about body weight need to be countered by a change in attitude. A reasonable weight must take into account a person's weight history, social circumstances, metabolic profile, and psychological well-being.

TIPS FOR TODAY AND THE FUTURE

Many approaches work, but the best recipe for weight management is the one that will work for you. This means that the results for a particular plan will vary from person to person based on individual metabolism, overall health, starting weight, age, physical activity level, and how prepared you are to follow the plan.

RIGHT NOW YOU CAN:

▪ Assess your weight management needs. Do you need to gain weight, lose weight, or stay at your current weight?
▪ List five things you can do to add more physical activity (not just exercise) to your daily routine.
▪ Identify the foods you regularly eat that may be sabotaging your ability to manage your weight.

IN THE FUTURE YOU CAN:

▪ Make an honest assessment of your current body image. Is it accurate and fair, or is it unduly negative and unhealthy? If your body image presents a problem, consider getting professional advice on how to view yourself realistically.
▪ Keep track of your energy needs to determine whether your energy balance equation is correct. Use this information as part of your long-term weight management efforts.

SUMMARY

• Body composition is the relative amounts of fat-free mass and fat in the body. *Overweight* and *obesity* refer to body weight or the percentage of body fat that exceeds what is associated with good health.

• Standards for assessing body weight and body composition include body mass index (BMI) and percent body fat.

• Too much or too little body fat is linked to health problems; the distribution of body fat can also be a significant risk factor for many kinds of health problems.

• Genetic factors help determine a person's weight, but the influence of heredity can be overcome with attention to lifestyle factors.

• Physiological factors involved in the regulation of body weight and body fat include metabolic rate, hormonal influences, and the size and number of fat cells.

• Nutritional guidelines for weight management include consuming a moderate number of calories; limiting portion sizes, energy density, and the intake of simple sugars, refined carbohydrates, and solid fats; and developing an eating schedule and rules for food choices.

• Activity guidelines for weight management emphasize daily physical activity and regular sessions of cardiorespiratory endurance exercise and strength training.

• Weight management requires developing positive self-talk and self-esteem, realistic weight and body composition goals, and a repertoire of appropriate techniques for handling stress and other emotional and physical challenges.

- People can be successful at long-term weight loss on their own by combining diet and exercise.

- Diet books, websites, social media programs, over-the-counter diet aids and supplements, and formal weight loss programs should be assessed for safety and efficacy.

- Professional help is needed in cases of severe obesity; medical treatments include prescription drugs and surgery.

- An inaccurate or negative body image is common and can lead to psychological distress.

- Dissatisfaction with weight and shape are common to all eating disorders.
- Anorexia nervosa is characterized by self-starvation, distorted body image, and an intense fear of gaining weight.
- Bulimia nervosa is characterized by recurrent episodes of uncontrolled binge eating and frequent purging.
- Binge-eating disorder involves binge eating without regular use of compensatory purging.
- People with other patterns of disordered eating have some symptoms of eating disorders but do not meet the full diagnostic criteria for anorexia, bulimia, or binge-eating disorder.

FOR MORE INFORMATION

American Diabetes Association. Provides information, a free newsletter, and referrals to local support groups; the website includes an online diabetes risk assessment.

http://www.diabetes.org

Calorie Control Council. Includes a variety of interactive calculators, including an Exercise Calculator that estimates the calories burned from various forms of physical activity.

http://www.caloriecontrol.org

Centers for Disease Control and Prevention: Obesity. The home page for accessing all the CDC's information about overweight and obesity, their health risks, statistics, and diet and exercise.

http://www.cdc.gov/obesity/index.html

FDA Center for Food Safety and Applied Nutrition: Dietary Supplements. Provides background facts and information on the current regulatory status of dietary supplements, including compounds marketed for weight loss.

http://www.fda.gov/Food/DietarySupplements/default.htm

National Heart, Lung, and Blood Institute (NHLBI): Aim for a Healthy Weight. Provides information and tips on diet and physical activity, as well as a BMI calculator.

http://www.nhlbi.nih.gov/health/educational/lose_wt/

National Institute of Diabetes and Digestive and Kidney Diseases (NIDDK): Weight Management. Provides information and referrals for problems related to obesity, weight control, and nutritional disorders.

https://www.niddk.nih.gov/health-information/weight-management

Resources for People Concerned about Eating Disorders:

Eating Disorder Referral and Information Center
http://www.edreferral.com

Eating Disorders Coalition for Research, Policy and Action
http://www.eatingdisorderscoalition.org

MedlinePlus: Eating Disorders
http://www.nlm.nih.gov/medlineplus/eatingdisorders.html

National Association of Anorexia Nervosa and Associated Disorders
630-577-1330 (help line)
http://www.anad.org

National Eating Disorders Association
800-931-2237
http://www.nationaleatingdisorders.org

National Institute of Mental Health: Eating Disorders
http://www.nimh.nih.gov/health/topics/eating-disorders/index.shtml
See also the listings in Chapters 13 and 14.

SELECTED BIBLIOGRAPHY

2018 Physical Activity Guidelines Advisory Committee. 2018 Physical Activity Guidelines Advisory Committee Scientific Report. Washington, DC: U.S. Department of Health and Human Services (https://health.gov/news-archive/blog-bayw/2018/03/2018-physical-activity-guidelines-advisory-committee-submits-scientific-report/index.html).

American Academy of Child and Adolescent Psychiatry. 2016. *Obesity in Children and Teens* (https://www.aacap.org/AACAP/Families_and_Youth/Facts_for_Families/FFF-Guide/Obesity-In-Children-And-Teens-079.aspx).

American Diabetes Association. 2018. *Statistics About Diabetes* (http://www.diabetes.org/diabetes-basics/statistics/).

Andreyeva, T., A. S. Tripp, and M. B. Schwartz. 2015. Dietary quality of Americans by Supplemental Nutrition Assistance Program participation status: A systematic review. *American Journal of Preventive Medicine* 49(4): 594–604.

Attia, P. 2016. Good science, bad interpretation. *The Eating Academy: The Personal Blog of Peter Attia* (http://eatingacademy.com/books-and-articles/good-science-bad-interpretation).

Bellissimo, N., and T. Akhavan. 2015. Effect of macronutrient composition on short-term food intake and weight loss. *Advances in Nutrition* 6(3): a302s–a308s.

Beleigoli, A. M., et al. 2019. Web-based digital health interventions for weight loss and lifestyle habit changes in overweight and obese adults: Systematic review and meta-analysis. *Journal of Medical Internet Research* 21(1): e298. DOI: 10.2196/jmir.9609.

Bentley, J. 2017. *US Trends in Food Availability and Dietary Assessment of Loss-Adjusted Food Availability* 1970–2014. USDA. A report summary from the Economic Research Service (https://www.ers.usda.gov/webdocs/publications/82220/eib166%20summary.pdf?v=0).

Boulangé, C. L., et al. 2016. Impact of the gut microbiota on inflammation, obesity, and metabolic disease. *Genome Medicine* 8(42). DOI: 10.1186/s13073-016-0303-2.

Bratland-Sanda, S. 2019. Defining compulsive exercise in eating disorders: Acknowledging the exercise paradox and exercise obsessions. *Journal of Eating Disorders* 7(1): 8.

Bratland-Sanda, S., et al. 2019. Defining compulsive exercise in eating disorders: Acknowledging the exercise paradox and exercise obsessions. *Journal of Eating Disorders* 7: 8.

Bray, G. A., et al. 2018. The science of obesity management: An Endocrine Society scientific statement. *Endocrine Reviews*, March 6. DOI: 10.1210

/er.2017-00253 (https://academic.oup.com/edrv/advance-article/doi/10.1210/er.2017-00253/4922247).

Bray, M. S., et al. 2016. NIH working group report—using genomic information to guide weight management: From universal to precision treatment. *Obesity* 24(1): 14–22.

Brown, P. 2016. Carbohydrate study leaves diet researchers divided. *MedPageToday*, July 11 (https://www.medpagetoday.com/primarycare/dietnutrition/59012).

Buttitta, M., A. Rousseau, and A. Guerrien. 2017. A new understanding of quality of life in children and adolescents with obesity: Contribution of the self-determination theory. *Current Obesity Reports* 6(4):432-437.

Calugi, S., G. Marchesini, M. El Ghoch, I. Gavasso, and R. Dalle Grave. 2020. The association between weight maintenance and session-by-session diet adherence, weight loss and weight-loss satisfaction. *Eating and Weight Disorders* 25(1): 127-133.

Centers for Disease Control and Prevention. 2015. *About Child & Teen BMI.* (https://www.cdc.gov/healthyweight/assessing/bmi/childrens_bmi/about_childrens_bmi.html).

Centers for Disease Control and Prevention. 2015. *Healthy Weight: Rethink Your Drink.* (https://www.cdc.gov/healthyweight/healthy_eating/drinks.html).

Centers for Disease Control and Prevention. 2017. National Center for Health Statistics. *Exercise or Physical Activity* (https://www.cdc.gov/nchs/fastats/exercise.htm).

Centers for Disease Control and Prevention. 2018 Behavior, environment, and genetic factors all have a role in causing people to be overweight and obese. *Public Health Genomics* (https://www.cdc.gov/genomics/resources/diseases/obesity/).

Centers for Disease Control and Prevention. 2018. *How Much Physical Activity Do Adults Need?* (https://www.cdc.gov/physicalactivity/basics/adults/index.htm).

Centers for Disease Control and Prevention. 2020. *National Diabetes Statistics Report, 2020 Estimates of Diabetes and Its Burden in the United States.* (https://www.cdc.gov/diabetes/pdfs/data/statistics/national-diabetes-statistics-report.pdf).

Centers for Disease Control and Prevention. 2020. *Overweight and Obesity* (https://www.cdc.gov/obesity/).

Centers for Disease Control and Prevention. 2020. *Physical Activity. Recommendations and Guidelines* (https://www.cdc.gov/physicalactivity/resources/recommendations.html).

Centers for Disease Control and Prevention. 2020. *Physical Activity Facts* (https://www.cdc.gov/healthyschools/physicalactivity/facts.htm).

Chambers, L., K. McCrickerd, and M. R. Yeomans. 2015. Optimising foods for satiety. *Trends in Food Science and Technology* 41(2): 149-160.

Cheung, P. C., et al. 2016. Childhood obesity incidence in the United States: A systematic review. *Childhood Obesity* 12(1): 1-11.

Christian, C., et al. 2020. Eating disorder core symptoms and symptom pathways across developmental stages: A network analysis. *Journal of Abnormal Psychology* 129(2):177-190.

Cobb, L. K., et al. 2015. The relationship of the local food environment with obesity: A systematic review of methods, study quality and results. *Obesity* 23(7): 1331-1344.

Cooper, C. B., et al. 2018. Sleep deprivation and obesity in adults: A brief narrative review. *British Medical Journal of Open Sport Exercise Medicine* 4(1): e000392.

Das, S. K., et al. 2017. Weight loss in videoconference and in-person iDiet weight loss programs in worksites and community groups. *Obesity* 25(6): 1033-1041.

Dashti, H. S., et al. 2015. Short sleep duration and dietary intake: Epidemiologic evidence, mechanisms, and health implications. *Advances in Nutrition* (6):648-659.

de Cabo, R., and M. P. Mattson MP. 2019. Effects of intermittent fasting on health, aging and disease. *New England Journal of Medicine* 381:2541-2551. DOI: 10.1056/NEJMra1905136.

Diabetes Prevention Program Research Group. 2015. Long-term effects of lifestyle intervention or metformin on diabetes development and microvascular complications over 15-year follow-up: The Diabetes Prevention Program Outcomes Study. *Lancet: Diabetes & Endocrinology* 3(11): 866–875.

Dues, K., et al. 2019. Adolescent body weight perception: Association with diet and physical activity behaviors. *Journal of School Nursing* 1-9. DOI: 10.1177/1059840518824386.

Dumas, A-A., and S. Desroches. 2019. Women's use of social media: What is the evidence about their impact on weight management and body image? *Current Obesity Reports* 8(1): 18-23.

Dyson, P. 2015. Low carbohydrate diets and type 2 diabetes: What is the latest evidence? *Diabetes Therapy* 6(4): 411–424.

Eating Disorders Coalition. *Facts about Eating Disorders* (http://eatingdisorderscoalition.org.s208556.gridserver.com/couch/uploads/file/fact-sheet_2016.pdf). Accessed March 16, 2020.

Eatright. Academy of Nutrition and Dietetics. 2018. *Orthorexia* (https://www.eatright.org/health/diseases-and-conditions/eating-disorders/orthorexia-an-obsession-with-eating-pure). Accessed March 28, 2020.

Ebbing, C. B., et al. 2018, November 14. Effects of a low carbohydrate diet on energy expenditure during weight loss maintenance: Randomized trial. *BMJ* 363: k4583. DOI: 10.1136/bmj.k4583.

Flegal, K., D. Kruszon-Moran, M. D. Carroll, C. D. Fryar, and C. L. Ogden. 2016. Trends in obesity among adults in the United States, 2005 to 2014. *JAMA* 315(21): 2284-2291.

Flemming, J. A., and P. M. Kris-Etherton. 2016. Macronutrient content of the diet: What do we know about energy balance and weight maintenance? *Current Obesity Reports* 5(2): 208-213.

Food and Drug Administration. 2017. *Dietary Supplements: What You Need to Know* (https://www.fda.gov/Food/ResourcesForYou/Consumers/ucm109760.htm).

Fothergill, E., et al. 2016. Persistent metabolic adaptation 6 years after "The Biggest Loser" competition. *Obesity* 24(8): 1612-1619.

Freedhoff, Y., and K. D. Hall. 2016. Weight loss diet studies: We need help not hype. *Lancet* 388(10047): 849–851.

Fryar, C. D., et al. Prevalence of overweight, obesity, and extreme obesity among adults aged 20 and over: United States, 1960-1962 through 2013-2014. Centers for Disease Control and Prevention (https://www.cdc.gov/nchs/data/hestat/obesity_adult_13_14/obesity_adult_13_14.htm) Accessed March 14, 2020.

Galmiche, M., et al. 2019. Prevalence of eating disorders over the 2000-2018 period: A systematic literature review. *American Journal of Clinical Nutrition* 109(5): 1402-1413.

GBD 2015 Obesity Collaborators. 2017. Health effects of overweight and obesity in 195 countries over 25 years. *New England Journal of Medicine.* DOI: 10.1056/NEJMoa1614362.

Gibson, A. A., and A. Sainsbury. 2017. Strategies to improve adherence to dietary weight loss interventions in research and real-world settings. *Behavioral Sciences (Basel).* 7(3). pii: E44.

Global BMI Mortality Collaboration. 2016. Body-mass index and all-cause mortality: Individual-participant-data meta-analysis of 239 prospective studies in four continents. *Lancet* 388(10046): 776-786.

Golden, N. H., M. Schneider, and C. Wood. Committee on Nutrition, Committee on Adolescence and Section on Obesity. 2016. Preventing obesity and eating disorders in adolescents. *Pediatrics* 138(3): e1-12.

Gray L. A., et al. 2018. Family lifestyle dynamics and childhood obesity: Evidence from the millennium cohort study. *BMC Public Health* 18: 500 (https://doi.org/10.1186/s12889-018-5398-5).

Hales, C. M., et al. 2018. Differences in obesity prevalence by demographic characteristics and urbanization level among adults in the United States, 2013-2016. *Journal of the American Medical Association* 319(23): 2419-2429.

Hales C. M., et al. 2020. *Prevalence of Obesity And Severe Obesity Among Adults: United States, 2017-2018.* NCHS Data Brief, No. 360. Hyattsville, MD: National Center for Health Statistics (https://www.cdc.gov/nchs/products/databriefs/db360.htm).

Hall, K. D., et al. 2016. Energy expenditure and body composition changes after an isocaloric ketogenic diet in overweight and obese men. *American Journal of Clinical Nutrition* 104(2): 324-333.

Harvard University T. H. Chan School of Public Health. 2015. *Toxic Food Environment: How Our Surroundings Influence What We Eat* (https://

www.hsph.harvard.edu/obesity-prevention-source/obesity-causes/food
-environment-and-obesity/).

Healthy People 2020. *Physical Activity,* Office of Disease Prevention and
Health Promotion, Centers for Disease Control and Prevention (https://
www.healthypeople.gov/2020/topics-objectives/topic/physical-activity).

Hills, R. D. et al. 2019. Gut Microbiome: Profound implications for diet and
disease. *Nutrients Open Access* 11(7): 1613. (https://doi.org/10.3390
/nu11071613).

Huang, T. T.-K., et al. 2015. Mobilisation of public support for policy actions
to prevent obesity. *Lancet* 385(9985): 2422–2431.

Hyde, P. N., et al. 2019. Dietary carbohydrate restriction improves metabolic
syndrome independent of weight loss. *JCI Insight* 4(12).

Jane, M., et al. 2018. Social media for health promotion and weight management: A critical debate. *BMC Public Health* 18: 932.

Jensen, M. D., et al. 2014. AHA/ACC/TOS guideline for the management of
overweight and obesity in adults: A report of the American College of
Cardiology/American Heart Association Task Force on Practice Guidelines and the Obesity Society. *Circulation* 129: S102–S138.

Jin, Y., C. Ha, H. Hong, and H. Kang. 2017. The relationship between depressive symptoms and modifiable lifestyle risk factors in office workers.
Journal of Obesity & Metabolic Syndrome 26(1): 52–60.

Johnson, S. S. 2019. The art of health promotion. Editor's desk: Masterful
Microbes: The gut microbiome and food as medicine. *American Journal
of Health Promotion* 35(5): 820 -834.

Karazsia, B. T., S. K. Murnen, and T. L. Tylka. 2017. Is body dissatisfaction
changing across time? A cross-temporal meta-analysis. *Psychological Bulletin* 143(3): 293–320.

Karl, J. P., et al. 2015. Effects of carbohydrate quantity and glycemic index
on resting metabolic rate and body composition during weight loss. *Obesity* 23(11): 2190–2198.

Kaur, J., M. M. Lamb, and C. L. Ogden. 2015. The association between food
insecurity and obesity in children—the National and Nutrition Examination
Survey. *Journal of the Academy of Nutrition and Dietetics* 115(5): 751–758.

Kenney, E. L., and S. L. Gortmaker. 2016. United States adolescents' television, computer, videogame, smartphone, and tablet use: Associations
with sugary drinks, sleep, physical activity, and obesity. *Journal of Pediatrics* S0022-3476(16): 31243–31244.

Khera, R., et al. 2016. Association of pharmacological treatments for obesity
with weight loss and adverse events: A systematic review and meta-analysis.
Journal of the American Medical Association 315(22): 2424–2434.

Kiviruusu, O., et al. 2016. Self-esteem and body mass index from adolescence
to mid-adulthood. A 26-year follow-up. *International Journal of Behavioral Medicine* 23(3): 355–363.

Krebs, G., L. Fernandez de la Cruz, and D. Mataix-Cols.2017. Recent advances in understanding and managing body dysmorphic disorder. *Evidence-Based Mental Health* 20(3):71–75.

Lane, R. 2015. Christina Roberto: Taking a broad view on combating obesity.
Lancet 385(9985): 2345.

LeBlanc, E. L., et al. 2018. *Behavioral and Pharmacotherapy Weight Loss In-
terventions to Prevent Obesity-Related Morbidity and Mortality in Adults: An
Updated Systematic Review for the U.S. Preventive Services Task Force.*
Rockville (MD): Agency for Healthcare Research and Quality (U.S.);
2018 Sep. Report No.: 18-05239-EF-1. U.S. Preventive Services Task
Force Evidence Syntheses, formerly Systematic Evidence Reviews.

Levis, L. 2016. Are all calories equal? *Harvard Magazine,* May–June 2016.

Ludwig, D. 2016. Lifespan weighed down by diet. *Journal of the American
Medical Association* 315(21): 2269–2270.

MacLean, P. S., et al. 2015. NIH working group report: Innovative research
to improve maintenance of weight loss. *Obesity* 23(1): 7–15.

Mayo Clinic. *Bariatric Surgery* (https://www.mayoclinic.org/tests-procedures
/bariatric-surgery/about/pac-20394258).

Mazidi, M., et al. 2016. Gut microbiome and metabolic syndrome. *Diabetes
and Metabolic Syndrome.* 10(2 Suppl. 1): S150–S157.

Mirror Mirror Eating Disorder Help. *Eating Disorder Statistics* (https://www
.mirror-mirror.org/eating-disorders-statistics.htm).

Moehlecke, M. et al. 2016. Determinants of body weight regulation in
humans. *Archives of Endocrinology and Metabolism* 60(2): 152–162.

Mozzafarian, D. 2016. Dietary and policy priorities for cardiovascular disease,
diabetes, and obesity: A comprehensive review. *Circulation* 133(2): 187–225.

National Association of Anorexia Nervosa and Associated Disorders
(ANAD). n.d. *Eating Disorders Statistics* (http://www.anad.org/education
-and-awareness/about-eating-disorders/eating-disorders-statistics/).

National Center of Diabetes and Digestive and Kidney Diseases. *Overweight
and Obesity Statistics.* (https://www.niddk.nih.gov/health-information
/health-statistics/overweight-obesity#prevalence).

National Center for Health Statistics. 2018. *Health, United States, 2018:*
Hyattsville, MD (https://www.cdc.gov/nchs/data/hus/hus18.pdf).

National Eating Disorders Association. n.d. *Other Specified Feeding or Eating
Disorders* (https://www.nationaleatingdisorders.org/learn/by-eating
-disorder/osfed).

National Eating Disorders Association. n.d. *What Are Eating Disorders?*
(https://www.nationaleatingdisorders.org/what-are-eating-disorders).

National Eating Disorders Association. 2017. *Statistics and Research on Eating
Disorders* (https://www.nationaleatingdisorders.org/statistics-research
-eating-disorders).

National Eating Disorders Association.2018. *Avoidant Restrictive Food Intake
Disorder (ARFID)* (https://www.nationaleatingdisorders.org/learn/by
-eating-disorder/arfid).

National Eating Disorders Collaboration. n.d. *Other Specified Feeding or Eating Disorders* (http://www.nedc.com.au/osfed).

National Institute of Diabetes and Digestive and Kidney Diseases. 2017.
Choosing a Safe and Successful Weight-Loss Program (https://www.niddk
.nih.gov/health-information/weight-management/choosing-a-safe
-successful-weight-loss-program#whatLook).

National Institutes of Health, National Institute of Diabetes and Digestive
and Kidney Diseases. *Definition and Facts for Bariatric Surgery* (https://
www.niddk.nih.gov/health-information/weight-management
/bariatric-surgery/definition-facts). Accessed March 24, 2020.

National Institutes of Health. Office of Dietary Supplements. *Dietary Supplement Fact Sheets* (https://ods.od.nih.gov/). Accessed March 24, 2020.

NCD Risk Factor Collaboration. 2016. Trends in adult body-mass index in
200 countries from 1975 to 2014: A pooled analysis of 1698 population-
based measurement studies with 19.2 million participants. *Lancet*
387(10026): 1377–1396.

Nunez, C., et al. 2017. Obesity, physical activity and cancer risks: Results
from the Cancer, Lifestyle and Evaluation of Risk Study (CLEAR). *Cancer Epidemiology* 47: 56–63

Ogilvie, R. P., et al. 2016. Actigraphy measured sleep indices and adiposity:
The Multi-Ethnic Study of Atherosclerosis (MESA). *Sleep* 39(9):
1701–1708.

Ogilvie, R. P., and S. R. Patel. 2017. The epidemiology of sleep and obesity.
Sleep Health 3(5): 383–388.

Patterson, R. E. and D. D. Sears. 2017, August. Metabolic effects of intermittent fasting. *Annual Review of Nutrition* 37:371-393.

Pearl, R. L., et al. 2020. Effects of a cognitive-behavioral intervention targeting weight stigma: A randomized controlled trial. *Journal of Consulting
and Clinical Psychology.* DOI: 10.1037/ccp0000480.

Pearson, N., et al.2020. Reducing screen time and unhealthy snacking in 9-11
year old children: The kids first pilot randomised controlled trial. *BMC
Public Health* 2(1):122.

Preston, S. H., Y. C. Vierboom, and A. Stokes. 2018. The role of obesity in ex-
ceptionally slow US mortality improvement. *Proceedings of the National
Academy of Sciences* 115(5): 957–961.

Rajan, T. M., and V. Menon. 2017. Psychiatric disorders and obesity: A
review of the association studies. *Journal of Postgraduate Medicine*
63(3):182–190.

Rejeski, W. J. et al. 2017. Community weight loss to combat obesity and disability in at-risk older adults. *Journals of Gerontology. Series A, Biological
Sciences and Medical Sciences* 72(11): 1547–1533.

Rinninella, E., et al. 2019. Food components and dietary habits: Keys for a
healthy gut microbiota composition. *Nutrients* 11(10): 2393.

Roberto, C. A., et al. 2015. Patchy progress on obesity prevention: Emerging
examples, entrenched barriers, and new thinking. *Lancet* 385(9985):
2400–2409.

Rouhani, M. H., et al. 2016. Associations between dietary energy density and obesity: A systematic review and meta-analysis of observational studies. *Nutrition.* 32(10): 1037–1047.

Schiller, J. S., T. C. Clarke, and T. Norris. 2018. Early release of selected estimates based on data from the January–September 2017 National Health Interview Survey. National Center for Health Statistics (https://www.cdc.gov/nchs/nhis.htm).

Sheikh, V. K., and H. A. Raynor. 2016. Decreases in high-fat and/or high-added-sugar food group intake occur when a hypocaloric, low-fat diet is prescribed within a lifestyle intervention: a secondary cohort analysis. *Journal of the Academy of Nutrition and Dietetics* 116(10): 1599–1605.

Shrestha, N., et al. 2019. Effectiveness of interventions for reducing non-occupational sedentary behaviour in adults and older adults: A systematic review and meta-analysis. *British Journal of Sports Medicine* 53(19): 1206–1213.

Sicat, M. 2018. Defining obesity's interplay among environment, behavior and genetics. *Obesity Medicine Association* (https://obesitymedicine.org/obesity-and-genetics/).

Siegel, K. R., et al. 2016. Association of higher consumption of foods derived from subsidized commodities with adverse cardiometabolic risk among US adults. *JAMA Internal Medicine* 176(8): 1124–1132.

Slomski A. 2019. Low-carb diets help maintain weight loss. *Journal of the American Medical Association* 321(4): 355.

Smethers, A. D., and B. J. Rolls. 2018. Dietary management of obesity: Cornerstones of healthy eating patterns. *Medical Clinics of North America* 102(1): 107–124.

Steiger, H., and L. Thaler 2016. Eating disorders, gene environment interactions and the epigenome: Roles of stress exposures and nutritional status. *Physiology and Behavior* 162: 181–185.

Thaler, L., and H. Steiger. 2017. Eating disorders and epigenetics. *Advances in Experimental Medicine and Biology* 978: 93–103.

Thomas, J. G., et al. 2017. Weight loss and frequency of body-weight self-monitoring in an online commercial weight management program with and without a cellular-connected "smart" scale: A randomized pilot study. *Obesity Science and Practice* 3(4): 365–372.

Thomas, J. G., et al. 2017. Weight loss in Weight Watchers Online with and without an activity tracking device compared to control. A randomized trail. *Obesity* 25(6): 1014–1021.

Todd, K. 2017. High-protein diet and weight loss. *Today's Dietitian* 19(12): 32. (https://www.todaysdietitian.com/newarchives/1217p32.shtml).

Trepanowski, J. F., et al. 2017. Effects of alternate day fasting on weight loss, weight maintenance and cardioprotection among metabolically healthy obese adults. A randomized clinical trial. *JAMA Internal Medicine* 177 (7): 930–938.

Tronieri, J. S., et al. 2019. Early weight loss in behavioral treatment predicts later rate of weight loss and response to pharmacotherapy. *Annals of Behavioral Medicine* 53(3): 290–295.

Udo, T., and C. M. Grilo. 2018. Prevalence and correlates of DSM-5 eating disorders in nationally representative sample of United States adults. *Biological Psychiatry* 84(5): 345–354.

USDA Nutrition.gov. n.d. *Online Tools* (https://www.nutrition.gov/topics/basic-nutrition/online-tools). Accessed March 18, 2020.

USDA Economic Research Service. 2016. *Recent Evidence on the Effects of Food Store Access on Food Choice and Diet Quality* (https://www.ers.usda.gov/amber-waves/2016/may/recent-evidence-on-the-effects-of-food-store-access-on-food-choice-and-diet-quality/). Accessed March 25, 2020.

U.S. Department of Health and Human Services. 2018. *Physical Activity Guidelines for Americans,* 2nd ed. Washington, DC: U.S. Department of Health and Human Services (https://health.gov/sites/default/files/2019-09/Physical_Activity_Guidelines_2nd_edition.pdf).

U.S. Department of Health and Human Services. 2020. *Healthy People 2020*: *Nutrition and Weight Status* (https://www.healthypeople.gov/2020/topics-objectives/topic/nutrition-and-weight-status).

U.S. Department of Health and Human Services and U.S. Department of Agriculture. 2015. *2015–2020 Dietary Guidelines for Americans,* 8th ed. (http://health.gov/dietaryguidelines/2015/guidelines).

Vaughan, K. L., and J. A. Mattison. 2018. Watch the clock, not the scale. *Cell Metabolism* 27(6): 1159–1160.

Ward, Z. J., et al. 2019. Estimation of eating disorders prevalence by age and associations with mortality in a simulated nationally representative US cohort. *JAMA Network Open* 2(10): e1912925.

World Health Organization. 2017. *10 Facts on Obesity* (https://www.who.int/features/factfiles/obesity/en/).

Yang, Q., et al. 2015. Predicted heart age and racial disparities in heart age among U.S. adults at the state level. *MMWR* 64(34): 950–958.

Yoon, C., et al. 2020. Disordered eating behaviors and 15-year trajectories in body mass index: Findings from Project Eating and Activity in Teens and Young Adults (EAT). *Journal of Adolescent Health* 66(2): 181–188.

Yu, D. E., et al. 2017. Weight history and all-cause and cause-specific mortality in three prospective cohort studies. *Annals of Internal Medicine* 166(9): 613–620.

Zheng, H., et al. 2013. Obesity and mortality risk: New findings from body mass index trajectories. *American Journal of Epidemiology* 178(11): 1591–1599.

Zuraikat, F. M., L. S. Roe, C. E. Sanchez, and B. J. Rolls. 2018. Comparing the portion size effect in women with and without extended training in portion control: A follow-up to the Portion-Control Strategies Trial. *Appetite* 123: 334–342.

The behavior management plan described in Chapter 1 provides an excellent framework for a weight management program. Following are some suggestions about specific ways you can adapt that general plan to control your weight.

Motivation and Commitment

Make sure you are motivated and committed before you begin. Failure at weight loss is a frustrating experience that can make it more difficult to lose weight in the future. Think about why you want to lose weight. Make a list of your reasons for wanting to lose weight, and post it in a prominent place.

Setting Goals

Choose a reasonable weight you think you would like to reach over the long term, and be willing to renegotiate it as you get further along. Break down your long-term weight and behavioral goals into a series of short-term action-oriented goals.

Creating a Negative Energy Balance

When your weight is constant, you are burning approximately the same number of calories as you are taking in. To tip the energy balance toward weight loss, you must consume fewer calories, or burn more calories through physical activity, or both. To generate a negative energy balance, it's usually best to begin by increasing activity level rather than decreasing your calorie consumption.

Physical Activity

Consider how you can increase your energy output simply by increasing routine physical activity, such as walking or taking the stairs. (Chapter 14 lists activities that use about 150 calories.) If you are not already involved in a regular exercise routine aimed at increasing endurance and building or maintaining muscle mass, seek help from someone who is competent to help you plan and start an appropriate exercise routine. If you are already doing regular physical exercise, evaluate your program according to the guidelines in Chapter 14.

Diet and Eating Habits

If you can't generate a large enough negative energy balance solely by increasing physical activity, you may want to supplement exercise with modest cuts in your calorie intake. Your goal is to make small changes in your diet that you can maintain for a lifetime. Focus on cutting your intake of added sugars, refined carbohydrates, and solid fats and on eating a variety of nutritious foods in moderation. Don't skip meals, fast, or go on a very-low-calorie diet or a diet that is unbalanced.

Making changes in eating habits is another important strategy for weight management. Refer to the box "Lifestyle Strategies for Successful Weight Management" for suggestions.

Self-Monitoring

Keep a record of your weight and behavior change progress. Try keeping a record of everything you eat. Record what you plan to eat, in what quantity, *before* you eat. You'll find that just having to record something that is not okay to eat is likely to stop you from eating it. Also, keep track of your daily activities and your formal exercise program so that you can monitor increases in physical activity.

Putting Your Plan into Action

- Examine the environmental cues that trigger poor eating and exercise habits, and devise strategies for dealing with them. Anticipate problem situations, and plan ways to handle them more effectively.

- Create new environmental cues that will support your new healthy behaviors. Move fruits and vegetables to the front of the refrigerator.

- Get others to help. Talk to friends and family members about what they can do to support your efforts. Find a buddy to join you in your exercise program.

- Give yourself lots of praise and rewards. Focus attention on your accomplishments and achievements and congratulate yourself. Plan special nonfood treats for yourself, such as a walk or a movie. Reward yourself often and for anything that counts toward success.

- If you slip, don't waste time on self-criticism. Think positively instead of getting into a cycle of guilt and self-blame.

- Don't get discouraged. Be aware that, although weight loss is bound to slow down after the first loss of body fluid, the weight loss at this slower rate is more permanent than earlier, more dramatic, losses.

- Remember that weight management is a lifelong project. You need to adopt reasonable goals and strategies that you can maintain over the long term.

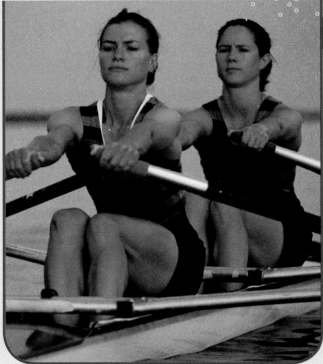
Dann Tardif/Getty Images

CHAPTER OBJECTIVES

- Identify the major components of the cardiovascular system
- Describe the risk factors associated with cardiovascular disease
- Discuss the major forms of cardiovascular disease
- List the steps you can take to protect yourself against cardiovascular disease

CHAPTER **16**

Cardiovascular Health

TEST YOUR KNOWLEDGE

1. **A sedentary lifestyle is an important risk factor for stroke.**
   True or False?

2. **Women are less likely to die of cardiovascular disease than they are to die of breast cancer.**
   True or False?

3. **On average, how much earlier does heart disease develop in people who don't exercise regularly than in people who do?**
   a. 6 months
   b. 2 years
   c. 6 years

4. **Healthy teenagers normally have no signs of cardiovascular disease.**
   True or False?

5. **Which of the following foods would be a good choice for promoting heart health?**
   a. Whole grains
   b. Salmon
   c. Bananas

ANSWERS

1. **TRUE.** Along with tobacco use, high blood pressure, unhealthy cholesterol levels, obesity, diabetes, and diet, a sedentary lifestyle is a major risk factor for stroke.

2. **FALSE.** Cardiovascular disease takes the lives of nearly one in four American women, which is more than all forms of cancer combined.

3. **C, 6 YEARS.** Both aerobic exercise and strength training significantly improve cardiovascular health.

4. **FALSE.** Autopsy studies of young trauma victims show that narrowing of the arteries that supply the heart with blood begins in adolescence in many people.

5. **ALL THREE.** Whole grains (such as whole wheat), foods with omega-3 fatty acids (salmon), and foods high in potassium and low in sodium (bananas) all improve cardiovascular health.

Cardiovascular disease (CVD) refers to the development of diseases that affect the heart and blood vessels: cardiomyopathy (weakness of heart muscle), heart attack (blockage of the coronary artery), stroke (blockage of blood flow to the brain), and angina (chest pain), as well as blood vessel diseases, arrhythmias (heart rhythm problems), and many other conditions affecting the heart's muscle, valves, or rhythms.

As the country's leading cause of death, CVD claims about 2300 American lives every day. More than 92 million American adults have one or more types of CVD, and of these, over half are estimated to be 60 years of age or younger. Heart disease, one form of CVD, is the leading cause of death for both U.S. men and women. Among the life-threatening manifestations of CVD, heart disease and strokes rank first and fifth on the list of the leading causes of death among Americans. Although CVD may seem like a disease that affects only adults, evidence has been mounting that atherosclerosis, the underlying cause of CVD, begins in childhood.

CVD is largely due to our lifestyle. Millions of Americans are overweight and sedentary; we smoke, manage stress ineffectively, have uncontrolled high blood pressure or high cholesterol levels, and don't know the signs of CVD. Not all risk factors for CVD are controllable—for example, some people have an inherited tendency toward high cholesterol levels—but many risk factors are within your control. This chapter introduces the workings of the cardiovascular system, explains CVD and its risks, and shows you how to keep your heart healthy for life.

THE CARDIOVASCULAR SYSTEM

The **cardiovascular system (CVS)** consists of the heart and blood vessels, which includes both arteries and veins. Together they transport blood throughout the body (Figure 16.1). When the lungs are included, the system is known as the *cardiorespiratory* or *cardiopulmonary system*.

The Heart

The heart is a four-chambered, fist-sized muscular organ located just beneath the sternum (breastbone). It pumps deoxygenated (oxygen-poor) blood to the lungs and delivers oxygenated (oxygen-rich) blood to the rest of the body.

Blood actually travels through two separate (but connected) circulatory systems. The right side of the heart pumps blood to the lungs in what is called **pulmonary circulation,**

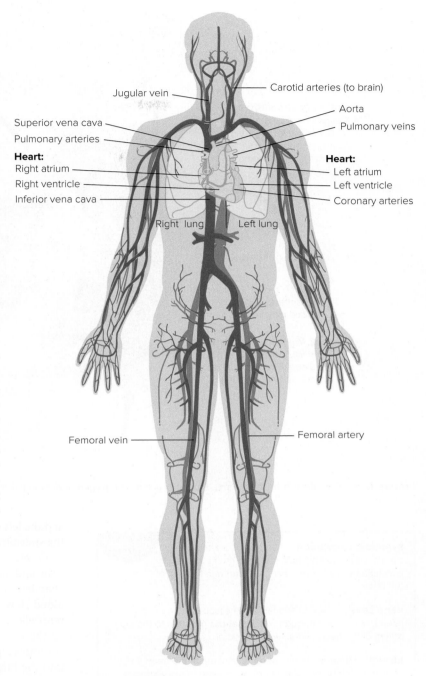

Jugular vein
Carotid arteries (to brain)
Aorta
Superior vena cava
Pulmonary veins
Pulmonary arteries
Heart:
Right atrium
Right ventricle
Inferior vena cava
Heart:
Left atrium
Left ventricle
Coronary arteries
Right lung
Left lung
Femoral vein
Femoral artery

FIGURE 16.1   The cardiorespiratory system.

---

cardiovascular disease (CVD)   The collective term for various diseases of the heart and blood vessels.

cardiovascular system (CVS)   The system that circulates blood through the body; consists of the heart and blood vessels.

pulmonary circulation   The part of the circulatory system controlled by the right side of the heart: the circulation of blood between the heart and the lungs.

TERMS

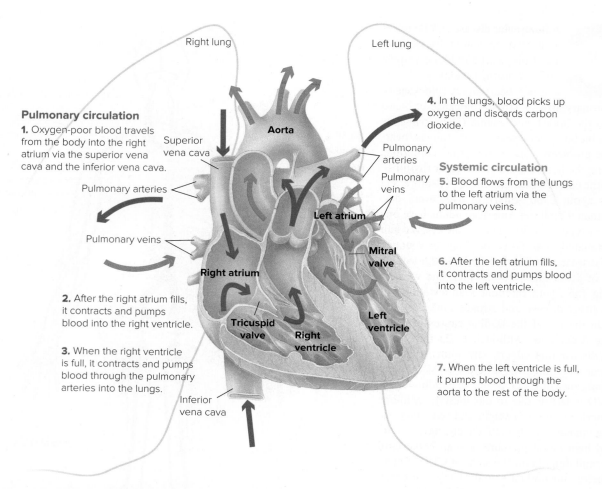

Pulmonary circulation

1. Oxygen-poor blood travels from the body into the right atrium via the superior vena cava and the inferior vena cava.

2. After the right atrium fills, it contracts and pumps blood into the right ventricle.

3. When the right ventricle is full, it contracts and pumps blood through the pulmonary arteries into the lungs.

4. In the lungs, blood picks up oxygen and discards carbon dioxide.

Systemic circulation

5. Blood flows from the lungs to the left atrium via the pulmonary veins.

6. After the left atrium fills, it contracts and pumps blood into the left ventricle.

7. When the left ventricle is full, it pumps blood through the aorta to the rest of the body.

Right lung · Left lung · Aorta · Superior vena cava · Pulmonary arteries · Pulmonary veins · Left atrium · Mitral valve · Right atrium · Tricuspid valve · Right ventricle · Left ventricle · Inferior vena cava

FIGURE 16.2 **Circulation in the heart.** Blue arrows indicate oxygen-poor blood; red arrows indicate oxygen-rich blood.

TERMS

systemic circulation The part of the circulatory system controlled by the left side of the heart: the circulation of blood between the heart and the rest of the body.

vena cava Either of two large veins (superior vena cava and inferior vena cava) through which blood is returned to the right atrium of the heart (plural, *venae cavae*).

atrium Either of the two upper chambers of the heart (left or right) in which blood collects before passing to the ventricles (plural, *atria*).

ventricle Either of the two lower chambers of the heart (left or right) that pump blood to the lungs and other parts of the body.

aorta The largest artery in the body; receives blood from the left ventricle and distributes it to the body.

systole The contraction phase of the heart.

diastole The relaxation phase of the heart.

blood pressure The force exerted by the blood on the walls of the blood vessels; created by the pumping of the heart and the resistance of the blood vessels.

and the left side pumps blood through the rest of the body in the **systemic circulation.**

Oxygen-poor blood travels through the **superior vena cava** and **inferior vena cava** into the heart's right upper chamber, the **right atrium.** After the right atrium fills, blood flows into the heart's right lower chamber, the **right ventricle.** The right atrium and right ventricle are separated by the tricuspid valve. When the right ventricle is full, it contracts and pumps blood through the pulmonary arteries into the lungs. There, blood picks up oxygen and discards carbon dioxide. The newly oxygenated blood flows from the lungs through the pulmonary veins into the heart's **left atrium.** When the left atrium fills, it contracts and pumps blood into the **left ventricle.** When the left ventricle fills, it pumps blood through the **aorta**—the body's largest artery—for distribution to the rest of the body. The path of blood flow through the heart and cardiorespiratory system is illustrated in Figure 16.2.

Each heartbeat consists of two basic parts: systole and diastole. During **systole,** the ventricles contract (ventricular systole) to pump blood out of the heart. During **diastole,** the heart relaxes and fills with blood.

Blood pressure, the force exerted by blood on the walls of the blood vessels, is created by the pumping action of the

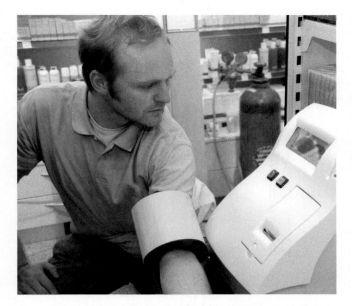

Monitoring blood pressure is a key strategy for the prevention of cardiovascular disease. Blood pressure can be measured during a health care visit, at home with a home blood pressure monitor, or at a drug store. Some newer technologies allow you to measure your blood pressure via wearable devices. Wakila/Stephan Zabel/Getty Images

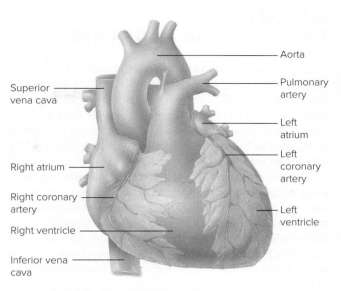

FIGURE 16.3 Blood supply to the heart.

heart and the resistance of the blood vessels. This is an important concept because high blood pressure is treated by medicines that work on relaxing cardiac contractions as well as on reducing the resistance of the blood vessels. Blood pressure is greater during systole (contraction) than during diastole (relaxation). Blood pressure is reported as systolic pressure over diastolic pressure; for example, 120 over 80 mm Hg (or 120/80). The numbers represent millimeters of mercury (mm Hg).

The heartbeat—the sequence of contractions of the heart's four chambers—is controlled by an ordered set of electrical impulses. These signals start in a bundle of specialized cells in the right atrium called the *sinoatrial node* or *pacemaker*. This pacemaker produces a steady heart rate that can be increased or decreased by a number of factors, including the brain's response to stimuli such as stress or the body's need for more oxygen (such as during exercise).

The Blood Vessels

Blood vessels are classified by size and function. **Veins** carry blood to the heart, whereas **arteries** carry blood away from the heart. In the systemic circulation, veins carry deoxygenated blood back to the heart from the body and arteries carry oxygenated blood from the heart to the body. This is reversed in the pulmonary circulation, as blood from the heart is deoxygenated and blood from the lungs to the heart

is oxygenated. Veins have thin walls, but arteries have thick elastic walls that enable them to expand and relax with the pressure of blood being pumped through them during ventricular contraction.

After leaving the heart, the aorta branches into smaller and smaller vessels. The smallest arteries branch still further into **capillaries**—tiny vessels with walls only one cell thick. The capillaries deliver oxygen- and nutrient-rich blood to the tissues, and then pick up oxygen-poor, carbon-dioxide-laden blood. From the capillaries, this blood empties into small veins (*venules*) and then into progressively larger veins that return it to the heart to repeat the cycle.

Blood pumped through the chambers of the heart does not reach the cells of the heart, so the organ has its own network of arteries, veins, and capillaries. Two large vessels, the right and left **coronary arteries,** branch off the aorta and supply the heart itself with oxygenated blood (Figure 16.3). Blockage of blood flow within a coronary artery is the leading cause of heart attacks.

> **vein**   A vessel that carries blood to the heart.   **TERMS**
>
> **artery**   A vessel that carries blood away from the heart.
>
> **capillary**   A small blood vessel that exchanges oxygen and nutrients between the blood and the tissues.
>
> **coronary artery**   A blood vessel branching from the aorta that provides blood to the heart muscle.

MAJOR FORMS OF CARDIOVASCULAR DISEASE

Although deaths from cardiovascular disease have declined dramatically over the past 60 years, it remains the leading cause of death in the United States. According to the CDC, heart disease killed approximately 650,000 Americans in 2017. Figure 16.4 shows the death rates among population groups due to heart disease in 2017, the most recent year for which data are available.

The main forms of CVD are atherosclerosis, coronary heart disease and heart attack, stroke, peripheral arterial disease, congestive heart failure, congenital heart disease, rheumatic heart disease, and heart valve disease. Many forms are interrelated and have elements in common; we treat them separately here for the sake of clarity. Hypertension, which is both a major risk factor and a form of CVD, is described later in the chapter.

Atherosclerosis

A major precursor to heart attacks and other CVD is atherosclerosis, or thickening and hardening of the arteries. **Atherosclerosis** is a disease process in which arteries become narrowed by deposits of fat, cholesterol, and other substances (Figure 16.5). The process begins when the endothelial cells (cells that line the arteries) become damaged, often through a combination of factors such as smoking, high blood pressure, high insulin or glucose levels, and deposits of oxidized cholesterol particles. The body's response to this damage results in inflammation and changes in the artery lining that create a magnet for cholesterol particles, platelets, and other cells. These cells build up and cause a bulge in the wall of the artery. As these deposits, called **plaques,** accumulate in artery walls, the arteries lose their elasticity and their ability to expand and contract, restricting blood flow. Once narrowed by a plaque, an artery is vulnerable to blockage by blood clots. The risk of life-threatening clots, or heart attacks, increases if the fibrous cap covering a plaque ruptures.

If the heart, brain, or other organs are deprived of blood and the oxygen it carries, the effects of atherosclerosis can be

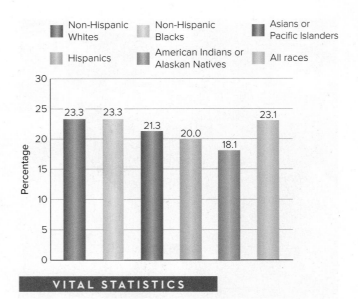

FIGURE 16.4 **Percentage of U.S. deaths due to heart disease, by race/ethnicity.**

SOURCE: National Center for Health Statistics. 2019. Deaths and percentage of total deaths for 10 leading causes of death, by race and Hispanic origin: United States, 2017 (https://www.cdc.gov/nchs/data/nvsr/nvsr68/nvsr68_06-508.pdf).

deadly. Coronary arteries, which supply the heart with blood, are particularly susceptible to plaque buildup, a condition called **coronary heart disease (CHD)** or *coronary artery disease (CAD)*. The blockage of a coronary artery causes a myocardial infarction, commonly described as a heart attack, and blockage of a cerebral artery (leading to the brain) causes a stroke. Blockage of an artery in a limb causes *peripheral arterial disease,* a condition that causes pain and may require amputation of the affected limb.

The main risk factors for atherosclerosis are tobacco use, physical inactivity, high blood cholesterol levels, high blood pressure, and diabetes. Atherosclerosis often begins in childhood: autopsy studies of young trauma victims have revealed atherosclerosis of the coronary arteries in adolescents. Healthy lifestyles can help delay progression of atherosclerosis, hopefully before it causes CHD and other potentially deadly conditions.

Coronary Artery Disease and Heart Attack

The most common form of heart disease is CHD caused by atherosclerosis. When one of the coronary arteries becomes blocked, the result is a **heart attack,** or *myocardial infarction* (*MI*). During a heart attack, the heart muscle (the myocardium) is damaged and may die from lack of oxygenated blood. Although a heart attack may come without warning, it usually results from a chronic disease process.

Myocardial infarctions are a significant cause of death in the United States, especially among people aged 65 and over. The average age for a first heart attack is 66 for men and 72 for women.

---

atherosclerosis A form of cardiovascular disease in which the inner layers of artery walls are made thick and irregular by plaque deposits; arteries become narrow, and blood supply can be reduced.

plaque A deposit of fatty (and other) substances on the inner wall of an artery.

coronary heart disease (CHD) Heart disease caused by atherosclerosis in the arteries that supply blood to the heart muscle; also called *coronary artery disease (CAD)*.

heart attack Damage to, or death of, heart muscle, resulting from a failure of the coronary arteries to deliver enough blood to the heart; also known as *myocardial infarction (MI)*.

TERMS

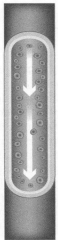 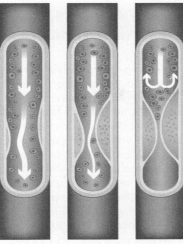 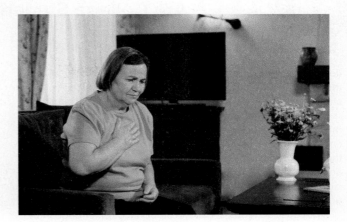

A healthy artery allows blood to flow freely.

As plaque builds up in the arteries, the inside of the arteries begins to narrow, which lessens or blocks the flow of blood. Plaques can also rupture, causing a blood clot to form on the plaque and blocking the flow of blood.

FIGURE 16.5 **Atherosclerosis: The process of cardiovascular disease.**

SOURCE: (left): Centers for Disease Control and Prevention. 2020. Heart Disease Facts. (https://www.cdc.gov/heartdisease/facts.htm) (right): Sanda Stanca/ EyeEm/Getty Images

Heart attack symptoms may include the following:

- Chest pain or pressure
- Arm, neck, or jaw pain
- Difficulty breathing
- Excessive sweating
- Nausea and vomiting
- Loss of consciousness

Most people having a heart attack suffer chest pain, but about one-third of heart attack victims do not. Women, older adults, and people with diabetes and certain forms of CVD are the most likely groups to experience heart attacks without chest pain. The American Heart Association estimates that 605,000 people have a first heart attack each year; 200,000 people have a recurrent attack. Each year, an estimated one in five heart attacks are symptomless or "silent" heart attacks; rates of silent heart attacks are higher among men than women and among blacks than whites.

Angina Arteries partially narrowed by disease may still be open enough to deliver sufficient amounts of oxygenated blood to the heart. However, during stress or exertion, the heart needs more oxygen than can be supplied by blood flow through narrowed arteries. When the need for oxygen exceeds the supply, chest pain, called **angina pectoris,** may occur.

Angina pain is usually felt as a tightness in the chest and heavy pressure behind the breastbone or in the shoulder,

neck, arm, hand, or back. The pain is usually relieved by rest or medicine called nitroglycerin. Although not actually a heart attack, angina is a warning that the load on the heart must be reduced. Any severe chest pain that lasts more than a few minutes should be considered life-threatening, and emergency medical help should be sought immediately.

Angina may be controlled in a number of ways (with drugs and medical procedures), but its course is unpredictable. Over a period ranging from hours to years, the narrowing may go on to full blockage and a heart attack.

Arrhythmias and Sudden Cardiac Death The pumping of the heart is controlled by electrical impulses from the sinus node that maintain a regular heartbeat of 60–100 beats per minute. If this electrical conduction system is disrupted, the heart may beat too quickly, too slowly, or in an irregular fashion. These conditions are known as **arrhythmias** and can cause symptoms ranging from imperceptible to severe and even fatal. Some new devices, such as wearable wristwatch heart-rate monitors, can allow for remote, real-time detection of cardiac arrhythmias.

TERMS

angina pectoris Pain in the chest, and often in the left arm and shoulder, caused by the heart muscle not receiving enough oxygenated blood. The pain is usually brought on by exercise or stress.

arrhythmia A change in the heartbeat's normal, regular pattern.

WELLNESS ON CAMPUS
Are College Students at Risk for Heart Attacks?

Do you know your blood pressure and cholesterol level? Are you prediabetic? If you don't know, you should find out. Although heart attack and strokes are rare events for college students, they do happen.

The college years are an important time to start looking at factors associated with cardiovascular disease. As adolescents, we think we are at low risk and engage in behaviors that worsen our risk factors. We may skip meals, avoid fruits and vegetables, sit on the couch or at a desk too much, smoke cigarettes, and drink alcohol. Young adults often lack knowledge about risk factors.

With busy schedules, college students often engage in behaviors that promote CVD risk. For some, studying and classes leave little time for physical activity. High-fat snack foods (cookies, cake, chips, and ice cream) often preempt nutrient-dense food (fruits, vegetables, and low-fat dairy foods). Dining halls have improved their nutritional outreach, posting signs about nutrition and offering healthy options, but many also offer all-you-can-eat buffets. College students also tend to gain weight. Men in college consume more fast food at lunch, which may explain why they gain more weight than women.

Men generally are at greater risk for CVD because they have lower HDL cholesterol and higher LDL cholesterol, blood pressure, fasting glucose, and BMI. Young adult males in college also engage in more of the behaviors that put them at risk.

College Athletes

Sudden cardiac death is the number-one cause of death among college athletes during sports activities. To determine whether they are at risk for CVD, college athletes must undergo a screening examination before they participate in sports. The screening may include a questionnaire about the student's personal and family history, a physical exam, and sometimes an electrocardiogram (ECG or EKG) to detect cardiac abnormalities.

One study analyzed the data from the screening examinations of 790 athletes at a National Collegiate Athletic Association (NCAA) Division I university. The most common reported complaints were fainting or near fainting (*syncope*) during or after exercise, chest discomfort/tightness/pressure during exercise, and a family history of a heart problem (including a pacemaker or an implanted defibrillator). During the physical exam, 26 athletes (3.3%) were found to have a heart murmur, and two athletes (0.3%) had physical signs of Marfan syndrome, a condition that strains the heart and aorta. ECG abnormalities were present in 22 athletes (2.8%).

The study found that a physical examination and the history questionnaires would not have been informative enough without the ECGs. The questionnaires are vague and too broad to catch all students whose risk for sudden cardiac death is high. Although this school did have experience using ECGs, others do not have the physician expertise and institutional resources to properly interpret such tests. The study also found that of all college athletes, male basketball players carry the highest risk for sudden cardiac death.

A heart attack can occur at any age. Because so many young people are overweight or obese, the chances of cardiovascular diseases are greater than in the past.

SOURCES: Abshire, D. A., et al. 2016. Perceptions related to cardiovascular disease risk in Caucasian college males. *American Journal of Men's Health* 10(6): N136–N144; ACLS. 2020. *Cardiac Disease in the Young* (https://www.acls.net/cardiac-disease-in-the-young.htm); De Young, W. 2018. College students may not be as heart-healthy as they think. *The Conversation* (https://theconversation.com/college-students-may-not-be-as-heart-healthy-as-they-think-91730); Drezner, J. A., et al. 2015. Cardiovascular screening in college athletes. *Journal of the American College of Cardiology* 65(21): 2353–2355.

Sudden cardiac death, also called *cardiac arrest,* is most often caused by an arrhythmia called *ventricular fibrillation,* a kind of heart rhythm that leads to ineffective blood flow. If ventricular fibrillation continues for more than a few minutes, it is generally fatal. Cardiac defibrillation, in which an electrical shock is delivered to the heart, can be effective in jolting the heart back into a normal rhythm. Emergency personnel typically carry defibrillators, and automated external defibrillators (AEDs) are becoming increasingly available in public places. AEDs monitor the heart's rhythm and, if appropriate,

deliver an electrical shock. (Training in the use of AEDs is available from organizations such as the American Red Cross and the American Heart Association.) Sudden cardiac death most often occurs in people with CHD, and it occasionally occurs in young people such as college athletes during sports activities (see the box "Are College Students at Risk for Heart Attacks?"). Serious arrhythmias frequently develop during or after a heart attack and are often the actual cause of death in cases of a fatal myocardial infarction.

Other potential causes of arrhythmia include congenital heart abnormalities, infections, drug use, abnormal concentrations of electrolytes, chest trauma, and congestive heart failure. Some arrhythmias cause no problems and resolve without treatment; more serious arrhythmias are usually treated with medication or a surgically implanted pacemaker or defibrillator that delivers electrical stimulation to the heart to create a more normal rhythm.

---

sudden cardiac death A nontraumatic, unexpected death from sudden cardiac arrest, most often due to arrhythmia; in most instances, victims have underlying heart disease.

TERMS

Helping a Heart Attack Victim   Most deaths from heart attacks occur within two hours of the first onset of symptoms. Unfortunately, many heart attack victims wait more than two hours before getting help. If you or someone you are with shows any of the signs of heart attack listed in the box "Warning Signs and Symptoms of Heart Attack, Stroke, or Cardiac Arrest," take immediate action. Call for help—even if the person denies something is wrong. Many experts also suggest that the heart attack victim *chew* and swallow one adult aspirin tablet (325 mg) as soon as possible after symptoms begin. Aspirin has an immediate anticlotting effect.

If the victim loses consciousness, a qualified person should immediately check for a pulse and, if no pulse is found, start administering emergency **cardiopulmonary resuscitation (CPR).** Another person should call 9-1-1 immediately. Damage to the heart muscle increases with time. If the person receives emergency care quickly enough, a clot-dissolving agent or emergency invasive procedure can be used to break up the clot in the coronary artery.

Detecting and Treating Heart Disease   Physicians have an expanding array of tools to evaluate the condition of the heart and its arteries. Currently the most common initial screening tool for CHD is the exercise stress test. During an exercise stress test, a patient runs or walks on a treadmill or pedals a stationary cycle while being monitored for abnormalities with an **electrocardiogram (ECG).** Changes in the heart's electrical activity while under stress can reveal heart problems and restricted blood flow. Exercise testing can also be performed in conjunction with imaging techniques such as nuclear medicine or echocardiography that provide pictures of the heart at or after stress, which can help pinpoint abnormal areas of the heart.

Many other imaging tests are also used for evaluating CHD. These tests include the following:

- *Computed tomography (CT)* scan uses a sweeping electron beam to produce computerized cross-sectional images of the heart and can pinpoint calcium in the arteries, which is a marker for atherosclerosis.

- *Echocardiography* utilizes ultrasound waves to examine the heart's pumping function and valves. This technology can identify rapidly moving heart muscles. For an exercise stress echocardiogram, echocardiography is performed after a patient exercises to evaluate the effect of stress on the heart.

- **Magnetic resonance imaging (MRI)** uses powerful magnets to look inside the body and generate pictures of the heart and blood vessels.

- *Nuclear myocardial perfusion imaging* injects radiotracers (such as thallium-201) into the bloodstream. The radiotracers' location and density in the heart can be imaged and quantified, which allows physicians to determine the blood flow to various areas of the heart and identify possible CHD.

- *Positron emission tomography (PET)* involves the use of positron-emitting isotopes to image and quantify regional blood flow in the heart and identify CHD. PET scans can also measure the metabolism of cells in the heart and therefore determine which parts of the heart are no longer alive.

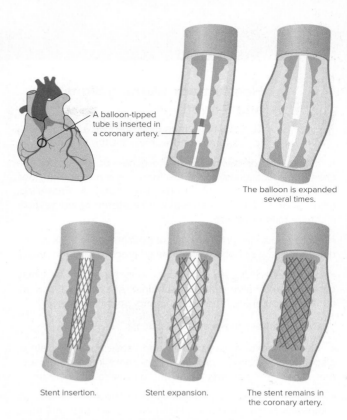

A balloon-tipped tube is inserted in a coronary artery.

The balloon is expanded several times.

Stent insertion.

Stent expansion.

The stent remains in the coronary artery.

FIGURE 16.6   Balloon angioplasty and stenting.

If symptoms or noninvasive tests suggest CHD, the next step is often a coronary **angiogram,** performed in a cardiac catheterization lab. In this test, a catheter (a small plastic tube) is threaded into an artery, usually in the wrist or groin, and advanced through the aorta to the coronary arteries. The catheter is then placed into the opening of the coronary artery and a special dye is injected. The dye can be seen moving through the arteries via X-ray, and any narrowing or blockage can be identified. If a problem is found, it is commonly treated with a metal stent or **balloon angioplasty,** which is performed by specially trained cardiologists (Figure 16.6).

cardiopulmonary resuscitation (CPR)   A technique involving mouth-to-mouth breathing and/or chest compressions to keep oxygen flowing to the brain.

electrocardiogram (ECG or EKG)   A test to detect cardiac abnormalities by evaluating the electrical activity in the heart.

magnetic resonance imaging (MRI)   A computerized imaging technique that uses a strong magnetic field to create detailed pictures of body structures.

angiogram   A picture of the arterial system taken after injecting a dye that is opaque to X-rays.

balloon angioplasty   A technique in which a catheter with a deflated balloon on the tip is inserted into an artery; the balloon is then inflated at the point of obstruction in the artery, pressing the plaque against the artery wall to improve blood supply.

TERMS

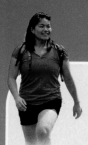

TAKE CHARGE
Warning Signs and Symptoms of Heart Attack, Stroke, or Cardiac Arrest

Heart Attack Warning Signs and Symptoms

The most common symptoms of a heart attack for both men and women are the following:

• *Chest pain or discomfort* in the center or left side of the chest that usually lasts for more than a few minutes or goes away and comes back. It can feel like pressure, squeezing, fullness, or pain. It also can feel like heartburn or indigestion. It can be mild or severe.

• *Upper body discomfort* in one or both arms, the back, shoulders, neck, jaw, or upper part of the stomach (above the navel).

• *Shortness of breath* may be the only symptom, or it may occur before or along with chest pain or discomfort. It can occur when you are resting or doing mild physical activity.

But remember these additional facts:

• Heart attacks can start slowly and cause only mild pain or discomfort. Symptoms can be mild or more intense and sudden. Symptoms also may come and go over several hours.

• People who have high blood sugar (diabetes) may have no symptoms or very mild ones. Heart attacks without symptoms or with very mild symptoms are called silent heart attacks.

• The most common symptom, in both men and women, is chest pain or discomfort.

• Women are somewhat more likely than men to experience shortness of breath; nausea and vomiting; unusual tiredness (sometimes for days); and pain in the back, shoulders, and jaw.

• Other possible symptoms include breaking out in a cold sweat, light-headedness or sudden dizziness, or a change in the pattern of usual symptoms.

The signs and symptoms of a heart attack can develop suddenly or slowly—within hours, days, or weeks of a heart attack. If you think you or someone you know might be having heart attack symptoms or a heart attack, don't ignore it or feel embarrassed to call for help. **Call 9-1-1 right away.** Here's why:

• Acting fast can save a life. Every minute matters. Never delay calling 9-1-1 to do anything you think might help.

• An ambulance is the best and safest way to get to the hospital. Emergency medical services (EMS) personnel start life-saving treatments right away. People who arrive at the hospital by ambulance often receive faster treatment.

• The 9-1-1 operator or EMS technician can give you advice. You might be told to chew (or crush) and swallow an aspirin, unless there is a medical reason for you not to take one.

Stroke Warning Signs and Symptoms

The symptoms of stroke are distinctive because they happen quickly:

• Sudden numbness or weakness of the face, arm, or leg (especially on one side of the body)

• Sudden confusion, trouble speaking, or understanding speech

• Sudden trouble seeing in one or both eyes

• Sudden trouble walking, dizziness, loss of balance or coordination

• Sudden severe headache with no known cause.

An acronym to help you remember the most common symptoms of a stroke is FAST (facial drooping, arm weakness, speech difficulty, and time to call 9-1-1). If you believe

---

This technique involves feeding a balloon-tipped catheter into the artery and inflating the balloon to flatten the fatty plaque and widen the arterial opening.

Balloon angioplasty is generally followed by placement of a *stent*—a small metal tube that helps keep the artery open.

Other treatments, ranging from medication to major surgery, are also available. Along with a low-fat diet, regular exercise, and smoking cessation, medical therapy can improve

> **coronary bypass surgery** Surgery in which a blood vessel is grafted from the aorta to a point below an obstruction in a coronary artery, improving the blood supply to the heart.
>
> **TERMS**

risk factors and biomarkers of health. A statin, or cholesterol-lowering medication, reduces lifetime risk of CHD by stopping or regressing plaque buildup in the heart arteries. Aspirin helps prevent platelets in the blood from sticking to arterial plaques and forming clots, and it also reduces inflammation.

Other prescription drugs can help control heart rate, dilate arteries, lower blood pressure, and reduce the strain on the heart—improving both the quality and length of life in heart patients.

In **coronary bypass surgery,** surgeons remove a healthy blood vessel—usually a vein from the patient's leg—and graft it from the aorta to one or more coronary arteries to bypass a blockage.

someone is having a stroke, call 9-1-1 immediately. Ischemic strokes, the most common type, can be treated with a drug called t-PA, which dissolves blood clots. The drug must be administered within three hours, but to be evaluated and receive treatment in time, patients must get to the hospital within 60 minutes.

A transient ischemic attack (TIA) has the same signs and symptoms as a stroke. However, TIA symptoms usually last less than 1–2 hours (although they may last up to 24 hours). A TIA may occur only once in a person's lifetime or more often and can be a warning sign for future strokes. At first, it may not be possible to tell whether someone is having a TIA or stroke. All stroke-like symptoms require medical care.

Sudden Cardiac Arrest Signs

In sudden cardiac arrest (SCA), the heart stops beating suddenly and unexpectedly, so blood stops flowing to the brain and other vital organs. The person suddenly becomes unresponsive and stops breathing, and if he or she does not receive treatment within minutes, death occurs. Usually, the first sign of SCA is loss of consciousness (fainting). At the same time, no heartbeat (or pulse) can be felt. Some people may have a racing heartbeat or feel dizzy or light-headed just before they faint. Within an hour before SCA, some people experience chest pain, shortness of breath, nausea, or vomiting.

If you are with someone who experiences these symptoms, begin CPR and call 9-1-1 immediately. Rapid treatment of SCA with a defibrillator can be lifesaving. A defibrillator is a device that sends an electric shock to the heart to restore its normal rhythm. Automated external defibrillators (AEDs) can be used by bystanders to save the lives of people who are having SCA. These portable devices often are found in public places, such as shopping malls, golf courses, businesses, airports, airplanes, convention centers, hotels, sports venues, and schools.

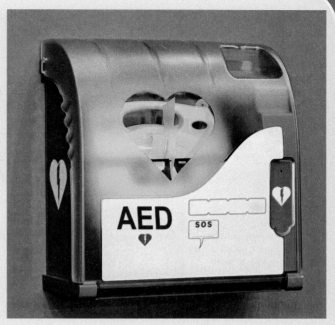

Baloncici/123RF

SOURCES: American Heart Association. 2020. *Heart Attack and Stroke Symptoms* (https://www.heart.org/en/about-us/heart-attack-and-stroke-symptoms); National Institute of Neurological Disorders and Stroke. 2013. *Know Stroke. Know the Signs. Act in Time* (http://stroke.nih.gov/materials/actintime.htm); National Heart, Lung, and Blood Institute. 2016. *What Is Sudden Cardiac Arrest?* (http://www.nhlbi.nih.gov/health-topics/sudden-cardiac-arrest).

Stroke

For brain cells to function, they require a continuous supply of oxygen-rich blood. If brain cells are deprived of oxygenated blood for more than a few minutes, they will die. A **stroke,** also called a *cerebrovascular accident (CVA),* occurs when the blood supply to the brain is interrupted and brain tissue subsequently dies. One study found that about 2 million brain cells die per minute and the brain ages about 3.5 years each hour during a stroke.

In the past, not much could be done for stroke victims. Today, however, prompt treatment can greatly decrease the risk of permanent disability. Once an angiogram detects a problem, medications and angioplasty can treat it. Everyone

should know the warning signs of a stroke and seek immediate medical help, just as they would at the first sign of a heart attack.

Types of Strokes There are two major types of strokes (Figure 16.7), described in the sections that follow.

> **stroke** Impeded blood supply to some part of the brain, resulting in the destruction of brain cells; also called a *cerebrovascular accident (CVA).*   **TERMS**

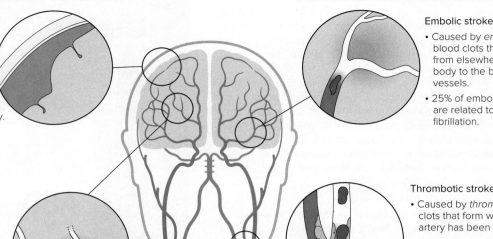

HEMORRHAGIC STROKE
- 13% of strokes.
- Caused by ruptured blood vessels followed by blood leaking into tissue.
- Usually more serious than ischemic stroke.

Subarachnoid hemorrhage
- A bleed into the space between the brain and the skull.
- Develops most often from an *aneurysm*, a weakened, ballooned area in the wall of an artery.

Intracerebral hemorrhage
- A bleed from a blood vessel inside the brain.
- Often caused by high blood pressure and the damage it does to arteries.

ISCHEMIC STROKE
- 87% of strokes.
- Caused by blockages in brain blood vessels; potentially treatable with clot-busting drugs.
- Brain tissue dies when blood flow is blocked.

Embolic stroke
- Caused by *emboli*, blood clots that travel from elsewhere in the body to the brain blood vessels.
- 25% of embolic strokes are related to atrial fibrillation.

Thrombotic stroke
- Caused by *thrombi*, blood clots that form where an artery has been narrowed.
- Usually due to formation of fatty deposits that build up and reduce blood flow (atherosclerosis) or to other artery conditions.

FIGURE 16.7   Types of stroke.

SOURCE: "Harvard Health Letter," Harvard University, April 2000. Artwork by Harriet Greenfield. Reprinted with permission.

ISCHEMIC STROKE   An **ischemic stroke** is caused by a blockage in a blood vessel. There are two types of ischemic strokes:

• A *thrombotic stroke* is caused by a **thrombus,** which is a blood clot that forms in a cerebral or carotid artery that has been previously narrowed or damaged by atherosclerosis.

• An *embolic stroke* is caused when an **embolus,** or a wandering blood clot, is carried through the bloodstream and becomes wedged in a cerebral artery. Many embolic strokes are linked to other diseases associated with forming blood clots. One common disease associated with blood clots is an abnormal heart rhythm called *atrial fibrillation.* When this arrhythmia occurs, the heart rhythm is irregular and blood may pool in the left atrium, which can cause a clot formation that can travel to the brain. Recent studies have shown some wearable technology, such as heart-rate monitors, can detect episodes of atrial fibrillation.

Ischemic strokes, which account for 87% of all strokes, are potentially treatable with clot-busting drugs, so immediate medical help is critical to improving the victim's chances of recovery.

HEMORRHAGIC STROKE   A **hemorrhagic stroke** occurs when a blood vessel in the brain bursts, spilling blood into the surrounding tissue. Cells normally nourished by the vessel are deprived of blood and cannot function. In addition, accumulated blood from the burst vessel may put pressure on surrounding brain tissue, causing damage and even death. There are two types of hemorrhagic strokes:

• In an *intracerebral hemorrhage,* a blood vessel ruptures within the brain. About 10% of strokes are caused by intracerebral hemorrhages.

• In a *subarachnoid hemorrhage,* a blood vessel on the brain's surface ruptures and bleeds into the space between the brain and the skull. About 3% of strokes are of this type.

Hemorrhages can be caused by head injuries or the bursting of a malformed blood vessel, or **aneurysm,** which

---

TERMS

ischemic stroke   Impeded blood supply to the brain caused by a clot obstructing a blood vessel.

thrombus   A blood clot that forms in a blood vessel that has already been damaged by plaque buildup; the clot may lead to stroke.

embolus   A blood clot that breaks off from its place of origin in a blood vessel and travels through the bloodstream.

hemorrhagic stroke   Impeded blood supply to the brain caused by the rupture of a blood vessel.

aneurysm   A sac or outpouching formed by a distention or dilation of the artery wall.

is a blood-filled pocket that bulges out from a weak spot in the artery wall. Aneurysms in the brain may remain stable and never break. But when they do, the result is a hemorrhagic stroke. Aneurysms may be caused or worsened by hypertension.

The Effects of a Stroke   The interruption of the blood supply to any area of the brain causes cell death in that region of the brain. Stroke survivors usually have some lasting disability. Which parts of the body are affected depends on the area of the brain that has been damaged. Brain cells control sensation and body movements, and so a stroke may cause paralysis, walking disability, speech impairment, memory loss, or changes in behavior. The severity of the stroke and how long the effects last depend on which brain cells have been injured, how widespread the damage is, how effectively the body can restore the blood supply, and how rapidly other areas of the brain can take over the functions of the damaged areas. Early treatment can significantly reduce the severity of disability resulting from a stroke—patients who arrive in the emergency room within three hours of onset of symptoms have less disability three months after a stroke compared to patients who receive delayed care.

Detecting and Treating Stroke   Death rates from stroke have declined significantly over the past decades—from nearly 90% in 1950 to about 18% today. Effective treatment requires the prompt recognition of symptoms and correct diagnosis of the type of stroke.

A quick way to recognize a stroke is to ask the person to do four simple things:

1. Ask the person to smile. If her smile droops on one side, or if she is unable to move or open one side of her mouth, she may be having a stroke.

2. Ask the person to hold his arms or legs out. If the person cannot move one arm/leg or hold one arm/leg still, it may be a sign of a stroke.

3. Ask the person to repeat a simple, short sentence, such as "Take me out to the ball game." If she has trouble speaking or cannot speak, a stroke is possible.

4. Ask the person whether he has any decreased sensation, numbness, or abnormal tingling in his legs, arms, or other body parts.

These are tests for Facial drooping, Arm weakness, and Speech difficulty, which stand for the first three letters of the acronym FAST; the T stands for *time to call 9-1-1*. If someone has difficulty performing any of these tests, follow the steps described in the box "Warning Signs and Symptoms of Heart Attack, Stroke, or Cardiac Arrest."

Many people have strokes without knowing it. These "silent strokes" do not cause any noticeable symptoms while they are occurring. Although they may be mild, silent strokes leave their victims at a higher risk for subsequent and more serious strokes. They also contribute to loss of mental and cognitive skills. In 2016, a study of MRI scans of over 1000 elderly people revealed that 6% of the subjects had brain damage from one or more strokes but did not realize they had ever had a stroke.

Some stroke victims have a **transient ischemic attack (TIA),** or "ministroke," days, weeks, or months before they have a full-blown stroke. A TIA produces temporary stroke-like symptoms, such as weakness or numbness in an arm or a leg, speech difficulty, or dizziness. These symptoms are brief, often lasting just a few minutes, and do not cause permanent damage. TIAs should be taken as warning signs of a stroke, however, and anyone with a suspected TIA should get immediate medical attention.

Strokes should be treated with the same urgency as heart attacks. A person with stroke symptoms should be rushed to the hospital. A **computed tomography (CT)** scan, which uses a computer to construct an image of the brain from X-rays, can assess brain damage and determine the type of stroke.

If tests reveal that a stroke is caused by a blood clot—and if help is sought within a few hours of the onset of symptoms—the blockage can be treated with the same kind of clot-dissolving drugs that are used to treat coronary artery blockages. If the clot is dissolved quickly enough, brain damage is minimized and symptoms may disappear. The longer the brain goes without blood, the greater the risk of permanent damage.

People who have had TIAs or who are at high risk for stroke due to narrowing of the carotid arteries (large arteries on either side of the neck, which carry blood to the head) may undergo a surgical procedure called *carotid endarterectomy,* in which plaque is removed. There is also a stent-based procedure, similar to coronary angioplasty and stenting, for patients who are at increased risk of surgical complications.

If tests reveal that a stroke was caused by a cerebral hemorrhage, drugs may be prescribed to lower the blood pressure, which will usually be high. Careful diagnosis is crucial, because administering clot-dissolving drugs to a person

TERMS

transient ischemic attack (TIA)   A small stroke; usually a temporary interruption of blood supply to the brain, causing numbness or difficulty with speech.

computed tomography (CT)   The use of computerized X-ray images to create a cross-sectional depiction (scan) of tissue density.

suffering a hemorrhagic stroke could cause more bleeding and potentially more brain damage.

If detection and treatment of stroke come too late, rehabilitation and prevention of further events is the mainstay of treatment. Although dead brain tissue does not regenerate, nerve cells in the brain can make new pathways and over time regain some motor or speech functions. Spontaneous recovery can start immediately after a stroke and continues for a few months.

Rehabilitation consists of physical therapy, which helps strengthen muscles and improve balance and coordination; speech and language therapy, which helps those whose speech has been damaged; and occupational therapy, which helps improve hand–eye coordination and everyday living skills. Some people recover completely in a matter of days or weeks, but many stroke victims who survive must adapt to some disability.

Peripheral Arterial Disease

Peripheral arterial disease (PAD) refers to atherosclerosis in the leg or arm arteries, which can eventually limit or completely obstruct blood flow. The same process that occurs in the heart arteries can occur in any artery of the body. In fact, patients with PAD frequently have coexisting coronary artery disease and cerebrovascular disease and have an increased risk of death from CVD. PAD affects approximately 8.5 million people in the United States.

The risk factors associated with coronary atherosclerosis, such as smoking, diabetes, hypertension, and high cholesterol, also contribute to atherosclerosis in the peripheral circulation. The risk of PAD is significantly increased in people with diabetes and people who use tobacco products.

Symptoms of PAD include claudication and a more difficult time fighting infections or healing ulcerations that can form in the leg or foot. *Claudication* is aching or fatigue in the affected leg with exertion, particularly walking, and often resolves with rest. Claudication occurs when leg muscles do not get adequate blood and oxygen supply. *Rest pain* occurs when the limb artery is unable to supply adequate blood and oxygen even when the body is not physically active. This occurs when the artery is significantly narrowed or completely blocked. If blood flow is not restored quickly,

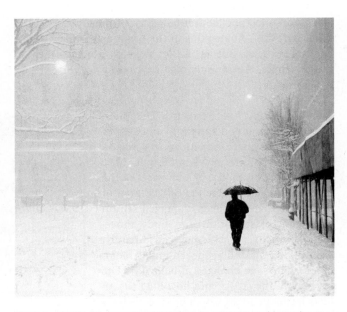

More heart attacks occur in winter than in summer, and more heart attacks occur in the morning than at other times of the day. Several explanations have been proposed for both phenomena. image 100/ Alamy Stock Photo

cells and tissues die; in severe cases, amputation may be needed. PAD is the leading cause of amputation in people over age 50. The likelihood of needing an amputation is increased in those who continue to use tobacco products, and PAD in people with diabetes tends to be extensive and severe.

Congestive Heart Failure

A number of conditions can damage the heart—high blood pressure, heart attack, atherosclerosis, alcoholism, illicit drug use, heart valve disease, viral infections, rheumatic fever, and birth defects. With weakening of the heart muscle, the heart cannot maintain its regular pumping rate and force, and this can cause fluid buildup, an indication of **congestive heart failure** or **cardiomyopathy**. When extra fluid seeps through capillary walls, edema (swelling) results, usually in the legs and ankles, but sometimes in other parts of the body as well. Fluid can collect in the lungs and interfere with breathing, particularly when a person is lying down. This condition is called **pulmonary edema.**

Treatment includes reducing the workload on the heart, modifying fluid and salt intake, and using drugs that help the body eliminate excess fluid. Drugs used to treat congestive heart failure improve the pumping action of the heart, lower blood pressure so that the heart doesn't have to work as hard, and help the body eliminate excess salt and water. When medical therapy is ineffective, heart transplant can be a solution for some patients with severe heart failure, but the need greatly exceeds the number of donor hearts available. About 5.7 million Americans suffer from heart failure.

---

peripheral arterial disease (PAD) **TERMS** Atherosclerosis in the arteries in the legs (or less commonly, the arms) that can impede blood flow and lead to pain, infection, and loss of the affected limb.

congestive heart failure A condition resulting from the heart's inability to pump enough blood to keep up with the body's metabolic needs; blood backs up in the veins leading to the heart, causing an accumulation of fluid in various parts of the body.

pulmonary edema The accumulation of fluid in the lungs.

The risk of heart failure increases with age, and being overweight is a significant independent risk factor. Experts suggest that the incidence of heart failure will increase dramatically over the next few decades as our population ages and becomes increasingly obese.

Other Forms of Heart Disease

Other, less common, forms of heart disease include congenital heart defects, rheumatic heart disease, and heart valve disorders.

Congenital Heart Defects   About 1% of births each year in America, equivalent to 40,000 children, have a defect or malformation of the heart or major blood vessels. These conditions are collectively referred to as **congenital heart defects**, and they cause nearly 13,500 deaths a year in children under 1 year of age. Most common congenital defects can be accurately diagnosed and treated with medication or surgery. The most common congenital defects are holes in the wall that divides the chambers of the heart, which can cause mixing of oxygenated and deoxygenated blood and ineffective circulation. Such defects can cause the heart to produce a distinctive sound, making diagnosis relatively simple. Another common defect is *coarctation of the aorta*—a narrowing, or constriction, of the aorta.

Hypertrophic cardiomyopathy occurs in approximately 1 out of every 500 people in the United States and is the most common cause of sudden death among athletes younger than age 35. This disease is visible in an unusually thick, or hypertrophied, heart muscle, which can lead to ineffective blood flow and abnormal heart rhythms. People with hypertrophic cardiomyopathy are at high risk for sudden death, mainly due to serious arrhythmias. Hypertrophic cardiomyopathy is most commonly diagnosed using echocardiography. Possible treatments include medications, surgery to reduce the thickened heart muscle, and even an implanted internal defibrillator for patients at high risk of sudden cardiac death.

Rheumatic Heart Disease   **Rheumatic fever,** a consequence of certain types of untreated streptococcal throat infections, is a leading cause of heart failure worldwide, but is relatively uncommon in the United States. Rheumatic fever can permanently damage the heart muscle and heart valves, a condition called *rheumatic heart disease (RHD).* Many of the approximately 100,000 operations on heart valves performed annually are related to RHD, and about 9500 Americans die each year from RHD. The incidence of rheumatic fever has declined significantly in the United States since the introduction of antibiotics.

Symptoms of strep throat include the sudden onset of a sore throat, painful swallowing, fever, swollen glands, headache, nausea, and vomiting. Careful laboratory diagnosis is important because strep throat is treated with antibiotics, which are not useful in the treatment of far more common viral sore throats. If left untreated, up to 3% of strep infec-

Ask Yourself

QUESTIONS FOR CRITICAL THINKING AND REFLECTION

Has anyone you know ever had a heart attack? If so, was the onset gradual or sudden? Were appropriate steps taken to help the person (for example, did anyone call 9-1-1, give CPR, or use an AED)? Do you feel comfortable dealing with a cardiac emergency? If not, what can you do to improve your readiness?

tions progress into rheumatic fever. Rheumatic fever affects primarily children between the ages of 5 and 15 years.

Heart Valve Disorders   Age, previous heart attacks, congenital defects, and certain types of infections can cause abnormalities in the valves between the chambers of the heart. Heart valve problems generally fall into two categories—the valve failing to open fully or failing to close completely. In either case, blood flow through the heart is impaired with decreased forward blood flow or occasional reversal of blood flow.

Treatment for heart valve disorders depends on their location and severity. Serious problems may be treated with surgery to repair or replace a valve. People with certain types of heart valve defects are advised to take antibiotics prior to some types of dental and surgical procedures in order to prevent bacteria, which may be dislodged into the bloodstream during the procedure, from infecting the defective valve.

The most common heart valve disorder is **mitral valve prolapse (MVP),** which occurs in about 3% of the population. MVP is characterized by a billowing of the mitral valve, which separates the left ventricle and left atrium, during ventricular contraction. In severe cases, blood leaks backward from the ventricle into the atrium and the heart has to work harder for the same amount of forward blood flow. Most people with MVP have no symptoms: They have the same ability to exercise and live as long as people without MVP. The condition is often

TERMS

congenital heart defect   A defect or malformation of the heart or its major blood vessels, present at birth.

hypertrophic cardiomyopathy   An inherited condition in which there is an enlargement of the heart muscle, especially the muscle between the two ventricles.

rheumatic fever   A disease, mainly of children, characterized by fever, inflammation, and pain in the joints. It often damages the heart valves and muscle, a condition called rheumatic heart disease.

mitral valve prolapse (MVP)   A condition in which the mitral valve billows out during ventricular contraction, allowing leakage of blood from the left ventricle into the left atrium.

diagnosed during a routine medical exam when an extra heart sound (a click) or murmur is heard. The diagnosis can be confirmed with echocardiography.

RISK FACTORS FOR CARDIOVASCULAR DISEASE

Factors associated with an increased risk of developing cardiovascular disease are grouped into two main categories: major risk factors and contributing risk factors. Some lifestyle risk factors can therefore be changed; these are called modifiable risk factors. Others are beyond our control, while some require more research to fully understand. To prevent heart disease later in life, it is very important to establish healthy eating and exercise habits at a young age.

Major Risk Factors That Can Be Changed

The American Heart Association (AHA) identifies certain factors that can increase the risk of developing CVD. Those that can be changed include tobacco use, high blood pressure, unhealthy blood cholesterol levels, physical inactivity, obesity, and diabetes. Although the AHA does not identify poor diet as a separate major risk factor, it contributes to several of the risk factors in this category; dietary recommendations are also discussed in this section. Most Americans, including young adults, have at least one major risk factor for CVD.

Tobacco Use   Annually, nearly one in five deaths can be attributed to smoking, equivalent to 1300 deaths per day. Smoking remains one of the leading preventable causes of CVD in the United States. People who smoke a pack of cigarettes a day have twice the risk of heart attack as nonsmokers; smoking two or more packs a day triples the risk. When smokers have heart attacks, they are two to three times more likely than nonsmokers to die from them. Cigarette smoking also doubles the risk of stroke.

High Blood Pressure   High blood pressure, or **hypertension,** is a risk factor for many forms of cardiovascular disease, including heart attacks and stroke.

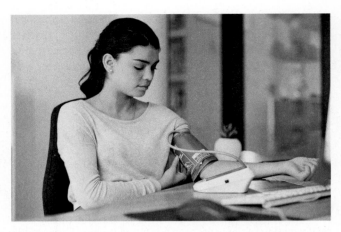

You can check your blood pressure in the time it takes some files to download. PeopleImages/E+/Getty Images

Blood pressure, the force exerted by the blood on the vessel walls, is created by the pumping action of the heart and the resistance of the arteries. High blood pressure occurs when too much force is exerted against the walls of the arteries. Many factors affect blood pressure, such as exercise or excitement. Short periods of high blood pressure are normal, but chronic high blood pressure is a health risk.

Health care professionals measure blood pressure with a stethoscope and an instrument called a *sphygmomanometer.* At home you can track your own blood pressure by using an electronic blood pressure monitor, and new technologies can measure blood pressure using wearable devices (see box "Digital Health Approach to Cardiovascular Disease"). A normal blood pressure reading for a healthy adult is below 120 mm Hg systolic and below 80 mm Hg diastolic. Blood pressure readings with systolic between 120 and 129 mm Hg and diastolic still less than 80 mm Hg are classified as elevated because they begin to carry risk. Stage 1 hypertension in adults is defined as systolic pressure between 130 and 139 mm Hg or diastolic pressure between 80 and 89 mm Hg, and stage 2 hypertension is defined as a systolic pressure of at least 140 mm Hg or a diastolic pressure of at least 90 mm Hg (Table 16.1); it is diagnosed based on the average of several readings taken at different times.

In about 90% of people with high blood pressure, the underlying cause is uncertain. This type of high blood pressure is called *primary* (or *essential*) *hypertension* and is probably due to a combination of genetic and environmental factors, including obesity, stress, excessive alcohol intake, inactivity, and a diet high in sodium and solid fats. Although primary hypertension often cannot be cured, it can be managed with lifestyle changes and medications. About 10% of people have secondary hypertension caused by an underlying illness.

HEALTH RISKS   High blood pressure is called a silent killer because it usually has no symptoms. A person may have high blood pressure for years without realizing it. But during that time, it slowly damages vital organs and increases the risk of heart attack, congestive heart failure, stroke, kidney failure, and blindness.

Ask Yourself

QUESTIONS FOR CRITICAL THINKING AND REFLECTION
How often do you think about the health of your heart? Do certain situations make you aware of your heart rate, or make you wonder how strong your heart is?

hypertension   Sustained abnormally high blood pressure.   **TERMS**

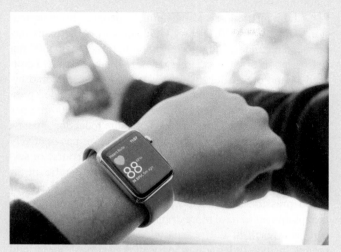

KANUT PHOTO/Shutterstock

Online Information

Online health information is changing the relationship between physicians and patients. Online references, patient communities, review sites, and electronic social networks have empowered patients to better understand their health and their health care choices.

Some cardiovascular diseases flare up quickly or allow but a brief time to attempt treatment, so a digital health approach could be especially useful. How can technology help detect diseases and make medical treatment more precise and individualized? A recent collaboration between Apple and Stanford University evaluated a smartwatch-based sensor for irregular heart rate and screening of atrial fibrillation. Because wearing a watch is convenient, the study could enroll over 400,000 participants in 8 months. When the algorithm detected an irregular heart rate, patients were immediately notified to see a physician about possible atrial fibrillation. This otherwise clinically silent condition could now be acted on immediately—patients could initiate treatment and reduce their risk of stroke.

Ambient Sensor Data

Managing chronic diseases also demands digital health interventions. We can keep tabs on our conditions through internet-connected scales, blood pressure cuffs, and other devices that are also available to health care professionals. They allow for more frequent checks to track progress and change. These devices also make measurements in our natural environments, instead of in a doctor's office. Currently, large health care systems such as the Veterans Health Administration and Kaiser Permanente Health Plan are implementing such devices for chronic disease management. In a national survey, one in four people reported conferencing with their physicians through video telemedicine.

Patient-Generated Health Data

Devices communicate with health care providers and also help us generate our own health data. Various smartphone applications, smartwatches, and other wearables provide information ranging from activity levels, ambient noise measurements, and menstrual cycle tracking to heart rate, food consumption, continuous blood glucose monitoring, and blood pressure measurements. Given the strong relationships among cardiovascular disease, lifestyle, and chronic disease, our self-generated data can be essential in making medical decisions and tracking progress in lifestyle modifications. In a national survey, 56% of individuals reported sharing their health tracking data with physicians.

SOURCE: Perez, M. V., et al. 2019. Large-scale assessment of a smartwatch to identify atrial fibrillation. *New England Journal of Medicine* 381: 1909–1917; Day, S., et al. 2019. Digital Health Consumer Adoption Report 2019. *Stanford Medicine Center for Digital Health and Rock Health Report.*

Recent research confirms the importance of lowering blood pressure to improve cardiovascular health. The risk of death from heart attack or stroke begins to rise even within the "normal" range when blood pressure is above 120 over 80 mm Hg, with a significant focus by doctors on targeting lower blood pressures than goals used in the past. People with blood pressure in the range referred to as elevated are at increased risk of heart attack and stroke.

An appropriate blood pressure target for risk reduction may depend on a person's age and other risk factors for cardiovascular disease. Traditionally, the treatment target was to reduce blood pressure below the cutoff for hypertension (140 over 90 mm Hg). However, a panel of experts recently reviewed all current trials and published updated guidelines in late 2017. Available data show that intensive blood pressure control with new, lower targets (systolic pressure below 120 mm Hg) reduces the risk of heart attack, stroke, and death. Future research may help identify criteria to set more individualized blood pressure targets for each person.

PREVALENCE Hypertension is common. Under the newly updated blood pressure guidelines, about 46% of adults have hypertension (defined as systolic pressure of 120–129 mm Hg and diastolic pressure of less than 80 mm Hg). The incidence of high blood pressure increases with age, but it does occur among overweight children and young adults. Women can sometimes develop hypertension during pregnancy (after which the blood pressure will usually return to normal). High blood pressure is also more common in women taking oral contraceptives, especially in obese and older women and women who have used oral contraceptives for a long time. The rate of hypertension is highest in African Americans

Table 16.1	Blood Pressure Classification for Healthy Adults		
CATEGORY[a]	SYSTOLIC (mm Hg)		DIASTOLIC (mm Hg)
Normal[b]	below 120	and	below 80
Elevated	120–129	and	below 80
Hypertension[c]			
Stage 1	130–139	or	80–89
Stage 2	at least 140	or	at least 90

[a]When systolic and diastolic pressures fall into different categories, the higher category should be used to classify blood pressure status.

[b]The risk of death from heart attack and stroke begins to rise when blood pressure is above 115/75.

[c]Based on the average of two or more readings taken at different physician visits. In people older than 50, systolic blood pressure greater than 140 mm Hg is a much more significant CVD risk factor than diastolic blood pressure.

SOURCE: Whelton, P. K. et al. 2017. 2017 ACC/AHA/AAPA/ABC/ACPM/AGS/APhA/ASH/ASPC/NMA/PCNA Guidelines for the Prevention, Detection, Evaluation, and Management of High Blood Pressure in Adults. A Report of the American College of Cardiology/American Heart Association Task Force on Clinical Practice Guidelines. *Journal of the American College of Cardiology* S0735–1097(17): 41519–1. Epub ahead of print.

(42–44%). Among African Americans, compared with other groups, the disorder is often more severe, more resistant to treatment, and more likely to be fatal at an early age.

TREATMENT Currently, primary hypertension cannot be cured, but it can be controlled and managed. Because hypertension has no early warning signs, it is crucial to have your blood pressure tested at least once every two years (and more often if you have other CVD risk factors). Experts advise anyone with elevated blood pressure to monitor their blood pressure several times each week. Self-monitoring is easy to do with a low-cost digital home blood pressure monitor, in the community at local pharmacies and grocery stores, and soon with wearable technology. Most important, those with hypertension must closely follow their physician's advice about lifestyle changes and medication.

Lifestyle changes are recommended for everyone with hypertension. These changes include weight reduction, regular exercise, a healthy diet, and moderation of salt and alcohol use. The DASH diet (see Chapter 13) is recommended specifically for people with high blood pressure. It emphasizes fruits, vegetables, and whole grains and increasing potassium

QUICK STATS

About half of U.S. adults have high blood pressure; only a quarter have it under control.

—Centers for Disease Control and Prevention, 2020

and fiber intake; it limits solid fats, sweets and added sugars, and salt. Even small increases in fruit and vegetable intake and small decreases in salt can create measurable drops in blood pressure.

Sodium restriction is also helpful for people with hypertension. The 2015–2020 Dietary Guidelines for Americans recommend restricting sodium consumption to less than 2300 mg (~1 teaspoon of table salt) per day for all adults and children aged 14 and over. Adults with elevated blood pressure and hypertension would particularly benefit from lowered blood pressure. For these individuals, further reduction to 1500 mg per day can result in even greater blood pressure reduction.

Over the short term, dietary salt restriction has relatively modest effects on blood pressure; but over the course of several decades, the reduction may be far more significant, in part because salt restriction minimizes the normal rise in blood pressure associated with aging. In addition, certain groups appear to have more dramatic decreases in blood pressure as a result of salt restriction. These more salt-sensitive groups include older adults, African Americans, obese individuals, people with metabolic syndrome, and those with chronic kidney disease. High dietary salt intake over many years probably plays a greater role in the development of hypertension in these groups.

Nearly 80% of dietary salt in the typical American diet is found in processed food and drinks. It follows, then, that the easiest way to achieve population-wide reduction is for the food industry to lower the amount of salt added to food products. Reductions in supplemental salt in restaurant food have also been suggested; some cities now require warnings listed on dishes with high amounts of sodium. Self-prepared meals offer the greatest control over dietary salt intake.

A recent study demonstrated that reducing salt in the American diet would significantly reduce the number of new cases of coronary heart disease, stroke, and heart attack in the United States. The benefits of reduced salt intake were estimated to be similar to the benefits of population-wide reductions in tobacco use, obesity, and cholesterol levels. For people whose blood pressure is not adequately controlled with lifestyle changes, medication can be prescribed.

High Cholesterol *Cholesterol* is a fatty, waxlike substance that circulates through the bloodstream. It is an important component of cell membranes, sex hormones, vitamin D, the fluid that coats the lungs, and the protective sheaths around nerves. Adequate cholesterol is essential for the proper functioning of the body. Excess cholesterol, however, can clog arteries and increase the risk of CVD. There are two primary sources of cholesterol: the liver, which manufactures it, and dietary sources.

GOOD VERSUS BAD CHOLESTEROL Cholesterol is carried in the blood in protein-and-lipid packages called **lipoproteins**

lipoproteins Protein and lipid substances in the blood that carry fats and cholesterol; classified according to size, density, and chemical composition.

TERMS

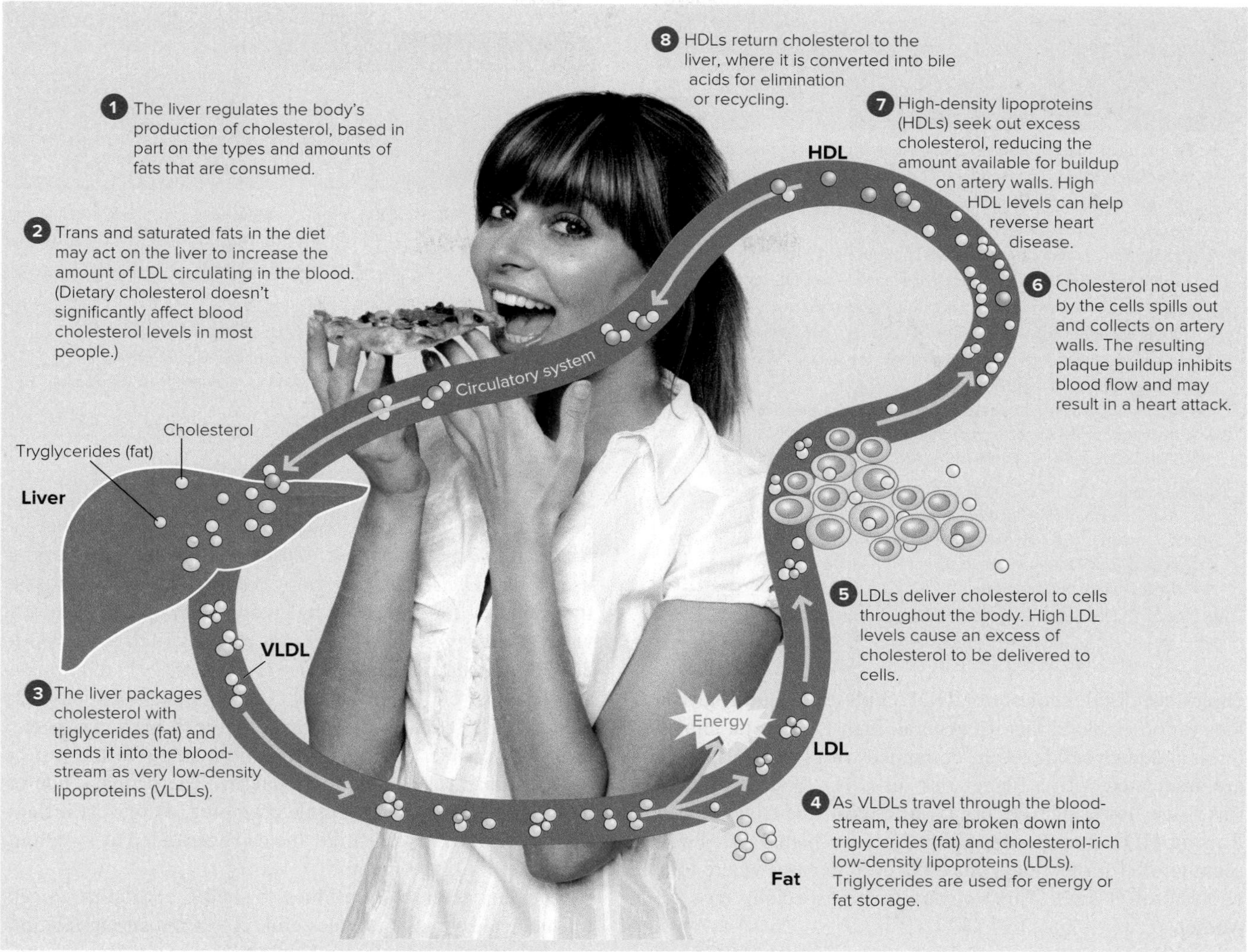

1 The liver regulates the body's production of cholesterol, based in part on the types and amounts of fats that are consumed.
2 Trans and saturated fats in the diet may act on the liver to increase the amount of LDL circulating in the blood. (Dietary cholesterol doesn't significantly affect blood cholesterol levels in most people.)
Cholesterol
Tryglycerides (fat)
Liver
VLDL
3 The liver packages cholesterol with triglycerides (fat) and sends it into the bloodstream as very low-density lipoproteins (VLDLs).
Circulatory system
8 HDLs return cholesterol to the liver, where it is converted into bile acids for elimination or recycling.
HDL
7 High-density lipoproteins (HDLs) seek out excess cholesterol, reducing the amount available for buildup on artery walls. High HDL levels can help reverse heart disease.
6 Cholesterol not used by the cells spills out and collects on artery walls. The resulting plaque buildup inhibits blood flow and may result in a heart attack.
5 LDLs deliver cholesterol to cells throughout the body. High LDL levels cause an excess of cholesterol to be delivered to cells.
Energy
LDL
Fat
4 As VLDLs travel through the bloodstream, they are broken down into triglycerides (fat) and cholesterol-rich low-density lipoproteins (LDLs). Triglycerides are used for energy or fat storage.

FIGURE 16.8 Cholesterol in the body. Westend61 - WEST/Getty Images

(Figure 16.8). Two types of lipoproteins influence an individual's risk of heart disease:

- **Low-density lipoproteins (LDLs)** (18–27 nm) shuttle cholesterol from the liver to the organs and tissues that require it. LDLs are known as "bad" cholesterol because, if the body has more than it can use, the excess cholesterol is deposited in the blood vessels. They can then be oxidized by free radicals, which speeds inflammation and damage to artery walls and increases the likelihood of a blockage. Recently discovered medications, called PCSK9 inhibitors, target the liver's handling of LDL cholesterol and greatly reduce blood LDL cholesterol levels, thus reducing the risk of heart attacks and strokes.

- **High-density lipoproteins (HDLs)** are "good" cholesterol. They shuttle unused cholesterol back to the liver for recycling. By removing cholesterol from blood vessels, HDLs help protect against atherosclerosis.

BLOOD CHOLESTEROL GUIDELINES Screening for cholesterol provides one part of the assessment of the risk of cardiovascular disease. This risk increases with higher LDL blood cholesterol levels. The National Cholesterol Education Program recommends lipoprotein testing at least once every five years for all adults, beginning at age 20, and once during adolescence for kids. The recommended test measures total

TERMS

low-density lipoprotein (LDL) A lipoprotein containing a moderate amount of protein and a large amount of cholesterol, which tends to become deposited on artery walls and increase the risk of heart disease; also known as "bad" cholesterol.

high-density lipoprotein (HDL) A lipoprotein containing relatively little cholesterol that helps transport cholesterol out of the arteries and thus protects against heart diseases; also known as "good" cholesterol.

Table 16.2	People Who Benefit from Treatment of High Cholesterol

1. People aged 75 and under with known cardiovascular disease, including previous heart attacks, chest pain due to partially clogged arteries, history of invasive treatment for clogged arteries, previous stroke, or previous clogged arteries in the limbs.
2. People aged 21 and over with high LDL levels, 190 mg/dl or greater.
3. People aged 40–75 with a history of diabetes, an LDL level 70–189 mg/dl, and no known history of cardiovascular disease.
4. People aged 40–75 without diabetes or known cardiovascular disease but with a high risk of developing it over the next 10 years and an LDL level over 70 mg/dl.*

*10-year cardiovascular risk is calculated using a tool available on the AHA website (https://professional.heart.org/professional/GuidelinesStatements /ASCVDRiskCalculator/UCM_457698_ASCVD-Risk-Calculator.jsp).

SOURCE: Stone, N. J., et al. 2013. ACC/AHA guideline on the treatment of blood cholesterol to reduce atherosclerotic cardiovascular risk in adults. A report of the American College of Cardiology/American Heart Association Task Force on Practice Guidelines. *Journal of the American College of Cardiology.*

VITAL STATISTICS

Table 16.3	Prevalence of High Cholesterol Levels ($\geq$ 200 mg/dl) in the United States by Race, Ethnicity, and Sex

RACIAL/ETHNIC GROUP	MEN, %	WOMEN, %
Non-Hispanic Blacks	32.6	36.1
Hispanics	43.1	41.2
Non-Hispanic Whites	37.0	43.4
Non-Hispanic Asians	39.9	40.5

SOURCE: Benjamin, E. J., et al. 2017. Heart disease and stroke statistics–2017 update. A report from the American Heart Association. *Circulation* 135: e146–e603.

cholesterol, LDL cholesterol, HDL cholesterol, and triglycerides (another blood fat). In general, high LDL, total cholesterol, and triglyceride levels, combined with low HDL levels, are associated with a higher risk for CVD. You can reduce this risk by lowering LDL, total cholesterol, and triglycerides. Raising HDL may be important because high HDL levels seem to offer protection from CVD even in cases where total cholesterol is high. This appears to be especially true for women.

In 2013, the American College of Cardiology (ACC) and the American Heart Association released updated guidelines on the treatment of high blood cholesterol. Assessing a person's risk of developing cardiovascular disease over the next 10 years, and treating this level, is now preferred. The ACC and AHA identified four groups of people, based on observations made during multiple published clinical trials, who would benefit from treatment of high blood cholesterol levels (see Table 16.2). An estimated 95 million American adults have total cholesterol levels of 200 mg/dl or higher (see Table 16.3).

The 2013 ACC/AHA guidelines also offer recommendations for people to modify their lifestyles either prior to developing or while already suffering from high cholesterol. These lifestyle guidelines include maintaining a healthy diet, engaging in regular aerobic exercise, avoiding tobacco products, and maintaining a healthy weight. These recommendations are vitally important in managing the risk of CVD and are often the first step in managing high cholesterol—before any medications are prescribed.

The updated cholesterol guidelines eliminate targeting specific levels of LDL and HDL. The new guidelines are based on overall cardiovascular risk and suggest statin therapy administered at different intensity doses if lifestyle

modifications have not adequately lowered cholesterol levels. *Statins* are the primary cholesterol-lowering medications used today. *High-intensity* therapy is defined as a statin dosage that reduces the LDL level by greater than or equal to 50%, whereas *moderate-intensity* therapy reduces LDL level by 30–50%. Statins dramatically reduce the risk of CVD in individuals with high cholesterol levels. These medications may also decrease CVD risk even in those without high cholesterol levels. Of course, with any medication, side effects must be weighed against the potential benefits. The primary side effect seen with statins is muscle cramping, or muscle inflammation, which is usually mild and can be avoided by switching to a different kind of statin.

Ongoing research continues to define additional targets for medical therapy of cholesterol. Given the strong relationship between high cholesterol and CVD, pharmaceutical companies are trying to identify ways to further reduce the risk of heart attacks and strokes.

BENEFITS OF CONTROLLING CHOLESTEROL Some studies have shown that people can cut their heart attack risk by about 2% for every 1% that they reduce their total blood cholesterol levels. Current research indicates that treating elevated LDL and raising HDL levels not only reduces the likelihood that arteries will become clogged but also may reverse deposits on artery walls.

See Chapter 13 for detailed information about nutrition and guidelines for heart-healthy eating.

Physical Inactivity An estimated 40–60 million Americans are sedentary and at high risk for developing CVD. Exercise is a key component in the fight against heart disease. Exercise lowers CVD risk by helping to decrease blood pressure and resting heart rate, increase HDL levels, maintain desirable weight, improve the condition of blood vessels, and prevent or control diabetes. One study found that women who accumulated at least three hours of brisk walking each week cut their risk of heart attack and stroke by more than 50%.

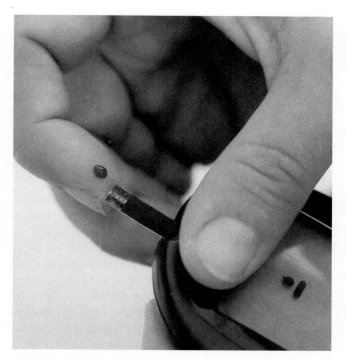

Blood glucose monitoring is important in managing diabetes and its associated risks. Michael Krasowitz/Photographer's Choice/Getty Images

Table 16.4	Characteristics of Metabolic Syndrome*
FACTOR	**CRITERIA**
Large waistline (abdominal obesity)	35 or more inches (88 cm) for women 40 or more inches (102 cm) for men
High triglyceride level	150 mg/dl or higher Or taking medication to treat high triglycerides
Low HDL level	Less than 50 mg/dl for women Less than 40 mg/dl for men Or taking medication to treat low HDL
High blood pressure	130/85 mm Hg or higher (one or both numbers) Or taking medication to treat high blood pressure
High fasting blood sugar	100 mg/dl or higher Or taking medication to treat high blood sugar

*A person having three or more factors listed here is diagnosed with metabolic syndrome.

SOURCE: Adapted from National Heart, Lung, and Blood Institute. 2015. *How Is Metabolic Syndrome Diagnosed?* (http://www.nhlbi.nih.gov /health/health-topics/topics/ms/diagnosis).

See Chapter 14 for detailed explanations of the benefits of physical activity and for help in creating your own exercise plan.

Obesity As your weight increases, your risk of CVD increases. Death from CVD is two to three times more likely in obese people (**body mass index, or BMI** ≥ 30) than it is in lean people (BMI = 18.5–24.9), and for every 5-unit increase in BMI, a person's risk of death from coronary heart disease increases by 30%. The higher your BMI at age 18, the more likely you will eventually die from CVD. Maintaining a healthy weight is also important. The Nurses' Health Study, in which Harvard researchers have followed more than 120,000 women since 1976, has found that even mildly to moderately overweight women have an 80% increased risk of developing coronary heart disease compared to leaner women. Researchers found that middle-aged women who had gained 22 pounds or more since age 18 had a significantly higher risk of subsequent death from CVD than those who maintained their weight over time.

As explained in Chapter 15, excess body fat is strongly associated with hypertension, high cholesterol levels, insulin resistance, diabetes, physical inactivity, and increasing age.

Insulin Resistance and Metabolic Syndrome When you consume carbohydrates, your blood glucose level increases. This stimulates the pancreas to secrete insulin, which allows body cells to pick up the consumed glucose to use for energy (see Chapter 15). The function of insulin is to maintain proper glucose levels in the body, which it does by regulating the uptake of glucose from the blood by muscle and fat tissue and by limiting the liver's production of glucose. As people gain weight and become less active, their muscles, fat, and liver become less sensitive to the effect of insulin—a condition known as *insulin resistance*. As the body becomes increasingly insulin resistant, the pancreas must secrete more and more insulin (hyperinsulinemia) to keep glucose levels within a normal range. Eventually even high levels of insulin may become insufficient, and blood glucose levels start to rise (hyperglycemia), setting the stage for prediabetes and, if not addressed, eventually for type 2 diabetes.

Those who have insulin resistance tend to have several other related risk factors. This cluster of abnormalities is called *metabolic syndrome* or *insulin resistance syndrome* (Table 16.4). Although several definitions of metabolic syndrome exist, someone is typically diagnosed with the condition if they have three or more of the following: high blood pressure, high triglyceride level, low HDL level, high fasting blood sugar, and a large waistline (a marker for abdominal obesity). Metabolic syndrome significantly increases the risk of CVD—more so in women than in men. It is estimated that about 34% of the adult U.S. population has metabolic syndrome.

To reduce your risk of developing metabolic syndrome, choose a healthy diet and get plenty of aerobic exercise. Regular physical activity increases your body's sensitivity to insulin, improves cholesterol levels, and decreases blood pressure. Reducing calorie intake to prevent weight gain or

body mass index (BMI) A calculated measure of human body shape; the ratio of mass (in kilograms) divided by height (in meters) squared: weight/height^2 **TERMS**

losing weight if needed also reduces insulin resistance. The amount and type of carbohydrate intake is also important. Diets high in simple carbohydrates, such as white sugar and white flour (high-glycemic-index foods), can raise levels of glucose and triglycerides while lowering HDL, thus contributing to metabolic syndrome and CVD. This is particularly true for people who are already sedentary and overweight. For people prone to insulin resistance, eating more protein, vegetables, and fiber while limiting fat, added sugars, and starches may be beneficial.

Diabetes   As described in Chapter 15, *diabetes mellitus* is a disorder characterized by elevated blood glucose levels due to an insufficient supply of insulin or inadequate response to insulin. Diabetes doubles the risk of CVD for men and triples the risk for women. The most common cause of death in adults with diabetes is CVD, and individuals with diabetes usually die at younger ages than people without diabetes. There is an estimated loss of 5–10 years of life in those with diabetes compared to those without.

People with diabetes have higher rates of other CVD risk factors, including hypertension, obesity, and unhealthy blood lipid levels (typically, high triglyceride levels and low HDL levels). The elevated blood glucose and insulin levels that occur in diabetes can damage the endothelial cells that line the arteries, making them more vulnerable to atherosclerosis. Diabetics also often have platelet and blood coagulation abnormalities that increase the risk of heart attack and stroke. People with prediabetes (when the blood sugar levels are elevated but not high enough to diagnose diabetes) also face an increased risk of CVD.

The number of people with diabetes (30.3 million) and prediabetes (84.1 million) in the United States continues to climb and is closely linked to obesity. It is estimated that for every kilogram (2.2 pounds) increase in weight, the risk of diabetes increases by approximately 9%. The largest increase in prevalence of type 2 diabetes over the past decade has been among people aged 30–39, and there has also been an alarming increase among children and adolescents. Children who are diagnosed with diabetes typically develop complications in their twenties or thirties.

Cardiovascular complications of diabetes primarily affect the arteries. When the larger arteries are affected, all forms of CVD may result, including heart attack, stroke, and peripheral vascular disease. Having diabetes is considered to be a heart disease risk equivalent, meaning that your CVD morbidity and mortality risk is the same as if you already had coronary heart disease. Diabetics who do have coronary artery disease fare even worse: They have accelerated atherosclerosis and benefit less from common forms of treatment than nondiabetics.

In people with prediabetes, a healthy diet and exercise are the most effective tools in preventing diabetes. For people with diabetes, a healthy diet, exercise, and careful control of glucose levels are recommended to reduce the chances of developing complications. Even people whose diabetes is under control face a high risk of CVD, so control of other risk factors is critical.

Contributing Risk Factors That Can Be Changed

Other cardiovascular disease risk factors that can be changed include triglyceride levels, metabolic syndrome, inflammation, psychological and social factors, and alcohol and drug use.

High Triglyceride Levels   Like cholesterol, **triglycerides** are blood fats that are obtained from food and manufactured by the body. High triglyceride levels are a reliable predictor of heart disease, especially if associated with other risk factors, such as low HDL levels, obesity, and diabetes. Factors contributing to elevated triglyceride levels include excess body fat, physical inactivity, cigarette smoking, type 2 diabetes, excessive alcohol intake, very high-carbohydrate diets, and certain diseases and medications.

High triglyceride levels may be a sign of poorly controlled type 2 diabetes, low levels of thyroid hormones, liver or kidney disease, or rare genetic conditions that affect how your body converts fat to energy. High triglycerides could also be a side effect of taking medications such as beta blockers, birth control pills, diuretics, or steroids.

For people with borderline high triglyceride levels, increased physical activity, reduced intake of added sugars, and weight reduction can help bring levels down into the healthy range. For people with high triglyceride levels, drug therapy may be recommended if initial strategies are ineffective. Fish oil and concentrated icosapent ethyl have been shown to significantly reduce triglyceride levels and reduce risk of heart attacks. Moderating alcohol intake and avoiding use of tobacco products are also important.

Inflammation   Inflammation plays a key role in the development of CVD. When an artery is injured by hypertension, smoking, cholesterol, or other factors, the body's response is to produce inflammation. A substance called *C-reactive protein (CRP)* is released into the bloodstream during the inflammatory response, and high levels of CRP indicate an elevated risk of heart attack and stroke. It has also been proposed that CRP by itself may harm the coronary arteries. Gum disease involves another type of inflammation that may moderately influence the progress of heart disease.

Lifestyle changes and certain drugs can reduce CRP levels. Statin drugs, widely prescribed to lower cholesterol, also have been shown to decrease inflammation and reduce CRP levels. Patients who receive intensive statin treatment fare better than patients who receive less aggressive treatment that primarily targets LDL levels—which is one of the

triglyceride   A type of blood fat that can be a predictor of heart disease.

TERMS

reasons the newly published guidelines have eliminated target LDL levels. The reduction in risk from decreased CRP levels is independent of changes in LDL levels.

The benefits of statins were reconfirmed in 2008, when findings were released from a study involving 18,000 patients in 26 countries. Volunteers who took statins reduced their risk of CVD by about 50% even if they had normal cholesterol levels. The patients had undergone a simple blood test that checked for inflammation by measuring levels of CRP; because statins lower CRP regardless of cholesterol levels, researchers concluded that CRP levels and inflammation are important markers of CVD risk.

Psychological and Social Factors

Many of the psychological and social factors that influence other areas of wellness are also important risk factors for CVD. The cardiovascular system is affected by both sudden, acute episodes of mental stress and the more chronic underlying emotions of anger, anxiety, and depression.

STRESS Excessive stress can strain the heart and blood vessels over time and contribute to CVD (Figure 16.9). When you experience stress, stress hormones activate the sympathetic nervous system. As described in Chapter 2, the sympathetic nervous system causes the fight-or-flight response. This response increases heart rate and blood pressure so that more blood is distributed to the heart and other muscles in anticipation of physical activity. Blood glucose concentrations and cholesterol also increase to provide a source of energy, and the platelets become activated so that they will be more likely to clot in case of injury. If you are healthy, you can tolerate the cardiovascular responses that take place during stress. But if you already have CVD, stress can lead to adverse outcomes such as abnormal heart rhythms (arrhythmias) and heart attacks.

Because avoiding all stress is impossible, having healthy mechanisms to cope with it is your best defense. Instead of adopting unhealthy coping habits such as smoking or overeating, use healthier strategies such as exercising, getting enough sleep, and talking to others.

CHRONIC HOSTILITY AND ANGER Certain traits in a hard-driving personality—hostility, cynicism, and anger—are associated with increased risk of heart disease. Men prone to anger have two to three times the heart attack risk of calmer men and are much more likely to develop CVD at young ages. In a 10-year study of young adults aged 18–30 years, those with high hostility levels were more than twice as likely to develop coronary artery calcification (a marker of early atherosclerosis) than were those with low hostility levels.

DEPRESSION Depression is common in people with coronary heart disease (CHD). Patients who are depressed tend to have worse outcomes than those who are not. Up to one-third of patients experience major depression within one year of having a heart attack, and those who are depressed after having a heart attack are more likely to have another heart attack or die of a cardiac cause.

The relationship between depression and CHD is complex and not fully understood. Depressed people may be more likely to smoke or be sedentary. They may not consistently take prescribed medications, and they may not cope well with having an illness or undergoing a medical procedure. Depression also causes physiological changes; for example, it elevates basal levels of stress hormones, which induce a variety of stress-related responses.

> ### QUICK STATS
> **85%** of people with type 2 diabetes also have metabolic syndrome.
> —National Heart, Lung, and Blood Institute, 2015

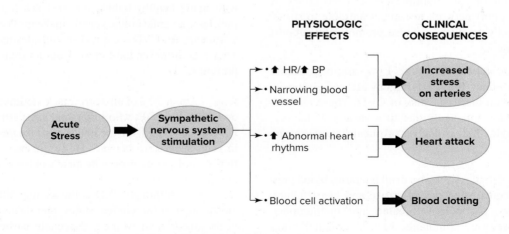

FIGURE 16.9 **The effects of stress and emotions on the cardiovascular system.**

SOURCE: Adapted from Rozanski, A., et al. 1999. Impact of psychological factors on the pathogenesis of cardiovascular disease and implications for therapy. *Circulation* 99: 2192–2217.

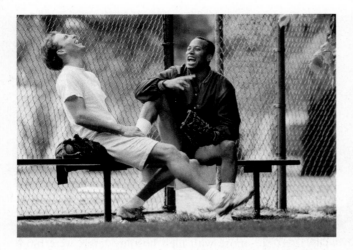

A strong social support network is a major antidote to stress and can help promote and support a healthy lifestyle that includes opportunities for exercise and relaxation. Corbis/Alamy Stock Photo

ANXIETY Evidence suggests that chronic anxiety and anxiety disorders (such as phobias and panic disorder) are associated with up to a threefold increased risk of CHD, heart attack, and sudden cardiac death. There is also some evidence that, similar to people with depression, people with anxiety are more likely to have a subsequent adverse cardiac event after having a heart attack. At the same time, people with anxiety and depression often have medically unexplained chest pain, meaning that no obvious CHD can be found. This can create difficulties in diagnosis and disease management, but it is important to seek medical attention if you experience any unexplained chest pain.

SOCIAL ISOLATION Social isolation and low social support (living alone, or having few friends or family members) are associated with an increased incidence of CHD and poorer outcomes after the first diagnosis of CHD. Elderly men and women who report less emotional support from others before they have a heart attack are almost three times more likely to die in the first six months after the heart attack. A strong social support network is a major antidote to stress. Friends and family members can also promote and support a healthy lifestyle.

LOW SOCIOECONOMIC STATUS Low socioeconomic status and low educational attainment are social factors associated with an increased risk of CVD. These associations are complex and likely due to a variety of factors, including lifestyle, diet, and access to health care, among others.

Alcohol and Drugs Excessive drinking raises blood pressure and can increase the risk of stroke and heart failure. Stimulant drugs, particularly cocaine and methamphetamines—and associated stimulants, such as designer drugs including Ecstasy (MDMA)—can also cause serious cardiac problems, including heart attack, stroke, and sudden cardiac death. For example, cocaine stimulates the nervous system, promotes platelet aggregation, and can cause spasms in the coronary arteries. Stimulant drugs can lead to heart attacks, rupture of arteries, inflammation of the heart muscle, and even stroke, among many other negative effects. Injection drug use can cause heart infections and stroke. See Chapters 10 and 11 for more information about the use of alcohol and drugs.

Major Risk Factors That Can't Be Changed

A number of major risk factors for cardiovascular disease cannot be changed. These include family history of CVD (genetics), aging, male gender, and ethnicity.

Genetics Multiple genes contribute to the development of CVD—and its associated risk factors, such as high cholesterol, hypertension, diabetes, and obesity. Having favorable genes decreases your risk of developing CVD; having an unfavorable set of genes increases your risk. This is a very active area of research, and new discoveries linking genes to cardiovascular disease are frequently made.

Because of the genetic complexity of CVD, genetic screening is recommended for only a few specific conditions (e.g., certain inherited cholesterol disorders), but you can learn more about your personal risk just by assessing your family history. If you have a first-degree relative (parent, sibling, child) who developed coronary heart disease before the age of 65, for example, you can have up to a twofold increased risk of developing CHD yourself. It is important to let your doctor know of any history of heart disease in your relatives.

Don't forget the role of lifestyle factors, however: risk may be modified by lifestyle factors such as whether you smoke, exercise, or eat a healthy diet. CHD is usually the result of the interaction of several unfavorable genetic and lifestyle factors, and people with the greatest number of both will face the highest risks. People with favorable genes may not develop CHD despite having an unhealthy lifestyle, and people with many healthy habits may still develop CHD because they have an unfavorable genetic makeup. People who inherit a tendency for CVD are not absolutely destined to develop it. They may, however, have to work harder than other people to prevent CVD.

Age About 70% of all heart attack victims are aged 65 and over, and about 80% who suffer fatal heart attacks are over 65. For people over 55, the incidence of stroke more than doubles in each successive decade. However, even people in their thirties and forties, especially men, can have heart attacks.

Gender Although CVD is the leading killer of both men and women in the United States, men face a greater risk of heart attack than women, especially earlier in life. Until age 55, men also have a greater risk of hypertension. The incidence of stroke is also higher for males than females, until age 65.

Risk factors for CVD are similar for men and women (age, family history, smoking, hypertension, high cholesterol, and diabetes), but gender differences do exist. HDL appears to be an even more powerful predictor of CHD risk in women than in men. Also, women with diabetes have a greater risk of having CVD events like heart attack and stroke than men with diabetes. Estrogen production, which is highest during the childbearing years, may protect against CVD in premenopausal women. By age 75, however, this gender gap nearly disappears.

Women who suffer heart attacks are more likely than men to die within a year. One reason is that, because women develop heart disease at older ages, they are more likely to have other health problems that complicate treatment. There also may be biological or psychosocial risk factors contributing to women's mortality.

Race and Ethnicity Rates of heart disease vary among racial and ethnic groups in the United States, with African Americans having much higher rates of hypertension, heart disease, and stroke than other groups (see the box "Gender, Race/Ethnicity, and Cardiovascular Disease"). Figure 16.10 compares overall rates of CVD among selected population groups in the United States. Patterns along ethnic lines can also be seen for specific forms of CVD. For example, in a comparison of rates for groups in the same communities, Mexican Americans were found to have a higher rate of stroke than non-Hispanic whites. Hispanic women have higher rates of angina (a warning sign of blocked coronary arteries) than non-Hispanic white women. Asian Americans historically have had far lower rates of CVD than white Americans.

Possible Risk Factors Currently Being Studied

In recent years, other possible risk factors for cardiovascular disease have been identified. These factors range from levels of various amino acids in the blood to infectious agents and even the season of the year. All of these risk factors are currently under study.

Homocysteine Having elevated levels of homocysteine, an amino acid circulating in the blood, is associated with an increased risk of CVD. Homocysteine levels track with stress and inflammation. Homocysteine appears to damage the lining of blood vessels, resulting in inflammation and the development of fatty deposits in artery walls. These changes can lead to the formation of clots and blockages in arteries. High homocysteine levels are also associated with cognitive impairment, such as memory loss. Homocysteine does not appear to play as large a role as hypertension, diabetes, tobacco use, and high cholesterol do in cardiovascular risk. Trials of lowering homocysteine levels have yet to show a proven benefit in preventing CVD.

Infectious Agents Several infectious agents have been identified as possible culprits in the development of CVD. *Chlamydia pneumoniae,* a common cause of flu-like respiratory infections, has been found in sections of clogged, damaged arteries but not in sections of healthy arteries. This effect may be secondary to the inflammation that many of these infectious agents produce in the body. People at risk are six times more likely to have a heart attack around the time of a flu infection than are individuals without the flu.

Lipoprotein(a) A high level of a specific type of LDL called lipoprotein(a), or Lp(a), may be a modest independent risk factor for CHD, especially when associated with high LDL or low HDL levels. Lp(a) is thought to contribute to CVD by promoting clots and delivering cholesterol to a site of vascular injury. Lp(a) levels have a strong genetic component and are difficult to treat. Lp(a) levels tend to increase with age and vary by race and ethnicity: African Americans have Lp(a) levels that are typically two to three times higher than those of whites; some Asian American populations have lower Lp(a) levels than do whites and Hispanics. Additionally, researchers have recommended a lower cutoff threshold for using Lp(a) to detect heart disease risk in African Americans.

Uric Acid Recent research suggests a link between high blood levels of uric acid and CVD mortality, particularly among postmenopausal women and African Americans. Uric acid may raise CVD risk by increasing inflammation and platelet aggregation or by influencing the development of hypertension. High uric acid levels also cause gout (a type of arthritis), kidney stones, and certain forms of kidney disease; they are also a risk factor in people with congestive heart failure. Medications to lower uric acid levels are available, but it is not yet known if they are useful in preventing CVD.

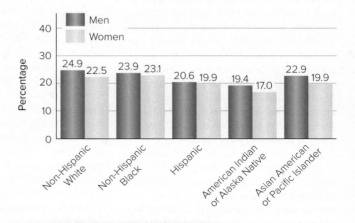

VITAL STATISTICS

FIGURE 16.10 **Percentage of adult Americans with cardiovascular disease.**

SOURCE: Heron, M. 2019. Deaths: Leading causes for 2017. *National Vital Statistics Reports* 68(6). Hyattsville, MD: National Center for Health Statistics.

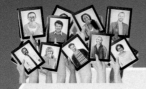
Cardiovascular disease is the leading cause of death for all Americans, but significant differences exist between men and women and among racial/ethnic groups in the incidence, diagnosis, and treatment of this deadly disease.

CVD in Women

CVD has been thought of as a "man's disease," but it actually kills more women than men. Polls indicate that women vastly underestimate their risk of dying of a heart attack and overestimate their risk of dying of breast cancer. In reality, approximately 1 in 4 women dies of CVD, whereas 1 in 38 dies of breast cancer. And although CVD typically does not develop in women younger than age 50, recent research suggests that the number of CVD deaths in women aged 35–45 may be increasing.

The hormone estrogen, produced naturally by a woman's ovaries until menopause, improves blood lipid concentrations and reduces other CVD risk factors. For several decades, many physicians encouraged menopausal women to take hormone replacement therapy (HRT), which includes estrogen, to relieve menopause symptoms and presumably to reduce their risk of CVD. However, some studies found that HRT may actually *increase* a woman's risk for heart disease and other health problems, including breast cancer. Some newer studies have found that the increased risk of CVD in women who start HRT may be age dependent; women in the early stages of menopause or ages 50–59 did not appear to have excess risk. These findings suggest that outcomes may depend on several factors, including the timing of hormone use. The U.S. Preventive Services Task Force and the American Heart Association recommend that HRT not be used to protect against CVD.

When women have heart attacks, they are more likely than men to die within a year and are less likely than men to report the usual symptoms of a heart attack, such as chest pain. Additionally, women are likely to report less specific symptoms, which may obscure the diagnosis. These symptoms include fatigue; weakness; shortness of breath; nausea; vomiting; and pain in the abdomen, neck, jaw, and back. Women are also more likely to have pain at rest, during sleep, or with mental stress. A woman who experiences these symptoms should be persistent in seeking accurate diagnosis and appropriate treatment.

Careful diagnosis of cardiac symptoms is also key in avoiding unnecessary invasive procedures in cases of stress cardiomyopathy ("broken heart syndrome"), which occurs much more commonly in women than in men. In this condition, hormones and neurotransmitters associated with a severe stress response stun the heart, producing heart-attack-like symptoms and decreased pumping function of the heart, but no damage to the heart muscle. Often, the condition reverses quickly.

Women should be aware of their CVD risk factors and consult with a physician to assess their risk and determine the best way to prevent CVD.

CVD in African Americans and Other Racial/Ethnic Groups

Although cardiovascular disease is the leading cause of death for all Americans, there is a higher prevalence of CVD in adult African Americans, and a higher prevalence of many associated risk factors in Mexican Americans, than in non-Hispanic whites and Asian Americans. The reasons for these disparities likely include both genetic and environmental factors.

African Americans are at substantially higher risk of death from CVD than other groups. The rate of hypertension among African Americans is among the highest in the world. African Americans tend to develop hypertension at an earlier age than non-Hispanic whites, and their average blood pressures are much higher. African Americans have a higher risk of stroke; have strokes at younger ages; and, if they survive, have more significant stroke-related disabilities. Some experts recommend that African Americans take antihypertensive drugs if their blood pressure reaches 130/80 rather than the typical 140/90 cutoff for hypertension—especially if they have diabetes or kidney disease.

A number of genetic and biological factors may contribute to CVD in African Americans. For instance, a higher sensitivity to dietary sodium may lead to elevated blood pressure. African Americans may also experience less dilation of blood vessels in response to stress, an attribute that also raises blood pressure for all racial/ethnic groups.

Heredity also plays a large role in the tendency to develop diabetes, another important CVD risk factor that is more common in blacks than whites. However, Latinos are even more likely to develop diabetes and insulin resistance, and at a younger age, than African Americans. There is variation within the Latino population, however; a higher prevalence of diabetes occurs among Mexican Americans and Puerto Ricans and a relatively lower prevalence among Cuban Americans.

Racial and ethnic minorities are more likely than non-Hispanic whites to be poor, and low income is associated with reduced access to health care and healthy dietary options for CVD prevention. People who live in low-income neighborhoods experience longer delays between the onset of heart attack symptoms and reaching a hospital. Lower educational attainment is associated with low income, which often means less access to information about preventive health care, such as diet and stress management. Populations with low incomes tend to smoke more, consume more salt, and exercise less than those with higher incomes.

Discrimination may also play a role in CVD. Physicians and hospitals may treat the medical problems of nonwhites differently from those of whites. Discrimination, low income, and other forms of deprivation may also increase stress, which is linked with hypertension and CVD. Lack of insurance coverage and less-advanced medical technologies in hospitals that serve minority and low-income neighborhoods may also play a role.

All Americans, regardless of background, are advised to have their blood pressure checked regularly, exercise on a regular basis, eat a healthy diet, manage stress, and avoid tobacco products. Tailoring your lifestyle to any risk factors that may be especially relevant for you can also be helpful in some cases. Discuss your particular risk profile with your physician to help identify the lifestyle changes most appropriate for you.

Ask Yourself

QUESTIONS FOR CRITICAL THINKING AND REFLECTION

What risk factors do you have for cardiovascular disease? Which ones are factors you control? If you have risk factors you cannot change (such as a family history of CVD), were you aware that you can make lifestyle adjustments to reduce your risk? Do you think you will make them?

Time of Day and Time of Year   Heart attacks and sudden cardiac deaths occur more frequently between 6:00 a.m. and noon than during other times of the day. This trend is possibly explained by the natural, physiologic increase in adrenaline and cortisol levels that occurs in the morning and by an increase in sympathetic nervous system activity at the beginning of the day. Blood pressure is often lowest during sleep and highest in the morning.

Heart attacks also follow a seasonal pattern, with up to 50% more occurring in winter months than in summer. Heart attacks that occur in winter are more often fatal than those during summer. Possible explanations include low temperatures, which can constrict blood vessels; bursts of exertion, such as snow shoveling; increased rates of smoking; increased stress and depression, including seasonal affective disorder (see Chapter 3); more frequent flu and viral illnesses causing inflammation; holiday-related episodes of high-fat eating and binge drinking; and physiological factors, including levels of cholesterol and C-reactive protein, which appear to rise in winter. People who have symptoms of heart trouble may also be more reluctant to seek help during the holidays.

PROTECTING YOURSELF AGAINST CARDIOVASCULAR DISEASE

You can take several important steps now to lower your risk of developing cardiovascular disease (Figure 16.11). CVD can begin very early in life. For example, fatty streaks (early atherosclerosis) can be seen on the aorta in children younger than age 10. Also, young adults with relatively low cholesterol levels go on to live substantially longer than those with higher levels. Reducing CVD risk factors when you are young can pay off with many extra years of life and health (see the box "Are You at Risk for CVD?").

Eat Heart-Healthy

For most Americans, eating a heart-healthy diet involves many of the changes suggested in the Dietary Guidelines for Americans. The following aspects of nutrition apply directly to heart health:

- Decrease saturated and trans-saturated fat intake.
- Eat a high-fiber diet.
- Reduce sodium intake.
- Avoid excessive alcohol consumption.
- Eat foods rich in omega-3 fatty acids.

In addition to these familiar guidelines, a few specifics pertain to heart health:

- ***Plant stanols and sterols.*** Plant stanols and sterols, found in some types of trans-fat-free margarines and other products, reduce the absorption of cholesterol in the body

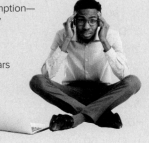

Do More

- Eat a diet rich in fruits, vegetables, whole grains, and low-fat or fat-free dairy products. Eat five to nine servings of fruits and vegetables each day.

- Eat several servings of high-fiber foods each day.

- Eat two or more servings of fish per week; try a few servings of nuts and soy foods each week.

- Choose unsaturated fats rather than saturated and trans fats.

- Be physically active; do both aerobic exercise and strength training on a regular basis.

- Achieve and maintain a healthy weight.

- Develop effective strategies for handling stress and anger. Nurture old friendships and family ties, and make new friends; pay attention to your spiritual side.

- Obtain recommended screening tests and follow your physician's recommendations.

Do Less

- Don't use tobacco in any form: cigarettes, smokeless tobacco, cigars and pipes, bidis and clove cigarettes.

- Limit consumption of trans fats and saturated fats.

- Limit consumption of salt to no more than 2300 mg of sodium per day (1500 mg if you have or are at high risk for hypertension).

- Avoid exposure to environmental tobacco smoke.

- Avoid excessive alcohol consumption— no more than one drink per day for women and two drinks per day for men.

- Limit consumption of added sugars and refined carbohydrates.

- Avoid excess stress, anger, and hostility.

FIGURE 16.11   **Strategies for reducing your risk of cardiovascular disease.** Jessica Peterson/Rubberball/Getty Images; Vladyslav Starozhylov/Alamy Stock Photo

ASSESS YOURSELF
Are You at Risk for CVD?

Your chances of suffering an early heart attack or stroke depend on a variety of factors, many of which are under your control. You can significantly affect your future health and quality of life if you adopt healthy behaviors when you are young.

To help identify your risk factors, circle the response for each risk category that best describes you:

1. Gender and age:

   0 Female aged 55 or younger, or male aged 45 or younger

   2 Female aged 55 or older, or male aged 45 or older

2. Heredity:

   0 Neither parent suffered a heart attack or stroke before age 60

   3 One parent suffered a heart attack or stroke before age 60

   7 Both parents suffered a heart attack or stroke before age 60

3. Smoking:

   0 Never smoked

   3 Quit more than two years ago, and lifetime smoking is less than five pack-years*

   6 Quit less than two years ago and/or lifetime smoking is greater than five pack-years*

   8 Smoke less than half a pack per day

   13 Smoke more than half a pack per day

   15 Smoke more than one pack per day

4. Environmental tobacco smoke (ETS):

   0 Do not live or work with smokers

   2 Exposed to ETS at work

   3 Live with a smoker

   4 Both live and work with smokers

5. Blood pressure—if available, average your last three readings:

   0 120/80 mm Hg or below

   1 121/81–130/85 mm Hg

   3 Don't know

   5 131/86–150/90 mm Hg

   9 151/91–170/100 mm Hg

   13 Above 170/100 mm Hg

6. Total cholesterol (mg/dl):

   0 Lower than 190

   1 190–210

   2 Don't know

   3 211–240

   4 241–270

   5 271–300

   6 Over 300

7. HDL cholesterol (mg/dl):

   0 Over 60

   1 55–60

   2 Don't know

   3 45–54

   5 35–44

   7 25–34

   12 Lower than 25

8. Exercise:

   0 Exercise three times a week

   1 Exercise once or twice a week

   2 Occasional exercise less than once a week

   7 Rarely exercise

9. Diabetes:

   0 No personal or family history

   2 One parent with diabetes

   6 Two parents with diabetes

   9 Non-insulin-dependent diabetes

   13 Insulin-dependent diabetes

10. Body mass index (using the formula provided in Chapter 15):

   0 <23.0

   1 23.0–24.9

   2 25.0–28.9

   3 29.0–34.9

   5 35.0–39.9

   7 ≥40

11. Stress:

   0 Relaxed most of the time

   1 Occasional stress and anger

   2 Frequently stressed and angry

   3 Usually stressed and angry

Scoring

Total your risk factor points. Refer to the following below to get an approximate rating of your risk of suffering an early heart attack or stroke.

Score	Estimated Risk
Less than 20	Low risk
20–29	Moderate risk
30–45	High risk
Over 45	Extremely high risk

*Pack-years can be calculated by multiplying the number of packs you smoked per day by the number of years you smoked. For example, if you smoked a pack and a half a day for five years, you would have smoked the equivalent of 1.5 × 5 = 7.5 pack-years.

NOTE: If you know your blood pressure and cholesterol numbers, a tool that estimates CVD lifetime risk percentage is available from the American College of Cardiology; for people over 40, it also provides a 10-year risk estimate (http://tools.acc.org/ASCVD-Risk-Estimator/).

and help lower LDL levels. For people with high LDL levels that do not respond to changes in fat intake, the National Cholesterol Education Program suggests an intake of 2 grams per day of plant stanols or sterols.

- **Folic acid, vitamin B-6, and vitamin B-12.** These vitamins lower homocysteine levels, and folic acid has also been found to reduce the risk of hypertension.

- **Calcium.** Diets rich in calcium may help prevent hypertension and possibly stroke by reducing insulin resistance and platelet aggregation. Good sources of calcium are low-fat and fat-free dairy products.

- **Vitamin D.** There appears to be a close association between vitamin D deficiency and cardiovascular disease. However, studies have failed to show benefits to replacement of low vitamin D levels with supplemental dietary vitamin D. Such findings remain controversial, and further studies may offer new information.

- **Soy protein.** Although soy itself doesn't seem to have much effect on cholesterol, replacing some animal proteins with soy protein (such as tofu) may help lower the effects of saturated fat.

- **Healthy carbohydrates.** Healthy carbohydrate choices include whole grains, fruits, and nonstarch vegetables. Healthy carbohydrates are important for people with insulin resistance, prediabetes, or diabetes.

- **Total calories.** Some studies have found that reducing energy intake can improve cholesterol and triglyceride levels. Reduced calorie intake also helps control body weight—an extremely important risk factor for CVD.

Most experts recommend against taking nutritional supplements in an effort to prevent heart disease. If you are concerned about your heart health and think you may not be getting the nutrition you need, ask your physician and/or a registered dietitian for guidance.

A diet plan that reflects many of the recommendations described here was released as part of a study called Dietary Approaches to Stop Hypertension, or DASH. The DASH study found that a diet low in fat and high in fruits, vegetables, and low-fat dairy products reduces blood pressure. It also follows the recommendations for lowering the risk of heart disease, cancer, and osteoporosis. See Chapter 13 for details about the DASH diet plan.

Exercise Regularly

You can significantly reduce your risk of CVD with a moderate amount of physical activity. Follow the guidelines for physical activity and exercise described in Chapter 14. In addition to aerobic exercise for building and maintaining cardiovascular health, strength training helps reduce body fat and improves lipid levels and glucose metabolism.

The more exercise you get, the less likely you are to develop or die from CVD. Compared to sedentary individuals,

people who engage in regular, moderate physical activity lower their risk of CVD by 20% or more. People who get regular, vigorous exercise reduce their risk of CVD by 30% or more. This positive benefit applies regardless of intensity of exercise, gender, age, race, or ethnicity.

The type of exercise performed is less important than the amount of energy expended during the activity. Weight loss can improve heart health by reducing the amount of stress on the heart. Changing body composition to a more positive ratio of fat to fat-free mass boosts resting metabolic rate. Exercise can also prevent metabolic syndrome and reverse many of its negative effects on the body. Exercise directly strengthens the heart muscle itself, and it improves the balance of fats in the blood by boosting HDL and reducing LDL and triglyceride levels.

One of the clearest positive effects of exercise is on hypertension. Many studies, involving thousands of people, have shown that physical activity reduces both systolic and diastolic blood pressure. These studies showed that people who did regular aerobic exercise lowered their resting blood pressure by 2–4% on average. Lowered blood pressure itself reduces the risk of other kinds of cardiovascular disease.

Avoid Tobacco Products

The number-one risk factor for CVD that you can control is smoking. If you smoke, quit. If you don't smoke, don't start. If you live or work with people who smoke, encourage them to quit—for their sake and yours. Exposure to environmental tobacco smoke raises your risk of CVD, and there is no safe level of exposure. If you find yourself breathing in smoke, take steps to prevent or stop the exposure. See Chapter 12 for detailed information about the effects of smoking and strategies for quitting. Recent research has shown that vaping, or smoking electronic cigarettes, carries substantial risks for lung injury and cardiovascular disease. The dose of nicotine in e-cigarettes is often considerably more than a standard cigarette. The American Heart Association has publicly spoken out against the vaping epidemic and the misleading marketing of e-cigarette companies.

Manage Your Blood Pressure, Cholesterol Levels, and Stress/Anger

If you have no CVD risk factors, have your blood pressure measured by a trained professional at least once every two years.

Yearly tests are recommended if you have risk factors. If your blood pressure is high, follow your physician's advice on how to lower it. For those with hypertension that is not readily controlled with lifestyle changes, an array of antihypertension medications is available. Drug stores or pharmacies often provide reliable automated blood pressure devices with detailed instructions. If you take your blood pressure on three occasions, you can average the result to approximate your risk of CVD.

All people aged 20 and over should have their cholesterol checked at least once every five years. The National Cholesterol Education Program recommends a fasting lipoprotein profile that measures total cholesterol, HDL, LDL, and triglyceride levels. Once you know your baseline numbers and overall risk of developing CVD, you and your physician can develop a lifestyle plan.

To reduce the psychological and social risk factors for CVD, develop effective strategies for handling the stress in your life. Shore up your social support network, and try some of the techniques described in Chapter 2 for managing stress.

TIPS FOR TODAY AND THE FUTURE

Because cardiovascular disease is a long-term process that can begin when you're young, it's important to develop heart-healthy habits early in life.

RIGHT NOW YOU CAN:

- Make an appointment to have your blood pressure and cholesterol levels checked.
- List the key stressors in your life, and decide what to do about the ones that bother you most.
- Plan to replace one high-fat and one high-sugar item in your diet with one that is high in fiber. For example, replace a doughnut with a bowl of whole-grain cereal.

IN THE FUTURE YOU CAN:

- Track your eating habits for one week and then compare them to the DASH eating plan. Make adjustments to bring your diet closer to the DASH recommendations.
- Sign up for a class in cardiopulmonary resuscitation (CPR). A CPR certification equips you with valuable lifesaving skills you can use to help someone who is choking, having a heart attack, or experiencing cardiac arrest.

SUMMARY

- The cardiovascular system circulates blood throughout the body. The heart pumps blood to the lungs via the pulmonary artery and to the body via the aorta.

- The exchange of nutrients and waste products takes place between the capillaries and the tissues.

- The six major risk factors for CVD that can be changed or controlled are tobacco use, high blood pressure, unhealthy cholesterol levels, inactivity, overweight or obesity, and diabetes.

- Effects of smoking include lower HDL levels, increased blood pressure and heart rate, and increased risk of blood clots.

- Hypertension occurs when blood pressure exceeds normal levels most of the time. It weakens the heart, scars and hardens arteries, and can damage the eyes and kidneys.

- High LDL and low HDL cholesterol levels contribute to clogged arteries and increase the risk of developing CVD.

- Physical inactivity, obesity, and diabetes are interrelated and are associated with high blood pressure and unhealthy cholesterol levels.

- Risk factors that can be changed include high triglyceride levels, metabolic syndrome, inflammation, and psychological and social factors.

- Risk factors that can't be changed include being over 65, being male, being African American, and having a family history.

- Atherosclerosis is a gradual hardening and narrowing of arteries that can lead to restricted blood flow and complete blockage.

- Heart attacks are usually the result of a long-term disease process. Warning signs of a heart attack include chest discomfort, shortness of breath, nausea, and sweating.

- A stroke occurs when the blood supply to the brain is cut off by a blood clot or hemorrhage. A transient ischemic attack (TIA) may be a warning sign of an impending stroke.

- Congestive heart failure occurs when the heart's pumping action becomes less efficient and fluid collects in the lungs or in other parts of the body.

- Dietary changes that can protect against CVD include decreasing your intake of fat and cholesterol, and increasing your intake of fiber by eating more fruits, vegetables, and whole grains.

- CVD risk can be reduced by exercising regularly, avoiding tobacco and environmental tobacco smoke, managing your blood pressure and cholesterol levels, and developing effective ways of handling stress and anger.

FOR MORE INFORMATION

American Heart Association (AHA). Provides information about hundreds of topics relating to cardiovascular disease.

http://www.heart.org

Dietary Approaches to Stop Hypertension (DASH). Provides information about the design, diets, and results of the DASH study, including tips on how to follow the DASH diet at home.

http://www.nhlbi.nih.gov/health-topics/dash-eating-plan

The Heart: The Engine of Life. An online museum exhibit containing information about the structure and function of the heart, how to monitor your heart's health, and how to maintain a healthy heart.

https://www.fi.edu/heart-engine-of-life

The American Heart Association recommends that no more than 1% of the calories in your diet come from trans fats. Similarly, the 2015–2020 Dietary Guidelines from the U.S. Department of Agriculture and U.S. Department of Health and Human Services recommend that Americans avoid trans fats from industrial sources completely and consume only small amounts from natural sources. Hydrogenated fats, products made with them, and deep-fried fast food can be high in trans fats. Although food manufacturers are phasing out trans fats, it's important to read labels to see how much a product contains. If a product contains less than 0.5% trans fat, the manufacturer is allowed to list trans fat content as 0%.

For saturated fats, the Dietary Guidelines for Americans recommend that intake be reduced to less than 10% of total calories. The American Heart Association recommends further reductions, down to less than 7% of total calories from saturated fat.

Monitor Your Current Diet

To see how your diet measures up, keep track of everything you eat for three days. Information about the calorie and fat content of foods is available on many food labels and online.

At the end of the monitoring period, record the calories and grams of trans and saturated fat for the foods you've eaten. Determine the percentage of daily calories as fat that you consumed for each day: Multiply grams of the type of fat by 9 (fat has 9 calories per gram) and then divide by total calories. For example, if you consumed 30 grams of saturated fats and 2100 calories on a particular day, then your saturated fat consumption as a percentage of total calories would be calculated as $30 \times 9 = 270$ calories of fat $\div$ 2100 total calories $= 0.13$, or 13%. If you have trouble obtaining all the data you need to do the calculations, you can still estimate whether your diet is high in saturated fat by seeing how many servings of foods high in unhealthy fats you typically consume on a daily basis. As described in Chapter 13, saturated fats are found in animal products, including meat and dairy products, as well as in tropical oils. Sources of healthy dietary fats that are most often recommended are liquid vegetable oils, fish, and nuts.

Make Healthy Changes

To reduce your intake of unhealthy fats, set a limit on the number of daily servings of foods high in saturated and trans fats that you have and continue to monitor your consumption. To plan healthy changes, take a close look at your food record. Do you choose many foods high in unhealthy fats? Do you limit your portion sizes to those recommended by MyPlate.gov? Try making healthy substitutions. Instead of a grilled ham and cheese sandwich, try a turkey sandwich with an oil-based dressing or sliced avocado. If you frequently eat in fast-food restaurants, find an appealing alternative—and recruit some friends to join you.

When you choose foods that are rich in saturated fat, *watch your portion sizes carefully*. Choose cuts of meat that have the least amount of visible fat, and trim off what you see. And balance your choices throughout the day. For example, if your lunch includes a cheeseburger and fries, choose a vegetarian pasta dish for dinner. Plan your diet around a variety of whole grains, vegetables, legumes, and fruits, which are nearly always low in unhealthy fats and high in nutrients; try nuts and fish for dietary sources of healthy fats. See Chapter 13 for more details about a heart-healthy diet and for a list of alternatives to some popular foods.

MedlinePlus: Blood, Heart, and Circulation Topics. Provides links to reliable sources of information on cardiovascular health.

> https://www.nlm.nih.gov/medlineplus/bloodheartandcirculation
> .html

National Heart, Lung, and Blood Institute. Provides information about and interactive applications for a variety of topics relating to cardiovascular health and disease, including cholesterol, smoking, obesity, hypertension, and the DASH diet.

> http://www.nhlbi.nih.gov/

National Heart, Lung, and Blood Institute—What Is Cholesterol? Provides information about cholesterol, the diagnosis of elevated cholesterol, and treatments.

> http://www.nhlbi.nih.gov/health-topics/high-blood-cholesterol

National Stroke Association. Provides information and referrals for stroke victims and their families as well as a stroke risk assessment.

> http://www.stroke.org

See also the listings for Chapters 2, 3, 4, and 13–15.

SELECTED BIBLIOGRAPHY

Adly, G., and R. Plakogiannis. 2013. Reinitiating aspirin therapy for primary prevention of cardiovascular events in a patient post–aspirin–induced upper gastrointestinal bleed: A case report and review of literature. *Annals of Pharmacotherapy* 47(2): e8.

American Cancer Society. 2016. *Cancer Facts and Figures, 2016.* Atlanta, GA: American Cancer Society.

American Heart Association. 2015. *What Is Metabolic Syndrome?* (https://www .heart.org/-/media/files/health-topics/answers-by-heart/what-is-metabolic -syndrome-300322.pdf?la=en).

American Heart Association. 2020. *2020 Heart Disease and Stroke Statistical Update Fact Sheet At-a-Glance* (https://www.heart.org/-/media/files /about-us/statistics/2020-heart-disease-and-stroke-ucm_505473 .pdf?la=en).

The ATLANTIS, ECASS, and NINDS rt-PA Study Group Investigators. 2004. Association of outcome with early stroke treatment: Pooled analysis of ATLANTIS, ECASS, and NINDS rt-PA stroke trials. *Lancet* 363: 768–774.

Benjamin, E. J., et al. 2019. Heart disease and stroke statistics–2019 update. A report from the American Heart Association. *Circulation* 139: e56–e528.

Bibbins-Doming, K., et al. 2010. Projected effect of dietary salt reductions on future cardiovascular disease. *New England Journal of Medicine* 362(7): 590–599.

Bønaa, K. H., et al. 2006. Homocysteine lowering and cardiovascular events after acute myocardial infarction. *New England Journal of Medicine* 354(15): 1578–1588.

Bucholz, E. M., et al. 2016. Life expectancy after myocardial infarction, according to hospital performance. *New England Journal of Medicine* 375(14): 1332–1342.

CDC, NCHS. Underlying Cause of Death 1999–2013 on CDC WONDER Online Database, released 2015. Data are from the Multiple Cause of Death Files, 1999–2013, as compiled from data provided by the 57 vital statistics jurisdictions through the Vital Statistics Cooperative Program. Accessed May 5, 2018.

Centers for Disease Control and Prevention. 2011. Prevalence, treatment, and control of high levels of low-density lipoprotein cholesterol–United States, 1999–2002 and 2005–2008. *MMWR* 60(4):109–114.

Centers for Disease Control and Prevention. 2017. *Vital Signs: E-Cigarette Ads and Youth* (http://www.cdc.gov/vitalsigns/ecigarette-ads/index.html).

Centers for Disease Control and Prevention. 2018. Current cigarette smoking among adults–United States, 2016. *MMWR* 67(2): 53–59.

Centers for Disease Control and Prevention. 2019. *Diabetes Home: Diabetes Quick Facts* (http://www.cdc.gov/diabetes/basics/quick-facts.html/).

Centers for Disease Control and Prevention. 2019. *Heart Disease Statistics and Maps* (http://www.cdc.gov/heartdisease/facts.htm).

Centers for Disease Control and Prevention. 2019. *National Diabetes Statistics Report: Estimates of Diabetes and Its Burden in the United States* (https://www.cdc.gov/diabetes/pdfs/data/statistics/national-diabetes-statistics-report.pdf).

Clark, R., et al. 2018. Plasma cytokines and risk of coronary heart disease in the PROCARDIS study. *Open Heart* 5(1): e000807.

de Torbal, A., et al. 2006. Incidence of recognized and unrecognized myocardial infarction in men and women aged 55 and older: The Rotterdam Study. *European Heart Journal* 27(6): 729–736.

Després, J.-P. 2012. Body fat distribution and risk of cardiovascular disease: An update. *Circulation* 126: 1301–1313.

Elliott, P., et al. 2006. Association between protein intake and blood pressure: The INTERMAP Study. *Archives of Internal Medicine* 166(1): 79–87.

Freeman, M. W., and C. E. Junge. 2005. *Harvard Medical School Guide to Lowering Your Cholesterol.* New York: McGraw Hill.

Gilboa, S. M., et al. 2010. Mortality resulting from congenital heart disease among children and adults in the United States, 1999–2006. *Circulation* 122: 2254–2263.

Giovannucci, E., et al. 2008. 25-hydroxyvitamin D and risk of myocardial infarction in men: A prospective study. *Archives of Internal Medicine* 168(11): 1174–1180.

Gommans, J., et al. 2009. Preventing strokes: The assessment and management of people with transient ischemic attack. *New Zealand Medical Journal* 122(1293): 50–60.

Guan, W., et al. 2015. Race is a key variable in assigning lipoprotein(a) cutoff values for coronary heart disease risk assessment: The Multi-Ethnic Study of Atherosclerosis. *Arteriosclerosis, Thrombosis, and Vascular Biology* 35(4): 996–1001.

Gurfinkel, E. P., et al. 2007. Invasive vs. non-invasive treatment in acute coronary syndromes and prior bypass surgery. *International Journal of Cardiology* 119(1): 65–72.

Haberg, A. K., et al. 2016. Incidental findings and their clinical impact; the HUNT MRI study in a general population of 1006 participants between 50–66 years. *PLoS One* 11(3): e0151080.

Heinl, R. E., et al. 2016. Comprehensive cardiovascular risk reduction and cardiac rehabilitation in diabetes and the metabolic syndrome. *Canadian Journal of Cardiology* 32(10S2): S349–S357.

Helfand, M., et al. 2009. Emerging risk factors for coronary heart disease: A summary of systematic reviews conducted for the U.S. Preventive Services Task Force. *Annals of Internal Medicine* 151(7): 496.

Jenkins, D. J., et al. 2006. Assessment of the longer-term effects of a dietary portfolio of cholesterol-lowering foods in hypercholesterolemia. *American Journal of Clinical Nutrition* 83(3): 582–591.

Kidambi, S., et al. 2009. Hypertension, insulin resistance, and aldosterone: Sex-specific relationships. *Journal of Clinical Hypertension* 11(3): 130–137.

Lipsky, M. S., et al. 2008. *American Medical Association Guide to Preventing and Treating Heart Disease.* New York: Wiley.

Lloyd-Jones, D. M., et al. 2016. 2016 ACC expert consensus decision pathway on the role of non-statin therapies for LDL-cholesterol lowering in the management of atherosclerotic cardiovascular disease risk: A report of the American College of Cardiology Task Force on Expert Consensus Documents. *Journal of the American College of Cardiology* 68(1): 92–125.

Lloyd-Jones, D. M., et al. 2017. 2017 focused update of the 2016 ACC expert consensus decision pathway on the role of non-statin therapies for LDL-cholesterol lowering in the management of atherosclerotic cardiovascular disease risk: A report of the American College of Cardiology Task Force on Expert Consensus Decision Pathways. *Journal of the American College of Cardiology* 70(14): 1785–1822.

Marchionni, N., et al. 2003. Improved exercise tolerance and quality of life with cardiac rehabilitation of older patients after myocardial infarction: Results of a randomized, controlled trial. *Circulation* 107(7): 2201.

Maron, M. S., et al. 2016. Occurrence of clinically diagnosed hypertrophic cardiomyopathy in the United States. *American Journal of Cardiology* 117(10): 1651-1654.

Marshall, D. A., et al. 2009. Achievement of heart health characteristics through participation in an intensive lifestyle change program (Coronary Artery Disease Reversal Study). *Journal of Cardiopulmonary Rehabilitation and Prevention* 29(2): 84–94.

Mendis, S., et al., eds. 2011. *Global Atlas on Cardiovascular Disease Prevention and Control.* Geneva, Switzerland: World Health Organization (in collaboration with the World Heart Federation and World Stroke Organization).

Mirmiran, P., et al. 2009. Fruit and vegetable consumption and risk factors for cardiovascular disease. *Metabolism* 58(4): 460–468.

Mora, S., et al. 2007. LDL particle subclasses, LDL particle size, and carotid atherosclerosis in the multi-ethnic study of atherosclerosis (MESA). *Atherosclerosis* 192: 211–217.

Mozaffarian, D., et al. 2016. Heart disease and stroke statistics—2016 Update: A report from the American Heart Association. *Circulation* 133: e38–e360.

Murphy, S. L., et al. 2015. Deaths: Final data for 2012. *National Vital Statistics Reports* 63(9).

National Center for Health Statistics. 2016. *Health, United States, 2015: With Special Feature on Racial and Ethnic Health Disparities.* Hyattsville, MD: National Center for Health Statistics.

National Heart, Lung, and Blood Institute. 2015. *How Is Metabolic Syndrome Diagnosed?* (http://www.nhlbi.nih.gov/health/health-topics/topics/ms/diagnosis).

Nita, C., et al. 2008. Hypertensive waist: First step of the screening for metabolic syndrome. *Metabolic Syndrome and Related Disorders* 7(2): 105–110.

Ostrom, M. P., et al. 2008. Mortality incidence and the severity of coronary atherosclerosis assessed by computed tomography angiography. *Journal of the American College of Cardiology* 52(16): 1335–1343.

Pham, T., et al. 2016. The effect of serum 25-hydroxyvitamin D on elevated homocysteine concentrations in participants of a preventive health program. *PLos One* 11(8): e061368.

Pickering, T. G., et al. 2008. Call to action on use and reimbursement for home blood pressure monitoring: A joint scientific statement from the American Heart Association, American Society of Hypertension, and Preventive Cardiovascular Nurses Association. *Hypertension* 52(1): 10–29.

Raggi, P., et al. 2008. Coronary artery calcium to predict all-cause mortality in elderly men and women. *Journal of the American College of Cardiology* 52(1): 17–23.

Refsum, H., et al. 2006. The Hordaland Homocysteine Study: A community-based study of homocysteine, its determinants, and associations with disease. *Journal of Nutrition* 136(Suppl. 6): 1731S–1740S.

Rho, R. W., and R. L. Page. 2007. The automated external defibrillator. *Journal of Cardiovascular Electrophysiology* 18: 1-4.

Ridker, P. M., et al. 2008. Rosuvastatin to prevent vascular events in men and women with elevated C-reactive protein. *New England Journal of Medicine* 359(21): 2195-2207.

Rothwell, P. M., et al. 2016. Effects of aspirin on risk and severity of early recurrent stroke after transient ischaemic attack and ischaemic stroke: time-course analysis of randomised trials. *Lancet* 388(10042): 365-375.

Schiller, J. S., et al. 2012. Summary health statistics for U.S. adults: National Health Interview Survey, 2010. National Center for Health Statistics. *Vital Health Stat* 10(252).

Semsarian, C., et al. 2015. New perspectives on the prevalence of hypertrophic cardiomyopathy. *Journal of the American College of Cardiology* 65(12): 1249-1254.

Shi, S., et al. 2017. Depression and risk of sudden cardiac death and arrhythmias: a meta-analysis. *Psychosomatic Medicine* 79(2): 153-161.

Sonnenburg, J. L., and F. Bäckhed. 2016. Diet-microbiota interactions as moderators of human metabolism. *Nature* 535: 56-64.

SPRINT Research Group. 2015. A randomized trial of intensive versus standard blood-pressure control. *New England Journal of Medicine* 373(22): 2103-2116.

Stone, N. J., et al. 2013. ACC/AHA guideline on the treatment of blood cholesterol to reduce atherosclerotic cardiovascular risk in adults: A report of the American College of Cardiology/American Heart Association Task Force on Practice Guidelines. *Journal of the American College of Cardiology*.

Suaya, J. A., et al. 2009. Cardiac rehabilitation and survival in older coronary patients. *Journal of the American College of Cardiology* 54(1): 25.

Sui, X., et al. 2007. Cardiorespiratory fitness and the risk of nonfatal cardiovascular disease in women and men with hypertension. *American Journal of Hypertension* 20(6): 608-615.

U.S. Department of Health and Human Services. 2014. *The Health Consequences of Smoking—50 Years of Progress: A Report of the Surgeon General.* Atlanta, GA: U.S. Department of Health and Human Services, Centers for Disease Control and Prevention, National Center for Chronic Disease Prevention and Health Promotion, Office on Smoking and Health.

U.S. Departments of Health and Human Services and Agriculture. 2015. *2015-2020 Dietary Guidelines for Americans* (http://health.gov/dietaryguidelines/2015/guidelines/).

Wang, X., et al. 2007. Efficacy of folic acid supplementation in stroke prevention: A meta-analysis. *Lancet* 369(9576): 1876-1882.

Watkins, D. A., et al. 2017. Global, regional, and national burden of rheumatic heart disease, 1990-2015. *New England Journal of Medicine* 377: 713-722.

Wenger, N. K., et al. 1995. *Cardiac Rehabilitation* (Clinical Practice Guideline No. 17, AHCPR Publication No. 96-0672). Rockville, MD: U.S. Department of Health and Human Services, Public Health Service, Agency for Health Care Policy and Research, and the National Heart, Lung, and Blood Institute.

Whelton, P. K., et al. 2017. 2017 ACC/AHA/AAPA/ABC/ACPM/AGS/APhA/ASH/ASPC/NMA/PCNA guideline for the prevention, detection, evaluation, and management of high blood pressure in adults. A report of the American College of Cardiology/American Heart Association Task Force on Clinical Practice Guidelines. *Journal of the American College of Cardiology* S0735-1097(17): 41519-1.

Widmer, R. J., et al. 2015. The Mediterranean diet, its components, and cardiovascular disease. *American Journal of Medicine* 128(3): 229-238.

Willershausen, I., et al. 2013. Association between chronic periodontal and apical inflammation and acute myocardial infarction. *Odontology,* April 21.

Xie, X., et al. 2015. Effects of intensive blood pressure lowering on cardiovascular and renal outcomes: Updated systematic review and meta-analysis. *Lancet* S0140-6736(15): 00805-3.

Zhang, Z. M., et al. 2016. Race and sex differences in the incidence and prognostic significant of silent myocardial infarction in the Atherosclerosis Risk in Communities (ARIC) study. *Circulation* 133(22): 2141-2148.

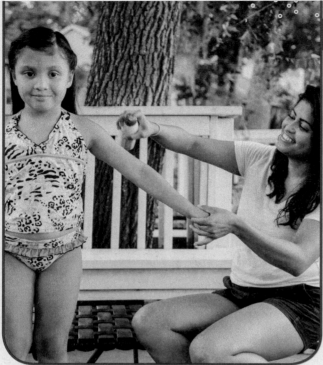

Jeff Greenough/Getty Images

CHAPTER 17

CHAPTER OBJECTIVES

- Explain the basic facts about cancer
- Discuss causes of cancer and how to avoid or minimize them
- Describe how cancer can be detected, diagnosed, and treated
- Describe common cancers as well as detection and treatment options for each
- List and describe new and emerging cancer treatments

Cancer

TEST YOUR KNOWLEDGE

1. **Which type of cancer kills the most women each year?**
   a. Breast cancer
   b. Lung cancer
   c. Ovarian cancer

2. **Which type of cancer kills the most men each year?**
   a. Prostate cancer
   b. Lung cancer
   c. Colon cancer

3. **Testicular cancer is the most common cancer in men under age 30.**
   True or False?

4. **The use of condoms during sexual intercourse can help prevent cervical cancer in women.**
   True or False?

5. **Eating which of these foods may help prevent cancer?**
   a. Chili peppers
   b. Broccoli
   c. Oranges

ANSWERS

1. **B.** There are more cases of breast cancer each year, but lung cancer kills more women. Smoking is the primary risk factor for lung cancer.

2. **B.** There are more cases of prostate cancer, but lung cancer kills more than twice as many men as prostate cancer does each year.

3. **TRUE.** Although rare, testicular cancer is the most common cancer in men under age 30. Regular self-exams may aid in its detection.

4. **TRUE.** The primary cause of cervical cancer is infection with human papillomavirus (HPV), a sexually transmitted pathogen. The use of condoms helps prevent HPV infection.

5. **ALL THREE.** These and many other fruits and vegetables are rich in phytochemicals, which are naturally occurring substances that may have anticancer effects.

Cancer is the second leading cause of death in the United States, after heart disease. Cancer is responsible for approximately 600,000 deaths in the United States annually.

Even as medical science struggles to find a cure for cancer, mounting evidence indicates that many cancers could be prevented by simple changes in lifestyle. Tobacco use, for example, is responsible for about 20% of all U.S. cancer diagnoses and 30% of all cancer deaths. Poor dietary and exercise habits, combined with heavy alcohol use, account for another 18% of cancer diagnoses and 20% of cancer deaths. Cancers caused by infectious agents could be prevented by lifestyle changes, vaccination, or treatment of the infections. Additional evidence indicates that individual behavior is a significant determinant of cancer risk.

This chapter explains how cancer progresses and identifies the factors that put people at risk for developing it.

BASIC FACTS ABOUT CANCER

Cancer is a group of diseases characterized by abnormal, uncontrolled multiplication of cells, which can ultimately cause death if left untreated.

Tumors

Most cancers take the form of tumors, although not all tumors are cancerous. A **tumor** (or *neoplasm*) is a mass of tissue that serves no physiological purpose. It can be benign, like a wart, or malignant, like most lung cancers.

Benign (noncancerous) **tumors** are made up of cells similar to the surrounding normal cells and are enclosed in a membrane that prevents them from penetrating neighboring tissues. They are dangerous only if their physical presence interferes with body functions. A benign brain tumor, for example, can cause death if it blocks the blood supply to the brain.

The term **malignant tumor** is synonymous with cancer. A malignant tumor can invade surrounding structures, including blood vessels, the **lymphatic system,** and nerves. It can also spread to distant sites via blood and lymphatic circulation, producing invasive tumors almost anywhere in the body. A few cancers, such as leukemia (cancer of the blood), typically do not produce a mass but still have the fundamental property of rapid, uncontrolled cell proliferation.

Cancer begins when a change (or mutation) in a cell allows the cell to grow and divide when it should not. In adults, cells normally multiply at a rate just sufficient to replace dying cells. In contrast, a malignant cell divides into new cells without regard for normal control mechanisms and gradually produces a mass of abnormal cells, or a tumor. A pea-sized mass is made up of about a billion cells, so a single tumor cell must divide many times before the tumor grows to a noticeable size (Figure 17.1).

Eventually a tumor becomes large enough to cause symptoms or to be detected directly. In the breast, for example, a tumor may be felt as a lump or seen on an X-ray called a mammogram. In less accessible locations, like the lung, a tumor may be noticed only after it has grown considerably and may then be detected only by an indirect symptom, such as a persistent cough or unexplained bleeding. In the case of leukemia, changes in the blood are eventually noticed as increasing fatigue, infection, or abnormal bleeding. Once there is a suspicion of cancer, a patient will have a **biopsy** to confirm the diagnosis.

Metastasis

Metastasis is the spread of cancer cells from one part of the body to another. Metastasis occurs because cancer cells do not cling to each other as strongly as normal cells do and therefore may migrate from the site of the *primary tumor* (the cancer's original location). After cancer cells break away, they can pass through the lining of lymph or blood vessels to invade nearby tissue. Once established, a tumor can recruit normal cells (such as bone marrow cells), modify them, and use them as "envoys" to travel to different parts of the body and prepare other sites to receive traveling cancer cells. The envoy cells work by creating proteins that attract the free-floating cancer cells, allowing them to gather at a new site and resume making copies of themselves. This traveling and seeding process is called *metastasizing,* and the new tumors are called *secondary tumors* or *metastases.*

The ability of cancer cells to metastasize makes early cancer detection critical. To cure cancer, every cancerous cell must be removed or destroyed. Once cancer cells enter either the lymphatic system or the bloodstream, it is extremely difficult to stop their spread to other organs of the body. In fact, counting lymph nodes that contain cancer cells is one of the principal methods of predicting the outcome of a disease: The probability of a cure is much greater when the lymph nodes do not contain cancer cells.

TERMS

cancer The abnormal, uncontrolled multiplication of cells.

tumor A mass of tissue that serves no physiological purpose; also called a *neoplasm*.

benign tumor A tumor that is not cancerous.

malignant tumor A tumor that is capable of spreading and thus is cancerous.

lymphatic system A system of vessels that returns proteins, lipids, and other substances from fluid in the tissues to the circulatory system.

biopsy The removal of a small piece of body tissue to allow for microscopic examination; a needle biopsy uses a needle to remove a small sample of tissue, but some biopsies require surgery.

metastasis The spread of cancer cells from one part of the body to another.

1. Tumor development begins when a cell (light orange) is altered so that it grows and divides when it normally would not. The altered cell and its descendants look normal but continue to reproduce too much, a condition called *hyperplasia*. Over time, new mutations may arise and cause even more cell proliferation (dark orange).

2. After additional mutations, the descendants of the altered cells may be abnormal in shape (purple), called *dysplasia*. Dysplasia may or may not develop into cancer.

3. Over time, the affected cells may become more abnormal in shape and behavior. *In situ cancer* is diagnosed if the abnormal cells are found only in the location where they first formed. The tumor may remain in this location or may acquire additional mutations (blue).

4. Abnormal cells may gain the ability to invade nearby tissues, causing *localized invasive cancer*. The function of the affected organ or tissue may be affected, but the tumor has not yet spread beyond the boundaries of the organ of origin.

5. If the tumor spreads so that it can shed malignant cells into a blood or lymphatic vessel, these cells can travel to distant sites and establish new tumors *(metastases)* throughout the body.

Altered cell   **Hyperplasia**

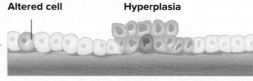

Dysplasia

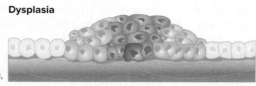

In situ cancer

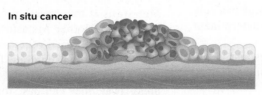

Localized invasive tumor

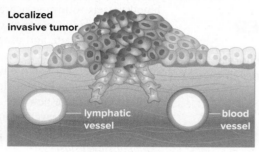

lymphatic vessel   blood vessel

Metastasis

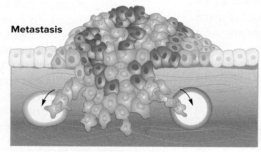

FIGURE 17.1   **Tumor development occurs in stages.**

SOURCES: Adapted from Mader/Windelspecht. 2016. *Human Biology*, 14e. New York: McGraw Hill; U.S. National Institutes of Health, National Cancer Institute.

The Stages of Cancer

Once a cancer has been diagnosed, physicians can classify the disease according to the extent of the cancer in the patient's body. This classifying process is called **staging,** and the extent or spread of the cancer is described in Table 17.1.

To identify a cancer's stage, physicians assess the size or extent of the primary tumor, whether the cancer has invaded nearby lymph nodes, and whether metastases are present. By judging the extent of each criterion, physicians can determine the cancer's stage, establish how severe it is, and choose the most appropriate treatment.

Remission

A significant number of cancer cases go into **remission,** which in some cases lasts for years, or indefinitely. In remission, signs and symptoms of cancer disappear, and the disease is considered to be under control. Remission typically results from treatment; rarely do cancer patients enter remission spontaneously.

The Incidence of Cancer

Each year more than 1.7 million people in the United States are diagnosed with cancer. Most will be cured or will live many years past their initial cancer diagnosis. In fact, the American Cancer Society (ACS) estimates that the **five-year survival rate** for all cancers diagnosed between 2007 and 2013 is 69%. These statistics exclude more than 1 million cases of the curable types of skin cancer. Figure 17.2 shows the number of new cases of cancer each year and the number of deaths by sex and by cancer site.

At current rates in the United States, nearly one in two people will develop cancer at some point in their lives. Men and women share most major risk factors for cancer, but they often have a different experience because more than one-third of all cancers occur in sex organs (prostate, testes, breasts, ovaries, uterus, and cervix). For both men and women, lung and colorectal cancers are among the three most common types. For men, prostate cancer, and for women, breast cancer account for the greatest number of new diagnoses. For women, in addition to lifestyle factors such as smoking, diet, and exercise, hormonal factors relating to their menstrual and childbearing history are also important risk considerations. Women may also have a greater biological vulnerability to specific carcinogens, such as those in cigarettes.

Table 17.1 Cancer Stages

STAGE	DESCRIPTION
0	Early cancer, present only in the layer of cells where it originated
I	More extensive cancer, with higher numbers
II	indicating greater tumor size and/or the degree
III	to which the cancer has spread to nearby lymph nodes or organs adjacent to the primary tumor
IV	Advanced cancer that has spread to another organ

SOURCE: American Joint Committee on Cancer. 2017. *AICC Cancer Staging Manual,* 8th ed. Chicago, IL: Springer.

Overall, however, men are more likely than women to die of cancer. For some cancers, the differences are especially significant. Here are some factors underlying the higher death rates among men:

• **Higher rates of tobacco use.** In the past, men had significantly higher rates of tobacco use than women, leading to much higher rates of the many cancers linked to smoking. This gap has been closing among white Americans as smoking prevalence for women (15%) grows closer to that of men

(17%); among Hispanics, blacks, and Asians, the gender gap remains larger.

• **Higher rates of alcohol use and abuse.** Alcohol abuse is more common in men and is a risk factor for several cancers, including oral and liver cancers.

• **Greater occupational exposure to carcinogens.** Men are more likely to work in jobs where they are exposed to chemicals—including asbestos, arsenic, coal tar, pitch, and dyes—or radiation, and such exposure is a risk factor for cancers of the bladder, lung, and skin. Men are also more likely to have outdoor jobs involving frequent sun exposure.

• **Less use of preventive measures and less contact with health care providers.** Traditional gender roles may make men more likely to minimize symptoms and less likely to seek help or to discuss cancer-related worries with a health care provider. Men may less frequently pursue preventive care, such as using sunscreen, and screenings such as self-exams.

For 60 years, the number of cancer deaths increased steadily in the United States, largely due to a wave of lethal lung cancers among men caused by smoking. As smoking rates declined, the cancer death rate fell 26% from its peak of 215 deaths per 100,000 people in 1991 to 159 deaths per 100,000 people in 2015; in other words, 2.3 million fewer cancer deaths occurred in this period. This trend suggests that efforts at prevention,

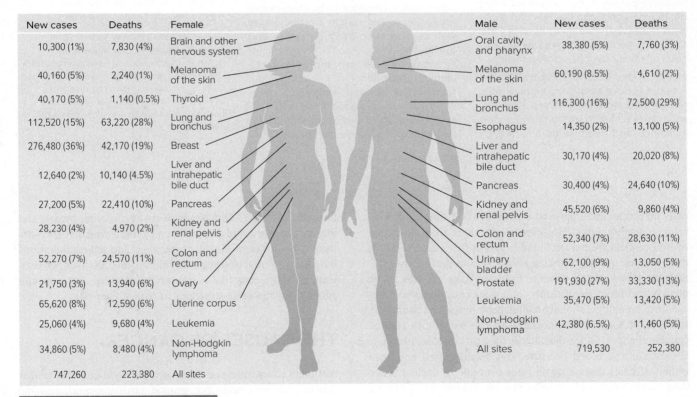

New cases	Deaths	Female		Male	New cases	Deaths
10,300 (1%)	7,830 (4%)	Brain and other nervous system		Oral cavity and pharynx	38,380 (5%)	7,760 (3%)
40,160 (5%)	2,240 (1%)	Melanoma of the skin		Melanoma of the skin	60,190 (8.5%)	4,610 (2%)
40,170 (5%)	1,140 (0.5%)	Thyroid		Lung and bronchus	116,300 (16%)	72,500 (29%)
112,520 (15%)	63,220 (28%)	Lung and bronchus		Esophagus	14,350 (2%)	13,100 (5%)
276,480 (36%)	42,170 (19%)	Breast		Liver and intrahepatic bile duct	30,170 (4%)	20,020 (8%)
12,640 (2%)	10,140 (4.5%)	Liver and intrahepatic bile duct		Pancreas	30,400 (4%)	24,640 (10%)
27,200 (5%)	22,410 (10%)	Pancreas		Kidney and renal pelvis	45,520 (6%)	9,860 (4%)
28,230 (4%)	4,970 (2%)	Kidney and renal pelvis		Colon and rectum	52,340 (7%)	28,630 (11%)
52,270 (7%)	24,570 (11%)	Colon and rectum		Urinary bladder	62,100 (9%)	13,050 (5%)
21,750 (3%)	13,940 (6%)	Ovary		Prostate	191,930 (27%)	33,330 (13%)
65,620 (8%)	12,590 (6%)	Uterine corpus		Leukemia	35,470 (5%)	13,420 (5%)
25,060 (4%)	9,680 (4%)	Leukemia		Non-Hodgkin lymphoma	42,380 (6.5%)	11,460 (5%)
34,860 (5%)	8,480 (4%)	Non-Hodgkin lymphoma		All sites	719,530	252,380
747,260	223,380	All sites				

VITAL STATISTICS

FIGURE 17.2 **Estimated number of new cancer cases and deaths by sex and by site, United States, 2020.** Estimated new cases are based on 2002–2016 incidence data reported by the North American Association of Central Cancer Registries (NAACCR). Estimated deaths are based on 2003–2017 US mortality data, National Center for Health Statistics.

SOURCE: American Cancer Society. 2020. *Cancer Facts and Figures, 2020.* Atlanta, GA: American Cancer Society.

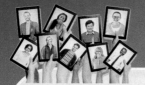

Rates of cancer have declined among all U.S. racial and ethnic groups in recent years, but significant disparities still exist:

• Among U.S. racial and ethnic groups, African American men have the highest incidence of and death rates from cancer.

• White women have a higher incidence of breast cancer, but African American women have the highest breast cancer death rate. African American women are more likely to have aggressive tumors, less likely to receive regular mammograms, and more likely to experience delays in follow-up.

• African American men have a higher rate of prostate cancer than any other U.S. group and more than twice the prostate cancer death rate of other groups. African American men are less likely than white men to undergo prostate-specific antigen (PSA) testing for prostate cancer.

• Latinas have the highest incidence of cervical cancer, but African American women have the highest cervical cancer death rate. Language barriers and problems accessing screening services are thought to particularly affect Latinas, who have relatively low rates of Pap testing.

• Asian Americans and Pacific Islander Americans have among the highest rates of liver and stomach cancers. Koreans, especially, suffer from stomach cancer; incidence and death rates are roughly twice as high as those among Japanese, who have the next-highest rates. Recent immigration helps explain these higher rates because these cancers are usually caused by infections that are more prevalent in Asian countries of origin.

Some of the disparities in cancer risks and rates may be influenced by genetic or cultural factors. For example, certain genetic/molecular features of aggressive breast cancer are more common among African American women with the disease, and breast cancer is more likely to be diagnosed at a later stage and with more aggressive tumors in these women. Genetic factors may also help explain the high rate of prostate cancer among black men. Women from cultures in which early marriage and motherhood are common are likely to have a lower risk of breast cancer.

Most of the differences in cancer rates and deaths, however, are thought to be the result of socioeconomic inequities, which influence the prevalence of many underlying cancer risk factors as well as access to early detection and quality treatment. People of low socioeconomic status are more likely to smoke, abuse alcohol, eat unhealthful foods, and be sedentary and overweight—all factors associated with cancer. High levels of stress associated with poverty may impair the immune system, which is the body's first line of defense against cancer.

People with low incomes are more likely to live in unhealthful environments. Low-income people may also have jobs in which they come into daily contact with carcinogenic chemicals. They may face similar risks in their homes and schools, where they may be exposed to asbestos or other carcinogens.

People with low incomes also have less exposure to information about cancer, are less aware of the early warning signs of cancer, and have less access to medical care when they have such symptoms. Lack of health insurance is a key factor explaining higher death rates among people with low incomes. Discrimination and language and cultural barriers can also affect patients' use of the health care system.

Public education campaigns that encourage healthy lifestyle habits, routine cancer screening, and participation in clinical trials may be one helpful strategy to reduce cancer disparities.

SOURCES: American Cancer Society. 2019. *Cancer Facts and Figures.* Atlanta, GA: American Cancer Society; Iqbal, J., et al. 2015. Differences in breast cancer stage at diagnosis and cancer-specific survival by race and ethnicity in the United States. *Journal of the American Medical Association* 313(2): 165–173.

early detection, and improved therapy are contributing to lowering mortality rates. However, death rates from smoking-related cancers are not declining as fast as heart disease death rates because quitting smoking affects various disease risks differently. Heart-related damage from smoking reverses more quickly and more significantly than does cancer-related damage from smoking. Smoking-related gene mutations cannot be reversed, although other mechanisms can sometimes control cellular changes. Other risk factors for heart disease, like high cholesterol and blood pressure, can be diagnosed and controlled. If heart disease death rates continue to decline faster than cancer death rates, cancer may overtake heart disease as the leading cause of death among Americans of all ages.

Still, many more people could be saved from cancer. The overwhelming majority of skin cancers could be prevented by protecting the skin from excessive sun exposure, and the majority of lung cancers could be prevented by avoiding exposure to tobacco smoke. Thousands of cases of colon, breast, and uterine cancers could be prevented by improving diet and controlling body weight. Regular screenings and self-examinations have the potential to save an additional 100,000 lives per year. Cancer may seem like a mysterious disease, but you can adopt many concrete strategies to reduce your risk.

THE CAUSES OF CANCER

Although scientists do not know everything about what causes cancer, they have identified genetic, environmental, and lifestyle factors that increase the risk of developing cancer (see the box "Race/Ethnicity, Poverty, and Cancer"). Around one-third of cancer deaths worldwide are due to five behavioral and dietary risks: high BMI, low fruit and vegetable intake, lack of physical activity, tobacco use, and alcohol use.

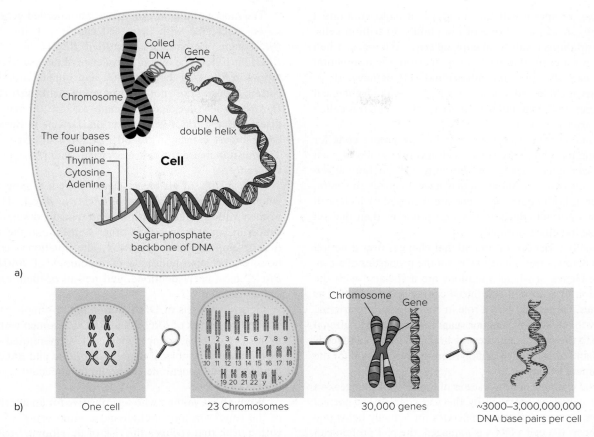

Coiled
DNA
Gene

Chromosome

DNA
double helix

The four bases
Guanine
Thymine
Cytosine
Adenine

Cell

Sugar-phosphate
backbone of DNA

a)

Chromosome
Gene

b) One cell 23 Chromosomes 30,000 genes ~3000–3,000,000,000
DNA base pairs per cell

1 2 3 4 5 6 7 8 9
10 11 12 13 14 15 16 17 18
19 20 21 22 y x

FIGURE 17.3 **(a) The double helix of DNA. (b) In each cell are 23 chromosomes; on each chromosome are 30,000 genes; each gene is made up of several thousand to several million base pairs, and in total, each genome contains 3 billion DNA base pairs.**

The Role of DNA

Heredity and genetics are important factors in a person's cancer risk. Certain genes may predispose some people to cancer, and specific genetic mutations have been associated with cancer. For the following DNA basics, it might be helpful to think of the genetic code as a set of instructions for building, operating, and repairing your body. The sections that follow explain how it works.

DNA Basics   The nucleus of each cell in your body contains 23 pairs of **chromosomes,** which are made up of tightly packed coils of **DNA** (deoxyribonucleic acid). DNA consists of two long strands wound around each other in a spiral structure, like a twisted ladder; scientists refer to this spiral as a *double helix* (Figure 17.3). The rungs of the ladder are made from four different nucleotide bases: adenine (A), thymine (T), cytosine (C), and guanine (G). Bases on opposite strands pair up specifically: A always with T, and C always with G. The arrangement of nucleotide bases along the double helix constitutes the genetic code.

A **gene** is a smaller unit of DNA made up of a specific sequence of nucleotide bases. Each chromosome contains hundreds, and in some cases thousands, of genes; you have about

30,000 genes in all. Each gene controls the production of a particular protein. Proteins build cells and make them work: They serve both as the structural material for your body and as the regulators of all chemical reactions and metabolic processes. By making different proteins at different times, genes can act as switches to alter the ways a cell works.

Cells reproduce by dividing in two, and your body makes billions of new cells every day. When a cell divides, the DNA replicates itself so that each new cell has a complete set of chromosomes. Genes that control the rate of cell division often play a critical role in the development of cancer.

DNA Mutations and Cancer   A *mutation* is any change in the normal makeup of a gene. Some mutations are inherited.

---

chromosomes   The threadlike bodies in a cell nucleus that contain molecules of DNA; most human cells contain 23 pairs of chromosomes.   **TERMS**

DNA   Deoxyribonucleic acid: a chemical substance that carries genetic information.

gene   A section of a chromosome that contains the nucleotide base sequence for making a particular protein; the basic unit of heredity.

If the egg or sperm cell that produces a child contains a mutation, so will every one of the child's 30 trillion cells. Other mutations result from copying errors that occur when DNA replicates itself as part of cell division. Environmental agents can also produce mutational cell damage; these **mutagens** include radiation, certain viruses, and chemical substances. (When a mutagen also causes cancer, it is called a *carcinogen*.)

A mutated gene no longer contains the proper code for producing its protein. Because a cell has two copies of each gene, it can sometimes get by with only one functioning version. In this case, the mutation may have no effect on health. However, if both copies of a gene are damaged or if the cell needs two normal copies to function properly, then the cell will cease to behave normally.

It usually takes several mutational changes over a period of years before a normal cell takes on the properties of a cancer cell. Genes in which mutations are associated with the conversion of a normal cell into a cancer cell are known as **oncogenes.** Genes that play a role in controlling or restricting cell growth are known as **tumor suppressor genes.** Mutational damage to these genes releases the brake on growth and leads to rapid and uncontrolled cell division—a precondition for the development of cancer.

A good example of how a series of mutational changes can produce cancer is provided by the *p53* gene. In its normal form, the protein that this gene codes for actually helps prevent cancer: If a cell's DNA is damaged, the p53 protein can either kill the cell outright or stop it from replicating until the damaged DNA is repaired. For example, if a skin cell's DNA is mutated by exposure to sunlight, the p53 protein activates the cell's "suicide" machinery. By preventing the replication of damaged DNA, the p53 protein keeps cells from progressing toward cancer. However, if the *p53* gene itself undergoes a mutation, these controls are lost, and the cell can become cancerous. In fact, the damaged version of *p53* can actually promote cell division and the spread of cancer. Researchers believe that damage to the *p53* gene and protein may be involved, directly and indirectly, in as many as 50–60% of cancers of all types.

Hereditary Cancer Risks   One way to obtain a mutated oncogene or tumor suppressor gene is to inherit it. The discovery of inherited disease-related genes is opening up a host of issues related to genetic testing and associated legal, financial, and ethical concerns.

> **mutagen**   Any environmental factor that can cause **TERMS** mutation, such as radiation and atmospheric chemicals.
>
> **oncogene**   A gene involved in the transformation of a normal cell into a cancer cell.
>
> **tumor suppressor gene**   A gene that normally functions to restrain cellular growth.

The most prominent example of an inherited genetic mutation associated with increased cancer risk involves the *BRCA* gene. Researchers identified *BRCA1* in 1994 and *BRCA2* in 1995. The overall prevalence of disease-related mutations in *BRCA1* is about 1 in 300, and 1 in 800 in *BRCA2*. In certain groups, most notably women of Ashkenazi (Eastern European) Jewish descent, as many as 3 in 100 may carry a disease-related *BRCA* gene mutation. Defects in these genes cause breast cancer in 50–80% of those affected women. They also increase the risk of ovarian, pancreatic, and prostate cancers.

Only 5–10% of all breast cancers occur among women who inherit an altered version of *BRCA1* or *BRCA2*. However, women with an altered *BRCA* gene tend to develop breast cancer at younger ages than other women, and the cancers that develop are more aggressive. The situation is complex, however, because hundreds of mutations of *BRCA1* and *BRCA2* have been identified, and not all of them carry the same risks.

Genetic analysis of DNA from a blood sample can identify mutant copies of *BRCA1* and *BRCA2*. Women with a family history of breast cancer must still be monitored closely, even if they carry normal versions of *BRCA1* and *BRCA2*. The cancer-causing genetic defect in the family could be located on another gene.

What about women who test positive for an altered copy of the gene? Options include close monitoring; treatment with a drug that reduces the risk of developing breast cancer, such as tamoxifen; and prophylactic surgical removal of breasts and/or ovaries. As shown in several studies, prophylactic bilateral mastectomy decreases the risk of developing breast cancer by at least 90% in *BRCA1* or *BRCA2* mutation carriers. When women with a *BRCA1* or *BRCA2* gene mutation have their ovaries and fallopian tubes removed as a preventive measure, their risk of breast cancer falls by approximately 50% and their risk of other gynecologic cancers falls by approximately 80%. Surgical removal of reproductive organs makes women infertile and needs to be considered carefully. However, none of these strategies eliminates risk completely, and they may expose a woman to a dangerous or drastic treatment that is potentially unnecessary. Men, too, can inherit the *BRCA* mutations, and they have a correspondingly higher rate of breast cancers than men without the mutation. However, in total, men develop less than 1% of all breast cancer cases in the United States.

Tests for hereditary mutations in breast cancer genes are now commercially available. The National Comprehensive Cancer Network developed specific risk assessment criteria that are recommended as part of the decision-making process in determining whether an individual should be considered for genetic testing. Some of these criteria include age at breast cancer diagnosis, presence of specific markers on breast cancer cells, presence of multiple breast cancers, diagnosis with other cancers, family history of cancers, and male breast cancer.

Although an area of active research, the science on this topic is still in its earliest stages. Patients who warrant genetic testing should first be referred to a cancer genetics professional, who can help them understand the role of genetic testing and interpret the results. In most cases, mutational damage occurs after birth. Lifestyle decisions are still important even for those who have inherited a damaged gene.

Cancer Promoters

Substances known as *cancer promoters* make up another important piece of the cancer puzzle. Carcinogenic agents, such as ultraviolet (UV) radiation, that cause mutational changes in the DNA of oncogenes are known as cancer *initiators*. Cancer *promoters,* by contrast, don't directly produce DNA mutations. Instead they accelerate the growth of initiated cells without damaging or permanently altering their DNA. However, a faster growth rate means less time for a cell to repair DNA damage caused by initiators, so errors are more likely to be passed on. Estrogen, which stimulates cellular growth in the female reproductive organs, is an example of a cancer promoter. Cigarette smoke is a complete carcinogen because it acts as both an initiator and a promoter.

Tobacco Use

Smoking is responsible for about one-third of all cancer deaths (see Figure 17.4), including 87% of lung cancer deaths for men and 76% of such deaths for women. The U.S. Surgeon General has reported that tobacco use is a direct cause of several types of cancer. In addition to lung and bronchial cancer (discussed later in this chapter and in Chapter 12), tobacco use is linked to cancers of the larynx, mouth, pharynx, esophagus, stomach, pancreas, liver, kidneys, bladder, and cervix, and directly causes acute myelogenous leukemia.

Dietary Factors

How important is diet in cancer prevention? The relationship between food and cancer risk is complex and controversial. There is no diet that completely eliminates the chance of developing cancer. However, experts are in virtually unanimous agreement that maintaining a healthy weight and eating a diet rich in fruits and vegetables will help lower the risk of cancer. The foods you eat contain many biologically active compounds, and your food choices may either increase your cancer risk by exposing you to potentially dangerous compounds or reduce your risk through consumption of potentially protective ones (Figure 17.5).

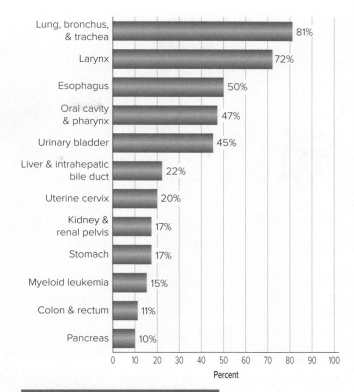

VITAL STATISTICS

FIGURE 17.4 **Number and percentage of cancer deaths attributable to cigarette smoking in U.S. adults age 30 and over, 2014.**

SOURCE: Islami, F., et al. 2017. Proportion and number of cancer cases and deaths attributable to potentially modifiable risk factors in the United States. *CA: A Cancer Journal for Clinicians* 68(1): 31–54.

These dietary factors may affect cancer risk:

• *Dietary fat and meat.* Diets high in fat and meat may contribute to colon, stomach, and prostate cancers. Certain types of fats may be riskier than others. Omega-6 polyunsaturated fats are associated with a higher risk of some cancers; omega-3 fats are not.

• *Alcohol.* Alcohol is associated with an increased incidence of several cancers. Women who have two to five drinks daily have about 1.5 times the cancer risk of women who drink no alcohol. Alcohol and tobacco interact as risk factors for oral cancer.

• *Foods cooked at high temperatures.* High levels of the chemical acrylamide (a probable human carcinogen) are found in starch-based foods that have been fried or baked at high temperatures, especially french fries and certain types of snack chips and crackers. Acrylamide is also found in high concentrations in tobacco.

• *Fiber.* Various potential cancer-fighting actions have been proposed for fiber, but none of these has been firmly established. Further study is needed to clarify the relationship between fiber intake and cancer risk, but experts still recommend a high-fiber diet for its overall positive effect on health.

Do More	**Do Less**

Do More

- *Eat a varied, plant-based diet that is high in fiber-rich foods such as legumes and whole grains.*

- *Eat 7–13 servings of fruits and vegetables every day, favoring foods from the following categories:*
  Cruciferous vegetables
  Citrus fruits
  Berries
  Dark green leafy vegetables
  Dark yellow, orange, or red fruits and vegetables

- *Be physically active.*

- *Maintain a healthy weight.*

- *Practice safer sex (to avoid HPV infection).*

- *Protect your skin from the sun with appropriate clothing and sunscreen.*

- *Perform regular self-exams (skin self-exam for all, testicular self-exam for men, breast self-awareness for women).*

- *Obtain recommended screening tests and discuss with your physician any family history of cancer.*

Do Less

- *Don't use tobacco in any form:*
  Cigarettes
  Smokeless tobacco
  Cigars and pipes
  Bidis and clove cigarettes

- *Avoid exposure to environmental tobacco smoke.*

- *Limit consumption of fatty meats and other sources of saturated fat.*

- *Avoid excessive alcohol consumption.*

- *Don't eat charred foods, and limit consumption of cured and smoked meats and meat and fish grilled in a direct flame.*

- *Avoid occupational exposure to carcinogens.*

- *Limit exposure to UV radiation from sunlight.*

- *Avoid tanning lamps or beds.*

FIGURE 17.5   Strategies for reducing your risk of cancer. MRS.Siwaporn/Shutterstock; Stockbyte/Stockdisc/Getty Images; Stockbyte/Stockdisc/Getty Images; Robyn Mackenzie/123RF

- *Fruits and vegetables.* Researchers have identified nutrients in food components that may act against cancer. Some may prevent carcinogens from forming in the first place or block them from reaching or acting on target cells. Others boost enzymes that detoxify carcinogens and render them harmless. Some essential nutrients help reduce the harmful effects of carcinogens; for example, vitamin C, vitamin E, selenium, and the **carotenoids** (vitamin A precursors) may help block cancer by acting as antioxidants.

Many other anticancer agents in the diet fall under the broader heading of **phytochemicals,** which are substances in plants that help protect against chronic diseases. One of the first to be identified was sulforaphane, a potent anticarcinogen found in broccoli. Sulforaphane induces the cells of the liver and kidney to produce higher levels of protective enzymes, which then neutralize dietary carcinogens. Most fruits and vegetables contain beneficial phytochemicals, and researchers are just beginning to identify them. Some of the most promising are listed in Table 17.2.

TERMS

carotenoid   Any of a group of yellow-to-red plant pigments that can be converted to vitamin A by the liver; many act as antioxidants or have other anticancer effects. The carotenoids include beta-carotene, lutein, lycopene, and zeaxanthin.

phytochemical   A naturally occurring substance found in plant foods that may help prevent chronic diseases such as cancer and heart disease; *phyto* means "plant."

Inactivity and Obesity

The American Cancer Society recommends maintaining a healthy weight throughout life with a balanced diet and physical activity. Obesity in middle and later age has been shown to increase risk for many cancers, and evidence suggests that weight gain in early adulthood also puts us at risk—in women, particularly for endometrial and postmenopausal breast cancers, and in men, for colorectal cancer (Figure 17.6). A higher body mass index at age 25 also increases one's risk of cancer later in life.

Carcinogens in the Environment

Some carcinogens occur naturally in the environment, like viruses and the sun's UV rays. Others are manufactured or synthetic substances that show up occasionally in the general environment but more often in the work environments of specific industries. The ACS estimates that about 6% of cancer deaths stem from exposure to carcinogens in the environment—about 4% from occupational exposure and about 2% from exposure to naturally occurring or human-made pollutants in the larger environment.

Microbes   It is estimated that 15–20% of the world's cancers are caused by microbes, including viruses, bacteria, and parasites, although the percentage is much lower in industrialized countries like the United States. Certain types of human papillomavirus are known to cause oropharyngeal cancer, cervical cancer, and other cancers, and the *Helicobacter pylori* bacterium has been linked to stomach cancer.

Table 17.2	Foods with Phytochemicals	
FOOD	**PHYTOCHEMICAL**	**POTENTIAL ANTICANCER EFFECTS**
Chili peppers (*Note:* Hotter peppers contain more capsaicin.)	Capsaicin	Neutralizes the effect of nitrosamines; may block carcinogens in cigarette smoke from acting on cells
Oranges, lemons, limes, onions, apples, berries, eggplant	Flavonoids	Act as antioxidants; block access of carcinogens to cells; suppress malignant changes in cells; prevent cancer cells from multiplying
Citrus fruits, cherries	Monoterpenes	Help detoxify carcinogens; inhibit spread of cancer cells
Cruciferous vegetables (broccoli, cabbage, bok choy, cauliflower, kale, brussels sprouts, collards)	Isothiocyanates	Boost production of cancer-fighting enzymes; suppress tumor growth; block effects of estrogen on cell growth
Garlic, onions, leeks, shallots, chives	Allyl sulfides	Increase levels of enzymes that break down potential carcinogens; boost activity of cancer-fighting immune cells
Grapes, red wine, peanuts	Resveratrol	Acts as an antioxidant; suppresses tumor growth
Green, oolong, and black teas (*Note:* Drinking burning hot tea may *increase* cancer risk.)	Polyphenols	Increase antioxidant activity; prevent cancer cells from multiplying; help speed excretion of carcinogens from body
Orange, deep yellow, red, pink, and dark green vegetables; some fruits	Carotenoids	Act as antioxidants; reduce levels of cancer-promoting enzymes; inhibit spread of cancer cells
Whole grains, flax seeds, nuts	Phytoestrogens	Block effects of estrogen on cell growth; lower blood levels of estrogen
Whole grains, legumes	Phytic acid	Binds iron, which may prevent it from creating cell-damaging free radicals

The Epstein-Barr virus, best known for causing mononucleosis, is also suspected of contributing to Hodgkin lymphoma, cancer of the nasopharynx, and some stomach cancers. Human herpes virus 8 has been linked to Kaposi's sarcoma and certain types of lymphoma. Hepatitis viruses B and C cause as many as 80% of the world's liver cancers.

Ingested Chemicals The food industry uses preservatives and other additives to prevent food from spoiling or becoming stale (see Chapter 13). Some of these compounds are antioxidants that may decrease cancer-causing properties of the foods.

Other compounds, like the nitrates and nitrites found in processed meat, are potentially more dangerous. Nitrites inhibit the growth of bacteria, which could otherwise cause food poisoning. They also preserve the pink color of the meat, which has no bearing on taste or safety but looks more appetizing to many people. Although nitrates and nitrites are not themselves carcinogenic, they can combine with substances in the stomach and be converted to nitrosamines, which are highly potent carcinogens. Foods cured with nitrites, or by salt or smoke, have been linked to esophageal and stomach cancer, and they should be eaten sparingly.

Environmental and Industrial Pollution Pollutants in the air have long been suspected of contributing to the incidence of lung cancer. Fossil fuels and their combustion products, such as complex hydrocarbons, have been of special concern.

The best available data indicate that less than 2% of cancer deaths is caused by general environmental pollution, such as substances in our air and water. Exposure to carcinogenic materials in the workplace is a more serious problem. Occupational exposure to specific carcinogens may account for about 4% of cancer deaths. Radon, for example, is a highly radioactive element that rises into the atmosphere from the ground in some regions of the country. A colorless, odorless, tasteless gas, radon is a by-product of the breakdown of uranium and radium within the earth. Exposure to radon is known to cause lung cancer and is the second-leading cause of lung cancer in the United States, second only to tobacco use. The National Cancer Institute estimates that radon is responsible for about 15,000 to 22,000 lung cancer deaths

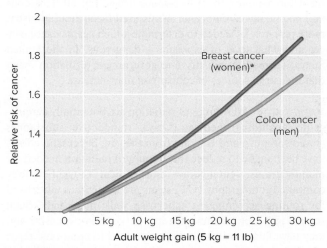

*Postmenopausal women not taking hormone replacement therapy.

FIGURE 17.6 **Adult weight gain and risk of cancer.** Gaining weight over time is a risk factor for several types of cancer, including cancers of the breast and colon. Preventing weight gain during adulthood is a key lifestyle cancer prevention strategy.

SOURCE: Keum, N., et al. 2015. Adult weight gain and adiposity-related cancers: A dose-response meta-analysis of prospective observational studies. *Journal of the National Cancer Institute* 107(2): djv088.

every year. Radon is present in many buildings and residences, especially in attics, basements, crawl spaces, and other underground areas, accumulating in such areas if they are not adequately ventilated. Radon poses a special threat to people who work underground, such as miners and construction workers who work in deep basements and tunnels.

Asbestos is another substance long known to cause cancer and other lung diseases. Asbestos was used for many years in home and building construction because of its fire-resistant properties. For decades, asbestos-containing insulation, tiles, and exterior sheathing were used in homes and commercial buildings. Asbestos was even used in special flame-retardant clothing for firefighters and factory workers. Asbestos use has been banned entirely in the European Union and is now highly restricted in the United States. When asbestos is uncovered in buildings, special abatement procedures must be taken to remove the material while protecting workers and surrounding areas. The human body is so sensitive to asbestos that inhaling even a few small asbestos fibers can result in lung damage, mesothelioma (a rare form of cancer caused almost exclusively by asbestos exposure), and lung cancer.

Carcinogens are encountered much more often in workplaces than in the home. Many chemicals, metals, and plastics used in industry are known or suspected carcinogens or cancer promoters. Ironically, many drugs used to treat cancer are known or suspected carcinogens, posing a risk of leukemia and other cancers to health care workers. Chemotherapy drugs can also cause skin rashes, infertility, miscarriage, and birth defects in people who work with or near these highly toxic substances without the appropriate personal protective equipment. The National Institute for Occupational Safety and Health publishes guidelines detailing proper procedures and equipment for handling these hazardous drugs. For all hazardous and potentially carcinogenic agents used throughout industry, more research is needed to determine which agents cause cancer and what level of exposure is dangerous. In the United States, decreasing industry and government regulation mean that industrial sources of cancer risk may increase.

Radiation All sources of radiation are potentially carcinogenic, including medical X-rays, radioactive substances (radioisotopes), and UV rays from the sun. Successful efforts have been made to reduce the amount of radiation needed for mammograms, dental X-rays, and medical X-rays. Full-body computed tomography (CT) scans are sometimes advertised for routine screening in otherwise well individuals. Such screening is not recommended; it is typically expensive and may have false positive findings that lead to additional tests, which may be unnecessary and invasive. Also, the radiation in these full-body X-rays may raise the risk of cancer; the radiation dose of one full-body CT scan is nearly 100 times that of a typical mammogram.

Sunlight is an important source of radiation, but because its rays penetrate only a millimeter or so into the skin, it could be considered a surface carcinogen. Most cases of skin cancer are highly curable, called basal cell carcinomas, but a

substantial minority are the potentially deadly malignant melanomas.

For a detailed discussion of environmental health—how the environment affects you and how you affect the environment—see Chapter 20.

DETECTING, DIAGNOSING, AND TREATING CANCER

Early cancer detection often depends on our willingness to be aware of changes in our own bodies and to make sure we keep up with recommended screening tests.

Detecting Cancer

Unlike signs of some diseases, early signs of cancer are usually not apparent to anyone but the person who has them. Even pain is not a reliable guide to early detection because initial stages of cancer are often painless. Self-monitoring is the first line of defense. By being aware of the risk factors in your own life, your immediate family's cancer history, and your own history, you may bring a problem to the attention of a physician long before it would have been detected at a routine physical.

In addition to self-monitoring, the ACS recommends routine cancer checkups, as well as specific screening tests for certain cancers (Table 17.3).

Diagnosing Cancer

Detecting a cancer by physical examination is only the beginning. Methods for determining the exact location, type, and extent of a cancer continue to improve. Knowledge of the exact location and size of a tumor is necessary for precise and effective surgery and/or radiation therapy. This is especially true in cases where the tumor may be hard to reach, as in the brain or viscera.

Imaging studies or exploratory surgery may help determine a cancer's stage. A biopsy may confirm the type of tumor. Several diagnostic imaging techniques have replaced exploratory surgery for some patients. Magnetic resonance imaging (MRI) uses a huge electromagnet to detect hidden tumors by mapping, on a computer screen, the vibrations of different atoms in the body. CT scanning uses X-rays to examine the brain and other parts of the body. The process allows

SITE/TESTS AND PROCEDURES	DESCRIPTION	LINKS FOR MORE INFORMATION
BREAST		
Mammography	Mammograms are the best way to find breast cancer early, when it is easier to treat. These imaging tests, which involve low-dose X-rays, are recommended every 1 to 2 years for women starting as early as age 40 and especially between 50 and 74, or as long as they are in good health.	CDC: www.cdc.gov/cancer/breast/basic_info/screening.htm NCI: www.cancer.gov/types/breast/mammograms-fact-sheet www.cancer.gov/types/breast/patient/breast-screening-pdq
Breast awareness	Routine examination of the breasts by health care providers or by women themselves starting in their 20s has not been shown to reduce deaths from breast cancer. However, any lump or other unusual change in the breast needs to be promptly reported to a doctor.	ACS: www.cancer.org/treatment/understandingyourdiagnosis /examsandtestdescriptions /mammogramsandotherbreastimagingprocedures/index
CERVIX		
Pap and HPV cytology tests	Pap tests can find abnormal cells in the cervix that may turn into cancer, and they can find cervical cancer early, when the chance of a cure is high. Testing every 3 to 5 years should begin at age 21 and end at age 65, if results have been normal. Women who have been vaccinated against HPV still need HPV tests.	CDC: www.cdc.gov/cancer/cervical/basic_info/screening.htm NCI: www.cancer.gov/types/cervical/pap-hpv-testing-fact-sheet www.cancer.gov/types/cervical/patient/cervical-screening-pdq
COLON		
Colonoscopy and sigmoidoscopy	A sigmoidoscopy every 5 years or a colonoscopy at least every 10 years between the ages of 45 and 75 can reduce the likelihood of death from colorectal cancer and can detect abnormal polyps that can be removed before they turn into cancer. The virtual colonoscopy has not been shown to reduce deaths from colorectal cancer.	CDC: https://www.cdc.gov/cancer/colorectal/pdf/QuickFacts -BRFSS-2016-CRC-Screening-508.pdf ACS: https://www.cancer.org/cancer/colon-rectal-cancer /detection-diagnosis-staging/acs-recommendations.html
High-sensitivity fecal occult blood test (FOBT)	This yearly multiple-stool, take-home test reduces death from colorectal cancer and is recommended for people between ages 50 and 75. If a positive result is found, the test is followed by a colonoscopy or sigmoidoscopy.	ACS: www.cancer.org/healthy/findcancerearly /examandtestdescriptions/faq-colonoscopy-and -sigmoidoscopy
LUNG		
Low-dose computed tomography (LDCT)	This imaging test has been shown to reduce lung cancer deaths among heavy smokers (30 pack-years*) between ages 55 and 74 who still smoke or have quit within the last 15 years.	CDC: www.cdc.gov/cancer/lung/basic_info/screening.htm NCI: www.cancer.gov/types/lung/patient/lung-screening-pdq
OVARY AND UTERUS		
CA-125 blood test, transvaginal ultrasound	There is no evidence that any screening test reduces deaths from ovarian cancer. However, these tests can help in diagnosing ovarian cancer. Women should report any unexpected bleeding or spotting to a doctor.	CDC: www.cdc.gov/cancer/ovarian/basic_info/screening.htm NCI: www.cancer.gov/types/ovarian/patient/ovarian-screening-pdq
PROSTATE		
Prostate-specific antigen (PSA)	Although this blood test, which is often done with a digital rectal exam, can detect prostate cancer at an early stage, it is more likely to lead to overdiagnosis and overtreatment than to reduce deaths from prostate cancer. Starting at age 50, men should talk to a doctor about the pros and cons of this test. African American men and men whose father or brother had prostate cancer before age 65 should talk to a doctor about this test starting at age 45.	CDC: www.cdc.gov/cancer/prostate/basic_info/screening.htm NCI: www.cancer.gov/types/prostate/psa-fact-sheet

*A pack-year is calculated by multiplying the number of packs of cigarettes smoked per day by the number of years the person has smoked. For example, smoking 2 packs per day for 10 years is equal to 20 pack-years; smoking one-half pack per day for 10 years is equal to 5 pack-years.

SOURCES: American Cancer Society (ACS). 2020. *Exams and Tests to Find and Diagnose Cancer* (http://www.cancer.org/healthy/findcancerearly /examandtestdescriptions/index); Centers for Disease Control and Prevention (CDC). 2020. *Cancer Prevention and Control: Cancer Screening Tests* (http:// www.cdc.gov/cancer/dcpc/prevention/screening.htm); National Cancer Institute (NCI). 2019. *Screening Tests* (http://www.cancer.gov/about-cancer/screening /screening-tests); American Cancer Society. 2020. *Cancer Facts and Figures, 2020*. Atlanta, GA: American Cancer Society (https://www.cancer.org/content /dam/cancer-org/research/cancer-facts-and-statistics/annual-cancer-facts-and-figures/2020/cancer-facts-and-figures-2020.pdf).

the construction of cross sections, which show a tumor's shape and location more accurately than possible with conventional X-rays.

Ultrasonography is also used to view tumors. It has several advantages: It can be used in the physician's office, it is less expensive than other imaging methods, and it does not expose the patient to radiation. Ultrasounds are commonly used to examine tumors of the breast and liver. Prostate ultrasound (a rectal probe using ultrasonic waves to produce an image of the prostate gland) is being investigated for its ability to detect small, hidden tumors that would be missed by a digital rectal exam.

Treating Cancer

The ideal cancer therapy would kill or remove all cancerous cells while leaving normal tissue untouched. This is possible, when superficial tumors of the skin are surgically removed. Usually the tumor is less accessible, and some combination of surgery, radiation therapy, and chemotherapy must be applied instead. Some patients choose to combine conventional therapies with alternative treatments (see the box "Choosing Cancer Treatments Wisely").

Surgery   For most cancers, surgery is a definitive treatment. Surgically removing all the cancerous cells from the body can result in a long-lasting cure. This is particularly true for early cancers of the breast, prostate, lung, and colon. When the cancer is more advanced or involves nearby lymph nodes, patients may require chemotherapy or radiation therapy in addition to surgery. Surgery is less effective when the tumor involves cells of the immune system, which are widely distributed throughout the body, or when the cancer has already metastasized.

Chemotherapy   **Chemotherapy,** or the use of medications to kill cancer cells, has been in use since the 1940s. Many of these drugs work by interfering with DNA synthesis and replication in rapidly dividing cells. Normal cells, which usually grow slowly, are not significantly destroyed by these drugs. However, some normal tissues such as intestinal, hair, and blood-forming cells are always growing, and damage to these tissues produces the unpleasant side effects of chemotherapy, including nausea, vomiting, diarrhea, and hair loss.

Chemotherapy can be used in a variety of settings, depending on the type of cancer and the timing of drug administration. When the goal of treatment is cure (that is, completely eradicating all cancer cells), chemotherapy is often given either before or after surgery. For example, in localized rectal cancer, studies have shown that chemotherapy

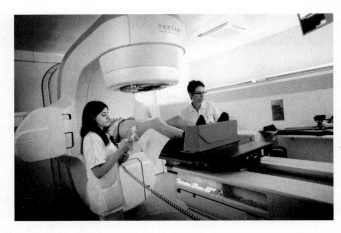

Radiation treatment for prostate cancer involves a machine that swings around the patient in a 360-degree fashion so that he gets beams of radiation from every direction. AMELIE-BENOIST/BSIP/Alamy Stock Photo

and radiation followed by surgery allows for a better cure rate and less toxicity than when surgery is done before chemotherapy and radiation. By contrast, most patients with localized breast cancers will have surgery first to remove their tumors and then will undergo chemotherapy in the hope of destroying any remaining cells, thereby reducing the chances that the cancer will recur. Patients with cancers that are not thought to be curable (that is, not all cancer cells can be destroyed) can still benefit from chemotherapy. This is often referred to as *palliative chemotherapy.*

Radiation   Radiation therapy uses a beam of X-rays or gamma rays directed at the tumor to kill tumor cells. With sophisticated techniques, the harmful rays are directed precisely at cancerous cells, in order to minimize damage to surrounding normal cells. Occasionally, when an organ is small enough, such as the prostate gland, radioactive seeds are surgically placed inside the cancerous organ to destroy the tumor. Radiation therapy can be performed on an outpatient basis.

COMMON TYPES OF CANCER

Because each cancer begins as a single, altered cell with a specific function in the body, the cancer retains some properties of the normal cell for a period of time. For instance, cancer of the thyroid gland may produce too much thyroid hormone and cause hyperthyroidism as well as cancer. Usually, however, cancer cells lose their resemblance to normal tissue as they continue to multiply, becoming groups of rogue cells with increasingly unpredictable behavior.

Cancers are classified according to the types of cells that give rise to them:

chemotherapy   The treatment of cancer with chemicals that selectively destroy cancerous cells.

TERMS

Sometimes conventional treatments for cancer are simply not enough. A patient may be told that conventional therapy can do little beyond easing pain. When therapy is available, it may be painful and even intolerable to some people. Not surprisingly, many cancer patients look for complementary and alternative therapies. As many as 80% of cancer patients report combining conventional treatments with some type of mind–body technique. A much smaller number of patients look for alternatives to the more conventional therapies. Such therapies may be within the bounds of legitimate medical practice but have not yet proven themselves in clinical trials. Or, at the extreme, alternative therapies may be scientifically unsound and dangerous, as well as expensive.

Complementary therapies such as yoga, massage, meditation, music therapy, tai chi, and prayer can have positive physical and psychological benefits for patients and help them improve their quality of life as they deal with illness and the often difficult treatments for cancer. Mind–body practices can reduce pain and anxiety, improve sleep, and give people a sense of control and participation in their treatment; such practices may also enhance the immune system. (See Chapter 2 for more about stress and relaxation techniques.) Mind–body practices typically can be used in combination with conventional cancer therapies.

For other types of therapies, the National Cancer Institute suggests that patients and their families consider the following questions when making decisions about cancer treatment:

- **Has the treatment been evaluated in clinical trials?** Advances in cancer treatment are made through carefully monitored clinical trials. If a patient wants to try a new therapy, participation in a clinical trial may be a treatment option.

- **Do the practitioners of an approach claim that the medical community is trying to keep their cure from the public?** No one genuinely committed to finding better ways to treat a disease would knowingly keep an effective treatment secret.

- **Does the treatment rely on nutritional or diet therapy as its main focus?** Although diet can be a key risk factor in the development of cancer, there is no evidence that diet alone can rid the body of cancer.

- **Do those who endorse the treatment claim that it is harmless and painless and that it produces no unpleasant side effects?** Reputable researchers are working to develop less toxic cancer therapies, but because effective treatments for cancer must be powerful, they frequently have unpleasant side effects.

- **Does the treatment have a secret formula that only a small group of practitioners can use?** Scientists who believe they have developed an effective treatment routinely publish their results in reputable journals so that they can be evaluated by other researchers.

Use special caution when evaluating cancer remedies promoted online. A recent study found that as many as one-third of cancer-related alternative medicine sites offered advice that was harmful or potentially dangerous.

One danger of alternative medicine is the very real possibility that a patient will neglect proven therapies while pursuing unproven, faddish alternatives; if alternative therapies delay proven therapies, lives may be lost. Another danger is that complementary therapies may affect conventional therapies. For example, some herbal supplements affect how cancer drugs are absorbed and used by the body. A recent study revealed that 70% of patients using complementary therapies do not inform their physicians. However, physicians must have this information so that they can address potential side effects or harmful interactions.

SOURCE: American Cancer Society. 2017. *Complementary and Alternative Therapies for Cancer Management* (https://www.cancer.org/treatment/treatments-and-side-effects/complementary-and-alternative-medicine/complementary-and-alternative-methods-and-cancer.html); National Cancer Institute. 2019. *Complementary and Alternative Medicine* (http://www.cancer.gov/cancertopics/cam).

- **Carcinomas** arise from *epithelia*—tissues that cover external body surfaces, line internal tubes and cavities, and form the secreting portion of glands. This type of cancer is the most common. Major sites include the skin, breast, uterus, prostate, lungs, and gastrointestinal tract.

- **Sarcomas** arise from connective and fibrous tissues such as muscle, bone, cartilage, and the membranes covering muscles and fat.

- **Lymphomas** are cancers of the lymph nodes, part of the body's infection-fighting system.

- **Leukemias** are cancers of the blood-forming cells, which reside chiefly in the bone marrow.

Cancers vary greatly in how easily they can be detected and how well they respond to treatment. For example, certain types of skin cancer are easily detected, grow slowly, and are easy to remove; virtually all of these cancers are cured. Cancer of the pancreas, by contrast, is difficult to detect or treat, and few patients survive the disease. In general,

carcinoma Cancer that originates in epithelial tissue (skin, glands, and lining of internal organs).

sarcoma Cancer arising from bone, cartilage, or striated muscle.

lymphoma A tumor originating from lymphatic tissue.

leukemia Cancer of the blood or the blood-forming cells.

TERMS

it is difficult for an **oncologist** or **hematologist** to predict how a specific cancer will behave because each one arises from a unique set of changes in a single cell.

In the sections that follow, we look more closely at the most common cancers and their causes, as well as how they are detected and treated.

Lung Cancer

Lung cancer accounts for about 14% of all new cancer diagnoses and is the most common cause of cancer death in the United States: It is responsible for about 136,000 deaths each year. Since 1987, lung cancer has surpassed breast cancer as the leading cause of cancer death in women.

Risk Factors The chief risk factor for lung cancer is tobacco smoke, which currently accounts for 32% of all cancer deaths and 80% of lung cancer deaths. When smoking is combined with exposure to other carcinogens, such as asbestos particles or certain pollutants, the risk of cancer can be multiplied by a factor of 10 or more.

The smoker is not the only one at risk. Environmental tobacco smoke (ETS) is a human carcinogen.

Detection and Treatment Lung cancer is difficult to detect at an early stage and hard to cure even when detected early. Symptoms of lung cancer do not usually appear until the disease has advanced to the invasive stage. Signs and symptoms such as a persistent cough, chest pain, or recurring bronchitis may be the first indication of a tumor's presence.

Studies have shown that spiral CT scans, a computer-assisted body imaging technique, can detect lung cancer in high-risk patients significantly earlier than chest X-rays. Screening with a CT scan is recommended in patients aged 55–74 years with a heavy smoking history.

Besides CT scanning, a diagnosis can usually be made by chest X-ray or by studying the cells in sputum. Because almost all lung cancers arise from the cells that line the bronchi, tumors can sometimes be visualized by fiber-optic bronchoscopy, a test in which a flexible lighted tube is inserted into the windpipe and the surfaces of the lung passages are inspected directly.

Treatment for lung cancer depends on the type and stage of the cancer. If caught early, localized cancers can be treated

with surgery alone. The majority of patients are diagnosed with advanced disease, however, and radiation and chemotherapy are often used in addition to surgery. Of patients with localized disease, 57% are alive five years after diagnosis. However, only about 16% of lung cancers are diagnosed at an early stage. The five-year survival rate for all stages combined is only 19%. In the past decade progress has occurred through identifying the key mutations that lead to lung cancer and using drugs to specifically target these cells. These targetable mutations have been identified in over 15% of patients, which has led to their greatly improved outcomes. Additional areas of research include phototherapy, gene therapy, and immunotherapy (vaccines).

Colon and Rectal Cancer

Another common cancer in the United States is colon and rectal cancer (also called *colorectal cancer*). Although effective screening methods exist, it is the fourth most common type of cancer, killing an estimated 53,000 Americans in 2020.

Risk Factors Age is a key risk factor for colon and rectal cancer; the vast majority of cases are diagnosed in people aged 45 and over. Heredity also plays a role. Many cancers arise from preexisting **polyps,** which are small growths on the wall of the colon that may gradually develop into malignancies. The tendency to form colon polyps appears to be determined by specific genes, so many colon cancers may be due to inherited gene mutations. Chronic bowel inflammation and type 2 diabetes increase the risk of colon cancer.

Lifestyle is also a risk factor for colon and rectal cancer. Excessive alcohol use and smoking may increase the risk of colorectal cancer. The World Health Organization has confirmed that processed meats (e.g., hot dogs, sausages, ham, jerky, corned beef, and smoked and canned meats) are carcinogenic and increase the risk of colorectal cancer. Consumption of red meat may also increase an individual's risk. Regular physical activity appears to reduce a person's risk, whereas obesity increases risk. A diet rich in fruits, vegetables, and whole grains is associated with lower risk. However, research findings on whether dietary fiber prevents colon cancer have been mixed. Studies have suggested a protective role for folic acid, magnesium, vitamin D, and calcium; in contrast, high intake of refined carbohydrates, simple sugars, and smoked meats and fish may increase risk.

Regular use of nonsteroidal anti-inflammatory drugs such as aspirin and ibuprofen may decrease the risk of colon cancer and other cancers of the digestive tract.

Detection and Treatment   If identified early, precancerous polyps and early-stage cancers can be removed before they become malignant or spread. Because polyps may bleed as they progress, common warning signs of colon cancer are bleeding from the rectum and a change in bowel habits.

Regular screening tests are recommended beginning at age 45 (earlier for people with a family history of the disease or who are otherwise at high risk). A yearly stool blood test can detect small amounts of blood in the stool long before obvious bleeding would be noticed. More involved screening tests are recommended at 5- or 10-year intervals. These tests include a sigmoidoscopy or colonoscopy (Figure 17.7), during which a flexible fiber-optic device is inserted through the rectum and the colon is examined and polyps biopsied or removed. Screening is effective, and studies demonstrate that it can prevent up to 76–90% of colon cancers. Still, only about half of U.S. adults have undergone any of these tests.

Surgery is the primary treatment for colon and rectal cancer. Radiation and chemotherapy may be used before surgery to shrink a tumor or after surgery to destroy any remaining cancerous cells. For advanced cancer, treatment with chemotherapy or monoclonal antibodies (discussed later in the chapter) is an option. This treatment inhibits the growth of new blood vessels (angiogenesis) in tumors. The five-year survival rate is 90% for colon and rectal cancers detected early and 64% overall.

Breast Cancer

Breast cancer is the most common cancer in women. In men, breast cancer occurs rarely. In the United States, about one woman in eight will develop breast cancer during her lifetime. In 2020, 276,480 new breast cancer diagnoses were expected in the United States, and about 42,700 were expected to die from it.

Fewer than 2% of breast cancer cases occur in women under age 35, but incidence rates increase quickly with age. About 50% of cases are diagnosed in women aged 45–65. Rates decrease slightly for women in their 70s and 80s, although this decrease could reflect a decrease in screening for this age population.

Risk Factors   Genetics plays a very important role in breast cancer. A woman who has two close relatives with breast cancer is about three times more likely to develop the disease than a woman who has no close relatives with it. Even though genetic factors are important, inherited mutations in breast cancer susceptibility genes account for only approximately 5–10% of all breast cancer cases.

Other risk factors include early onset of menstruation, late onset of menopause, having no children or having a first child after age 30, current use of hormone replacement therapy, obesity, and alcohol use. Estrogen exposure can increase the risk for breast and uterine cancer. Estrogen circulates in a woman's body in high concentrations between puberty and menopause. Fat cells also produce estrogen, and estrogen levels are higher in obese women. Alcohol can interfere with estrogen metabolism in the liver and increase estrogen levels in the blood. A dramatic drop in rates of breast cancer from 2001 to 2004 was attributed in part to reduced use of hormone replacement therapy by women over age 50. Millions of women stopped taking the hormones after research from the Women's Health Initiative linked hormone replacement therapy with an increased risk of breast cancer and heart disease.

Although some of the risk factors for breast cancer cannot be changed, important lifestyle risk factors can be controlled. Eating a low-fat, vegetable-rich diet, exercising regularly, limiting alcohol intake, and maintaining a healthy body weight can minimize the chance of developing breast cancer, even for women at risk from family history or other factors. Despite some popular myths, studies have shown that breast

QUICK STATS

86% of diagnosed cancers occur in people aged 50 and over.
—American Cancer Society, 2016

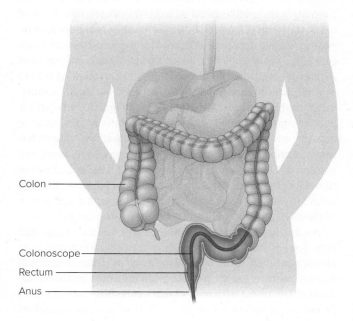

Colon

Colonoscope

Rectum

Anus

FIGURE 17.7   Colonoscopy.

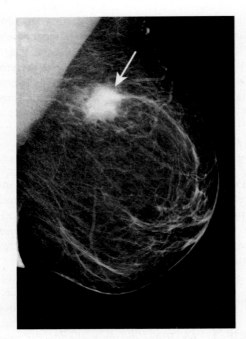

FIGURE 17.8   Mammogram image depicting a breast cancer tumor. ksass/E+/Getty Images

cancer incidence is not increased by underwire bras, antiperspirants, breast implants, or abortions.

Early Detection   A cure is most likely if breast cancer is detected early, so regular screening is a good investment, even for younger women. The ACS recommends the following for the early detection of breast cancer:

• *Mammography.* A **mammogram** is a low-dose breast X-ray that can identify about 80–90% of breast cancers at an early stage, before physical symptoms develop (Figure 17.8). The ACS recommends that women at average risk for breast cancer begin annual mammograms at age 40; between age 45 and 54, women should have mammograms every year. Women over the age of 55 may choose to have mammograms every year or two. Some controversy surrounds the best age to start mammographic screening. Some groups have argued that the rates of false-positive mammograms are higher between ages 40 and 50; thus, the U.S. Preventive Services Task Force, for example, advises that women should wait until age 50 to begin routine screening.

• *Breast awareness.* The ACS no longer recommends breast self-exams (BSEs) or clinical breast exams, but many

---

mammogram   A low-dose X-ray of the breasts used to check for early signs of breast cancer.

ultrasonography   An imaging method in which sound waves are bounced off body structures to create an image on a TV monitor; also called *ultrasound*.

monoclonal antibody   An antibody designed to bind to a specific cancer-related target.

TERMS

---

doctors still do, and a woman should be familiar with her breasts and alert her health care provider to any changes right away. The following are warning signs of breast cancer but can also be caused by other conditions (most breast lumps and changes are benign but should be checked by a health care provider):

A new lump in the breast or underarm

Thickening or swelling of part of the breast

Irritation or dimpling of breast skin

Redness or flaky skin in the nipple area or the breast

Pulling in of the nipple or pain in the nipple area

Nipple discharge other than breast milk, including blood

Any change in the size or the shape of the breast

Pain in any area of the breast

Women who choose to perform BSE should review the recommended technique with their health care provider.

Additional screenings may be recommended for women at increased risk for breast cancer. Studies show that MRI may be better than mammography at detecting breast abnormalities in some women. The ACS recommends both an annual mammogram and an annual MRI for women who are at high risk for breast cancer, such as those who carry a *BRCA* mutation. **Ultrasonography** (use of sound waves to create images of soft tissue) is not a standard screening tool for breast cancer, but it is often used as a follow-up test if a mammogram reveals an abnormality in breast tissue. A number of factors determine a woman's risk for developing breast cancer, and every woman should discuss her risk factors with a physician to determine what kinds of screening tests are warranted and how frequently screening is recommended.

Treatment   If a lump is detected, it may be scanned by ultrasonography and biopsied to see if it is cancerous. In most cases, the lump is found to be a cyst or other harmless growth, and no further treatment is needed. If the lump contains cancer cells, a variety of surgeries may be indicated, ranging from a lumpectomy (removal of the lump and surrounding tissue) to a mastectomy (removal of the breast). For small tumors, many studies have demonstrated that long-term survival for lumpectomy combined with radiation therapy is similar to that for mastectomy. To determine whether the cancer has spread, lymph nodes from the underarm may be removed and examined. Depending on the stage of the cancer and tumor characteristics, additional therapy—such as hormone therapy, antibody therapy, radiation, chemotherapy, or a combination of these—may be recommended before or after surgery.

Analyzing the tumor specimen with special stains can help predict the risk of breast cancer recurrence and help identify women who will benefit most from additional therapy; women can then make more informed treatment decisions. Treatment with **monoclonal antibodies,** such as trastuzumab, is an option for about 15–20% of patients diagnosed with breast cancer. Antibodies, discussed in Chapter 18, are proteins produced by the immune system that recognize and bind to foreign substances such as bacteria. A monoclonal antibody is a special type of antibody that is produced in a laboratory and designed to bind to a specific cancer-related target. Many other monoclonal antibodies are currently in development for breast cancer treatment.

Survival of breast cancer varies, depending on the nature of the tumor and whether it has metastasized. If the tumor is discovered before it has spread to the adjacent lymph nodes or outside the breast, the patient has a 99% chance of surviving more than five years. The relative survival rate for all stages is 90% at five years.

Strategies for Prevention A number of drugs have been proposed for the prevention of breast cancer, especially in high-risk patients. A family of drugs called *selective estrogen receptor modulators* (*SERMs*) acts like estrogen in some tissues of the body but blocks estrogen's effects in others. One SERM, tamoxifen, has long been used in breast cancer treatment because it blocks the action of estrogen in breast tissue. In 1998, the U.S. Food and Drug Administration (FDA) approved the use of tamoxifen to reduce the risk of breast cancer in healthy women who are at high risk for the disease. However, the drug has serious potential side effects, including increased risk of blood clots and uterine cancer. Another SERM, raloxifene, was approved in 2007 for the reduction of invasive breast cancer risk in postmenopausal women at high risk for breast cancer. Compared to tamoxifen, raloxifene has been shown to pose a slightly lower risk of blood clots and uterine cancer, but the risk is still higher than that of a placebo. Raloxifene has also been shown to improve bone mineral density.

Prostate Cancer

The prostate gland is located at the base of the bladder in men and completely surrounds the male's urethra; if enlarged, it can block the flow of urine. Prostate cancer is the most common cancer in men and the second leading cause of cancer death in men. In the United States in 2020, nearly 192,000 new cases and more than 33,000 deaths were estimated.

Risk Factors Age is the strongest predictor of risk, with approximately 60% of cases of prostate cancer diagnosed in men over age 65. Inherited genetic predisposition may be responsible for 5–10% of cases, and men with a family history of the disease should be particularly vigilant about screening. African American men and Jamaican men of African descent have the highest rates of prostate cancer of any groups in the world. Both genetic and lifestyle factors may be involved.

Diets that are high in calories, dairy products, and animal fats and also low in plant foods have been implicated as possible culprits, as have obesity, inactivity, and a history of sexually transmitted diseases. Type 2 diabetes and insulin resistance are also associated with prostate cancer. Soy foods, tomatoes, and cruciferous vegetables are being investigated for their possible protective effects.

Detection Early prostate cancer usually has no symptoms. Warning signs of prostate cancer can include changes in urinary frequency, weak or interrupted urine flow, painful urination, and blood in the urine.

Techniques for early detection include a digital rectal examination and the **prostate-specific antigen (PSA) test.** The PSA screening test has been controversial because of too many false-positive results, especially in men over age 75. In older men, most prostate cancers are not deadly, making treatment pointless and potentially harmful. The test may detect an elevated level or a rapid increase in PSA, which can indicate early prostate cancer, but it also can be associated with benign conditions (more than half of men over age 50 have benign prostate disease) and very slow-growing cancers that are unlikely to kill affected individuals. The ACS recommends that men be provided information about the benefits and limitations of the tests and that both the exam and the PSA test be offered annually, beginning at age 50, for men who are at average risk of prostate cancer, do not have any major medical problems, and have a life expectancy of at least 10 years. Men at high risk, including African Americans and those with a family history of the disease, should consider beginning screening at age 45. Men with multiple family members who have been diagnosed with the disease should consider beginning screening at age 40.

A digital rectal exam (DRE) is less effective than a PSA test but may find cancer in men with normal PSA levels. During a DRE, a physician inserts a finger into the rectum to feel the prostate gland and determine if the gland is enlarged or if lumps are present.

Treatment Treatments vary based on the stage of the cancer and the patient's age. A small, slow-growing tumor in an older man may be treated with watchful waiting and no initial therapy because he is more likely to die from another cause before his cancer becomes life-threatening. More aggressive treatment would be indicated for younger men or those with more advanced cancers. Treatment may involve *radical prostatectomy* (surgical removal of the prostate). Although this has an excellent cure rate, it is major surgery and often results in **incontinence** or erectile dysfunction. Minimally invasive surgery, which utilizes a laparoscopic or robotic approach, can sometimes be performed with fewer complications and quicker recovery.

A less invasive alternative involves surgical implantation of radioactive seeds. Radiation from the seeds destroys the tumor and much of the normal prostate tissue but leaves surrounding tissue relatively untouched. Alternative or additional treatments include external radiation, hormonal therapy, cryotherapy, and chemotherapy. Several new treatments for

TERMS

prostate-specific antigen (PSA) test A screening test for prostate cancer that measures blood levels of prostate-specific antigen (PSA).

incontinence The inability to control the flow of urine.

advanced prostate cancer have recently been approved by the FDA. A cancer vaccine, known as sipuleucel-T, was approved for some men with hormone-refractory advanced prostate cancer. Drugs recently approved for the treatment of metastatic prostate cancer that is resistant to hormonal therapy and chemotherapy include abiraterone and enzalutamide.

Survival rates for all stages of this cancer have improved steadily since 1940; the five-year survival rate is nearly 100%.

Cancers of the Female Reproductive Tract

Several types of cancer can affect the female reproductive tract, and a few of these cancers are relatively common.

Cervical Cancer Cancer of the cervix can occur in women in their twenties and thirties. In the United States, approximately 13,000 women are diagnosed with cervical cancer each year, and the disease kills more than 4000 women annually.

Cervical cancer is largely a sexually transmitted infection or disease. Virtually all cases of cervical cancer stem from infection by the human papillomavirus (HPV), a group of about 100 related viruses that also cause common warts and genital warts. When certain types of HPV are introduced into the cervix, usually by an infected sex partner, the virus infects cervical cells, causing them to divide and grow. If unchecked, this growth can develop into cervical cancer. Cervical cancer is associated with multiple sex partners and is extremely rare in women who have not had heterosexual intercourse. Smoking, immunosuppression, and prolonged use of oral contraceptives also have been associated with increased risk.

Screening for the changes in cervical cells that precede cancer is done chiefly by means of the **Pap test.** During a pelvic exam, loose cells are scraped from the cervix and examined under a microscope to see whether they are normal. If cells are abnormal but not yet cancerous, the patient has a condition commonly referred to as *cervical dysplasia.* Sometimes such abnormal cells spontaneously return to normal, but in about one-third of cases the cellular changes progress toward malignancy. If this happens, the abnormal cells must be removed, either surgically or with a cryoscopic (ultra-cold) probe or localized laser treatment. When abnormal cells are in a precancerous state, the small patch of dangerous cells can be removed completely.

Without timely surgery, the malignant cells invade the cervical wall and spread to the uterus and adjacent lymph nodes. At this stage, chemotherapy and radiation may be used to kill the cancer cells, but chances for a complete cure are reduced. Even when a cure can be achieved, it often requires surgical removal of the uterus.

Because the Pap test is highly effective, all women between ages 21 and 65 should be tested. The recommended schedule for testing depends on risk factors, the type of Pap test performed, and whether the Pap test is combined with HPV testing.

Three HPV vaccines have been approved by the FDA for the prevention of cervical cancer. According to a 2018 study, following the introduction of the HPV vaccine in 2006, the rates of invasive cervical cancer dropped by 29% in younger women. Women who receive one of the vaccines should continue to receive routine Pap tests because the vaccines do not protect against all types of the virus.

Uterine, or Endometrial, Cancer Cancer of the lining of the uterus (the *endometrium*) most often occurs after the age of 55. Uterine cancer strikes approximately 65,000 American women annually and kills about 12,000 women each year.

The risk factors are similar to those for breast cancer, including prolonged exposure to estrogen, early onset of menstruation, late menopause, never having been pregnant, and obesity. Type 2 diabetes is also associated with increased risk. The use of oral contraceptives or hormone therapies that contain estrogen plus progestin does not appear to increase risk.

Endometrial cancer often presents with abnormal vaginal bleeding in a postmenopausal woman. It is treated surgically, commonly by *hysterectomy,* or removal of the uterus. Radiation treatment, hormones, and chemotherapy may be used in addition to surgery. The 5-year relative survival rate for uterine cancer is 84% for white women and 62% for black women, partly because white women are more likely to be diagnosed with early-stage disease; however, survival is substantially lower for black women for every stage of diagnosis.

Ovarian Cancer Although ovarian cancer is rare compared with cervical or uterine cancer, it causes more deaths than the other two combined. In 2020, an estimated 21,750 new cases of ovarian cancer will be diagnosed in the United States and 13,940 women will die from it. There are often no warning signs of ovarian cancer. Early symptoms may include increased abdominal size and bloating, urinary urgency, and pelvic pain. It cannot be detected by Pap tests or any other simple screening method and is often diagnosed late in its development, when surgery and other therapies are unlikely to be successful.

The risk factors are similar to those for breast and endometrial cancers: increasing age (most ovarian cancer occurs after age 60), never having been pregnant, a family history of breast or ovarian cancer, obesity, and specific genetic mutations including *BRCA1* and *BRCA2.* A high number of ovulations appears to increase the chance that a cancer-causing genetic mutation will occur, so anything that lowers the number of lifetime ovulation cycles—pregnancy, breastfeeding, or use of oral contraceptives—reduces a woman's risk of ovarian cancer.

There is currently no accurate screening test to detect ovarian cancer. Women with symptoms or who are at high risk because of family history or because they harbor a mutant gene may be offered screening with a pelvic exam, ultrasound, and blood test. The latter test can be used to search for the tumor marker CA125. The use of these tests remains controversial because no data have demonstrated an improvement in mortality when these tests are used for screening.

Pap test A scraping of cells from the cervix for examination under a microscope to detect cancer. TERMS

Your risk of skin cancer from the ultraviolet radiation in sunlight depends on several factors. Take this quiz to see how sensitive you are. The higher your UV risk score, the greater your risk of skin cancer—and the greater your need to take precautions against too much sun.

Score 1 point for each true statement:

_____ 1. I have had skin cancer before.

_____ 2. I have a family history of skin cancer.

_____ 3. I have a lot of moles.

_____ 4. I have fair skin and burn before tanning.

_____ 5. I have blue, green, or gray eyes.

_____ 6. I have blond, red, or light brown hair.

_____ 7. I live or vacation at high altitudes.

_____ 8. I live or vacation in tropical or subtropical climates.

_____ 9. I work indoors all week but spend a lot of time in the sun on weekends.

_____ 10. I spend a lot of time outdoors.

_____ 11. I am currently taking medication that makes my skin more sensitive to sunlight.

_____ 12. I sometimes go to a tanning parlor or use a sunlamp.

Total Score: _____

Score	Risk of Skin Cancer from UV Radiation
0	Low
1–3	Moderate
4–7	High
8–12	Very high

For a detailed assessment of your skin type and how your skin behaves in response to sun exposure, complete the Skin Cancer Foundation's skin type assessment (http://www.skincancer.org/prevention/are-you-at-risk/fitzpatrick-skin-quiz).

SOURCES: Adapted from Centers for Disease Control and Prevention; American Cancer Society, 2015.

Ovarian cancer is treated by surgical removal of both ovaries, the fallopian tubes, and the uterus. Radiation and chemotherapy are sometimes used in addition to surgery. When the tumor is localized to the ovary, the five-year survival rate is more than 90%. However, it is diagnosed this early only 15% of the time. For all stages, the five-year survival rate is only 47%.

Skin Cancer

Skin cancer is the most common type of cancer, but it is often not included in cancer incidence and mortality statistics because many types of skin cancer are easily curable. Of the approximate 3.5 million cases of skin cancer diagnosed each year, about 1% are of the most serious type, **melanoma.**

Risk Factors Almost all cases of skin cancer can be traced to excessive exposure to **ultraviolet (UV) radiation** from the sun, including longer-wavelength ultraviolet A (UVA) and shorter-wavelength ultraviolet B (UVB) radiation. UVB radiation causes sunburns and can damage eyes and the immune system. UVA is less likely to cause an immediate sunburn, but it damages connective tissue and leads to premature aging of the skin, giving it a wrinkled, leathery appearance. (Tanning lamps and tanning salon beds emit mostly UVA radiation.) Both UVA and UVB radiation have been linked to the development of skin cancer, and the National Toxicology Program has declared both solar and artificial sources of UV radiation, including sunlamps and tanning beds, to be known human carcinogens.

Both severe, acute sun reactions (sunburns) and chronic low-level sun reactions (suntans) can lead to skin cancer. People with fair skin have less natural protection against skin damage from the sun and a higher risk of developing skin cancer, whereas people with naturally dark skin have a considerable degree of protection (see the box "What's Your UV Risk?"). Lighter-skinned people are about 10 times more likely to develop melanoma, but darker-skinned people are still at risk. Before age 40, incidence rates are higher in women than in men. After age 40, rates are nearly twice as high in men as in women.

Severe sunburns in childhood have been linked to a significantly increased risk of skin cancer in later life, so children in particular should be protected. According to the Skin Cancer Foundation, the risk of skin cancer doubles in people who have had five or more sunburns in their lifetime. Because of damage to the ozone layer of the atmosphere (discussed in Chapter 20), there is a chance that we may all be exposed to increased UV radiation in the future. Melanoma rates have been rising for the past 30 years.

Other risk factors for skin cancer include having many moles (particularly large ones), spending time at high altitudes

> **melanoma** A malignant tumor of the skin that arises from pigmented cells, usually a mole. **TERMS**
>
> **ultraviolet (UV) radiation** Light rays of a specific wavelength emitted by the sun; most UV rays are blocked by the ozone layer in the upper atmosphere.

(fewer layers of atmosphere filter UV radiation), and a family history of the disease. Skin cancer may also be caused by exposure to coal tar, pitch, creosote, arsenic, and radioactive materials. Compared to sunlight, however, these agents account for only a small proportion of skin cancers.

Types of Skin Cancer   There are three main types of skin cancer, named for the types of skin cells from which they develop. **Basal cell carcinoma** and **squamous cell carcinoma** together account for about 95% of the skin cancers diagnosed each year. They are usually found in chronically sun-exposed areas, such as the face, neck, hands, and arms. They usually appear as pale, waxlike, pearly nodules or red, scaly, sharply outlined patches. These cancers are often painless, although they may bleed, crust, and form an open sore on the skin.

Melanoma is by far the most dangerous skin cancer because it spreads so rapidly. It can occur anywhere on the body, but the most common sites are the back, chest, abdomen, and lower legs. A melanoma usually appears at the site of a preexisting mole. The mole may begin to enlarge, become mottled or varied in color (colors can include blue, pink, and white), or develop an irregular surface or irregular borders. Tissue invaded by melanoma may also itch, burn, or bleed easily.

Prevention   One major step you can take to protect yourself against all forms of skin cancer is to avoid lifelong overexposure to sunlight. Blistering, peeling sunburns from unprotected sun exposure are particularly dangerous, but suntans—whether from sunlight or from tanning lamps—also increase your risk of developing skin cancer later in life. People of every age, especially babies and children, need to be protected from the sun with **sunscreens** and protective clothing. For a closer look at sunlight and skin cancer, see the box "Sunscreens and Sun-Protective Clothing."

Detection and Treatment   The only sure way to avoid a serious outcome from skin cancer is to make sure it is recognized and diagnosed early. The majority of melanomas are brought to a physician's attention by patients themselves. Make it a habit to examine your skin regularly. Most spots, freckles, moles, and blemishes on your body are normal; you were born with some of them, and others appear and disappear throughout your life. But if you notice an unusual growth, discoloration, sore that does not heal, or mole that undergoes a sudden or progressive change, see your physician or dermatologist immediately.

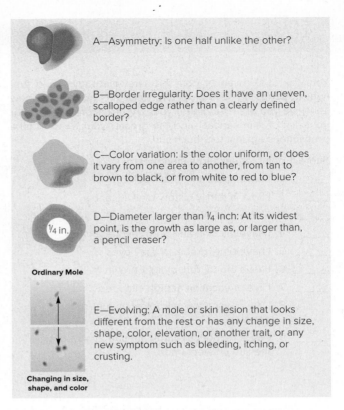

FIGURE 17.9   **The ABCDE test for melanoma.** To see a variety of photos of melanoma and benign moles, visit the National Cancer Institute's Visuals Online site (http://visualsonline.cancer.gov).

Figure 17.9 illustrates the characteristics of a possible melanoma—asymmetry; border irregularity; color variations; a diameter greater than ¼ inch; and changes in the size, shape, or color of the mole. If someone in your family has had multiple skin cancers or melanomas, consult a dermatologist for a complete skin examination and discussion of your particular risk. Don't depend on a smartphone application promoted for the detection of melanoma; initial studies of such apps have not found them to be consistently accurate.

If you have an unusual skin lesion, your physician will examine it and possibly perform a biopsy. If the lesion is cancerous, it is usually removed surgically, a procedure that can almost always be performed in the physician's office using a local anesthetic. Other forms of treatment may also be used.

If cancer has spread from the skin to the lymph nodes or internal organs, local surgical treatment is inadequate. Since 2011, the FDA has approved several new therapies for metastatic melanoma. For example, ipilimumab is a monoclonal antibody that activates the body's anticancer immune response and was approved for patients with previously untreated metastatic melanoma. Since then, other immune therapies have also proven to be beneficial. These newer therapies have revolutionized the treatment of melanoma. For melanoma, the five-year survival rate is 99% if the tumor is localized but only 63% if the cancer has spread to adjacent lymph nodes. Improvements in survival are anticipated with the use of these new immune-based treatments.

---

basal cell carcinoma   Usually benign skin cancer of the base of the outermost layer of the skin.

squamous cell carcinoma   Malignant cancer of the surface of the outermost layer of the skin.

sunscreen   A substance used to protect the skin from UV rays; usually applied as a lotion, cream, or spray.

TERMS

CRITICAL CONSUMER
Sunscreens and Sun-Protective Clothing

With consistent use of proper clothing, sunscreens, and common sense, you can lead an active outdoor life *and* protect your skin against most sun-induced damage.

Clothing

• Wear long-sleeved shirts and long pants. Dark-colored, tightly woven fabrics provide reasonable protection from the sun. Another good choice is clothing made from special sun-protective fabrics; these garments have an ultraviolet protection factor (UPF) rating, similar to the sun protection factor (SPF) rating for sunscreens.

• Wear a hat. A good choice is a broad-brimmed hat or a legionnaire-style cap that covers the ears and neck. Wear sunscreen on your face even if you are wearing a hat.

• Wear sunglasses. Exposure to UV rays can damage the eyes and cause cataracts.

Sunscreen

• Use a sunscreen and lip balm with an SPF of 15 or higher. An SPF rating refers to the amount of time you can stay out in the sun before you burn, compared with not using sunscreen. For example, a product with an SPF of 30 would allow you to remain in the sun without burning 30 times longer, on average, than if you didn't apply sunscreen. If you're fair-skinned, have a family history of skin cancer, are at high altitude, or will be outdoors for many hours, use a sunscreen with an even higher SPF. A higher SPF does not mean you can use less.

• Choose a broad-spectrum sunscreen that protects against both UVA and UVB radiation. The SPF rating of a sunscreen currently applies only to UVB, but a number of ingredients, especially titanium dioxide and zinc oxide, are effective at blocking most UVA radiation.

• Use a water-resistant sunscreen if you swim or sweat a great deal. Under FDA regulations, sunscreens cannot be labeled as "waterproof" or "sweatproof" because these claims overstate the products' actual effectiveness. Labels for "water resistant" must specify whether they provide the labeled SPF protection for 40 or 80 minutes of swimming or sweating. Also be sure to reapply sunscreen after activities, such as swimming, that could remove sunscreen.

• If you have acne, look for a sunscreen that is labeled "noncomedogenic," which means that it will not cause pimples.

• Shake sunscreen before applying. Apply it 30 minutes before exposure to allow it time to bond to the skin. Reapply sunscreen frequently and generously to all sun-exposed areas (many people overlook their temples, ears, and sides and backs of their necks). Most people use less than half as much as they need to attain the full SPF rating. One ounce of sunscreen is enough to cover an average-size adult in a swimsuit. Reapply sunscreen every two hours.

• If you're taking medications, ask your physician or pharmacist about possible reactions to sunlight or interactions with sunscreens. Medications for acne, allergies, and diabetes are just a few of the products that can trigger reactions. If you're using sunscreen and an insect repellent containing DEET, use extra sunscreen (DEET may decrease sunscreen effectiveness).

Time of Day and Location

• Avoid sun exposure between 10:00 a.m. and 2:00 p.m., when the sun's rays are most intense. Clouds allow as much as 80% of UV rays to reach your skin. Stay in the shade when you can.

• Consult the day's UV Index, which predicts UV levels on a 0–11+ scale, to get a sense of the amount of sun protection you'll need. Take special care on days with a rating of 5 or above. You can download a free UV index app from the U.S. Environmental Protection Agency or find index ratings from the National Weather Service.

• UV rays can penetrate at least 3 feet below the surface of water, so swimmers should wear water-resistant sunscreens. Snow, sand, water, concrete, and white-painted surfaces are also highly reflective of UV rays.

Tanning Salons

• Stay away from tanning salons! Despite advertising claims to the contrary, the lights used in tanning parlors are damaging to your skin. Tanning beds and lamps emit mostly UVA radiation, increasing your risk of premature skin aging (such as wrinkles) and skin cancer.

Testicular Cancer

Testicular cancer is relatively rare, accounting for only 1% of cancers in U.S. men (about 9600 cases and 440 deaths per year), but it is the most common cancer in men aged 20–35. It is much more common among European Americans than among Latinos, Asian Americans, or African Americans. It is also relatively common among men whose fathers had testicular cancer. Men with undescended testicles are at in-

creased risk for testicular cancer, and for this reason that condition should be corrected in early childhood.

Self-examination may help in the early detection of testicular cancer (see the box "Testicle Self-Examination"). Tumors are treated by surgical removal of the testicle and, if the tumor has spread, by chemotherapy; radiation treatment is used only rarely. The five-year survival rate for testicular cancer is 96% if *regional*, beyond the primary tumor and reaching nearby tissues, organs, or lymph nodes.

Testicle Self-Examination

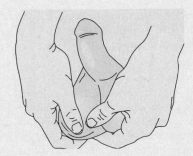

The best time to perform a testicular self-exam is after a warm shower or bath, when the scrotum is relaxed.

First, stand in front of a mirror and look for any swelling of the scrotum. Then examine each testicle with both hands. Place the index and middle fingers under the testicle and the thumbs on top. Roll the testicle gently between the fingers and thumbs. Don't worry if one testicle seems slightly larger than the other; that's common. Also, expect to feel the epididymis, which is the soft, sperm-carrying tube at the rear of the testicle.

Perform a self-exam each month. If you find a lump, swelling, or nodule, see a physician right away. The abnormality may not be cancer, but only a physician can make a diagnosis.

Other possible signs of testicular cancer include a change in the way a testicle feels, a sudden collection of fluid in the scrotum, a dull ache in the lower abdomen or groin, a feeling of heaviness in the scrotum, or pain in a testicle or the scrotum.

SOURCES: Testicular Cancer Resource Center. 2012. *How to Do a Testicular Self Examination* (http://tcrc.acor.org /tcexam.html); National Cancer Institute. 2013. *General Information about Testicular Cancer* (http://www .cancer.gov/cancertopics/pdq/treatment/testicular/Patient).

Other Cancers

Several other cancers affect a significant number of people each year. Some have identifiable risk factors, particularly smoking and obesity, that are controllable. Causes of others are still under investigation.

Pancreatic Cancer   The pancreas, a gland found deep within the abdomen behind the stomach, produces both digestive enzymes and insulin. Because of the gland's hidden location, pancreatic cancer is usually well advanced before symptoms become noticeable. In the United States, about 57,600 new cases and over 47,000 deaths occur annually.

Incidence rates are approximately twice as high for cigarette smokers as for nonsmokers. Other risk factors include being male, African American, obese, sedentary, or over age 60; having a family history of pancreatic cancer; having diabetes; and eating a diet high in fat and meat and low in vegetables. Fewer than 20% of patients are candidates for potentially curative surgeries because pancreatic cancer is usually detected only after it has spread outside the pancreas or is locally advanced. Even for those who have potentially curative surgeries to remove their tumors, the cancer often returns. Chemotherapy and radiation provide only modest benefits.

Head and Neck Cancers   Head and neck cancers—cancers of the oral cavity, pharynx, larynx, and nasal cavity—can be traced principally to tobacco smoking; the use of smokeless tobacco; and excessive alcohol consumption. These risk factors work together to multiply a person's risk of oral cancer. The incidence of head and neck cancer is twice as great in men as in women, and the disease is most frequent in men over age 40. Prominent sufferers of oral cancer include Sigmund Freud and Fidel Castro, both notorious cigar smokers. Sports figures who use smokeless tobacco are also increasingly diagnosed with oral cancer. Among long-term snuff users, the excess risk of cancers of the cheek, tongue, and gum is nearly 50-fold (see Chapter 12 for more about tobacco). Additionally, cancers of the tonsils and tongue base are commonly related to HPV infection.

Chemotherapy, radiation, and surgery are the primary methods of treatment for head and neck cancers. Patients often endure intense mouth and throat inflammation and some require invasive surgeries, but many can be cured. Among those who survive, a significant number will develop another primary cancer of the head and neck.

Stomach Cancer   Stomach cancer is the most common form of cancer in many parts of the world, but it is relatively rare in the United States, with over 27,000 new cases and 11,000 deaths each year. Approximately two-thirds of people with stomach cancer are 65 or older, and it is slightly more common in men than women.

Risk factors include infection with the bacterium *Helicobacter pylori*—which has also been linked to the development of ulcers—and a diet high in smoked, salted, or pickled fish or meat. Bacteria, including *H. pylori,* can convert the nitrites in preserved foods into carcinogenic amines, and salt can break down the normal protective stomach coating, allowing these carcinogenic compounds access to the cells of the stomach wall. However, the great majority of people with *H. pylori* infection do not develop stomach cancer, particularly if they eat a low-salt diet with plenty of fruits, vegetables, and whole grains.

There is no screening test for stomach cancer. It is usually recognized only after it has spread, and the overall five-year survival rate is only 30% for all stages.

Bladder Cancer   This cancer is about three times as common in men as in women, and smoking is the key risk factor. (Smokers are twice as likely to develop bladder cancer as nonsmokers.) People living in urban areas and workers exposed to chemicals used in the dye, rubber, and leather industries are also at increased risk.

There is no screening test for bladder cancer. The first symptoms are likely to be blood in the urine and/or increased frequency of urination. These symptoms can also signal a urinary infection but should trigger a visit to a physician, who can evaluate the possibility of cancer. With early detection, more than 90% of cases are curable. There are about 80,000 new cases and 18,000 deaths each year in the United States.

Kidney Cancer   Although this cancer usually occurs in people over age 50, anyone can develop it, and few risk factors are controllable. Smoking and obesity are mild risk factors, as is a family history of the disease. Symptoms may include fatigue, pain in the side, and blood in the urine. Kidney cancer is difficult to treat, with a five-year survival rate of only 75% for all stages. Recently, immune cell therapies and targeted agents such as angiogenesis inhibitors have shown some promise in the disease's advanced stage. In the United States, there are about 73,800 new cases each year and about 14,830 deaths.

Brain Cancer   Tumors can arise from most of the many types of cells found in the brain. The vast majority of brain cancers develop for no apparent reason. One of the few established risk factors is ionizing radiation, such as X-rays. Before the risks were recognized, children with ringworm of the scalp (a fungal infection) often received low-dose radiation therapy, which substantially increased their risk of brain tumors later in life. Symptoms are often nonspecific and include headaches, fatigue, behavioral changes, and sometimes seizures. There has been a slight increase in the incidence of tumors over the past 20 years, but this may be due to improved methods of diagnosis. Some brain tumors are curable by surgery or by radiation and chemotherapy, but most are not. Survival time varies with the type of the tumor. In the United States each year there are about 24,000 new cases and 18,000 deaths.

Leukemia   Leukemia, cancer of the white blood cells, can affect both children and adults. It starts in the bone marrow but can spread to the lymph nodes, spleen, liver, other organs, and central nervous system. It is a complex disease with many different types and subtypes. Most people with leukemia have no known risk factors. Some possible risk factors include smoking, exposure to radiation and certain chemicals, and infections. Most symptoms occur because leukemia cells crowd out the production of normal blood cells; the result can be fatigue, anemia, weight loss, and increased risk of infection. Treatment and survival rates vary depending on the exact type and other factors. There are about 60,000 new cases and 23,000 deaths each year in the United States.

Lymphoma   Lymphoma begins in the lymph nodes and then may spread to almost any part of the body. There are two types—Hodgkin lymphoma and non-Hodgkin lymphoma (NHL). NHL is the more common and more deadly form of the disease. It is the sixth most common cancer in the United States, with about 86,000 people diagnosed annually and almost 21,000 deaths. Risk factors for NHL are not well understood, but people with compromised immune systems are at increased risk, especially when exposed to radiation or certain infections and chemicals. The monoclonal antibody rituximab has greatly improved therapy in the last decade. Survival

Ask Yourself   ?

QUESTIONS FOR CRITICAL THINKING AND REFLECTION
Has anyone you know had cancer? If so, what type of cancer was it? What were its symptoms? Based on the information presented so far in this chapter, did the person have any of the known risk factors for the disease?

rates for Hodgkin lymphoma have improved significantly over the past few decades, and there are now about 8400 new cases and nearly 1000 deaths each year in the United States.

Multiple Myeloma   Normal plasma cells play an important role in the immune system, producing antibodies. Malignant plasma cells may produce tumors in several sites, particularly in the bone marrow, and when they grow in multiple sites, they are referred to as multiple myeloma (MM). By crowding out normal bone marrow cells, MM can lead to anemia, excessive bleeding, and decreased resistance to infection. Age is the most significant risk factor: Most patients diagnosed with MM are over age 65. Other risk factors are not well understood, although MM is about twice as common among African Americans as among whites. In the United States, over 32,000 new cases and almost 13,000 deaths occur each year.

NEW AND EMERGING CANCER TREATMENTS

As we understand more about how cancers develop, new targets have become available that allow more focused therapies with less severe side effects. Here are some specialized treatments beyond those of surgery, radiation, and chemotherapy.

Beyond Traditional Treatments

The cure can be worse than the disease, so many researchers look for biological therapy alternatives, such as immunotherapies, hormone therapies, and stem cell therapies.

- *Immunotherapies* boost the immune system's response to cancer and help mark cancer cells so that it is easier for the immune system to find, identify, and destroy them. One example of an immunotherapy is monoclonal antibodies, which are used to fight cancer in a way that is similar to how the immune system fights an infection. All cells in the body have markers on their surfaces, and the immune system develops antibodies, or special proteins, that can recognize these markers, bind to them, and trigger destruction. Scientists carefully select cell-surface markers that are displayed on cancer cells and then administer antibodies to the patient. These monoclonal antibodies target the cancer cells and enlist the help of the body's own immune system to selectively kill them. (*Monoclonal* means they bind to only one particular cell-surface marker.)

  CAR-T-cell therapy is another form of immunotherapy. A patient's T cell lymphocytes, which are part of a normal immune system, are biochemically engineered to attack the cancer cells. Specifically, the T cells are removed and then engineered to have chimeric antigen receptors (CARs) on their surface. These engineered cells, now known as CAR T cells, are then injected back into the patient. The CARs recognize antigens on the tumor cells, thereby bringing immune T cells in close proximity to cancer cells so that the immune system can try to eliminate the cancer.

• *Hormone therapies* are used to treat some cancers for which hormones promote the growth and spread of cancer cells, such as prostate and breast cancers. Hormone therapies usually work by blocking the body's ability to produce hormones or by interfering with how hormones act in the body. Tumor cells can be tested for the presence of hormone receptors or monitored in other ways to help determine if a hormone therapy is potentially beneficial for a particular patient.

• *Stem cell transplants* restore blood-forming cells in people who have had their own cells destroyed by high-dosage radiation therapy or chemotherapy. They are most often used for cancers that affect the immune system or the blood, such as leukemia or lymphoma. Stem cells are taken from the patient (prior to radiation or chemotherapy) or from a compatible donor and then transplanted into the patient. Once they enter the bloodstream, stem cells travel to the bone marrow, where they take the place of the cells that were destroyed by prior cancer treatment; they start producing the blood cells the patient needs.

Experimental Techniques

Many exciting possibilities for cancer therapy come from genomic and genetic research. Completion of the sequencing of the human genome in 2003 was a landmark achievement for scientists and opened a treasure chest of new insights into cancer. The Cancer Genome Atlas (TCGA) has identified common genetic mutations in dozens of cancer types, creating a huge database for this valuable information. Many important new subtypes of tumors for breast cancer, melanoma, leukemia, and lymphomas have been identified based on patterns of gene expression. Drugs are being designed to specifically attack genetic changes in tumors; this approach is known as **targeted therapy**. Patients often undergo genomic testing in the hope of finding a targetable mutation in their cancer cells.

A particularly exciting possibility for genomic therapy involves the ability to detect cancer mutations through a liquid biopsy. This method involves simply drawing a sample of urine or blood, or maybe cerebrospinal fluid or saliva. Compared with today's typical biopsy, a process involving open surgery, or an endoscope or a large needle, the liquid biopsy is less invasive and can be repeated multiple times to track a patient's progress or response to treatment.

targeted therapy The use of specially designed **TERMS** drugs to attack genetic changes in tumors.

stem cells Unspecialized cells that can divide and produce cells that differentiate into the many types of specialized cells in the body (brain cells, muscle cells, skin cells, blood cells, and others).

Liquid biopsies are possible due to the discovery that all cells, including cancer cells, continuously shed a very small amount of DNA into the bloodstream and other body fluids (known as *cell-free DNA*). Due to the development of highly sensitive DNA detection tests, it may be possible to diagnose and track cancers by monitoring their DNA levels in blood and other fluids.

Genomic research is also the basis for the Precision Medicine Initiative. By gathering and analyzing the genetic profiles of hundreds of thousands of individuals, researchers hope to understand which mutations place individuals at higher risk of developing diseases.

Starve or Feed the Tumors? In the 1990s, a prevalent idea for treating malignant tumors was to starve them of oxygen, which every living thing needs to survive. Researchers knew that when cancer cells became *hypoxic* (low on oxygen), cancer cells—like healthy cells—grow new blood vessels. This replenishing of the blood and oxygen supply is called angiogenesis. If this process could be blocked (using anti-angiogenesis drugs), it seemed logical that the tumor would stop growing and eventually die. Accordingly, doctors started treating tumors with new anti-angiogenesis drugs.

But most researchers and doctors did not understand how resilient tumors are. Although lack of oxygen kills some tumor cells, other hypoxic tumor cells kick into panic mode, turning on a "subcommittee" of proteins to ensure their survival. In addition to forming new blood vessels, the stressed cells lay down highways of collagen—a stringy web that provides links over which cancer cells can move away from the "toxic neighborhood," or metastasize. The tumor cells also develop properties like **stem cells** to repopulate the tumor. And they become more resistant to chemotherapy. Thus, what had seemed like the obvious answer—anti-angiogenesis drugs—failed in many cases. The tumors soon grew back and even more aggressively.

Cancer researcher Rakesh Jain tried a contrarian idea: Rather than deprive cancer cells of oxygen, he suggested infusing them with it. Trained as an engineer and now a Harvard professor of tumor biology, Jain noticed that the capillaries of tumors resembled leaky pipes, inefficient at delivering blood. His idea was to boost oxygen levels to keep tumors from entering panic mode and becoming super-tumors. Instead, they would remain inefficient at best. Jain's experiments showed that well-oxygenated tumor cells could be more efficiently killed by chemotherapy. In 2001, many opposed Jain's ideas, but they are now gaining momentum. In 2016 President Barack Obama commemorated Jain's accomplishment with the National Medal of Science.

David Cheresh, a research pathologist from the University of California at San Diego, established that nutrient deprivation, like oxygen deprivation, makes tumors more aggressive and resistant to drugs. Cheresh and his team explained that tumor cells respond to stress by converting themselves into a kind of chemotherapy-resistant stem cell. These cells are not naturally powerful; their strength is their ability to reprogram themselves. This discovery has prompted the development of drugs, still under trial, that would block the tumor's stem-cell-like adaptation.

Another avenue of research in cancer control involves blocking tumor cell migration and metastasis. To do so, oncology professor Daniele Gilkes at Johns Hopkins University is targeting the protein that first responds to the hypoxic tumor's emergency calls and gets activated to form collagen. Stopping this process, Gilkes's lab hopes, will stop metastasis.

These ideas are still in experimental stages and need time and money to continue down their innovative paths. A more complete understanding of tumor cell responses will eventually enable researchers to stop cancer.

Support during Cancer Therapy

Receiving cancer therapy can be very difficult, physically and emotionally. Some cancer treatments cause serious side effects, which can make patients more vulnerable to infections. Common side effects of chemotherapy include fatigue, nausea, and vomiting. Individuals who suffer pain from their cancer can be given a variety of pain control medications, but these too may have side effects such as sleepiness or constipation. Individuals undergoing cancer treatment may expect to experience disruptions in their daily lives. For example, many cancer patients are unable to work, which may result in finan-

cial hardship. Others find that their schedules are no longer routine due to frequent and required visits to the hospital or cancer center for chemotherapy or radiation treatment.

Fortunately, many support services are available for patients undergoing treatment and for their families, and it is vital that the patient take advantage of the psychological support that is available. Although some patients do well with the support of family and friends and a caring physician or nurse, others seek more communal comfort. Organized groups comprising other patients with the same type of cancer can help provide needed social and psychological support. Non-patient-focused support groups are also available for friends and family members. Visit www.cancer.org to find support programs and services groups in your area.

SUMMARY

• Cancer is the abnormal, uncontrolled multiplication of cells; it can cause death if untreated.

• A malignant tumor can invade surrounding structures and spread to distant sites via the blood and lymphatic system, producing additional tumors.

• A malignant cell divides without regard for normal growth. As tumors grow, they produce signs or symptoms that are determined by their location in the body.

• Mutational damage to a cell's DNA can lead to rapid and uncontrolled growth of cells; mutagens include radiation, viral infection, and chemical substances in food and air.

• Cancer-promoting dietary factors include meat, especially red and processed meat; certain types of fats; and alcohol.

• Diets high in fruits and vegetables are linked to a lower risk of cancer.

• Other possible causes of cancer include inactivity and obesity, certain viruses and chemicals, and radiation.

• Self-monitoring and regular screening tests are essential to early cancer detection.

• Methods of cancer diagnosis include MRI scanning, CT scanning, and ultrasound.

• Treatment methods usually consist of some combination of surgery, chemotherapy, and radiation.

• Lung cancer kills more people than any other type of cancer. Tobacco smoke is the primary cause.

• Colon and rectal cancers are linked to age, heredity, obesity, and a diet rich in processed meat and low in fruits and vegetables. Most colon cancers arise from preexisting polyps.

• Breast cancer affects about one in eight women in the United States. Although there is a genetic component to breast cancer, diet and hormones are also risk factors.

• Prostate cancer is chiefly a disease of aging; diet and lifestyle probably are factors in its occurrence. Early detection is possible through rectal examinations and PSA blood tests.

Ask Yourself

QUESTIONS FOR CRITICAL THINKING AND REFLECTION

For men, do you know how to perform self-examinations, such as testicular exams? For women, do you have breast self-awareness, which means familiarity with the appearance and feel of your breasts? Has your doctor ever given you instructions on self-exams? Given what you know about yourself and your family's medical history, do you think self-exams could be important for you?

TIPS FOR TODAY AND THE FUTURE

A growing body of research suggests that you can take an active role in preventing many cancers by adopting a wellness-focused lifestyle.

RIGHT NOW YOU CAN:

▪ Buy multiple bottles of sunscreen and put them in places where you will most likely need them, such as your backpack, gym bag, or car.
▪ Check the cancer screening guidelines in this chapter and make sure you are up-to-date on your screenings.
▪ If you are a woman, develop breast self-awareness. If you are a man, do a testicular self-exam.

IN THE FUTURE YOU CAN:

▪ Learn where to find information about daily UV radiation levels in your area, and learn how to interpret the information. Many local newspapers and television stations (and their websites) report current UV levels every day.
▪ Gradually add foods with abundant phytochemicals to your diet.

- Cancers of the female reproductive tract include cervical, uterine, and ovarian cancers. The Pap test is an effective screening test for cervical cancer.

- Abnormal cellular changes in the skin, often a result of exposure to the sun, cause skin cancer, as does chronic exposure to certain chemicals. Skin cancers include basal cell carcinoma, squamous cell carcinoma, and melanoma.

- Testicular cancer can be detected early through self-examination.

- Newer treatments such as immunotherapies, hormone therapies, and stem cell transplants have greatly improved outcomes. Research continues to show promise in these and other areas.

FOR MORE INFORMATION

American Academy of Dermatology. Provides information about skin cancer prevention.

http://www.aad.org

American Cancer Society. Provides a wide range of free materials on the prevention, diagnosis, and treatment of cancer.

http://www.cancer.org

American Institute for Cancer Research. Provides information about lifestyle and cancer prevention, especially nutrition.

http://www.aicr.org

Clinical Trials. Information about clinical trials for new cancer treatments can be accessed at the following sites:

http://www.cancer.gov/clinicaltrials

http://www.centerwatch.com

EPA/Sunwise. Provides information about the UV index and the effects of sun exposure, with links to sites with daily UV index ratings for cities in the United States and other countries.

http://www.epa.gov/sunwise/uvindex.html

MedlinePlus Cancer Information. Provides news and links to reliable information on a variety of cancers and cancer treatment.

http://www.nlm.nih.gov/medlineplus/cancers.html

National Cancer Institute. Provides information about treatment options, screening, and clinical trials.

http://www.cancer.gov

National Comprehensive Cancer Network (NCCN). Presents treatment guidelines for physicians and patients related to the treatment of various cancers; these guidelines were developed by a group of leading cancer centers.

http://www.nccn.org

National Toxicology Program. The federal program that creates regular reports listing the substances known or reasonably assumed to cause cancer in humans.

http://ntp.niehs.nih.gov

Oncolink/The University of Pennsylvania Cancer Center Resources. Contains information about different types of cancer and answers to frequently asked questions.

http://www.oncolink.org

See also the listings in Chapters 11–15.

SELECTED BIBLIOGRAPHY

American Cancer Society. 2020. *About Breast Cancer.* Atlanta, GA: American Cancer Society (https://www.cancer.org/cancer/breast-cancer.html).

American Cancer Society. 2020. *Cancer Facts and Figures 2020.* Atlanta, GA: American Cancer Society (https://www.cancer.org/content/dam/cancer-org/research/cancer-facts-and-statistics/annual-cancer-facts-and-figures/2020/cancer-facts-and-figures-2020.pdf).

American Cancer Society. 2020. *Key Statistics for Basal and Squamous Cell Skin Cancers.* Atlanta, GA: American Cancer Society.

American Cancer Society. 2020. *Key Statistics for Melanoma Skin Cancer.* Atlanta, GA: American Cancer Society (https://www.cancer.org/cancer/basal-and-squamous-cell-skin-cancer.html).

American Cancer Society. 2020. *Key Statistics for Testicular Cancer.* Atlanta, GA: American Cancer Society (https://www.cancer.org/cancer/testicular-cancer.html).

American Cancer Society. 2020. *Special Section: Ovarian Cancer.* Atlanta, GA: American Cancer Society (https://www.cancer.org/cancer/ovarian-cancer.html).

Arana, J. E., et al. 2018. Post-licensure safety monitoring of quadrivalent human papillomavirus vaccine in the Vaccine Adverse Event Reporting System (VAERS), 2009–2015. *Vaccine* 36(13): 1781–1788.

Beil, L. 2017. Deflating cancer: New approaches to low oxygen may thwart tumors. *Science News* 191(4): 24–27.

Bouvard, V., et al. 2015. Carcinogenicity of consumption of red and processed meat. *Lancet Oncology* 16(16): 1599–1600.

Cao, S., et al. 2015. The health effects of passive smoking: An overview of systematic reviews based on observational epidemiological evidence. *PLoS One* 10(10): e0139907.

Castellsaqué, X., et al. 2016. HPV involvement in head and neck cancers: Comprehensive assessment of biomarkers in 3680 patients. *Journal of the National Cancer Institute* 108(6): djv403.

Demeyer, D., et al. 2015. Mechanisms linking colorectal cancer to the consumption of (processed) red meat: A review. *Critical Reviews in Food Science and Nutrition*, May 15.

Farvid, M. S., et al. 2016. Fruit and vegetable consumption in adolescence and early adulthood and risk of breast cancer: Population based cohort study. *British Medical Journal* 353: i2343.

Gilkes, D. M. 2016. Implications of hypoxia in breast cancer metastasis to bone. *International Journal of Molecular Sciences* 17(10): 1669. DOI:10.3390/ijms17101669.

Guo, F., L. E. Cofie, and A. B. Berenson. 2018. Cervical cancer incidence in young U.S. females after Human Papillomavirus Vaccine introduction. *American Journal of Preventive Medicine* 55(2): 197–204.

Han, X., et al. 2015. Body mass index at early adulthood, subsequent weight change and cancer incidence and mortality. *International Journal of Cancer* 135(12): 2900–2909.

Holyoake, T. L., and D. Vetrie. 2017. The chronic myeloid leukemia stem cell: Stemming the tide of persistence. *Blood* 129(12): 1595–1606.

Jones, K. L., et al. 2009. Evolving novel anti-HER2 strategies. *Lancet Oncology* 10(12): 1179–1187.

Kaiser, J. 2016. Tests of blood-borne DNA pinpoint tissue damage: Assays spot cell death from diabetes, cancer, and more. *Science* 351(6279): 1253.

Kassianos, A. P., et al. 2015. Smartphone applications for melanoma detection by community, patient and generalist clinician users: A review. *British Journal of Dermatology* 172(6): 1507–1518.

Li, X., et al. 2016. Effectiveness of prophylactic surgeries in *BRCA1* or *BRCA2* mutation carriers: A meta-analysis and systematic review. *Clinical Cancer Research* DOI: 10.1158/1078-0432.CCR-15-1465.

McKee, S. J., A. S. Bergot, and G. R. Leggatt GR. 2015. Recent progress in vaccination against human papillomavirus-mediated cervical cancer. *Reviews in Medical Virology* 25(1): 54–71.

McNeil, J. J., et al. 2018. Effect of aspirin on disability-free survival in the healthy elderly. *The New England Journal of Medicine* DOI: 10.1056/NEJMoa1800722.

Moore, S. C., et al. 2016. Leisure-time physical activity and risk of 26 types of cancer in 1.44 million adults. *JAMA Internal Medicine* 176(6): 816–825.

Mpekris, F., et al. 2017. Role of vascular normalization in benefit from metronomic chemotherapy. *Proceedings of the National Academy of Sciences of the United States of America* 114(8): 1994–1999.

Myers, E. R., et al. 2015. Benefits and harms of breast cancer screening: A systematic review. *Journal of the American Medical Association* 314(15): 1615–1634.

National Cancer Institute, National Institutes of Health. 2011. *Radon and Cancer* (http://www.cancer.gov/cancertopics/factsheet/Risk/radon).

National Cancer Institute. 2017. Liquid biopsy: Using DNA in blood to detect, track, and treat cancer. *Cancer Currents Blog* (https://www.cancer.gov/news-events/cancer-currents-blog/2017/liquid-biopsy-detects-treats-cancer).

National Human Genome Research Institute. 2014. *A Brief Guide to Genomics Fact Sheet* (http://www.genome.gov/18016863).

National Toxicology Program. 2014. *Report on Carcinogens,* 13th ed. Research Triangle Park, NC: USDHHS Public Health Service.

Planchard, D., and B. Besse. 2015. Lung cancer in never-smokers. *European Respiratory Journal* 45(5): 1214–1217.

Razdan, S. N., et al. 2016. Quality of life among patients after bilateral prophylactic mastectomy: A systematic review of patient-reported outcomes. *Quality of Life Research* 25(6): 1409–1421.

Roura, E., et al. 2014. Smoking as a major risk factor for cervical cancer and pre-cancer: Results from the EPIC cohort. *International Journal of Cancer* 135(2): 453–466.

Siegel, R. L., K. D. Miller, and A. Jemal. 2018. Cancer statistics, 2018. *CA: A Cancer Journal for Clinicians* 68(1) (https://onlinelibrary.wiley.com/doi/abs/10.3322/caac.21442).

Torre, L. A., et al. 2016. Cancer statistics for Asian Americans, Native Hawaiians, and Pacific Islanders, 2016: Converging incidence in males and females. *CA: A Cancer Journal for Clinicians* 66(3): 182–202.

Wilson, R., et al. 2016. MicroRNA regulation of endothelial TREX1 reprograms the tumour microenvironment. *Nature Communications* 7(13597). DOI: 10.1038/ncomms13597.

Wolf, A. M. D., et al. 2018. Colorectal cancer screening for average-risk adults: 2018 guideline update from the American Cancer Society. *CA: A Cancer Journal for Clinicians.* DOI: 10.3322/caac.21457.

World Health Organization. 2018. *Fact Sheet: Cancer* (http://www.who.int/en/news-room/fact-sheets/detail/cancer).

BEHAVIOR CHANGE STRATEGY
Incorporating More Fruits and Vegetables into Your Diet

You know that fruits and vegetables are good for you, but did you know that they help fight cancer? They contain specific cancer-fighting compounds (phytochemicals) that help slow, stop, or even reverse the process of cancer. The National Cancer Institute (NCI) reports that people who eat five or more servings a day of fruits and vegetables have half the risk of cancer compared to those who eat fewer than two. According to the NCI, at least seven to nine servings per day is optimal.

Most Americans need to double the amount of fruits and vegetables they eat every day. Monitor your diet for one or two weeks to assess your current intake. Here are some tips to help you incorporate these foods into your diet.

Breakfast

- Drink pure fruit juice every morning.
- Add raisins, berries, or sliced fruit to cereal, pancakes, or waffles. Top bagels with tomato slices.
- Try a fruit smoothie made from fresh or frozen fruit and orange juice or low-fat yogurt.

Lunch

- Choose vegetable soup or salad with your meal.
- Replace potato chips or french fries with carrots, cucumbers, celery, bell pepper, or jicama.
- Add extra fruits or vegetables to salads—oranges, melons, tomatoes, dried cranberries.
- Add vegetables such as roasted peppers, cucumber slices, shredded carrots, avocado, or salsa to sandwiches.
- Drink tomato or vegetable juice instead of soda (watch for excess sodium and sugar).

Dinner

- Choose a vegetarian main course, such as stir-fry or vegetable stew. Have at least two servings of vegetables with every dinner.
- Microwave vegetables and sprinkle them with a little olive oil and fresh garlic.
- Substitute vegetables for meat in casseroles, pasta, and chili.
- At the salad bar, pile your plate with steamed or raw vegetables and use low-fat or nonfat dressing.

Snacks and On the Go

- Keep ready-to-eat fruits and vegetables on hand (apples, plums, pears, and carrots).
- Keep small packages of dried fruit in the car (try dried apples, apricots, peaches, pears, and raisins).
- Make ice cubes from pure fruit juice and drop them into regular or sparkling water.
- Freeze grapes for a cool summer treat.

The All-Stars

Different fruits and vegetables contribute different vitamins, phytochemicals, and other nutrients, so be sure to get a variety. The following types of produce are particularly rich in nutrients and phytochemicals:

- Cruciferous vegetables (e.g., broccoli, cauliflower, cabbage, bok choy, brussels sprouts, kohlrabi, turnips)
- Citrus fruits (e.g., oranges, lemons, limes, grapefruit, tangerines)
- Berries (e.g., strawberries, raspberries, blueberries)
- Dark green leafy vegetables (e.g., spinach, chard, collards, beet greens, kale, mustard greens, romaine and other dark lettuces)
- Deep yellow, orange, and red fruits and vegetables (e.g., carrots, pumpkin, sweet potatoes, winter squash, red and yellow bell peppers, apricots, cantaloupe, mangoes, papayas)

Design Elements: Assess Yourself icon: Aleksey Boldin/Alamy Stock Photo; Diversity Matters icon: Rawpixel Ltd/Getty Images; Wellness on Campus icon: Rawpixel Ltd/Getty Images; Take Charge icon: VisualCommunications/Getty Images; Critical Consumer icon: pagadesign/Getty Images.

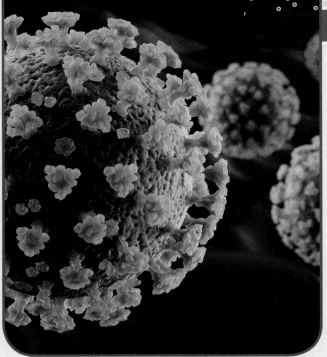

- Explain the body's physical and chemical defenses against infection
- Describe the step-by-step process by which infectious diseases are transmitted
- Identify the major types of pathogens, the diseases they cause, and possible treatments for them
- Discuss steps you can take to support your immune system

Andriy Onufriyenko/Getty Images

CHAPTER **18**

Immunity and Infection

TEST YOUR KNOWLEDGE

ANSWERS

1. Which of the following can transmit disease-causing pathogens (such as bacteria or viruses) from one person to another?
   a. Mosquitoes
   b. Doorknobs
   c. Soil

2. When taking a prescription antibiotic, you should always finish all the medication, even if you start feeling better before running out of medicine. True or False?

3. Which of the following can recognize and eliminate specific microbes (such as bacteria) that invade the body?
   a. Antigens
   b. Antibodies
   c. Antidotes

4. Patients rarely catch bacterial infections in hospitals. True or False?

5. You can reduce your chances of getting sick by doing which of the following?
   a. Washing your hands frequently
   b. Keeping your immunizations up-to-date
   c. Getting enough sleep

1. **ALL THREE.** Pathogens can be transmitted directly (by contact with a sick person) or indirectly (by contact with an infected animal or insect or a contaminated object like a doorknob).

2. **TRUE.** Failing to take all your medication can lead to a relapse of the illness; taking antibiotics incorrectly also contributes to the development of antibiotic-resistant bacteria.

3. **B.** Antibodies are specialized proteins produced by the immune system that can target specific invading organisms.

4. **FALSE.** Thousands of people die each year from infections contracted in health care settings.

5. **ALL THREE.** Frequent hand washing prevents the spread of many disease-causing agents. Immunizations prime the body to tackle an invading organism. Sleep helps support a healthy immune system.

Countless microscopic organisms live around, on, and in us. Although most microbes are beneficial, many of them can cause **infections.** But the constant vigilance of our immune system keeps them at bay and our bodies healthy. The immune system protects us not just from **pathogens** (disease-causing organisms) but also from cancers, some of which are linked to persistent infections and chronic inflammation.

In the past decade, the reemergence of old scourges such as tuberculosis and the appearance of new viruses such as Coronavirus Disease 2019 (COVID-19) highlight the importance of understanding both the immune system and the pathogens that can cause us harm. This chapter introduces you to the mechanisms of immunity and infection; we also discuss strategies for keeping ourselves healthy.

THE BODY'S DEFENSE SYSTEM

Our bodies have very effective ways of protecting themselves against invasion by foreign organisms. The immune system is the body's collective set of defenses that includes surface barriers as well as the specialized cells, tissues, and organs that carry out the immune response. The first line of defense is a formidable array of physical and chemical barriers. When these barriers are breached, cellular processes of the immune system come into play. Together these defenses provide an effective response to nearly all the invasions that our bodies experience.

Physical and Chemical Barriers

The skin, the body's largest organ, prevents many microorganisms from entering the body. Although many bacterial and fungal organisms live on the surface of the skin, few can penetrate it except through a cut or break.

All body cavities and passages that are exposed to the external environment are lined with mucous membranes, which secrete mucus and contain cells designed to prevent unwanted organisms and particles from passing through or penetrating them. These areas include the mouth, nostrils, eyelids, bronchioles, vagina, and other organs of the respiratory, digestive, and urogenital tracts. Skin and mucous membranes are made of epithelial tissue, which consists of one or more layers of closely packed cells. They act as both physical and chemical barriers to potential invaders. The fluids that cover epithelial tissue, such as tears, saliva, and vaginal secretions, are rich in enzymes and other proteins that break down and destroy many microorganisms.

The respiratory tract is lined not only with mucous membranes but also with cells having hairlike protrusions called *cilia.* The cilia sweep foreign matter up and out of the respiratory tract. Particles that are not caught by this mechanism may be expelled from the system by a cough.

The Immune System: Cells, Tissues, and Organs

Beyond surface barriers, the **immune system** operates through a remarkable information network involving billions of white blood cells that protect the body when a threat arises. We produce these white blood cells continuously throughout life.

The immune system is actually two interacting systems; both consist of cells that can recognize pathogenic microorganisms. The cells of the *innate immune system* are the first to respond to those pathogens. The T cells and B cells of the *adaptive immune system* have the remarkable ability both to accelerate and to improve the effectiveness of their responses. The complete elimination of a pathogen involves the coordinated activities of both systems.

Cells of the Innate Immune System   The cells of the innate immune system recognize pathogens as "foreign" and kill them, but unlike cells of the adaptive immune system, they have no memory of these pathogens. Thus, they respond the same way no matter how many times a pathogen invades. The innate immune system includes the following types of cells:

- *Neutrophils* are white blood cells that ingest and destroy pathogens.
- *Eosinophils* are white blood cells that fight parasitic infections. Eosinophils occur not so much in the blood but rather in the lower intestinal tract and in lymphoid organs.
- *Macrophages* are scavenger cells that engulf and destroy bacteria and dying cells. Macrophages exist in many tissues. They are mobile and can home in on chemicals released by bacterial and dying cells.
- *Natural killer cells* are cells that directly destroy virus-infected cells and cells that have turned cancerous.
- *Dendritic cells* are cells that reside in tissues in contact with the external environment, such as the skin and the mucosa of the respiratory and digestive tracts. They are called dendritic cells because in the immature state they have long branches, or *dendrites.* When they encounter pathogens, they engulf them and migrate to lymph nodes where they can activate T and B cells. Thus, dendritic cells initiate the adaptive immune response.

Cells of the Adaptive Immune System   The cells of the adaptive immune system are white blood cells called **lymphocytes.** The two main types of lymphocytes are T cells and B cells. They are always ready to attack an invader.

TERMS

infection   Invasion of the body by a microorganism.

pathogen   An organism that causes disease.

immune system   The body's collective system of defenses that includes surface barriers as well as the specialized cells, tissues, and organs that carry out the immune response.

lymphocyte   A type of white blood cell that carries out important functions in the immune system.

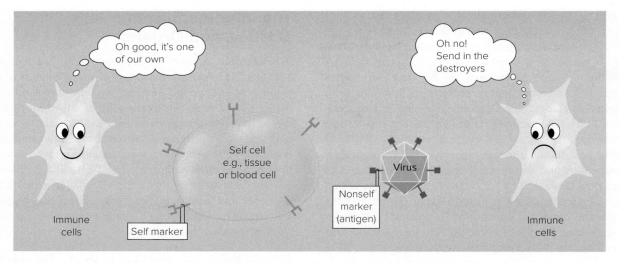

FIGURE 18.1 Immune cells learn to ignore cells marked "self" and to attack nonself antigens introduced into the body.

Antigens All your body cells display "self" markers that tell lymphocytes: *I belong to this body.* Invading microbes display markers that identify them as "nonself" or foreign (Figure 18.1). Nonself markers that trigger an immune response are called **antigens**. Each bacterial cell or virus has many antigens.

Antibodies **Antibodies** are specialized proteins that can recognize and neutralize specific invaders such as viruses and bacteria.

T Cells and B Cells Each T and B cell has receptors that allow it to recognize one specific antigen. The immune system produces T and B cells with many receptor types, each capable of recognizing a different antigen. Thus the immune system can recognize nearly all disease-causing microbes. When a B cell lymphocyte or T cell lymphocyte encounters the antigen for which it is specific, they attack the invading organisms. **B cells** become plasma cells that secrete antibodies. **T cells** differentiate into helper T cells, killer T cells, or suppressor T cells (also called regulatory T cells). B and T cells can mount a rapid and powerful response should they encounter the same invader months or even years in the future.

The Inflammatory Response When injured or infected, the body reacts by producing an inflammatory response.

> **TERMS**
>
> **antigen** A substance that triggers the immune response.
>
> **antibody** A specialized protein, produced by plasma cells, that can recognize specific antigens.
>
> **B cell** A type of lymphocyte that produces antibodies.
>
> **T cells** Cells responsible for cell-mediated adaptive immune reactions. Helper T cells activate macrophages and promote activation of B cells and killer T cells. Killer T cells kill cells infected with viruses, other intracellular pathogens, and tumor cells.

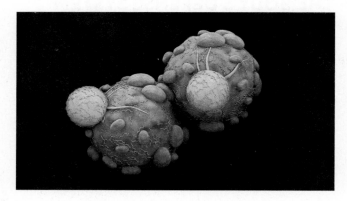

A dendritic cell is a white blood cell that engulfs foreign cells and displays their antigens in a way that makes these antigens recognizable by B and T cells. This process activates the B and T cells, signaling them to proliferate and respond to the specific invader. The dendritic cell shown in this scanning electron micrograph is magnified 2700 times. luismmolina/Getty Images

Macrophages engulf the invading microbe and produce substances that signal danger to other immune system cells. The resulting inflammatory response causes blood vessels to dilate and fluid to flow out of capillaries into the injured tissue. White blood cells are drawn to the area and attack the invaders, in many cases destroying them. At the site of infection there may be *pus*—a collection of dead white blood cells and debris resulting from the encounter.

The Immune Response The activities of the innate and adaptive immune systems are integrated to generate a coordinated and usually highly effective immune response. Figure 18.2 illustrates how this happens:

• *Phase 1: Recognition.* If a pathogen breaches the body's physical and chemical barriers (e.g., skin, cilia, and mucus), it initiates the first phase of the immune response by arousing dendritic cells at the site of pathogen entry. They engulf the pathogen and migrate to nearby lymphoid tissue. There the den-

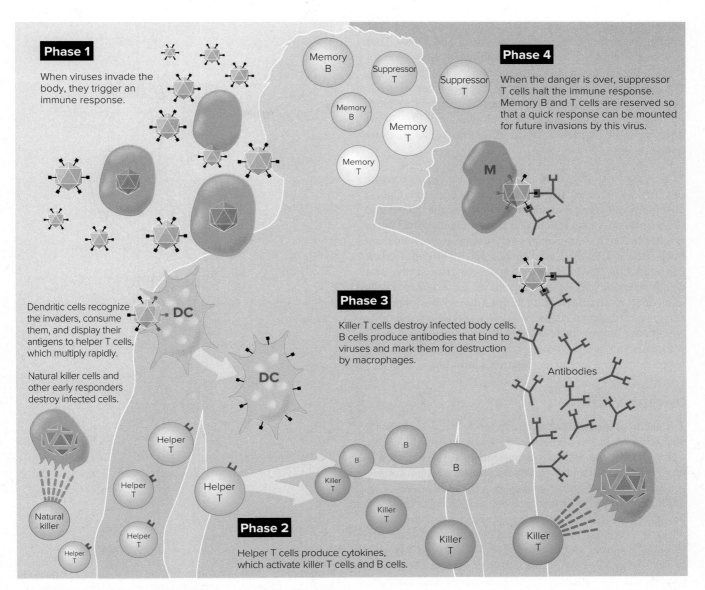

Phase 1

When viruses invade the body, they trigger an immune response.

Dendritic cells recognize the invaders, consume them, and display their antigens to helper T cells, which multiply rapidly.

Natural killer cells and other early responders destroy infected cells.

DC

DC

Natural killer

Helper T

Helper T

Helper T

Helper T

Helper T

Phase 2

Helper T cells produce cytokines, which activate killer T cells and B cells.

Killer T

Killer T

Killer T

Killer T

Killer T

B

B

B

Memory B

Suppressor T

Memory B

Memory T

Memory T

Phase 3

Killer T cells destroy infected body cells. B cells produce antibodies that bind to viruses and mark them for destruction by macrophages.

Antibodies

Suppressor T

Phase 4

When the danger is over, suppressor T cells halt the immune response. Memory B and T cells are reserved so that a quick response can be mounted for future invasions by this virus.

M

FIGURE 18.2 **The immune response.** Once invaded by a pathogen, the body mounts a complex series of reactions to destroy the invader. Pictured here are the phases of the immune response as the body works to destroy a virus.

dritic cells activate helper and killer T cells by presenting fragments of pathogen proteins to T cells. Antigen carried into lymphoid tissue also activates B cells, which can produce plasma cells to attack a specific type of invader.

• *Phase 2: Proliferation.* The activated helper and killer T cells multiply, amplifying the immune response to the pathogen. Helper T cells produce special growth stimulants called cytokines, signaling molecules that regulate immunity, inflammation, and production of blood cells and platelets; they further stimulate the activation and proliferation of killer T cells and B cells.

• *Phase 3: Elimination.* The activated T and B cells then become either memory cells or effector cells. The effector cells eliminate the pathogen. If the infecting pathogen is a virus or an intracellular bacterium, then killer T cells destroy body cells that are infected with that pathogen. Activated B cells become

memory B cells or antibody-producing plasma cells. The antibodies bind to extracellular pathogens (those outside body cells) and mark them for destruction by macrophages and natural killer cells.

• *Phase 4: Slowdown.* Regulatory T cells inhibit lymphocyte proliferation and induce lymphocyte death, causing a slowdown of the immune response. This process restores memory T and B cells, which can initiate a rapid response if the same pathogen reappears.

Immunity Usually, after an infection, a person is immune to the same pathogen. This **immunity,** or insusceptibility,

| immunity | Resistance to infection. | **TERMS** |

occurs because lymphocytes created during phase 2 of the immune response are reserved as memory T and B cells. They continue to circulate in the blood and lymphatic system for years. If the same antigen enters the body again, the memory T and B cells recognize and destroy it before it can cause illness. The ability of memory lymphocytes to remember previous infections and improve immune defenses if the same microbe is encountered in the future is called **adaptive immunity.**

The Lymphatic System   The lymphatic system consists of a network of vessels that carry a clear fluid called lymph. It also includes organs and structures, such as the spleen and the lymph nodes, that function as part of the immune system (Figure 18.3). The lymphatic vessels pick up excess fluid from body tissues. This fluid may contain microbes and dead or damaged body cells. Macrophages, dendritic cells, and lymphocytes congregate in the lymph nodes. If immune cells in a lymph node recognize an antigen, the adaptive immune response is triggered. As the immune response progresses, a lymph node actively involved in fighting an infection may fill with cells and swell. Physicians use the location of swollen lymph nodes as a clue to an infection's location.

Immunization

The ability of the immune system to remember previously encountered organisms and retain its ability to destroy or neutralize them is the basis for **immunization.** When a person is immunized, the immune system is primed with an antigen similar to the pathogenic organism. The body responds by producing antibodies, which prevent serious infection if the person is exposed to the disease organism itself. Thus, immunization (vaccination) activates the immune system and launches a natural immune response. The preparations used to alert the immune system are known as **vaccines.** Table 18.1 summarizes the vaccines currently recommended for most adults. Visit the Centers for Disease Control and Prevention (CDC) Vaccines & Immunizations website (www.cdc.gov /vaccines) for updates and the recommendations for children, travelers, pregnant women, and adults with special health risks. Some vaccines require multiple doses or periodic booster shots to maintain effectiveness, so it is important to keep up with the recommended vaccine schedule.

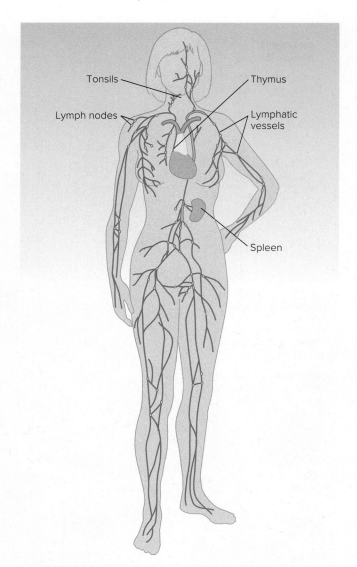

FIGURE 18.3   The lymphatic system. The lymphatic organs are production centers for infection-fighting cells and sites for some immune responses.

Immunization has become a source of public debate among people who question whether vaccinations do more harm than good. They worry in particular about the efficacy and safety of certain types of vaccinations. Public health officials are concerned because decreases in vaccination rates can result in outbreaks of dangerous infectious diseases, especially since international travel makes it easy for pathogens to cross borders from countries with low vaccination rates. Large outbreaks have occurred in other countries in recent years. For example, France had an outbreak of measles in 2008–2011 (more than 20,000 cases; 5000 hospitalizations; and 10 deaths), and U.S. travelers to France brought measles home with them. Vaccine-preventable diseases still exist around the world. If vaccination rates drop, diseases can become much more common.

Types of Vaccines   Vaccines can be made in several ways. In some cases, microbes are cultured in the laboratory in a way

adaptive immunity   Immunity to infection acquired by the activation of antigen-specific lymphocytes in response to infection or immunization. Adaptive immunity results in immunological memory.

TERMS

immunization   The process of conferring immunity to a pathogen by administering a vaccine to a person.

vaccines   A preparation of killed or weakened microorganisms, inactivated toxins, or components of microorganisms that is administered to stimulate an immune response; a vaccine protects against future infection by the pathogen.

Table 18.1	Immunizations Recommended for Adults (Aged 19 and Over)*

VACCINE	RECOMMENDATION
Flu	All adults, every year
Td/Tdap (tetanus, diphtheria, pertussis)	All adults, Td booster every 10 years, substitute Tdap for Td once
HPV (human papillomavirus)	Women up to age 26, men up to age 21, and men aged 22–26 who have sex with men who have not already completed the vaccine series; 2 or 3 doses (depending on age at series initiation)
Shingles (Shingrix vaccine)	Adults aged 50+, including those who have had shingles, are not sure if they have had chickenpox, or were immunized with Zostavax, in two doses 4–8 weeks apart
Pneumococcal	Adults aged 65+
Meningococcal	Adults at risk, including unvaccinated college students living in dormitories; every 5 years
MMR (measles, mumps, rubella)	Adults born after 1957 who were not vaccinated as children and who lack evidence of past infection
Chickenpox	Adults not vaccinated as children who lack evidence of past infection
Hepatitis A	Adults with specific health conditions or risk factors who were not vaccinated as children
Hepatitis B	Adults with specific health conditions or risk factors who were not vaccinated as children

*For international travelers, all standard childhood immunizations should be up-to-date and additional vaccines considered. Information for travelers and adults with special health concerns is available from the CDC's national immunization program (800-232-2522; www.CDC.gov/vaccines/) and the CDC's travelers' health resources (877-394-8747; www.cdc.gov/travel). The CDC has interactive tools (at www.cdc.gov/vaccines) to help individuals decide which vaccines they need.

SOURCE: Centers for Disease Control and Prevention. 2020. *2020 Immunization Schedules and Resources.* (http://www.cdc.gov/vaccines/schedules/index.html).

that attenuates (weakens) them. These live, attenuated organisms are used in vaccines against diseases such as measles, mumps, and rubella (German measles). In other cases, when it is not possible to generate attenuated organisms, vaccines are made from pathogens that have been killed but that still retain their ability to stimulate the immune system to produce antibodies. Vaccines composed of killed viruses are used against influenza viruses, among others.

Vaccine Efficacy   In the past century, vaccines have helped to increase the average American life span by approximately 30 years—and they have done so with an excellent safety record. Nevertheless, misinformation about vaccines has spread (particularly on the internet and in popular media), raising concerns about their efficacy and safety. The success of vaccines in preventing disease has been well established, but their role in human health is underappreciated.

Most childhood vaccines are effective enough to prevent disease in most people. For a small proportion of people, a vaccine is not effective—that is, the vaccine does not provoke a strong enough immune response. For example, for measles, an estimated 3 of 100 vaccinated people are not fully protected, although if infected, they are likely to have milder illness and are less likely to spread the disease compared to someone who is not vaccinated. Protection from infection is provided by those around them, as long as they live, work, and travel around people who have been vaccinated and are themselves protected. The same is true for people who cannot be vaccinated due to young age or underlying medical conditions (such as cancer treatment).

Keeping vaccination rates consistently high over time is necessary to maintain protection. Before the development of the measles vaccine in 1963, nearly everyone in the United States got measles, and hundreds died from measles every year. In the five years before the vaccine was introduced, about 400–500 deaths and 48,000 hospitalizations from measles occurred annually. Following widespread vaccination, the United States was declared measles-free in 2000, meaning measles is not constantly present. However, outbreaks have continued to occur, with infection brought into the United States by unvaccinated travelers (Americans or foreign visitors) who get measles while they are in other countries. People with measles can easily spread it to others who are not vaccinated or otherwise protected (e.g., from past infection). In an outbreak in 2011, over 70% of cases were traced to travel abroad by U.S. citizens, nearly half of whom acquired measles in Europe. In 2019, over 1200 cases of measles occurred in 31 states, the biggest outbreak since 1992. The majority of cases occurred among people who were not vaccinated, and they resulted in 128 hospitalizations. Globally, measles affects more than 7 million people each year and causes more than 100,000 deaths. Reduced vaccination rates have led to a nearly 300% increase in measles infections since 2018.

Vaccine Safety   Vaccines are approved by the Advisory Committee on Immunization Practices—the advisors for the CDC—and the Committee on Infectious Diseases—the advisors for the American Academy of Pediatrics (AAP). Both the AAP and the CDC advisory committees have expert knowledge in virology, microbiology, statistics, epidemiology, and pathogenesis—knowledge necessary for reviewing and evaluating studies on vaccine efficacy and safety.

To further ensure their safety, vaccines are tested before being licensed in greater numbers of people for longer periods of time than are drugs. For example, the human papillomavirus (HPV) vaccine was tested in 30,000 women, pneumococcal vaccine was tested in 40,000 children, and each of the current rotavirus vaccines was tested in 70,000 children before being licensed. No other type of medication receives this degree of scrutiny.

Additionally, safety mechanisms such as the Vaccine Adverse Event Reporting System (VAERS) and the Vaccine Safety Datalink Project monitor adverse events reported after licensure. Side effects from immunization are usually mild, such as soreness at the injection site. It is estimated that an allergic reaction may occur in 1 in 1.5 million doses. Any risk from a vaccine must be balanced against the risk posed by the diseases it prevents. For example, the last major U.S. epidemic of rubella in 1964–1965 infected 12.5 million Americans, caused 11,000 miscarriages, killed 2000 infants, and resulted in 20,000 infants being born with rubella-caused birth defects. Since the introduction of the vaccine and the maintenance of high vaccination rates, U.S. rubella cases have dropped to an average of about 10 per year. Worldwide, however, an estimated 100,000 babies are born each year with birth defects due to rubella infection in pregnant women.

Recent studies on children suggest that long-term measles damage is far worse than previously imagined: Measles wipes out the immune system's memory of some previous illnesses and leaves the body less equipped to fight off new infections long after the initial illness has passed. Measles survivors may gradually (months to years) regain their previous immunity to other viruses and bacteria as they are re-exposed to them.

For more on the safety, efficacy, and testing of vaccines, visit the CDC Vaccines & Immunizations website (www.cdc.gov/vaccines) and the website for the American Academy of Pediatrics (www.aap.org).

Allergy: A Case of Mistaken Identity

Allergies affect an estimated 50 million Americans. In a person with an allergy, the immune system reacts to a harmless

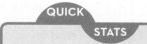

QUICK STATS

Since the HPV vaccine's introduction, HPV infections that cause most HPV cancers and genital warts among young adult women have dropped 71%.

—CDC, 2019

TERMS

allergy An immune response to normally innocuous foreign chemicals and proteins that is characterized by specific symptoms such as sneezing, rash, and swelling; also called *hypersensitivity*.

allergen A substance, such as pollen, that triggers an allergic reaction.

histamine A chemical responsible for the dilation and increased permeability of blood vessels in the allergic and inflammatory responses.

asthma A disease in which chronic inflammation and periodic constriction of the airways cause wheezing, shortness of breath, and coughing.

substance as if it were a harmful pathogen. Allergy symptoms—stuffy nose, sneezing, wheezing, skin rashes, and so on—usually result from the immune response.

Allergens An **allergen** is a molecule that elicits an exaggerated immune response. The best scenario would be for the body to work a foreign substance out of the body over time without such an exaggerated response, as is the case when a splinter sometimes slowly works its way out on its own. Common allergens include the following:

- **Pollen.** Referred to as hay fever or allergic rhinitis, pollen allergies are widespread. Weeds, grasses, and trees commonly produce allergenic pollen.

- **Animal dander.** People with animal allergies are usually allergic not to fur but to dander (dead skin flakes), urine, or a protein found in saliva. Allergies to mice, dogs, and cats are common.

- **Dust mites and cockroaches.** The droppings of cockroaches and microscopic dust mites can trigger allergies. Mites live in carpets, upholstered furniture, and bedding.

- **Molds and mildew.** The small spores produced by these fungi can trigger allergy symptoms. Molds and mildew thrive in damp areas of buildings.

- **Foods.** The most common food allergens for adults include peanuts, tree nuts, fish, and shellfish.

- **Insect stings.** The venom of insects such as yellow jackets, honeybees, hornets, paper wasps, and fire ants causes allergic reactions in some people.

People may also be allergic to certain medications, plants such as poison oak, latex, metals such as nickel, and compounds found in cosmetics.

The Allergic Response Allergies are an adverse response to environmental antigens that are not pathogenic. The body's response is to release large amounts of **histamine,** a chemical involved in some cases of inflammation as well as allergy. In the nose, histamine may cause congestion and sneezing; in the eyes, itchiness and tearing; in the skin, redness, swelling, and itching; in the intestines, bloating and cramping; and in the lungs, coughing, wheezing, and shortness of breath.

In some people, an allergen can trigger an **asthma** attack (see the box "Poverty, Ethnicity, and Asthma"). Symptoms—wheezing, tightness in the chest, shortness of breath, and coughing—often occur immediately, within minutes of exposure, but inflammatory reactions may take hours or days to develop and then may persist for several days. The symptoms may be mild and occur only occasionally, or they may be severe and occur daily.

Asthma affects around 25 million people in the United States. Since 1980, the number of Americans with asthma has been increasing steadily, despite better treatments and cleaner air.

Prevalence

The prevalence of asthma is higher among children, women, African Americans, Puerto Ricans, and people whose family income is below the poverty line. African Americans are four times more likely to be hospitalized with asthma than are other ethnic groups and five times more likely to die from it. People with low incomes are especially at risk; they are more often exposed to the environmental factors that contribute to asthma, such as air pollutants, allergens indoors, and air pollution from highways, incinerators, and waste facilities outdoors.

Treatment and Prevention of Attacks

The symptoms of an asthma attack can be relieved by the use of a bronchodilator—a fast-acting medication, delivered through an inhaler, that opens the airways. Inhaled corticosteroids and other prescribed medications are needed to treat the underlying inflammation of the airways. People with asthma can monitor their condition by self-testing their peak airflow, the speed at which they can exhale, using a special device. A drop in peak airflow can signal an upcoming attack.

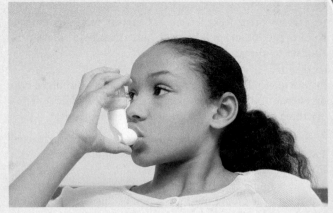

moodboard/Getty Images

Some simple measures can help people avoid allergens and triggers. These measures include using HEPA (high-efficiency particulate air) filters in vacuum cleaners and room air purifiers, covering mattresses and pillows with special covers, avoiding tobacco smoke, and using professional pest control.

SOURCES: Centers for Disease Control and Prevention. 2018. *Most Recent Asthma Data: National Data* (http://www.cdc.gov/asthma/most_recent _data.htm); Akinbami, L. J., A. E. Simon, and K. C. Schoendorf. 2015. Trends in allergy prevalence among children aged 0–17 years by asthma status, United States, 2001–2013. *Journal of Asthma* 15: 1–21.

Asthma is caused by both chronic inflammation of the airways and spasm of the muscles surrounding the airways. The spasm causes constriction, and the inflammation causes the airway linings to swell and secrete extra mucus, which further obstructs the passages.

An asthma attack is initiated by an irritating stimulus in the bronchial tubes. The stimulus may be an inhaled allergen, such as pollen, dust mites, mold, animal dander, or cockroach droppings, or it can be a nonallergen stimulus, such as exercise, cold air, pollutants, tobacco smoke, infection, or stress. In women with asthma, hormonal changes that occur as menstruation starts may increase vulnerability to attacks. Both environmental and genetic factors contribute to the development of asthma.

Anaphylaxis is the most serious—although rare—acute allergic reaction to an antigen that the body has become hypersensitive to (e.g., a bee sting). Anaphylaxis results from a release of histamine throughout the body that can be life threatening. Symptoms may include swelling of the throat, extremely low blood pressure, fainting, heart arrhythmia, and

> **QUICK STATS**
>
> About **8%** of U.S. children and **8%** of U.S. adults currently have asthma.
>
> —Centers for Disease Control and Prevention, 2018

seizures. Anaphylaxis is a medical emergency, and treatment requires immediate injection of epinephrine. People at risk for anaphylaxis should wear medical alert identification and keep self-administrable epinephrine readily available.

Climate Change and Allergies The predicted global changes in climate are likely to exacerbate allergies, including allergic rhinitis and asthma. Global warming is influencing plant and fungal reproduction and thus is influencing both spatial and temporal production of allergens. If warm weather periods lengthen, then the period of pollen release also will be prolonged and the amount of pollen released may increase. Thus, politicians and policymakers must become involved in

anaphylaxis A severe systemic hypersensitive reaction to an allergen characterized by difficulty breathing, low blood pressure, heart arrhythmia, seizure, and sometimes death. **TERMS**

reducing the impact of climate change on human health. As a first step, in 2006 the World Health Organization (WHO), governments of some countries, scientific organizations, and patient advocacy groups formed the Global Alliance against Chronic Respiratory Disease (GARD). One goal of GARD is to prevent or at least lessen risk factors (such as tobacco smoke and other pollutants) that exacerbate allergic responses to allergens.

Dealing with Allergies   If you suspect you might have an allergy, visit your physician or an allergy specialist. There are three general strategies for dealing with allergies:

- *Avoidance.* You may be able to avoid or minimize exposure to allergens by changing your environment or behavior. For example, removing carpets from the bedroom and using special bedding can reduce dust mite contact. Limit pollen exposure by avoiding outdoor activities during peak pollination times, keeping windows shut, and showering and changing clothes following outdoor activities. If you can't part with a pet, keep pets out of bedrooms and frequently vacuum or damp-mop floors.

- *Medication.* A variety of medications are available for allergy sufferers. Many over-the-counter antihistamines are effective at controlling symptoms such as blocked nasal, sinus, or middle ear passages. Prescription corticosteroids delivered by aerosol markedly reduce allergy symptoms by reducing the inflammatory response to the allergen.

- *Immunotherapy.* Referred to as "allergy shots," immunotherapy desensitizes a person to a particular allergen through the administration of gradually increasing doses of the allergen over a period of months or years.

THE SPREAD OF DISEASE

The immune system is operating at all times, maintaining its vigilance when you're well and fighting invaders when you're sick. How does it all feel to you, the host? And how do diseases spread from one person to another, sometimes resulting in epidemics or pandemics? These questions are addressed in this section.

Symptoms and Contagion

The symptoms you experience during an illness are related to the phase of infection and the actions of your immune system. During the first phase of infection, or **incubation period,** when viruses or bacteria are actively multiplying before the immune system has gathered momentum, you may not have

> **incubation period**   The period when bacteria or viruses are actively multiplying inside the body's cells; usually a period without symptoms of illness.   **TERMS**

any symptoms of the illness, but you may be contagious. During the second and third phases of the immune response, you may still be unaware of the infection, or you may "feel a cold coming on." Symptoms first appear during the *prodromal period,* which follows incubation. If you have acquired immunity, the infection may be eradicated during the incubation period or the prodromal period. In this case it does not develop into a full-blown illness.

Many symptoms of an illness are actually due to the body's immune response rather than to the actions or products of the invading organism. For example, fever is caused by the release of certain cytokines by macrophages and other cells during the immune response. These cytokines travel in the bloodstream to the brain and cause the body's thermostat to be reset to a higher level. The resulting elevated temperature helps the body fight against pathogens by enhancing immune responses. (During an illness, it is necessary to lower a fever only if it is uncomfortably high [over 101.5°F] or if it occurs in an infant who is at risk for seizures from fever.) Similarly, you get a runny nose when your lymphocytes destroy infected mucosal cells, leading to increased mucus production. The malaise and fatigue of the flu are caused by pro-inflammatory cytokines.

You may be contagious before you experience any symptoms, and you are contagious as long as your body is releasing infectious microbes. For example, adults who have contracted the flu can infect other people beginning one day *before* symptoms develop and up to five to seven days *afterward.* Children may pass the flu virus for longer than seven days. Symptoms appear one to four days *after* infection.

Some people can be infected with the flu virus and yet perceive no symptoms. These individuals who are asymptomatic are difficult to identify and study, so we do not know why they do not develop disease. The basis is likely to be in their innate and adaptive immune systems. The numerous genes that regulate and mediate immune responses can vary from person to person.

Regardless of the reasons for the asymptomatic state, mathematical models suggest that asymptomatic carriers contribute to the spread of a variety of diseases, such as influenza, Ebola, and others. The possibility that asymptomatic people can be infectious is an important reason that everyone should remain up to date on vaccines.

The Chain of Infection

Infectious diseases are transmitted from one person to another through a series of steps (Figure 18.4). New infections can be prevented by interfering with any step in this process.

Links in the Chain   The chain of infection has six major links:

1. *Pathogen.* The infectious disease cycle begins with a pathogen that enters the body. Many pathogens cause illness by invading body cells; others cause illness by producing toxins that harm tissue.

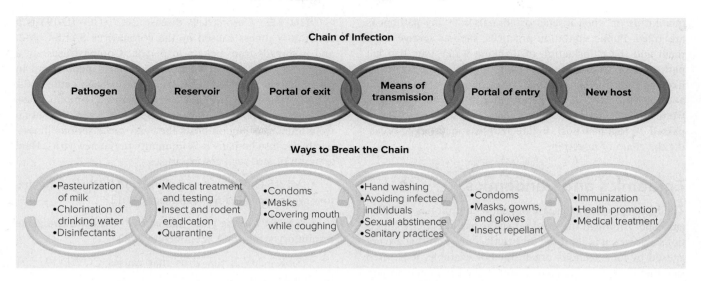

FIGURE 18.4 **The chain of infection.** Any break in the chain of infection can prevent disease.

2. *Reservoir.* The pathogen has a natural environment—called a **reservoir**—in which it typically lives. This reservoir can be a person or an animal. A person who is the reservoir for a pathogen may be ill or may be an asymptomatic carrier who, although having no symptoms, can spread infection.

3. *Portal of exit.* To transmit infection, the pathogen must leave the reservoir through some portal of exit. In the case of a human reservoir, portals of exit include saliva, the mucous membranes, blood, feces, and nose and throat discharges.

4. *Means of transmission.* Transmission can occur directly or indirectly. In *direct transmission,* the pathogen is passed from one person to another without an intermediary. Most common respiratory infections and many intestinal infections are passed directly—for example, when a person with an infectious agent on his or her hands touches someone else. Other means of direct transmission include sexual contact and contact with blood. In *indirect transmission,* animals or insects such as rats, ticks, and mosquitoes serve as **vectors,** carrying the pathogen from one host to another. Pathogens can also be transmitted via contaminated soil, food, or water or from inanimate objects, such as eating utensils, doorknobs, and handkerchiefs. Some pathogens float in the air for long periods, suspended on tiny particles of dust or droplets that can travel long distances before they are inhaled and cause infection.

5. *Portal of entry.* To infect a new host, a pathogen must have a portal of entry into the body. Pathogens can enter through direct contact with or penetration of the skin or mucous membranes, inhalation, or ingestion. Pathogens that enter the skin or mucous membranes can cause a local infection of the tissue, or they may penetrate into the bloodstream or lymphatic system, thereby causing a **systemic infection.** Agents that cause

sexually transmitted infections usually enter the body through the mucous membranes lining the urethra (in males) or the cervix (in females). Organisms that are transmitted via respiratory secretions may cause upper respiratory infections or pneumonia, or they may enter the bloodstream and cause systemic infection. Foodborne and waterborne organisms enter the mouth and travel to the tissue that will best support their reproduction. They may attack the cells of the small intestine or the colon, causing diarrhea, or they may enter the bloodstream via the digestive system and travel to other parts of the body.

6. *The new host.* Once in the new host, a variety of factors determine whether the pathogen will establish itself and cause infection. People with a strong immune system or resistance to a particular pathogen are less likely to become ill than are people with poor immunity. If conditions are right, the pathogen will multiply and produce disease in the new host. In such a case, the new host may become a reservoir from which a new chain of infection can be started.

Breaking the Chain   Interrupting the chain of infection at any point can prevent disease. Strategies for breaking the chain include both public health measures and individual action. For example, a pathogen's reservoir can be isolated or destroyed, as when a sick individual is placed under

---

reservoir   A long-term host in which a pathogen typically lives.

vector   An insect, rodent, or other organism that carries and transmits a pathogen from one host to another.

systemic infection   An infection spread by the blood or lymphatic system to large portions of the body.

TERMS

quarantine or when insects or animals carrying pathogens are killed. Public sanitation practices, such as sewage treatment and the chlorination of drinking water, can also kill pathogens. Transmission can be disrupted through strategies like hand washing and the use of face masks. Immunization and the treatment of infected hosts can stop the pathogen from multiplying, producing a serious disease, and being passed on to a new host. Figure 18.4 lists methods of breaking the chain of infection.

Epidemics and Pandemics

The rapid spread of a disease or health condition is called an **epidemic.** Although the word is usually used to refer to infectious diseases, it is also used for health conditions that are not caused by an infectious organism. For example, it is often said that obesity and diabetes have reached epidemic proportions in the United States.

An important underlying premise of the concept of "epidemic" is that the occurrence of the disease is greater than what is expected normally. Thus, the common cold, which occurs with great frequency, is never classified as an epidemic. Conversely, the term *epidemic* is used to refer to outbreaks of diseases that are not widespread. For example, when 10 infants died in California in 2010 from whooping cough, the incident was referred to as an epidemic.

A **pandemic** is an epidemic that has spread across a large area, such as an entire nation, a continent, or even the world. The term *pandemic* refers exclusively to infectious disease. Human history has been punctuated by numerous pandemics of various diseases, including bubonic plague, smallpox, and influenza. One of the most severe influenza pandemics occurred in 1918–1919, following World War I, when 20–40% of the world's population became ill and as many as 40 million people died. The probability of pandemics has increased over the past century because people have engaged in more global travel and integration, migrated to cities, changed land use, and exploited the natural environment more. These trends will probably continue and intensify. At the time of writing, September 2020, the number of worldwide deaths projected from the coronavirus disease 2019 is in the millions.

Not all widespread infectious diseases are pandemics. An infectious disease is said to be *endemic* when it habitually exists in a certain region. Endemic diseases generally occur at low frequency in particular populations or regions. For example, malaria is endemic to low-altitude areas of northern and eastern South Africa. Seasonal epidemics of malaria can occur in these areas where malaria is endemic.

COVID-19 Coronavirus disease 2019 (COVID-19) is a respiratory illness caused by the coronavirus SARS-CoV-2, and it spreads from person to person. Coronaviruses are a large, diverse family of viruses common in people and in different species of animals, including camels, cattle, cats, dogs, ferrets, and bats. Some coronaviruses commonly cause mild upper-respiratory tract illnesses. But when they jump from animal to human hosts they can cause serious illness, partly because humans lack immunity to the new virus. Here are examples of such coronaviruses:

- MERS-CoV, the virus that caused Middle East respiratory syndrome (MERS), identified in 2012

- SARS-CoV, the virus that caused SARS (severe acute respiratory syndrome), identified in 2003

- SARS-CoV-2, the virus that causes COVID-19, first identified in 2019

COVID-19 and SARS are similar in many ways: They linger in air and on surfaces, and they can lead to potentially serious illness, pneumonia sometimes requiring oxygen or mechanical ventilation, and fatal blood clotting throughout the body. Both viruses can build to worsening symptoms later on in the illness, and they have similar at-risk groups to which they present a more serious threat, such as older adults and those with underlying health conditions. They have no specific proven treatments or vaccines. The receptor binding site of SARS-CoV-2 binds to the host cell receptor with a higher affinity than does that of SARS-CoV, and that may explain its rapid spread. COVID-19 cases can range from mild to severe, whereas SARS cases, in general, were more severe.

COVID-19 symptoms vary tremendously: fever, cough, fatigue, shortness of breath; and less routinely, headache, muscle aches and pains, sore throat, nausea, diarrhea, chills, loss of taste, loss of smell. About half of patients report neurological symptoms. At the time of writing, biotech companies are racing to invent vaccines for COVID-19.

H1N1 Influenza Before the COVID-19 outbreak, the last global pandemic was the 2009 outbreak of H1N1 influenza A virus. Initially called swine flu, this new strain of virus had never before been identified as a cause of human illness. Like COVID-19, H1N1 is an infectious respiratory illness. But it comes from any of several different types and strains of influenza viruses, rather than the single, novel virus that causes COVID-19. The influenza A virus mutates frequently

---

epidemic A rapidly spreading disease or health-related condition.

pandemic A widespread epidemic.

TERMS

Ask Yourself

QUESTIONS FOR CRITICAL THINKING AND REFLECTION

Think about the last time you were sick with a cold, the flu, or an intestinal infection. Can you identify the reservoir from which the infection came? What vector, if any, transmitted the illness to you? Did you pass the infection to anyone else? If so, how?

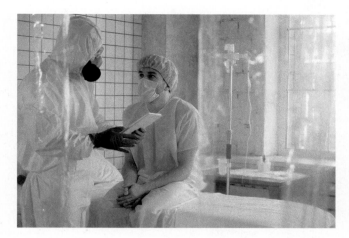

Treating someone with the highly infectious COVID-19 virus involves a careful and meticulous process of putting on and taking off protective gear. The use of protective gear is one strategy for breaking the chain of infection. FunKey Factory/Getty Images

VITAL STATISTICS

Table 18.2 Estimated Annual Deaths Due to Top Infectious Diseases Worldwide

DISEASE	DEATHS
Tuberculosis	1.5 million
Vaccine-preventable diseases	1.5 million
COVID-19	950,000
Pneumonia in children	808,694
HIV/AIDS	770,000
Diarrheal diseases in children	525,000
Malaria	405,000

SOURCES: World Health Organization. 2020. *Tuberculosis* (https://www.who.int/news-room/fact-sheets/detail/tuberculosis); World Health Organization. 2019. *Pneumonia* (https://www.who.int/news-room/fact-sheets/detail/pneumonia); World Health Organization. 2020. *Malaria* (https://www.who.int/news-room/fact-sheets/detail/malaria); Johns Hopkins University and Medicine. 2020. *Maps: Tracking Global Cases* (https://coronavirus.jhu.edu/map.html). World Health Organization. 2020. *Immunization* (http://www.who.int/news-room/fact-sheets/detail/immunization-coverage); World Health Organization. 2017. *Fact Sheet: Diarrhoeal Disease* (http://www.who.int/en/news-room/fact-sheets/detail/diarrhoeal-disease);

during replication, and it can also exchange genes with other influenza A viruses, including strains that infect domestic and wild animals. The H1N1 strain resulted from a combination of genes from four viruses: two from swine flu viruses, one from an avian (bird) flu virus, and one from a human flu virus. The addition of the gene from a human virus meant that humans could be infected with it, and, because it was new, they had no prior immunity.

In June 2009, with cases reported in 74 countries, the World Health Organization declared that a flu pandemic was under way. By February 2010, the WHO reported up to 86 million cases and nearly 18,000 deaths. By May of that year, flu activity had tapered off and declined to normal levels, but the same influenza A (H1N1) virus was the predominant strain during the 2013–2014 influenza season. The WHO continues to track trends globally, and the CDC continues to recommend H1N1 vaccination for persons aged 6 months to 24 years and people aged 25–64 years who are at high risk.

PATHOGENS, DISEASES, AND TREATMENTS

Most microorganisms do not cause disease at all. Some that potentially can cause disease are readily dealt with by the body's defenses discussed earlier in the chapter. However, some microorganisms cause infectious disease even in a healthy person. Worldwide, infectious diseases are responsible for more than 11 million deaths each year. Table 18.2 provides data on some of the more deadly infectious diseases. The pathogens that cause infectious diseases include bacteria, viruses, fungi, protozoa, and parasitic worms (Figure 18.5). Infections can occur almost anywhere in or on the body. Examples of common infections are bronchitis, which is an infection of the airways (bronchi); meningitis, infection of the tissue surrounding the brain and spinal cord; and conjunctivitis (pinkeye), infection of the layer of cells surrounding the eyes.

Bacteria

The most abundant living things on earth are **bacteria.** Bacteria are often classified by their shape: bacilli (rod-shaped), cocci (spherical), spirochete (spiral-shaped), or vibrios (comma-shaped).

Bacteria play very important roles in human health. For example, our gut microbiota include at least a thousand different species of bacteria. Remarkably, the genetic material of all these bacteria adds up to more than 150 times as many genes as appear in our genome. These bacteria have several important functions, including assisting the digestion of certain foods and the production of vitamin K and some B vitamins, and controlling the growth of pathogenic bacteria by stimulating the mucosal immune system. In addition, there is evidence from studies of mice that gut microbiota influence the development of autoimmune disease. We also have bacteria in our skin and in our reproductive tracts. About 100 species of bacteria can cause disease in humans.

> **bacterium** A microscopic single-celled organism with a cell wall (plural, *bacteria*). Bacteria may be helpful or harmful to humans.. **TERMS**

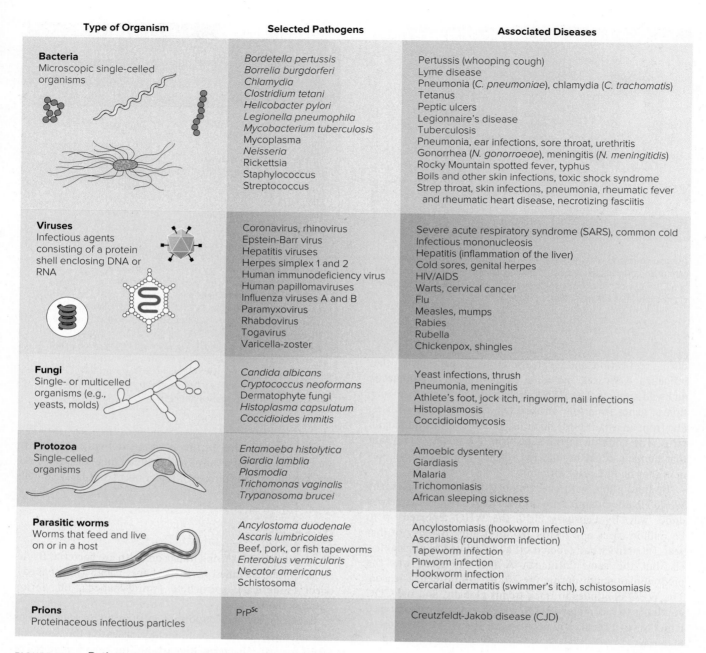

Type of Organism	Selected Pathogens	Associated Diseases
Bacteria Microscopic single-celled organisms	*Bordetella pertussis* *Borrelia burgdorferi* *Chlamydia* *Clostridium tetani* *Helicobacter pylori* *Legionella pneumophila* *Mycobacterium tuberculosis* Mycoplasma *Neisseria* Rickettsia Staphylococcus Streptococcus	Pertussis (whooping cough) Lyme disease Pneumonia (*C. pneumoniae*), chlamydia (*C. trachomatis*) Tetanus Peptic ulcers Legionnaire's disease Tuberculosis Pneumonia, ear infections, sore throat, urethritis Gonorrhea (*N. gonorroeae*), meningitis (*N. meningitidis*) Rocky Mountain spotted fever, typhus Boils and other skin infections, toxic shock syndrome Strep throat, skin infections, pneumonia, rheumatic fever and rheumatic heart disease, necrotizing fasciitis
Viruses Infectious agents consisting of a protein shell enclosing DNA or RNA	Coronavirus, rhinovirus Epstein-Barr virus Hepatitis viruses Herpes simplex 1 and 2 Human immunodeficiency virus Human papillomaviruses Influenza viruses A and B Paramyxovirus Rhabdovirus Togavirus Varicella-zoster	Severe acute respiratory syndrome (SARS), common cold Infectious mononucleosis Hepatitis (inflammation of the liver) Cold sores, genital herpes HIV/AIDS Warts, cervical cancer Flu Measles, mumps Rabies Rubella Chickenpox, shingles
Fungi Single- or multicelled organisms (e.g., yeasts, molds)	*Candida albicans* *Cryptococcus neoformans* Dermatophyte fungi *Histoplasma capsulatum* *Coccidioides immitis*	Yeast infections, thrush Pneumonia, meningitis Athlete's foot, jock itch, ringworm, nail infections Histoplasmosis Coccidioidomycosis
Protozoa Single-celled organisms	*Entamoeba histolytica* *Giardia lamblia* *Plasmodia* *Trichomonas vaginalis* *Trypanosoma brucei*	Amoebic dysentery Giardiasis Malaria Trichomoniasis African sleeping sickness
Parasitic worms Worms that feed and live on or in a host	*Ancylostoma duodenale* *Ascaris lumbricoides* Beef, pork, or fish tapeworms *Enterobius vermicularis* *Necator americanus* Schistosoma	Ancylostomiasis (hookworm infection) Ascariasis (roundworm infection) Tapeworm infection Pinworm infection Hookworm infection Cercarial dermatitis (swimmer's itch), schistosomiasis
Prions Proteinaceous infectious particles	PrP^{Sc}	Creutzfeldt-Jakob disease (CJD)

FIGURE 18.5 **Pathogens and associated infectious diseases.**

Pathogenic bacteria cause disease when they release toxins or grow in tissues that are normally sterile, such as the bladder. They can enter the body through a cut in the skin, an insect bite, contaminated food or drink, sexual activity, or any of several other means. (See the box "Strategies for Avoiding Illnesses.")

pneumonia Inflammation of the lungs, typically caused by infection or exposure to chemical toxins or irritants.

TERMS

Pneumonia **Pneumonia** is an inflammation of the lungs. Although it can be caused by viruses or fungi, bacterial pneumonia is the most common and the most treatable. Pneumonia often follows another illness, such as a cold or the flu, but the symptoms are typically more severe—fever, chills, shortness of breath, increased mucus production, and cough. Pneumonia is one of the 10 leading causes of death for Americans; people most at risk for severe infection include those under age 2 or over age 75 and those with chronic health problems such as heart disease, asthma, or HIV. Worldwide, pneumonia is the leading cause of death for children under 5 years of age.

The most common cause of bacterial pneumonia is *Streptococcus pneumoniae*, or pneumococcus. A vaccine is available for pneumococcal pneumonia and is recommended for all adults age 65 and over and others at risk. Other bacteria that may cause pneumonia include *Haemophilus influenzae, Chlamydia pneumoniae,* and *Mycoplasma pneumoniae.* Mycoplasma is a very small bacterium; *M. pneumoniae* causes a mild form of pneumonia often called "walking pneumonia." Outbreaks of infection with mycoplasmas are relatively common among young adults, especially in crowded settings such as dormitories. Bacterial pneumonia can be treated with antibiotics, discussed below.

Meningitis Inflammation of the *meninges,* the protective membranes covering the brain and spinal cord, is called **meningitis.** Inflammation is usually caused by infection of the fluid surrounding the brain. Most cases of meningitis are viral. Viral meningitis is usually mild and resolves without medical intervention. Bacterial meningitis, however, can be life threatening and requires immediate treatment with antibiotics. Symptoms of meningitis include fever, a severe headache, stiff neck, sensitivity to light, and confusion. Symptoms can appear quickly or over a few days. Immediate treatment is needed because death can occur within hours. Before the 1990s, *Haemophilus influenzae* type b (Hib) was the leading cause of bacterial meningitis, but routine vaccination of children has reduced the occurrence of Hib meningitis. Today *Neisseria meningitidis* (meningococcus) and *Streptococcus pneumoniae* (pneumococcus) are the leading causes of bacterial meningitis, particularly in adolescents and young adults.

In the United States, between 8000 and 9000 cases of meningitis are reported each year, although the actual numbers are probably higher. The disease is fatal in 10-15% of cases, and 10–20% of people who recover have permanent disabilities, including brain damage, seizures, and hearing loss. Worldwide, meningitis kills about 170,000 people each year, particularly in the so-called meningitis belt in sub-Saharan Africa.

A vaccine is available, but it is not effective against all strains of meningitis-causing bacteria. The CDC recommends routine vaccination of children aged 11–18 years, previously unvaccinated adolescents at high school entry, and first-year college students who live in dormitories.

Strep Throat and Other Streptococcal Infections **Streptococcus** is the genus name of a group of bacteria that cause several diseases in humans. Streptococcal pharyngitis, or strep throat, is characterized by a red, sore throat with white patches on the tonsils, swollen lymph nodes, fever, and headache. Typically the streptococcus bacterium is spread from an infected individual through close contact via respiratory droplets that are released when the infected person sneezes or coughs. If left untreated, strep throat can develop into the more serious rheumatic fever (see Chapter 16). Other streptococcal infections include scarlatina (scarlet fever), characterized by a sore throat, fever, bright red tongue, and rash over the upper body; impetigo, a

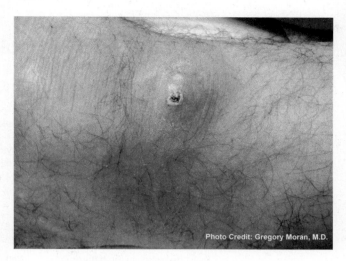

Photo Credit: Gregory Moran, M.D.

Skin infections caused by methicillin-resistant *Staphylococcus aureus* (MRSA) can be very hard to treat.

SOURCE: Gregory Moran, M.D./Centers for Disease Control and Prevention

superficial skin infection most common among children; and erysipelas, which causes inflammation of skin and underlying tissues. Streptococcal infections are treated with antibiotics. If you have a streptococcal infection, you can minimize the risk of spreading it by washing your hands well, especially before preparing foods, and by staying home until at least 24 hours after starting a course of antibiotics.

A particularly virulent type of streptococcus can invade the bloodstream, spread to other parts of the body, and produce dangerous systemic illness. It can also cause a serious but rare infection of the deeper layers of the skin, a condition called necrotizing fasciitis or "flesh-eating strep." This dangerous infection is characterized by tissue death and is treated with antibiotics and removal of the infected tissue or limb. Other species of streptococci are implicated in pneumonia, endocarditis (infection of the heart lining and valves), and serious infections in pregnant women and newborns.

Toxic Shock Syndrome and Other Staphylococcal Infections **Staphylococcus** (staph) bacteria are commonly found on the skin and in the nasal passages of healthy people. For example, *Staphylococcus aureus* occurs on 15–40% of people who show no signs of disease. Occasionally, however, staphylococci enter the body and cause an infection, ranging

TERMS

meningitis Infection of the meninges (membranes covering the brain and spinal cord).

streptococcus Any of a genus (*Streptococcus*) of spherical bacteria; streptococcal species can cause skin infections, strep throat, rheumatic fever, pneumonia, scarlet fever, and other diseases.

staphylococcus Any of a genus (*Staphylococcus*) of spherical, clustered bacteria commonly found on the skin or in the nasal passages; staphylococcal species may enter the body and cause conditions such as boils, pneumonia, toxic shock syndrome, and severe skin infections.

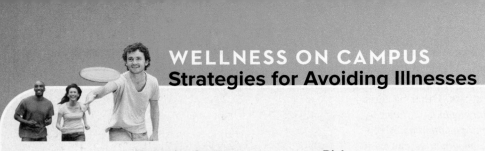

WELLNESS ON CAMPUS
Strategies for Avoiding Illnesses

Where	Behavior Strategy	Risk	Tips
Dormitory/Shared Living	Don't share: • Deodorant • Makeup • Towels • Sponges • Razors • Toothbrushes	Anything that contacts skin or body fluids can spread viruses and bacteria	Keep hand towels and personal items separate from others' items Disinfect and dry out bathroom and kitchen areas frequently
	Don't do dishes in the bathroom	Bathroom surfaces are quickly contaminated with pathogens like norovirus and *Salmonella*	Use food preparation area sink. If unavailable, use a clean plastic dish pan or disinfect bathroom sink
	Routinely clean the dorm room: sweep, dust, vacuum, disinfect The dirtiest areas of a dorm room include: • Desk and dresser surfaces • Door handles • Light switches • Bed sheets	Pathogens and allergens like mold can cause respiratory problems Bed sheets and pillowcases collect dead skin cells, body oils and fluids, which can cause acne; allergens and dust mites can cause allergies, eczema, and asthma. Bed linens can also house *Staphylococcus* bacteria and viruses that cause the common cold and stomach flu	Hire a cleaner with fees from roommates who don't clean
	Get vaccines and flu shot before school and flu season begin	Unvaccinated college students increase risk for everyone else during flu season Vaccines protect from other infections that thrive in close living conditions, like meningitis	Prepare for illness with OTC medications and a first-aid kit instead of having to hunt for them when you're sick Rally roommates to share costs for items you all may need
	Seek medical evaluation and treatment for prolonged symptoms Avoid coughing and sneezing on, and touching others	What may appear to be a common cold can be more serious and, if left untreated, can require an emergency room visit You can contract the flu from someone 6 feet away	Ask friends to help each other rest by bringing food and running errands If your roommate is ill, wash hands, surfaces, handles, use separate towels, and stay on your side of the room
Gym or swimming pool	Wipe away sweat and disinfect exercise equipment at the gym	Sweat and spittle can spread pathogens like staphylococcus bacteria and influenza virus	Stock a dedicated gym bag with disinfectant wipes, clean towels, and flip-flops. Regularly clean the bag!
	Wear flip-flops or waterproof sandals in locker rooms, bathrooms, and communal showers; dry feet well afterward	Warmth and moisture help *tinea pedis* thrive and promote fungal infections like athlete's foot and nail fungus and HPV, which can cause viral infections like plantar warts	Forgot your flip-flops? Clean and thoroughly dry your feet after contact with floors. Avoid contact with floors if your feet have open cuts or wounds
Classroom	Don't go to class sick	You may infect other students, teachers, and staff	Know the attendance policies of your university and classes Save absences for when you're actually sick Know how to access health services and where the health center or clinic is

Where	Behavior Strategy	Risk	Tips
Dining halls or other food environments	Don't share cups, water bottles, or eating utensils	Viruses spread easily through saliva	
	Don't eat old food or food that's been sitting out long	Resist that old slice of pizza. Food left out at temperatures between 40°F and 140°F (the temperature range known as the "danger zone") allow the rapid growth of bacteria like *Staphylococcus aureus*, *Salmonella enteritidis*, *E. coli*, and *Campylobacter* within two hours	Cool and store leftovers within two hours
		Bacteria such as *Listeria monocytogenes* can grow on foods in the refrigerator	
	Don't eat food in classrooms, libraries, computer labs, or study areas	Surfaces in rooms not meant for eating are likely more contaminated than those in dining halls, which are washed and disinfected more regularly	Disinfect surfaces with wipes if you must eat in a communal non-eating room
On you	Frequently clean and disinfect your germiest objects: • Cell phone • Computer keyboard • Bookbag, purse • Headphones (earbuds)	These items tend to come with us everywhere we go, but don't get cleaned or disinfected nearly as often as they should. One in six cell phones tested positive for *E. coli* (from fecal matter); one in four had *Staphylococcus aureus*	Sanitize cell phones and earbuds daily with sanitation wipes; throw your bookbag in the washing machine; disinfect purses
		Computer keyboards commonly house *E. coli* and *Staphylococcus aureus*; viruses may also be transmitted on keyboards. Crumbs found in keyboards encourage bacterial growth	
		Bookbags and purses come in frequent contact with floors—even restroom floors; avoid laying them on beds, surfaces where you eat, or near your face and mouth	
		Potential pathogens like *Staphylococcus* and others can greatly multiply on headset devices after one hour of use	
	Greetings: Offer an "elbow-bump" over a handshake or high-five, or just say hello	Handshakes transmit lots of germs, and students who regularly shake hands have been shown to get sick more often than those who don't. High-fives transmit half the germs of a handshake, and fist bumps 1/20th	Carry a small bottle of hand sanitizer in your bookbag supplies

from minor skin infections such as boils to very serious conditions such as blood infections and pneumonia. The risk of a serious staph infection is higher in persons with certain medical conditions, including people suffering from malnutrition, alcoholism, intravenous drug use, diabetes, or kidney failure.

Staphylococcus aureus is responsible for many cases of toxic shock syndrome (TSS). The bacteria produce a toxin that causes a massive proliferation of T cells that can bind to it. The staphylococcus toxins are referred to as "super antigens" because the massive proliferation of T cells results in excessive production of pro-inflammatory cytokines. This "cytokine storm" causes tissue damage, widespread coagulation of blood in the blood vessels, and ultimately organ failure. TSS was first diagnosed in women using highly absorbent tampons, which appear to allow the growth of staphylococci; however, about half of all cases occur in men and in women not using tampons. (See Chapter 7 for information about toxic shock syndrome as it relates to contraception.)

A serious antibiotic-resistant infection is caused by a staphylococcus bacterium known as methicillin-resistant *Staphylococcus aureus* (MRSA). Many cases of MRSA infection occur in hospitalized patients, and these infections tend to be severe. They include infections of surgical wounds, pneumonia, urinary tract infections, and blood infections. MRSA is also common in the community (outside hospital settings), where it usually infects the skin, causing painful lesions that resemble infected spider bites. The spread of MRSA infection is associated with places where people are in close contact with one another, such as locker rooms and playing fields. Athletes are particularly at risk and should keep any cuts or abrasions covered. The best defense against MRSA, whether in health care settings or in the community, is good hygiene and frequent hand washing.

Tuberculosis   Caused by the bacterium *Mycobacterium tuberculosis,* **tuberculosis (TB)** is a chronic bacterial infection that usually affects the lungs, though it can affect other organs as well. TB is spread via the respiratory route. Symptoms include coughing, fatigue, night sweats, weight loss, and fever.

Between 10 and 15 million Americans have been infected with *M. tuberculosis* and continue to carry it. The immune system usually prevents the disease from becoming active. In the United States, active TB is most common among people infected with HIV, recent immigrants from countries where TB is endemic, and those who live in inner cities. In 2019, a total of 8920 new cases of TB were reported—an incidence of 2.7 cases per 100,000 population. This is the lowest rate since national tracking began in 1953, but the rate of decline has slowed. Across the world, the COVID-19 lockdowns have exacerbated TB treatment by raising barriers to patients who must travel to get diagnoses and treatment. The longer a person goes undiagnosed, the more likely the disease will spread.

TB is a leading cause of death in people with HIV infection. Many strains of tuberculosis respond to antibiotics, but only over a course of treatment lasting 6–12 months. Failure to complete treatment can lead to relapse and the development of strains of antibiotic-resistant bacteria. Multidrug-resistant TB (MDR TB) is resistant to at least two of the best anti-TB drugs. Extensively drug-resistant TB (XDR TB) is resistant to those drugs as well as some second-line drugs. XDR TB is relatively rare, but patients with this form of TB have fewer and less effective treatment options.

Tick-Borne Infections   Some diseases are transmitted via insect vectors. Lyme disease is one such infection, and it accounts for more than 30,000 reported cases per year, although the actual number may be as high as 300,000. It is spread by the bite of a tick that is infected with the spiral-shaped bacterium *Borrelia burgdorferi.* Ticks acquire the bacterium by ingesting the blood of an infected animal. They can then transmit the microbe to their next host. The deer tick is responsible for transmitting Lyme disease bacteria to humans in the northeastern and north-central United States; on the Pacific Coast, the culprit is the western black-legged tick. Lyme disease has been reported in 48 states, but significant risk of infection is found in only about 100 counties in 10 states located in the northeastern and mid-Atlantic seaboard, the upper north-central region, and parts of northern California.

Symptoms of Lyme disease vary but typically occur in three stages. In the first stage, about 80% of victims develop a bull's-eye-shaped red rash expanding from the area of the bite, usually about two weeks after the bite occurs. The second stage occurs weeks to months later in 10–20% of untreated patients. Symptoms may involve the nervous and cardiovascular systems and can include impaired coordination, partial facial paralysis, and heart rhythm abnormalities. These symptoms usually disappear within a few weeks. Lyme disease can also cause fetal damage or death at any stage of pregnancy. Lyme disease is treatable at all stages, although arthritis symptoms arising in the third stage may not resolve completely. Lyme disease is preventable by avoiding contact with ticks, for example by wearing tick-repellent clothing or applying tick-repellent sprays, or by removing a tick before it has had the chance to transmit the infection.

Rocky Mountain spotted fever and typhus are caused by the *rickettsia* bacterium and are also transmitted via tick bites. Rocky Mountain spotted fever is characterized by sudden onset of fever, headache, and muscle pain, followed by development of a spotted rash. Ehrlichiosis, another tick-borne disease, typically causes less severe symptoms.

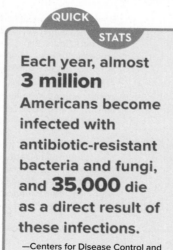

tuberculosis (TB)   A chronic bacterial infection that usually affects the lungs.   TERMS

Ulcers   About 25 million Americans suffer from *ulcers*, which are sores in the lining of the stomach or the first section of the small intestine (duodenum). Long-term use of nonsteroidal anti-inflammatory drugs (NSAIDs) can contribute to the development of ulcers. However, up to 90% of ulcers are caused by infection with the bacterium *Helicobacter pylori*. If tests show the presence of *H. pylori*, antibiotics often cure the infection and the ulcers. Individuals who take NSAIDs and contract ulcers should be tested for *H. pylori* because they are likely infected, and termination of NSAIDs alone will not cure the ulcers.

Other Bacterial Infections   The following are a few of the many other infections caused by bacteria:

• **Tetanus.** Also known as lockjaw, tetanus is caused by the bacterium *Clostridium tetani*, which thrives in deep puncture wounds and produces a deadly toxin. The toxin causes muscular stiffness and spasms, and infection is fatal in about 30% of cases. Due to widespread vaccination, tetanus is rare in the United States. Worldwide, however, approximately 31,000 newborns die each year through infection by unsterile cutting of the umbilical cord.

• **Clostridium difficile.** Another type of *Clostridium* bacteria, called *Clostridium difficile* (*C. diff*), has joined MRSA as a major emerging threat in American health care settings, particularly hospitals. Considered a health-care-associated infection, *C. diff* occurs in patients with conditions requiring prolonged use of antibiotics. It causes inflammation of the colon, resulting in diarrhea, fever, and nausea. Bacterial spores can live outside the body for long periods and can be found on objects like medical equipment, bathroom fixtures, and bed linens, as well as on people's hands. Most cases of *C. diff* infection respond to a new class of antibiotics that selectively kills *C. diff* without affecting the many bacterial species that populate the normal, healthy intestine. Nevertheless, about 13,000 people die each year from this infection. The CDC recommends that doctors, nurses, and other health care providers wash their hands frequently to reduce the spread of the bacterium.

• **Pertussis.** Also known as whooping cough, pertussis is a highly contagious respiratory illness caused by the bacterium *Bordetella pertussis*. Pertussis is characterized by bursts of rapid coughing, followed by a long attempt at inhalation that is often accompanied by a high-pitched whoop. Symptoms may persist for two to eight weeks. The number of pertussis cases in the United States has alternately risen and fallen over the past two decades; in 2019 there were close to 15,700 cases. Those at high risk include infants and children who are too young to be fully vaccinated and those who have not completed the primary vaccination series. Adolescents and adults become susceptible when immunity from vaccination wanes, so a booster shot is recommended at 11–12 years or during adolescence and thereafter every 10 years. Adults account for about 24% of whooping cough cases.

• **Urinary tract infections (UTIs).** Infection of the bladder and urethra is most common among sexually active women, but UTIs can occur in anyone. The bacterium *Escherichia coli* (*E. coli*) is the most common infectious agent, responsible for about 80% of all UTIs. Infection most often occurs when bacteria from the digestive tract that live on the skin around the anus get pushed toward the opening of the urethra during sexual intercourse; the bacteria then travel up the urethra and into the bladder. Urinating before and after intercourse may help prevent UTIs.

• **Travelers' diarrhea (TD).** Symptoms include abdominal cramps, nausea, vomiting, and fever. The most common cause of TD are bacterial pathogens. If left untreated, bacterial TD lasts about 3–7 days. Protozoa account for approximately 10% of TD cases and can last weeks or even months if left untreated. Intestinal viruses account for 5–8% of cases and last 2–3 days. Treatments include fluid and electrolyte replenishment and antimotility drugs such as loperamide. Antibiotic treatment of bacterial TD is discouraged because of the possibility of triggering a different infection.

Other illnesses caused by bacteria include foodborne illness, discussed in Chapter 13, and sexually transmitted infections, discussed in Chapter 19.

Antibiotic Treatments   The body's immune system can fight off many, if not most, bacterial infections. However, even as the body musters its defenses, some bacteria can cause a great deal of damage. Antibiotics can help the body deal with these infections. **Antibiotics** are drugs that either inhibit the growth of bacteria or kill them. Some antibiotics have also been developed to inhibit fungi and protozoa, but antibiotics with antibacterial activity are the most widely used, and these are the ones we will discuss here.

ACTIONS OF ANTIBIOTICS   Antibiotics both naturally occur and are manufactured synthetically. Antibacterial antibiotics are categorized based on their mechanism of action. The majority of antibiotics inhibit the synthesis of the bacterial cell wall. The second largest group interferes with the production of bacterial proteins. A third class prevents the replication of the bacterial DNA.

ANTIBIOTIC RESISTANCE   Antibiotics have saved millions of lives. However, their overuse and misuse has led to the emergence of antibiotic-resistant bacteria. A bacterium can become resistant from a chance genetic mutation or through the transfer of genetic material from one bacterium to another. When exposed to antibiotics, resistant bacteria can grow and flourish while the antibiotic-sensitive bacteria die off. Antibiotic-resistant strains of many common bacteria, including strains of gonorrhea, salmonella, and tuberculosis, have developed. Antibiotic resistance is a major factor contributing to the rise in problematic infectious diseases. The CDC estimates that about 30% of antibiotic prescriptions in the United States are unnecessary.

---

antibiotic   A synthetic or naturally occurring substance that kills or inhibits the growth of bacteria, fungi, or protozoa.   **TERMS**

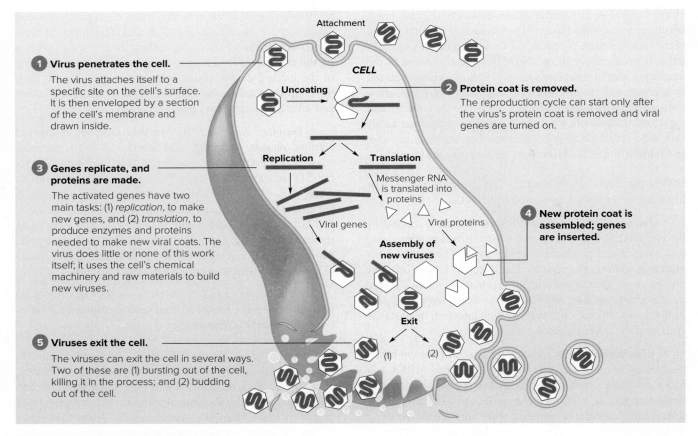

FIGURE 18.6 **Life cycle of a virus.**

① **Virus penetrates the cell.**
The virus attaches itself to a specific site on the cell's surface. It is then enveloped by a section of the cell's membrane and drawn inside.

③ **Genes replicate, and proteins are made.**
The activated genes have two main tasks: (1) *replication*, to make new genes, and (2) *translation*, to produce enzymes and proteins needed to make new viral coats. The virus does little or none of this work itself; it uses the cell's chemical machinery and raw materials to build new viruses.

⑤ **Viruses exit the cell.**
The viruses can exit the cell in several ways. Two of these are (1) bursting out of the cell, killing it in the process; and (2) budding out of the cell.

Attachment

CELL

Uncoating

② **Protein coat is removed.**
The reproduction cycle can start only after the virus's protein coat is removed and viral genes are turned on.

Replication   Translation

Messenger RNA is translated into proteins

Viral genes   Viral proteins

④ **New protein coat is assembled; genes are inserted.**

Assembly of new viruses

Exit
(1)   (2)

The more often bacteria encounter antibiotics, the more likely they are to develop resistance. Resistance is promoted when people fail to take the full course of an antibiotic or when they inappropriately take antibiotics for viral infections. Another possible source of resistance is the use of antibiotics in agriculture, which is estimated to account for 50–80% of the 25,000 tons of antibiotics used annually in the United States. At least four species of antibiotic-resistant bacteria have been transmitted from food animals to humans, leading the U.S. Food and Drug Administration (FDA) to issue guidelines to the pharmaceutical industry regarding the use of new antibiotics in food-producing animals. Recent studies show that antibiotics cause long-term changes to the protective bacteria in our bodies and may cause an increased susceptibility to infections and disease.

You can help prevent the development of antibiotic-resistant strains of bacteria by using antibiotics properly:

• Don't ask your doctor for an antibiotic every time you get sick. Antibiotics are helpful for bacterial infections but are ineffective against viruses.

• Use antibiotics as directed, and finish the full course of medication even if you begin to feel better. Doing so helps ensure that all targeted bacteria are killed off.

• Never take an antibiotic without a prescription. If you take an antibiotic for a viral infection, your illness will not improve.

WHY THE FDA BANNED SOME ANTIBACTERIAL SOAPS In 2019, the FDA banned additives found in many antibacterial soap products. Beyond manufacturers' failing to prove that the products were more effective than regular soap, the banned additives were found to harm humans and the environment; they also increased the risk of generating drug-resistant bacteria. When regular handwashing is not available, however, hand sanitizers, wipes, or antibacterial products without the 19 banned additives are still used, especially in healthcare settings.

Viruses

A **virus** is a microscopic organism consisting of genetic material covered by a protein coat. Visible only with an electron (high-magnification) microscope, viruses are about one one-hundredth of the size of a typical bacterium. Viruses lack the enzymes essential to energy production and protein synthesis in normal animal cells, and they can replicate only inside the cells of another organism—acting as a parasite. Once a virus is inside the host cell, it sheds its protein covering and exploits

virus A very small infectious agent composed of nucleic acid (DNA or RNA) surrounded by a protein coat; lacks an independent metabolism and reproduces only within a host cell.

TERMS

Table 18.3	Is It a Cold or the Flu?	
SYMPTOMS	COLD	FLU
Fever	Rare	Usual; high (100–102°F; occasionally higher, especially in young children); lasts 3–4 days
Headache	Rare	Common
General aches, pains	Slight	Usual; often severe
Fatigue, weakness	Sometimes	Usual; can last up to 2–3 weeks
Extreme exhaustion	Never	Usual; at the beginning of the illness
Stuffy nose	Common	Sometimes
Sneezing	Usual	Sometimes
Sore throat	Common	Sometimes
Chest discomfort, cough	Mild to moderate; hacking cough	Common; can become severe
Treatment	Antihistamines, decongestants, nonsteroidal anti-inflammatory medicines	Antiviral medicines—see your health care provider
Prevention	Wash your hands often with soap and water; avoid close contact with anyone who has a cold	Annual vaccination; antiviral medicines—see your health care provider
Complications	Sinus infection; middle ear infection; asthma	Bronchitis; pneumonia; can worsen chronic conditions; can be life-threatening (complications are more likely in the elderly, those with chronic conditions, young children, and pregnant women)

SOURCE: Centers for Disease Control and Prevention. 2019. *Cold Versus Flu* (https://www.cdc.gov/flu/symptoms/coldflu.htm).

the host's cellular machinery to produce more viruses like itself (Figure 18.6). The immune system of the host responds by producing substances called *interferons*—the first line of defense against viral infection. Interferons block the spread of virus infection to other cells in the body and can stimulate the immune system to kill infected cells.

But sometimes the immune system gets hijacked, as in the case of SARS-CoV-2, a trickster that causes COVID-19. It recruits host cells to replicate viral proteins instead of its own, lops off needed cell markers that direct the cell to clean away its debris, camouflages its own viral genes so that host proteins don't chop up viral RNA, and pokes a hole in the infected cell membrane to ease viral escape. The virus even generates proteins to tell the infected host cell to commit suicide—a real-life blueprint for a horror movie.

Most contagious diseases are caused by viruses. Different viruses infect different kinds of cells, and the seriousness of the disease they cause depends greatly on which kind of cell is infected. The viruses that cause colds, for example, attack upper respiratory tract cells; because these cells are constantly replaced, the disease is mild in otherwise healthy individuals. In contrast, SARS-CoV-2 attacks both upper and lower respiratory tract cells, wreaking heavy damage. HIV, a virus that attacks the cells of the immune system, can destroy the body's ability to fight infectious diseases and is thus extremely serious.

The Common Cold Although generally brief, lasting only one to two weeks, colds often interfere with your normal activities. A cold may be caused by any of more than 200 viruses. Rhinoviruses and coronaviruses cause a large percentage of all colds among adults. Cold viruses have been with us forever, but their DNA mutates frequently and requires us to

produce new immunity and vaccines to the new strands. In contrast, the SARS-CoV-2 virus mutates relatively slowly.

Cold viruses are almost always transmitted by hand-to-hand contact. To lessen your risk of contracting a cold, wash your hands frequently.

If you catch a cold, over-the-counter (OTC) cold remedies may relieve your symptoms, but they do not eliminate the virus (see the box "Preventing and Treating Contagious Respiratory Virus Infections: The Common Cold and COVID-19"). Sometimes it is difficult to determine whether your symptoms are due to a virus (as in colds, flu, and some sinus infections), a bacterium (as in other sinus infections), or an allergy, but this information is important for appropriate treatment (Table 18.3). For example, antibiotics will not affect a viral infection but will help treat a bacterial sinus infection.

Influenza Commonly called the flu, **influenza** is an infection of the respiratory tract caused by the influenza virus. (Many people use the term "stomach flu" to describe gastrointestinal illnesses, but these infections are actually caused by organisms other than influenza viruses.) Influenza is more serious than the common cold, usually including a fever and extreme fatigue. Most people who get the flu recover within one to two weeks, but some develop potentially life-threatening complications, such as pneumonia. The highest rates of infection occur in children. Influenza is highly contagious and is spread via respiratory droplets.

> **influenza**   Infection of the respiratory tract by the influenza virus, which is highly infectious and prone to variation; the form changes rapidly; commonly known as the flu.   **TERMS**

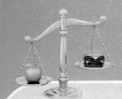

CRITICAL CONSUMER
Preventing and Treating Contagious Respiratory Virus Infections: The Common Cold and COVID-19

Prevention

Colds and other respiratory virus infections are usually spread by hand-to-hand contact with an infected person or with doorknobs and remote controls that an infected person has handled. Averting both the common cold—sometimes caused by a coronavirus—and the recently discovered coronavirus, SARS-CoV-19, requires similar practices, though their histories vary.

Vaccines and Antiviral Drugs

At the time of writing, we have neither a vaccine nor an antiviral drug able to combat COVID-19 spread. Strategies for vaccines vary, but they mainly aim to train the immune system to interfere with the replication of viruses or to make antibodies that recognize and block the spike protein that the SARS-CoV-19 uses to enter human cells. Vaccines also work to prompt the body to generate antibodies that block other viral proteins, or to make T cells that can recognize and kill infected cells. Essential regions of a virus that have few mutations over generations appear to make especially good targets to attack with antiviral drugs because the drugs could deprive the virus of speedy mutations that help it evade our immune systems.

Since each infected person normally infects at least two others—unless social distancing and preventive strategies are practiced—and almost no one has immunity to a new virus, epidemiologists suggest that the virus may continue to spread to more than a billion people. Averting this great danger demands our focused effort.

While we wait for a therapeutic solution to coronavirus disease, we can adopt sensible preventive practices as advised by the CDC and WHO. These precautions will help protect you and others against COVID-19 and other virus diseases, like the common cold and influenza.

Public Practices

• Wear a mask in public settings and when around people who don't live with you.

• Do not shake hands. Keep your distance—six feet is not too far. Replace greetings with noncontact routines.

• In public spaces, avoid touching surfaces with your bare hands.

• Wash your hands thoroughly (20–30 seconds) and frequently with soap and water. Soap dissolves the lipid (fatty) membrane around the virus.

• Take pains not to touch your eyes, nose, mouth, or face with unwashed hands. A mask can remind you.

• Don't open doors with your bare hand: instead use your foot, the back of your hand, your elbow, or your shoulder.

• Use a disposable rag or wipe for handling railings and dial pads.

• Turn away from people when you cough or sneeze, and do so into a tissue; in a pinch, use your elbow.

• Stay home if you are sick.

• Avoid crowds.

The most effective way to prevent the flu is through annual vaccination. Because flu viruses are constantly changing, the influenza vaccine composition is revised every year. More than 100 national influenza centers in over 100 countries conduct year-round influenza surveillance by testing thousands of influenza virus samples from patients. Although the WHO recommends specific vaccine viruses (usually three or four) to be included in the flu vaccines, each country decides its own vaccine composition. In the United States, the FDA makes the final decision. The CDC recommends vaccination for all people aged 6 months and over. Residents of nursing homes and long-term care facilities, health care workers, and household contacts and caregivers of children up to age 5 years are particularly at risk. A nasal aerosol vaccine is available for healthy nonpregnant people aged 2–49 years.

Measles, Mumps, and Rubella Due to effective vaccines, three viral childhood illnesses that have decreased in the United States are measles, mumps, and rubella. Measles and rubella are generally characterized by rash and fever. Measles can occasionally cause more severe illness, including liver or brain infection or pneumonia. Worldwide, more than 140,000 people die each year from measles. Measles is a highly contagious disease. Before the introduction of vaccines, more than 90% of Americans contracted measles by age 15.

Rubella can be transmitted by a pregnant woman to her fetus, causing miscarriage, stillbirth, or severe birth defects, including deafness, eye and heart defects, and mental impairment.

Mumps generally causes swelling of the parotid (salivary) glands, located just below and in front of the ears. This virus can also cause meningitis and, in males, inflammation of the testes.

Home Treatments

- Get extra rest so that your body can work on healing itself.
- If you have a bad cough or fever or feel unwell, stay home from school and work. This may hasten your recovery and reduce the risk of infecting others.
- Drink plenty of liquids, and avoid alcoholic beverages to prevent dehydration. Hot liquids such as herbal tea and clear chicken soup will soothe a sore throat and loosen secretions.
- Gargle with slightly salty water.
- Use a humidifier to help eliminate nasal stuffiness and soothe inflamed membranes.
- Use a personal steam inhaler for 20 minutes when you suspect that you have been in contact with someone who has a cold. This treatment can abort a cold in its early stages but is not so effective if the infection is beyond the sore throat stage.

Over-the-Counter Treatments

Avoid multisymptom cold remedies, unless you need to address all symptoms they affect. Otherwise you risk experiencing side effects from medications you don't need. It's better to treat each symptom separately:

- Analgesics—aspirin, acetaminophen (Tylenol), ibuprofen (Advil or Motrin), and naproxen sodium (Aleve)—all help lower fever and relieve muscle aches. Aspirin should be taken only by adults to avoid the risk of a serious condition called Reye's syndrome, which increases for children and teenagers.
- Decongestants shrink nasal blood vessels, relieving swelling and congestion. However, they may dry out mucous membranes in the throat and make a sore throat worse. Nasal sprays shouldn't be used for more than two or three days to avoid rebound congestion.
- Cough medicines may be helpful when your cough is nonproductive (not bringing up mucus) or if it disrupts your sleep or work. Expectorants make coughs more productive by increasing the volume of mucus and decreasing its thickness, thereby helping remove irritants from the respiratory airways. Cough suppressants (antitussives) reduce the frequency of coughing.
- Antihistamines decrease nasal secretions caused by the effects of self-produced histamine, so they are much more useful in treating allergies than in treating colds. Many antihistamines can make you drowsy.

Other remedies, including zinc gluconate lozenges, echinacea, and vitamin C, relieve symptoms or shorten the duration of a cold. Researchers are also studying antiviral drugs that target the most common types of cold viruses.

Sometimes a cold leads to a more serious complication, such as bronchitis, pneumonia, or strep throat. If a fever of 102°F or higher persists, or if cold symptoms don't abate after two weeks, see your physician.

Chickenpox, Cold Sores, and Other Herpesvirus Infections The **herpesviruses** are a large group of viruses. Once infected, the host is never free of the virus. The virus lies latent within certain cells and becomes active periodically, producing symptoms. Herpesviruses are particularly dangerous for people with a depressed immune system. The family of herpesviruses includes the following:

- *Varicella-zoster virus,* which causes chickenpox and shingles. Chickenpox is a highly contagious disease characterized by an itchy rash made up of small blisters. The infection is usually mild, although complications are more likely to occur in young infants and adults. After the rash resolves, the virus becomes latent, living in sensory nerves. Many years later, the virus may reactivate and cause shingles. One in three people who had chickenpox develop shingles. Some people have long-lasting pain called postherpetic neuralgia (PHN). In 2017 the FDA licensed a new, highly effective shingles vaccine called Shingrix. The CDC recommends that healthy adults 50 years and older get two doses of Shingrix, 2–6 months apart.

- *Herpes simplex virus (HSV) types 1 and 2,* which cause cold sores and the sexually transmitted infection herpes (see Chapter 19). Herpes infections are characterized by small, painful ulcers in the area around the mouth or genitals, at the site where a person first contracts the virus. Following the initial infection, HSV becomes latent and may reactivate again and again over time. Many infected people do not know they are infected, and the virus can be transmitted even when sores are not apparent. Antiviral medications are available to prevent recurrences of genital herpes.

- *Epstein-Barr virus (EBV),* which causes infectious mononucleosis. Mono, as it is commonly called, is characterized by fever, sore throat, swollen lymph nodes, and fatigue. It is usually spread by intimate contact with the saliva

herpesvirus A large family of viruses responsible for cold sores, mononucleosis, chickenpox, shingles, and the sexually transmitted infection herpes; causes latent infections. **TERMS**

of an infected person—hence the nickname "kissing disease." Mono most often affects adolescents and young adults. EBV can reactivate throughout life with a recurrence of symptoms. In some people, especially those with HIV infection, EBV is associated with the development of cancers of the lymph system.

Two herpesviruses that can cause severe infections in people with AIDS or who have a suppressed immune system are cytomegalovirus (CMV), which infects the lungs, brain, colon, and eyes, and human herpesvirus 8 (HHV-8), which has been linked to Kaposi's sarcoma, a cancer of the connective tissue.

Viral Encephalitis
HSV type 1 is a possible cause of viral **encephalitis**—inflammation of brain tissue. Other possible causes include HIV and several mosquito-borne viruses, including Japanese encephalitis virus, equine encephalomyelitis virus, and West Nile virus. Mild cases of encephalitis may cause fever, headache, nausea, and lethargy. Severe cases are characterized by memory loss, delirium, diminished speech function, and seizures, and even permanent brain damage or death.

Viral Hepatitis
Hepatitis is inflammation of the liver. Hepatitis is usually caused by one of the three most common hepatitis viruses:

- *Hepatitis A virus (HAV)* causes the mildest form of the disease and is usually transmitted by food or water contaminated by sewage or an infected person.

- *Hepatitis B virus (HBV)* is usually transmitted sexually (see Chapter 19).

- *Hepatitis C virus (HCV)* can also be transmitted sexually, but it is much more commonly passed through direct contact with infected blood via injection drug use or—prior to the development of screening tests—blood transfusions. HBV and, to a lesser extent, HCV can also be passed from a pregnant woman to her child.

Symptoms of acute hepatitis infection can include fatigue, **jaundice,** abdominal pain, loss of appetite, nausea, and diarrhea. Most people recover from hepatitis A within a month or so. However, 5–10% of people infected with HBV and 70–85% of people infected with HCV become

chronic carriers of the virus, capable of infecting others. Some chronic carriers remain asymptomatic, while others slowly develop chronic liver disease, cirrhosis, or liver cancer. An estimated 4 million Americans and 500 million people worldwide may be chronic carriers of hepatitis. Each year in the United States, HBV and HCV are responsible for more than 15,000 deaths.

The extent of HCV infection has been recognized only recently. The WHO estimates that in 2015, worldwide, 71 million people had hepatitis C. Most infected people are unaware of their condition. To ensure proper treatment and prevention, testing for HCV may be recommended for people who have injected drugs (even once); received a blood transfusion or a donated organ prior to July 1992; engaged in high-risk sexual behavior; or had body piercing, tattoos, or acupuncture involving unsterile equipment (see the box "Tattoos and Body Piercing"). There are effective vaccines for hepatitis A and B, but more than 150,000 new cases of hepatitis occur in the United States each year. In 2017, the FDA approved a new drug combination for treating hepatitis C called Epclusa, which results in a cure (<1% probability of relapse) in 98–99% of treated individuals. The good news is that all types of viral hepatitis can be controlled or prevented.

Poliomyelitis
An infectious viral disease that affects the nervous system, **poliomyelitis** (polio) can cause irreversible paralysis and death in some people. As with other vaccine-preventable diseases, the incidence of polio declined dramatically in the United States following the introduction of the vaccine. North and South America are now considered free of the disease. It has also been eradicated from most countries of the world and remains endemic only in Afghanistan and Pakistan.

Rabies
Caused by a rhabdovirus that infects both humans and animals, the rabies virus infects the nervous system and is fatal if untreated. Humans become infected by rabies when they are bitten by a rabies-infected animal. U.S. rabies-related deaths among humans declined dramatically during the 20th century due to the widespread vaccination of domestic animals and the development of a highly effective vaccine regimen that provides immunity following exposure (post-exposure prophylaxis, or PEP). PEP consists of one dose of immunoglobulin and five doses of rabies vaccine over a 28-day period.

Human Papillomavirus (HPV)
The more than 200 types of HPV cause a variety of warts (noncancerous skin tumors), including common warts on the hands, plantar warts on the soles of the feet, and genital warts around the genitalia. Depending on their location, warts may be removed using OTC preparations or professional methods such as laser surgery or cryosurgery. Because HPV infection is chronic, warts can reappear despite treatment. As described in Chapter 17, HPV causes the majority of cases of cervical cancer. Three vaccines are available, targeting the types of HPV linked to the majority of HPV-caused cancers.

---

encephalitis Inflammation of the brain; fever, headache, nausea, and lethargy are common initial symptoms, followed in some cases by memory loss, seizures, brain damage, and death.   **TERMS**

hepatitis Inflammation of the liver, which can be caused by infection, drugs, or toxins.

jaundice Increased bile pigment levels in the blood, characterized by yellowing of the skin and the whites of the eyes.

poliomyelitis A disease of the nervous system, sometimes crippling; vaccines now prevent most cases of polio.

Because tattooing and body piercing involve the use of needles, they carry health risks. Tattoos are permanent marks applied with an electrically powered instrument that injects dye into the second layer of the skin. A tattoo typically takes a week or two to heal and should be protected from sun exposure until then. In piercing, the artist pushes a needle through the skin; a piece of jewelry holds the piercing open. Healing time varies depending on the site of the piercing and other factors.

Potential Health Complications

• **Infection.** There is a risk of transmission of blood-borne infectious agents, such as hepatitis, if instruments are not sterilized properly. In 2006, the CDC reported an outbreak of methicillin-resistant *Staphylococcus aureus* among customers of tattoo parlors in several states. Due to the potential risks of infection, people currently cannot donate blood for 12 months following application of body art, including tattoos and some body piercings. People with heart valve problems should check with a physician prior to body piercing to determine if they should take antibiotics before the procedure.

• **Allergic reactions.** Some people may be allergic to pigments used in tattooing or to metals used in body-piercing jewelry. All jewelry should be made of noncorrosive materials such as stainless steel or titanium; avoid jewelry that contains nickel.

• **Nodules and scars.** Some people may develop granulomas (nodules) or keloids (a type of scar) following tattooing or body piercing.

Choosing a Body Artist and Studio

A body art studio should be clean and have an autoclave for sterilizing instruments. Needles should be sterilized and disposable; piercing guns should not be used because they cannot be sterilized adequately. The body artist should wear disposable latex gloves throughout the procedure. Ask if the studio and/or artist are members of the Alliance of Professional Tattooists (www.safe-tattoos.com) or the Association of Professional Piercers (www.safepiercing.org); these organizations have developed infection control and other guidelines for their members to follow.

The National Institute for Occupational Safety and Health issues guidelines designed to protect both tattoo artists and customers from blood-borne infections. They cover such practices as washing hands, changing gloves, disinfecting surfaces, cleaning and sterilizing tools and equipment, and receiving training. Regulations and recommended practices vary from state to state; for more information, contact your state's public health department.

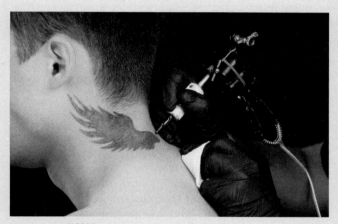

blueskyimage/123RF

Initial vaccination is recommended for all girls and boys aged 11 or 12; women can get the HPV vaccine through age 26 and men, through age 21. HPV is discussed in detail in Chapters 17 and 19. An analysis of a four-year clinical trial showed that an HPV vaccine is 100% effective in preventing the abnormal proliferation of cervical cells that precedes the development of cervical cancer.

Treating Viral Illnesses   Antiviral drugs typically work by interfering at some segment of the viral life cycle; for example, they may prevent a virus from entering body cells or from successfully reproducing within cells. Antivirals are currently available to fight infections caused by HIV, influenza, herpes simplex, varicella-zoster, HBV, and HCV. A six-month disruption in antiviral treatment because of a pandemic such as COVID-19 could lead to more than 500,000 extra deaths from AIDS-related illnesses, including tuberculosis, in sub-Saharan Africa.

Fungi

A **fungus** is an organism that reproduces by spores. Only about 50 of the many thousands of species of fungi cause disease in humans. Some fungal diseases are extremely difficult to treat. First, our normal defenses must contend with fungal infections to skin, nails, and the respiratory tract. Second, external treatments are difficult because, unlike bacteria, fungi are similar enough in their cellular chemistry to humans that it is difficult to kill fungi without harming the infected human.

> **fungus**   A single-celled or multicelled organism that reproduces by spores and feeds on organic matter; examples include molds, mushrooms, and yeasts. Fungal diseases include yeast infections, athlete's foot, and ringworm.   **TERMS**

Candida albicans is a common fungus found naturally in the vagina of most women. When excessive growth occurs, the result is itching and discomfort, commonly known as a yeast infection. Factors that increase the growth of *C. albicans* include the use of antibiotics, clothing that keeps the vaginal area excessively warm and moist, pregnancy, oral contraceptive use, and certain diseases, including diabetes and HIV infection. The most common symptom is a thick white or yellowish discharge. Prescription and OTC treatments are available. Women should not self-treat unless they are certain from a past medical diagnosis that they have a yeast infection. (Misdiagnosis could mean that a different and more severe infection goes untreated.) *C. albicans* overgrowth can occur in other areas of the body, especially in the mouths of infants (a condition known as thrush).

Other common fungal conditions, including athlete's foot, jock itch, and ringworm, affect the skin. These three conditions are usually mild and easy to cure.

Fungi can also cause systemic diseases that are severe, life threatening, and extremely difficult to treat. Histoplasmosis, or valley fever, causes pulmonary and sometimes systemic disease and is most common in the Mississippi and Ohio River Valleys. Coccidioidomycosis is also known as valley fever because it is most frequent in the San Joaquin Valley of California. Fungal infections can be especially deadly in people with impaired immune systems.

Protozoa

Protozoa are single-celled organisms that can cause a range of diseases in humans. Millions of people in developing countries suffer from protozoal infections.

Malaria, caused by a parasitic protozoan of the genus *Plasmodium,* is characterized by recurrent attacks of severe chills, fever, headache, nausea, and vomiting; it may also cause anemia. The protozoan is injected into the bloodstream via a mosquito bite. Although now relatively rare in the United States, malaria is a major killer worldwide. Over 3 billion people in 92 countries and territories (half the world's population) live in areas where malaria is a problem. In 2018, 228 million people had malaria, and 405,000 people died of it. Insecticide-treated bed nets reduce malarial infections, and they have reduced the deaths of children under age 5 by about 20%. Children under 5 account for 61% of all malaria deaths. Several antimalarial drugs can prevent or treat the disease, but drug resistance is an increasing problem.

Giardiasis is caused by *Giardia intestinalis,* a protozoan responsible for most cases of protozoal travelers' diarrhea.

---

protozoan A microscopic single-celled organism that often produces recurrent, cyclical attacks of disease; plural, *protozoa.*

malaria A severe, recurrent, mosquito-borne infection caused by the parasitic protozoan *Plasmodium.*

giardiasis An intestinal disease caused by the parasitic protozoan *Giardia lamblia.*

TERMS

Giardiasis is characterized by nausea, diarrhea, bloating, and abdominal cramps, and it is among the most common waterborne diseases in the United States. People may become infected with *Giardia* if they consume contaminated food or water or pick up the parasite from the contaminated surface of an object such as a bathroom fixture, diaper pail, or toy. People at risk include child care workers, children who attend day care, international travelers, and hikers and campers who drink untreated water. Giardiasis is rarely serious and can be treated with prescription medications.

Water Treatment The need for water treatment was recognized as long ago as 2000 BC, when ancient Greeks initiated the most primitive water treatment processes. In the United States, the 1974 Safe Drinking Water Act authorizes the Environmental Protection Agency (EPA) to set health guidelines for the public wells, reservoirs, and springs that are the sources of our drinking water.

Modern water treatments remove bacteria, parasites, pesticides, and other harmful contaminants. The success of these procedures is manifest in the low incidence of water-associated diseases in the United States. For example, in 2013–2014 there were only an estimated 42 drinking water–associated outbreaks. Even this small number caused 1006 cases of illness, 124 hospitalizations, and 13 deaths. By contrast, in the developing world, access to clean water is a serious public health problem. Waterborne diseases such as cholera are still threats. In 2017 in Yemen alone, 1 million people were made ill by cholera. The problems experienced by Flint, Michigan, residents with contaminated public water supplies demonstrate that our government must be more diligent in keeping our infrastructure up to date. Even seemingly pristine mountain streams can be contaminated with the protozoan *Giardia lamblia,* as many unwary hikers and campers have discovered.

Other protozoal infections include the following:

• **Trichomoniasis,** a common vaginal infection. Although usually mild and treatable, trich may increase the risk of HIV transmission (see Chapter 19).

• **Trypanosomiasis** (African sleeping sickness), which is transmitted through the bite of an infected tsetse fly and causes extreme fatigue, fever, rash, severe headache, central nervous system damage, and death.

• **Amoebic dysentery,** a severe form of amebiasis—infection of the intestines with the parasite *Entamoeba histolytica.* It is characterized by bloody diarrhea, stomach pain, and fever.

• **Toxoplasmosis,** a disease caused by *Toxoplasma gondii*, a protozoan parasite. About 11% of people in the United States over the age of 6 have been infected with *Toxoplasma.* In some parts of the world, particularly in hot, humid climates, up to 95% of the population has been infected. The principal route of transmission is from undercooked, contaminated meat. When a pregnant woman eats the meat, infection of the fetus can lead to miscarriage, stillbirth, or a baby who suffers from vision loss, mental disability, and seizures.

Parasitic Worms

Parasitic worms are the largest organisms that can enter the body to cause infection. Intestinal parasites, such as the tapeworm and hookworm, cause a variety of relatively mild infections. Pinworm, the most common worm infection in the United States, primarily affects young children.

Emerging Infectious Diseases

Emerging infectious diseases are infections that have increased in incidence or may increase in the near future. They include both known diseases that have experienced a resurgence, such as tuberculosis and cholera, and diseases that were previously unknown or confined to specific areas, such as the Zika and Ebola viruses.

Selected Infections of Concern Although the chances of the average American contracting an exotic infection are very low, emerging infections are a concern to public health officials and represent a challenge to all nations in the future.

ZIKA DISEASE Zika virus is transmitted by several species of *Aedes* mosquitoes. It can also spread through sex with an infected partner, and it can pass from a pregnant woman to her fetus.

In most people, Zika symptoms are very mild, lasting a week or less, and may include fever, rash, and joint pain. However, a small proportion of people infected with Zika develop a neurological condition called Guillain-Barré syndrome, usually characterized by muscle weakness. This condition typically resolves within a few weeks or several months. Zika can also cause birth defects including microcephaly (small head size), impaired growth, eye defects, hearing loss, and possibly other problems.

The specific geographic areas where Zika virus is spreading are likely to change over time, and research is ongoing into its effects and the best strategies for testing and prevention. The mosquitoes that carry Zika are found in many parts of the world, including much of the United States. But no local mosquito-borne Zika virus transmission was reported in the United States in 2018 and 2019.

EBOLA Ebola virus disease (EVD) is caused by Ebola virus, which is transmitted to people from wild animals. Infected people can then transmit the virus to others through direct contact with blood or body fluids or objects that have been contaminated. EVD is a severe infection with an average fatality rate of about 50%. Ebola is rare, but outbreaks have occurred periodically since it was first identified in 1976. There is no vaccine; it is treated with supportive care (including providing intravenous fluids and electrolytes, maintaining oxygen and blood pressure, and treating other infections if they occur). The spread of the infection is controlled by identifying and isolating the sick and their close contacts. The outbreak in West Africa that raged 2014-2016 was the largest in history, with 11,310 deaths. The WHO declared the end of the 10th Ebola outbreak in the Democratic Republic of Congo in June 2020.

WEST NILE VIRUS West Nile virus (WNV) is carried by birds and then passed to humans when mosquitoes bite first an infected bird and then a person. In the United States, West Nile virus has caused infections in humans in 47 states and the District of Columbia. Eighty percent of infected people do not develop a serious condition. However, those who develop WNV disease have serious, long-lasting problems. In 2019, 917 cases of WNV disease in people were reported to the CDC. Of those, 607 (66%) had neuroinvasive disease (meningitis or encephalitis) and 310 (34%) had non-neuroinvasive disease.

PATHOGENIC *ESCHERICHIA COLI* *E. coli* bacteria live in the intestines of humans and animals and are an essential component of gut immunity. However, some strains of *E. coli* cause diarrhea; six types cause disease. Since 2006, there have been 38 multistate outbreaks of *E. coli*–caused disease. These outbreaks have been caused by contaminated foods including lettuce, spinach, sprouts, hazelnuts, processed meats, frozen foods, poultry, and beef sold both in grocery store chains and in restaurants. However, people also can become infected in other ways, such as by swallowing contaminated swimming pool water and through contact with an infected animal—for example, by petting an animal and then not washing hands before eating. Pets and animals at exhibits such as petting zoos can be healthy but carry pathogens on their bodies that can be passed to humans. The CDC website has guidelines for preventing infection.

HANTAVIRUS Hantavirus infection can cause a deadly disease called hantavirus pulmonary syndrome (HPS). In North America, the deer mouse, the white-footed mouse, the rice rat, and the cotton rat are carriers of hantaviruses. People can become infected when rodent urine and droppings that contain the virus get into the air, for example, after they dry out. Between 1993 and 2017, 728 cases of HPS have been counted in 36 states.

Factors Contributing to Emerging Infections What's behind this rising tide of infectious diseases? Contributing factors are complex and interrelated.

DRUG RESISTANCE New or increasing drug resistance has been found in organisms that cause malaria, tuberculosis, gonorrhea, influenza, AIDS, and pneumococcal and staphylococcal infections. Infections caused by drug-resistant organisms prolong illness, and—if not treated in time—they can cause death. Some bacterial strains now appear to be resistant to all available antibiotics.

> **parasitic worm** **TERMS** A pathogen that causes intestinal and other infections; includes tapeworms, hookworms, pinworms, and flukes.

POVERTY More than 1 billion people live in extreme poverty, and half the world's population has no regular access to essential drugs. Population growth, urbanization, overcrowding, and migration (including the movement of refugees) also spread infectious diseases.

BREAKDOWN OF PUBLIC HEALTH MEASURES A poor public health infrastructure is often associated with poverty and social upheaval, but problems such as contaminated water supplies can occur even in industrial countries. Inadequate vaccination has led to the reemergence of diseases such as diphtheria, pertussis, measles, and mumps. Natural disasters such as hurricanes also disrupt the public health infrastructure, leaving survivors with contaminated water and food supplies and no shelter from disease-carrying insects.

TRAVEL AND COMMERCE International tourism and trade open the world to infectious agents. Consider the global spread of COVID-19. COVID-19 was reported to WHO on December 31, 2019, based on an unknown illness affecting workers at a seafood market in the city of Wuhan, China. By January 17, the United States, Nepal, France, Australia, Malaysia, Singapore, South Korea, Vietnam, and Taiwan had confirmed cases of the virus. WHO declared the situation a "global emergency" on January 30, and by March 11, a pandemic. It took over three months to reach the first 100,000 confirmed cases of the virus, and only 12 days to reach the next 100,000.

MASS FOOD PRODUCTION AND DISTRIBUTION Food now travels long distances to our table, and microbes are transmitted along with it. Mass production of food increases the likelihood that a chance contamination can lead to mass illness.

HUMAN BEHAVIORS The widespread use of injectable drugs rapidly transmits HIV infection and hepatitis. Changes in sexual behavior over the past 40 years have led to a proliferation of old and new sexually transmitted infections. The use of day care facilities for children has led to increases in the incidence of several infections that cause diarrhea.

CLIMATE CHANGE The lengthening of warm periods and a change to shorter or milder winters may enable pathogenic species and, for some pathogens, their insect vectors to expand their range into countries or states where they once had not existed or had been rare.

Immune Disorders

Considering the complexity of the immune system, it is not surprising that the system sometimes fails to operate properly, resulting in disease.

Autoimmune Diseases As discussed earlier, the immune system can recognize the body's cells and tissues as "self" and foreign organisms as "nonself." When this ability breaks down, "self" may be misread and attacked as "nonself," and the result is an autoimmune disease. In most autoimmune diseases, the immune system targets or destroys specific tissues. For example, in type 1 diabetes, the insulin-producing cells

of the pancreas are destroyed. In multiple sclerosis, the protective coating around nerves is destroyed. In Hashimoto's thyroiditis, the thyroid gland is destroyed. In rheumatoid arthritis, the membranes lining the joints are destroyed. In systemic lupus erythematosus, destructive inflammation affects the joints, blood vessels, heart, lungs, brain, and kidneys.

The Immune System and Cancer As discussed in Chapter 17, cancer cells are cells that mutate and multiply uncontrollably. The immune system detects cells that have recently become abnormal and destroys them just as it would a foreign cell. However, some types of cancer cells actually suppress immune responses.

In recent years, conventional cancer treatments use immunotherapy to stimulate the patient's immune system to attack tumor cells. Because some strains of HPV are linked to cervical, anal, and some throat cancers, the commercially available Gardasil and Cervarix vaccines can prevent cancer by stimulating immunity to HPV.

SUPPORTING YOUR IMMUNE SYSTEM

The immune system does an amazing job of protecting you from illness, but you can help ensure its optimal functioning by choosing healthy behaviors. Here are some general guidelines for supporting your immune system:

• Get more sleep: People who sleep fewer than six hours per night have compromised immune function, according to scientific studies. For example, people who operate on insufficient sleep are more susceptible to the common cold. They also do not respond as well to immunizations. See Chapter 4 for more on sleep.

• Maintain regular eating patterns. Recent research suggests that eating—even anticipating eating—switches on immune cell activity to potentially incoming pathogens or "bad" bacteria. This activity may explain why disruptions to circadian rhythms and regular eating patterns could increase chronic inflammation in the gut.

• Wash your hands frequently. Use regular soap and wash thoroughly by scrubbing at least 20–30 seconds. When soap and water are not available, use hand sanitizer. Make sure the product is at least 60% alcohol, but avoid sanitizers that contain *triclosan* or more than 630 ppm methanol.

Ask Yourself

QUESTIONS FOR CRITICAL THINKING AND REFLECTION
Have you ever had any of the illnesses described in the preceding sections? How were you exposed to the disease? Could you have taken any precautions to avoid it?

- Avoid contact with people who are contagious with an infectious disease.

- Make sure you drink water only from clean sources. Unpurified water from lakes and streams can carry pathogens, even if it appears pristine.

- Avoid contact with disease carriers such as rodents, mosquitoes, and ticks. Never touch or feed wild animals.

- Make sure you have received all your recommended vaccinations, and keep them up to date. Your physician can tell you exactly what immunizations you need and when you should have them.

TIPS FOR TODAY AND THE FUTURE

Your immune system is a remarkable germ-fighting network, but it needs your help to work at its best.

RIGHT NOW YOU CAN:
- Make sure that you have plenty of soap in your bathroom and kitchen. It should not be antibacterial soap.
- Launder your dirty hand towels and bath towels. It's a good practice to hang towels unfolded to let them air dry and to replace them with clean towels after three uses. Make sure everyone you live with has his or her own towels; sharing can spread germs.
- Start getting at least 15 more minutes of sleep each night.

IN THE FUTURE YOU CAN:
- Stock up on hand sanitizer and tissues. Put them in your backpack, car, locker, and other places where you might need to wash your hands when soap and water won't be available.
- Make an appointment with your physician to ensure your immunizations are up to date.
- Create an immunization record; it can be helpful in the future (e.g., if you are ever injured and must decide whether you need a tetanus booster).

SUMMARY

- The immune system includes both surface barriers and the cells that mount the immune response.

- Physical and chemical barriers to microorganisms include skin, mucous membranes, and the cilia lining the respiratory tract.

- The immune response is carried out by white blood cells that are continuously produced in the bone marrow. Cells of the innate immune system include neutrophils, eosinophils, macrophages, dendritic cells, and natural killer cells. Cells of the adaptive immune system are lymphocytes—in particular, T cells and B cells.

- The immune response has four stages: recognition of the invading pathogen; replication of T cells and B cells; attack by killer T cells and macrophages; and suppression of the immune response.

- Immunization is based on the body's ability to remember previously encountered organisms. Measles wipes out some of the immune system's memory of previous illnesses.

- Allergic reactions occur when the immune system responds to harmless substances as if they were dangerous pathogens.

- The step-by-step process by which infections are transmitted from one person to another involves a pathogen, its reservoir, a portal of exit, a means of transmission, a portal of entry, and a new host. Infection can be prevented by breaking the chain at any point.

- The spread of disease may result in epidemics or pandemics.

- Bacteria are single-celled organisms; some cause disease in humans. Significant bacterial infections include pneumonia, meningitis, strep throat, toxic shock syndrome, MRSA, tuberculosis, Lyme disease, and ulcers.

- Most antibiotics work by interrupting the production of new bacteria; they do not work against viruses. Bacteria can become resistant to antibiotics.

- Viruses cannot grow or reproduce themselves; viruses cause the common cold, influenza, measles, mumps, rubella, chickenpox, cold sores, mononucleosis, encephalitis, hepatitis, polio, and warts.

- Other infectious diseases are caused by certain types of fungi, protozoa, and parasitic worms.

- Autoimmune diseases occur when the body identifies its own cells as foreign.

- A healthy immune system can destroy mutant cells that may become cancerous.

- The immune system needs adequate nutrition and rest, moderate exercise, and protection from excessive stress. Vaccinations also help protect against disease.

FOR MORE INFORMATION

Alliance for the Prudent Use of Antibiotics. Provides information about the proper use of antibiotics and tips for avoiding infections.

https://apua.org

American Academy of Allergy, Asthma & Immunology. Provides information and publications; pollen counts are available from the website.

http://www.aaaai.org

American Autoimmune-Related Diseases Association. Provides background information, coping tips, and an online knowledge quiz about autoimmune diseases.

http://www.aarda.org

American College of Allergy, Asthma & Immunology. Provides information for patients and physicians; website includes an extensive glossary of terms related to allergies and asthma.

http://www.acaai.org

American Society for Microbiology. Includes a library of images and an introduction to microbes.

http://www.asm.org

CDC National Center for Emerging and Zoonotic Infectious Diseases. Provides extensive information on a wide variety of infectious diseases.

http://www.cdc.gov/ncezid/

CDC: Vaccines & Immunizations. Provides information and answers to frequently asked questions about vaccines and immunizations.

http://www.cdc.gov/vaccines

National Foundation for Infectious Diseases. Provides information about a variety of diseases and disease issues.

http://www.nfid.org

National Institute of Allergy and Infectious Diseases. Includes fact sheets about many topics relating to allergies and infectious diseases, including tuberculosis and sexually transmitted infections.

http://www.niaid.nih.gov

World Health Organization: Infectious Diseases. Provides fact sheets about many emerging and tropical diseases as well as information about current outbreaks.

http://www.who.int/topics/infectious_diseases/en

SELECTED BIBLIOGRAPHY

Barry, J. 2005. *The Great Influenza: The Epic Story of the Deadliest Plague in History.* New York: Penguin.

Blaser, M. 2011. Antibiotic overuse: Stop the killing of beneficial bacteria. *Nature* 476: 393–394.

Callaway, E. 2020. Coronavirus vaccines: Five key questions as trials begin. Some experts warn that accelerated testing will involve some risky trade-offs (https://www.nature.com/articles/d41586-020-00798-8).

Centers for Disease Control and Prevention. 2020. *Influenza (Flu)* (https://www.cdc.gov/flu/index.htm).

Centers for Disease Control and Prevention. 2019. *Measles (Rubeola)* (https://www.cdc.gov/measles/).

Centers for Disease Control and Prevention. 2020. *2020 Immunization Schedules and Resources* (https://www.cdc.gov/vaccines/schedules/downloads/adult/adult-combined-schedule.pdf).

Centers for Disease Control and Prevention. 2020. *West Nile Virus* (https://www.cdc.gov/westnile/).

Centers for Disease Control and Prevention. 2019. *Lyme Disease* (https://www.cdc.gov/lyme/datasurveillance/index.html?CDC_AA_refVal=https%3A%2F%2Fwww.cdc.gov%2Flyme%2Fstats%2Findex.html).

Centers for Disease Control and Prevention. 2019. Clostridioides difficile *Infection* (https://www.cdc.gov/hai/organisms/cdiff/cdiff_infect.html).

Centers for Disease Control and Prevention. 2019. *Antibiotic Use in the United States, 2018 Update: Progress and Opportunities.* Atlanta, GA: U.S. Department of Health and Human Services (https://www.cdc.gov/antibiotic-use/stewardship-report/pdf/stewardship-report-2018-508.pdf).

Centers for Disease Control and Prevention. 2019. *Zika Virus* (https://www.cdc.gov/zika/index.html).

Centers for Disease Control and Prevention. 2017. *Asthma* (https://www.cdc.gov/nchs/fastats/asthma.htm).

Centers for Disease Control and Prevention. 2019. *Human Papillomavirus (HPV)* (https://www.cdc.gov/hpv/parents/vaccine.html).

Chhabra, N., et al. 2012. Pharmacotherapy for multidrug resistant tuberculosis. *Journal of Pharmacology and Pharmacotherapy* 3(2): 98–104.

Cohen, S, et al. 2009. Sleep habits and susceptibility to the common cold. *Archives of Internal Medicine* 169: 62–67.

Corum, J., and C. Zimmer. 2020. Bad news wrapped in protein: Inside the coronavirus genome. *The New York Times*, 3 April (https://www.nytimes.com/interactive/2020/04/03/science/coronavirus-genome-bad-news-wrapped-in-protein.html).

D'Amato, G., et al. 2015. Effects on asthma and respiratory allergy of climate change and air pollution. *Multidisciplinary Respiratory Medicine* 10: 39.

Do Prado, M. F., et al. 2012. Antimicrobial efficacy of alcohol-based gels with a 30-s application. *Letters in Applied Microbiology* 54(6): 564–567.

Food and Drug Administration. 2019. FDA issues final rule on safety and effectiveness of consumer hand sanitizers. (https://www.fda.gov/news-events/press-announcements/fda-issues-final-rule-safety-and-effectiveness-consumer-hand-sanitizers).

Frieri, M., and A. Valluri. 2011. Vitamin D deficiency as a risk factor for allergic disorders and immune mechanisms. *Allergy and Asthma Proceedings* 32(6): 438–444.

Kamidani, S., and L. K. Pickering. 2019. Tetanus spores lie in wait for unvaccinated children. *American Academy of Pediatrics* (https://www.aappublications.org/news/2019/07/03/mmwr070319).

Lamb, A. K., et al. 2011. Reducing asthma disparities by addressing environmental inequities: A case study of Regional Asthma Management and Prevention's advocacy efforts. *Family & Community Health* 34: S54–S62.

Larru, B., and P. Offit. 2014. Communicating vaccine science to the public. *Journal of Infection* 69 (Suppl. 1): S2–S4.

Lehtinen, M., et al. 2012. Overall efficacy of HPV-16/18 AS04-adjuvanted vaccine against grade 3 or greater cervical intraepithelial neoplasia: 4-year end-of-study analysis of the randomised, double-blind PATRICIA trial. *Lancet Oncology* 13(1): 89–99.

Markowitz, L. E., et al. 2016. Prevalence of HPV after introduction of the vaccination program in the United States. *Pediatrics* 137(3): e20151968.

McKenzie, J. F., and R. R. Pinger. 2015. *Introduction to Community and Public Health,* 8th ed. Burlington, MA: Jones & Bartlett Learning.

Murray, K. A., et al. 2015. Global biogeography of human infectious diseases. *Proceedings of the National Academy of Sciences* 112(41): 12746–12751.

National Institute of Allergy and Infectious Disease. 2020. *COVID-19, MERS & SARS* (https://www.niaid.nih.gov/diseases-conditions/covid-19).

National Institute of Allergy and Infectious Diseases. 2014. *Immune Cells* (https://www.niaid.nih.gov/research/immune-cells).

National Institute of Neurological Disorders and Stroke. 2020. *Meningitis and Encephalitis Fact Sheet* (https://www.ninds.nih.gov/Disorders/Patient-Caregiver-Education/Fact-Sheets/Meningitis-and-Encephalitis-Fact-Sheet).

National Notifiable Disease Surveillance System. 2020. *Provisional 2019 Reports of Notifiable Diseases,* Week 52. Unpublished. Atlanta, GA: U.S. Department of Health and Human Services (https://www.cdc.gov/pertussis/downloads/pertuss-surv-report-2019-508.pdf).

Pennell, L. M., et al. 2012. Sex affects immunity. *Journal of Autoimmunity* 38(2): 1282–1291.

Petrova, V. N., et al. 2019. Incomplete genetic reconstitution of B cell pools contributes to prolonged immunosuppression after measles. *Science Immunology* 4(4): eaay6125.

Porkka-Heiskanen, T., et al. 2013. Sleep, its regulation and possible mechanisms of sleep disturbances. *Acta Physiologica (Oxford)* 208(4): 311–328.

Rockefeller University Press. 2019. How sleep can fight infection. *ScienceDaily*, 12 February (www.sciencedaily.com/releases/2019/02/190212094839.htm).

Schwartz, N. G., et al. 2020. Tuberculosis—United States, 2019. *MMWR* 69(11): 286–289.

Seehan, M. D., and W. Phipatanaul. 2015. Difficult to control asthma: Epidemiology and its link with environmental factors. *Current Opinion in Allergy and Clinical Immunology* 15(5): 397–401.

Seillet, C. et al. 2019. The neuropeptide VIP confers anticipatory mucosal immunity by regulating ILC3 activity. *Nature Immunology* 21(2): 168.

Sompayrac, L. M. 2012. *How the Immune System Works,* 4th ed. Malden, MA: Blackwell Science.

Tamimi, A. H., et al. 2015. Impact of the use of an alcohol-based hand sanitizer in the home on reduction in probability of infection by respiratory and enteric viruses. *Epidemiology and Infection* 143(15): 3335–3341.

Taniguchi, K., and M. Karin. 2018. NF-κB, inflammation, immunity and cancer: Coming of age. *Nature Reviews Immunology* 18: 309–324.

Taylor, D. J. 2016. Is insomnia a risk factor for decreased influenza vaccine response? *Behavioral Sleep Medicine* 14: 1–18.

Toh, Z. Q., et al. 2015. Reduced dose human papillomavirus vaccination: An update of the current state-of-the-art. *Vaccine* 33: 5042–5050.

Wadman, M., et al. 2020. How does coronavirus kill? Clinicians trace a ferocious rampage through the body, from brain to toes. *Science*, 17 April (https://www.sciencemag.org/news/2020/04/how-does-coronavirus-kill-clinicians-trace-ferocious-rampage-through-body-brain-toes).

World Health Organization. 2020. The cost of inaction: COVID-19-related service disruptions could cause hundreds of thousands of extra deaths from HIV. (https://www.who.int/news-room/detail/11-05-2020-the-cost-of-inaction-covid-19-related-service-disruptions-could-cause-hundreds-of-thousands-of-extra-deaths-from-hiv).

World Health Organization. 2020. WHO Director-General's opening remarks at the media briefing on COVID-19, 11 March https://www.who.int/dg/speeches/detail/who-director-general-s-opening-remarks-at-the-media-briefing-on-covid-19—11-march-2020

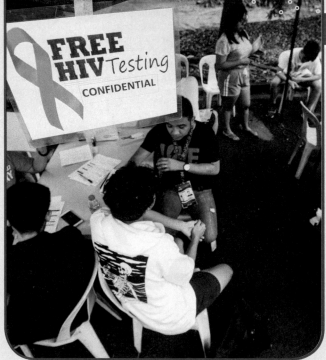

MARIA TAN/Getty Images

- Discuss the symptoms, risks, and treatments for the major sexually transmitted infections
- List strategies for protecting yourself from sexually transmitted infections

CHAPTER **19**

Sexually Transmitted Infections

TEST YOUR KNOWLEDGE

1. Most people who have sexually transmitted infections (STIs) have symptoms.
   True or False?

2. Worldwide, which of the following is the primary means of spreading HIV infection?
   a. Injection drug use
   b. Sex between men
   c. Mother-to-child transmission
   d. Heterosexual sex

3. All sexually active women aged 25 or younger should be screened for gonorrhea and chlamydia at least annually.
   True or False?

4. Few STIs in the United States are diagnosed in men and women ages 15–24.
   True or False?

5. After you have had an STI once, you become immune to that disease and cannot get it again.
   True or False?

ANSWERS

1. **FALSE.** Many people with sexually transmitted infections (STIs) have no symptoms and do not know they are infected; however, they can still pass an infection to their partners.

2. **D.** The vast majority of HIV infection cases worldwide result from heterosexual contact, and the majority of new cases occur in teenage girls and young women.

3. **TRUE.** The CDC recommends yearly gonorrhea and chlamydia screening for all sexually active women aged 25 or younger, as well as older women with risk factors such as new or multiple sex partners, or a sex partner who has a sexually transmitted infection.

4. **FALSE.** Young people in the United States account for half the newly diagnosed cases of STIs.

5. **FALSE.** Reinfection with STIs is common. For example, if you receive treatment for and are cured of chlamydia and then you have unprotected sex with your untreated partner, the chances are very good that you will be infected again.

Sexually transmitted infections (STIs) spread from person to person mainly through sexual activity. STIs are a particularly insidious group of illnesses because a person can be infected and be able to transmit the disease, yet not look or feel sick. The Centers for Disease Control and Prevention (CDC) estimates that the cost of STIs to the health care system in the United States is almost $16 billion per year.

STIs can be prevented. Many STIs can also be cured if treated early and properly. This chapter introduces the major forms of STIs. It also provides information about safer sexual behavior that protects you from infection and helps to reduce the spread of these diseases.

THE MAJOR SEXUALLY TRANSMITTED INFECTIONS

The following seven STIs pose major health threats: HIV/AIDS, chlamydia, gonorrhea, human papillomavirus (HPV), herpes, hepatitis, and syphillis.

STIs are caused by a number of organisms, including bacteria, viruses, protozoa, and parasites (Table 19.1). STIs can cause serious complications if left untreated and can result in long-term consequences, including chronic pain, infertility, stillbirths, genital cancers, and death. Additionally, women exposed to STIs while pregnant may place their fetus and newborn at risk for infection if untreated. The rates of many STIs in the United States have reached record highs—in some instances, much higher than those of other industrialized nations.

In 2018, the number of chlamydia, gonorrhea, and syphilis cases collectively reached an all-time high (Table 19.2). There are many possible reasons behind this: health and wealth disparities, declining condom use in vulnerable populations such as men who have sex with men, and lack of access to STI diagnostic, treatment, and preventive services. Certain STIs such as syphilis are affecting more women, and therefore more babies; and better detecting methods in certain populations are revealing higher incidence rates. Public health funding for STI clinics has also been severely cut over the past decade. Lack of effective sexual health education and educational policies results in less healthy choices.

Young people especially need more education: Those aged 15–24 account for half of STI cases in the United States. With the rise of dating apps, the increasing anonymity of sexual encounters, coupled with the stigma of STIs and our reluctance to talk about them, may also play a role in higher STI rates. The National Health Statistics Report indicates an overall decline beginning in the late 1980s in sexually active youth. Trends also show increased condom use with first sexual activity. Condom use at nongenital sites (anal and oral), however, is reported in some studies to be less consistent, thus increasing the possibility of STI exposure at those sites.

> **sexually transmitted infection (STI)** An infection that is transmitted mainly by sexual contact; some can also be transmitted by other means.
>
> **TERMS**

Table 19.1	Sexually Transmitted Pathogens and Associated Infections	
PATHOGEN	INFECTIONS	COMMON SYNDROMES AND DISEASE MANIFESTATIONS
BACTERIA		
Chlamydia trachomatis	Chlamydia	Pelvic inflammatory disease, epididymitis, urethritis, proctitis
Chlamydia trachomatis	Lymphogranuloma venereum	Proctitis
Haemophilus ducreyi	Chancroid	
Neisseria gonorrhoeae	Gonorrhea	Pelvic inflammatory disease, epididymitis, urethritis, proctitis
Treponema pallidum	Syphilis	Primary, secondary, tertiary, neurological, ocular, congenital syphilis
VIRUSES		
Hepatitis B virus (HBV)		Hepatitis, cirrhosis, liver cancer
Hepatitis C virus (HCV)		Hepatitis, cirrhosis, liver cancer
Herpes simplex virus (HSV)		Genital herpes, proctitis, oral–labial herpes (cold sores)
Human immunodeficiency virus (HIV)		HIV/AIDS
Human papillomavirus (HPV)		Genital warts; cervical, anal, penile, vaginal, vulvar, and oral cancers
PROTOZOA		
Trichomonas vaginalis	Trichomoniasis	Vaginitis, urethritis, cervicitis
ECTOPARASITES		
Phthirus pubis	Pubic lice	
Sarcoptes scabiei	Scabies	

Table 19.2	Estimated Annual New Cases of Selected STIs in the United States

SEXUALLY TRANSMITTED INFECTION	NEW CASES
Human papillomavirus (HPV)	*14,000,000
Chlamydia	1,758,668
Trichomoniasis	*1,090,000
Herpes simplex virus (HSV 2)	*776,000
Gonorrhea	583,405
HIV infection	37,377
Hepatitis B	^22,200
Hepatitis C	^44,700
Syphilis (all stages)	115,045

* Nonreportable diseases; statistics are estimated.

^ Adjusted statistics includes actual and estimated numbers of acute hepatitis cases.

SOURCES: Centers for Disease Control and Prevention. 2019. *Sexually Transmitted Disease Surveillance 2018*. Atlanta, GA: U.S. Department of Health and Human Services; Centers for Disease Control and Prevention. Centers for Disease Control and Prevention. 2019. *HIV Surveillance Report, 2018* (Preliminary); vol. 30 (http://www.cdc.gov /hiv/library/reports/hiv-surveillance.html. Centers for Disease Control and Prevention. 2019. *Viral Hepatitis Surveillance United States, 2017* (https://www.cdc.gov/hepatitis/statistics/2017surveillance /pdfs/2017HepSurveillanceRpt.pdf); Satterwhite, C. L., et al. 2013. Sexually transmitted infections among U.S. women and men: Prevalence and incidence estimates, 2008. *Sexually Transmitted Diseases* 40(3): 187–193.

HIV Infection and AIDS

HIV causes AIDS. With recent advances in the treatment of **human immunodeficiency virus (HIV),** people infected with the virus are now living almost as long as people not infected with it. Adequate treatment is not accessible, however, for most people worldwide. Untreated HIV infection may advance to **acquired immunodeficiency syndrome (AIDS)** within 8-10 years of diagnosis. This stage of HIV infection is

QUICK STATS

HIV/AIDS is ranked as the ninth leading cause of death among Americans aged 25–34 years.

—National Center for Health Statistics, 2019

TERMS

human immunodeficiency virus (HIV) The virus that causes HIV infection and AIDS.

acquired immunodeficiency syndrome (AIDS) An advanced stage of HIV infection.

HIV infection A chronic, progressive viral infection that damages the immune system.

CD4 T cell A type of white blood cell that helps coordinate the activity of the immune system; the primary target of HIV infection. A decrease in the number of these cells correlates with the severity of HIV-related illness.

defined by a severely compromised immune system and the presence of opportunistic infections.

An estimated total of 78 million people have been infected since the HIV/AIDS epidemic began—nearly 1% of the world's population—and tens of millions of those people have died (see the box "HIV/AIDS around the World"). In 2018, about 37.9 million people were infected with HIV worldwide; nearly two-thirds of them lived in sub-Saharan Africa. Overall trends demonstrate the number of people living with HIV continues to level off. Many experts believe that the global HIV epidemic peaked in the late 1990s, at about 3.5 million new infections per year, compared with an estimated 1.7 million new infections in 2018. Despite a slowing of the epidemic, AIDS remains a primary cause of death in Africa and continues to be a major cause of mortality around the world. Disparities exist for incident infections and access to treatment in youth, women, and key populations. Youth aged 15–24 represent 16% of the global population and one-third of incident HIV infections. Thus, despite a slowing of the epidemic, HIV continues to be a major cause of morbidity and mortality around the world.

In the United States, about 1 million people are living with HIV; 15% of these people are not aware of their HIV status. In 2018, there were 37,832 HIV cases in the United States, 52% of which occurred in the South. Men who have sex with men, transgender women, persons of color, and youth are also disproportionately burdened with HIV.

What Is HIV Infection? **HIV infection** is a chronic disease that progressively damages the body's immune system, making an otherwise healthy person less able to resist a variety of infections and disorders. Normally, when a virus or other pathogen enters the body, it is targeted and destroyed by the immune system. But HIV attacks the immune system itself, invading and taking over **CD4 T cells** (white blood cells that fight infection), macrophages, and other essential elements of the immune system (see Chapter 18). HIV enters a human cell and converts its own genetic material, RNA, into DNA. It then inserts this DNA into the chromosomes of the host cell. The viral DNA is not only instrumental in producing new copies of HIV, but it also seriously reduces immune functions.

Immediately following infection with HIV, billions of infectious particles are produced every day. For a time, the immune system keeps pace, also producing billions of new cells. Unlike the virus, however, the immune system cannot make new cells indefinitely; as long as the virus keeps replicating, it wins in the end. The destruction of the immune system is signaled by the loss of CD4 T cells (Figure 19.1). As the number of CD4 cells declines, an infected person may begin to experience mild to moderately severe symptoms. A person is diagnosed with AIDS when the number of CD4 cells in the blood drops below a certain level (200/μl).

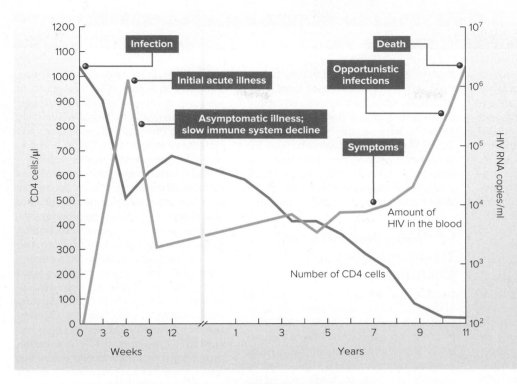

During the initial acute illness, CD4 levels fall sharply and HIV RNA levels increase; 60–90% of infected people experience flulike symptoms during this period. Antibodies to HIV usually appear 2–12 weeks after the initial infection. During the asymptomatic phase that follows, CD4 levels gradually decline, and HIV RNA levels again increase. Due to declines in immunity, infected individuals eventually begin to experience symptoms; when CD4 levels drop very low, people become vulnerable to serious opportunistic infections characteristic of full-blown AIDS. Chronic or recurrent illnesses continue until the immune system fails and death results.

FIGURE 19.1 **The general pattern of untreated HIV infection.** The blue line represents the number of CD4 cells in the blood, a marker for the status of the immune system. The orange line shows the amount of HIV RNA in the blood.

SOURCE: Adapted from Fauci, A. S., and G. Pantaleo. 1996. Immunopathogenic mechanisms of HIV infection. *Annals of Internal Medicine* 124(7): 654–663, Figure 1.

People with AIDS are vulnerable to several serious **opportunistic (secondary) infections**.

The first weeks after being infected with HIV are called the *primary infection* phase. Most, but not all, infected people develop flulike symptoms about two to four weeks after being exposed to the virus. During primary HIV infection, people have large amounts of HIV in the bloodstream and genital fluids, making it easier to transmit the virus. Several months later, infected people develop antibodies to the virus, so commonly available tests will show a positive result. The next phase of HIV infection is the chronic **asymptomatic** (symptom-free) stage, also called the *latency* phase. This period can last from 2 to 20 years, averaging 11 years in untreated adults. During this time, the virus progressively infects and destroys the cells of the immune system. Even if they are symptom-free, people infected with HIV can transmit the disease to others if untreated.

Transmitting the Virus HIV lives only within cells and body fluids, not outside the body. It is transmitted by blood and blood products, semen, vaginal and cervical secretions, and breast milk. It cannot live in air, in water, or on objects or surfaces such as toilet seats, eating utensils, or telephones. A person is not at risk of HIV infection by being in the same classroom, dining room, or even household with someone who is infected.

There are three main routes of HIV transmission:

- Specific kinds of sexual contact
- Direct exposure to infected blood

- Contact between an HIV-positive woman and her child during pregnancy, childbirth, premastication (prechewing food for a child) or breastfeeding

SEXUAL CONTACT HIV is more likely to be transmitted by unprotected anal or vaginal intercourse than by other sexual activities. During vaginal intercourse, male-to-female transmission is more likely to occur than female-to-male transmission. HIV has been found in preejaculatory fluid, which means that transmission can occur before ejaculation. Being the receptive partner during unprotected anal intercourse is the riskiest of all sexual activities. Oral–genital contact carries some risk of transmission, although less than anal or vaginal intercourse. HIV can be transmitted through tiny tears, traumatized points, or irritated areas in the lining of the vagina, cervix, penis, anus, mouth, and throat and through direct infection of cells in these areas. Sexual assault is a major factor in the transmission of HIV throughout the world. Barrier protection is almost never used during sexual assault, and tissue trauma is generally greater than in unforced sexual activity.

opportunistic (secondary) infection An infection caused when organisms take the opportunity presented by a primary (initial) infection to multiply and cause a new, different infection. **TERMS**

asymptomatic Showing no signs or symptoms of a disease.

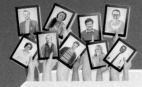

DIVERSITY MATTERS
HIV/AIDS around the World

We are nearly four decades removed from the first reports of cases of what we now know as AIDS. Those cases appeared in gay men in California and New York, hemophiliacs, individuals who had received blood transfusions, injection drug users, infected women, and their newborn infants. To date, between 58.3 million and 98.1 million people have been infected, and tens of millions have died from HIV/AIDS.

Global Disparities in HIV/AIDS

The vast majority of cases have occurred in economically emerging countries, where heterosexual contact is the primary means of transmission. Sadly, HIV continues to disproportionately affect nonwhite racial and ethnic populations and the poor. Approximately 6000 women ages 15–24 are infected with HIV weekly. The gender imbalance is even more pronounced in sub-Saharan Africa, the hardest-hit region, where four in five new infections appear in adolescent girls ages 15–19, despite their comprising only 10% of the population. For adolescents, HIV falls among the top 10 causes of death overall and among the top five causes for younger adolescent girls aged 10–14. Factors at the root of this disparity include harmful gender norms and inequalities, violence, poverty, and lack of access to sexual and reproductive health services.

Other key populations at risk worldwide include gay men and other men who have sex with men, people who inject drugs, sex workers, transgender people, prisoners, clients of sex workers, and other sex partners of at-risk populations. These groups are often marginalized and stigmatized, reducing their access to services, which in turn increases rates of infection. Outside of sub-Saharan Africa, key populations and their partners accounted for up to 95% of new HIV infections in 2018. The risk of HIV infection was 22 times higher among men who have sex with men and persons who inject drugs, 21 times higher among sex workers, and 12 times higher among transgender people.

HIV/AIDS Prevention and Treatment Gains and Challenges

Despite the ongoing tragedy of the epidemic, strides have been made in treatment and prevention measures. In 2018, an estimated 79% of people living with HIV knew their status, 62% were on treatment, and 63% were virally suppressed. Due to these scaled-up efforts, the rate of new infections and deaths has declined in some regions. AIDS-related deaths have decreased 56% since they peaked in 2004. Treating HIV with effective drugs not only prolongs life and decreases suffering, but it also reduces the spread of the virus because individuals who have received treatment are generally much less infectious than those who have not.

Efforts to combat AIDS are complicated by political, economic, and cultural barriers. Education and prevention programs are often hampered by resistance from social and religious institutions and by the taboo on openly discussing sexual issues. Moreover, approximately 50% of adolescents cannot make decisions about their health. Condoms are not commonly used in many countries, and even when they are, women may not have agency to negotiate their use. Empowering women is a crucial priority in reducing the spread of HIV. In particular, reducing sexual violence against women, promoting financial independence, and increasing women's education and employment opportunities are essential.

Successful prevention approaches include STI treatment and education, public education campaigns about safer sex, and syringe exchange programs for injection drug users. Efforts are ongoing to improve access to barrier protective devices such as condoms. Male circumcision has been shown to reduce the risk of heterosexually acquired HIV infection in men by about 60%; voluntary adult male circumcision is recommended by the World Health Organization (WHO) as part of HIV prevention programs in regions with HIV epidemics among heterosexuals and with high HIV and low male circumcision prevalence. The partial protection provided by circumcision does not eliminate the need for condom use. The effectiveness for HIV prevention of consistent condom use is estimated to be about 70–80%.

Despite progress, according to the Joint United Nations Programme on HIV/AIDS (UNAIDS), without a scale-up in prevention and treatment efforts, the epidemic will continue to outrun the response. There is a historic obligation to end the AIDS epidemic. UNAIDS launched a fast-track strategy in 2014 that aimed to greatly step up the response in low- and middle-income countries, with the goal of ending the epidemic by 2030. For 2020, UNAIDS set a 90-90-90 treatment target:

- 90% of people living with HIV know their status.

The presence of lesions, blisters, or inflammation from other STIs in the genital, anal, or oral areas makes it two to nine times easier for the virus to be passed. Spermicides may also cause irritation and increase the risk of HIV transmission. Studies of the widely used spermicide nonoxynol-9 (N-9) have found that frequent use may cause vaginal and rectal irritation, increasing the risk of transmission of HIV and other STIs. The WHO recommends that spermicides containing N-9 not be used for protection against HIV and STIs. Condoms or lubricants with N-9 should never be used during anal intercourse because N-9 damages the lining of the rectum, providing an entry point for HIV and other STIs. Recent studies show that some other commonly used lubricants can also cause rectal irritation (see the box "Playing It Safe").

The risk of HIV transmission during oral sex is generally considered to be low but may be increased if a person has oral sores or other damage to the gums or tissues in the mouth.

Studies in economically emerging nations with high rates of HIV infection have found that circumcised males have a lower risk of HIV infection than uncircumcised males. Circumcision is uncommon in most parts of the world, but these findings are

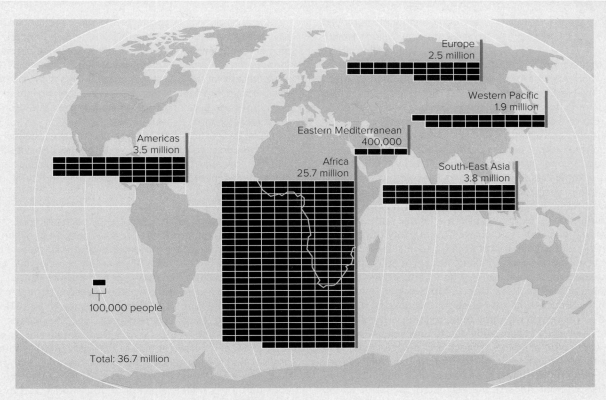

Europe
2.5 million

Western Pacific
1.9 million

Eastern Mediterranean
400,000

Americas
3.5 million

Africa
25.7 million

South-East Asia
3.8 million

100,000 people

Total: 36.7 million

Approximate number of people living with HIV/AIDS in 2018.

- 90% of people living with HIV who know their status are receiving treatment.

- 90% of people on treatment have suppressed viral loads. However, we still have miles to go.

The United States continues to be involved in the global strategy for closing treatment and prevention gaps. The President's Emergency Plan for AIDS Relief (PEPFAR), the Global Fund, and other organizations helped save more than 21.7 million lives, with PEPFAR supporting the provision of lifesaving antiretrovirals to over 14.6 million people. In 2019 the Office of the President put forth a renewed effort to reduce new HIV infections by 90% over the next 10 years domestically. This strategy will focus on four main areas: early diagnosis of HIV infections, striving for undetectable viral loads in individuals undergoing HIV treatment, optimizing HIV prevention strategies such as PrEP in communities where there is high risk for HIV, and rapidly identifying and responding to clusters of HIV infection to reduce transmission. Key to addressing these areas will be collaboration with multiple stakeholders in the community and addressing wealth, geographic, and racial disparities associated with HIV.

SOURCES: UNAIDS. 2018. *Global AIDS Update 2018: Miles to Go: Closing Gaps, Breaking Barriers, Righting Injustices* (https://www.unaids.org/en/20180718 _GR2018); Joint United Nations Programme on HIV/AIDS. 2016. *On the Fast-Track to End AIDS: 2016–2021 Strategy*. Geneva: UNAIDS; UNAIDS. 2019. *Women and HIV: A Spotlight on Adolescent Girls and Young Women* (https://www.unaids.org/sites/default/files/media_asset/2019_women-and-hiv_en.pdf).

heightening interest in the practice. In the United States, where HIV infection rates are much lower, circumcision does not appear to offer any significant protection against HIV.

DIRECT CONTACT WITH INFECTED BLOOD Direct contact with the blood of an infected person is another major route of HIV transmission. Needles and syringes used to inject drugs (including heroin, cocaine, anabolic steroids, and opioid medications) are usually contaminated with the user's blood. If needles are shared, small amounts of one person's blood are injected directly into another person's bloodstream. HIV may be transmitted through subcutaneous and intramuscular injection as well, from needles or blades used in acupuncture, tattooing, body piercing, and ritual scarring.

In the past, before effective screening was available, some people were infected with HIV through blood transfusions and other medical procedures involving blood products. All blood in licensed U.S. blood banks and plasma centers is now screened thoroughly for bloodborne pathogens, including HIV. However, the blood supply is much less safe in the rest of the world due the prevalence of HIV in the donor pool, type/risk of donors, and access to education and screening

WELLNESS ON CAMPUS
Playing It Safe

College-age students surveyed by the American College Health Association–National College Health Assessment in spring 2019 reported on what types of sex they had. About 68% of women and 62% of men reported vaginal sex. Extragenital sex or sex at oral or anal sites is also more common than you might think: Oral sex was reported by about 70% of women and 68% of men; anal sex by 29% of male students and about 25% of female students.

Sexual practices among individuals are diverse and may change across one's life span. If you are sexually active or planning to be, know that depending on the sites of exposure (oral, penile-vaginal, anal), the type of sexual activity you engage in may have unique risks for sexually transmitted infections.

Although some people associate anal sex with gay sex, heterosexual anal sex is common. The majority of gay men and transgender women report having had anal sex, although the practice is not universal. Taking into account the fact that heterosexuals far outnumber gay and transgender people, the vast majority of anal sex is occurring between heterosexual couples. Educational efforts about the risks of anal sex have been geared toward gay men, missing a much larger group at risk for STI transmission due to anal sex.

Like every type of sexual contact, anal sex can have serious health consequences. Unprotected anal sex (without using a condom) is the riskiest of *all* sexual behaviors. For every act of unprotected anal sex, the estimated risk for acquiring HIV from an infected person is 11 (insertive) and 138 (receptive) out of 10,000 exposures. For penile-vaginal intercourse, the risk is 4 (insertive) and 8 (receptive). Anal sex is associated with high transmission levels of all the common STIs. Even if a condom is used, some STIs such as syphilis and herpes can be transferred through skin-to-skin contact.

Why is anal sex so risky? Anal tissues are much more delicate and easily damaged than vaginal tissue. The vaginal opening is more elastic and wider than the anal opening. The natural fluids that provide lubrication in the vagina are absent in anal tissue. Even gentle penetration of the anus tends to create small tears that infectious agents can enter easily. Bacteria and parasites in feces can also be easily passed to both sexual partners. Health risks are generally greatest for the receptive partner, but the insertive partner is also at high risk for transmission of infection at the opening at the tip of the penis (urethra), the foreskin (if uncircumcised), and nicks, cuts, or scratches where HIV can enter the body. HIV can also be found in pre-seminal fluid (pre-ejaculate) such that the risk for HIV exposure exists even if the penis is withdrawn prior to ejaculation. Condom use reduces the risk, but only a minority of people use condoms consistently for anal sex. Some heterosexual couples use anal sex as a form of contraception when they don't have a condom available. Although condoms provide some protection, it is not uncommon for condoms to break due to increased friction and stress during anal sex.

If people choose to have anal sex, how can it be made safer? Traditionally, health providers have recommended that plenty of non-oil-based lubricant should be used along with a condom to avoid tissue trauma, which increases the likelihood of STI transmission.

Currently only male condoms are approved for use in anal sex, but some experts believe that the female condom could also be effective and could provide the receptive partner with more control in protecting himself or herself against STIs. The currently available FC2 female condom was not designed for this purpose, but several researchers are looking into the possibility of reengineering the female condom and testing its effectiveness for anal intercourse.

Given the health risks, the choice to abstain from anal sex is reasonable and should be respected by partners. Besides the risk of STIs, repeated or forceful anal intercourse can cause anal fissures, ulcers, hemorrhoids, rectal prolapse, and stool incontinence.

Oral sex, the practice of using the mouth or tongue to stimulate a sex partner's penis (fellatio), vagina (cunnilingus), or anus (anilingus), is a common form of sex. It is possible to get an STI in your mouth or throat by giving oral sex to your partner if they have a genital or anal/rectal STI. Similarly, it is possible to give your partner an STI at the genitals or anus/rectum if infected. The risk of acquiring sexually transmitted infections through oral sex depends on the type of STI, the prevalence of the STI in the population, the sexual acts performed, and the number of the exposures.

Additionally, certain strains of HPV may be transmitted by oral sex and lead to cancer of the neck or throat. Many infections are asymptomatic, and you cannot reliably predict if your partner is infected or not. If you choose to have oral sex, you can decrease your chances of getting an STI of the mouth, throat, genitals, or anus/rectum by making sure that you and your partner use barrier protection consistently. For performing oral sex on the penis, use nonlubricated latex or, if you have a latex allergy, polyurethane condoms. For performing oral sex on the vagina or anus, use a dental dam as a protective barrier between the mouth and partner's vagina or anus.

So which is safer: oral, vaginal, or anal sex? When it comes to HIV, the risk of acquisition is lower for insertive and receptive oral sex than for vaginal or anal sex. But several bacterial STIs such as syphilis, gonorrhea, and chlamydia still pose a serious threat. The only way you can avoid an STI is to not have sex or remain in a mutually monogamous sexual relationship with a partner who is not infected with an STI (tested with negative results). The choice to have sexual intercourse is very personal and should be made with the knowledge of its inherent risks. If you choose to have sex, play it safe!

SOURCES: American College Health Association. 2018. *American College Health Association–National College Health Assessment II: Reference Group Executive Summary Spring 2019*. Hanover, MD: American College Health Association; Centers for Disease Control and Prevention. 2019. *HIV Risk Behaviors* (http://www.cdc.gov/hiv/risk/estimates/riskbehaviors.html); Centers for Disease Control and Prevention. 2019. *Anal Sex and HIV Risk* (https://www.cdc.gov/hiv/risk/analsex.html); Crosby, R. A., et al. 2018. A comparison of HIV-risk behaviors between young black cisgender men who have sex with men and young black transgender women who have sex with men. *International Journal of STD & AIDS* 29(7): 665–672; Centers for Disease Control and Prevention. *Condom Use and STDs* (https://www.cdc.gov/condomeffectiveness/docs/Condoms_and_STDS.pdf).

technologies. The WHO estimates that 0.003% of high- and 1.08% of low-income countries have transfusion transmissible HIV in their blood donor supply.

A small number of health care workers have acquired HIV on the job. Most of these cases involve needle sticks, in which a health care worker is accidentally stuck with a needle used on an infected patient. The likelihood of a patient's acquiring HIV infection from a health care worker is almost negligible; the risk of health care workers' acquiring HIV from infected patients is much greater.

MOTHER-TO-CHILD TRANSMISSION The final major route of HIV transmission is mother-to-child transmission (MCT), also called *vertical* or *perinatal transmission.* MCT can occur during pregnancy, childbirth, breastfeeding, or premastication. Without intervention, the likelihood of HIV transmission from mother to child is 15–45%; with intervention, the likelihood is reduced to less than 1%. This intervention commonly occurs for women in the United States and other industrialized countries. In the United States, it is estimated that less than 5000 women live with HIV and give birth every year. Interrupting the transmission includes continued access to HIV care and antiretroviral medications for both the pregnant woman and the child during those stages in which transmission is known to occur. The mother should avoid breastfeeding and premastication. Before conception, counseling should involve a discussion of risk behaviors including substance abuse, and treatment and prevention services such as needle exchange, if relevant.

Populations of Special Concern for HIV Infection

The populations most vulnerable to HIV infection include the youngest sexually active people (aged 13–24), people who inject drugs, and men who have sex with other men. Young people are more likely to report that they have never been tested for HIV. In 2018, this age group made up 21% of all new HIV diagnoses in the United States. Young African American and Latino gay and bisexual men were especially affected.

Among Americans newly diagnosed with HIV infection, the most common means of HIV exposure is sexual activity between men (Figure 19.2). Men who have sex with men (MSM) represent about 2% of the male population in the United States but they account for most cases of HIV. Drug and alcohol use has also been associated with risky sexual behavior and is directly or indirectly associated with HIV acquisition in this population. Use of methamphetamine and club drugs, as well as the recreational use of erectile dysfunction drugs, has been associated with risky sexual behavior and HIV infection in MSM.

Data from the 2018 HIV Surveillance Report indicate that 7% of newly diagnosed HIV cases are attributable to injection drug use. People who inject drugs are particularly at risk from unsafe injection practices and high-risk sex, including condomless sex with casual partners and exchang-

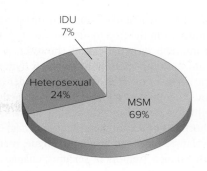

* MSM = Men who have sex with men
IDU = Injection drug users

FIGURE 19.2 **Routes of HIV transmission among Americans newly diagnosed with HIV infection in 2018.**

SOURCE: Centers for Disease Control and Prevention. 2020. *HIV in the United States and Dependent Areas* (https://www.cdc.gov/hiv/statistics/overview/ataglance.html).

ing sex for money or drugs. These findings highlight the importance of educating people who inject drugs about HIV acquisition. Topics should include safe injection practices, how to get substance abuse counseling, and medication-assisted treatment.

In the United States, high rates of HIV infection occur in males, certain racial and ethnic groups, and poor people. In 2018, blacks and Latinos represented 42% and 27% of new HIV cases even though they make up only 12% and 18% of the U.S. population, respectively. The majority of these infections occurred among men, particularly those reporting male-to-male sexual contact.

These patterns of HIV infection reflect complex social, economic, and behavioral factors. Reducing the rates of HIV transmission and AIDS death in nonwhite racial and ethnic groups, women, and high-risk groups requires addressing problems of poverty, discrimination, and drug abuse. HIV prevention programs must be tailored to meet the special needs of high-risk underserved communities and include testing, education, and equal access to health care.

Symptoms As described earlier, in the days or weeks following infection with HIV, most people develop symptoms, which can include fever, fatigue, rashes, headache, swollen lymph nodes, body aches, night sweats, sore throat, nausea, and ulcers in the mouth. Symptoms of primary infection can last from a few days to more than a month. Because these symptoms are similar to those of many common viral illnesses, the condition often goes undiagnosed.

Diagnosis of HIV at this very early stage of infection is extremely beneficial. People with early-stage HIV can make lifestyle changes to improve their overall health during this period. They can also protect their partners during this phase, when viral levels are high—by initiating antiretroviral therapy and using condoms correctly and consistently.

QUICK STATS

46% of Americans aged 18–64 have been tested for HIV at least once.
—Kaiser Family Foundation, 2019

Other than the initial flulike symptoms, most people have few if any symptoms in the first months or years of HIV infection. As the immune system weakens, however, a variety of symptoms can develop—persistent swollen lymph nodes; lumps, rashes, sores, or other growths on or under the skin or on the mucous membranes; persistent yeast infections; unexplained weight loss; fever and drenching night sweats; dry cough and shortness of breath; persistent diarrhea; easy bruising and unexplained bleeding; profound fatigue; memory loss; difficulty with balance; tremors or seizures; changes in vision, hearing, taste, or smell; changes in mood and other psychological symptoms; and persistent or recurrent pain. Many of these symptoms can also occur with a variety of other illnesses.

Because the immune system is weakened, people with HIV infection are highly susceptible to opportunistic infections, as noted earlier. The infection most often seen in the United States among people with HIV is *Pneumocystis* **pneumonia,** a fungal infection. **Kaposi's sarcoma,** a previously rare form of cancer, is common in HIV-positive men. Women with HIV infection often have frequent and difficult-to-treat vaginal yeast infections. Cases of tuberculosis (TB) are increasingly being reported in people with HIV, and the CDC recommends TB testing for anyone with HIV infection.

Diagnosis   Three general types of HIV diagnostic tests are currently available:

- **HIV antibody tests,** performed on blood or oral fluids, check whether the body is producing antibodies against the HIV virus; these tests usually detect infection within 3–12 weeks after exposure.
- **Combination HIV antigen/antibody tests** look both for antibodies and for an HIV antigen known as p24 (part of the virus itself). Because the antigen is produced before antibodies develop, combination blood tests can detect HIV earlier in the course of infection (usually 2-6 weeks after exposure), compared to antibody-only tests.

TERMS

***Pneumocystis* pneumonia**   A fungal infection common in people infected with HIV.

Kaposi's sarcoma   A form of cancer characterized by purple or brownish lesions that are generally painless and occur anywhere on the skin; usually appears in persons infected with HIV.

HIV antibody test   A blood test to determine whether a person has been infected with HIV; becomes positive within weeks or months of exposure.

combination HIV antigen/antibody test   A blood test that detects the presence of HIV p24 antigen, an early marker for HIV infection, as well as HIV antibodies.

HIV nucleic acid test (NAT)   A test used to detect the presence of HIV RNA and to determine the viral load (the amount of HIV in the blood).

HIV positive   A diagnosis resulting from the presence of HIV in the bloodstream; also referred to as *seropositive*.

- **Nucleic acid tests (NATs)** test directly for HIV RNA in the blood and can usually detect HIV within 1-4 after infection; the test is expensive and not routinely used for initial screening.

If you get an HIV test within three months after a potential HIV exposure and the result is negative, get tested again in three months, or earlier if at greater risk for HIV. Testing for HIV is recommended for everyone (see the box "Getting an HIV Test").

If a person is diagnosed as **HIV positive,** the next step is to determine the disease's severity. The infection itself can be monitored by tracking the viral load (the amount of virus in the body) with blood tests that measure HIV RNA (NAT tests).

A diagnosis of AIDS, the most severe form of HIV infection, is given if a person is HIV positive and either has developed an infection defined as an AIDS indicator or has a severely damaged immune system (as measured by CD4 T cell counts).

The CDC recommends that states provide opportunities for people to receive confidential HIV testing and counseling services. In the United States, every state has laws that require doctors, clinics, and laboratories to report all diagnosed cases of HIV and AIDS to public health authorities, who use this information to track and prevent the spread of the disease. Despite efforts to safeguard confidentiality and prohibit discrimination, mandatory reporting of HIV infection remains controversial. If people believe they are risking their jobs, friends, or social acceptability, they may be less likely to get tested or disclose partners to public health authorities. Resources are available to help you tell others the news: https://www.cdc.gov/hiv/basics/livingwithhiv/telling-others.html.

Treatment   Although there is no known cure for HIV infection, medications can significantly alter the course of the disease and extend life. The drop in the number of U.S. AIDS deaths since 1996 is in large part due to the increasing use of combinations of new drugs.

The main types of antiviral drugs used against HIV/AIDS are reverse transcriptase inhibitors, protease inhibitors, integrase inhibitors, and entry inhibitors. These drugs either block HIV from replicating itself or prevent it from infecting other cells (Figure 19.3). Research has shown that using combinations of antiviral drugs can sometimes reduce HIV in the blood to undetectable levels. A healthy person infected with HIV who takes HIV medications as prescribed and has achieved HIV virus suppression, or undetectable levels of HIV in the blood, has effectively no risk of transmitting HIV to an uninfected partner. More than 30 drugs are now available to treat HIV, including several once-a-day tablets (containing a combination of HIV medications). Patients with low CD4 T cell counts can take a variety of antibiotics to help prevent opportunistic infections such as pneumonia, tuberculosis, and other bacterial and fungal infections.

HIV treatment is also challenging because taking the combination drugs is complicated, and the drugs have short-term side

Who and How Often?

The CDC recommends that everyone between the ages of 13 and 64 be tested for HIV at least once as part of routine health care. The CDC hopes that routine HIV testing will increase the likelihood that people with HIV will be diagnosed earlier. People with certain risk factors should be tested more often. The CDC recommends testing at least once a year for anyone who answers yes to any of the following:

- Are you a man who has had sex with another man?

- Have you had sex—anal or vaginal—with an HIV-positive partner?

- Have you had more than one sex partner since your last HIV test?

- Have you injected drugs and shared needles or "works" (e.g., water or cotton) with others?

- Have you exchanged sex for drugs or money?

- Have you been diagnosed with or sought treatment for another STI?

- Have you been diagnosed with or received treatment for hepatitis or TB?

- Have you had sex with someone who could answer yes to any of the above questions or someone whose sexual history you don't know?

In addition, CDC guidelines state that sexually active gay and bisexual men may benefit from more frequent testing (e.g., every three to six months).

Physician or Clinic Testing

Your physician, student health clinic, Planned Parenthood, or public health department can arrange your HIV test. Testing usually costs $50–$100, but public clinics often charge little or nothing. The standard test involves drawing a sample of blood that is sent to a lab, where it is checked using one or more of the available test types. For accuracy and early diagnosis, the CDC recommends laboratory tests done in the following sequence:

1. Combination test; if it is positive for antibodies and/or p24 antigen, this is followed by

2. Specialized antibody test, which confirms which type of HIV is present

3. If findings from the second test are indeterminate or contradictory, a NAT test is done to confirm if HIV RNA is present

It may take a week or more for the results of these tests to become available, and you'll be asked to call or come in personally to obtain your results, which should also include appropriate counseling.

Alternative tests are available at some clinics. Rapid oral tests use oral fluid, which is collected by swabbing the inside of the mouth. Rapid tests are available at some locations. These tests involve the use of blood or oral fluid and can provide results in as little as 20 minutes. If a rapid test is positive for HIV infection, a confirming test will be performed. Most rapid tests are antibody tests, which may be less likely than

combination tests to detect HIV infection in the first few weeks following exposure. Similarly, blood tests may detect infection earlier than oral fluid tests, because the level of antibodies in oral fluid is lower than in blood.

Before you get an HIV test, be sure you understand what will be done with the results. Results from confidential tests may still become part of your medical record and are required to be reported to state and federal public health agencies. If you decide you want to be tested anonymously, ask your physician about an anonymous test, or use a home test.

Home Testing

Home test kits vary in cost; however, you should be able to purchase a kit for $40–$70. Avoid test kits sold on the internet that are not approved by the U.S. Food and Drug Administration (FDA). As of this printing, two HIV home-testing devices were approved by the FDA: Home Access and OraQuick. Positive results with either test kit need to be confirmed with follow-up testing. To use the Home Access test, you prick a finger with a supplied lancet, blot a few drops of blood onto blotting paper, and mail it to the company's laboratory. In about a week (or within three business days for more expensive "express" tests), you call a toll-free number to find out your results. Anyone testing positive is routed to a trained counselor, who can provide emotional and medical support. The OraQuick HIV test, manufactured by Orasure, was approved by the FDA in July 2012. This home test is the first rapid HIV test approved for home use. Like the Orasure test available to clinics, the OraQuick home test uses a sample taken from the mouth and returns results in 20 minutes. The results of home test kits are completely anonymous. Anyone testing positive should call a medical doctor or the OraQuick Consumer Support Center for counseling and routes to care.

Understanding the Results

A negative test result means that no evidence of infection was found—no antibodies or, if you had a combination test, p24 antigens. However, as noted earlier, it may take three weeks or even longer for the infection to be detectable. Therefore, an infected person may get a false-negative result. If you test negative but your risk of infection is high, ask about obtaining an NAT test, which allows for very early diagnosis. If you engage in any risky behaviors, get retested frequently.

A positive result means that you are infected. Seek medical care and counseling immediately. Rapid progress is being made in treating HIV, and treatments are potentially much more successful when started early. For more information about testing, visit the CDC National HIV, STD, and Hepatitis Testing website (www.hivtest.org).

SOURCES: Centers for Disease Control and Prevention. 2020. *HIV Basics: Testing* (http://www.cdc.gov/hiv/basics/testing.html); HIV.gov. 2020. *HIV Testing Overview* (https://www.hiv.gov/hiv-basics/hiv-testing/learn-about -hiv-testing-overview); Centers for Disease Control and Prevention and Association of Public Health Laboratories. 2014. *Laboratory Testing for the Diagnosis of HIV Infection: Updated Recommendations* (http://dx.doi .org/10.15620/cdc.23447); U.S. Food and Drug Administration. 2018. *Testing for HIV* (http://www.fda.gov/BiologicsBloodVaccines /SafetyAvailability/HIVHomeTestKits/ucm126460.htm).

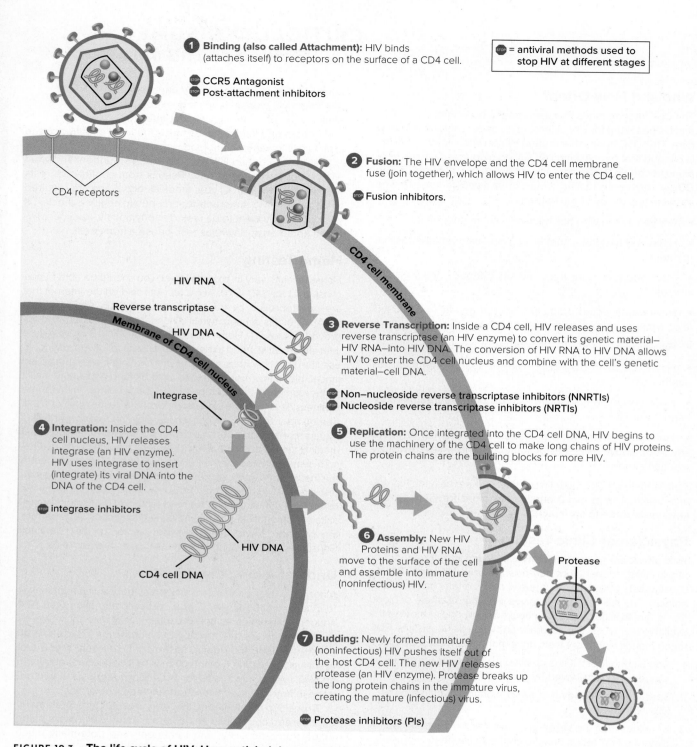

1 Binding (also called Attachment): HIV binds (attaches itself) to receptors on the surface of a CD4 cell.

■ CCR5 Antagonist
■ Post-attachment inhibitors

■ = antiviral methods used to stop HIV at different stages

CD4 receptors

2 Fusion: The HIV envelope and the CD4 cell membrane fuse (join together), which allows HIV to enter the CD4 cell.

■ Fusion inhibitors.

CD4 cell membrane

HIV RNA
Reverse transcriptase
HIV DNA
Membrane of CD4 cell nucleus
Integrase

3 Reverse Transcription: Inside a CD4 cell, HIV releases and uses reverse transcriptase (an HIV enzyme) to convert its genetic material—HIV RNA—into HIV DNA. The conversion of HIV RNA to HIV DNA allows HIV to enter the CD4 cell nucleus and combine with the cell's genetic material—cell DNA.

■ Non–nucleoside reverse transcriptase inhibitors (NNRTIs)
■ Nucleoside reverse transcriptase inhibitors (NRTIs)

4 Integration: Inside the CD4 cell nucleus, HIV releases integrase (an HIV enzyme). HIV uses integrase to insert (integrate) its viral DNA into the DNA of the CD4 cell.

■ integrase inhibitors

5 Replication: Once integrated into the CD4 cell DNA, HIV begins to use the machinery of the CD4 cell to make long chains of HIV proteins. The protein chains are the building blocks for more HIV.

HIV DNA
CD4 cell DNA

6 Assembly: New HIV Proteins and HIV RNA move to the surface of the cell and assemble into immature (noninfectious) HIV.

Protease

7 Budding: Newly formed immature (noninfectious) HIV pushes itself out of the host CD4 cell. The new HIV releases protease (an HIV enzyme). Protease breaks up the long protein chains in the immature virus, creating the mature (infectious) virus.

■ Protease inhibitors (PIs)

FIGURE 19.3 **The life cycle of HIV: How antiviral drugs work.** Different classes of drugs block the replication of HIV at different points in the virus's life cycle.

SOURCE: National Institutes of Health. 2019. *The HIV Life Cycle* (http://aidsinfo.nih.gov/understanding-hiv-aids/infographics/7/hiv-life-cycle).

effects that may cause people to stop taking them. Drug resistance develops quickly if the medicines are taken inconsistently. The drugs can also have long-term side effects, including serious health problems in some individuals. The National Institutes of Health (NIH) has issued guidelines for HIV treatment that help patients and their doctors with decisions about the optimal retroviral treatment. Data from randomized, controlled clinical trials have demonstrated a clinical benefit to early initiation of antiretroviral therapy for the treatment of HIV. Moreover, the reduced likelihood that an infected individual receiving early treatment will transmit HIV to others highlights the potential public health advantage to this approach.

Over the past few years, there have been attempts to eradicate HIV and to effectively produce a functional cure. The case of Timothy Brown, the Berlin Patient, is the most famous example: Because Brown had leukemia, in addition to HIV, he received a stem cell transplant while living in Berlin in 2007 and 2008. The donor had two copies of a unique genetic mutation that blocks HIV entry into the cell. After Brown received the transplant, HIV was no longer detectable.

Recently, a similar case of sustained HIV remission was reported in an HIV-infected patient with Hodgkin's lymphoma who received a stem cell transplant for treatment of his malignancy. Although this process appears to have been successful, due to the inherent risk and cost of this procedure, it cannot be routinely recommended.

Prevention Research on the development of a safe, effective, and inexpensive vaccine to stop the spread of HIV worldwide has been ongoing. Currently researchers are investigating **microbicides** that could be used to prevent HIV and other STIs. A microbicide in the form of a cream, gel, sponge, or suppository could function as a kind of chemical condom.

Effective approaches to prevention include abstinence, correct and consistent condom use with all sexual acts, and needle exchange programs for persons who use intravenous drugs. Another prevention method is called a preexposure prophylaxis (PrEP), meaning that it is intended to be used with other methods for reducing HIV risk. The FDA has approved PrEP, a drug to be taken by people who do not have HIV but are at high risk for it. In some cases, medications are also used to prevent infection in people who have been exposed to HIV, such as victims of sexual assault and health care workers with potential exposure to HIV-positive blood or other body fluids. This type of treatment, called PEP, should begin as soon as possible after exposure, but always within 72 hours. PEP treatment usually lasts 28 days. The out-of-pocket costs for PrEP and PEP can be high. But talk to your provider—financial help is sometimes available.

Decreasing the amount of HIV virus in the body to prevent transmission—whether from mother to child, during birth, breastfeeding, sex, or needle sharing—is a treatment that is often referred to as prevention. Several large studies have demonstrated that HIV virus suppression or undetectable levels of HIV in the blood can effectively prevent the transmission of HIV to an uninfected partner.

The cost of treatment for HIV continues to be an area of major concern. Costs are tremendous even for relatively wealthy countries, but 95% of people with HIV infection live in poor countries, where treatments are unlikely to be available to anyone except the wealthiest few. Pharmaceutical companies, the World Bank, and the international community are working to lower drug costs and provide aid for developing regions. Improved access and increased use of HIV treatment as a form of prevention is a game changer, furthering our progress toward the goal of zero HIV transmission in the near future.

How Can You Protect Yourself? Although AIDS cannot be cured, infection can be prevented. You can protect

High Risk

Unprotected anal sex is the riskiest sexual behavior, especially for the receptive partner.

Unprotected vaginal intercourse is the next riskiest, especially for women, who are much more likely to be infected by an infected male partner than vice versa.

Oral sex is probably considerably less risky than anal and vaginal intercourse but can still result in HIV transmission.

Sharing of sex toys is considered low risk but carries a theoretical risk of transmission because they can carry blood, semen, or vaginal fluid.

Use of a condom reduces risk considerably but not completely for any type of intercourse. Anal sex with a condom is riskier than vaginal sex with a condom; oral sex with a condom is less risky, especially if the man does not ejaculate.

Hand-genital contact and deep kissing are less risky but could still theoretically transmit HIV; the presence of cuts or sores increases risk.

Sex with only one uninfected and totally faithful partner is without risk, but effective only if both partners are uninfected and completely monogamous.

Activities that don't involve the exchange of body fluids carry no risk: hugging, massage, closed-mouth kissing, masturbation, phone sex, and fantasy.

Abstinence is completely without risk. For many people, it can be an effective and reasonable method of avoiding HIV infection and other STIs during certain periods of life.

No Risk

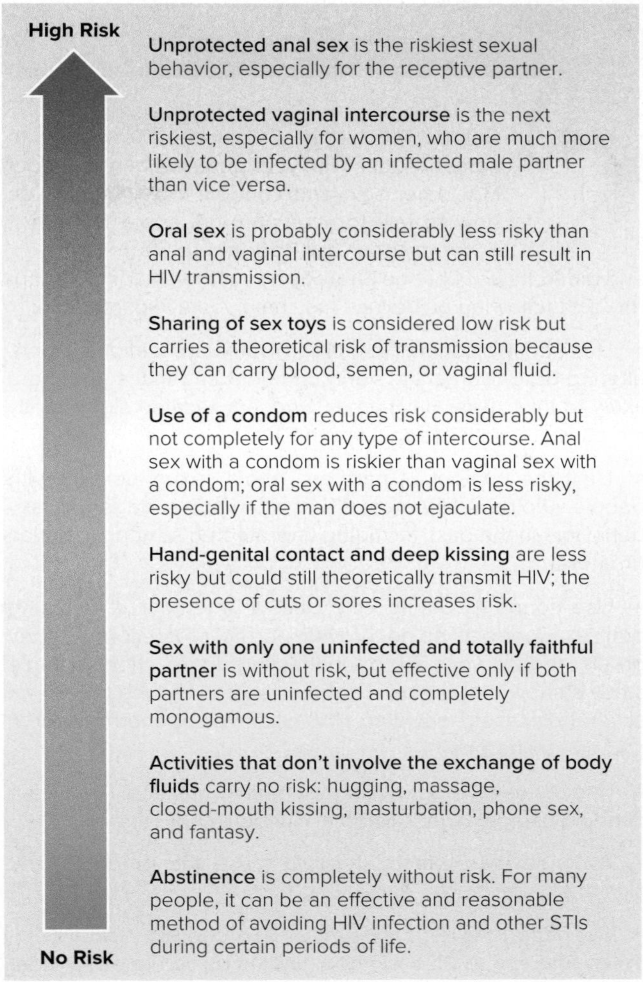

FIGURE 19.4 **What's risky and what's not: The approximate relative risk of HIV transmission in various sexual activities.** (For additional information about the risk of acquiring HIV from certain types of exposures, visit https://www.cdc.gov/hiv/risk/index.html.)

yourself by avoiding behaviors that may bring you into contact with HIV. This means making careful choices about sexual activity and not sharing needles if you inject drugs.

In a sexual relationship, the current and past behaviors of you and your partner determine the amount of risk involved. If you are uninfected and in a mutually monogamous relationship with another uninfected person, you are not at risk for HIV. For anyone not involved in a long-term, mutually monogamous relationship, abstinence from any sexual activity that involves the exchange of body fluids is the only sure way to prevent HIV infection (Figure 19.4).

Use of a condom reduces the risk of transmitting HIV during all forms of intercourse. Condoms are not perfect, and they do not ensure risk-free sex; however, used properly, a

microbicide A disinfectant that kills microorganisms and their spores.

TERMS

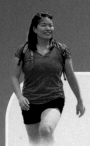

TAKE CHARGE
Preventing STIs

Before you begin a sexual relationship with someone, talk with your potential partner about HIV, safer sex, and condom use. (For tips on how to talk to your partners about STIs, visit www.gytnow.org/talking-to-your-partner/ and the Behavior Change Strategy box at the end of this chapter). The following guidelines may help you avoid infection:

• Don't drink alcohol or use drugs in sexual situations. Mood-altering drugs can affect your judgment and make you more likely to take risks. Having sex when intoxicated significantly increases the risk of exposure to STIs.

• Limit the number of partners. Avoid sexual contact with people who have HIV or an STI or who have engaged in risky behaviors in the past, including unprotected sex and injection drug use.

• Use condoms during every act of intercourse including oral sex. Condoms do not provide perfect protection, but they greatly reduce your risk of contracting an infection. Multiple studies show that regular condom use can reduce the risk of several diseases, including HIV, chlamydia, gonorrhea, HPV, and genital herpes.

• Use condoms properly for maximum protection. Follow the condom use guidelines listed in Chapter 7.

• Avoid sexual contact that could cause cuts or tears in the skin or tissue.

• Get periodic screening tests for STIs and HIV. Sexually active women aged 25 and under should be screened for gonorrhea and chlamydia at least annually, and older women at risk for STIs should be offered screening. MSM should be tested for STIs at least annually or more frequently depending on risk behaviors. As described in Chapter 17, a Pap test is recommended at age 21 and every three to five years thereafter, depending a woman's age and on whether a Pap test is combined with HPV screening. More frequent screening may be recommended for women who have compromised immune systems or abnormal screening results.

• Get vaccinated. All sexually active men and women should be vaccinated against hepatitis B. All MSM should be vaccinated against hepatitis A. Young men and women aged 26 years and under should consider getting vaccinated against HPV; the vaccine protects against the strains that cause most (but not all) cases of cervical cancer and genital warts.

• Get prompt treatment for any STIs you contract. Make sure your partner gets tested and receives treatment, too. In some parts of the country, expedited partner therapy may allow your health care provider to give you a prescription or medications for your partner (consult your health care provider to see if this is available in your area). Don't have sex until both of you have completed your treatment.

• If you inject drugs of any kind, don't share needles, syringes, or anything that might have blood on it. If your community has a syringe exchange program, use it. Seek treatment.

• If you are at risk for HIV infection, don't donate blood, sperm, or body organs. Don't have unprotected sex or share needles or syringes. Consider talking to your provider to see if PrEP is right for you. Get tested for HIV soon, and get treatment. HIV-positive people who receive early treatment generally feel better and live longer than those who delay.

---

condom provides a high level of protection against HIV. Experts also suggest the use of latex squares and dental dams as barriers during oral–genital or oral–anal sexual contact. As mentioned earlier, avoid using nonoxynol-9 lubricants because of the risk of tissue irritation, which can make STI transmission more likely.

People who inject drugs should avoid sharing needles, syringes, filters, or anything that might have blood on it. Needles can be decontaminated with a solution of bleach and water, but this is not a foolproof procedure, and HIV can survive in a syringe for a month or longer. HIV can also survive boiling. As described in Chapter 10, obtaining sterile syringes through a syringe exchange program is much more effective than attempting to sterilize used syringes.

If you have an ongoing risk for HIV exposure, talk to a health care provider about PrEP. Other measures to take in addition to safe injection practices include substance abuse counseling, treatment programs, and opioid replacement; these may be useful in decreasing HIV-risk-associated behaviors. Until an effective vaccine and a cure are found, HIV infection will remain one of the biggest challenges of this generation. Once you know your status, education on risk reduction and individual responsibility can lead the way to ending this epidemic (see the box "Preventing STIs"). Learn more about ways to stop the spread of HIV at www.cdc.gov/stophivtogether.

Chlamydia

Chlamydia trachomatis causes **chlamydia,** the most prevalent bacterial STI in the United States. According to the CDC, almost 1.8 million new cases of chlamydia were officially reported in 2018—a near 3% increase from the previous year. Many experts believe, however, that chlamydia is vastly underreported because infections are often asymptomatic, and screening may not occur. *C. trachomatis* can be transmitted by sexual contact with the penis, vagina, mouth, or anus of

chlamydia An STI transmitted by the bacterium *Chlamydia trachomatis*.

| Table 19.3 | Rates of Common STIs in the United States, per 100,000 Population, by Race/Ethnicity, 2018 |

	CHLAMYDIA	GONORRHEA	SYPHILIS*
American Indians/ Alaska Natives	784.8	329.5	15.5
Asians	132.1	35.1	4.6
Hispanics	392.6	115.9	13.0
Multirace	184.9	94.4	9.4
Native Hawaiians/ Other Pacific Islanders	700.8	181.4	16.3
Non-Hispanic Blacks	1,192.5	548.9	28.1
Non-Hispanic Whites	212.1	71.1	6.0

*Primary and secondary stages.

SOURCES: Centers for Disease Control and Prevention. 2019. *Sexually Transmitted Disease Surveillance 2018*. Atlanta, GA: Centers for Disease Control and Prevention.

an infected partner. If a mother has untreated chlamydia, it can be transmitted to the newborn perinatally (during the birthing process), leading to neonatal conjunctivitis (a type of eye infection) and pneumonia. Having a chlamydia infection increases the risk of HIV transmission.

Both men and women are susceptible to chlamydia, but, as with most STIs, women bear the greater burden because of possible complications and consequences of the disease. Rates of chlamydia in women were about two times those in men in 2018. For women, the highest rates of infection occur among 15- to 24-year-olds. For men, the highest rates occur among 20- to 24-year-olds. Black men and women have chlamydia infection rates nearly six times higher than those of white men and women (Table 19.3).

Symptoms Most people experience few or no symptoms from chlamydia infection, increasing the likelihood that they will inadvertently spread the infection to their partners. The exact time from chlamydia infection to symptomatic disease is unknown, though it may range up to 12 weeks. If they notice any symptoms, women may experience increased vaginal discharge, burning with urination, pain or bleeding with intercourse, and lower abdominal pain. Symptomatic chlamydia may show up as syndromes, including **urethritis**, inflammation of the urethra resulting in pain with urination; *cervicitis*, inflammation of the cervix characterized by discharge and bleeding on contact; and *proctitis*, inflammation of the rectum characterized by anorectal pain, the sensation of incomplete bowel movements, and discharge. Untreated urethral and cervical infections in women can lead to pelvic inflammatory disease (PID), which is discussed later in this chapter. Chlamydia also greatly increases a woman's risk for infertility and ectopic (tubal) pregnancy. The CDC currently recommends annual chlamydia testing for all sexually active women aged 25 and under and for older women. Older women who are at increased risk such as those with one or more partners that are new, concurrent, or have a history of STI, should be tested.

Symptoms for men can include painful urination, watery discharge from the penis, and pain around the testicles. Chlamydia can also lead to infertility in men. For those under age 35, chlamydia is the most common cause of epididymitis, which is inflammation of the sperm-carrying ducts. Up to half of all cases of urethritis in men are caused by chlamydia.

Infants of infected mothers can acquire the infection through contact with the pathogen in the birth canal during delivery; this exposure leads to infections in the mucous membranes of the eye, oropharynx, urogenital tract, and rectum, which may be asymptomatic. Symptomatic infection may include chlamydia conjunctivitis in up to 50% and pneumonia in up to 30% of infants born to women with untreated chlamydia.

Diagnosis and Treatment Chlamydia can be diagnosed through laboratory tests on the parts of the body that were exposed to the bacteria. Depending on the test, samples of urine, urethral, vaginal, cervical, throat, or rectal fluids may be collected by the patient or provider. Once chlamydia has been diagnosed, the infected person and his or her partner(s) are given antibiotics—usually doxycycline for a week or azithromycin in a single dose, which can cure uncomplicated infection. Testing and treatment of partners is important. When it is unlikely that a partner will seek medical treatment, the CDC recommends that extra medication or an extra prescription be given to the patient to provide to his or her partner. This strategy, called *expedited partner therapy,* is legal and encouraged in some states under certain circumstances. It is important that both partners complete their treatment before resuming sexual activity. If a one-dose treatment is given, couples should wait for seven days after taking their medication to resume sexual activity. Treatment for epididymitis and proctitis may involve more than one antibiotic and a longer duration of treatment. It is recommended that women and men who have received treatment for chlamydia be retested three months later, regardless of whether their partner received treatment, because of the likelihood of reinfection. Women who are pregnant should be retested earlier, at three to four weeks posttreatment and if at high risk should be rescreened later in pregnancy. All persons diagnosed with an STI should be tested for HIV.

Gonorrhea

Gonorrhea is caused by the bacterium *Neisseria gonorrhoeae,* which flourishes in mucous membranes and is transmitted

> **urethritis** Inflammation of the tube that carries urine from the bladder to the outside opening. **TERMS**
>
> **gonorrhea** A sexually transmitted bacterial infection caused by the bacterium *Neisseria gonorrhoeae* that usually affects mucous membranes.

through sexual contact with the penis, vagina, mouth, or anus of an infected partner. The microbe cannot thrive outside the human body and dies within moments of exposure to light and air.

In 2018, 583,405 new cases of gonorrhea were reported to the CDC, a significant increase from the previous year, mostly in men. Because the infection often causes no symptoms, many cases go undetected, and the number of new infections may be much higher. The incidence rates peak among 15- to 24-year-olds. Like chlamydia, gonorrhea can cause the syndromes urethritis, cervicitis, PID, epididymitis, and proctitis. It can also cause eye infections. Being infected with gonorrhea increases the likelihood that HIV will be acquired and transmitted. An infant passing through the birth canal of an infected mother may contract *gonococcal conjunctivitis*, an eye infection that can cause blindness if not treated. Newborn babies are routinely given antimicrobial eye drops to prevent gonorrhea infection.

Symptoms   In males, the incubation period for gonorrhea is generally two to seven days. The first symptoms are due to urethritis, which causes urinary discomfort and discharge from the penis. The lips of the urethral opening may become inflamed and swollen. In some cases, the lymph glands in the groin become enlarged and swollen. Up to half of infected males have very minor symptoms or none at all.

Most females with gonorrhea are asymptomatic. Those who have symptoms often experience pain with urination, increased vaginal discharge, pain or bleeding with intercourse, and lower abdominal pain. Women may also develop painful abscesses in the Bartholin glands, located on either side of the vaginal opening. Up to 40% of women with untreated gonorrhea develop PID.

Rectal gonorrhea infections in men and women may be associated with pus or blood in the feces or rectal pain and itching. Pharyngeal infections in men and women often do not cause symptoms; however, they may be associated with sore throat or pus on the tonsils.

Diagnosis and Treatment   Gonorrhea is detectable by several tests, which are performed at the sites of sexual exposure. Depending on the test, samples of urine, urethral, vaginal, cervical, throat, or rectal fluids may be collected by the patient or provider. Antibiotics are used to treat gonorrhea, but increasing drug resistance is a major concern.

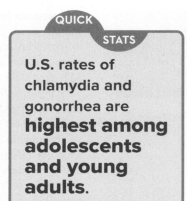

---

pelvic inflammatory disease (PID)   An ascending infection that progresses from the vagina and cervix to the uterus, oviducts, and pelvic cavity.

laparoscopy   A method of examining the internal organs by inserting a tube containing a small light through an abdominal incision.

TERMS

Pelvic Inflammatory Disease

Pelvic inflammatory disease (PID) is a major complication in 10–40% of women who have been infected with either gonorrhea or chlamydia and have not received treatment. PID occurs when the initial infection travels upward beyond the cervix into the uterus, oviducts, ovaries, and pelvic cavity. PID may be serious enough to require hospitalization and sometimes surgery. Even if the disease is treated successfully, about 25% of affected women will have long-term problems, such as a continuing susceptibility to infection, ectopic pregnancy, infertility, and chronic pelvic pain.

PID is the leading cause of infertility in young women, often going undetected until the inability to become pregnant leads to further evaluation. Infertility occurs in 8% of women after one episode of PID, 20% after two episodes, and 40% after three episodes. The risk of ectopic pregnancy, a medical emergency that can be fatal if not treated quickly, increases significantly in women who have had PID.

Women under age 25 are much more likely to develop PID than are older women. Risk factors include having a new or multiple sex partners, having a sex partner who has other sex partners at the same time, inconsistent use of condoms, prior history of an STI, vaginal douching, and intrauterine device use in the first three weeks after insertion. Smokers have twice the risk of PID compared to nonsmokers. Using an intrauterine device for contraception increases the risk of PID, though this is primarily confined to the first three weeks after insertion, and risk of an STI-related cause is greatly reduced for women with only one uninfected sexual partner.

Symptoms   Symptoms of PID vary greatly. Some women may be asymptomatic; others may have abdominal pain, fever, chills, nausea, and vomiting. Early symptoms are essentially the same as those described for chlamydia and gonorrhea. Symptoms often begin or worsen during or soon after a woman's menstrual period. Many women have abnormal vaginal bleeding—either bleeding between periods or heavy and painful menstrual bleeding.

Diagnosis and Treatment   Diagnosis of PID is made on the basis of symptoms, physical examination, ultrasound, and laboratory tests. Chlamydia and gonorrhea are bacteria associated with PID in sexually active women, and diagnosis of these infections may support the PID diagnosis. Other bacteria from within the vagina, such as those associated with bacterial vaginosis, may also be involved in some infections. **Laparoscopy** may be used to confirm the diagnosis and obtain material for cultures.

Treatment should begin as quickly as possible to minimize damage to the reproductive organs. Antibiotics are usually started immediately; in severe cases, the woman may be hospitalized and given intravenous antibiotics. It is especially

Why Do College Students Have High Rates of STIs?

- Risky sexual behavior is common. The National College Health Association found that fewer than half of college students used condoms consistently, and nearly a quarter of students reported more than one sex partner.

- College students underestimate their risk of STIs. Although students may have considerable knowledge about STIs, they often feel the risks do not apply to them—a dangerous assumption.

- Students may be infected but don't know it. Surveys by the National College Health Association found that despite reported access to sexual health services, a college survey found less than a quarter of women under age 26 received STI screening, and only 29% of students reported ever being tested for HIV.

What About Dating Apps?

- In this digital age, dating applications have expedited partner access with the click of a button or swipe.

- Some studies have shown an increase in risky sexual contacts and STIs with the use of dating apps for partner meetups. A number of factors are likely at play, including the ability to access new partner networks with varying levels of risk, which may increase the likelihood of STI exposure.

- Some apps allow users to disclose their STI, HIV, and PrEP use status upfront; however, this is not a reliable way to screen your partners.

What Can Students Do to Protect Themselves against STIs?

- Take charge of your sexual health. The only person you can count on to stay safe is you!

- Limit your number of sex partners. Even people who are always in a monogamous relationship can end up with extensive potential exposure to STIs if, over the years, they have many relationships.

- Use barrier protection consistently, and don't assume it's safe to stop after you've been with a partner for several months. HIV infection, HPV infection, herpes, and chlamydia can be asymptomatic for months or years and can be transmitted at any time. If you haven't been using condoms with your current partner, start now.

- Stay healthy, and follow up with a provider regularly. If you are at risk for HIV, talk to your provider about PrEP. If there is a possibility that you have been exposed to HIV, talk to your doctor about post-exposure prophylaxis (PEP). Get tested for HIV and STIs regularly, and know your status.

- Enjoy sexuality on your own terms. Don't let the expectations of friends and partners cause you to ignore your own feelings. Let your own wellness be your first priority. If you choose to be sexually active, learn about safer sex practices.

- Get to know your partner, and talk to him or her before becoming intimate. Be honest about yourself, and encourage your partner to do the same. But practice safer sex no matter what.

SOURCES: Beymer, M. R., R. E. Weiss, R. K. Bolan, et al. 2014. Sex on demand: Geosocial networking phone apps and risk of sexually transmitted infections among a cross-sectional sample of men who have sex with men in Los Angeles County. *Sexually Transmitted Infections* 90: 567–572; Cabecinha, M., C. H. Mercer, K. Gravningen, et al. 2017. Finding sexual partners online: Prevalence and associations with sexual behaviour, STI diagnoses and other sexual health outcomes in the British population. *Sexually Transmitted Infections* 93: 572–582.

important that an infected woman's partners receive treatment. As many as 60% of the male contacts of women with PID are infected, up to half of whom are asymptomatic.

Human Papillomavirus

Human papillomavirus (HPV) infection can cause several diseases, including common warts, **genital warts** (Figure 19.5), and genital cancers. HPV causes virtually all cervical cancers, as well as anal, penile, vulvar, vaginal, and some forms of oropharyngeal cancers (the oropharynx includes the back of the mouth and the throat). Genital HPV is usually spread through sexual activity, including oral sex.

HPV is the most common STI in the United States. About 14 million Americans become infected with HPV each year. In all, more than 80% of sexually active people will have been infected with HPV by age 50. HPV is especially common in young people, with some of the highest infection rates among college students (see the box "College Students and STIs"). Many young women contract HPV infection within three months of becoming sexually active.

There are more than 100 different strains of HPV, and different strains cause different types of infection. More than 40 types are likely to cause genital infection. Types 6 and 11

> **TERMS**
>
> **human papillomavirus (HPV)** The pathogen that causes human warts, including genital warts, as well as anal and genital cancers.
>
> **genital warts** A sexually transmitted viral infection characterized by growths on the genitals; also called *genital HPV infection* or *condyloma*. Persistence of HPV infection predisposes the infected person to some forms of genital cancers.

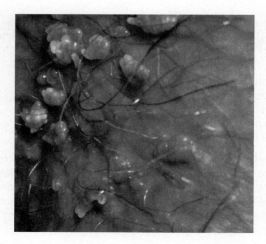

FIGURE 19.5 **Genital warts caused by HPV infection.** Genital warts are found on the shaft of the penis; on the vagina, vulva, or cervix; and around the anus. Dr. P. Marazzi/Science Source

Symptoms Most people infected with HPV have no visible warts or other symptoms and are not aware that they are infected and contagious to others. The good news is that the immune system usually clears the virus on its own, and infection disappears without any treatment. But in some cases, the infection persists and causes genital warts or cancers.

The types of HPV that cause cervical cancer do not produce any visible changes on the external genitals. The types that cause genital warts can produce anything from a small bump to a large, warty growth. Untreated warts can grow together to form a cauliflower-like mass. In males, they appear anywhere on the genitals, including the penis and urethra, appearing first at the opening and then spreading inside. The growths may cause irritation and bleeding, leading to painful urination and a urethral discharge. Warts may also appear around the anus or within the rectum. In women, warts may appear on the labia or vulva and may spread to the *perineum*, the area between the vagina and the rectum. They may also appear on the cervix.

The incubation period ranges from one month to two years from the time of contact. People can be infected with the virus and be capable of transmitting it to their sex partners without having any symptoms at all. The vast majority of people with HPV infection have no visible warts or symptoms of any kind.

cause 90% of visible genital warts. There are at least 13 other HPV strains, including 16 and 18, that are considered high-risk strains for cancer and most often implicated in anogenital cancers (anal, cervical, penile, vaginal, and vulvar cancers). Most HPV infections clear in one to two years in individuals with a normal immune system; however, infections with high-risk strains of HPV that persist may lead to precancer and cancer. Persons living with HIV may be more likely to have persistent HPV infections, cancer-causing strains, and symptoms that are harder to manage. As of June 2016, three HPV vaccines were licensed in the United States. Each protects against HPV 16 and 18, the most common cancer-causing HPV types. In addition, the 4vHPV vaccine protects against HPV 6 and 11, two common wart-causing HPV types. The 9vHPV vaccine has the added benefit of protection from five different cancer-causing strains of the HPV virus.

All three vaccines are licensed for use in females, and two (4vHPV and 9vHPV) are licensed for use in males. The CDC recommends vaccination for all girls and boys aged 11–12, although the vaccine can be given as early as age 9. The vaccine is most effective when given prior to exposure to genital HPV, as this virus is so common that many young people will be exposed to it shortly after becoming sexually active. For people not vaccinated as children, or those who are inadequately vaccinated, catch-up vaccination is recommended up to age 26. Individuals ages 27–45 who have not previously been vaccinated and are at risk for HPV or have been inadequately vaccinated may benefit from HPV vaccination. For this age group, the decision should be made together with your physician. Immunized women should continue to receive cervical cancer screening according to current guidelines (for more about HPV, see Chapter 17).

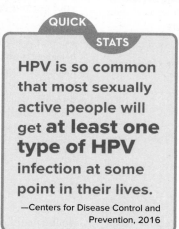

QUICK STATS

HPV is so common that most sexually active people will get **at least one type of HPV** infection at some point in their lives.

—Centers for Disease Control and Prevention, 2016

Diagnosis and Treatment Genital warts are usually diagnosed based on the appearance of the lesions. HPV infection of the cervix is often detected on routine Pap tests. Special tests are now available to detect the presence of cancer-causing HPV infections and to distinguish among the more common strains of HPV, as a part of cervical cancer screening.

Treatment of genital warts focuses on reducing the number and size of warts, although most warts disappear eventually, even without treatment. The currently available treatments do not eradicate HPV infection. Warts may be removed by cryosurgery (freezing), electrocautery (burning), or laser surgery. Direct applications of cytotoxic acids may be used, and there are treatments that patients can use at home. Even after treatment and the disappearance of visible warts, the individual may continue to carry HPV in healthy-looking tissue and can probably still infect others.

Cervical abnormalities that are cancerous or precancerous are treated surgically or with other techniques such as electrical excision, freezing, and laser. See Chapter 17 for more information about cervical cancer.

Anyone who has ever had HPV infection should inform all partners and use condoms, even though they do not provide total protection. Whether or not they have had the vaccine, women should have regular pelvic exams and Pap tests according to current guidelines.

Genital Herpes

Up to one in eight adults aged 14–49 in the United States has **genital herpes.** Worldwide, genital herpes is extremely common, and it is a major factor in HIV transmission. Most people with HIV are also infected with one form of herpes, and their herpes lesions contain large amounts of HIV, making it more likely that the virus will be transmitted. The presence of herpes lesions in an HIV-negative person increases the likelihood that she or he will be infected by an HIV-positive partner.

Two types of herpes simplex viruses, HSV 1 and HSV 2, cause genital herpes and oral–labial herpes. HSV 1 is usually associated with oral herpes (infection of the mouth) and genital herpes can be caused by HSV 1 or HSV 2. Many people wrongly assume that they are unlikely to pick up an STI if they limit their sexual activity to oral sex, but this is not true, particularly in the case of genital herpes. These infections are commonly acquired through oral sex, particularly among young people (infection from kissing is uncommon, though still possible). HSV can also cause rectal lesions, usually transmitted through anal sex. Infection with HSV is generally lifelong. After infection, the virus lies dormant in nerve cells and can reactivate at any time. The type of virus may determine how frequently genital outbreaks occur. Compared to individuals with HSV 1 genital infections, those with HSV 2 infections tend to have more frequent outbreaks of genital lesions and shed more virus without having symptoms.

Forty-eight percent of U.S. adults have antibodies to HSV 1, indicating that they have had previous exposure to the virus. Most people are exposed to HSV 1 during childhood. HSV 2 infection usually occurs during adolescence and early adulthood.

HSV 2 is almost always sexually transmitted. However, changes in sexual behaviors, specifically oral–genital contact, have contributed to increased incidence of anogenital HSV 1 infections in young adults. HSV infections spread readily whether people have active sores or are completely asymptomatic. Because HSV is asymptomatic in 80–90% of people, the infection is often acquired from a person who does not know that he or she is infected.

It is possible to transmit herpes in the absence of symptoms, so talk to your partners if you have ever had an outbreak of genital herpes. Tips on talking about your STI status are available on http://www.itsyoursexlife.com/stds-testing-gyt/article/talk-to-your-partner. Avoid intimate contact when any sores are present, and use condoms during all sexual contact. One study showed that using condoms for every act of intercourse results in a 30% decrease in the transmission of herpes, compared with no condom use. Condoms are more effective in preventing the transmission of other STIs than herpes, but the same study showed that they can make a significant difference in preventing the spread of genital herpes.

Newborns can occasionally be infected with HSV, usually during passage through the birth canal of an infected mother. Such transmission is more likely to occur when HSV 2 infection was acquired by the mother during the third trimester of pregnancy.

Treatment with acyclovir improves survival. However, up to 50% of newborns who have central nervous system infection with HSV 2 (seizures, abnormal imaging of the brain, nervous system abnormalities) but who survive will have some degree of brain damage at one year. Neonates with disseminated disease (multiple organ dysfunction) face the highest risk of death at up to 30%, even with treatment. The morbidity and mortality associated with neonatal HSV infection highlights the importance of disclosing HSV status to your medical provider team during pregnancy.

The risk of mother-to-child HSV transmission during pregnancy and delivery is low (less than 1%) in women with long-standing herpes infection. A woman whose partner has herpes should practice safer sex and abstain from sex in the late stages of pregnancy.

Precautions mothers can take to protect their babies from infection include medications to prevent or treat outbreaks and a cesarean section if active lesions are present at the time of delivery.

Symptoms   Up to 90% of people who are infected with HSV have no symptoms. Those who develop symptoms often first notice them within 2–20 days of having sex with an infected partner. (However, it is not unusual for the first outbreak to occur months or even years after initial exposure.) The first episode of genital herpes frequently causes flulike symptoms in addition to genital lesions. The lesions tend to be painful or itchy and can occur anywhere on the genitals, inner thighs, or anal area. Depending on their location, they can cause considerable pain with urination. Lymph nodes in the groin may become swollen and tender. The sores usually heal within three weeks.

On average, people with a new diagnosis will experience five to eight outbreaks per year, with a decrease in the frequency of outbreaks over time. Recurrent episodes are usually less severe than the initial one, with fewer and less painful sores that heal more quickly. Outbreaks can be triggered by a number of events, including stress, illness, fatigue, sun exposure, sexual intercourse, and menstruation.

Diagnosis and Treatment   Routine screening for HSV in asymptomatic adults and adolescents, including females who are pregnant, is not currently recommended. Genital herpes can be diagnosed on the basis of

> **QUICK STATS**
>
> In the United States, about **one out of every eight people aged 14–49** years has genital herpes.
>
> —Centers for Disease Control and Prevention, 2018

genital herpes   A sexually transmitted infection caused by the herpes simplex virus.

TERMS

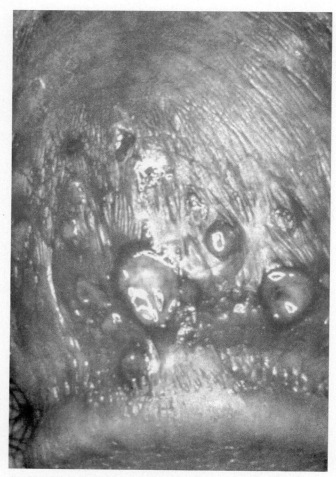

Genital herpes can be caused by either HSV 1 or HSV 2 infections.

SOURCE: Dr. N.J. Flumara and Dr. Gavin Hart/Centers for Disease Control and Prevention

clinical findings, but laboratory testing is helpful if there is any question about the diagnosis. Lesions can be tested directly by viral culture or polymerase chain reaction (PCR). Several blood tests can detect the presence of HSV antibodies in the blood.

There is no cure for herpes. Once infected, a person carries the virus for life. Antiviral drugs such as acyclovir can be taken at the beginning of an outbreak to shorten the severity and duration of symptoms. Support groups are available to help people learn to cope with herpes. There is no vaccine to prevent herpes, but research is ongoing.

Hepatitis A, B, and C

Hepatitis (inflammation of the liver) can cause serious and sometimes permanent damage to the liver, which can result in death in severe cases (see Table 19.4). One of the many types of hepatitis is caused by hepatitis B virus (HBV). Like HIV, HBV is found in most body fluids, including blood and

hepatitis Inflammation of the liver, which can be caused by infection, drugs, or toxins; some forms of infectious hepatitis can be transmitted sexually.

Table 19.4	Estimated Number of U.S. New Cases and Deaths from Hepatitis in 2017		
HEPATITIS TYPE	NEW CASES	CHRONIC INFECTIONS	DEATHS
HAV	6700	*	91
HBV	22,000	862,000	1,727
HCV	44,700	2,400,000	17,253

*HAV is usually a short-term infection and does not become chronic.

blood products, semen, saliva, urine, and vaginal secretions. Hepatitis B is much more contagious than HIV infection; it is easily transmitted through any sexual activity that involves the exchange of body fluids. HBV is not usually spread by hugging, coughing, food or water, sharing eating utensils or drinking glasses, or casual contact. The primary risk factors for HBV infection are sexual exposure and injection drug use (IDU); having multiple sex partners greatly increases risk. HBV can also be transmitted through sharing needles, razor blades, and toothbrushes contaminated with blood. Vaccination against HBV is recommended for incoming college students.

Other forms of viral hepatitis can also be sexually transmitted. Hepatitis A (HAV) is of particular concern for people who engage in anal sex; a vaccine is available and is recommended for all people at risk. There are no chronic infections associated with HAV.

Large population-based studies have demonstrated an association between hepatitis C virus (HCV) and individuals who engage in high-risk sexual encounters (multiple sex partners, unprotected sex, or sex with an HCV-infected person or injection drug user). Individuals born between 1945 and 1965 are also at risk for HCV infection if they received blood products or solid organ transplantation before screening of the blood supply was implemented in 1992 or if they had risk factors decades prior. The recommendation is for individuals with high-risk behaviors to be screened and individuals born between 1945 and 1965 to receive a one-time screening. HIV-positive individuals should be screened when they first appear for care with one or more follow-up screenings 6-12 months based on risk for HCV acquisition. Though fewer people in the United States acquire acute HCV infection annually, more chronic cases of HCV infection and subsequent deaths are noted than for cases of HBV. Most U.S. cases of HCV are associated with IDU. Other risks include receipt of infected blood products, needle-stick injuries in health care settings, and birth from a mother with HCV infection. Additionally, high-risk sexual exposure; sharing needles, razor blades, and toothbrushes contaminated with blood; high-risk health care procedures involving injections; and receipt of an unregulated tattoo are risk factors. Unlike HAV and HBV, there are no vaccines available to protect against HCV. If you inject drugs, talk to your doctor about counseling, treatment services, and safe injection practices.

Symptoms Many people infected with HBV never develop symptoms; they have what are known as silent infections. The normal incubation period is 30–180 days. Mild cases of hepatitis cause flulike symptoms such as fever, body aches, chills, and loss of appetite. As the illness progresses, there may be nausea, vomiting, dark-colored urine, abdominal pain, and jaundice. Some people with hepatitis also develop a skin rash and joint pain or arthritis. Acute HBV infection can sometimes be severe, resulting in prolonged illness or even death.

Most adults who have acute HBV infection recover completely within a few weeks or months. But about 5% of adults who are infected with HBV become chronic carriers of the virus, capable of infecting others for the rest of their lives. Some chronic carriers remain asymptomatic, whereas others develop chronic liver disease. Chronic hepatitis can cause cirrhosis, liver failure, and liver cancer.

Diagnosis and Treatment Hepatitis is diagnosed by blood tests used to analyze liver function, detect the infecting organism, and detect antibodies to the virus. Over the past few years, there has been a surge in safe and effective treatments to cure HCV; thus, testing and managing the care of infected individuals may help to curb this problem. See Chapter 18 for more about these forms of hepatitis. There is no cure for HBV infection and no specific treatment for acute infections; antiviral drugs and immune system modulators may be used for chronic HBV infection.

Since 1990, the number of cases of acute HBV infection in the United States continues to decrease, likely due to HBV vaccine practices. In addition, mother-to-child transmission has been greatly reduced because of routine HBV screening of pregnant women.

Vaccination against HBV is recommended for all infants and children as well as previously unvaccinated adults, high-risk groups such as people who have more than one sex partner in six months, men who have sex with other men, those who inject illegal drugs, health care workers who are exposed to blood and body fluids, and individuals with a compromised immune system, such as people with HIV, diabetes, or advanced liver or kidney disease.

Syphilis

Syphilis, a disease that once caused death and disability for millions, can now be treated effectively with antibiotics. In 2018, there were nearly 35,063 new cases of primary and secondary syphilis (early syphilis) reported in the United States, and nearly 115,045 people received new diagnoses for any stage of syphilis.

By 2016, syphilis rates were higher than they had been in the previous 20 years. Specifically, rates in young men who have sex with men were high; rates of co-infection with HIV were also high in this group. In 2018, 86% of reported early cases of syphilis were among men. When data on the partners of these men were available, 78% of those indicated infections among MSM.

Individuals newly diagnosed with syphilis are also at high risk for HIV. An additional alarming trend are rising rates of congenital syphilis concurrent with increases in primary and secondary syphilis in reproductive-aged women.

Syphilis is caused by a spirochete called *Treponema pallidum,* a thin, corkscrew-shaped bacterium. It requires warmth and moisture to survive and dies quickly outside the human body. The disease is usually acquired through sexual contact, although infected pregnant women can transmit it to their fetuses. The pathogen passes through any break or opening in the skin or mucous membranes and can be transmitted by vaginal or anal intercourse or oral contact with a syphilitic lesion. Although easy to treat, syphilis can be difficult to recognize, and if left untreated the disease can cause devastating damage to almost any system of the body.

Symptoms Syphilis progresses through several stages, though not always in sequence. *Primary syphilis* is characterized by an ulcer called a **chancre** that appears within 10–90 days after exposure. The chancre is usually found at the site where the organism entered the body, such as the genital area, but it may also appear in other sites such as the mouth, breasts, or fingers. Chancres contain large numbers of bacteria and make the disease highly contagious when present; they are often painless and typically heal on their own within a few weeks. If the disease is not treated during the primary stage, about a third of infected individuals progress to chronic stages of infections.

Secondary syphilis is usually characterized by a skin rash that appears three to six weeks after the chancre. The rash may cover the entire body or only a few areas, but the palms of the hands and soles of the feet are usually involved. The rash is highly contagious but usually heals within several weeks or months. Other symptoms include patchy hair loss, weight loss, and symptoms that may resemble flulike illness such as fever, swollen lymph glands, sore throat, headaches, muscle aches, and fatigue.

If the disease remains untreated, the symptoms of secondary syphilis may recur over a period of several years; affected individuals may then lapse into an asymptomatic latent stage in which they experience no further consequences of infection. However, in about 15–30% of untreated syphilis cases, the individual develops *late,* or *tertiary, syphilis,* with symptoms that can appear 10–20 years after infection. Late syphilis can damage many organs of the body (brain, nerves, eyes, heart, blood vessels, liver, bones, and joints), possibly

---

syphilis A sexually transmitted bacterial infection **TERMS** caused by the spirochete *Treponema pallidum.*

chancre The sore produced by syphilis in its earliest stage.

causing severe dementia, cardiovascular damage, blindness, and death.

Neurosyphilis, syphilis that invades the nervous system, can occur at any stage of the infection. Symptoms vary but may include headaches, vision or hearing loss, alterations in behavior, and disorders of movement. It is also possible that the patient has no overt symptoms at the time of diagnosis. *Ocular syphilis* is a clinical manifestation of neurosyphilis that can affect nearly any part of the eye structure. Symptoms may include decreased vision and the potential for permanent blindness. More than 200 cases of ocular syphilis were reported in 20 states in 2014–2015. Most of these cases were found in HIV-infected men who have sex with men, and few were found among heterosexual men and women not infected with HIV.

In infected pregnant women, syphilis can cross the placenta. If the mother does not receive treatment, the probable result is stillbirth, prematurity, or congenital deformity. In many cases, the infant is also born infected (*congenital syphilis*) and requires treatment.

Diagnosis and Treatment   Syphilis is diagnosed by examination of infected tissues and with blood tests. Penicillin is the preferred antibiotic for treating syphilis at all stages, but damage from neurosyphilis and late syphilis can be permanent.

Trichomoniasis

Trichomoniasis (often called *trich*) is the most prevalent nonviral STI in the United States; it is estimated to affect some 3.7 million individuals. The actual number of new infections is unknown; however, there were 222,000 office-

trichomoniasis   A protozoal infection caused by *Trichomonas vaginalis*, most commonly transmitted sexually.   **TERMS**

bacterial vaginosis (BV)   A condition that may be linked to sexual activity; caused by an overgrowth of certain bacteria inhabiting the vagina.

pubic lice   Parasites that infest the hair of the pubic region; commonly called crabs.

scabies   A contagious skin disease caused by a type of burrowing parasitic mite.

related visits for trich in 2016. The parasite that causes trich, *Trichomonas vaginalis,* is highly transmissible during penile–vaginal sex. Nonsexual transmission is rare. Up to 85% of those infected may have no or minimal symptoms. Untreated infections might last for years. Women who become symptomatic with trich develop a yellowish-green, diffuse, or foul-smelling vaginal discharge and severe itching and vulvar irritation. Men may develop inflammation of the urethra, epididymis, or prostate. *T. vaginalis* is not visible to the naked eye; however, a physician can check urine or urethral specimens and vaginal secretions for the presence of this organism. Prompt treatment with oral metronidazole or tinidazole is important because studies suggest that trich may increase the risk of HIV acquisition and transmission and, in pregnant women, premature delivery. If you or your partner has trich, you should both receive treatment.

Other Sexually Transmitted Infections

A number of other diseases are also transmitted sexually.

Bacterial vaginosis (BV) is the most common cause of abnormal vaginal discharge in women of reproductive age. BV occurs when healthful bacteria that normally inhabit the vagina become displaced by unhealthful species. BV is generally not considered an STI but may be associated with sexual activity—for example, change in partners, multiple partners, and female same-sex relationships. Symptoms of BV include vaginal discharge with a fishy odor, and sometimes vaginal irritation. BV can place women at risk for other STIs, complications after some gynecological surgical procedures, and complications during pregnancy. BV is treated with topical and oral antibiotics.

Pubic lice (commonly known as *crabs*) and **scabies** are highly contagious parasitic infections. They are usually treated with topical medicines, but oral medications are sometimes needed as well. Lice infestation can require repeated treatment.

WHAT YOU CAN DO ABOUT SEXUALLY TRANSMITTED INFECTIONS

Take responsibility for your health and contribute to a reduction of STIs in three major areas: education, diagnosis and treatment, and prevention.

Education

Many schools have STI counseling and education programs. These programs allow students to practice communicating with potential sex partners and negotiating for safer sex, among other skills. You can find free pamphlets and literature about STIs at health clinics, physicians' offices, and Planned Parenthood. National hotlines provide free,

If you have had a recent risky sexual encounter, visit your physician, student health center, or local STI clinic and ask for testing. Don't wait for symptoms to develop—you may never have any. Permanent damage from STIs, including infertility, can occur even if you have no symptoms. Treating STIs like chlamydia and gonorrhea within a few days of infection is very likely to prevent complications such as PID and infertility. You will also be much less likely to pass the infection on to anyone else.

When a person has sex without a condom with a person who is HIV-positive, they might be a candidate for PEP treatment described earlier in the chapter; if you receive treatment within 72 hours of possible exposure, PEP will significantly reduce your risk of HIV infection. If you develop flulike symptoms in the days or weeks following risky sexual or drug-taking behavior, see your physician and ask for an HIV RNA test in addition to standard STI tests. (HIV antibody tests may not register primary HIV infection.) If HIV treatment is begun within the first weeks of the infection, chances are good that damage to the immune system can be reduced or even prevented. Many physicians will not think of primary HIV infection when you describe flulike symptoms, so be sure to speak up about your recent risky activities and your concerns about HIV.

If tests come back positive for a particular STI, you need to be tested for others, including HIV infection. Infection with any STI means that you are at higher risk for all others. Women should also have STI testing and a Pap test.

If you are given medication to treat an STI, take all of it as directed. Incomplete treatment can result in an incomplete cure, thereby contributing to the development of drug-resistant organisms. Do not share your medication with a partner; he or she should see a physician for testing and treatment.

Do not have sexual intercourse for at least a week until your treatment—and your partner's treatment—is complete. If your partner still carries the infection, you are likely to be reinfected when you resume sexual activity. If you have an incurable (viral) STI such as herpes or HPV infection, always use a condom and talk to your partner to make sure they are fully informed of the potential risks of being intimate with you, even if you are using condoms.

---

confidential information and referral services to callers anywhere in the country (see For More Information at the end of the chapter).

Educational campaigns about HIV/AIDS and other STIs have paid off in changing attitudes and sexual behaviors. Levels of awareness about HIV infection among the general population are quite high, although some segments of the population are harder to reach and continue to engage in high-risk behaviors. Learning about STIs is still up to every person individually, as is applying that knowledge to personal situations.

Diagnosis and Treatment

Early diagnosis and treatment of STIs can help you avoid complications and help prevent the spread of infection. The following actions are important:

- *Be alert for symptoms.* If you are sexually active, be alert for any sign or symptom of disease, such as a rash, a discharge, sores, or pain. Although only a physician can make a proper diagnosis of an STI, you can perform a genital self-examination between checkups to look for early warning signs of disease, such as bumps, sores, blisters, warts, or unusual discharge. Use a mirror to view your entire genital area. Remember, though, that many STIs can be asymptomatic, so a professional exam and testing are recommended following any risky sexual encounter.

- *Get vaccinated.* Every young, sexually active person should be vaccinated against hepatitis B; vaccines are available for all age groups. The CDC also recommends that men who have sex with men be vaccinated against hepatitis A, and males and females aged 9–26 be vaccinated against HPV.

- *Get tested.* Everyone aged 13–64 should be tested for HIV. If you are a sexually active woman aged 25 or younger, you should be receiving annual gonorrhea and chlamydia screening. MSM and other high-risk men should also receive annual or more frequent STI testing depending on risk, even if no symptoms are present. If you have a risky sexual encounter, see a physician as soon as possible (see the box "Don't Wait—Early Treatment of STIs Really Matters").

- *Inform your partners.* Telling a partner that you have exposed him or her to an STI isn't easy. Despite the awkwardness and difficulty, it is crucial that your sex partner or partners be informed and urged to seek testing and/or treatment as quickly as possible. You can get help telling your partner if you need it. Public health departments will notify sex partners of their possible exposure while maintaining your confidentiality and anonymity. There are also apps that can assist with anonymous partner notification.

- *Get treatment.* Treatments for STIs are safe, and most are inexpensive. If you are receiving treatment, follow instructions carefully and complete all the medication as prescribed. Don't stop taking the medication just because you

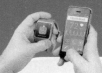

To identify your STI risk factors, read the following statements and identify whether each one is true or false for you.

True or False?

1. I have never been sexually active. (If false, continue. If true, you are not at risk; respond to the remaining statements based on how you realistically believe you would act.)

2. I am in a mutually monogamous relationship with an uninfected partner or am not currently sexually active. (If false, continue. If true, you are at minimal risk now; respond to the remaining statements according to your attitudes and past behaviors.)

3. I have only one sex partner.

4. I always use a condom for each act of intercourse, even if I am fairly certain my partner has no infections.

5. I do not use oil-based lubricants or other products with condoms.

6. I discuss STIs and prevention with new partners before having sex.

7. I do not use alcohol or another mood-altering drug in sexual situations.

8. I would tell my partner if I thought I had been exposed to an STI.

9. I am familiar with the signs and symptoms of STIs.

10. I regularly perform genital self-examinations.

11. When I notice any sign or symptom of any STI or if I engage in risky sexual behavior, I consult my physician immediately.

12. I obtain screening for HIV and STIs regularly. In addition (if female), I obtain pelvic exams and Pap tests at recommended intervals.

13. When diagnosed with an STI, I inform all recent partners.

14. When I have a sign or symptom of an STI that goes away on its own, I still consult my physician.

15. I do not use drugs prescribed for friends or partners or left over from other illnesses to treat STIs.

16. I do not share syringes or needles to inject drugs.

False answers indicate attitudes and behaviors that may put you at risk for contracting STIs or for suffering serious medical consequences from them. (For a more detailed self-assessment, take the quiz at www.thebody.com/surveys/sexsurvey.html.)

feel better or your symptoms have disappeared. If you have an STI, your partner needs to be tested and, if necessary, receive treatment. It is recommended that you return for follow-up testing to make sure that you have not been reinfected and that your infection is cured. There are safe and effective drugs for the management of HIV/AIDS. Many of these drugs are expensive; however, insurance and patient assistance programs are available to assist with medication coverage.

Prevention

STIs *are* preventable. As discussed earlier, the only sure way to avoid exposure to STIs is to abstain from sexual activity. But if you choose to be sexually active, think about prevention *before* you have a sexual encounter or find yourself in the heat of the moment. To identify your STI risk factors, see the box "Do Your Attitudes and Behaviors Put You at Risk for STIs?" Find out what your partner thinks before you become sexually involved. By thinking and talking about responsible sexual behavior, you are expressing a sense of caring for yourself, your potential partner, and your future children.

TIPS FOR TODAY AND THE FUTURE

Because STIs can have serious, long-term effects, it's important to be vigilant about exposure, treatment, and prevention.

RIGHT NOW YOU CAN:

- Make an appointment with your health care provider if you are worried about possible STI infection.
- Resolve to discuss condom use with your partner if you are sexually active and are not already using condoms.

IN THE FUTURE YOU CAN:

- Learn how to communicate effectively with a partner who resists safer sex practices or is reluctant to discuss his or her sexual history. Support groups and educational classes can help.
- Make sure all your vaccinations are up-to-date; ask your doctor if you should be vaccinated against hepatitis A or B, HPV, or any other diseases. If you are at high risk for HIV, ask your doctor if you are a candidate for pre-exposure prophylaxis (PrEP).

SUMMARY

- *Sexually transmitted infection (STI)* is used interchangeably with the term *sexually transmitted disease (STD)* and is gradually replacing it.

- Human immunodeficiency virus (HIV) affects the immune system, making an otherwise healthy person less able to resist a variety of infections.

- HIV is carried in blood and blood products, semen, vaginal and cervical secretions, and breast milk. HIV is transmitted through the exchange of these fluids.

- There is currently no cure or vaccine for HIV infection. Drugs have been developed to slow the course of the disease and to prevent or treat certain secondary infections.

- HIV infection can be prevented by making careful choices about sexual activity and not sharing drug needles.

- If you have been exposed to HIV, it is very important that you are seen by a provider. There are medications that can prevent HIV infection if given in a timely manner.

- If you are at high risk for acquiring HIV, talk to your provider about PrEP for HIV prevention.

- Chlamydia causes epididymitis and urethritis in men; in women, it can lead to urethritis, cervicitis, pelvic inflammatory disease (PID), and infertility if untreated. Patients and their partners should be treated. In infants born to mothers with untreated chlamydia, it cause eye infections and pneumonia.

- Untreated gonorrhea can cause PID in women and epididymitis in men, leading to infertility. Patients and their partners should be treated. In infants born to mothers with untreated gonorrhea, infections of the eyes and other serious complications can occur.

- PID, usually a complication of untreated gonorrhea or chlamydia, is an ascending infection that progresses from the vagina and cervix to the uterus, oviducts, and pelvic cavity. It can lead to infertility, ectopic pregnancy, and chronic pelvic pain. Both the infected woman and her partners must receive treatment.

- Human papillomavirus (HPV) can cause genital warts and cervical cancer. The virus can be transmitted by asymptomatic people. Even after treatment, a person may continue to carry the virus in healthy-looking tissue. The immune system often clears HPV on its own.

- Genital herpes is a common viral infection that can cause painful blisters on the genitals. The virus remains in the body for life and causes recurrent outbreaks.

- Hepatitis B (HBV) and C (HCV) are inflammation of the liver caused by two of the many types of hepatitis virus. Both are transmitted through sexual and nonsexual contact. Following an initial infection, people can recover, but some become carriers and may develop serious complications.

- Vaccines are available to prevent HBV.

- Most U.S. HCV infections are found in persons who inject drugs. No vaccines are available to prevent HCV infection. Safe and effective medications are now available to cure hepatitis C.

- Syphilis is a highly contagious infection caused by the spirochete *T. pallidum*. It can be treated with antibiotics. The disease progresses through three stages. Untreated, it can lead to organ damage, deterioration of the central nervous system, and death. Patients and their partners should be treated. Untreated pregnant women with syphilis can pass on the infection to their unborn child, leading to serious complications and even death.

- Trichomoniasis is a protozoal infection that is readily transmitted by penile–vaginal sex.

- Other diseases that can be transmitted sexually or are linked to sexual activity include bacterial vaginosis, pubic lice, and scabies. Any STI that causes sores or inflammation can increase the risk of HIV transmission.

- Individuals can contribute to a reduction in the incidence of STIs by educating themselves, having any infections diagnosed and treated, and practicing preventive strategies.

FOR MORE INFORMATION

American College Health Association (ACHA). Offers free brochures on STIs, alcohol use, acquaintance rape, and other health issues.

http://www.acha.org/ACHA/Resources/Topics/Sexual
_Health.aspx

American Social Health Association (ASHA). Provides written information on STIs and referrals for those infected; sponsors support groups for people with herpes and HPV infections.

http://www.ashastd.org

Black AIDS Institute. Provides public health information about a variety of topics including testing, treatment, vaccines, and health care access; focuses on black people and the black community.

http://www.blackaids.org

The Body: The Complete HIV/AIDS Resource. Provides information about prevention, testing, and treatment and includes an online risk assessment.

http://www.thebody.com

CDC Female Condom Use. Shows how to use a female condom.

https://www.cdc.gov/condomeffectiveness/Female-condom-use
.html

CDC Male Condom Use. Shows the right way to use a male condom.

https://www.cdc.gov/condomeffectiveness/male-condom-use.html

CDC National Prevention Information Network. Provides extensive information and links for HIV/AIDS and other STIs.

http://www.cdcnpin.org

CDC National STD and AIDS Hotlines. Callers can obtain information, counseling, and referrals for testing and treatment. The hotlines offer information on more than 20 STIs and include Spanish and TTY services.

800-342-AIDS *or* 800-227-8922

800-344-SIDA (Spanish)

800-243-7889 (TTY, deaf access)

BEHAVIOR CHANGE STRATEGY
Talking about Condoms and Safer Sex

The time to talk about safer sex is before you begin a sexual relationship. But even if you've been having unprotected sex with your partner, you can still start practicing safer sex now.

There are many ways to bring up the subject of safer sex and condom use with your partner. Be honest about your concerns, and stress that protection against STIs means that you care about yourself and your partner. You may find that your partner shares your concerns and also wants to use condoms. He or she may be happy and relieved that you have brought up the subject of safer sex.

However, if he or she resists the idea of using condoms, you may need to negotiate (see the dialogue suggestions). Stress that you both deserve to be protected and that sex will be more enjoyable when you aren't worrying about STIs. If you and your partner haven't used condoms before, buy some and familiarize yourselves with how to use them. Once you feel more comfortable handling condoms, you'll be able to use them correctly and incorporate them into your sexual activity. Consider trying the female condom as well.

If your partner still won't agree to use condoms, think carefully about whether you want to have a sexual relationship with this person. Maybe he or she is not the right partner for you.

IF YOUR PARTNER SAYS . . .	TRY SAYING . . .
"They're not romantic."	"Worrying about AIDS isn't romantic, and with condoms we won't have to worry." or "If we put one on together, a condom could be fun."
"I don't have any kind of disease! Don't you trust me?"	"Of course I trust you, but anyone can have an STI and not even know it. This is just a way to take care of both of us."
"I forgot to bring a condom. Let's just do it without a condom this time."	"It only takes one time to get pregnant or to get an STI. I just can't have sex unless I know I'm as safe as I can be." or "I never have sex without a condom. Let's go get some." or "I have some right here."
"I don't like sex as much with a rubber. It doesn't feel the same."	"This is the only way I feel comfortable having sex, but believe me, it'll still be good even with protection! And it lets us both just focus on each other instead of worrying about all that other stuff." or "They might feel different, but let's try." or "Sex won't feel good if we're worrying about diseases." or "How about trying the female condom?"
"But I love you."	"Being in love can't protect us from diseases." or "I love you, too. We still need to use condoms."
"But we've been having sex without condoms."	"I want to start using condoms now so we won't be at any more risk." or "We can still prevent infection or reinfection."
"I don't know how to use them."	"I can show you—want me to put it on for you?"
"No one else makes me use a condom!"	"This is for both of us . . . and I won't have sex without protection. Let me show you how good it can be—even with a condom."
"I'm [or you're] on the pill."	"But that doesn't protect us from STIs, so I still want to be safe, for both of us."

SOURCES: KidsHealth. 2019. *Talking to Your Partner About Condoms* (https://kidshealth.org/en/teens/talk-about-condoms.html); American Sexual Health Association. 2020. *Talking to a Partner* (http://www.ashasexualhealth.org/sexual-health/talking-about-sex/).

HIV InSite: Gateway to AIDS Knowledge. Provides information about prevention, education, treatment, statistics, clinical trials, and new developments; from the University of California, San Francisco.

http://hivinsite.ucsf.edu

It's Your Sex Life (IYSL). Provides information on prevention, education related to STIs, and messages to support making responsible decisions related to sexual health.

http://www.itsyoursexlife.com

Joint United Nations Programme on HIV/AIDS (UNAIDS). Provides information on the international HIV/AIDS situation.

http://www.unaids.org

Know the HIV Risk. CDC's online tool for estimating your risk for HIV with each sexual act.

https://wwwn.cdc.gov/hivrisk/estimator.html

MedlinePlus: Sexually Transmitted Diseases. Provides a clearinghouse of links and information on STIs and other sexual health topics; maintained by the CDC.

https://medlineplus.gov/sexuallytransmitteddiseases.html

The NAMES Project Foundation, AIDS Memorial Quilt. Includes the story behind the quilt, images of quilt panels, and information and links relating to HIV infection.

http://www.aidsquilt.org

National STD Curriculum. Gives information about the epidemiology, pathogenesis, clinical manifestations, diagnosis, management, and prevention of STDs.

https://www.std.uw.edu/

National HIV Curriculum. Updates health care providers about HIV prevention, screening, diagnosis, and ongoing treatment and care.

https://www.hiv.uw.edu/

Planned Parenthood Federation of America. Provides information about STIs, family planning, and contraception.

http://www.plannedparenthood.org

World Health Organization (WHO): Sexually Transmitted Infections. Provides information on international statistics and prevention efforts.

http://www.who.int/topics/sexually_transmitted_infections/en

See also the listings for Chapters 7 and 18.

SELECTED BIBLIOGRAPHY

Abma, J. C., and G. M. Martinez. 2017. Sexual activity and contraceptive use among teenagers in the United States, 2011–2015. *National Health Statistics Reports*; no 104. Hyattsville, MD: National Center for Health Statistics (https://www.cdc.gov/nchs/data/nhsr/nhsr104.pdf).

AIDS.gov. 2020. *The Basics of HIV Prevention* (https://aidsinfo.nih.gov/understanding-hiv-aids/fact-sheets/20/48/the-basics-of-hiv-prevention).

AIDS.gov. 2020. *Pre-Exposure Prophylaxis (PrEP)* (https://aidsinfo.nih.gov/understanding-hiv-aids/fact-sheets/20/85/pre-exposure-prophylaxis-prep-).

AIDS.gov. 2020. *Recommendations for the Use of Antiretroviral Drugs in Pregnant Women with HIV Infection and Interventions to Reduce Perinatal HIV Transmission in the United States* (https://aidsinfo.nih.gov/guidelines/html/3/perinatal/224/whats-new-in-the-guidelines).

American Association of Blood Banks. 2020. *Blood FAQ* (http://www.aabb.org/tm/Pages/bloodfaq.aspx).

American College Health Association. 2019. *American College Health Association National College Health Assessment II: Reference Group Executive Summary Spring 2019.* Hanover, MD: American College Health Association (https://www.acha.org/documents/ncha/NCHA-II_SPRING_2019_US_REFERENCE_GROUP_DATA_REPORT.pdf).

American College of Gynecology. 2016. *Cervical Cancer Screening and Prevention* (https://www.acog.org/clinical/clinical-guidance/practice-bulletin/articles/2016/10/cervical-cancer-screening-and-prevention).

American Sexual Health Association. 2020. *How Does Herpes Testing Work?* (https://www.ashasexualhealth.org/herpes-testing-work/).

Bernstein, D. I., et al. 2013. Epidemiology, clinical presentation, and antibody response to primary infection with herpes simplex virus type 1 and type 2 in young women. *Clinical Infectious Diseases* 56(3): 344–351.

Beymer, M. R., et al. 2014. Sex on demand: Geosocial networking phone apps and risk of sexually transmitted infections among a cross-sectional sample of men who have sex with men in Los Angeles County. *Sexually Transmitted Infections* 90: 567–572.

Buchbinder, S. 2010. HIV epidemiology, testing strategies and prevention interventions. *Topics in HIV Medicine* 18(2): 38–44.

Cabecinha, M., et al. 2017. Finding sexual partners online: Prevalence and associations with sexual behaviour, STI diagnoses and other sexual health outcomes in the British population. *Sexually Transmitted Infections* 93: 572–582.

Cantor, A. G., et al. 2016. Screening for syphilis: Updated evidence report and systematic review for the U.S. Preventive Services Task Force. *Journal of the American Medical Association* 315(21): 2328–2337.

Centers for Disease Control and Prevention. 2017. *Pelvic Inflammatory Disease (PID): CDC Fact Sheet* (https://www.cdc.gov/std/pid/stdfact-pid-detailed.htm).

Centers for Disease Control and Prevention. 2017. *Sexually Transmitted Disease Surveillance 2016.* Atlanta: U.S. Department of Health and Human Services.

Centers for Disease Control and Prevention. 2019. *HIV Surveillance Report, 2018* (Preliminary); vol. 30 (https://www.cdc.gov/hiv/library/reports/hiv-surveillance.html).

Centers for Disease Control and Prevention. 2020. *HIV: Testing* (https://www.cdc.gov/HIV/Basics/testing.html).

Centers for Disease Control and Prevention. 2019. *HIV Surveillance Supplemental Report 24(6)* (http://www.cdc.gov/hiv/library/reports/hiv-surveillance.html).

Centers for Disease Control and Prevention. 2020. *HIV in the United States: At a Glance* (https://www.cdc.gov/hiv/statistics/overview/ataglance.html).

Centers for Disease Control and Prevention. 2020. *Expedited Partner Therapy* (http://www.cdc.gov/std/ept/).

Centers for Disease Control and Prevention. 2020. *Surveillance for Viral Hepatitis-United States, 2018* (https://www.cdc.gov/hepatitis/statistics/2018surveillance/index.htm).

Centers for Disease Control and Prevention and Association of Public Health Laboratories. 2014. *Laboratory Testing for the Diagnosis of HIV Infection: Updated Recommendations.* doi: 10.15620/cdc.23447.

Centers for Disease Control and Prevention, National Center for HIV/AIDS, Viral Hepatitis, STD and TB prevention, Division of HIV/AIDS Prevention. 2017. *HIV in the United States: At a Glance* (https://www.cdc.gov/hiv/statistics/overview/ataglance.html).

Copen, C. E., A. Chandra, and I. Febo-Vazquez. 2016. *Sexual Behavior, Sexual Attraction, and Sexual Orientation among Adults Aged 18–44 in the United States: Data from the 2011–2013 National Survey of Family Growth* (National Health Statistics Reports No. 88). Hyattsville, MD: National Center for Health Statistics.

Dean, L. T., et al. 2018. The affordability of providing sexually transmitted disease services at a safety-net clinic. *American Journal of Preventive Medicine* 54(4): 552–558.

Edward, L., and P. J. Lynch. 2011. *Genital Dermatology Atlas,* 2nd ed. Philadelphia, PA: Lippincott Williams & Wilkins.

Fauci, A. S. 2019. Ending the HIV epidemic: A plan for the United States. *Journal of the American Medical Association* 321(9): 844–845.

Febo-Vazquez, I., C. E. Copen, and J. Daugherty. 2018. Main reasons for never testing for HIV among women and men aged 15–44 in the United States, 2011–2015. *National Health Statistics Reports*; no 107. Hyattsville, MD: National Center for Health Statistics.

Food and Drug Administration. 2020. Women and HIV: *Get the Facts on HIV Testing, Prevention, and Treatment* (https://www.fda.gov/consumers/free-publications-women/women-and-hiv-get-facts-hiv-testing-prevention-and-treatment).

Ginocchio, C. C., et al. 2012. Prevalence of *Trichomonas vaginalis* and coinfection with *Chlamydia trachomatis* and *Neisseria gonorrhoeae* in the United States as determined by the Aptima *Trichomonas vaginalis* nucleic acid amplification assay. *Journal of Clinical Microbiology* 50(8): 2601–2608.

Goulder, P. J., S. R. Lewin, and E. M. Leitman. 2016. Paediatric HIV infection: The potential for cure. *Nature Reviews Immunology* 16: 259–271.

Gradison, M. 2012. Pelvic inflammatory disease. *American Family Physician* 85(8): 791–796.

Hay, P. E., et al. 2016. Which sexually active young female students are most at risk of pelvic inflammatory disease? A prospective study. *Sexually Transmitted Infections* 92(1): 63–66.

Henry J. Kaiser Family Foundation. 2020. *The HIV/AIDS Epidemic in the United States* (https://www.kff.org/hivaids/fact-sheet/the-hivaids-epidemic-in-the-united-states-the-basics/).

Henry J. Kaiser Family Foundation. 2019. *The Global HIV/AIDS Epidemic* (https://www.kff.org/global-health-policy/fact-sheet/the-global-hivaids-epidemic/).

Hutton, H. E., et al. 2013. Alcohol use, anal sex, and other risky sexual behaviors among HIV-infected women and men. *AIDS and Behavior* 17(5): 1694.

James, A. B., T. Y. Simpson, and W. A. Chamberlain. 2008. Chlamydia prevalence among college students: Reproductive and public health implications. *Sexually Transmitted Diseases* 35(6): 529-532.

Jemal, A., et al. 2013. Annual report to the nation on the status of cancer, 1975-2009, featuring the burden and trends in human papillomavirus (HPV)-associated cancers and HPV vaccination coverage levels. *Journal of the National Cancer Institute* 105: 175-201.

Joint United Nations Programme on HIV/AIDS (UNAIDS). 2017. *UNAIDS Ending AIDS Progress towards the 90-90-90 targets* (http://www.unaids.org/sites/default/files/media_asset/Global_AIDS_update_2017_en.pdf)

Kreisel, K., et al. 2017. Prevalence of pelvic inflammatory disease in sexually experienced women of reproductive age—United States, 2013-2014. *MMWR* 66(3): 80-83.

Lam, C. B., and E. S. Lefkowitz. 2013. Risky sexual behaviors in emerging adults: Longitudinal changes and within-person variations. *Archives of Sexual Behaviors* 42(4): 523-532.

Markowitz, L. E., et al. 2016. Prevalence of HPV after introduction of the vaccination program in the United States. *Pediatrics* 137(3): e20151968.

Martin, E. T., et al. 2009. A pooled analysis of the effect of condoms in preventing HSV-2 acquisition. *Archives of Internal Medicine* 169(13):1233-1240.

Mathers, C. D., and D. Loncar. 2006. Projections of global mortality and burden of disease from 2002 to 2030. *PLOS Medicine* 3(11): 2011-2030.

McQuillan, G., et al., 2018. *Prevalence of Herpes Simplex Virus Type 1 and Type 2 in Persons Aged 14-49: United States, 2015-2016.* NCHS Data Brief no. 304 (https://www.cdc.gov/nchs/products/databriefs/db304.htm).

McRee, A. L., et al. 2012. Human papillomavirus vaccine discussions: An opportunity for mothers to talk with their daughters about sexual health. *Sexually Transmitted Diseases* 29(5): 394-401.

Meites, E., et al. 2019. Human papillomavirus vaccination for adults: Updated recommendations of the Advisory Committee on Immunization Practices. *Morbidity and Mortality Weekly Report* 68: 698-702.

Moreira, E. D., Jr., et al. 2016. Safety profile of the 9-valent HPV vaccine: A combined analysis of 7 phase III clinical trials. *Pediatrics* 138(2): e20154387.

National Institutes of Health. 2019. *The HIV Life Cycle* (https://aidsinfo.nih.gov/understanding-hiv-aids/infographics/7/hiv-life-cycle).

Oswalt, S., and T. Wyatt. 2013. Sexual health behaviors and sexual orientation in a U.S. national sample of college students. *Archives of Sexual Behavior* 42(8): 1561-1572.

Patel, P., et al. 2012. Prevalence and risk factors associated with herpes simplex virus-2 in a contemporary cohort of HIV-infected persons in the United States. *Sexually Transmitted Diseases* 3(2): 154-160.

Perillo, R. P., and J. W. Ward. 2012. *A Silent Epidemic: Why Chronic Hepatitis B Matters.* Web video. Medscape Education Family Medicine (http://www.medscape.org/viewarticle/759762).

Petrosky, E., et al. 2015. Use of 9-valent human papillomavirus (HPV) vaccine: Updated HPV vaccination recommendations of the Advisory Committee on Immunization Practices. *MMWR* 64: 300-304.

Piot, P., and T. Quinn. 2013. The AIDS pandemic—A global health paradigm. *New England Journal of Medicine* 368(23): 2210-2218.

Poole, C. L., and D. W. Kimberlin. 2018. Antiviral approaches for the treatment of herpes simplex virus infections in newborn infants. *Annual Review of Virology* 5: 407-425.

Price, M. J., et al. 2016. Proportion of pelvic inflammatory disease cases caused by *Chlamydia trachomatis*: Consistent picture from different methods. *Journal of Infectious Diseases* 214(4): 617-624.

Satterwhite, C. L., et al. 2013. Sexually transmitted infections among U.S. women and men: Prevalence and incidence estimates, 2008. *Sexually Transmitted Diseases* 40(3): 187-193.

Smith, D. K., et al. 2015. Condom effectiveness for HIV prevention by consistency of use among men who have sex with men in the United States. *Journal of Acquired Immune Deficiency Syndrome* 68(3): 337-344.

Tobian, A., et al. 2009. Male circumcision for the prevention of HSV-2 and HPV infections and syphilis. *New England Journal of Medicine* 360: 1298-1309.

United Nations. 2019. *AIDS* (https://www.un.org/en/sections/issues-depth/aids/index.html).

U.S. Department of Health and Human Services. 2019. *HIV Overview: The HIV Life Cycle* (https://aidsinfo.nih.gov/understanding-hiv-aids/fact-sheets/19/73/the-hiv-life-cycle).

U.S. Food and Drug Administration. 2020. *Facts About In-Home HIV Testing* (https://www.fda.gov/consumers/consumer-updates/facts-about-home-hiv-testing).

U.S. Food and Drug Administration. 2020. *Patient Information—Gardasil 9* (http://www.fda.gov/downloads/BiologicsBloodVaccines/Vaccines/ApprovedProducts/UCM426460.pdf).

U.S. Preventive Services Task Force. 2019. *Screening for Hepatitis C Virus Infection in Adults* (https://www.uspreventiveservicestaskforce.org/Page/Document/draft-recommendation-statement/hepatitis-c-screening).

U.S. Preventive Services Task Force. 2016. *Serologic Screening for Genital Herpes Infection US Preventive Services Task Force Recommendation Statement* (https://jamanetwork.com/journals/jama/fullarticle/2593575).

Vásquez-Otero, O., et al. 2016. Dispelling the myth: Exploring associations between the HPV vaccine and inconsistent condom use among college students. *Preventive Medicine* (http://dx.doi.org/10.1016/j.ypmed.2016.10.007).

World Health Organization. 2017. *Global Status Report on Blood Safety and Availability 2016.* (https://apps.who.int/iris/bitstream/handle/10665/254987/9789241565431-eng.pdf;jsessionid=05E320DB42B1AB0A8BDE00A533E5C3EE?sequence=1).

World Health Organization. 2020. *HIV/AIDS: Mother-to-Child Transmission of HIV* (https://www.who.int/hiv/topics/mtct/about/en/).

World Health Organization. 2020. *Male Circumcision for HIV Prevention* (http://www.who.int/hiv/topics/malecircumcision/en).

World Health Organization. 2020. (http://www.who.int/en/news-room/fact-sheets/detail/blood-safety-and-availability).

World Health Organization. 2019. *Number of People (All Ages) Living with HIV Estimates by WHO Region* (https://apps.who.int/gho/data/view.main.22100WHO?lang=e).

World Health Organization. 2020. Pre-Exposure Prophylaxis (http://www.who.int/hiv/topics/prep/en/).

- Explain the concept of environmental health and how it has developed
- Explain how population growth affects the earth's environment
- Explain the impact of energy use and production on the environment
- Describe the causes and effects of air and water pollution
- Describe the problem of solid waste disposal
- Identify environmental issues related to chemical pollution and hazardous waste
- Identify environmental issues related to radiation pollution
- Explain the concept of noise pollution and its impacts

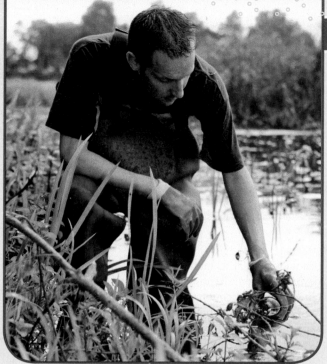

BartCo/Getty Images

CHAPTER 20

Environmental Health

TEST YOUR KNOWLEDGE

1. **Which figure is closest to the world's current population size?**
   a. 6.7 billion
   b. 7.7 billion
   c. 77 billion

2. **Air pollution can occur naturally as well as result from human activities.**
   True or False?

3. **Worldwide, how many people do not have consistent access to safe drinking water?**
   a. 20 million
   b. 200 million
   c. 2 billion

4. **Light-emitting diode (LED) bulbs can last 50 times longer than standard incandescent lightbulbs.**
   True or False?

ANSWERS

1. **B.** The world's current population is 7.7 billion and is expected to reach 9.7 billion people by 2050, according to the United Nations Population Division.

2. **TRUE.** There are many types of naturally occurring air pollution, such as smoke from forest fires and dust from dust storms.

3. **C.** According to the World Health Organization, at least 2 billion people worldwide do not have reliable access to safe drinking water. 4.5 billion do not have access to safe sanitation.

4. **TRUE.** Compared to regular lightbulbs, LED bulbs use 10% as much energy and last up to 50 times longer.

We are constantly reminded of our intimate relationship with everything that surrounds us—our **environment**. Although the planet provides us food, water, air, and everything else that sustains life, it also provides us with natural occurrences—earthquakes, tsunamis, hurricanes, drought, and changes in climate—that destroy life and disrupt society. Humans have always had to contend with the environment to survive. Today, in addition to dealing with natural disasters, we also have to find ways to protect the environment and our health from harmful by-products of our way of life.

This chapter introduces the concept of environmental health and explains how the environment affects us. It also discusses the ways humans affect the planet and its resources—focusing in particular on energy use and production, air and water pollution, solid waste disposal, chemical and radiation pollution, and noise pollution. The chapter also describes steps you can take to improve your personal environmental health while reducing your impact on the earth.

ENVIRONMENTAL HEALTH DEFINED

The field of **environmental health** grew out of efforts to control communicable diseases. When certain insects and rodents were found to carry microorganisms that cause disease in humans, campaigns were undertaken to control these animal vectors. It was also recognized that pathogens (i.e., microorganisms that cause diseases) could be transmitted in sewage, drinking water, and food. These discoveries led to systematic garbage collection, sewage treatment, filtration and chlorination of drinking water, food inspection, and the establishment of public health enforcement agencies.

These efforts to control and prevent communicable diseases changed the health profile of the industrialized world. Americans rarely contract cholera, typhoid fever, plague, diphtheria, or other diseases that once killed large numbers of people; but these diseases have not been eradicated worldwide.

In the United States, a complex public health system is constantly at work behind the scenes attending to the details of these critical health concerns. Every time the system is disrupted, danger recurs. After any disaster that damages a community's public health system—whether a natural disaster such as a hurricane or a human-made disaster such as a terrorist attack—prompt restoration of basic health services

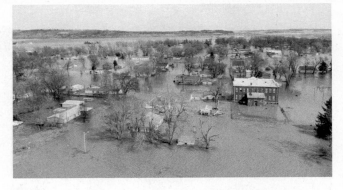

Natural events—such as the great flooding of 2019 across the Midwest and South—can impact many essential services, pollute water, and facilitate the spread of disease. ChrisBoswell/Getty Images

becomes crucial to human survival. Every time we venture beyond the boundaries of our everyday world, whether traveling to a poorer country or camping in a wilderness area, we are reminded of the importance of these basics: clean water, sanitary waste disposal, safe food, and insect and rodent control.

Over the past few decades, the focus of environmental health has expanded and become more complex, for several reasons. We now recognize that environmental pollutants contribute not only to infectious diseases and immediate symptoms, but to many chronic diseases as well. In addition, technological advances have increased our ability to affect and damage the environment. Further, rapid population growth (more than doubling in the past 50 years), which has resulted partly from past environmental improvements, means that ever more people are consuming and competing for resources, increasing human environmental impact.

Environmental health encompasses all the interactions of humans with their environment and the health consequences of these interactions. Fundamental to this definition is a recognition that we hold the world in trust for future life on earth. Our responsibility is to pass on a world no worse, and preferably better, than the one we live in today. Although many environmental problems are complex and seem beyond the control of the individual, there are ways that every person can make a difference to the future of the planet (see the box "Environmental Health Checklist").

environment   The natural and human-made surroundings in which we spend our lives.

environmental health   The collective interactions of humans with the environment and the short-term and long-term health consequences of those interactions.

TERMS

Ask Yourself

QUESTIONS FOR CRITICAL THINKING AND REFLECTION

How often do you think about the environment's impact on your personal health? In what ways do your immediate surroundings (your home, neighborhood, school, workplace) affect your well-being? In what ways do you influence the health of your personal environment?

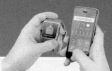

The following list of statements relates to your impact on the environment. Put a check mark next to the statements that are true for you:

_____ I ride my bike, walk, carpool, or use public transportation whenever possible.

_____ I keep my car tuned up and well maintained.

_____ My residence is well insulated and energy efficient.

_____ I use LEDs or compact fluorescent bulbs instead of incandescent bulbs.

_____ I turn off lights and unplug appliances and electronics when they are not in use.

_____ I avoid turning on heat or air conditioning whenever possible.

_____ I run the washing machine, clothes dryer, and dishwasher only when they have full loads.

_____ I use cold water when washing clothes in the washing machine.

_____ I run the clothes dryer only as long as it takes my clothes to dry.

_____ I dry my hair with a towel rather than a hair dryer.

_____ I keep my car's air conditioner in good working order and have it serviced by a service station that recycles chlorofluorocarbons (CFCs).

_____ When shopping, I choose products with the least amount of packaging.

_____ I choose reused, recycled, and recyclable products.

_____ I avoid products packaged in plastic and unrecycled aluminum.

_____ I store food in reusable/glass containers.

_____ I take my own bags along when I go shopping.

_____ I recycle newspapers, glass, cans, and other recyclables.

_____ When shopping, I read labels and try to buy the least toxic products available.

_____ I eat organically and limit meat consumption.

_____ I dispose of household hazardous wastes properly.

_____ I take showers instead of baths.

_____ I take short showers and switch off the water when I'm not actively using it.

_____ I do not run the water while brushing my teeth, shaving, or washing dishes.

_____ My faucets have aerators installed in them.

_____ My shower has a low-flow showerhead.

_____ I have a water-saving toilet or a water displacement device in my toilet.

_____ I snip or rip plastic six-pack rings before I throw them out.

_____ When hiking or camping, I never leave anything behind.

Statements you have not checked can help you identify behaviors you can change to improve environmental health.

For an estimate of how much land and water your lifestyle requires, take the Ecological Footprint quiz at www.myfootprint.org. You can also determine your "carbon footprint" at the Global Footprint Network website (www.footprintnetwork.org/en/index.php /GFN/page/calculators) or at the Nature Conservancy website (www.nature.org/greenliving/carboncalculator/index.htm).

POPULATION GROWTH AND CONTROL

Throughout most of history, humans have been a minor pressure on the planet. About 300 million people were alive in the year 1 CE (Common Era); by the time Europeans were settling in the Americas 1600 years later, the world population had increased gradually to a little over half a billion. But then it began rising exponentially—zooming to 1 billion by about 1800, more than doubling by 1930, and then doubling again in just 40 years (Figure 20.1).

The world's human population, currently around 7.7 billion, is increasing at a rate of about 80 million per year—approximately 150 people every minute. The average number of children per woman fell from 5 in 1950 to half that (2.5) in 2019. This decline in fertility has been happening in Western countries for decades and is now also happening in many of today's poor countries. In sub-Saharan Africa, Asia, and Latin

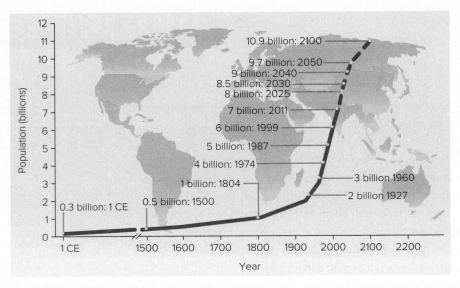

FIGURE 20.1 World population growth. The United Nations estimates that the world population will reach 8.5 billion in 2030, 9.7 billion in 2050, and 10.9 billion in 2100.

SOURCE: United Nations. 2019. *World Population Prospects: The 2019 Revision* (https://population.un.org/wpp/).

America, women with more education are having fewer children; these regions nevertheless contribute the most to population size. Changes are also projected for the world's age distribution: For the first time in history, there are more older people than young children. By 2050, there will be 3.4 times more people aged 60 and over than children aged 4 and under.

Despite a slowing rate of expansion, the population is still always expanding. This expansion, particularly in the past 50 years, is believed to be responsible for most of the stress humans put on the environment. A large and rapidly growing population makes it more difficult to provide the basic components of environmental health, including clean and disease-free food and water. It is also a driving force behind many of the relatively more recent environmental health concerns, including chemical pollution, global climate change, and the thinning of the atmosphere's ozone layer—all topics covered in this chapter.

How Many People Can the World Hold?

No one knows how many people the world can support, but most scientists agree that there is a limit. A 2011 report from the United Nations' Convention on Biological Diversity states that the population's demand for resources already exceeds the earth's capacity by 20%. The primary factors that may eventually put a cap on human population are the following:

• **Food.** Enough food is currently produced to feed the world's entire population, but economic and sociopolitical factors have led to food shortages and famine. Food production can be expanded in the future, but better distribution of food will be needed to prevent even more widespread famine with the growing population. For all people to receive adequate nutrition, the makeup of the world's diet may also need to change. The use of "golden rice," a crop genetically modified to contain vitamin A, could provide extra nutrition to economically emerging countries. Although many people oppose the use of genetically modified organisms (GMOs), others believe that GMOs can help solve the food crisis. The use of insects for food and to feed livestock has also been promoted as a sustainable protein source. Insects have been commonly eaten for centuries, but recent movements have sought to increase consumer acceptance in the Western world.

• **Available land and water.** Rural populations rely on local trees, soil, and water for their direct sustenance, and a growing population puts a strain on these resources. Forests are cut for wood, soil is depleted, and water is used at ever-increasing rates. These trends contribute to local hardships and to many global environmental problems, including habitat destruction and species extinction.

• **Energy.** Currently most of the world's energy comes from nonrenewable sources: oil, coal, natural gas, and nuclear power. As these sources are depleted, the world will have to shift to renewable (*sustainable*) energy sources, such as hydropower and solar, geothermal, wind, biomass, and ocean power. Supporting a growing population, maintaining economic productivity, and stemming environmental degradation will

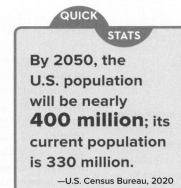

QUICK STATS

By 2050, the U.S. population will be nearly **400 million**; its current population is 330 million.

—U.S. Census Bureau, 2020

require both greater energy efficiency and an increased use of renewable energy sources.

- **Minimum acceptable standard of living.** The mass media have exposed the entire world to the American lifestyle and raised people's expectations of living at a comparable level. But such a lifestyle is supported by levels of energy consumption that the earth cannot support indefinitely. The United States has about 5% of the world's population but uses 25% of the world's energy. In contrast, India has 16% of the world's population but uses only 3% of its energy. China's energy consumption is increasing rapidly, and that nation accounts for 20% of the world's population. If *all* people are to enjoy a minimally acceptable standard of living, the population must be limited to a number that available resources can support.

Factors That Contribute to Population Growth

Although it is apparent that population growth must be controlled, population trends are difficult to influence and manage. A variety of interconnecting factors fuel the current population explosion:

- **High birth rates.** The combination of poverty, high child mortality rates, and a lack of social provisions of every type is associated with high birth rates in the developing world. Families have more children to ensure that enough survive childhood to work for the household and to care for parents in old age. Most countries, whether economically emerging or stable, have experienced significant reductions in birth rates as contraceptive use has increased. However, the majority of economically emerging countries still have birth rates that ensure substantial population growth. In a small number of countries, most of which are classified as the poorest, birth rates continue to be very high.

- **Lack of family planning resources.** Half the world's couples don't use any form of family planning or contraceptives.

- **Lower death rates.** Although death rates remain relatively high in the developing world, they have decreased in recent years because of public health measures and improved medical care.

Changes in any of these factors can affect population growth, but the issues are complex. Increasing death rates through disease, famine, or war might slow population growth, but few people would argue in favor of these as methods of population control. Although the increased availability of family planning services is a crucial part of population management, cultural, political, and religious factors also need to be considered.

To be successful, population management policies must change the condition of people's lives, especially poverty, to remove the pressures to have large families. Research indicates that the combination of improved health, better education, and increased literacy and employment opportunities for women work together with family planning to decrease birth rates.

ENVIRONMENTAL IMPACTS OF ENERGY USE AND PRODUCTION

The United States and China are the biggest energy consumers (Figure 20.2). We use energy to create electricity, transport us, power our industries, and run our homes. About 81% of the energy we use comes from fossil fuels—oil, coal, and natural gas. The remainder comes from nuclear power and

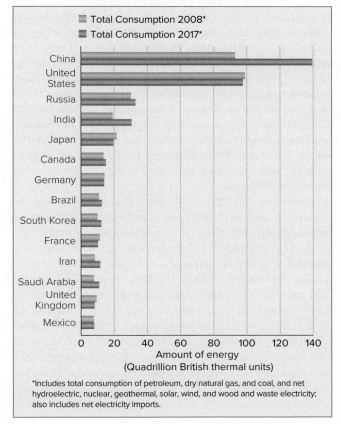

Energy Consumption of Selected Countries

■ Total Consumption 2008*
■ Total Consumption 2017*

(China, United States, Russia, India, Japan, Canada, Germany, Brazil, South Korea, France, Iran, Saudi Arabia, United Kingdom, Mexico)

Amount of energy
(Quadrillion British thermal units)

*Includes total consumption of petroleum, dry natural gas, and coal, and net hydroelectric, nuclear, geothermal, solar, wind, and wood and waste electricity; also includes net electricity imports.

FIGURE 20.2 Energy Consumption of Selected Countries.

SOURCE: U.S. Energy Information Administration. 2020. *International Energy Statistics: Total Primary Energy Consumption (Quadrillion BTU): All Countries, 2017* (http://www.eia.gov/international/rankings/world?pa= 44&u=2&f=A&v=none&y=01%2F01%2F2017&ev=false).

renewable energy sources such as hydroelectric, wind, and solar power.

Energy consumption is at the root of many environmental problems. Automobile exhaust and the burning of oil and coal by industry and by electric power plants are primary causes of the greenhouse effect, smog, and acid precipitation (discussed in detail in later sections of the chapter). The mining of coal and the extraction and transportation of oil and natural gas cause pollution on land and in the water. Several studies have shown birth defects and other health effects in people living near natural gas extraction (i.e., "fracking") sites.

More than 75% of commuters drive alone to work, and low-fuel-economy sport-utility vehicles (SUVs) remain popular. Every gallon of gas burned puts about 20 pounds of carbon dioxide into the atmosphere. The largest SUVs emit at least six more tons of greenhouse gases each year than an average car.

Environmental Threats of Extreme Energy Sources

Despite improvements in energy efficiency, the combination of increasing global population and economic growth is expected to continue to drive up worldwide energy demand over time. At the same time, supplies of easily accessible oil will decline. In response, some energy companies have turned to what are often called "extreme energy sources." This term describes fossil fuels that are relatively difficult to access and extract from the environment. Technologies needed to access extreme energy sources include deepwater oil rigs, tar sands oil extraction, and drilling and hydraulic fracturing for natural gas extraction. Critics worry that these new technologies have been insufficiently studied and regulated and may pose significant new environmental risks.

Deepwater rigs extract oil that is buried deep under the ocean floor and can be difficult to manage. A tragic example was the Deepwater Horizon rig that exploded in April 2010 in the Gulf of Mexico. Oil gushed into the water at an estimated rate of 60,000 barrels a day. It took BP three months to plug the leak, after nearly 5 million barrels of oil escaped into the Gulf. Chemical dispersants used to break up the oil had possible toxic effects and may have caused much of the oil to remain beneath the surface where it cannot be reached for cleanup. The disaster killed thousands of birds, hundreds of endangered sea turtles, and many dolphins and other marine mammals. The long-term health effects to the remaining wildlife are not known. The Gulf's ecosystems may need generations to recover fully, and some parts of it may never recover. Researchers have discovered trace amounts of oil in some fish and shellfish, leading to concerns that oil could reach the human food chain.

Tar sands (or oil sands) are sand deposits that are saturated with a dense form of petroleum called bitumen. The largest deposits are found in Canada, Kazakhstan, and Russia. Making liquid fuel from the oil in tar sands is an energy-intensive process. The resulting product yields two to four times the amount of greenhouse gases per barrel compared to conventional oils. Canada has placed a priority on tar sands development, but critics note that these "dirty" deposits contain 240 gigatons of carbon, representing twice the amount of carbon dioxide emitted by all oil ever used. In addition, Canada's tar sands oil will need to travel through thousands of miles of leak-prone pipelines across pristine wildlife habitats in both Canada and the United States, and when it reaches shipping terminals, huge increases in oil tanker ship traffic will endanger fragile marine habitats in both countries.

Hydraulic fracturing, or fracking, uses pressurized mixes of fluids to create cracks in rock formations deep underground, releasing natural gas. The term *fracking* is commonly used to describe both the drilling and fracturing processes in natural gas extraction. Health experts have raised concerns about the safety of the technique, especially since many of these wells are in residential areas, near homes and schools. Companies are not required to publicly disclose the specific chemicals used. In addition, the disposal of wastewater from the fracking process (which is done by injecting the fluid deep in the ground) can induce earthquakes and has been linked to a dramatic increase in earthquakes in the central United States. A 2019 review of hundreds of studies shows that fracking pollutes the air, water, and soil and can cause noise and physical disturbances. This pollution is linked to preterm births, high-risk pregnancies, asthma, and other health problems. Despite this, there are few regulations in place to protect people from the effects of fracking.

Renewable Energy

With fossil fuels becoming increasingly problematic politically, economically, and environmentally, interest and investment in renewable energy sources have grown in recent years. Renewable energy sources are sources that are naturally replenished and essentially inexhaustible, such as wind and sunlight. Together with technologies that improve energy efficiency, renewable energy sources contribute to sustainability—the capacity of natural or human systems to endure and maintain well-being over time. A common definition of *sustainable development* is development that meets society's present needs without compromising the ability of future generations to meet their needs. Here are some of our best sources of renewable energy:

- *Wind power* uses the wind to turn blades that run a turbine, which spins an electricity-producing generator.

- **Solar power** uses the heat and light of the sun to produce energy via a variety of technologies. One solar technology is the concentrating solar power (CSP) system, which uses mirrors, dishes, or towers to reflect and collect solar heat to generate steam, which runs a turbine to produce electricity. Another solar technology is the photovoltaic (solar cell) system, which converts sunlight directly into electricity by means of semiconducting materials.

- **Geothermal power** taps the heat in the earth's core. It may be in the form of hot water or steam, which can be used to run a turbine to produce electricity.

- **Biomass** is plant material, including trees. When burned, it produces energy. If the plants are produced and harvested sustainably, they are a renewable source of energy.

- **Biofuels** are fuels based on natural materials—either alcohol or oil. They can be used as fuel or added to fossil fuels to reduce emissions. These alternative fuels are described in more detail in the next section.

In 2011, President Barack Obama called for a new energy future, embracing alternative and renewable energy, ending the United States' dependence on foreign oil, and addressing the global climate crisis. In 2018, however, President Donald Trump initiated efforts to cut funding for renewable energy research.

Worldwide, renewable energy sources were around a third of total installed electricity capacity in 2019. World renewable energy production capacity increased by 56% from 2008 to 2010 (Figure 20.3). By 2011, more than 118 countries had enacted some type of policy target or promotion policy related to renewable energy. Many of these targets call for 15–26% of energy or electricity to be provided by renewable sources by 2020. The pursuit of renewable energy sources is seen as having the potential to create new industries and generate jobs, in addition to benefiting the environment.

Alternative Fuels

The U.S. Department of Energy (DOE) is encouraging researchers and automobile manufacturers to produce vehicles that can run on alternative fuels such as ethanol.

Ethanol Ethanol, a form of alcohol, is a renewable and largely domestic transportation fuel produced from fermenting plant sugars such as corn, sugarcane, and other starchy agricultural products. Ethanol use reduces the amount of imported oil required to produce gasoline, reduces overall greenhouse gas emissions from automobiles, and supports the U.S. agricultural industry.

Another type of alternative fuel is E85, which is a mixture of 85% ethanol and 15% gasoline. E85 is becoming popular in the Midwest region (the "corn belt") of the United States. E85 generates lower mileage than gasoline, though it typically costs less than regular gasoline.

Ethanol's critics say it may do more harm than good. Some reports show that corn-based ethanol requires more energy to produce than it yields when burned as fuel. Other reports dispute this point, and improvements in manufacturing processes may reduce the amount of energy required to make the fuel. Regardless, some experts point out that ethanol made from sugarcane and other "woody crop" plant matter like switch grass may be far more energy efficient than corn.

One huge potential drawback of ethanol is the diversion of corn crops from the food supply to produce the fuel. This practice has been blamed for skyrocketing food prices and food shortages around the world. At the same time, the federal government has given billions of dollars in subsidies to farmers to grow corn for ethanol production, even as grain prices have soared. However, ethanol production continues to increase in the United States, with more than 16 billion gallons produced in 2018.

Biodiesel Fuel Biodiesel, like ethanol, can be problematic depending on its material source. It is carbon neutral when the plants that are used to make it, such as soybeans and palm oil trees, absorb carbon dioxide as they grow and offset the carbon dioxide produced while making and using biodiesel. Most of the biodiesel used in the United States is made from soybean oil that is a by-product of processing soybeans for animal feed and numerous other food and non-food products, and from waste animal fat and grease. However, in some parts of the world, natural vegetation and forests have been cleared and burned to grow soybeans and palm oil trees to make biodiesel, and these negative environmental and social effects can outweigh any benefit. Biodiesel is the fastest-growing alternative fuel in the United States,

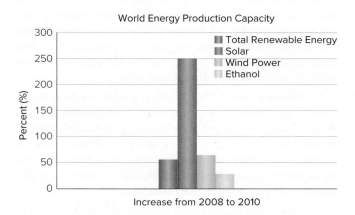

FIGURE 20.3 World Renewable Energy Production Capacity

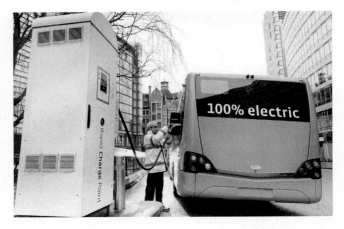

In many areas, public transit buses use alternative fuels or hybrid technology to reduce polluting emissions.

SOURCE: Monty Rakusen/Getty Images

and it produces lower levels of most air pollutants than petroleum-based products.

Hybrid and Electric Vehicles

Hybrid electric vehicles (HEVs) use two or more distinct power sources to propel the vehicle, such as an onboard energy storage system (e.g., batteries), a traditional internal combustion engine, and an electric motor. Hybrid vehicles typically have greater fuel economy than conventional cars do, and they produce fewer polluting emissions. Hybrids also tend to run with less noise than conventional vehicles. Several hybrid models are currently available in the United States, but they typically cost several thousand dollars more than their conventional gas-powered counterparts. Still, hybrids are gaining popularity with consumers and are being used more commonly in both corporate and government vehicle fleets.

A second generation of all-electric vehicles (EVs) has recently been introduced to consumer markets, taking advantage of better battery storage performance and more "quick-charging" stations, and changing consumer perceptions of the convenience of EVs.

Hybrid and electric technology has been extended to all types of vehicles, including SUVs, pickup trucks, buses, and big rigs, and the technology is continually improving.

TERMS

Air Quality Index (AQI) A measure of local air quality and what it means for health.

fossil fuels Buried deposits of decayed animals and plants that are converted into carbon-rich fuels by exposure to heat and pressure over millions of years; oil, coal, and natural gas are fossil fuels.

AIR QUALITY AND POLLUTION

Air pollution is not a human invention or even a new problem. The air is polluted naturally by forest fires, pollen, dust storms, and other natural pollutants. Humans contribute to pollution with the by-products of their activities.

Air pollution is linked to a wide range of health problems, and the very young and the elderly are among the most susceptible to its effects. For people with chronic ailments such as diabetes or heart failure, even relatively brief exposures to particulate air pollution increases the risk of death by nearly 40%, with air pollution (combustion emissions) causing about 200,000 deaths per year in the United States. Recent studies have linked exposure to air pollution to reduced lung capacity in teens and atherosclerosis (thickening of the arteries) in adults. Further, the children of pregnant women exposed to air pollution in urban environments have reduced birth weight, reduced IQ, and increased incidence of obesity.

Air Quality and Smog

The U.S. Environmental Protection Agency (EPA) uses a measure called the **Air Quality Index (AQI)** to indicate whether air pollution levels pose a health concern. The AQI is used for five major air pollutants:

- *Carbon monoxide (CO).* An odorless, colorless gas, CO forms when the carbon in **fossil fuels** does not burn completely. The primary sources of CO are vehicle exhaust and fuel combustion in industrial processes. CO binds to blood cells in place of oxygen (O_2), depriving the body of O_2 and causing headaches, fatigue, and impaired vision and judgment.

- *Sulfur dioxide (SO_2).* SO_2 is produced by the burning of sulfur-containing fuels such as coal and oil, during metal smelting, and by other industrial processes; power plants are a major source. In humans, SO_2 narrows the airways (vasoconstriction), which may cause wheezing, chest tightness, and shortness of breath, and it may aggravate symptoms of cardiovascular disease and asthma.

- *Nitrogen dioxide (NO_2).* NO_2 is a reddish-brown, highly reactive gas formed when nitric oxide combines with oxygen in the atmosphere; major sources include motor vehicles and power plants. In people with respiratory diseases such as asthma, NO_2 affects lung function and causes symptoms such as wheezing and shortness of breath. NO_2 exposure may also increase the risk of respiratory infections.

- *Particulate matter (PM).* Particles of different sizes are released into the atmosphere from sources including combustion of fossil fuels, crushing or grinding operations, industrial processes, and roadway dust. PM can accumulate in the respiratory system, aggravate cardiovascular and lung diseases, and increase the risk of respiratory infections.

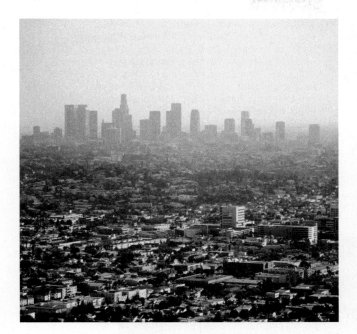

Smog tends to form over Los Angeles because of the natural geographic features of the area and because of the tremendous amount of motor vehicle exhaust in the air. Ocean/Corbis

• **Ground-level ozone.** At ground level, ozone is a harmful pollutant. Where it occurs naturally in the upper atmosphere, it shields the earth from the sun's harmful ultraviolet (UV) rays. (The health hazards from the thinning of this protective ozone layer are discussed later in the chapter.) Ground-level ozone is formed when pollutants emitted by cars, power plants, industrial plants, and other sources react chemically in the presence of sunlight (photochemical reactions). Ozone can irritate the respiratory system, reduce lung function, aggravate asthma, increase susceptibility to respiratory infections, and damage the lining of the lungs. Short-term increases in ozone levels have also been linked to increased death rates.

AQI values run from 0 to 500; the higher the AQI, the greater the level of pollution and associated health danger. When the AQI exceeds 100, air quality is considered unhealthful for groups sensitive to pollution, and for everyone as AQI values rise over 150. For local areas, AQI values are calculated for each of the five pollutants just listed, and the highest value becomes the AQI rating for that day. Depending on the AQI value, local officials may issue precautionary health advice.

The term **smog** was first used in the early 1900s in London to describe the combination of smoke and fog. What we typically call *smog* today is a mixture of pollutants, with ground-level ozone being the key ingredient. Major smog occurrences are linked to the combination of several factors: Heavy motor vehicle traffic, high temperatures, and sunny weather (UV radiation) can increase the production of ozone. Pollutants are also more likely to build up in areas with little wind or where a topographic feature such as a mountain range or valley prevents the wind from pushing out stagnant air.

The Greenhouse Effect and Global Warming

Life on earth depends on a process known as the **greenhouse effect,** which allows for a warm atmosphere. The temperature of the earth's atmosphere depends on the balance between the amount of energy the planet absorbs from the sun (mainly as high-energy UV radiation) and the amount of energy lost back into space (as lower-energy infrared radiation). Key components of temperature regulation are carbon dioxide, water vapor, methane, and other **greenhouse gases**—so named because, like the glass panes in a greenhouse, they let through visible light from the sun but trap some of the resulting infrared radiation and reradiate it back to the earth's surface. This process causes a buildup of heat (i.e., the greenhouse effect) that raises the temperature of the lower atmosphere (Figure 20.4).

There is scientific consensus that this natural process has been disrupted by human activity, causing **global warming** or *climate change*. The concentration of greenhouse gases is increasing because of human activity, especially the combustion of fossil fuels (Table 20.1). Carbon dioxide levels in the atmosphere have increased rapidly in recent decades and, for the first time in recorded history, exceeded 400 parts per million in 2015, and they continue to rise. Many scientists say that 350 parts per million is the target number for the safe upper limit. The use of fossil fuels pumps more than 20 billion tons of carbon dioxide into the atmosphere every year. Experts believe carbon dioxide may account for about 60% of the greenhouse effect. Analysis of ice core samples drilled from glaciers shows that carbon dioxide levels are now about 30% higher than the atmospheric levels spanning at least 800,000 years before the Industrial Revolution. The United States is responsible for one-third of the world's total emissions of carbon dioxide. Deforestation, often by burning, also releases carbon dioxide into the atmosphere and reduces the number of trees available to convert carbon dioxide into oxygen.

With rising temperatures, events such as droughts, floods, and wildfires have become much more common. More than ever previously recorded, the fires this past decade have burned more acres, spread more particulate matter and other

smog   Hazy atmospheric conditions resulting from increased concentrations of ground-level ozone and other pollutants.   **TERMS**

greenhouse effect   A warming of the earth due to a buildup of greenhouse gases in the atmosphere.

greenhouse gas   A gas (such as carbon dioxide) or vapor that traps infrared radiation instead of allowing it to escape through the atmosphere, resulting in a warming of the earth (the *greenhouse effect*).

global warming   An increase in the earth's atmospheric temperature when averaged across seasons and geographic regions; also called *climate change*.

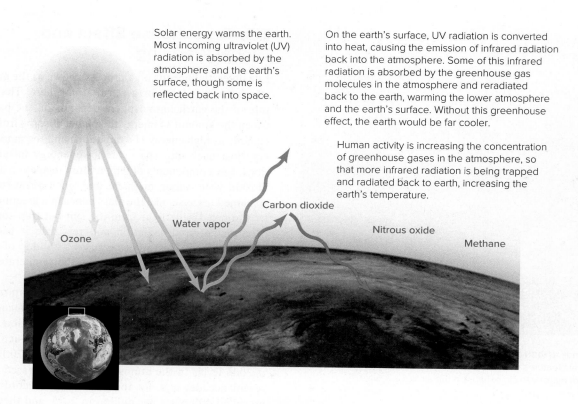

Solar energy warms the earth. Most incoming ultraviolet (UV) radiation is absorbed by the atmosphere and the earth's surface, though some is reflected back into space.

On the earth's surface, UV radiation is converted into heat, causing the emission of infrared radiation back into the atmosphere. Some of this infrared radiation is absorbed by the greenhouse gas molecules in the atmosphere and reradiated back to the earth, warming the lower atmosphere and the earth's surface. Without this greenhouse effect, the earth would be far cooler.

Human activity is increasing the concentration of greenhouse gases in the atmosphere, so that more infrared radiation is being trapped and radiated back to earth, increasing the earth's temperature.

Carbon dioxide

Water vapor

Nitrous oxide

Methane

Ozone

FIGURE 20.4 **The greenhouse effect.** Key greenhouse gases that help trap heat energy in the lower atmosphere are carbon dioxide, methane, nitrous oxide, ozone, and water vapor. titoOnz/Alamy Stock Photo

Table 20.1	Sources of Greenhouse Gases
GREENHOUSE GAS	SOURCES
Carbon dioxide	Fossil fuel and wood burning, factory emissions, car exhaust, deforestation
Chlorofluorocarbons (CFCs)	Refrigeration and air conditioning, aerosols, foam products, solvents
Methane	Cattle, wetlands, rice paddies, landfills, gas leaks, coal and gas industries
Nitrous oxide	Fertilizers, soil cultivation, deforestation, animal feedlots and wastes
Ozone and other trace gases	Photochemical reactions, car exhaust, power plant emissions, solvents

debris, and destroyed forests, buildings, and human and animal life. Fires have ravaged the United States West Coast, the Brazilian Amazon, and parts of Australia, the Arctic, Indonesia, Siberia, Portugal, and Argentina.

According to estimates from the EPA, the earth's average surface temperature is likely to increase 4–8°F (7.2–14.4°C) by the end of the 21st century (Figure 20.5). Warming will not be evenly distributed around the globe. Land areas will warm more than oceans in part due to water's ability to store heat. High latitudes will warm more than low ones in part due to the effects of melting ice.

If global warming persists, experts say the impact may be devastating (Figure 20.6). Possible consequences include the following:

• Increased rainfall and flooding in some regions, and increased drought in others. Coastal zones, where half the world's people live, would be severely affected.

• Increased mortality from heat stress, urban air pollution, and tropical diseases. Deaths from extreme weather events such as hurricanes, tornadoes, droughts, and floods might also increase.

• A poleward shift of about 50–350 miles (150–550 km) in the location of vegetation zones, affecting crop yields, irrigation demands, and forest productivity.

• Alterations of ecosystems, resulting in possible species extinction.

• Increasingly rapid and drastic melting of the earth's polar ice caps. Arctic ice melts to some extent during the summer each year, but melting has increased by 20% since 1979. Many decades earlier than originally predicted by the last Intergovernmental Panel on Climate Change (IPCC), the Arctic sea ice's melting away could occur completely during the summer as soon as 2030, though it would return in the winter months.

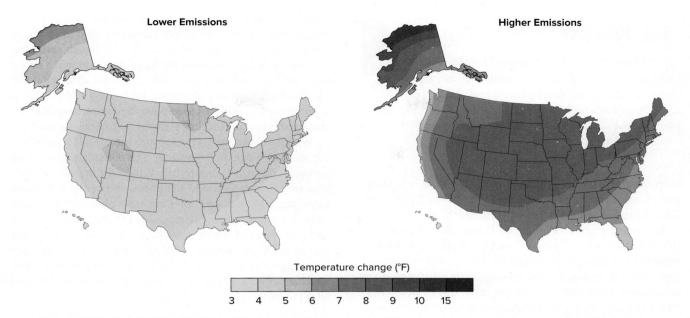

Temperature change (°F)

3 4 5 6 7 8 9 10 15

FIGURE 20.5   Projected temperature change. The maps show the possible rise in average surface air temperature in the period 2071–2099 compared to 100 years earlier (1970–1999), under two scenarios. The map at the left assumes substantial reductions in greenhouse gases; the map at the right assumes continued increases in global emissions.

SOURCE: Melillo, J. M., T. C. Richmond, and G. W. Yohe, Eds. 2014. *Climate Change Impacts in the United States: The Third National Climate Assessment* (http://nca2014.globalchange.gov).

At the 2015 United Nations Climate Change Conference in Paris, France, 195 countries made a landmark agreement to limit average global warming to 2°C above preindustrial temperatures, striving for a limit of 1.5°C. According to the Paris Agreement, each country is in charge of setting its own greenhouse emissions limits, so countries must pledge sufficient reductions in order for the Agreement to be effective. In 2017, President Trump withdrew the United States

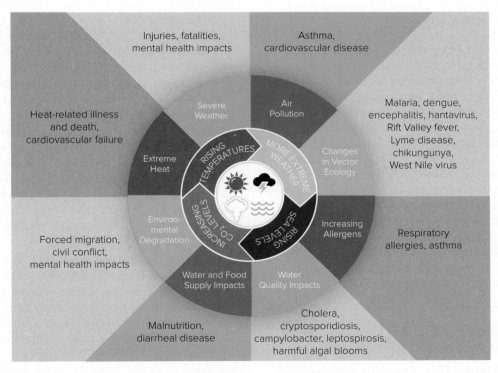

FIGURE 20.6   Impact of climate change on human health. Climate change can influence health and disease in many ways; the effects may vary based on location, age, socioeconomic status, and other factors.

SOURCE: Centers for Disease Control and Prevention. 2020. *Climate Effects on Health* (http://www.cdc.gov/climateandhealth/effects).

from the Agreement. Although many individual U.S. states and cities pledged to continue to abide by the Agreement, federal support will be necessary to meet the goals.

Increasing research on climate change has revealed that significant amounts of greenhouse gases come from sources other than manufacturing industries. The United Nations has reported, for example, that raising cattle produces more greenhouse gases than does driving cars, due to both cattle methane production and deforestation needed for cattle grazing and feed. So far, agriculture has not been included in global climate change agreements.

Thinning of the Ozone Layer

Another air pollution problem is the thinning of the atmosphere's **ozone layer,** a fragile, invisible layer about 10–30 miles above the earth's surface that shields the planet from the sun's hazardous UV rays. Since the mid-1980s, scientists have observed the seasonal appearance and growth of a hole in the ozone layer over Antarctica. Thinning over other areas has been noted more recently.

The ozone layer is being destroyed primarily by **chlorofluorocarbons (CFCs),** which are industrial chemicals used as coolants in refrigerators and air conditioners, as agents in some rigid foam products, as propellants in some aerosol sprays (most of which were banned in 1978), and as solvents. When CFCs rise into the atmosphere, winds carry them toward the polar regions. During winter, circular winds form a vortex that keeps the air over Antarctica from mixing with air from elsewhere. CFCs react with airborne ice crystals, destroying ozone. When the polar vortex weakens in the summer, winds richer in ozone from the north replenish the lost Antarctic ozone.

The largest and deepest ozone hole on record occurred in 2000. At over 26 million square kilometers (over 10 million square miles), it was larger than the entire continent of North America. About 30 years ago, an international agreement, the Montreal Protocol, engendered regulations on the pro-

TERMS

ozone layer   A layer of ozone molecules in the upper atmosphere that screens out UV rays from the sun.

chlorofluorocarbons (CFCs)   Chemicals used as spray can propellants, refrigerants, and industrial solvents, which have been implicated in the destruction of the ozone layer.

duction of ozone-depleting chemicals. Because of this, overall atmospheric ozone is no longer decreasing, and in 2019, the ozone hole was the smallest since 1982 (although variations in weather helped account for this). The Antarctic ozone layer has begun to show signs of healing, and although it will likely not return to its early-1980s state until about 2070, this is an example of science-based policy and international cooperation successfully tackling a global environmental issue.

Without the ozone layer to absorb the sun's UV radiation, life on earth would be impossible. The potential effects of increased long-term exposure to UV light for humans include skin cancer, cataracts and blindness, and reduced immune response. UV light may interfere with photosynthesis and cause lower crop yields; it may also kill phytoplankton and krill—the bases of the ocean food chain. And because heat generated by the absorption of UV rays in the ozone layer helps create stratospheric winds, the driving force behind weather patterns, a drop in the concentration of ozone could alter the earth's climate systems.

Indoor Air Quality (IAQ)

Although most people associate air pollution with the outdoors, homes and other buildings can harbor potentially dangerous pollutants. Some of these compounds trigger allergic responses, and others have been linked to cancer and developmental problems in children. Common indoor pollutants include the following:

• **Environmental tobacco smoke (ETS)** is a human carcinogen that also increases the risk of asthma, bronchitis, and cardiovascular disease (see Chapter 12). The definition of ETS has broadened recently to include the toxic residues of thirdhand smoke, chemicals that linger on indoor surfaces and in dust long after smoking stops.

• **Carbon monoxide and other combustion by-products** can cause chronic bronchitis, headaches, dizziness, nausea, fatigue, and even death. Common sources in the home are woodstoves, fireplaces, kerosene heaters and lamps, and gas ranges. Gas stoves produce nitrogen dioxide, carbon monoxide, and formaldehyde, which can cause health problems. In poverty-stricken areas, especially in Asia and Africa, people commonly burn solid fuels like coal for cooking and heating their homes. The World Health Organization says the smoke and by-products from these indoor fires kill about 4 million people annually—mostly children.

• **Volatile organic compounds (VOCs)** are gases emitted from certain solids and liquids. VOCs are responsible for the smell of fresh paint, the creosote-soaked smell of a beach boardwalk, and even the otherwise satisfying "new car smell." The concentration of many organic compounds is up to 10 times higher indoors than outdoors and can be over 1000 times higher after activities like paint stripping. VOCs are found in paints, lacquers, cleaning supplies, aerosols, building materials, furnishings, and office equipment. A recent article reported a finding that VOCs produced half the pollution in urban areas. Although these VOCs are widely considered a major health risk, no regulatory standards have been set for VOCs in nonindustrial environments. Leadership in Energy and Environmental Design (LEED) standards from the U.S. Green Building Council, however, do address building material composition and adequate ventilation.

• *Biological pollutants* include bacteria, dust mites, mold, and animal dander, which can cause allergic reactions and other health problems. These allergens are typically found in bathrooms, damp or flooded basements, humidifiers, air conditioners, and even some carpets and furniture.

• *Indoor mold* is fungus that grows in damp places, such as on shower tiles and damp basement walls. More than 100 common indoor molds have been classified as potentially hazardous to people, but only a few are serious threats to human health. One of the most common of these is *Stachybotrys* mold, commonly known as "toxic black mold." It is greenish black in color and appears slimy when wet. Toxic mold spores permeate the air and can cause health problems when inhaled, especially for people with asthma and other respiratory conditions.

Preventing Air Pollution

Here are a few ideas for how you can reduce air pollution:

• Cut back on driving. Ride your bike, walk, use public transportation, or carpool in a fuel-efficient vehicle. When air pollutants (CO, NO, and PM) were reduced in Los Angeles County, the number of hospitalizations for asthma decreased.

• Keep your car tuned up and well maintained. Keep your tires inflated at recommended pressures to reduce tailpipe emissions of carbon dioxide. To save energy when driving, avoid quick starts, stay within the speed limit, limit the use of air conditioning, and don't let your car idle unless absolutely necessary. Have your car's air conditioner checked and serviced by a station that uses environmentally friendly refrigerants.

• Buy energy-efficient appliances and use them only when necessary. Run the washing machine, clothes dryer, and dishwasher only when you have full loads, do laundry in cold water, and don't overdry your clothes. Clean refrigerator coils and clothes dryer lint screens frequently. Towel or air-dry your clothes and hair rather than using a dryer.

• Use energy-efficient lighting: halogen, light-emitting diode (LED), or compact fluorescent bulbs (not fluorescent tubes). For more information, see the box "High-Efficiency Lighting."

• Make sure your home is well-insulated with ozone-safe agents; use insulating shades and curtains to keep heat in during winter and out during summer. A home energy audit can pinpoint air leakage and where the most useful changes can be made for increased energy efficiency.

• Plant and care for trees in your yard and neighborhood. Trees recycle carbon dioxide, and in so doing, trees work against global warming. They also provide shade and cool the air so that less air conditioning is needed.

• Before discarding a refrigerator, air conditioner, or humidifier, check with the waste hauler or your local government to ensure that ozone-depleting refrigerants will be removed prior to disposal.

• Keep your house adequately ventilated, and buy some houseplants—they have a natural ability to rid the air of harmful pollutants.

• Keep paints, cleaning agents, and other chemical products tightly sealed in their original containers.

• Don't smoke, and don't allow others to smoke in your home. If these rules are too strict for your situation, limit smoking to a single, well-ventilated room.

• Clean and inspect chimneys, furnaces, and other appliances regularly. Install carbon monoxide detectors.

• Always use an outside-venting hood when cooking.

• Use paints with low or no VOCs, and ventilate well when using high-VOC products. Pregnant women should avoid painting (for example, the nursery).

• Keep areas mold free by fixing any leaks from the bathroom, roof, or basement.

• Use a HEPA air filter.

WATER QUALITY AND POLLUTION

Few parts of the world have enough safe, clean drinking water, and yet few things are as important to human health.

Water Contamination and Treatment

Many cities rely at least in part on wells that tap local groundwater, but often it is necessary to tap lakes and rivers to supplement wells. Because such surface water is more likely to be contaminated with both organic matter and pathogenic microorganisms, it is purified in water treatment plants before being piped into the community. At treatment facilities, the water is subjected to various physical and chemical processes, including screening, filtration, and disinfection (often with chlorine), before it is introduced into the water supply system. **Fluoridation,** a water treatment process that reduces tooth decay by 15–40%, has been used successfully in the United States for more than 60 years. However, there is controversy regarding its safety for human health, and many towns have banned its use in public water.

In most areas of the United States, water systems have adequate, dependable supplies; are able to control waterborne disease; and provide water with acceptable color, odor,

fluoridation The addition of fluoride to the water supply to reduce tooth decay. **TERMS**

TAKE CHARGE
High-Efficiency Lighting

Lighting accounts for about 15% of all residential electricity use. Switching to energy-efficient lighting is a good way to cut your home's energy use, lower your energy bills, and reduce your environmental footprint.

The Energy Independence and Security Act (EISA) of 2007 set national performance standards for lightbulbs for the first time, requiring that basic bulbs be at least about 25% more efficient; the standards were phased in by 2014. Traditional incandescent lightbulbs did not meet these new efficiency standards, so the use of other lighting choices has grown:

- **Halogen incandescents.** More energy-efficient incandescent bulbs that also last up to three times longer than traditional bulbs.

- **Compact fluorescent lightbulbs (CFLs).** Long-lasting fluorescents that work in many types of household fixtures. These bulbs contain a very small amount of mercury and require special handling if they are broken (visit www.epa.gov/cfl for specific cleanup and recycling instructions).

- **Light-emitting diodes (LEDs).** Rapidly expanding in household use, LEDs use only about 10% of the energy and last up to 50 times longer, compared to traditional bulbs.

Although the newer styles of lightbulbs are more expensive than traditional incandescents, they save money because they require less energy to produce light. For example, a 17-watt (W) LED bulb produces as much light as a 75 W incandescent lightbulb. The new lightbulbs also last longer: CFLs last up to 10 times longer than conventional lightbulbs, and some LED bulbs last longer than 22 years. However, it is important to continue to actively conserve energy, even when using more energy-efficient technology. A "rebound effect" occurs when behavioral or other factors cause less gain in conservation than expected (for example, when people needlessly leave on lights because they know them to be more energy efficient).

To aid consumers in selecting bulbs, the Federal Trade Commission mandated Lighting Facts labels on all bulbs. Using these labels, you can compare types of bulbs and select the most appropriate one for your planned use. The brightness comparison is based on lumens rather than watts, because energy-efficient bulbs produce a brighter light with less energy—more lumens per watt than does a traditional incandescent bulb.

SOURCES: U.S. Energy Information Administration. 2020. *How Much Electricity Is Used for Lighting in the United States?* (http://www.eia.gov/tools/faqs/faq.cfm?id=99&t=3); Office of Energy Efficiency & Renewable Energy. 2014. *How Energy-Efficient Light Bulbs Compare with Traditional Incandescents* (http://energy.gov/energysaver/save-electricity-and-fuel/lighting-choices-save-you-money/how-energy-efficient-light)

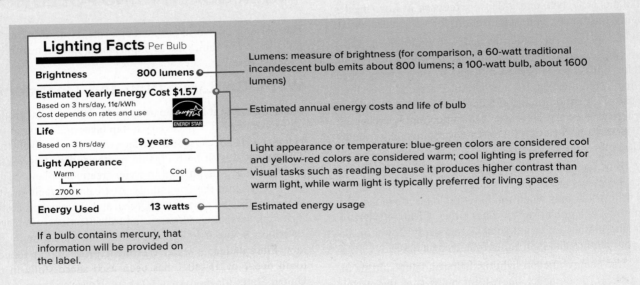

Lighting Facts Per Bulb

Brightness	800 lumens
Estimated Yearly Energy Cost $1.57 Based on 3 hrs/day, 11¢/kWh Cost depends on rates and use	ENERGY STAR
Life Based on 3 hrs/day	9 years
Light Appearance Warm — Cool 2700 K	
Energy Used	13 watts

If a bulb contains mercury, that information will be provided on the label.

Lumens: measure of brightness (for comparison, a 60-watt traditional incandescent bulb emits about 800 lumens; a 100-watt bulb, about 1600 lumens)

Estimated annual energy costs and life of bulb

Light appearance or temperature: blue-green colors are considered cool and yellow-red colors are considered warm; cool lighting is preferred for visual tasks such as reading because it produces higher contrast than warm light, while warm light is typically preferred for living spaces

Estimated energy usage

and taste. However, problems occur. In 2014, over 100,000 Flint, Michigan, residents were exposed to high levels of lead and other contaminants, and the waterborne illness Legionnaires' disease spiked, due to insufficient treatment of water from the Flint River. Residents were instructed to drink bottled water until the infrastructure could be repaired, no sooner than 2020. The Centers for Disease Control and Prevention (CDC) estimates that 1 million Americans become ill and 900–1000 die each year from microbial illnesses from drinking water. Pollution by hazardous chemicals from manufacturing, agriculture, household wastes, and other sources is another concern. (Chemical pollution is discussed later in the chapter.) Worldwide, more than 1.6 million people, mostly children, die from water-related diseases each year.

Water Shortages

Water shortages are a growing concern in many regions of the world. Some parts of the United States, such as the desert West, are experiencing rapid population growth that outstrips the ability of local systems to provide adequate water to all. Many proposals are being discussed to relieve these shortages, including long-distance transfers; conservation; the recycling of some water, such as the water in office building air conditioners; and the sale of water by regions with large supplies to areas with less available water.

According to the World Health Organization, 2 billion people do not have safe drinking water, and 4.5 billion do not have access to safely managed sanitation. Less than 1% of the world's fresh water—about 0.007% of all the water on earth—is readily accessible for direct human use.

Groundwater pumping and the diversion of water from lakes and rivers for irrigation are further reducing the amount of water available to local communities. In some areas, groundwater is being removed at twice the rate at which it is replaced. Due to agricultural diversions, in 1972 the Yellow River ran dry for the first time in China's 3000-year history, failing to reach the sea for 15 days that year; now the dry period extends for more than half of each year. In the United States, the Colorado River has been diverted to the extent that it no longer flows into the ocean. (In 2014, there was a joint effort between Mexico and the United States to send a temporary pulse flow to the Colorado River Delta. Although short-lived, it represents more potential future collaborations to manage resources.)

Sewage

Prior to the mid-19th century, many people contracted diseases such as typhoid, cholera, and hepatitis A by direct contact with human feces, which were disposed of at random. After the links between sewage and disease were discovered, practices began to change. People learned how to build sanitary outhouses and how to locate them so that they would not contaminate water sources. As plumbing moved indoors, sewage disposal became more complicated. In rural areas, the **septic system,** a self-contained sewage disposal system, worked quite well. Today many rural homes still rely on septic systems; however, many old septic systems leak contaminants into the environment.

Different approaches became necessary as urban areas developed. Most cities have sewage treatment systems that separate fecal matter from water in huge tanks and ponds and stabilize it so that it cannot transmit infectious diseases. After it is treated and biologically safe, the water is released back into the environment. The sludge that remains behind is often contaminated with **heavy metals** and is handled as hazardous waste. If incorporated into the food chain, heavy metals—such as lead, cadmium, copper, and tin—can cause illness or death. Therefore, these chemicals must not be released into the environment when sludge is burned or buried.

In addition to regulating industrial discharge, many cities have expanded sewage treatment measures to remove heavy metals and other hazardous chemicals. This action has resulted from many studies linking exposure to chemicals such as mercury, lead, and **polychlorinated biphenyls (PCBs)** with long-term health consequences, including cancer and damage to the central nervous system. The technology to effectively

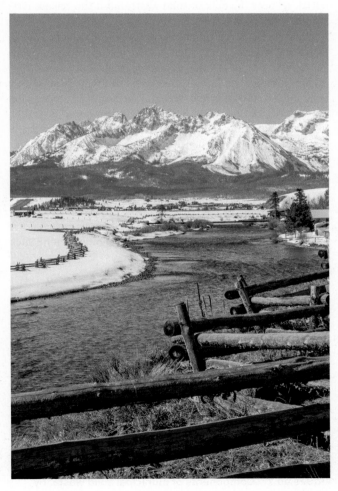

Most communities in the United States draw on surface water for their drinking water supply. Unlike groundwater, surface water is never free of contaminants and has to be treated before it is safe for humans to drink. Steve Smith/Blend Images

TERMS

septic system   A self-contained sewage disposal system, often used in rural areas, in which waste material is decomposed by bacteria.

heavy metal   A metal with a high specific gravity, such as lead, copper, or tin.

polychlorinated biphenyl (PCB)   An industrial chemical used as an insulator in electrical transformers and linked to certain human cancers; banned worldwide since 1977 but persistent in the environment. Humans are exposed mainly through consumption of meat, fish, and dairy.

remove heavy metals and chemicals from sewage is still developing, and the costs involved are immense.

Protecting the Water Supply

By reducing your own water use, you help preserve your community's valuable supply and lower your monthly water bill. By taking steps to keep the water supply clean, you reduce pollution overall and help protect the land, wildlife, and other people from illness. Here are some simple steps you can take to protect your water supply:

• Take showers, not baths, to minimize your water consumption. Don't let water run when you're not actively using it while brushing your teeth, shaving, or hand-washing clothes or dishes. Don't run a dishwasher or washing machine until you have a full load.

• Install sink faucet aerators and water-efficient showerheads, which use two to five times less water with no noticeable decrease in performance.

• Replace old toilets; modern ones are much more efficient.

• Fix leaky faucets in your home. Leaks can waste thousands of gallons of water per year.

• Don't pour toxic materials such as cleaning solvents, bleach, or motor oil down the drain. Store them until you can take them to a hazardous waste collection center.

• Don't pour old medicines down the drain or flush them down the toilet. A 2014 study found active pharmaceutical ingredients in 90% of drinking water samples. The EPA is working on strategies to remove medicines from drinking water, but for now the EPA says the drugs appear only in trace amounts and generally are not considered a health hazard, although scientists believe they may cause problems for fish and other aquatic organisms. Experts suggest that the best way to discard old medicines is to mix them with coffee grounds or cat litter, seal them in a container, and put them in the trash. Some pharmacies will take back unused or expired medications for disposal, and many communities have drop-off days for these drugs.

SOLID WASTE POLLUTION

Humans living in the industrialized world generate huge amounts of waste, which must be handled appropriately if the environment is to be kept safe.

The bulk of the organic food garbage produced in American kitchens is now dumped into the sewage system by way of the mechanical garbage disposal. The garbage that remains is not hazardous from the standpoint of infectious disease because there is very little food waste in it, but it does represent an enormous disposal and contamination problem.

> **sanitary landfill** A disposal site where solid wastes are buried.
>
> **TERMS**

Ask Yourself

QUESTIONS FOR CRITICAL THINKING AND REFLECTION

How would you describe the quality of the water where you live? Are there lakes or streams where you can safely swim or fish? What local information sources can you find about water quality in your area?

What's in Our Garbage?

In 2017, Americans generated about 268 million tons of trash and recycled and composted about 94 million tons of materials. The biggest single component of household trash by weight is paper products, including junk mail, glossy mail-order catalogs, and computer printouts (Figure 20.7). Yard waste, plastic, metals, and glass are other significant components. About 1% of the solid waste is toxic; a new source of toxic waste is the disposal of computer components in both household and commercial waste. Burning, as opposed to burial, reduces the bulk of solid waste, but it can release hazardous material into the air.

Solid waste is not limited to household products. Manufacturing, mining, and other industries all produce large amounts of potentially dangerous materials that cannot simply be dumped. At Love Canal (near Buffalo, New York), toxic industrial wastes had been dumped into a waterway for years until, in the 1970s, nearby residents began to suffer from associated birth defects and cancers. The government had to step in, people had to move from their homes, and huge costs were incurred.

Disposing of Solid Waste

Since the 1960s, billions of tons of solid waste have been buried in **sanitary landfill** disposal sites. Potential landfill sites

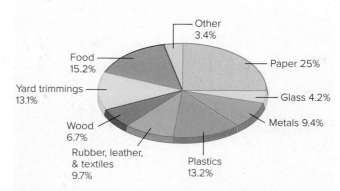

FIGURE 20.7   Components of municipal solid waste, by weight, before recycling.

SOURCE: U.S. Environmental Protection Agency. 2019. *Advancing Sustainable Materials Management: 2017 Fact Sheet* (Pub. No. 530-F-19-007). Washington, DC: EPA.

are studied thoroughly to ensure that they are not near sources of water that could be contaminated by leakage from the landfill. Sometimes protective liners are used around the site, and nearby monitoring wells are now required in most states. Layers of solid waste are regularly covered with thin layers of dirt until the site is filled. Some communities then plant grass and trees and convert the site into a park. Landfill is relatively stable; almost no decomposition occurs in the solidly packed waste.

Burying solid waste in landfills has several disadvantages. Burial is expensive and requires huge amounts of space. Waste can also contain chemicals such as pesticides, paints, and oils, which should not be released into the environment. Despite precautions, buried contaminants sometimes leak into the surrounding soil and groundwater.

Biodegradability

Biodegradation is the process by which organic substances are broken down naturally by living organisms. These organic materials—including plant and animal matter, substances originating from living organisms, or artificial materials similar in nature to plants and animals—are put to use by microorganisms. The term **biodegradable** means that certain products can break down naturally, safely, and quickly into the raw materials of nature and then disappear back into the environment. If a product is **compostable,** it may break down through *biotic* processes—those involving living organisms—as well as *abiotic* processes, which involve nonliving factors such as climate and natural disasters. Table 20.2 shows the amount of time required for materials to biodegrade.

Recycling   Because of the expense and potential chemical hazards of any form of solid waste disposal, many communities encourage individuals and businesses to recycle their trash. In **recycling,** many kinds of waste materials are collected and used as raw materials in the production of new products. For example, waste paper can be recycled into new paper products, or an old bicycle frame can be melted down and used in the production of appliances. The number of recycling opportunities is almost limitless. Recycling is a good idea for two reasons. First, it puts unwanted objects to good use. Second, it reduces the amount of solid waste sitting in landfills, some of which takes decades to decay naturally. Some cities offer curbside pickup of recyclables; others have recycling centers where people can bring their waste. These materials include paper, glass, cans, and things such as discarded tires and used oils. Recycling uses energy and resources, so waste reduction is still important.

Even as recycling grows in popularity, however, the total amount of garbage Americans generate will probably continue to rise as the population increases. Researchers estimate that 80% of the nation's existing landfills will be filled within 20 years.

Discarded Technology: E-waste   A newer solid waste disposal problem involves the discarding of old computers, televisions, cell phones, and other electronic devices. Americans scrap about 400 million consumer electronic devices each year. This "e-waste" is the fastest-growing portion of our waste stream. Junked electronic devices are toxic because they contain varying amounts of lead, mercury, and other heavy metals. Many components of electronic devices are valuable, however, and can be recycled and reused. Local and state e-waste recycling programs are becoming more common, and private companies are also getting into the e-waste recycling business. If you recycle your electronic devices, look for a "green" program or one that is certified by e-stewards, an organization that advocates for responsible e-waste recycling (www.e-stewards.org).

Table 20.2	How Long Items Take to Biodegrade

ITEM	TIME REQUIRED TO BIODEGRADE
Banana peel	2–10 days
Paper	2–5 months
Rope	3–14 months
Orange peel	6 months
Wool sock	1–5 years
Cigarette butt	1–12 years
Plastic-coated milk carton	5 years
Aluminum can	80–100 years
Plastic bottle	450 years
Plastic six-pack holder ring	450 years
Disposable diapers	500 years
Plastic bag	1000 years
Glass bottle	1 million years
Styrofoam	Does not biodegrade

QUICK STATS

The average American generates **4.5 pounds** of trash per day; about 1.5 pounds of this is recycled.

—U.S. Environmental Protection Agency, 2017

TERMS

biodegradable   The ability of materials to break down via biotic processes—consumption by bacteria or fungi, or other biological processes.

compostable   The ability of materials to break down via abiotic and biotic processes.

recycling   The use of waste materials as raw materials in the production of new products.

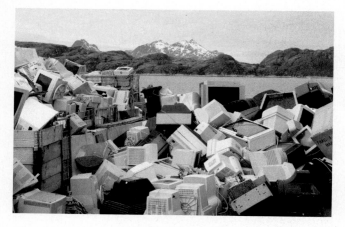

If you have an electronic device to dispose of, look for an e-waste recycling program in your area. Many communities have recycling facilities that handle e-waste or host special e-waste collection events. Philip Laurell/Getty Images

Ask Yourself

QUESTIONS FOR CRITICAL THINKING AND REFLECTION

What are your own waste-disposal habits? Do you recycle everything you can? Do you reuse items? Even if you are conscientious about the way you deal with waste, how could you improve your habits?

Reducing Solid Waste

By reducing your consumption, recycling more, reusing, and throwing away less, you can conserve landfill space. Here are some ideas to help you reduce solid waste:

- Limit your purchase and use of plastic products, including micro plastics, which can be present in soaps (microbeads).

- Buy products with the least amount of packaging, or buy products in bulk. For example, buy large jars of juice, not individually packaged juice drinks. Buy products packaged in recyclable containers.

- Buy recycled or recyclable products. Avoid disposables; instead use long-lasting or reusable products such as refillable pens and rechargeable batteries.

- Bring your own reusable ceramic coffee mug and metal spoon to work or wherever you drink coffee or tea. Use a reusable straw. Pack your lunch in reusable containers.

- To store food, use reusable plastic or glass containers and reusable wrap.

- Recycle your newspapers, glass, cans, paper, and other recyclables. If you receive something packaged with foam pellets, take them to a commercial mailing center that accepts them for recycling.

- Do not throw electronic items, batteries, or fluorescent lights into the trash. Take these to state-approved recycling centers; check with your local disposal service for more information.

- Start a compost pile for your organic garbage if you have a yard. If you live in an apartment, you can take your organic wastes to a community composting center, or use an indoor worm composting bin. Many communities now offer curbside collection of kitchen scraps for recycling into compost, which is sold to farms.

CHEMICAL POLLUTION AND HAZARDOUS WASTE

Chemical pollution is by no means a new problem. The ancient Romans were plagued by lead poisoning, and industrial chemicals have claimed countless lives over the past few centuries.

Today new chemical substances are continually being introduced into the environment as pesticides, herbicides, solvents, and hundreds of other products. More people and wildlife are exposed to them than ever before.

The pivotal publication of Rachel Carson's *Silent Spring* in 1962 drew attention to the problems of chemical pollution and prompted the formation of the EPA. In the 1970s, the EPA established the Superfund program to clean up the nation's uncontrolled hazardous waste sites. A national list prioritizes over 1300 sites for cleanup. To date, the EPA has completed cleanups of 375 sites. As the Superfund program matures, so do the size, complexity, and cost of cleanup work. The EPA also pushes industrial polluters to pay the costs of cleanup, as in the case of General Electric's cleanup of PCBs from the Hudson River.

Asbestos

A mineral-based compound, asbestos was widely used for fire protection and insulation in buildings until the late 1960s. As described in Chapter 17, microscopic asbestos fibers can be released into the air when this material is applied or when it later deteriorates or is damaged. These fibers can lodge in the lungs, causing **asbestosis,** lung cancer, and other serious lung diseases. Similar conditions expose workers to risk in the coal mining industry, from coal and silica dust (black lung disease), and in the textile industry, from cotton fibers (brown lung disease). The EPA has no general ban on asbestos.

Asbestos can pose a danger in homes and apartment buildings, about 25% of which are thought to contain some. Areas where it is most likely to be found are insulation around

> **QUICK STATS**
>
> **The Superfund National Priorities List includes 1335 sites as of June 2020.**
> —U.S. Environmental Protection Agency, 2020

> **asbestosis**   A lung condition caused by inhalation of microscopic asbestos fibers, which inflame the lung and can lead to lung cancer. **TERMS**

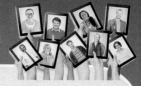

Residents of low-income and minority communities are often exposed to more environmental toxins than residents of wealthier communities and they are more likely to suffer from health problems caused or aggravated by pollutants.

Poor neighborhoods are often located near highways and industrial areas that have high levels of air and noise pollution; they are also common sites for hazardous waste production and disposal. Residents of substandard housing are more likely to come into contact with lead, asbestos, carbon monoxide, pesticides, and other hazardous pollutants associated with peeling paint, old plumbing, and poorly maintained insulation and heating equipment. In addition, low-income people are more likely to have jobs that expose them to asbestos, silica dust, and pesticides, and they are more likely to catch and consume fish contaminated with PCBs, mercury, and other toxins.

In the case of lead poisoning in children, the link among poverty, the environment, and health is abundantly clear. Because children may be at higher risk and more biologically vulnerable to lead exposure, elevated levels of lead show up in their test results. The CDC and the American Academy of Pediatrics recommend annual testing of blood lead levels for all children under age 6, with more frequent testing for children at special risk. In the Flint, Michigan, water crisis, the highest blood lead levels in children were found in the most socioeconomically disadvantaged neighborhoods. Causes include aging infrastructure, neglect by city officials, and the targeting of industry looking for cheap property. Additionally, poor residents suffer the consequences of lead exposure exponentially: even when diagnosed with high levels of poisoning and told how to improve the problem, families often cannot afford the medical treatments and the costs of repainting their houses.

Asthma is another health threat that appears to be linked with both environmental and socioeconomic factors. Although the number of Americans with asthma has been rising for 20 years, a recent study found a leveling and even decrease of incidence in children since 2013. Unfortunately, rates are still increasing in the poorest families. Researchers are not sure what causes asthma, but suspects include household pollutants, pesticides, air pollution, cigarette smoke, and allergens like cockroaches. These risk factors are likely to cluster in poor urban areas where inadequate health care may worsen the effects of asthma.

Gender also influences exposure to environmental hazards. In many societies, women are more often involved in day-to-day activities associated with the environment, including food preparation, agricultural work, and tasks around the home. These activities can expose women to indoor air pollution, water pollution, foodborne pathogens, agricultural chemicals, and waste contamination. Indoor pollutants, especially soot from burning wood, charcoal, and other solid fuels used for home heating and cooking, are a particular risk. Exposure to this particulate pollution increases the risk of respiratory diseases, lung cancer, and reproductive problems.

All humans are exposed to chemicals in air, food, and drinking water, and we all carry a load of chemicals in our bodies. Some of these chemicals accumulate in our bones, blood, or fatty tissues. Women are smaller than men, on average, and have a higher percentage of body fat, so chemicals that accumulate in fatty tissue may pose a relatively greater risk for women. By contrast, men may be more likely to work in industries that involve significant occupational exposures to disease-related toxins. For example, coal miners have an increased risk of lung cancer (black lung disease).

Although any chemical exposure can be a concern for health, women face the added risk of passing pollutants to a developing fetus during pregnancy or to an infant through breastfeeding. Even relatively low exposure to pollutants can result in a significant chemical body load in an infant or young child because of their small body size. And because infants and children are still developing, the effects of chemical exposure can be significant and devastating. It is not unusual for dangerous toxin exposures to be recognized first through noticeable effects on infants or children.

SOURCES: Muller, C., R. J. Sampson, and A. S. Winter. 2018. Environmental inequality: The social causes and consequences of lead exposure. *Annual Review of Sociology* 44 (https://doi.org/10.1146/annurev-soc-073117-041222); Akinbami, L. J., A. E. Simon, and L. M. Rosen. 2016. Changing trends in asthma prevalence among children. *Pediatrics* 137(1); Aelion, C. M., et al. 2013. Associations between soil lead concentrations and populations by race/ethnicity and income-to-poverty ratio in urban and rural areas. *Environmental Geochemistry and Health* 35(1): 1–12.

water and steam pipes, ducts, and furnaces; boiler wraps; vinyl flooring; floor, wall, and ceiling insulation; roofing and siding; and fireproof board.

Lead

The CDC estimates that approximately half a million U.S. children aged 1–5 have blood lead levels above the cutoff at which the CDC recommends public health action. Many of these children live in poor, inner-city areas (see the box "Poverty, Gender, and Environmental Health"). No safe blood lead level has been identified for children. When lead is ingested or inhaled, it can permanently damage the central nervous system, cause mental impairment, hinder oxygen transport in the blood, and create kidney and digestive problems. Severe lead poisoning may cause coma or death. Lead exposure has been linked to attention-deficit/hyperactivity disorder (ADHD) in children. Lead can also build up in bones, where it may be released into the bloodstream during pregnancy or when bone mass is lost from osteoporosis.

Most environmental lead comes from lead-based paints. Lead paints were banned from residential use in 1978, but as many as 57 million American homes still contain them. In 2010, new guidelines were implemented requiring contractors to take special lead-containment measures when doing renovations, repairs, or painting. The use of lead in plumbing is now also banned, but some old pipes and faucets contain it; if these pipes and fixtures corrode, lead can leach into the water. The presence of lead pipes contributed to the drinking water crisis in Flint, Michigan. In 2014, the city changed water suppliers to one that produced higher levels of corrosive compounds but failed to add a required anticorrosive agent; lead from aging pipes leached into the drinking water. Researchers found that the incidence of elevated blood lead levels doubled in children in Flint after the water source change.

Pesticides

Pesticides are chemicals that kill unwanted pests. Herbicides (plant killers) and insecticides (insect killers) are used extensively in agriculture, and they often have toxic effects in unwanted targets, such as beneficial insects and birds. Pesticide use has risks and benefits. For example, DDT was extremely effective in controlling mosquito-borne diseases in tropical countries and in increasing crop yields throughout the world, but it was found to harm wildlife. DDT also builds up in the food chain, increasing in concentration as larger animals eat smaller ones—a process known as **biomagnification** or *bioaccumulation.* DDT bioaccumulation was linked to eggshell thinning in predatory birds, contributing to the decline of species such as the peregrine falcon. DDT was banned in the United States in 1972.

Glyphosate (Roundup) is an herbicide that is widely used with genetically modified crops such as corn and soybeans ("Roundup-ready" crops). Glyphosate has been found in the majority of oat and wheat-based foods tested (i.e. cereal, pasta, breads, etc). In 2015, the World Health Organization listed glyphosate as a "probable human carcinogen." Organophosphate and organochlorine pesticides have been linked to mental problems in children, such as ADHD and low IQ. Pesticide exposure has also been linked to Alzheimer's and Parkinson's diseases, cancers, reproductive problems, depression, and respiratory problems.

Conventionally grown produce (i.e., grown using synthetic pesticides and herbicides) can have higher or lower levels of pesticide residue depending on the type of fruit and vegetable and the country of origin. *Consumer Reports* has created a tool to indicate which types of conventional produce are safer than others and when to opt for organic products (see For More Information). Washing conventional produce in water and rubbing or scrubbing produce to remove dirt and residues is recommended.

Mercury

A naturally occurring metal, mercury is a toxin that affects the brain and nervous system and may damage the kidneys and gastrointestinal tract, and increase blood pressure, heart rate, and heart attack risk. Mercury slows fetal and child development and causes irreversible deficits in brain function. Coal-fired power plants are the largest producers of mercury; other sources include mining and smelting operations and the disposal of consumer products containing mercury.

Mercury persists in the environment and bioaccumulates. In particular, large, long-lived fish may carry high levels of mercury. Chapter 13 includes information about safe fish consumption.

Other Chemical Pollutants

There are tens of thousands of chemical pollutants, and the extent of their toxic effects is just beginning to be understood (see the box "Endocrine Disruption: A 'New' Toxic Threat"). As mentioned earlier, hazardous wastes are commonly found in the home and should be handled and disposed of properly. They include automotive supplies (motor oil, antifreeze, transmission fluid), paint supplies (turpentine, paint thinner, mineral spirits), art and hobby supplies (oil-based paint, solvents, acids and alkalis, aerosol sprays), insecticides, batteries, computer and electronic components, and household cleaners containing sodium hydroxide (lye) or ammonia. These chemicals are dangerous when inhaled or ingested, when they contact the skin or the eyes, or when they are burned or dumped. Many cities provide guidelines about approved disposal methods and have hazardous waste collection days.

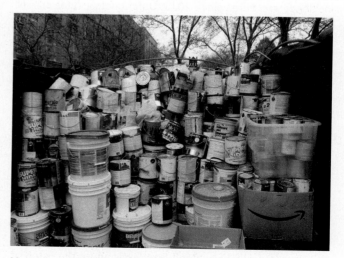

Many communities offer household hazardous waste drop-off programs for safe disposal of potentially harmful household chemicals. Zoran Milich/Moment Mobile/Getty Images

In the 1970s and 1980s, scientists began to document strange occurrences in wildlife: disrupted reproduction, birth defects, tumors, and behavioral changes in birds, fish, and reptiles. The wildlife in and around the Great Lakes, an area with a history of industrial spills and contamination, was particularly affected. It was also becoming apparent that a drug given to pregnant women in the 1950s (a potent synthetic estrogen, DES) was causing infertility and rare reproductive cancers in their adult daughters.

In the mid-1990s, the influential book *Our Stolen Future* by Theo Colborn was published. Colborn suggested that toxic chemicals can cause effects other than acute toxicity (i.e., death), and that low amounts of these chemicals, over a long period of time, can cause disease. Even more concerning was the evidence that a fetus's exposure to chemicals during gestation can cause lasting changes and possible future disease in adulthood.

These chemicals, known also as **endocrine-disrupting chemicals (EDCs)** were altering the hormone systems of organisms. Most systems in the body rely on hormones, such as the immune, metabolic, and brain/nervous systems. A *hormone* is a chemical signal that is made in one area or organ of the body and travels to another to initiate effects. Estrogen, testosterone, and thyroid hormones are well-known examples.

Low levels of EDCs can disrupt these systems by mimicking or blocking natural hormones, causing abnormal effects. EDC exposure before and after birth may cause lifelong effects, including fertility problems, cancers, cardiovascular diseases, obesity, and mental disorders. These effects have been proven in laboratory animals and supported by observational (epidemiological) studies in humans.

Various manufactured chemicals, some in everyday products such as plastics, cosmetics, food packaging, flame retardants, pesticides, and others, are EDCs. These chemicals are known to contaminate household dust, drinking water, and food (especially meat and dairy products). Bisphenol A (BPA) is a chemical present in #7 plastic—in water bottles, the lining of canned foods, dental fillings, and cash register receipts.

The chemical has been banned in children's products in California and the European Union, and many scientists believe it should be regulated more stringently in the United States.

Traditional methods of determining chemical toxicity usually test "gross" effects: death, deformities, and tumors. These methods typically do not test low (environmental) doses of chemicals; rather, they test at high doses and extrapolate down to find "safe" exposure levels. Often, EDCs have detrimental effects at low doses but not higher ones. Therefore, a new testing paradigm must be employed that addresses physiological effects at low doses. The modern environmental movement is new, and as our scientific knowledge of these chemicals evolves and improves, so must government testing and policies surrounding the issues of EDCs, for the continued protection of human health.

What can you do?

- Avoid personal and household products that contain EDCs (see https://www.ewg.org)

- Eat organic foods. Eat lower on the food chain.

- Avoid plastics, especially in contact with food and drinks. Do not microwave plastic containers.

- Dust, vacuum, and wipe down surfaces often.

- Avoid nonstick cookware and products.

- Avoid flame-retardant clothes and furniture.

- Avoid handling cash-register receipts. If you must, use gloves or wash your hands after handling receipts.

- Be especially cautious about exposing pregnant women, infants, and children to EDCs.

- Support legislation that will provide adequate testing and regulation of potential EDCs.

For more information and a list of EDCs visit www.endocrinedisruption.org.

Preventing Chemical Pollution

You can take steps to reduce the chemical pollution in your community. Just as important, by reducing and eliminating the number of chemicals in your home, you may save the life of a child or animal who might encounter one of those chemicals.

• When buying products, read the labels. Choose nontoxic, nonpetrochemical cleansers, disinfectants, polishes, and other personal and household products. Visit https://EWG.org. Check out the Green America website (https://www.greenamerica.org) for how to purchase nontoxic personal care, household, and food items. Also available is the "Detox Me" app (https://www.silentspring.org/detoxme/) to assist in ridding your home of toxic chemicals.

Ask Yourself

QUESTIONS FOR CRITICAL THINKING AND REFLECTION

Are there any hazardous chemicals in your home, such as those found in cleaning products, solvents, paint, or batteries? Would you know what to do if one of these chemicals spilled? How would you clean it up?

---

endocrine-disrupting chemicals (EDCs)   TERMS
Chemicals that disrupt the hormone systems of organisms.

- Eat and live organically. Avoid using chemical pesticides (weed, insect, and rodent killers) in the home and garden.

- Dispose of your household hazardous wastes properly. If you are not sure whether something is hazardous or don't know how to dispose of it, contact your local environmental health office or health department.

- Buy organic produce and produce that has been grown locally.

- If you must use pesticides or toxic household products, store them in a locked place where children and pets can't get to them. Don't measure chemicals with food preparation utensils, and wear gloves whenever handling them.

- If you have your house fumigated for pest control, be sure to hire a licensed exterminator. Keep everyone, including pets, out of the house while the crew works and, if possible, for a few days after.

RADIATION POLLUTION

Radiation comes in several forms, such as UV rays, microwaves, or X-rays, and from several sources, such as the sun, electronics, uranium, and nuclear weapons (Figure 20.8).

> **TERMS**
>
> **radiation** Energy transmitted in the form of rays, waves, or particles.
>
> **radiation sickness** An illness caused by excess radiation exposure, marked by low white blood cell counts and nausea; possibly fatal.
>
> **nuclear power** The use of controlled nuclear reactions to produce steam, which in turn drives turbines to produce electricity.

These forms of electromagnetic radiation differ in wavelength and energy, with shorter waves having the highest energy levels.

Of most concern to health are gamma rays, which are produced by radioactive sources such as nuclear weapons, nuclear energy plants, and radon gas. These high-energy waves are powerful enough to penetrate objects and break molecular bonds. Gamma radiation cannot be seen or felt, and its effects at high doses can include **radiation sickness** and death. At lower doses, chromosome damage, sterility, tissue damage, cataracts, and cancer can occur. Other types of radiation can also affect health. For example, exposure to UV radiation from the sun or from tanning salons can increase the risk of skin cancer. The effects of some sources of radiation, such as cell phones, remain controversial.

Nuclear Weapons and Nuclear Energy

Nuclear weapons pose a health risk of the most serious kind to all species. Public health associations have stated that in the event of an intentional or unintentional discharge of these weapons, there could be millions of casualties. Reducing the stockpiles of nuclear weapons is a challenge and a goal for the 21st century.

Power-generating plants that use nuclear fuel also pose health problems. When **nuclear power** was first developed as an alternative to oil and coal, it was promoted as clean, efficient, inexpensive, and safe. In general, these claims have proven to be the case. Power systems in several parts of the world rely on nuclear power plants. However, despite safeguards and regulating agencies, accidents in nuclear power plants happen, many due to human error (as at Three Mile Island in Pennsylvania), and the consequences of such accidents are far more serious than those of similar accidents in other types of power-generating plants.

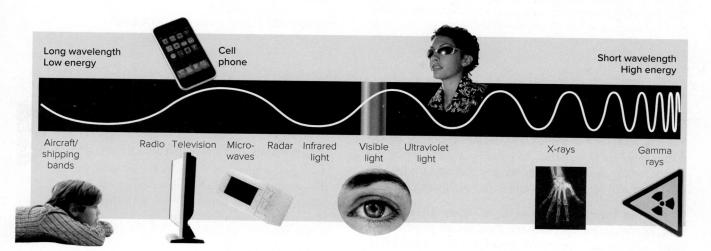

FIGURE 20.8 Electromagnetic radiation. Electromagnetic radiation takes the form of waves that travel through space. The length of the wave determines the type of radiation: The shortest waves are high-energy gamma rays; the longest are radio waves and extremely low-frequency waves used for communication between aircraft, ships, and submarines. Different types of electromagnetic radiation have different effects on health. McGraw Hill; Stockbyte/Getty Images; Imagery Majestic/Cutcaster; Stockbyte/Getty Images; Barbara Penoyar/Photodisc/Getty Images; Mega Pixel/Shutterstock; Martin Diebel/fStop/Getty Images.

The 1986 fire and explosion at the Chernobyl nuclear power station in Ukraine caused hundreds of deaths and increased rates of genetic mutation and cancer; the long-term effects are not yet clear. The zone around Chernobyl has been sealed off to human habitation and could be unsafe for the next 24,000 years. On March 11, 2011, a 9.0 magnitude earthquake 15 miles below Japan's Honshu Island, followed by a powerful tsunami, rocked Japan's northern Fukushima Prefecture and severely damaged the Fukushima Daiichi nuclear power plant complex. Seawater was used to cool the damaged reactors, resulting in the largest release of radiation into the Pacific Ocean in history. All nuclear plants in Japan were shut down until August 2015. Fisheries in the nearby area were also closed due to concern about exposure to radiation.

An additional enormous problem is disposing of the radioactive wastes these plants generate. They cannot be dumped in a sanitary landfill because the amount and type of soil used to cap a sanitary landfill are not sufficient to prevent radiation

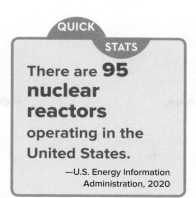

QUICK STATS

There are **95 nuclear reactors** operating in the United States.

—U.S. Energy Information Administration, 2020

from escaping. Deposit sites have to be developed that will be secure for tens of thousands of years—longer than the total recorded history of human beings on this planet. To date, no storage method has been devised that can provide infallible, infinitely durable shielding for nuclear waste. Despite these problems, nuclear power is gaining favor again as an alternative to fossil fuels.

Medical Uses of Radiation

Another area of concern is the use of radiation in medicine. The development of machines that could produce images of internal bone structures was a major advance in medicine. Chest X-rays were routinely used to screen for tuberculosis, and children's feet were even X-rayed in shoe stores to make sure their new shoes fit properly. However, as time passed, studies revealed that X-ray exposure is cumulative and that no level of exposure is absolutely safe.

Early X-ray machines are no longer used, because of the high amounts of radiation they gave off. Each new generation of X-ray machines has used less radiation more effectively. From a personal health point of view, no one should ever have a "routine" X-ray examination; each such exam should have a definite purpose, and its benefits and risks should be weighed carefully.

Radiation in the Home and Workplace

Recently there has been concern about electromagnetic radiation associated with common modern devices such as microwave ovens, computer monitors, and even high-voltage power lines. These forms of radiation do have effects on health, but research results are inconclusive.

Another controversial issue today is the effect of radiation from cell phones on health. The California Department of Public Health recently issued a fact sheet on the possible risks of cell phone use and how to reduce radiation exposure. Cell phones use electromagnetic waves (radio frequency radiation) to send and receive signals. This radiation is not directional, meaning that it travels in all directions equally, including toward the user. Factors such as the type of digital signal coding in the network, the antenna and handset design, and the position of the phone relative to the head all determine how much radiation is absorbed by a user.

Specific absorption rate (SAR) is a way of measuring the quantity of radio frequency energy that is absorbed by the body. If you're concerned about limiting your exposure to possible radiation from your cell phone, look for a phone with a low SAR. You can also text instead of calling, use a wired headset or speakerphone whenever possible, and carry your phone at least one inch from your body. Studies to date have not provided conclusive evidence that cell phone use exposes users to harmful levels of radiation.

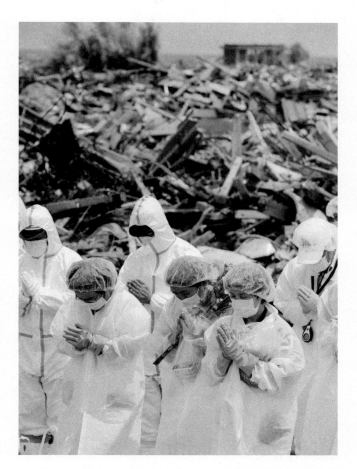

The 2011 Fukushima Daiichi nuclear disaster occurred when a tsunami, following a massive earthquake, flooded the low-lying rooms in which the plant's emergency generators were housed. The plant overheated, causing full meltdown in three of the six reactors.
Kyodo/AP Images

Another area of concern is **radon,** a naturally occurring radioactive gas found in certain soils, rocks, and building materials (see Chapter 17).

Avoiding Radiation

The following steps can help you avoid unneeded exposure to radiation:

• Get only X-rays that you need, and keep a record of the date and location of every X-ray exam. Don't have a full-body CT (computed tomography) scan for routine screening; the radiation dose of one full-body CT scan is nearly 100 times that of a typical mammogram.

• Follow government recommendations for radon testing.

• Use sunscreen to protect yourself from the sun's UV radiation.

NOISE POLLUTION

We are increasingly aware of the health effects of loud or persistent noise in the environment. Concerns focus on two areas: hearing loss and physical and mental stress. Prolonged exposure to sounds above 80–85 **decibels** (a measure of the intensity of a sound wave) can cause permanent hearing loss (Figure 20.9). Hearing damage can occur after eight hours of exposure to sounds louder than 80 decibels. Regular exposure for longer than one minute to more than 100 decibels can cause permanent hearing loss. Children may suffer damage to their hearing at lower noise levels than those at which adults suffer damage. Toys that make noise can also be a problem; they are typically loud, and children are usually close to the toys during play.

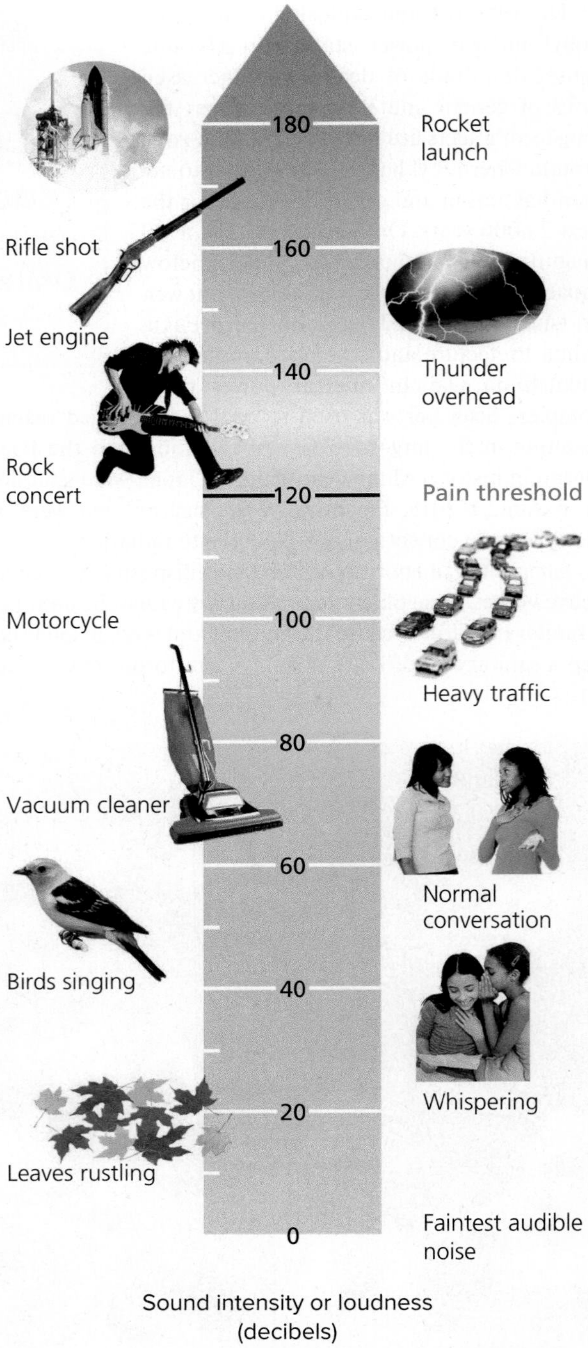

Noise pollution can cause chronic stress: it affects productivity and memory, increases stress hormone levels, and causes health effects such as cardiovascular problems and reduced immune function. Two common sources of excessive noise are the workplace and large gatherings of people at sporting events, rock concerts, and movie theaters. The Occupational Safety and Health Administration (OSHA) sets

radon A naturally occurring radioactive gas emitted from rocks and natural building materials that can become concentrated in insulated homes, causing lung cancer.

decibel A unit for expressing the relative intensity of sounds on a scale from 0 for the average least-perceptible sound to about 120 for the average pain threshold.

TERMS

Sound intensity or loudness
(decibels)

FIGURE 20.9 The intensity of selected sounds. Stocktrek/age fotostock; Stockbyte/Getty Images; Daxiao Productions/Shutterstock; Brand X Pictures/Getty Images; Pacific Northwest Photo/Shutterstock; Siede Preis/Photodisc/Getty Images; JupiterImages/Comstock Images/Getty Images; Stockbyte/Getty Images; Ken Karp/McGraw Hill; Jupiterimages/Getty Images

legal standards for noise in the workplace, but no laws exist regulating noise levels at concerts, which can be much louder than most workplaces.

Here are some ways to avoid exposing yourself to excessive noise:

• Wear ear protectors when working around noisy machinery.

How often do you listen to loud music? Do you ever use headphones? At what volume level do you like to listen? Do you think your listening habits pose a threat to your hearing? Would you let a child listen at the same volume level?

• When listening to music on a headset with a volume range of 1–10, keep the volume no louder than 6. Your headset is too loud if you are unable to hear people around you speaking in a normal tone of voice. Earmuff-style headphones may be easier on the ears than earbuds, which are inserted into the ear canal. Experts warn that earbuds should not be used more than 30 minutes a day unless the volume is set below 60% of maximum; headphones can be used up to one hour. Putting covers over your earbuds can reduce the dB level. Do not push your earbuds in too far. Keep the volume quite a bit lower than you think you need.

• For children, avoid toys that make loud noise.

• Avoid loud music. Don't sit or stand near speakers or amplifiers at a concert, and don't play a car radio or stereo so high that you can't hear the traffic.

• Avoid exposure to painfully loud sounds, and avoid repeated exposure to any sounds above 80 decibels.

TIPS FOR TODAY AND THE FUTURE

*

Environmental health involves protecting yourself from environmental dangers and protecting the environment from the dangers created by humans.

RIGHT NOW YOU CAN:

- Turn off the lights, televisions, and stereos in any unoccupied rooms.
- Turn off power strips when not in use.
- Turn down the heat a few degrees and put on a sweater, or turn off the air conditioner and change into cooler clothes.
- Check your trash for recyclable items and take them out for recycling. If your town does not provide curbside pickup for recyclable items, find out the location of the nearest community recycling center.

IN THE FUTURE YOU CAN:

- Replace burned-out lightbulbs with halogen, LED, or compact fluorescent lightbulbs.
- Have your car checked to make sure it runs as well as it can and puts out the lowest amount of polluting emissions possible.
- Go online and find one of the many calculators available that can help you estimate your environmental footprint. After calculating your footprint, figure out ways to reduce it.

SUMMARY

• Environmental health encompasses all the interactions of humans with their environment and the health consequences of those interactions.

• The world's population is increasing rapidly, especially in developing countries. Factors that may eventually limit human population are food, availability of land and water, energy, and a minimum acceptable standard of living.

• Environmental damage from energy use and production can be limited through energy conservation and the development of nonpolluting, renewable sources of energy.

• Increased amounts of air pollutants are especially dangerous for children, older adults, and people with chronic health problems.

• Factors contributing to the development of smog include heavy motor vehicle traffic, hot weather, and stagnant air.

• Carbon dioxide and other natural gases act as a greenhouse around the earth, increasing the temperature of the atmosphere. Levels of these gases are rising through human activity; as a result, the world's climate is changing.

• The ozone layer that shields the earth's surface from the sun's UV rays has thinned and developed holes in certain regions.

• Indoor pollutants can trigger allergies and illness in the short term and chronic disease in the long term.

• Concerns with water quality focus on pathogenic organisms and hazardous chemicals from industry and households, as well as on water shortages.

• Sewage treatment prevents pathogens from contaminating drinking water; it often must also deal with heavy metals and hazardous chemicals.

• The amount of garbage is growing all the time; paper is the biggest component. Recycling can help reduce solid waste disposal problems.

• Potentially hazardous chemical pollutants include asbestos, lead, pesticides, mercury, and many household products. Proper handling and disposal are critical.

• Radiation can cause radiation sickness, chromosome damage, and cancer, among other health problems.

• Loud or persistent noise can lead to hearing loss, elevated blood pressure, and/or stress.

FOR MORE INFORMATION

California Department of Public Health: How to Reduce Exposure to Radiofrequency Energy from Cell Phones. Fact sheet.

https://www.cdph.ca.gov/Programs/CCDPHP/DEODC/EHIB/CDPH%20Document%20Library/Cell-Phone-Guidance.pdf

CDC National Center for Environmental Health. Provides brochures and fact sheets about a variety of environmental issues.

http://www.cdc.gov/nceh/default.htm

Clean Label Project. Tests a variety of consumer foods and products for toxic chemicals.

https://cleanlabelproject.org

DetoxMe. Free smartphone app that helps reduce your exposure to potentially harmful chemicals where you live and work.

https://www.silentspring.org/detoxme/

Earth Times. An international online newspaper devoted to global environmental issues.

http://www.earthtimes.org

Environmental Working Group. Provides several consumer guides for reducing toxic chemical exposures.

https://ewg.org/consumer-guides

Fuel Economy. Provides information about the fuel economy of cars made since 1985 and tips on improving gas mileage.

http://www.fueleconomy.gov

Global Footprint Network. Calculates your personal ecological footprint based on your diet, transportation patterns, and living arrangements.

http://www.footprintcalculator.org/

Indoor Air Quality Information Hotline. Answers questions, provides publications, and makes referrals.

800-438-4318

National Lead Information Center. Provides information packets and specialist advice.

http://www.epa.gov/lead

National Oceanic and Atmospheric Administration (NOAA): Climate. Provides information about a variety of issues related to climate, including global warming, drought, and El Niño and La Niña.

http://www.noaa.gov/climate.html

National Safety Council. Provides information about lead, radon, indoor air quality, hazardous chemicals, and other environmental issues.

http://www.nsc.org/pages/home.aspx

Pesticides in Produce: Consumer Reports Special Report. Guidelines on how to minimize exposure to pesticides.

https://www.consumerreports.org/cro/health/natural-health/pesticides/index.htm

The Post Carbon Institute: The Post Carbon Reader. A collection of diverse and provocative articles on pressing environmental problems and what can be done about them.

http://www.postcarbon.org/pcr

TEDX, The Endocrine Disruption Exchange. Information about endocrine-disrupting chemicals, the prenatal origins of diseases, natural gas extraction, and pesticides.

http://endocrinedisruption.org

United Nations. Several UN programs are devoted to environmental problems on a global scale; the websites provide information about current and projected trends and about international treaties developed to deal with environmental issues.

https://www.un.org/en/sections/issues-depth/population/

http://www.unep.org (Environment Programme)

U.S. Department of Energy: Energy Efficiency and Renewable Energy (EERE). Provides information about alternative fuels and tips for saving energy at home and in your car.

http://energy.gov/eere/office-energy-efficiency-renewable-energy

U.S. Environmental Protection Agency (EPA). Provides information about EPA activities and many consumer-oriented materials. The website includes special sites devoted to global warming, ozone loss, pesticides, and other areas of concern.

http://www.epa.gov

Yale Environment 360. An online magazine offering opinion, analysis, reporting, and debate on global environmental issues.

http://e360.yale.edu

There are many national and international organizations working on environmental health problems. A few of the largest and best known are listed here:

Greenpeace: 800-326-0959; http://www.greenpeace.org

National Audubon Society: 212-979-3000; http://www.audubon.org

National Resources Defense Council: 212-727-2700; http://www.nrdc.org

National Wildlife Federation: 800-822-9919; http://www.nwf.org

Nature Conservancy: 800-628-6860; http://www.nature.org

Sierra Club: 415-977-5500; http://www.sierraclub.org

U.S. Green Building Council: 800-795-1747; http://www.usgbc.org

World Wildlife Fund—U.S.: 800-960-0993; http://www.worldwildlife.org

SELECTED BIBLIOGRAPHY

Aelion, C. M., et al. 2013. Associations between soil lead concentrations and populations by race/ethnicity and income-to-poverty ratio in urban and rural areas. Environmental Geochemistry and Health 35(1): 1–12.

Almukhtar, S., et al. 2019. The Great Flood of 2019: A complete picture of a slow-motion disaster. The New York Times, 11 September (https://www.nytimes.com/interactive/2019/09/11/us/midwest-flooding.html).

American Lung Association. 2020. State of the Air, 2018 (http://www.lung.org/our-initiatives/healthy-air/sota/).

Centers for Disease Control and Prevention. 2017. Childhood blood lead levels in children aged <5 years—United States, 2009–2014. Surveillance Summaries/MMRW 66(3): 1–10.

Centers for Disease Control and Prevention. 2017. Surveillance for water-borne disease outbreaks associated with drinking water—United States, 2013–14. MMWR 66(44): 1216–1221.

Centers for Disease Control and Prevention. 2020. Lead (http://www.cdc.gov/nceh/lead).

Cooper, T. 2010. Longer Lasting Products: Alternatives to the Throwaway Society. Burlington, VT: Ashgate Publishing Co.

Gore, A. C., et al. 2015. Executive summary to EDC-2: The endocrine society's second scientific statement on endocrine-disrupting chemicals. Endocrine Reviews 36(6): 593.

Gorski, I., et al. 2019. Environmental health concerns from unconventional natural gas development. Oxford Research Encyclopedia of Global Public Health.

Grasso, M., et al. 2012. The health effects of climate change: A survey of recent quantitative research. International Journal of Environmental Research and Public Health 9(5): 1523–1547.

Griffith, G. P., et al. 2012. Predicting interactions among fishing, ocean warming, and ocean acidification in a marine system with whole-ecosystem models. Conservation Biology 26(6): 1145–1152.

Hatta-Attisha, M., et al. 2016. Elevated blood lead levels in children associated with the Flint drinking water crisis: A spatial analysis of risk and public health response. American Journal of Public Health 106(2): 283–290.

Hegarty, M. J. 2012. Invasion of the hybrids. Molecular Ecology 21(19): 4669–4671.

Lovell, J. 2016. Q&A: What really happened to the water in Flint, Michigan? Scientific American (http://www.scientificamerican.com/article/q-a-what-really-happened-to-the-water-in-flint-michigan/).

Maslin, M. 2014. *Climate Change: A Very Short Introduction*, 3rd ed. New York: Oxford University Press.

McDonald, B. C., et al. 2018. Volatile chemical products emerging as largest petrochemical source of urban organic emissions. *Science* 359(6377): 760–764.

Melillo, J. M., T. C. Richmond, and G. W. Yohe (eds.). 2014. *Climate Change Impacts in the United States: The Third National Climate Assessment* (http://nca2014.globalchange.gov).

Nadakavukaren, A. 2011. *Our Global Environment: A Health Perspective,* 7th ed. Prospect Heights, IL: Waveland Press.

National Oceanic and Atmospheric Administration. 2020. *Billion Dollar U.S. Weather Disasters, 1980–2016* (http://www.ncdc.noaa.gov/billions/).

Newell, K., et al. 2017. Cardiorespiratory health effects of particulate ambient air pollution exposure in low-income and middle-income countries: A systematic review and meta-analysis. *The Lancet: Planetary Health* 1(9): e368–e380 (https://www.thelancet.com/journals/lanplh/article/PIIS2542-5196(17)30166-3/fulltext?code=lancet-site).

Petersen, M. D., et al. 2016. *One-Year Seismic Hazard Forecast for the Central and Eastern United States from Induced and Natural Earthquakes.* U.S. Geological Survey (https://pubs.er.usgs.gov/publication/ofr20161035).

REN21. 2018. *Renewables 2018 Global Status Report.* Paris: REN21 (http://www.ren21.net/status-of-renewables/global-status-report/).

Solomon, S., et al. 2016. Emergence of healing in the Antarctic ozone layer. *Science* 353(6296): 269–274.

United Nations Population Division, Department of Economic and Social Affairs. 2019. *World Population Prospects: Highlights.* New York: United Nations (https://www.un.org/development/desa/publications/world-population-prospects-2019-highlights.html).

U.S. Census Bureau. 2018. *National Population Projections* (https://www.census.gov/programs-surveys/popproj/data/tables.html).

U.S. Energy Information Administration. 2020, August 10. *Gasoline and Diesel Fuel Update* (https://www.eia.gov/petroleum/gasdiesel/).

U.S. Energy Information Administration. 2020. *How Many Nuclear Power Plants Are in the United States, and Where Are They Located?* (https://www.eia.gov/tools/faqs/faq.cfm?id=207&t=3).

U.S. Energy Information Administration. 2020. *How Much Oil Is Consumed in the United States?* (https://www.eia.gov/tools/faqs/faq.cfm?id=33&t=6).

U.S. Energy Information Administration. 2019. *International Energy Outlook 2019* (www.eia.gov/outlooks/ieo).

U.S. Environmental Protection Agency. 2020. *Superfund: National Priorities List* (https://www.epa.gov/superfund/).

U.S. Environmental Protection Agency. 2019. *Advancing Sustainable Materials Management: 2017 Fact Sheet* (https://www.epa.gov/sites/production/files/2019-11/documents/2017_facts_and_figures_fact_sheet_final.pdf).

World Health Organization. 2017. Cholera vaccines: WHO position paper. *Weekly Epidemiological Record* 34(92): 477–500.

World Health Organization. 2018. *A Global Overview of National Regulations and Standards for Drinking-Water Quality.* Geneva: WHO.

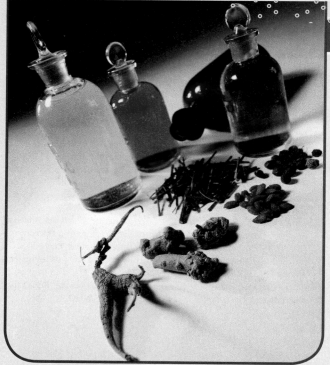

Corbis/Alamy Stock Photo

CHAPTER OBJECTIVES

- Understand options for self-care
- Understand options for professional care
- Describe the practices of conventional medicine
- Learn about integrative health practices
- Understand the costs of health care and how to pay for it

CHAPTER **21**

Conventional and Complementary Medicine

TEST YOUR KNOWLEDGE

1. The people most likely to use complementary and alternative medicine are those who do not have a conventional primary health care provider.
   True or False?

2. Which of the following are shared by both conventional Western medicine and complementary and alternative medicine practitioners?
   a. Careful observation of symptoms
   b. Treatment with remedies derived from plants
   c. Concern with the patient–practitioner relationship

3. Herbal remedies and dietary supplements like St. John's wort must meet FDA standards for safety and effectiveness before they are on the market.
   True or False?

4. Generic drugs are often less effective than brand-name drugs.
   True or False?

5. After historic gains in numbers of Americans covered by health insurance since 2008, those numbers have been dropping since 2017, especially among which of these groups:
   a. Young adults
   b. Blacks and Latinos
   c. People making less than $36,000 a year

ANSWERS

1. **FALSE.** The more often a person visits a conventional primary care provider, the more likely he or she is to use complementary and alternative medicine.

2. **ALL THREE.** Although there are profound philosophical differences between the approaches, they share many characteristics.

3. **FALSE.** Manufacturers are responsible for the safety of the dietary supplements they sell; however, the FDA has the power to restrict a product if it is found to pose a health safety risk after it is on the market. Manufacturers are not required to prove that their products are effective.

4. **FALSE.** Price is often the only difference. The generic version of a drug has the same active ingredient or combination of ingredients as the brand-name drug, but it may have different inactive ingredients.

5. **ALL THREE.** Of the 27.5 million Americans without health coverage in 2017, the most vulnerable populations were those that the Affordable Care Act had focused enrollment efforts on.

Today people are becoming more empowered and confident in their ability to solve personal health problems on their own. People who effectively manage their own health care gather information and learn skills from a variety of resources. They solicit opinions and advice in order to practice safe, effective self-care, and to make decisions about seeking professional medical care—whether conventional Western medicine or complementary and alternative medicine.

This chapter helps you develop skills needed to identify and manage medical problems and to make the health care system work effectively for you.

SELF-CARE

Effectively managing medical problems involves developing several skills. First, you need to learn to closely examine your own body and assess your symptoms. You also must be able to decide when to seek professional advice and when you can safely deal with a problem on your own. You need to know how to safely and effectively self-treat common medical problems. Finally, you need to know how to develop a partnership with physicians and other health care providers and how to implement treatment plans.

Self-Assessment

Symptoms are often the body's attempt to heal itself. For example, the pain and swelling that occur after an ankle injury immobilize and protect the injured joint so that healing can take place. A fever works to inhibit growth and reproduction of infectious agents. A cough can help clear the airways and protect the lungs. Understanding what a symptom means and what is happening in your body helps reduce anxiety about symptoms and enables you to practice safe self-care that supports your own healing mechanisms.

Carefully observing symptoms also helps you identify signals that indicate you need professional help. You should begin by noting when a symptom begins, how often and when it occurs, what makes it worse, what makes it better, and whether you have any associated symptoms or illnesses. You can also monitor your body's vital signs, such as temperature and heart rate. Medical self-tests for blood pressure, blood sugar, pregnancy detection, and urinary tract infections can also help you make more informed decisions about when to seek medical help and when to self-treat.

Knowing When to See a Physician

Human responses to symptoms of injury and illness range from total denial to constant worry. In general, you should see a physician for symptoms that you would describe as follows:

• *Severe.* If a symptom is severe or intense, medical assistance is advised. Examples include significant pain, major injury and other emergencies.

• *Unusual.* If a symptom is peculiar and unfamiliar, it is wise to check it out with your physician. Examples include unexpected lumps, changes in a mole, problems with vision, difficulty swallowing, numbness, weakness, unexplained weight loss, or blood in the sputum (spit), urine, or stool.

• *Persistent.* If a symptom lasts longer than expected, seek medical advice. Examples in adults include fever for more than five days, a cough lasting longer than two weeks, a sore that doesn't heal within a month, and hoarseness lasting longer than three weeks.

• *Recurrent.* If a symptom returns again and again, medical evaluation is advised. Examples include recurring headaches, persistent abdominal pain, and backache.

Sometimes a single symptom is not a cause for concern, but when the symptom is accompanied by other symptoms, the combination suggests a more serious problem. For example, a fever accompanied by neck pain can suggest meningitis.

If you evaluate your symptoms and think you need professional help, you must decide how urgent the problem is. If it is a true emergency, you should go (or ask someone to take you) to the nearest hospital emergency department. Emergencies include the following:

• Major trauma or injury especially to the head, a suspected broken bone, deep wound, severe burn, eye injury, or animal bite

• Uncontrollable bleeding or internal bleeding, as indicated by blood in the sputum, vomit, or stool

• Intolerable and uncontrollable pain or severe chest pain

• Severe shortness of breath

• Persistent abdominal pain, especially if associated with nausea and vomiting

• Poisoning or drug overdose

• Sudden numbness, weakness, or loss of function involving an arm or leg, speech difficulty, or drooping of the face

• Seizure or loss of consciousness

• Stupor, drowsiness, or disorientation that cannot be explained

• Severe or worsening reaction to an insect bite or sting, or to a medication or food, especially if accompanied by swelling of the lips, mouth, or throat, or difficulty breathing

If your problem is not an emergency but still requires medical attention, call your physician's office or contact the office's online interactive website, if available. Often you can be given medical advice over the phone or online without needing a clinical visit. To help you make wise medical decisions, "A Self-Care Guide for Common Medical Problems" is provided in Appendix B.

Self-Treatment

When confronted with a new symptom, many people try to find a medication that will relieve or cure the illness. However, other self-treatment options are available.

Watchful Waiting In most cases, your body can relieve your symptoms and heal the disorder. The prescriptions filled by your body's "internal pharmacy" are frequently the safest and most effective treatment, so patience and careful self-observation are often the best choices in self-treatment.

Nondrug Options Nondrug options are often easy, inexpensive, safe, and highly effective. For example, ice packs, massage, gentle yoga stretching, and neck exercises may at times be more helpful than drugs in relieving headaches and other pains. Getting adequate rest, increasing exercise, drinking more water, eating more or less of certain foods, using humidifiers, and changing ergonomics when sitting or working are some of the hundreds of nondrug options for preventing or relieving many common health problems. For a variety of disorders caused or aggravated by stress, the treatment of choice may be relaxation or other stress management strategies (see Chapter 2).

> **over-the-counter (OTC) medication** A medication or product that can be purchased by a consumer without a prescription.
>
> **TERMS**

Self-Medication Self-treatment with nonprescription medications is an important part of health care. Nonprescription medications, also called **over-the-counter (OTC) medications**, are medicines that the U.S. Food and Drug Administration (FDA) has determined are safe to take without a prescription when used according to label directions.

Many OTC drugs are highly effective in relieving symptoms and sometimes in helping to cure illnesses. In fact, many OTC drugs were formerly prescription drugs. Hundreds of OTC products today use ingredients or dosage strengths that were available only by prescription a generation ago. With this increased consumer choice, however, consumers have an increased responsibility for using OTC drugs safely.

Consumers also need to be aware of the barrage of OTC drug advertising aimed at them. The implication of such advertising is that every symptom can and should be relieved by a drug. Although many OTC products are effective, others are unnecessary or divert attention from better ways of coping. Many ingredients in OTC drugs—an estimated 70%—have not been proven to be effective, a fact the FDA recognizes. And any drug may have risks and side effects.

Follow these simple guidelines to self-medicate safely:

- Always read labels and follow directions carefully. The information on most OTC drug labels now appears in a standard format developed by the FDA (Figure 21.1). Ingredients, directions for safe use, and warnings are clearly indicated. If you have any questions, ask a

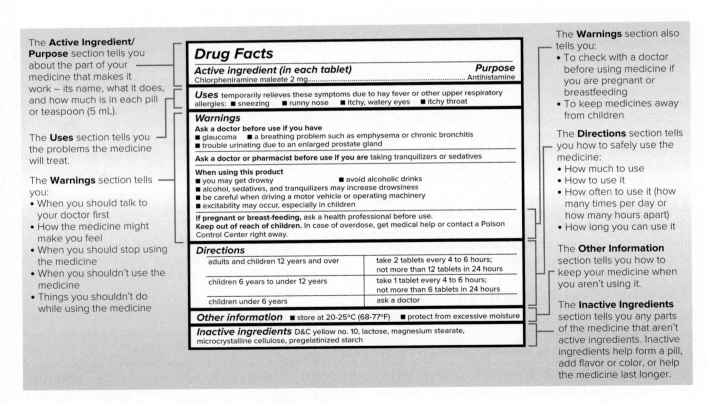

FIGURE 21.1 **Reading and understanding OTC drug labels.**

SOURCE: U.S. Food and Drug Administration. 2017. *Protecting and promoting your health.*

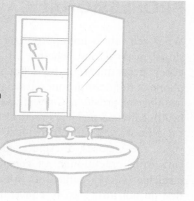

Closet

- Analgesic (relieves pain)
- Antacid (relieves upset stomach)
- Antihistamine (relieves allergy symptoms)
- Antibiotic ointment (reduces risk of infection)
- Antiseptic (helps stop infection)
- Fever reducer (adult and child)
- Decongestant (relieves stuffy nose and other cold symptoms)
- Hydrocortisone (relieves itching and inflammation)

Medicine Cabinet

- Adhesive bandages
- Adhesive tape
- Alcohol wipes
- Calibrated measuring spoon
- Disinfectant
- Gauze pads
- Thermometer
- Tweezers

FIGURE 21.2 **Your home medical care kit.** A cool, dark, and dry place such as the top of a linen closet, preferably in a locked container and out of a child's reach, is best for storing medicines. Showers and baths create heat and humidity that can cause some drugs to deteriorate rapidly. Use your bathroom medicine cabinet for supplies that aren't affected by heat and humidity.

SOURCE: Lewis, C. 2000. Your medicine cabinet needs an annual checkup, too. *FDA Consumer*, March/April.

pharmacist or a qualified health care provider before using a product.

- Do not exceed the recommended dosage or length of treatment unless you discuss this with your health care provider.

- Use caution if you are taking other medications or supplements because OTC drugs and herbal supplements can interact with some prescription drugs. If you have questions about drug interactions, ask your health care provider or pharmacist *before* you take medicines in combination.

- Try to select medications with one active ingredient rather than a combination. A product with multiple ingredients is likely to include drugs for symptoms you don't have, which can increase side effects. Using single-ingredient products also allows you to adjust the dosage of each medication separately for optimal symptom relief with minimal side effects.

- When choosing medications, look for **generic drugs,** which contain the same active ingredient as brand-name products but generally at a much lower cost.

- Use a drug only if it is labeled clearly on its container, never when you can't read the label.

- If you are pregnant or nursing or have a chronic condition such as kidney or liver disease, consult your health care provider before self-medicating.

- The expiration date marked on many medications only estimates how long the medication is likely to be safe and effective. However, an extensive study by the FDA found that 90% of all prescription and OTC medications are potent well after their stated expiration dates. Exceptions include tetracycline and other antibiotics, nitroglycerine, and insulin. Expiration dates are very conservative. If a medicine is expired by more than a few months and you need to be certain that the medication

is completely effective, you should purchase new medication. Because of environmental and safety concerns, never flush medicine down the toilet or sink, and do not discard medicine directly into the trash. You can dispose of old medicine by placing it in a sealed container with coffee grounds or cat litter, but the safest way to get rid of outdated medicines is to take them to a pharmacy or hospital. If you have any questions about a medicine's expiration date, ask a pharmacist.

- Store your medications in a cool, dry place away from direct light and out of the reach of children (Figure 21.2).

- Use special caution with aspirin. Because of an association with a rare but serious problem known as Reye's syndrome, aspirin should not be used by children or adolescents who may have the flu, chickenpox, or any other viral illness. Outdated aspirin that has an acidic odor should be discarded.

Ask Yourself

QUESTIONS FOR CRITICAL THINKING AND REFLECTION

Do you often self-medicate for common medical problems, such as headaches or colds? If so, how careful are you about reading product labels and following directions? For example, would you know if you were taking two OTC medications that contained the same ingredient (such as acetaminophen or ibuprofen) at the same time?

generic drug A drug that is not registered or protected by a commercial trademark; a drug that does not have an exclusive brand name. **TERMS**

PROFESSIONAL CARE

When self-care is not appropriate or sufficient, seek professional medical care, whether by going to a hospital emergency department or by scheduling an appointment by phone or online with your physician or another conventional health care provider. **Conventional medicine** is mainstream health care and medical practices taught in most U.S. medical schools and offered in most U.S. hospitals. In recent years, the majority of Americans have also sought health care from practitioners of **complementary and alternative medicine (CAM)**—defined as those therapies and practices that do not form part of conventional medicine. The most frequently used CAM therapies are nonvitamin, nonmineral dietary supplements, yoga, meditation, chiropractic, and massage therapy. (Table 21.1 shows that popularity among some of these therapies is increasing.) According to the most recent Centers for Disease Control and Prevention (CDC) report, 33.2% of adults in the United States use some form of CAM. Among those who do, at least 83% use it together with conventional medicine, not in place of it.

The term *CAM* includes both the terms **complementary** and **alternative medicine:** "Complementary" means an approach that combines nonmainstream and conventional medicine. "Alternative" refers to an approach that replaces conventional medicine. For example, when a conventional drug such as penicillin (an antibiotic) is used to fight an infection together with an unconventional remedy such as the herb echinacea (which enhances immunity to an infection), these treatments are considered complementary. However, if an unconventional remedy, such as a wrist band designed to apply pressure to an acupressure point, is used to prevent motion sickness *instead* of taking a conventional medication such as Dramamine (a drug used for motion sickness), the wrist bracelet is considered *alternative.* When an alternative practice is used, it should have a high level of proof that it is safe and as effective as a conventional method, especially if the condition being treated or prevented is serious or life-threatening.

Table 21.1	Complementary and Alternative Therapies Commonly Used by U.S. Adults

TYPE OF THERAPY	PERCENTAGE WHO USED THERAPY	
	2012	2017
Yoga	9.5	14.3
Meditation	4.1	14.2
Chiropractic	9.1	10.3

SOURCE: Clark, T. C., et al. 2018. Use of yoga, meditation, and chiropractors among U.S. adults aged 18 and over. NCHS Data Brief, No. 325. Hyattsville, MD: National Center for Health Statistics.

Ask Yourself

QUESTIONS FOR CRITICAL THINKING AND REFLECTION

What are your views about the use of CAM therapies? What events or information has shaped those views? Would you consider using complementary or alternative medicine?

Another term, *integrative medicine,* has become widely accepted in the United States. In integrative health it is understood that conventional methods are given priority, and a CAM *modality* (technique or form) may be included if it could have additional benefits.

Consumers turn to integrative health or CAM for a variety of purposes related to health and well-being, such as boosting the immune system, lowering cholesterol levels, losing weight, quitting smoking, or enhancing memory. People with chronic conditions, including cancer, asthma, autoimmune diseases, and HIV infection, are particularly likely to try CAM therapies. Despite their popularity, many CAM practices remain controversial, and consumers need to be critically aware of safety issues. The National Center for Complementary and Integrative Health (NCCIH), formerly called the National Center for Complementary and Alternative Medicine, was established in 1992 to apply rigorous scientific methodology and standards for proving or disproving the safety and effectiveness of CAM.

The following sections examine the principles used by providers of both conventional medicine—the dominant medical system in the United States and Europe, also referred to as *standard Western medicine* or *biomedicine*—and integrative health and CAM, with particular attention to consumer issues.

CONVENTIONAL MEDICINE

Referring to conventional medicine as "standard Western medicine" draws attention to the fact that it differs from various traditional medical systems that have developed in China,

---

TERMS

conventional medicine   A system of medicine emphasizing biological and physical scientific principles; diseases are thought to be caused by identifiable physical factors and characterized by a representative set of signs and symptoms; also called *biomedicine* or *standard Western medicine.*

complementary and alternative medicine (CAM)   Health care practices and products that are not considered part of conventional, mainstream medical practice as taught in most U.S. medical schools and that are not available at most U.S. health care facilities; examples of CAM practices include acupuncture and herbal remedies.

complementary medicine   Unconventional medical practices that are used together with conventional ones.

alternative medicine   Unconventional medical practices that are used instead of conventional methods.

Japan, India, and other parts of the world. Calling it "biomedicine" reflects conventional medicine's foundation in the biological and physical sciences.

Premises and Assumptions of Conventional Medicine

An important characteristic of Western medicine is the belief that disease is caused by identifiable and reproducible factors. Western medicine identifies the causes of disease as pathogens (such as bacteria and viruses), physical factors (such as trauma or toxins), genetic factors, or unhealthy lifestyles that result in changes at the cellular and molecular levels. In most cases, the focus of conventional medicine is primarily on the physical causes of illness rather than on mental or spiritual imbalance, which is more central to traditional medical systems, sometimes known as whole medical systems.

Another feature that distinguishes Western biomedicine from other medical systems is the concept that almost every disease is defined by a certain set of signs (*objective* physical manifestations) and symptoms (*subjective* effects perceived by a person), and that they are similar in most patients suffering from the disease. Western medicine tends to treat diseases as biological disturbances occurring in a patient rather than as the result of mind, body, and spirit interactions.

A disease can be caused by either internal or external factors. Internal factors include anatomic or physiologic abnormalities, and defective genetic, hormonal, and immune mechanisms. External causes include infections by bacteria and viruses, and some cases of traumatic injury. The public health measures of the 19th and 20th centuries—chlorination of drinking water, sewage disposal, food safety regulations, vaccination programs, education about hygiene, and so on—were an outgrowth of this orientation.

The implementation of public health measures is one way to control diseases; others include preventive lifestyle measures and the use of drugs and surgery. The discovery and development of sulfa drugs, antibiotics, and steroids in the 20th century, along with advances in chemistry that made it possible to identify the active ingredients in common plant-derived remedies, paved the way for the current close identification of Western medicine with **pharmaceuticals** (medical drugs, both prescription and over-the-counter). Western medicine also relies heavily on surgery and advanced medical technology to discover the physical cause of an individual's disease and to correct, remove, or destroy it.

Western medicine is based on the scientific method for obtaining knowledge and explaining health-related phenomena. The resulting scientific explanations build on these kinds of evidence:

- *Empirical.* They are based on the evidence of the senses and on objective and systematic observation, often carried out under carefully controlled conditions; they

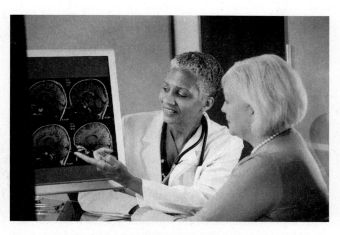

One feature that distinguishes Western biomedicine from other medical systems is the concept that almost every disease is defined by a certain set of signs and symptoms and that they are similar in most patients suffering from the disease. Ariel Skelley/Blend Images/Getty Images

must be capable of verification by others through objective observation, which may include the use of technology (such as lab tests and physical measurement, such as blood pressure).

- *Rational.* They follow the rules of logic and are consistent with known facts.
- *Testable.* Either they are verifiable through objective observation or they lead to predictions about what should occur under defined, controlled conditions (as in randomized controlled trials).
- *Parsimonious.* They explain phenomena using the fewest causes (for example, symptoms are attributed to the simplest explanation as supported by evidence).
- *Generality.* They explain phenomena among other patients who have similar signs and symptoms. (Most of the time, people with the same disease will have similar symptoms.)
- *Rigorously evaluated.* They are continuously evaluated for agreement with the evidence and known principles of parsimony and generality.
- *Tentative.* Scientists are willing to entertain the possibility that their conclusions may be faulty if new and better evidence becomes available.

The scientific method is both a way of acquiring knowledge and a method of problem solving that includes carefully defining the parameters of a problem, seeking relevant evidence, and subjecting proposed solutions to rigorous testing.

Western medicine uses the scientific method in health care practice by applying the research process, a highly refined and well-established approach to exploring the causes

pharmaceuticals Medical drugs, both prescription and over-the-counter.

TERMS

of disease and ensuring the safety and efficacy of treatments. Research ranges from case studies—descriptions of a single patient's illness and treatment—to **randomized controlled trials (RCTs)** conducted on large populations. RCTs are considered the highest level of evidence for treatment outcomes. Conclusions made based on an RCT may be enhanced by a relatively new standard of evidence, a **meta-analysis,** which mathematically combines data from two or more methodologically similar RCTs. If several RCTs show marginal or questionable conclusions, a meta-analysis determines which way "the scale will tip" by statistically combining the data from the studies.

The process of drug development is an example of rigorous scientific investigation. Drugs are developed and tested through an elaborate process that typically begins with preliminary research in a laboratory and continues through trials with human participants, review and approval by the FDA, and monitoring of the drug's effects even after it is on the market. The process may take several years or more, and only about 20% of drugs are eventually approved for marketing. The FDA now has new tracks to speed up the approval process, but the time for approval varies widely. Fast track, for example, is designated for an unmet medical need for a serious condition.

When results of research studies are published in medical journals, the community of scientists, physicians, researchers, and scholars has the opportunity to share the findings and enter a dialogue about the subject. Publication of research often prompts further research designed to replicate and confirm the findings, challenge the conclusions, or pursue related lines of thought or experimentation. (For guidelines on how to interpret research when it is reported in the popular media, see the box "Evaluating Health News.")

Pharmaceuticals and the Placebo Effect

In medical research, a placebo is often used when evaluating a new drug in a controlled trial (see Figure 21.3). A *placebo* is a biologically inactive substance that the subject cannot distinguish from the experimental drug. (For studies that don't involve drugs, such as surgery or acupuncture, a *sham* procedure may be used.) Either the experimental treatment or a placebo or sham procedure is administered randomly to subjects who are unaware which they are receiving (a "blinded" trial). By

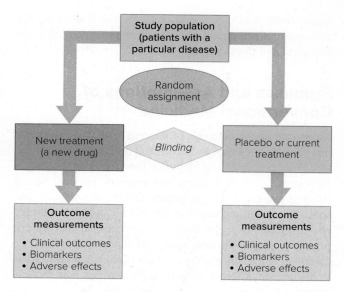

FIGURE 21.3 **How a randomized control trial works.**

comparing the effects of the experimental treatment with the effects of the placebo or sham, researchers can evaluate whether the experimental treatment is more effective than the placebo.

Researchers have consistently found that 30–40% of all patients given a placebo show some improvement. A *placebo effect* occurs when a research subject improves after receiving a placebo; the placebo effect is the difference in outcome compared to no intervention at all (no placebo and no experimental treatment). The *treatment effect* is the difference in outcome between the placebo and the experimental treatment. If the subject does not respond better to the experimental treatment than to the placebo, then the improvement cannot be attributed to the specific actions or properties of the drug or procedure. The new science of psychoneuroimmunology (PNI) helps explain why and how the body responds to placebos, which were once considered neutral non-interventions (see Chapter 2 for more about PNI).

A placebo effect has been observed in treatment of a wide variety of conditions or symptoms, including coughing, seasickness, depression, migraines, and angina. In some cases, people given a placebo even report having the side effects associated with an actual drug. Studies have shown that placebos are particularly effective when they are administered by someone the patient likes and believes in. Experimental studies have shown that placebos that are thought to be expensive are more effective than an identical "cheap" placebo, and placebos administered by injection are more effective than ones taken orally.

An example of the placebo effect occurred in a study that examined the effectiveness of a drug used to treat benign enlargement of the prostate. The men who participated were randomly assigned to one of two groups: One group received the medication while the other received a placebo. More than half the men who received the placebo pills reported significant relief from their symptoms, including faster urine

Health-related research published in scientific medical journals is often summarized for the public in the popular media, which may oversimplify, exaggerate, distort, or sensationalize the results. The following questions can help you evaluate the health information about conventional medicine and CAM that you will likely encounter in popular media:

1. *Is the report based on scientific studies?* Information or advice based on carefully designed research studies has more validity than opinions, anecdotes, or casual observations.

2. *What is the source of the information?* A study published in a respected peer-reviewed scientific journal has been examined by editors and researchers who are professionally prepared to evaluate the merits of a study and its results, and its application to actual patients. Most journals include information on the funding source and the authors' affiliations that may introduce a bias or conflict of interest. Studies sponsored by drug companies or other commercial groups are suspect. Sources sponsored by universities, government agencies, professional groups (such as MayoClinic.org and MedlinePlus.gov), and others that are rigorously peer-reviewed typically base their reports on scientific information and are considered more valid than commercial websites. Wikipedia is not considered a scientifically valid resource. When health information is critical, the consumer should review the original reference rather than rely solely on secondary interpretations.

3. *How many subjects were included in the study?* A study involving many subjects—hundreds or thousands of people—is more likely to yield reliable results than a study involving only a few subjects. Most quality studies include a "statistical power analysis" section that specifies how many subjects were necessary in order for the findings to be meaningful.

4. *Who were the subjects?* Research findings are more likely to apply to you if you share important characteristics with the study participants. For example, the results of a study on male smokers over age 60 may not be particularly meaningful for a 25-year-old female nonsmoker.

5. *What kind of study was it?* Randomized controlled trials (RCTs) and meta-analyses are considered the most valid. Epidemiological studies (which involve noncontrolled observations) may suggest useful information, but they cannot always establish cause-and-effect relationships. The following questions may help you to decide whether a study's results should be considered valid:

   • *Were the treatment group results compared to those of a control group or an already accepted therapy?*

   • *Were the subjects randomly assigned to the experimental groups?*

   • *Was the study blinded (to the subjects, the experimenters/evaluators, or both)?*

   • *Was it a multicenter study?* The results of several studies conducted in different places at different times can be mathematically combined as a meta-analysis. A well-conducted meta-analysis is considered one of the most valid types of studies.

6. *What do the statistics really say?* Are the results statistically significant? Statistical significance is usually reported as a p-value; when it is less than or equal to 0.05 or 5%, it is considered "statistically significant," meaning there is a 5% or lower probability that the findings were the result of chance. Does the study have the required number of subjects according to a statistical power analysis? Some studies report the effect size—the statistical difference in outcome between the treatment being tested and the control—instead of or in addition to a p-value. Most of the time the effect size is more revealing than the p-value.

   If study results are given in terms of relative risk—for example, a 50% reduction in the risk of developing a disorder—you should also consider the absolute risk of the condition. For example, if the absolute risk of developing a disorder is 2%, then a medication that reduced that risk by 50% (relative risk) would lower the risk to 1%: Out of 100 people *not taking* the medication, two on average would develop the disorder; out of 100 people *taking* the medication, one would develop the disorder.

7. *Is new health advice being offered?* If the media report new guidelines for health behavior or medical treatment, examine the source. Be suspicious of absolutes and overstated claims that use words such as "certainty," "always," and "never." Scientifically accurate reports use words such as "results show," "for many people," and "the evidence suggests." Reliable information sources should present the limitations of a study's results, describe how the results compare with those of other studies, and consider a great deal of evidence before offering health advice. Above all, use common sense, and check with your physician before making a major change in your health habits based on news reports.

For additional tips, visit NCCIH, *9 Questions to Help You Make Sense of Scientific Research* (https://nccih.nih.gov/health/know-science/make-sense-health-research), and NIH, *Understanding Risk: What Do Those Headlines Really Mean?* (https://permanent.access.gpo.gov/gpo64263/understanding_risk_0.pdf).

flow—even though these men experienced an *increase* in the size of their prostates.

Why did the men in the study experience fewer symptoms despite no actual improvement in their condition? Researchers hypothesize that the patients' positive expectations for the medication may have generated changes in nervous activity and muscle relaxation affecting the bladder, prostate, and urethra.

Studies of people with depression or Parkinson's disease have found that treatment with a placebo results in documented changes in brain function. These changes in the electrical or chemical activity of the brain may help explain the positive result of the placebo effect.

As noted, in research, a placebo is used to evaluate and control for the added benefit of a physiologically active treatment. However, a placebo effect can be exploited by unscrupulous people who knowingly misrepresent and sell otherwise worthless treatments to the public. But the effects of placebos can also be harnessed for a patient's benefit. The way medical practitioners interact with patients may also bring about a positive placebo response independent of any specific treatment.

When a skilled and compassionate doctor or nurse can provide patients with confidence and hope, the positive aspects of the placebo effect can add to the benefits of treatment. Getting well, like getting sick, is a complex process. Anatomy, physiology, emotions, hope, beliefs, expectations, and prior experiences can contribute to the way the body reacts to medical treatments.

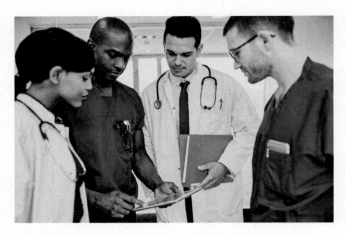

In Western medicine, treatment is usually provided by a team of health care professionals, often with different areas of specialization but with shared ideas and beliefs about the causes of illness. langstrup/123RF

The Providers of Conventional Medicine

Conventional medicine is practiced by a wide range of health care professionals in the United States. Several kinds of health care professionals are licensed to open their own practices, including medical doctors, osteopaths, dentists, podiatrists, psychologists, and optometrists.

• **Medical doctors** are practitioners who hold a doctor of medicine (MD) degree from an accredited medical school. With proper postgraduate education (residency), they are licensed to practice medical or surgical specialties such as family medicine, internal medicine, orthopedics, ophthalmology, pathology, and others. They are commonly called "allopathic" physicians because of their historical practice philosophy: Treatment with opposites (the Greek prefix *allo-* means "difference," or "opposition"). For example, if the body is too cold, add heat; if it's too warm, cool it down; if a patient is too stimulated, administer a tranquilizer; too tranquil, give a stimulant. In the United States, becoming a practicing physician has several stages: premedical education in a college or university to earn a bachelor's degree; usually four years of medical school, which teaches basic medical skills and awards

the doctor of medicine degree; and three to eight years of graduate medical study that includes an internship and a residency and possibly a specialty fellowship. The American Board of Medical Specialties currently recognizes and approves over 145 medical specialties and subspecialties.

• **Doctors of osteopathic medicine** (DO) receive formal premedical education to earn a bachelor's degree; four years of osteopathic medical school leading to the DO degree; and residency and fellowship education similar to that of allopathic medical doctors over a comparable time frame. The osteopathic philosophy emphasizes structural and functional relationships and a whole-person approach to medicine. Like allopathic physicians, osteopathic physicians practice in all of the medical and surgical specialties and subspecialties, but osteopathic physicians may also practice and specialize in osteopathic manipulative treatment (manipulation of muscles and joints using stretching, pressure, and resistance). MDs and DOs often complete their postgraduate education and practice medicine in the same hospitals and medical centers.

• **Dentists** focus on the care of the teeth and mouth. They are graduates of four-year dental schools and hold the doctor of dental surgery (DDS) or doctor of medical dentistry (DMD) degree; dental specialists such as oral surgeons and orthodontists receive additional education. Dentists can perform surgery and prescribe drugs within the scope of their training.

• **Podiatrists** are practitioners who specialize in the medical and surgical care of the feet. They hold a doctor of podiatric medicine (DPM) degree. The length of training is similar to that of MDs and DOs. They can prescribe drugs and perform surgery on the feet.

• **Psychologists** work with individuals, couples, families, or groups in many settings, such as private offices, hospitals, mental health organizations, schools, businesses, and nonprofit agencies. Many clinical and counseling psychologists hold a Doctor of Psychology (PsyD) or a Doctor of Philosophy (PhD) degree; they may be faculty members in colleges and engage in research and teaching. Clinical psychologists, like psychiatrists, treat mental health problems but, unlike psychiatrists, are not medical doctors and usually do not prescribe medications.

- **Optometrists** are practitioners trained to examine the eyes, detect eye diseases, and treat certain vision problems, most often through the use of corrective lenses. They hold a doctor of optometry (OD) degree. All states permit optometrists to use certain drugs for diagnostic purposes, and most permit them to use drugs to treat minor eye problems. **Ophthalmologists** have an MD or DO degree and serve a residency or fellowship specializing in diseases of the eye. They care for all types of eye problems using drugs and surgery.

- **Nurses** or *registered nurses (RNs)* are practitioners concerned with the diagnosis and treatment of human responses to actual or potential health problems. They act to promote, maintain, or restore health. A nurse may receive advanced education to become a nurse practitioner (NP), a certified registered nurse anesthetist (CRNA), or a certified nurse midwife (CNM).

- **Physician assistants** (PAs) are nationally certified and state-licensed health care professionals who practice medicine as part of a team with physicians.

In addition to these practitioners, highly educated health care professionals work in over a hundred other medical professions (or specialties or disciplines), including physical therapists, pharmacists, medical social workers, and registered dietitians.

QUICK STATS

More than 12 million health care professionals of all types work in the United States, including more than 3 million registered nurses (the largest health care occupation).

—U.S. Bureau of Labor Statistics, 2020

To select a PCP, begin by making a list of possible choices. If your insurance limits the health care providers you can see, check the plan's list first to see which doctors its network includes. Student health services or health maintenance organizations (discussed later) may assign you a physician. If your health plan lets you choose a physician, ask for recommendations from family, friends, coworkers, local medical societies, and the physician referral service at a local clinic or hospital. Any health care provider you know, such as a physician assistant, nurse, nurse practitioner, or physical therapist who will provide impartial information or a recommendation, can be an excellent resource for choosing a physician. Some clinics provide brief biographies of physicians on staff who are accepting new patients. Once you have a list of possible physicians, find out if a consumer or other independent group has rated doctors in your area; such a rating system may help you check on the quality of care they provide. You might also want to check online or call the offices of those on your list to find out the following:

- Is the physician covered by your health plan and accepting new patients?

- What are the office hours, and when is the physician or office staff available?

- What do patients do if they need urgent care or have an emergency?

- Which hospitals does the physician use?

- How many other physicians are available to cover when your PCP isn't available, and who are they?

Choosing a Primary Care Physician

Most experts believe it is best to have a primary care physician (PCP) who gets to know you, coordinates your medical care, and refers you to specialists when you need them. Some health care insurance plans require you to identify a PCP. The primary care disciplines include family practice, internal medicine, pediatrics, and gynecology. These physicians are able to diagnose and treat the vast majority of common health problems and provide many preventive health services. The best time to look for a physician is before you become sick.

Many physicians coordinate your care through highly trained medical professionals such as physician assistants and nurse practitioners. These professionals perform many services that have traditionally been provided by physicians, including taking medical histories, performing physical exams, ordering laboratory and imaging studies, prescribing medications, and performing minor surgery. They work as part of a team with your doctor and are frequently able to spend more time to provide patient education and answer detailed questions about your concerns, preventive measures, and lifestyle choices.

TERMS

podiatrist A practitioner who holds a doctor of podiatric medicine (DPM) degree and specializes in the medical and surgical care of the feet.

psychologist Health care provider who holds a PsyD or PhD degree; they treat mental health problems and usually do not prescribe medicine.

optometrist A practitioner who holds a doctor of optometry (OD) degree and is trained to examine the eyes, detect eye diseases, and prescribe corrective lenses.

ophthalmologist A practitioner who holds an MD or DO degree, has served a residency or fellowship specializing in diseases of the eye, and cares for all types of eye problems using drugs and surgery.

nurse A licensed health provider who is concerned with the diagnosis and treatment of human responses to actual or potential health problems and acts to promote, maintain, or restore health. Registered nurses (RNs) complete a bachelor of nursing degree. Licensed practical and vocational nurses complete a one- or two-year training program (LPN, LVN).

physician assistant A health provider who is nationally certified and licensed by his or her state to practice medicine as part of a team with physicians.

- How long does it usually take to get a routine appointment?
- Does the office send reminders about preventive services and tests such as Pap tests?
- Does the physician (or a nurse or physician assistant) give advice online or over the phone for common problems and continued care of a diagnosed problem?

A physician's practice philosophy is another important factor; most clinics provide their physicians' personal statements in brochures or online. Schedule a visit with the physician you think you would most like to use. During that first visit, you'll get a sense of how well matched you are and how well he or she might meet your medical needs.

Choosing a Specialist

Compared to finding your PCP, your choices in finding a specialist are more limited. If you need emergency care, you may have few or no options, although you may be able to go to an accredited emergency department of a hospital you trust. If possible, go to one your PCP recommends or in which he or she has hospital privileges. For non-emergencies you may be limited to specialists covered by your insurance plan. When you do have choices, look for the same qualities you used for selecting your PCP, including their ability to communicate with you using terminology you understand and their willingness to answer your questions.

You should be referred to a specialist when the services you need are outside the scope of your PCP's practice. The specialist may not be a physician but rather a physical therapist, audiologist, psychologist, or another type of practitioner. In most cases, your PCP will recommend the type of specialist you need based on your clinical findings; unless it's obvious, most of the time patients cannot accurately identify the appropriate medical discipline needed, since there are 145 medical specialties and subspecialties. In general, physician specialists are from the internal medicine subdisciplines, such as dermatology, gastroenterology, and neurology, or from the surgical subdisciplines, such as thoracic surgery, orthopedics, and neurosurgery. Some subdisciplines involve both internal medicine and surgery (gynecology, urology, and ophthalmology).

By the time of your visit, the specialist should have received a referral note from your PCP, your complete medical record, and access to all your recent lab tests and imaging studies as well as past tests that may be significant (e.g., MRIs of the spine years earlier). If your specialist refers you to another specialist, you should visit your PCP first, to keep him or her up to date on your symptoms and to discuss any questions you have about the next step in your specialized care.

Getting the Most Out of Your Medical Care

The key to making the health care system work for you lies in good communication with your physician and other members of the health care team. Studies show that patients who interact more with physicians and ask more questions enjoy better health outcomes (see the box "Health Care Visits and Gender").

The Physician–Patient Partnership The physician–patient relationship is undergoing an important transformation. The image of the all-knowing physician and the passive patient is fading. What is emerging is a physician–patient *partnership* in which the physician acts more like a consultant and the patient participates more actively (see the box "Creating Your Own Health Record"). You should expect your physician to be attentive, caring, and able to listen and clearly explain health care matters to you. You also must do your part. You need to be assertive in a firm but nonaggressive manner. You need to express your feelings and concerns, ask questions, and, if necessary, be persistent. If your physician is unable to communicate clearly with you despite your best efforts, you probably need to change physicians.

Your Physician Appointments You may be offered the opportunity to see a physician assistant or nurse practitioner who works with your physician. This option may result in an earlier appointment where you may have more time to discuss your health concerns. Physicians are often pressed for time, so prepare for office visits by writing down your key concerns and questions, along with notes about your symptoms (when they started, how long they last, what makes them better or worse, what treatments you have already tried, and so on). Even well-informed, proactive patients often forget important information and questions during the dynamics of an office visit. If you're uncomfortable asking certain questions, practice discussing them ahead of time. Bring a list of all the medications you're taking—prescription, nonprescription, and herbal. Also bring any medical records or test results your physician may not already have.

Present your concerns at the beginning of the visit to set the agenda. Be specific and concise about your symptoms, and be open and honest about your concerns. Share your hunches with your physician—your guesses can provide vital clues. Ask questions if you don't understand something he or she says to you. Let your physician know if you are taking any drugs, are allergic to any medications, are breastfeeding, or may be pregnant.

At the end of the visit, briefly repeat the physician's diagnosis, prognosis, the purpose of any tests, and instructions you have received to make sure you understand your next steps, such as making another appointment, phoning for test results, watching for new symptoms, and so on.

Ask Yourself

QUESTIONS FOR CRITICAL THINKING AND REFLECTION
What sort of relationship do you have with your physician? Do you think he or she understands your needs and is familiar enough with your history? Are you satisfied with this relationship?

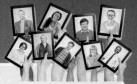

Women are more likely than men to visit a health care provider. According to data from the National Center for Health Statistics covering all age groups, 20% of men report no health care visits in the past 12 months—nearly twice the 11% rate for women. A Kaiser Family Foundation survey of adults aged 18–64 found that 25% of men had not seen a provider within the past two years, compared to only 9% of women. Men also have lower rates of many preventive health services, including flu vaccinations and colon cancer screening, and are less likely than women to have a usual source of health care.

Women also seek a wider variety of health care alternatives. A study found that more women than men in 2017 used yoga, meditation, and chiropractors in the past year. One explanation for this gender disparity may lie in the prenatal care and childbirth visits made by women of reproductive age. They may also need to make health care vis-its to obtain prescription contraceptives and have pelvic exams and Pap tests. Still, even when physician visits related to reproductive care are discounted, American men are less likely to report their symptoms and seek medical help.

Perhaps the way boys in the United States (and many other countries) are raised has something to do with their reluctance to seek preventive care (when no symptoms are present). One study of boys aged 15–19 in the United States reveals that they equated health with physical fitness. They saw no reason for preventive care and justified seeking any care only when a person was physically and severely ill. This belief system correlates with ideas of men as strong, tough, and able to ignore pain or symptoms of illness.

Ideally, everyone, regardless of gender or socioeconomic status, would get recommended health care screenings and immunizations. Without them, people may be unaware of asymptomatic conditions such as high cholesterol levels or high blood pressure. Preventive care throughout life is important for maximum wellness.

SOURCES: Clark, T. C., et al. 2018. Use of yoga, meditation, and chiropractors among U.S. adults aged 18 and over. *NCHS Data Brief* 325. Hyattsville, MD: National Center for Health Statistics (https://www.cdc.gov/nchs/data/databriefs/db325-h.pdf). Kaiser Family Foundation. 2015. *Gender Differences in Health Care, Status, and Use* (http://kff.org/womens-health-policy/fact-sheet/gender-differences-in-health-care-status-and-use-spotlight-on-mens-health); World Health Organization. 2010. *Gender, Women and Primary Health Care Renewal: A Discussion Paper.* Geneva, Switzerland: World Health Organization; Harvard Men's Health Watch. 2010. Mars vs. Venus: The gender gap in health. *Harvard Health Letter* (http://www.health.harvard.edu/newsletter_article/mars-vs-venus-the-gender-gap-in-health); Westwood, M., and J. Pinzon. 2008. Adolescent male health. *Paediatrics and Child Health* 13(1): 31–36.

The Diagnostic Process   The first step in the diagnostic process is the medical history, which includes primary reason for the visit, current symptoms, past medical history, and social history (job, family life, major stressors, living conditions, and health habits). Keeping up-to-date records of your medical history can help you provide your physician with key facts about your health.

The next step is usually the physical exam, which begins with a review of vital signs: blood pressure, heart rate (pulse), breathing rate, and temperature. Depending on your primary complaint, your physician may give you a complete physical or instead focus on specific areas, such as your ears, nose, and throat.

Additionally, your physician may order medical tests. Diagnostic testing provides a wealth of information to help solve medical problems. Physicians can order imaging studies (e.g., X-rays, MRIs, or CT scans), biopsies, blood and urine tests, or **endoscopies** to view, probe, or analyze almost any part of the body.

If your physician orders a test for you, be sure you know why you need it, what the risks and benefits are for you, how you should prepare for it (e.g., by fasting or discontinuing medications or herbal remedies), and what the test will involve. Also ask what the test results mean because no test is 100% accurate—**false positives** and **false negatives** can occur—and interpretation of some tests is subjective. You may want to obtain a second opinion, especially for serious conditions or major surgical procedures, or if you have significant unmet needs related to your medical care. When there are good reasons for obtaining a second opinion, most physicians welcome them; if they resist, it could be a sign that you should find another physician.

Medical and Surgical Treatments   Many conditions can be treated in a variety of ways; in some cases, lifestyle changes are sufficient. When starting any treatment, make sure you know the possible risks and side effects as well as the potential benefits.

PRESCRIPTION MEDICATIONS   Each month, about half of Americans use at least one prescription medication. Among those aged 65 and over, 80–90% use prescription drugs. Thousands of lives are saved each year by antibiotics, insulin,

TERMS

endoscopy   A medical procedure in which a viewing instrument is inserted into a body cavity or opening.

false positive   A test result that incorrectly detects a disorder or condition in a person who does not have the disorder or condition.

false negative   A test result that fails to correctly detect a disease or condition.

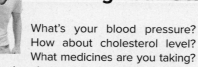

WELLNESS ON CAMPUS
Creating Your Own Health Record

What's your blood pressure? How about cholesterol level? What medicines are you taking? Many Americans believe that their medical records are compiled and maintained by some mysterious entity (probably called "them"), but this is not the case. The expanding use of computerized medical records may be useful within a particular clinic or health care system, but this does not mean that every person's individual medical history has been automatically collated into a single, easy-to-find source. Computerized health records maintained by one hospital or medical care system might not be accessible by another. We each need to be responsible for compiling our important medical records and keeping them safe and easily available to us or a caregiver in case we need the records for an emergency, or when traveling, moving, or looking for a new primary care provider. College is a good time to start doing this for yourself, and by sharing your health knowledge and assisting family members to do the same, you are playing a more active role in your family's health care.

Personal health records should be readily accessible in case of an emergency. Some personal computerized health record systems can be purchased online, or one can be devised individually. (You can find out about various personal health records on the U.S. government's HealthIT.gov website: http://www.healthit.gov/how-do-i/individuals.) Whether purchased or created individually, here's what your personal health record should contain:

- Your name, emergency contact, birth date, blood type, religious preference (if any), and the date this record was compiled or updated.

- All known allergies (including medications).

- A list of all chronic conditions and the dates of their diagnosis (e.g., diabetes, high blood pressure, asthma, emphysema).

- Any hereditary diseases.

- The names and dosages of all medications you take and reasons for taking them.

- The results of tests or procedures such as blood pressure, cholesterol, vision, and others.

- The dates and reasons for all past hospitalizations and operations. If the reasons were serious or may affect future treatments (e.g., major organ involvement; devices or materials implanted surgically), a hospital discharge summary should be included.

- The dates of physical exams and any major findings.

- Vaccination schedules.

- A print-out of all laboratory test results, and a written report of any imaging studies (e.g., X-rays, CT scans, MRIs), electrocardiograms (ECGs), and special tests such as audiograms and exercise stress tests. Check to verify that dates are included.

You have the right to all of your medical records—that is, to view them or request a copy or a summary of the information. To request copies, ask for an "authorization for the release of information form." Any fee should include only the cost of copying and postage (if you request mailing). If you see something in your medical record that you believe is incorrect or incomplete, you can request an amendment through your physician or a medical information professional, and you have the right for your amendment to be permanently included in your record.

SOURCES: MedlinePlus. *Personal Health Records* (www.nlm.nih.gov/medlineplus/personalhealthrecords.html); AHIMA Foundation. *myPHR* (http://www.ahimafoundation.org/).

---

and other drugs, but we pay a price for having such powerful tools. A report from the National Academy of Medicine estimates that 1.5 million prescription-drug-related errors—called adverse drug events, or ADEs—occur each year in the United States. ADEs happen for several reasons:

- *Medication errors.* Physicians may overprescribe drugs, sometimes in response to pressure by patients. ADEs can occur if a physician prescribes the wrong drug or a dangerous combination of drugs. Such problems are especially prevalent among older adults, who typically take multiple medications. The risk of ADEs increases greatly with the number of medicines you take. At the pharmacy, patients may receive the wrong drug or may not be given complete information about drug risks, side effects, and interactions. Problems can occur because of a physician's poor handwriting, misinterpretation of an abbreviated drug name, or similarities between the names and packaging of different drugs.

- *Off-label drug use.* Another potential problem is off-label use of drugs. Once a drug is approved by the FDA for one purpose, it can legally be prescribed (although not marketed) for purposes not listed on the label. Many off-label uses are safe and supported by some research, but both consumers and health care providers need to take special care with off-label use of medications. Physicians should explain their reason for prescribing an off-label drug.

- *Online pharmacies.* Although convenient, some online pharmacies may sell products or engage in practices that are illegal in the offline world, putting consumers at risk for receiving adulterated, expired, ineffective, or counterfeit drugs. The FDA recommends that consumers avoid sites that prescribe drugs for the first time without a physical exam, sell prescription drugs without a prescription, or sell medications not approved by the FDA. You should also avoid sites that do not provide access to a registered pharma-

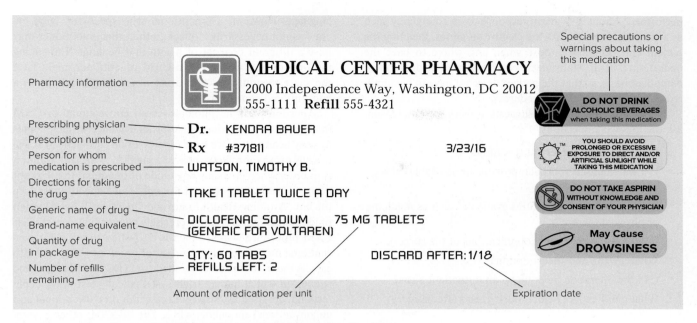

Pharmacy information

MEDICAL CENTER PHARMACY
2000 Independence Way, Washington, DC 20012
555-1111 **Refill** 555-4321

Special precautions or warnings about taking this medication

Prescribing physician
Prescription number
Person for whom medication is prescribed
Directions for taking the drug
Generic name of drug
Brand-name equivalent
Quantity of drug in package
Number of refills remaining

Dr.   KENDRA BAUER
Rx   #371811   3/23/16
WATSON, TIMOTHY B.

TAKE 1 TABLET TWICE A DAY

DICLOFENAC SODIUM   75 MG TABLETS
(GENERIC FOR VOLTAREN)

QTY: 60 TABS   DISCARD AFTER: 1/18
REFILLS LEFT: 2

DO NOT DRINK ALCOHOLIC BEVERAGES when taking this medication

YOU SHOULD AVOID PROLONGED OR EXCESSIVE EXPOSURE TO DIRECT AND/OR ARTIFICIAL SUNLIGHT WHILE TAKING THIS MEDICATION

DO NOT TAKE ASPIRIN WITHOUT KNOWLEDGE AND CONSENT OF YOUR PHYSICIAN

May Cause DROWSINESS

Amount of medication per unit

Expiration date

FIGURE 21.4   Reading and understanding prescription medication labels.

cist to answer questions or that do not provide a U.S. address and phone number to contact if there's a problem. The National Association of Boards of Pharmacy sponsors a voluntary certification program for internet pharmacies. To be certified, a pharmacy must have a state license and allow regular inspections. Many experts recommend that consumers use online pharmacies only to obtain medicines prescribed by their usual health care providers.

• *Costs.* Spending on prescription drugs is rising faster than the rate of inflation and is now the fastest-growing portion of U.S. health care spending. Many Americans have no or limited insurance coverage for prescription drug costs. Consumers may be able to lower their drug costs by using generic versions of medications; by joining a drug discount program sponsored by a company, organization, or local pharmacy; or by investigating mail-order or internet pharmacies.

Importing lower-cost drugs from Canada may be problematic. Canada imports U.S. drugs, and Health Canada–which provides regulation similar to the U.S. FDA–helps ensure the quality of Canadian-produced drugs, so safety should theoretically not be a concern for medicines from Canada. However, companies in Canada may make drugs for export only, thus avoiding standard regulation, and online pharmacies may claim they are operating in Canada but may be located in another country with little or no regulation. U.S. regulators have found online sites advertising Canadian drugs but shipping fake or substandard versions of medications, and shipping costs can be high. The safety of medications purchased in-person in Canada is comparable to that of those purchased in the United States. However, a prescription from a Canadian physician may be required.

Patients share responsibility for their use of prescription drugs. Many people don't take their medications properly—skipping doses, taking incorrect doses, stopping too soon, or not taking the medication at all. An estimated 30–50% of the 4 billion prescriptions dispensed annually in the United States are not taken correctly and thus may not produce the desired results. Consumers can increase the safety and effectiveness of their treatment by carefully reading any prescription label (Figure 21.4) and fact sheets or brochures that come with the medication. Whenever you are given a prescription, ask the following questions:

• Are there nondrug alternatives?

• What is the name of the medication, and what is it supposed to do, within what period of time?

• Can I take a generic drug rather than a brand-name one?

• Is there written information about the medication?

If written information is provided, check it for the following:

• How and when do I take the medication, how much do I take, and for how long? What should I do if I miss a dose?

• What medications, foods, drinks, or activities should I avoid when taking this drug?

• What are the side effects, and what do I do if they occur?

Remember to store your medications in a cool, dry place, out of direct light. Never share your prescription medications with anyone else, and never use an old prescription for a new ailment.

SURGERY   Surgical procedures are performed more often in the United States than anywhere else in the world. Each year more than 70 million operations and related procedures are performed. About 20% are in response to an emergency such as a severe injury, and 80% are **elective surgeries,** meaning the patient can generally choose when and where to have the operation, if at all. Many elective surgeries can be done on an **outpatient** basis, so that the patient does not have to be admitted to a hospital for the procedure.

If a health care provider suggests surgery for any reason, ask the following questions:

- Why do I need surgery at this time?
- Is a wait-and-see approach possible or advisable? If so, what are the risks?
- Are any nonsurgical options available, such as medicine or physical therapy?
- What are the risks and complications of the surgery?
- What are the anesthesia options?
- Can the operation be done on an outpatient basis?
- What can I expect before, during, and after surgery?

INTEGRATIVE HEALTH

Increasingly, more conventional Western medical providers are receptive to integrative health, and they may approve or recommend safe and effective CAM in addition to conventional treatment. Whereas conventional Western medicine tends to focus on the body, on the physical causes of disease, and on ways to eradicate pathogens in order to restore health, CAM tends to focus on the mind, body, and spirit in seeking ways to prevent diseases and restore the whole person to balance so that he or she can regain health. This is referred to as **holistic health care**—considering the whole person as a mind–body–spirit entity when diagnosing, treating, or preventing any illness or disorder. The opposite of holistic is dualistic, which refers to treating the mind and body separately. Under dualism, it is believed that treating an individual's physical body is separate and different from treating an individual's mental state. Under holistic approaches, health is not achieved if the mental state is ignored, if the individual is spiritually isolated, or if the body has a disease; holistic health means that the needs of the body, mind, and spirit are balanced and in harmony.

Many alternative medical systems with long-standing traditions have concepts and theories that once differed dramatically from those of conventional Western medical thought. Some people consider CAM quackery and tell you that you can recognize a quack by the use of pseudoscientific

language. However, a practitioner who speaks of "vital energy" is not necessarily a quack; rather, this practitioner may have a different concept of health and healing. "Enhancing the flow of vital energy" to a CAM practitioner might have the same meaning as "improving a neurologic deficit" to a conventional neurologist.

Anecdotes and testimonials—about conventional or CAM treatments—are not adequate levels of evidence when it comes to your health. Nor are case reports alone sufficient to scientifically prove the effectiveness of a medical treatment. Caution is in order when choosing any mode of treatment that has not been scientifically evaluated for safety and effectiveness (see the box "Avoiding Health Fraud and Quackery"). Even though practitioners may not know precisely why or how a particular CAM procedure works—which is also often the case for conventional modalities—the standard of proof for safety and efficacy is the randomized controlled trial (RCT). RCT outcome studies, in which human trials systematically test how people respond, are used extensively in research on conventional and unconventional modalities alike. The NCCIH, other governmental agencies, national foundations, and universities are sponsoring numerous outcome studies on CAM interventions.

CAM practices can be classified into several broad categories: alternative medical systems, mind–body medicine, natural products, manipulative and body-based practices, and other CAM practices (Figure 21.5). Here is a general introduction to the five categories of CAM and a brief description of some of the more widely used therapies.

Alternative Medical Systems

The nonconventional systems best known in the United States include traditional Chinese medicine, also known as traditional Oriental medicine, and homeopathy. Traditional, or whole, medical systems have developed in many regions of the world, including in the Americas; the Middle East, India, Tibet, and Australia. These cultures formed complete systems of medical philosophy, theory, and practice. In many countries, these medical approaches continue to be used—frequently alongside Western medicine and often by physicians trained in Western medicine.

Alternative medical systems tend to have a number of concepts in common. For example, the concept of life force or energy exists in many cultures. In traditional Chinese medicine, the life force contained in all living organisms is called qi (sometimes spelled "chi"). Qi resembles the vis vitalis (Latin for "life force") of Greek, Roman, and European medical systems, and prana of ayurveda, a traditional medical system of India. Most traditional medical systems think of disease as a disturbance or imbalance not just of physical processes but also of forces or energies within the body, the mind, and the spirit. In traditional Chinese medicine, for example, the principle of balance is expressed as yin and yang, which are opposites that complement each other. Disease is often defined as a disturbance of qi reflecting an imbalance between yin and yang. Treatment aims at reestablishing equilibrium, balance, and harmony.

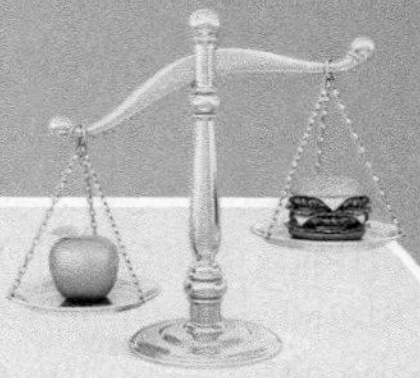

According to the Federal Trade Commission, consumers waste billions of dollars on unproven, fraudulently marketed, and sometimes useless health care products and treatments. In addition, individuals with serious medical problems may waste valuable time before seeking proper treatment. Worse yet, some of the products they're buying and using may cause serious harm. Health fraud often targets people with diseases that have no medical cure, and people who want shortcuts to improved health, weight loss, or enhanced personal appearance.

To help evaluate a product, you may talk to a physician or other licensed health professional who is impartial and knowledgeable about CAM modalities. Be wary of treatments offered by people who advise you to avoid seeking additional information or consulting others. Check with the Better Business Bureau or the local attorney general's office to see if other consumers have lodged complaints about a product or a product's marketer. You can also check with the appropriate health professional group such as the American Diabetes Association, American Cancer Society, or National Arthritis Foundation. Take special care with products and devices sold on television or online; the broad reach of the internet, combined with the ease of setting up and removing websites, makes online sellers particularly difficult to regulate.

If you think you have been a victim of health fraud or if you have an adverse reaction that you think is related to a particular supplement, you can report it to the appropriate agency:

- *False advertising claims.* Contact the FTC by phone (877-FTC-HELP), by mail (Consumer Response Center, Federal Trade Commission, Washington, DC 20580), or online (http://www.ftc.gov). You can also contact your state attorney general's office, your state department of health, or the local consumer protection agency (check a website or your local telephone directory).

- *False labeling on a product.* Contact the FDA district office consumer complaint coordinator for your geographic area. The FDA regulates safety, manufacturing, and product labeling.

- *Adverse reaction to a supplement.* If a health risk appears serious, call your physician immediately or go to an emergency clinic. You can also report your adverse reaction to FDA MedWatch by calling 800-FDA-1088 or by visiting the MedWatch website (http://www.fda.gov/Safety/MedWatch/).

- *Unlawful internet sales.* If you find a website that you think is misrepresenting or illegally selling drugs, medical devices, dietary supplements, or cosmetics, report it to the FDA. Problems can be reported to MedWatch or via the FDA website (http://www.fda.gov/ForConsumers/ProtectYourself).

Domain	Characteristics	Examples
Alternative medical systems 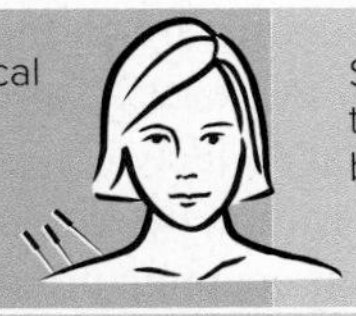	Systems of health/healing theory and practice that have evolved independently and long before conventional biomedical approaches.	Traditional Chinese medicine, ayurvedic medicine, homeopathy, naturopathy.
Mind–body medicine	Practices that use thoughts, beliefs, and other mental activities to affect the health and functioning of the physical body (including the brain).	Meditation, hypnosis, prayer, guided imagery, art therapy, music therapy, emotive writing. 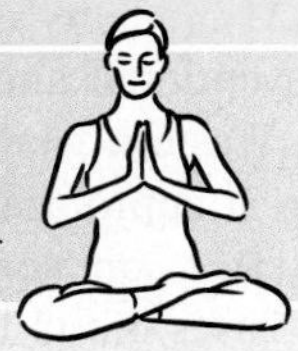
Natural biologic products	Plant (herbals) and animal products used as medicinals and dietary supplements. 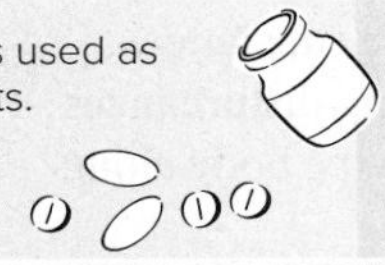	Ginko biloba, shark cartilage, probiotics (live bacteria that may have beneficial health effects when ingested).
Manipulative and body-based practices	Methods for adjusting, moving, or touching the body to promote health and healing.	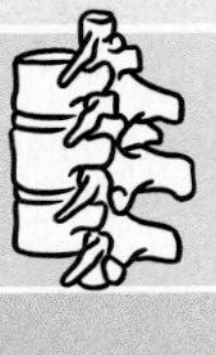 Chiropractic, osteopathic manual therapy, massage.
Other CAM practices 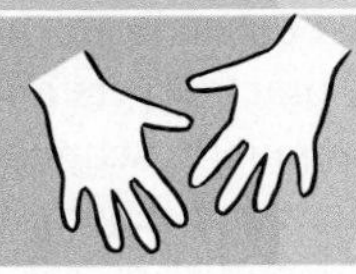	Therapeutic methods involving energy modalities.	Magnet therapy, light therapy, Reiki, qigong, therapeutic touch.

FIGURE 21.5 **The categories of CAM.**

Because the whole patient, rather than an isolated body part or disease, is treated in most comprehensive alternative medical systems, it is rare that only a single treatment approach is used. Most commonly, multiple remedies and techniques are employed together and are adjusted according to the changes in the patient's health status.

Traditional Chinese Medicine

Traditional Chinese medicine (TCM) is based on complex, abstract concepts; a sophisticated set of techniques and methods; and individualized diagnosis, treatment, and prevention. Typically, no two diseases are alike in the TCM perspective. Two patients with the same diagnosis in Western medicine may be diagnosed differently in TCM and given different treatments.

In TCM the free and harmonious flow of qi defines health of the body, mind, and spirit. Illness occurs when qi is deficient or the flow of qi is blocked or disturbed. TCM is believed to restore the flow of blocked qi, treating illness by balancing energy, preventing disease, and supporting immunity.

Two major TCM treatment methods include **herbal remedies** and **acupuncture.** Chinese herbal remedies number about 5800 (compared with about 6800 prescription and many other OTC medications). In addition to herbs, plant products, fungi (mushrooms), animal parts, and minerals may be used. These remedies, like everything else, have yin and yang properties or qi. When a disease is perceived to be due to a yin deficiency, remedies with more yin characteristics might be used for treatment. The use of a single medicinal substance is rare in Chinese herbal medicine; rather, several substances are combined in precise proportions, often to make a tea or soup. For example, a remedy might include a primary herb that targets the main symptom, a second herb that enhances the effects of the primary herb, a third that lessens side effects, and a fourth that helps deliver ingredients to a particular body site.

An accumulating body of scientific evidence supports the medical use of acupuncture, expanding the acceptance of this CAM modality in the West and placing it on the border of conventional and nonconventional health care practice. In the Western view, acupuncture needles inserted through the skin at appropriate sites by highly trained professionals have an effect on nerves, muscles, and connective tissues that increases blood flow and stimulates the body's natural production of painkillers, hormones, and immune substances.

In TCM, acupuncture is viewed as correcting disturbances in the flow of qi. Qi is believed to flow through the body along

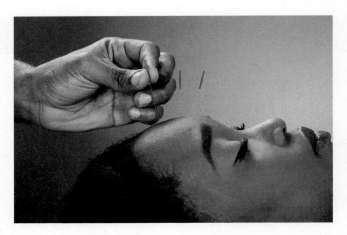

Acupuncture involves the insertion of needles at appropriate points in the skin to treat a variety of illnesses. andreypopov/123RF

several meridians, or pathways, and there are hundreds of acupuncture points located along these meridians. Acupuncturists use a variety of diagnostic techniques to identify the nature of the imbalance in a patient and to choose the points where acupuncture needles are placed. Acupuncturists trained in either TCM or conventional Western health care disciplines insert approximately 4–16 needles at these points and leave them in for 15 minutes or longer. Other means of stimulating acupuncture points include heat, pressure, friction, suction, or electrical stimulation. The points chosen for acupuncture are highly individualized for each patient, and they change during treatment as the patient's health status changes. For acupuncture to be effective, its practitioners require special training. In the United States, some physicians, physician assistants, nurse practitioners, physical therapists, dentists, and other licensed health professionals add acupuncture to their practice. Most states require licensure and evidence of proper acupuncture training, but requirements vary widely.

The World Health Organization has compiled a list of more than 40 conditions for which acupuncture may be beneficial. At a conference called by the National Institutes of Health (NIH), a panel of experts analyzed the available information on the scientific evidence for the efficacy of acupuncture for the treatment of many of these conditions. These experts cited evidence that acupuncture was effective in relieving nausea and vomiting after chemotherapy and pain after surgery, including dental surgery. Newer studies show that acupuncture may help relieve the painful symptoms of fibromyalgia and reduce the joint pain and stiffness of osteoarthritis. There is insufficient evidence showing that acupuncture is effective for menstrual cramps, tennis elbow, carpal tunnel syndrome, asthma, and certain other conditions. Acupuncture is considered very safe, and over decades, few side effects have been reported. Although rare, problems can occur from the improper insertion of needles by untrained practitioners and from the use of unsterile needles. The FDA regulates acupuncture needles like other standard medical devices and requires that they be sterile. If you are considering acupuncture, ask your practitioner about the safety practices he or she follows.

> **TERMS**
>
> **traditional Chinese medicine (TCM)** The traditional medical system of China, which views illness as the result of a problem in the quality, quantity, balance, or flow of qi, the life force; therapies include acupuncture, herbal medicine, and massage.
>
> **herbal remedy** A medicine prepared from plants.
>
> **acupuncture** Insertion of thin needles through the skin at points along meridians—pathways through which qi is believed to flow.

Homeopathy As a CAM system of medical practice that has unconventional origins in Germany, **homeopathy** involves treating an individual with highly diluted substances intended to trigger the body's natural system of healing. The theory is that when given in very diluted, minute quantities, substances that produce symptoms of an illness in a healthy person will help bring about a cure in someone who is ill, and it will do this by stimulating the body's healing processes. A primary principle of homeopathy is "like cures like." Based on a patient's specific signs and symptoms, a homeopathic practitioner determines the most appropriate treatment; diluted remedies are typically administered in liquid form or applied to sweetened pellets. Although most homeopathic remedies are highly diluted, some products may be labeled as homeopathic but contain substantial amounts of active ingredients that can cause side effects or drug interactions.

Because treatments are highly individualized for each patient and difficult to explain using the conventional laws of chemistry, randomized controlled trials on homeopathy are difficult. Most clinical trials have concluded that at best there is only weak evidence of efficacy. Nevertheless, some states require homeopaths to be licensed and fulfill certain requirements before they are permitted to practice.

Naturopathy **Naturopathy** is based on the premise that the body has the ability to maintain and restore optimal health. Naturopathy should not be confused with homeopathy. Naturopathic doctors (NDs) use both CAM and conventional approaches holistically for prevention, diagnosis, and treatment and for helping their patients minimize risks and barriers to good health. They work in hospitals, clinics, and community health centers and are licensed to practice in 22 states, the District of Columbia, Puerto Rico, the U.S. Virgin Islands, and five Canadian provinces. The number of states granting licensure is expected to increase. The ND degree is granted after completing a four-year professional program in naturopathic medicine from an accredited naturopathic medical school. In addition, the Naturopathic Physicians Licensing Exam (NPLEX) must be passed for state licensure. Content includes basic medical sciences, clinical nutrition, acupuncture, homeopathic medicine, herbology, psychology, and counseling. The scope of practice varies according to state and provincial regulations; in states currently without licensure, NDs often practice under the legal provisions of licensed physicians (MDs and DOs). The most frequently treated conditions include allergies, chronic pain, obesity, heart disease, fertility problems, and cancer. Naturopaths can perform minor surgery such as cyst removal and skin suturing. They are also trained to use prescription medications, although their education emphasizes natural modalities for healing.

Mind–Body Medicine

Mind–body interventions make use of the integral connection between mind and body and the effect each can have on the other. They include many of the stress management techniques discussed in Chapter 2, including meditation, yoga, visualization, tai chi, and biofeedback. Psychotherapy, support groups, prayer, and music and art therapy are mind–body interventions. The placebo effect is one of the most widely known examples of mind–body interdependence. Many studies have shown evidence that mind–body interventions such as imagery, support groups, friendships, strong family relationships, meditation, prayer, and hypnotherapy can all have a positive impact on health.

Clinical hypnosis is a focused state of awareness, perception, or consciousness that professionally trained practitioners use to treat a variety of physical and psychological conditions. **Hypnotherapy** is considered to be a CAM modality, although its use for certain conditions was accepted more than 40 years ago by the American Medical Association. Relatively few individuals have experienced clinical hypnotherapy or are knowledgeable about it, but many have been exposed to "stage hypnosis" and may believe that it has no legitimate clinical utility and no valid, evidence-based support. However, numerous evidence-based outcome studies have demonstrated its clinical usefulness, and brain-imaging technologies are helping to explain possible neurologic mechanisms.

Hypnotherapy involves the induction of a state of deep relaxation during which the patient is more likely to accept suggestions that can influence health and overcome conditions such as chronic pain, pain during surgery or childbirth, unhealthy habits, and anxiety and phobias. A number of NIH-sponsored reports found strong evidence for the effectiveness of hypnosis in reducing chronic pain stemming from a variety of medical conditions.

Health professionals who are properly trained in hypnotherapy use this modality to augment their conventional treatments. Training and certification are offered by several hypnotherapy associations or agencies. Many states require hypnotherapists to be licensed, but the requirements for licensing vary substantially. There is little regulation of practitioners of other relaxation techniques, but such techniques rarely produce adverse events.

TERMS

homeopathy An alternative system of practice that uses a holistic approach to diagnosis and treatment; involves administering minute doses of remedies that would, in larger quantities, produce symptoms similar to those of the illness.

naturopathy An alternative medical system based on supporting the body's ability to heal itself and maintain optimal health by removing barriers and creating an internal and external environment that promotes health and healing.

hypnotherapy A mind–body technique that uses relaxation and imagery to help a patient imagine specific health outcomes and establish a belief that they can be achieved; commonly used for managing pain, phobias, and addictions.

Natural Products

Natural products, also known as *biologically based therapies*, include substances derived from plant or animal sources. They consist primarily of herbal therapies or remedies, botanicals, and extracts from animal tissues (such as shark cartilage). A majority of the world's population relies on herbal remedies and other components of traditional, or indigenous, forms of medicine. Some countries and cultures make concerted efforts to document their use of traditional medicine, especially because the knowledge and skills that native peoples have gathered for centuries are dwindling, and organisms used in traditional medicine are going extinct.

Well-designed clinical studies have been conducted on a number of natural products. A few commonly used herbals, their uses, and the evidence supporting their efficacy are presented in Table 21.2. Clinical trials with herbals such as

> **TERMS**
>
> **natural products** CAM therapies that include biologically based interventions and products; examples include herbal remedies, extracts from animal tissues, and dietary supplements.

Table 21.2	Commonly Used Herbals, Their Uses, Evidence for Their Effectiveness, and Contraindications		
BOTANICAL	**USE**	**EVIDENCE**	**EXAMPLES OF ADVERSE EFFECTS AND INTERACTIONS**
Cranberry (*Vaccinium macrocarpon*)	Prevention or treatment of urinary tract infections	Some evidence of a modest preventive effect in some women	None known
Dandelion (*Taraxacum officinale*)	As a "tonic" against liver or kidney ailments	No conclusive evidence	May cause diarrhea in some users; people with gallbladder or bile duct problems should not take dandelion
Echinacea (*Echinacea purpurea, E. angustifolia, E. pallida*)	Stimulation of immune functions; to prevent colds and flulike diseases; to lessen symptoms of colds and flu	Some trials showed that it prevents colds and flu and helps patients recover faster from colds	Might cause liver damage if taken over long periods of time (more than 8 weeks); because it is an immune stimulant, it is not advisable to take it with immune suppressants (e.g., corticosteroids) or during chemotherapy
Evening primrose oil (*Oenothera biennis L.*)	Reduction of inflammation	Long-term supplementation effective in reducing symptoms of rheumatoid arthritis	None known
Feverfew (*Tanacetum parthenium*)	Prevention of headaches and migraines	Most trials indicate that it is more effective than placebo	Should not be used by people allergic to other members of the aster family; has the potential to increase the effects of warfarin and other anticoagulants
Garlic (*Allium sativum*)	Reduction of cholesterol	Short-term studies have found a modest effect	May interact with some medications, including anticoagulants, cyclosporine, and oral contraceptives
Ginkgo (*Ginkgo biloba*)	Improvement of circulation and memory	Improves cerebral insufficiency and slows progression of senile dementia in some patients; improves blood flow	Could increase bleeding time; should not be taken with nonsteroidal anti-inflammatory drugs (NSAIDs) like aspirin or with anticoagulants; may cause gastrointestinal disturbance
Ginseng (*Panax ginseng*)	Improvement of physical performance, memory, immune function, and glycemic control in diabetes; treatment of herpes simplex 2	No conclusive evidence exists for any of these uses	Interacts with warfarin and alcohol in mice and rats, so should probably not be used with these drugs; may cause liver damage
St. John's wort (*Hypericum perforatum*)	Treatment of depression	There is evidence that it is significantly more effective than placebo, is as effective as some standard antidepressants for mild to moderate depression, and causes fewer adverse effects	Known to interact with a variety of pharmaceuticals and should not be taken together with digoxin, theophylline, cyclosporine, indinavir, and serotonin reuptake inhibitors
Saw palmetto (*Serenoa repens*)	Improvement of benign prostatic hypertrophy	Studies show that saw palmetto may reduce mild prostate enlargement	Has no known interactions with drugs, but should probably not be taken with hormonal therapies
Valerian (*Valeriana officinalis*)	Treatment of insomnia	May help with some sleep disorders	Interacts with thiopental and pentobarbital and should not be used with these drugs

St. John's wort, ginkgo biloba, and echinacea have shown only a few minor side effects. New studies are also evaluating the efficacy of varying dosages and their interactions with conventional drugs.

Although most drug–herb interactions are relatively minor compared to conventional drug–drug interactions, some can be potentially serious. Because of reports of bleeding, a popular herb, ginkgo biloba, although generally well tolerated, should be used cautiously in people suffering from clotting disorders or taking blood thinners, or prior to surgical or dental procedures involving any bleeding. St. John's wort interacts with drugs used to treat HIV infection and heart disease, and the herb may also reduce the effectiveness of oral contraceptives, antirejection drugs used in patients receiving organ transplants, and some medications used to treat infections, depression, asthma, and seizure disorders. Supplements containing kava kava have been linked to liver damage, and anyone who has liver problems, drinks large amounts of alcohol, or takes medications that can affect the liver is advised to consult a physician or pharmacist before using kava kava–containing supplements.

Another potential problem is the possibility of contaminants. In a sample of ayurvedic herbal medicine products, 20% were found to contain potentially harmful levels of lead, mercury, or arsenic. The content and potency of herbal preparations is also variable. Herb producers do not have complete control over natural products any more than farmers have control over the vitamin content of fruit.

As an attempt toward standardization, many herb producers identify the analysis results of selected active ingredients. Some responsible retailers check the safety and purity standards of the herbal preparations they sell. Informed consumers should always examine containers for analysis results, lot numbers, and a website, and they should purchase products only from reputable sources and avoid those that are questionable or discounted.

In the United States, because natural products are considered supplements rather than drugs, they are currently not required to meet FDA food and drug standards for safety or effectiveness, nor are they required to meet any manufacturing standards. Still, the Dietary Supplement Health and Education Act of 1994 requires that dietary supplement labels list the name and quantity of each ingredient. The manufacturer is responsible for ensuring that a supplement is safe before it is marketed; the FDA has the power to restrict a substance if it is found to pose a health risk after it is on the market.

Studies have shown that most people do not reveal their use of CAM therapies to their conventional health care providers, a problem that can have significant health consequences. Any herbs that are used in combination with conventional drugs should be evaluated for safety by a knowledgeable health care provider such as a pharmacist.

Manipulative and Body-Based Practices

These modalities are based on manipulating or moving one or more body parts. Touch and body manipulation are long-standing forms of health care. Manual healing techniques include the concept that misalignment or dysfunction in one part of the body can cause pain or dysfunction in that or another part. Correcting these misalignments can help restore optimal health.

Chiropractic Many manipulative and body-based practices are integral components of physical therapy and osteopathic medicine, although certain techniques fit the definition of CAM because they are not a part of conventional health care practice. Unconventional healing methods include massage, acupressure, and numerous other techniques. The most commonly used CAM manual healing method is **chiropractic,** a method that focuses on the relationship between structure and function, primarily of the spine, joints, muscles, and the nervous system, to maintain or restore health. An important therapeutic procedure is the manipulation of joints, particularly those of the spinal column. However, chiropractors also use a variety of other techniques, including exercise, patient education and lifestyle modification, nutritional supplements, and orthotics (mechanical supports and braces). They do not use conventional drugs or surgery, although many chiropractors may recommend conventional drugs or surgery in addition to chiropractic care.

Chiropractors, or doctors of chiropractic, are trained for a minimum of four years at accredited chiropractic colleges and can go on to postgraduate training in many countries. Although specifically listed by NCCIH as one of the manipulative and body-based practices of CAM, chiropractic is accepted by many health care and health insurance providers to a far greater extent than are many other types of CAM therapies. Based on research showing the efficacy of chiropractic management in acute lower-back pain, spinal manipulation has been included in the federal guidelines for the treatment of this condition, and electrodiagnostic tests show that chiropractic is effective in controlling back pain. Promising results have also been reported with the use of chiropractic techniques in neck pain and headaches.

A word of caution: Spinal manipulation must be performed only by a properly trained professional such as a chiropractor, osteopathic physician, or physical therapist who is specially trained and certified in orthopedic manual physical therapy (OMPT). Your state's medical and osteopathic board

chiropractic A CAM manipulative, body-based **TERMS** practice that focuses on disorders of the spine, and musculoskeletal and nervous systems, and the effects of these disorders on general health; the primary treatment is manipulation of the spine and other joints.

or a local health service locator will help you find qualified practitioners near you.

Exercise Exercise for health maintenance, promotion, and disease prevention currently fits the definition of a CAM modality. However, this is changing due to an active campaign, Exercise Is Medicine (EIM), co-launched in 2007 by the American College of Sports Medicine and the American Medical Association. A study has found that 65% of Americans would be more interested in exercising to stay healthy if advised to do so by their physicians.

The EIM initiative encourages physicians to record a patient's exercise level as a routine vital sign during clinical visits, along with pulse, respiratory rate, temperature, and blood pressure. Those who are able will be advised to exercise for at least 30 minutes and to stretch and engage in light muscle training for an additional 10 minutes five days each week. The EIM website (www.exerciseismedicine.org) advises physicians, other health care providers, medical educators, and the public about the benefits of exercise. Through efforts such as this, exercise is likely to transition from a CAM modality to a conventional modality and to be taught in more U.S. medical schools and to be recommended and used as a treatment in U.S. health care institutions.

Other CAM Practices

CAM practices also include traditional healing practices and energy therapies. Traditional healers may rely on touch as well as other senses, for example, sound—the clanging of a bell or the quality of a singing voice. These healers may incorporate counseling or psychological therapy in addition to prescribing herbal remedies.

Energy therapies are forms of treatment that use energy interactions between living organisms, energies produced by the organism itself, and those produced by outside sources such as electromagnetic energy. The recognition that the body produces electromagnetic fields has led to the development of many diagnostic procedures in Western medicine, including electroencephalography (EEG), electromyography (EMG), electrocardiography (ECG), and nuclear magnetic resonance imaging (NMRI). Energy therapies are

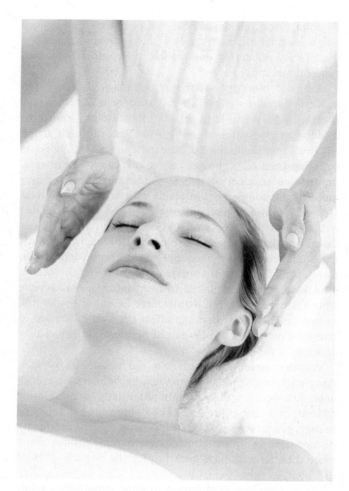

One of several energy therapies, Reiki has both energy and manual contact components. Wavebreakmedia/Getty Images

based on the concept that energy surrounds and penetrates the body and can be influenced by movement, touch, pressure, or the placement of hands in or through the fields. Some evidence supports energy theory because the body's electromagnetic energy can be measured through ECG, EMG, and EEG technologies.

Reiki is an example of energy therapy; it is intended to correct disturbances in the flow of life energy (ki in the Japanese tradition) and enhance the body's healing powers through the use of specific hand positions on or near the patient's body. **Therapeutic touch** is derived from ancient techniques involving using the hands to detect and transmit energy (electromagnetic energy). It is based on the premise that healers can identify and correct energy imbalances by passing their hands over the patient's body.

Magnetic therapies include the application of therapeutic magnets to the body to manage pain, increase blood flow, and treat conditions such as arthritic pain. One animal study reported an increased rate of wound healing using magnets, but comprehensive literature reviews of studies on therapeutic magnets report little or no supporting evidence.

---

energy therapies   Forms of CAM treatment that use varying sources of energy originating either within the body or from outside sources to promote health and healing. **TERMS**

Reiki   A CAM practice intended to correct disturbances in the flow of life energy and enhance the body's healing powers through the use of various hand positions on the patient.

therapeutic touch   A CAM practice based on the premise that healers can identify and correct energy imbalances by passing their hands over the patient's body.

magnetic therapies   A form of alternative medicine that uses magnets to treat pain and other health problems.

When Does CAM Become Conventional Medicine?

From a Western point of view, when ancient healers used the foxglove plant for medicinal purposes, it could be considered "alternative"—or even superstition. But when the plant's content, digitalis, was scientifically shown to be a useful pharmaceutical, it became a conventional medication for the treatment of heart disease. Because of modern research sponsored mostly by the NIH, we are seeing a number of therapeutic alternatives become mainstream medicine.

People of all backgrounds use CAM; use is greater among women than men and among those with higher levels of education and higher incomes. More than 42% of hospitals offer one or more CAM therapies, and 57 major U.S. universities have added integrative medical centers to their facilities. In addition, because of the widespread use of CAM among patients, U.S. medical schools include integrative medicine in their curricula, and the American Board of Physician Specialties recognizes integrative medicine as a distinct medical discipline.

In 2016, Americans spent 9% of all out-of-pocket expenditures on complementary health approaches. In 2017, yoga was the most practiced CAM in the United States—14% of adults, according to an NCCIH survey. Meditation also soared in popularity, tripling from 4% to 14% over five years. Other increasingly common CAM therapies in the United States include the following examples.

Tai Chi and Fibromyalgia

A once mysterious and misunderstood disorder, fibromyalgia causes chronic pain throughout the body and general fatigue. It can be partially treated with drugs, but exercise is an important component of fibromyalgia therapy because it helps maintain or improve muscle strength and function.

Tai chi, a CAM practice with origins in ancient China, uses slow, meditative movements for maintaining and restoring health. Tai chi has long been known to offer many benefits, including gains in strength and flexibility, and it has also been shown to be helpful in pain management. A study published in the *New England Journal of Medicine* tracked the symptoms of two groups of fibromyalgia patients: one that learned a variety of tai chi movements and another that practiced stretching exercises and received wellness counseling. Over the course of the study, the patients who practiced tai chi reported significantly less pain than the other group, and the benefits lasted well beyond the study's end.

In another study, researchers undertook a comprehensive review of existing studies involving tai chi and **qigong** (a related CAM energy practice) to determine whether evidence consistently supported claims that the two practices yield health benefits. In more than 60 studies involving nearly 6500 participants, those who engaged in tai chi or qigong demonstrated improved blood pressure, bone density, balance, immune function, and overall quality of life. The researchers concluded that tai chi and qigong may be

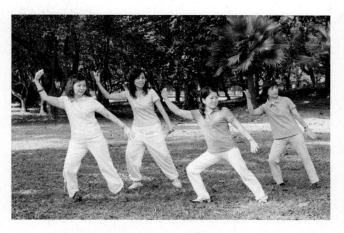

Tai chi combines gentle movements with mental focus, breathing, and relaxation. It has been shown to improve balance and stability and to help people with chronic conditions cope with pain. Phil Date/123RF

excellent alternatives to conventional forms of exercise for some people.

CAM Therapies and Back Pain

CAM therapies are used more often for back pain than for any other condition. Over 80% of adults suffer from low-back pain at some point in their lives. A wide survey found that people tended to try chiropractic, massage, and acupuncture therapies for more severe cases and yoga, tai chi, and qigong for milder cases. Respondents said they elected to try CAM because conventional medical treatments weren't providing adequate pain relief. Nearly two-thirds said they experienced significantly reduced pain as a result of CAM therapy.

Chiropractic and Headaches

A new study shows that a specific type of chiropractic technique—called spinal manipulative therapy (SMT)—can be particularly helpful for people who suffer from chronic headaches, especially headaches related to neck problems. The study compared the effects of SMT to those of light massage between two groups of patients who suffered frequent, severe headaches. The group who underwent SMT from an experienced chiropractor reported less pain and fewer headaches than the group who had light massages. Significantly, the SMT group reported half as many headaches as the massage group during a 24-week period of follow-up.

> **TERMS**
>
> **tai chi** An ancient Chinese philosophy adapted as a CAM energy modality and practiced as exercise involving slow, continuous, meditative movements accompanied by deep breathing, and used for maintaining and restoring health.
>
> **qigong** A CAM energy modality from ancient China that is related to tai chi. Qigong exercises integrate physical postures, breathing techniques, and focused intention for health maintenance, healing, and increased vitality.

Evaluating Complementary and Alternative Therapies

Compared to conventional medical therapies, CAM has less scientific information available about it and less regulation of associated products and providers. CAM therapies are more difficult to investigate than conventional therapies for several reasons. One problem is that of effect size—the statistical difference in outcome between the treatment being tested and the control. Most CAM therapies have a smaller effect size than conventional treatments, making experimental outcomes difficult to detect. Meta-analysis can sometimes be used to overcome the problem of small effect size by combining the results of multiple small trials.

Other difficulties include delayed effects (CAM therapies require longer studies and therefore more funding), variable effects (not all CAM therapies work equally well on everybody), and combination effects (several approaches used together may produce results not seen in a single approach—violating the traditional scientific tenet of parsimony). Traditional Chinese medicine is by design not parsimonious. Health-promoting modalities—such as lifestyle change, exercise, and dieting to control heart disease, cancer, and obesity—face similar obstacles in research. The bottom line is that it is important to take an active role when you are seeking medical information and advice in any modality, conventional or unconventional.

Working with Your Physician   When a health issue might be serious, the NCCIH advises consumers not to seek complementary therapies without first consulting a conventional health care provider. Become informed and discuss conventional treatments that have been shown to be beneficial for your condition. If you are thinking of trying any complementary or alternative therapies, discuss these with your physician, pharmacist, or other conventional provider who is knowledgeable about your health status and is also informed about CAM or is willing to learn by consulting proper resources. If they are not informed about CAM, it may be helpful to share information from reliable, evidence-based sources with them. Areas to discuss with your physician or pharmacist include the following:

* **Safety.** Whether or not the treatment is effective, it must be safe. Is something about the treatment unsafe for you specifically? Should you be aware of safety issues, such as drug–herb interactions?

* **Effectiveness.** Is there evidence-based research about the use of the therapy for your condition? If definitive evidence about effectiveness is lacking, but the treatment is safe and causes no interaction with your conventional treatment, make an informed decision in consultation with your physician.

* **Timing.** Is the immediate use of a conventional treatment indicated?

* **Cost.** Is the therapy likely to be expensive, especially in light of the potential benefit?

If appropriate, schedule a follow-up visit with your physician to assess your condition and your progress after a certain amount of time using a complementary therapy. Keep a symptom diary to track your symptoms and gauge your progress. Symptoms such as pain and fatigue are difficult to recall with accuracy, so an ongoing symptom diary is an important tool. If your physician advises against CAM and can support the advice with good evidence, you should probably not use it. If your physician is simply unreceptive or uninformed about CAM, you may need to find another physician whose health beliefs are compatible with your own (see the box "Exploring What You Know about CAM"). If you plan to pursue a therapy against your physician's advice, tell him or her.

For supplements, particularly botanicals, pharmacists can also be an excellent source of information; inform them about any other unconventional or conventional medications you are taking.

Questioning the CAM Practitioner   You can also get information from individual practitioners, educational programs, professional organizations, and state licensing boards. Ask about education, training, licensing, and certification. If appropriate, check with local or state regulatory agencies or the consumer affairs department to determine if any complaints have been lodged against the practitioner. Some guidelines for talking with a CAM practitioner include the following:

* Ask the practitioner why he or she thinks the therapy will be beneficial for your condition. Ask for a full description of the therapy and any potential side effects. In all cases, demand an evidence-based approach.

* Describe in detail any conventional treatments you are receiving or plan to receive.

* Ask how long the therapy should continue before it can be determined if it is beneficial.

* Ask about the expected cost of the treatment. Does it seem reasonable? Will your health insurance pay some or all of the costs?

If anything an unconventional practitioner says or recommends directly conflicts with advice from your physician, discuss it with your physician before making any major changes in your current treatment regimen or lifestyle. You may wish to consult authoritative websites such as NCCIH.nih.gov or WebMD.com for new information that you can print out and discuss with your physician.

Ask Yourself

QUESTIONS FOR CRITICAL THINKING AND REFLECTION
Have you ever considered using a complementary or alternative treatment? If so, was it in addition to conventional treatment or instead of it? What kind of research did you do before having the treatment? What advice did your conventional health care provider give you about it?

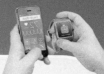

Before talking to your physician about using a CAM modality, explore your own attitudes and knowledge base by responding "true" or "false" to the following statements:

T   F   1. You are the exception; most patients rarely use CAM.

T   F   2. Most physicians are familiar with CAM through their extensive medical training.

T   F   3. Before trying any CAM modality for an illness, it's better to try a conventional remedy.

T   F   4. CAM modalities are based on folk remedies, so there is no scientific information available about their effectiveness.

T   F   5. CAM modalities are safe and natural, so they can only help or do nothing at all.

T   F   6. Because herbal preparations are derived from plants and are not regulated by the FDA, there are no purity assurances.

T   F   7. Acupuncture has few risks.

T   F   8. If you have a CAM modality in mind, find a scientifically based article about it and share it with your physician.

T   F   9. If you experience any improvement after using CAM, it is probably a placebo effect.

T   F   10. Routine medical assessments such as physical exams and lab tests cannot be used to show how your body is responding to CAM interventions.

T   F   11. After discussing your ideas about using CAM with your physician, you should choose between using either CAM or a conventional modality.

T   F   12. CAM is not covered by most health insurance policies.

Answers

1. False. Scientific studies show that more than one-third of Americans use CAM.

2. False. Most physicians have been introduced to CAM only through a single lecture or course. CAM is not yet a significant part of most medical school curricula, although its coverage is increasing.

3. False. It is generally advantageous to choose the treatment that is most likely to work, has the fewest side effects, and has the highest benefit-to-risk ratio. The treatment(s) of choice may be conventional or unconventional.

4. False. Numerous studies on CAM have been conducted and more are under way, sponsored mostly by the NCCIH.

5. False. Not all CAM modalities are completely safe, and many have synergistic or opposing effects when used together with conventional treatments.

6. False. Even though these products are plant derived and not regulated in the United States as they are in some other countries, industry self-regulation can be effective.

7. True. When administered by trained professional acupuncturists, any risk is exceedingly rare.

8. True. Evidence-based studies published in peer-reviewed scientific journals are likely to be helpful for many physicians. Articles and CAM guidelines are also published online by governmental agencies, universities, and reputable hospitals and clinics.

9. False. Through randomized controlled trials, many CAM modalities have been shown to be efficacious compared to placebo or sham modalities. All treatments, conventional and unconventional, have a placebo effect component.

10. False. Many of the assessments that are used to evaluate conventional interventions are also used to evaluate CAM.

11. False. The best modalities should be chosen from among conventional and unconventional ones available; choices should be based on safety, efficacy, risk-to-benefit ratio, and cost. Conventional and CAM modalities can be used in combination.

12. True. Most CAM is not covered. However, some modalities that are part of physical therapy, such as chiropractic and massage, may be covered.

If you answered 10 or more questions correctly, you are probably ready to have an informed discussion about CAM use with your physician or to find a physician who is at least receptive to your inquiry.

PAYING FOR HEALTH CARE

The U.S. health care system is one of the most advanced and comprehensive in the world, but it is also the most expensive (Figure 21.6). In 2018, Americans spent $3.5 trillion on health care, or more than $11,000 per person. Many factors contribute to the high cost of health care in the United States, including the cost of advanced equipment and new technology, expensive treatments for some illnesses, aging of the population, and the demand for profits by many commercial health enterprises. When we look at what rich countries spend on health per person and life expectancy in those countries, Americans spend far more money and live shorter lives (see Figure 21.7).

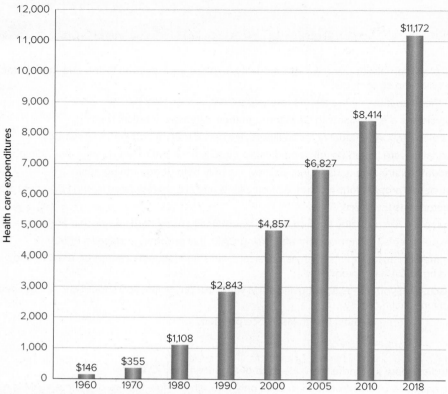

FIGURE 21.6 **Per-capita national health care expenditures, 1960–2018.**

SOURCE: Centers for Medicare & Medicaid Services. 2019. *National Health Expenditure Data: Historical* (https://www.cms.gov/Research-Statistics-Data-and-Systems/Statistics-Trends-and-Reports/NationalHealthExpendData/NationalHealthAccountsHistorical).

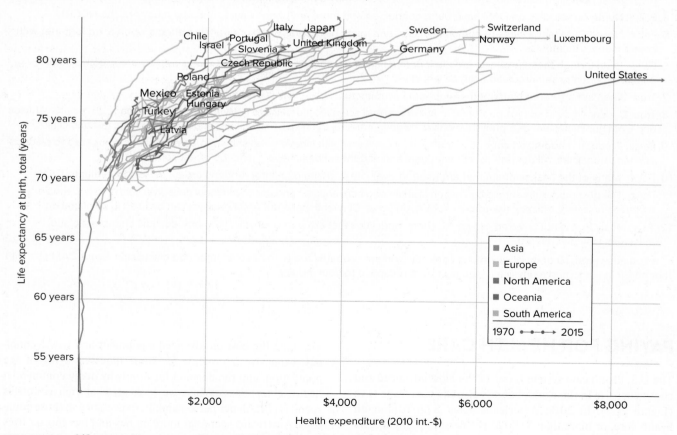

FIGURE 21.7 **Life expectancy versus health expenditure, 1970–2015.**

SOURCE: World Bank. 2019. WDI, Health Expenditure and Financing, OECDstat (https://ourworldindata.org).

The Affordable Care Act

Health care in the United States is financed by private and public insurance plans, patient out-of-pocket payments, and government assistance. The **Affordable Care Act (ACA)**, also called Obamacare, aimed to tackle expanding health care costs, regulate the way insurance companies provide medical coverage, and encourage as many Americans as possible to get health coverage.

Uninsured and underinsured people use primary health services less often than they need and less than insured people do. When they do use health services, they receive lower-quality care, often only after becoming seriously ill, and usually in hospital emergency departments. Children without insurance are less likely to receive screening tests and immunizations. They have fewer checkups, are less likely to receive treatment for injuries and chronic conditions such as asthma, and are more likely to go without eyeglasses and prescribed medications.

The ACA encourages healthy people to purchase insurance because more people paying into plans helps insurance companies keep **premiums** lower. An individual mandate had required that everyone buy a minimal insurance plan or pay a tax penalty. Opponents of this penalty argued that the government was overstepping its reach, and Congress repealed the individual mandate in 2017.

Two key provisions of the ACA are that it increases preventive services and it forbids insurance companies from discriminating on the basis of preexisting medical conditions. Preventive services include doctors' services, inpatient and outpatient hospital care, prescription drug coverage, pregnancy and childbirth, and mental health services.

Before the ACA, a preexisting condition such as depression or diabetes—even pregnancy—could be the basis for insurance companies' rejecting a new patient. By some estimates, as many as 50 million Americans—the vast majority of them employed—had no health insurance. Private insurance and individual patients paid about 55% of the total spent on health care; the government paid the rest, mainly through Medicare and Medicaid. Most nonelderly Americans receive health insurance through their employers, but as medical costs increase, the number of Americans with private insurance has decreased by approximately 10% over the past two decades.

Since the ACA came into effect, insurance companies have needed to publicly justify rate hikes. Historic gains in the number of insured Americans have been made, especially among young adults, blacks and Latinos, and people making less than $36,000 a year. The government has given payments to health insurers known as cost-sharing reductions, which compensate them for reducing costs for their lowest-income patients. In 2017, the Trump administration announced it would no longer fund the ACA's cost-sharing reduction payments, which would increase the price of health insurance for the country's poorest citizens. In that year, 3.2 million people lost their insurance. Because insurance companies must still offer these discounted rates for low-income customers, insurers have been making up the difference by raising premiums for other customers. Uninsured rates grew again in 2018—largely among blacks, Hispanics, poorer people, and young adults.

How Health Insurance Works

Health insurance as required under the ACA protects you against costs incurred for medical expenses due to illness or injury. Depending on the policy, coverage may also include preventive services such as yearly exams; other physician services; medications; hospital stays; emergency department visits; physical, occupational, and speech therapy; vision care; dental coverage; and other expenses. Some insurance policies provide riders for specific CAM coverage for an additional charge. Policies differ based on the services covered, the amount of the **deductible** and **copayment,** and the limit of coverage. Of course, with many plans, the more services you add to the policy, the higher the premium. Coverage may be provided as an employment benefit or through a government-sponsored plan such as Medicaid (for certain disabled and low-income individuals) or Medicare (typically for individuals aged 65 and over and those with certain illnesses). See the box "Choosing a Health Insurance Plan."

Health insurance enables people to receive health care they might not otherwise be able to afford. Hospital care costs hundreds of dollars a day, and surgical fees can cost thousands. A serious illness or accident can cost over $1 million. Health insurance is important for everyone.

Health insurance plans are either fee-for-service (indemnity) or managed care. With both types, the individual or his or her employer pays a basic premium, usually on a monthly basis; there are often other payments as well. Insurance policies are sold to both groups and individuals; group plans tend to cover more services and cost less. Group coverage is often available through employers to workers and their families. People who are self-employed or whose employers don't offer

---

Affordable Care Act   A U.S. law requiring most **TERMS** health insurance plans to include certain rights and protections (e.g., mental health and preventive services, no penalties for preexisting conditions, and the right to appeal health service charges). The law attempts to make health care more affordable for individuals and families.

premium   The amount you pay each month for your insurance.

deductible   The amount you pay for services before your insurance coverage begins. For example, if your deductible is $1000, the insurance company won't pay anything for services until your expenses total $1000. The insurance company may fully cover certain services before you've reached your deductible amount.

copayment   The amount you pay for a particular health care service; your insurance provider pays the balance. For example, for a physical exam that costs $150, you might pay your doctor's office $25 at the time of service (your copayment), and the insurance company would pay $125. The copayment amount may vary according to the type of service you received.

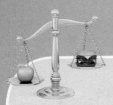

CRITICAL CONSUMER
Choosing a Health Insurance Plan

Under the Affordable Care Act (ACA), a health insurance marketplace, also called a health exchange, facilitates the purchase of health insurance. But choosing a plan can be a complicated matter—confusing and intimidating. To organize your thinking about this decision, look for answers to the three questions discussed here.

1. What Does the Plan Cover?

These are the 10 categories of health care services that health plans must cover to meet requirements of the ACA:

- Ambulatory patient services (care you get without being admitted to a hospital)
- Emergency services
- Hospitalization
- Maternity and newborn care
- Mental health and substance use disorder services including behavioral health treatment
- Prescription drugs
- Rehabilitative and habilitative services and devices (to help people with injuries, disabilities, or chronic conditions gain or recover mental and physical skills)
- Laboratory services
- Preventive services and chronic disease management
- Pediatric services, including oral and vision care

Insurance provided by large employers may differ slightly. You can ask for a summary of benefits and coverage to see what is covered.

2. How Much Does the Plan Cost?

You pay for health insurance in two ways—through (1) your monthly premium and (2) the out-of-pocket expenses you pay when you receive care. Out-of-pocket expenses include deductibles, coinsurance, and copayments (see text for definitions). The higher the monthly premium you pay, the lower will be your out-of-pocket expenses.

For the ACA, the "metal categories"—bronze, silver, gold, and platinum—were created to help people choose a plan by simplifying the differences between costs and levels of coverage. As you consider your choices, note what the total cost of care includes: your premium plus out-of-pocket costs.

Generally, your monthly insurance payment is lowest in the bronze category, but deductibles are higher and you may have more out-of-pocket costs. Platinum plans typically have the highest premiums, but deductibles and out-of-pocket costs are low. If your income qualifies you for cost-sharing reductions, you can enroll in a silver plan where you get the best of both worlds: a lower premium and a lower deductible. Out-of-pocket costs will be lower as well.

PLAN CATEGORY	THE INSURANCE COMPANY PAYS	YOU PAY
Bronze	60%	40%
Silver	70%	30%
Gold	80%	20%
Platinum	90%	10%

The "metal categories" help you determine how you and your insurance plan share total costs.

SOURCE: https://www.healthcare.gov/choose-a-plan/plans-categories/.

3. Which Doctors and Hospitals Are in Your Plan?

Every health insurance plan has a network of providers who agree to provide services to plan members for specific prices. As you've learned, plans vary in how restricted members are in relation to these networks. Some only allow members to receive services provided by doctors, specialists, or hospitals in the plan's network. Others are more flexible: They may charge less when plan members use doctors, hospitals, and other health care providers that belong to the plan's network; require members to get referrals to go outside the network; or allow members to use doctors, hospitals, and providers outside their network without a referral for an additional cost. It makes sense, then, to check the health plan and your doctor's office to make sure your desired providers are in the network of the plan you are considering.

You can get more information, browse plans, and apply for coverage at HealthCare.gov.

---

group policies may need to buy individual plans. As part of the ACA, states now provide interactive online exchanges that supply information about various insurance plans, which can be adapted to fit an individual's needs and income level. Most insurance is provided by and can be purchased from private companies using the online exchanges.

Traditional Fee-for-Service (Indemnity) Plans In a fee-for-service plan, or **indemnity plan,** you can go to any physician or hospital you choose. You or the provider sends the bill to your insurance company, which pays part of it. Usually you have to pay a deductible amount each year, and then the

> **indemnity plan** A health insurance plan based on a fee for each service provided; the cost is shared between you and the insurance company, and you can go to any physician or hospital you choose.
>
> TERMS

plan will pay a percentage—often 80%—of what it considers the "usual and customary" charge for covered services. You pay the remaining 20%, which is known as *coinsurance.*

Freedom of choice is a major benefit of indemnity plans. You can see any physician you choose, including specialists. Your physician is paid based on the services he or she provides. Critics point to the fee-for-service payment system as a contributing factor in the rapid growth of U.S. health care costs because physicians have a financial incentive to order more tests and treatments for their patients. However, the vast majority of working Americans are covered by managed care plans.

Managed Care Plans   **Managed care plans** have agreements with a network of specified physicians, hospitals, and health care providers to offer a range of services to plan members at reduced cost. In general, you have lower out-of-pocket costs and less paperwork with a managed care plan than with an indemnity plan, but you also have less freedom in choosing your health care providers. Most Americans with job-based insurance are covered by managed care plans. These include health management organizations (HMOs), preferred provider organizations (PPOs), and point of service (POS) plans:

  • **Health maintenance organizations (HMOs)** offer members a range of services for a set monthly fee. You choose a primary care physician who manages your care and refers you to specialists if you need them. If you go outside the HMO, you have to pay for the service yourself. Physicians participating in the HMO agree to accept a monthly per-patient fee, or **capitation,** or to charge less than standard fees for services. Out-of-network services generally aren't covered except for emergencies. You may be required to live or work within the HMO's service area to be eligible for coverage, and you will typically need to visit a PCP before going to a specialist. HMOs often focus on prevention and wellness.

  • **Preferred provider organizations (PPOs)** have arrangements with physicians and other providers who have agreed to accept lower fees. If you go outside the PPO, you have to pay more.

  • **Point-of-service (POS) plans** are options offered by many HMOs in which you can see a specialist or a physician outside the plan, but you will have to pay most or all of the cost unless your primary care physician referred you.

Many managed care plans try to reduce costs over the long term by paying for routine preventive care, such as regular checkups and screening tests and prenatal care; they may also encourage prevention by offering health education and lifestyle modification programs for members.

Other cost-cutting measures under managed care plans are less consumer oriented. Consumers' choice of physicians is limited, and they may have to wait longer for appointments and travel farther to see participating physicians or receive specialized tests. Managed care plans may also try to discourage overtreatment through the use of gatekeepers: In many plans, patients must get preapproval through their PCP or a plan representative for diagnostic tests, referrals to specialists, or

Ask Yourself   ?

QUESTIONS FOR CRITICAL THINKING AND REFLECTION
What type of health insurance coverage do you have? If you are covered by your parents' or guardians' insurance, what are the plan's benefits? If you have coverage, do you know what types of medical services are fully or partially covered? What are your copayments and deductibles? If you were faced with a medical emergency, would you know how to contact and work with your insurer to make sure your costs were covered?

hospital treatments. If a patient goes outside the rules for obtaining services, the plan typically will not cover the cost. Nonemergency visits to emergency departments are usually not covered.

Government Programs   Americans aged 65 and over and younger people with certain disabilities can be covered by **Medicare,** a federal health insurance program that helps pay for hospitalization, physician services, and prescription drugs. As a result of limits placed on payments, however, some physicians and managed care programs have stopped accepting Medicare patients. **Medicaid** is a joint federal–state health insurance program that covers some low-income people, especially children, pregnant women, and people with certain disabilities. The number of people and the number and cost of services covered by government programs has grown in recent years, challenging the ability of these programs to provide needed coverage.

TERMS

managed care plan   A health insurance plan that contracts with providers and health care facilities (the plan's "network") to provide care at reduced costs. There are three types of managed care plans: health management organizations (HMOs), preferred provider organizations (PPOs), and point of service (POS).

health maintenance organization (HMO)   A type of prepaid health insurance plan that covers services within a network of physicians and other professionals who are contracted with the HMO.

capitation   A payment made to a health care provider per person, rather than a payment per service provided.

preferred provider organization (PPO)   A prepaid health insurance plan that contracts with physicians, other professionals, and hospitals to provide services for discounted fees. You can go to any provider including specialists without a PCP referral. Using nonparticipating providers results in higher costs to the patient.

point-of-service (POS) plan   A type of plan where you pay less if you use physicians, other professionals, and hospitals that belong to the plan's network, but you are required to get a referral from a PCP before going to a specialist. A POS plan combines some of the essentials of both HMO and PPO plans.

Medicare   A federal health insurance program for people aged 65 and over and for younger people with certain disabilities.

Medicaid   A federally subsidized state-run plan of health care for people with low income.

Most of the time, you can take care of yourself without consulting a health care provider. When you need professional care, you can still take responsibility for yourself by making informed decisions.

RIGHT NOW YOU CAN:

- Make sure that you have enough of your prescription medications on hand and that your prescriptions are up-to-date.
- If you take any supplements (dietary or herbal), ask your pharmacist if they can interact with any prescription drugs you are taking.
- Stock your home and car with basic first aid supplies.

IN THE FUTURE YOU CAN:

- Use professional and authoritative internet resources to thoroughly research complementary or alternative medical treatments you are using or considering to make sure they are considered safe and effective.
- Review your medical insurance needs by checking your coverage under your parents' or guardians' policy if you are under age 26 or by checking your state's online health insurance exchange, and contact your insurance agent if you have questions about your coverage.

SUMMARY

- Informed self-care requires knowing how to evaluate symptoms. You should see a physician if symptoms are severe, unusual, persistent, or recurrent.

- Self-treatment doesn't necessarily require medication, but over-the-counter (OTC) drugs can be a helpful part of self-care.

- Conventional medicine is characterized by a focus on the physical causes of disease, the identification of signs and symptoms, the use of drugs and surgery for treatment, and the use of scientific thinking and research to understand diseases.

- Conventional practitioners include medical doctors, doctors of osteopathic medicine, podiatrists, optometrists, and dentists, as well as other highly trained professionals.

- The diagnostic process involves a medical history, a physical exam, and medical tests. Patients should ask questions about tests and treatments recommended by their providers.

- Safe use of prescription drugs requires knowledge of what the medication is supposed to do, how and when to take it, and the possible side effects.

- All surgical procedures carry risk; patients should ask many questions, including about alternatives.

- Complementary and alternative medicine (CAM) is defined as those therapies and practices that are not part of conventional health care and medical practice as taught in most U.S. medical schools and offered in most U.S. hospitals.

- *Integrative health* is a term used when CAM methods are added to conventional practice—conventional methods are considered first, and CAM may be included if it could have additional benefits. The term *integrative health* or *integrative medicine* should be used in discussions with conventional providers.

- CAM is a view of health as a balance and integration of body, mind, and spirit; a focus on ways to restore the individual to optimal functioning using methods from the five fields of CAM practice as defined by the National Institutes of Health; and a body of knowledge based on the accumulated observations and experience of practitioners, often over decades or centuries, and, more recently, on the scientific evaluation of safety and efficacy.

- CAM practices can be classified into several broad categories: alternative medical systems, mind–body medicine, natural products, manipulative and body-based practices, and other CAM practices.

- Alternative medical systems such as traditional Chinese medicine and homeopathy are complete systems of medical philosophy, theory, and practice.

- Mind–body medicine includes meditation, biofeedback, group support, hypnosis, and prayer.

- Natural products include herbal remedies, botanicals, animal tissue products, and dietary supplements.

- Manipulative and body-based practices include massage and other healing techniques; the most frequently used is chiropractic.

- Other CAM practices include traditional healing practices and energy therapies.

- Because there is currently less information available about CAM and less regulation of its providers and modalities, consumers should be proactive in researching and choosing treatments, using critical thinking skills, examining the available evidence-based information available, and exercising caution.

- The Affordable Care Act and other recent government reforms of the health care system (particularly the insurance industry) aim to make affordable health insurance coverage available to more Americans.

- Health insurance plans are usually described as either fee-for-service (indemnity) or managed care plans. Indemnity plans allow consumers more choice in medical providers, but managed care plans are less expensive.

- Government programs include Medicaid for the poor and Medicare for those aged 65 and over or chronically disabled.

BEHAVIOR CHANGE STRATEGY
Adhering to Your Physician's Instructions

Even though you sometimes have to entrust yourself to the care of medical professionals, you are still responsible for your own behavior. Following medical instructions and advice often requires the same kind of behavioral self-management that's involved in quitting smoking, losing weight, or changing eating patterns. For example, if you have an illness or injury, you may be instructed to take medication at certain times of the day, do special exercises or movements, or change your diet.

The medical profession recognizes the importance of patient adherence and encourages different strategies to support it, such as the following:

1. Use reminders placed at home, in the car, at work, on your computer screensaver, or elsewhere that improve follow-through in taking medication and keeping scheduled appointments. To help you remember to take medications:

   - Use one of the many quality apps available for your phone or computer. (Several of the best ones are listed and reviewed at http://www.singlecare.com /blog/best-medication-reminder-apps/)

   - Link taking the medication with some well-established routine, like brushing your teeth or eating breakfast.

   - Use a medication calendar, and check off each pill.

   - Use a medication organizer or pill dispenser.

   - Plan ahead; don't wait until you take the last pill to get a prescription refilled.

2. Use a journal or another form of self-monitoring to keep a detailed account of your health-related behaviors, such as taking pills on schedule, following dietary recommendations, following an exercise program, and so on.

3. Use a self-reward system so that desired behavior changes are encouraged, with a focus on short-term rewards.

4. Develop a clear image or explanation of how the medication or behavior change will improve your health, how you will look and feel, and your long-term well-being.

If these strategies don't help you stick with your treatment plan, you may need to consider other possible explanations for your lack of adherence. For example, are you confused about some aspect of the treatment? Do you find the schedule for taking your medications too complicated, or do the drugs have bothersome side effects that tempt you to avoid them? Do you feel that the recommended treatment is unnecessary or unlikely to help? Are you afraid of becoming dependent on a medication or that you'll be judged negatively if people know about your condition or treatment? A follow-up discussion with a health professional (your physician, physician assistant, nurse practitioner, dietitian, or physical therapist) and an examination of your attitudes and beliefs about your condition and treatment plan can also help improve your adherence.

FOR MORE INFORMATION

Affordable Care Act. Provides information on the Affordable Care Act and the Health Insurance Marketplace.

   https://www.healthcare.gov

Exercise Is Medicine. Provides information on the initiative to promote physical activity, as well as a series of factsheets with guidelines on exercise for people many different chronic conditions.

   https://exerciseismedicine.org

HealthIT. Presents tips and tools related to health information technology.

   https://www.healthit.gov

National Center for Complementary and Integrative Health (NCCIH). Provides background information and research results on many forms of CAM.

   https://nccih.nih.gov

U.S. Food and Drug Administration: For Consumers. Provides materials about supplements, prescription and OTC drugs, and other FDA-regulated products.

   http://www.fda.gov/consumers/

SELECTED BIBLIOGRAPHY

Academic Consortium for Integrative Medicine & Health. 2016. *Member Listing* (https://www.imconsortium.org/).

Agency for Healthcare Research and Quality. 2012. *The 10 Questions You Should Know* (http://www.ahrq.gov).

American Academy of Family Physicians. 2020. *Patient Protection and Affordable Care Act (ACA)* (https://www.aafp.org/advocacy/informed/coverage /aca.html).

American Academy of Pediatrics. 2017. Off-label use of medical devices in children. Policy statement, Section on Cardiology and Cardiac Surgery, Section on Orthopaedics. *Pediatrics* 139(1).

American Association of Naturopathic Physicians. 2020. *About Naturopathic Medicine* (http://www.naturopathic.org/medicine).

American Board of Medical Specialties. 2020. *Specialty and Subspecialty Certificates* (http://www.abms.org/member-boards/specialty-subspecialty -certificates/).

American Chiropractic Association. 2019. *Facts about Chiropractic* (www .acatoday.org/News-Publications/News/Facts-About-Chiropractic).

American College of Physicians. 2009. *The ACP Evidence-Based Guide to Complementary and Alternative Medicine.* Washington, DC: American College of Physicians.

American Hospital Association. 2015. *Hospital Emergency Room Visits per 1,000 Population by Ownership Type* (http://kff.org/other/state-indicator /emergency-room-visits-by-ownership/).

Ayers, S. L., and J. J. Kronenfeld. 2012. Delays in seeking conventional medical care and complementary and alternative medicine utilization. *Health Services Research* 47(5): 2081–2096.

Baer, H. A., et al. 2012. A dialogue between naturopathy and critical medical anthropology: What constitutes holistic health? *Medical Anthropology Quarterly* 26(2): 241–256.

Berchick, E. R., J. C. Barnett, and R. D. Upton. 2019. Health insurance coverage in the United States: 2018. (https://www.census.gov/library /publications/2019/demo/p60-267.html).

Bryan, S., G. P. Zipp, and R. Parasher. 2012. The effects of yoga on psycho-social variables and exercise adherence: A randomizved, controlled pilot study. *Alternative Therapies in Health and Medicine* 18(5): 50–59.

Buenz, E. J., R. Verpoorte, and B. A. Bauer. 2018. The ethnopharmacologic contribution to bioprospecting natural products. *Annual Review of Pharmacology and Toxicology* 58: 509–530.

Clarke, T. C., et al. 2015. Trends in the use of complementary health approaches among adults: United States, 2002–2012. *National Health Statistics Reports* 79: 1–16.

Clark, T. C., et al. 2018. Use of yoga, meditation, and chiropractors among U.S. adults aged 18 and over. NCHS Data Brief, No. 325. Hyattsville, MD: National Center for Health Statistics. (https://www.cdc.gov/nchs /data/databriefs/db325-h.pdf).

Commonwealth Fund. 2015. *The Problem of Underinsurance and How Rising Deductibles Will Make It Worse* (http://www.commonwealthfund.org /publications/issue-briefs/2015/may/problem-of-underinsurance).

Cowen, V. S., and V. Cyr. 2015. Complementary and alternative medicine in US medical schools. *Advances in Medical Education and Practice* 6: 113–117.

Cramer, H., et al. 2012. Mindfulness-based stress reduction for low back pain: A systematic review. *BMC Complementary and Alternative Medicine* 12(1): 162.

Del Prete, A., et al. 2012. Herbal products: Benefits, limits, and applications in chronic liver disease. *Evidence-Based Complementary and Alternative Medicine*. doi: 10.1155/2012/837939.

D'Silva, S., et al. 2012. Mind–body medicine therapies for a range of depression severity: A systematic review. *Psychosomatics* 53(5): 407–423.

Exercise Is Medicine. 2016. *Getting Started* (http://www.exerciseismedicine .org/support_page.php?p56).

Fronstin, P. 2012. Employment-based health benefits: Recent trends and future outlook. *Inquiry* 49(2): 101–115.

Ghildayal, N., et al. 2016. Complementary and alternative medicine use in the US adult low back pain population. *Global Advances in Health and Medicine* 5(1): 69–78.

Greene, J. A. 2010. What's in a name? Generics and the persistence of the pharmaceutical brand in American medicine. *Journal of the History of Medicine and Allied Sciences* 66(4): 468–506.

Harris, P., et al. 2012. Prevalence of complementary and alternative medicine (CAM) use by the general population: A systematic review and update. *International Journal of Clinical Practice* 66(10): 924–939.

Health Canada. 2016. *Drugs and Health Products* (http://www.hc-sc.gc.ca /index-eng.php).

Jahnke, R., et al. 2010. A comprehensive review of health benefits of qigong and tai chi. *American Journal of Health Promotion* 24(6): e1–e25.

Johns Hopkins Medicine 2020. *Types of Complementary and Alternative Medicine* (https://www.hopkinsmedicine.org/health/wellness-and-prevention/types-of-complementary-and-alternative-medicine).

Levey, N. N. 2018. Number of Americans without health insurance grows in Trump's first year, new figures show. *Los Angeles Times*, January 16 (http://www.latimes.com/politics/la-na-pol-health-insurance-survey -20180116-story.html).

Litscher, G., et al. 2012. High-tech acupuncture and integrative laser medicine. *Evidence-Based Complementary and Alternative Medicine*. doi: 10.1155/2012/363467.

Micozzi, M. S. 2015. *Fundamentals of Complementary and Alternative Medicine*, 5th ed. New York: Saunders.

National Center for Complementary and Integrative Health. 2020. *Complementary, Alternative or Integrative Health: What's In a Name?* (https://www.nccih .nih.gov/health/complementary-alternative-or-integrative-health-whats-in-a -name).

National Center for Complementary and Integrative Health. 2020. *Placebo Effect* (https://nccih.nih.gov/health/placebo).

National University of Natural Medicine. 2019. Licensing and scope of practice: How it affects your career as a naturopathic physician. (https:// nunm.edu/2019/05/nd-licensing-and-scope/).

O'Malley, P. A. 2012. Preventing and reporting adverse drug events: Pharmacovigilance for the clinical nurse specialist. *Clinical Nurse Specialist* 26(3): 136–137.

Physicians' Desk Reference. 2014. *PDR for Nonprescription Drugs*, 35th ed. Montvale, NJ: Thomson Healthcare.

Sarris, J., et al. 2012. Complementary medicine, exercise, meditation, diet, and lifestyle modification for anxiety disorders: A review of current evidence. *Evidence-Based Complementary and Alternative Medicine*. doi: 10.1155/2012/809653.

Scott, D. 2019. The uninsured rate had been steadily declining for a decade. But now it's rising again. *Vox* 10 September (https://www.vox.com /policy-and-politics/2019/9/10/20858938/health-insurance-census -bureau-data-trump).

Shen, P. F., et al. 2012. Acupuncture intervention in ischemic stroke: A randomized controlled prospective study. *American Journal of Chinese Medicine* 40(4): 685–693.

Society of Homeopaths. 2020. *What Is Homeopathy?* (https://homeopathy -soh.org/homeopathy-explained/what-is-homeopathy/).

Tariq, R. A., and Y. Scherbak. 2020. Medication Errors. *National Center for Biotechnology Information* (https://www.ncbi.nlm.nih.gov/books /NBK519065/).

U.S. Food and Drug Administration. 2016. *Information for Consumers* (http://www.fda.gov/drugs/resourcesforyou/consumers/).

U.S. Food and Drug Administration. 2018. *Understanding Unapproved Use of Approved Drugs "Off-Label"* (https://https://www.fda.gov/patients/learn -about-expanded-access-and-other-treatment-options/understanding -unapproved-use-approved-drugs-label).

Wang, C., et al. 2010. A randomized trial of tai chi for fibromyalgia. *New England Journal of Medicine* 363(8): 743–754.

Wong, C. 2019. 5 Types of Complementary and Alternative Medicine *VeryWellHealth* (https://www.verywellhealth.com/types-of-complementary-and-alternative-medicine-88741).

Zhao, X. F., et al. 2012. Mortality and recurrence of vascular disease among stroke patients treated with combined TCM therapy. *Journal of Traditional Chinese Medicine* 32(2): 173–178.

Zhuang, L. X., et al. 2012. An effectiveness study comparing acupuncture, physiotherapy, and their combination in poststroke rehabilitation: A multicentered, randomized, controlled clinical trial. *Alternative Therapies in Health and Medicine* 18(3): 8–14.

CHAPTER OBJECTIVES

- List the most common unintentional injuries and strategies for preventing them
- Discuss violence and intentional injuries, and how to protect yourself
- List strategies for helping others in an emergency

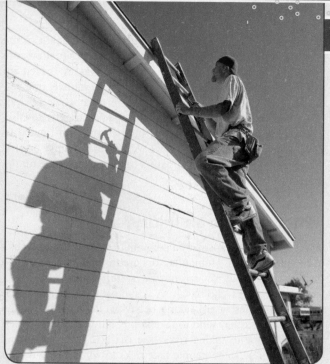

Brand X Pictures/Getty Images

CHAPTER 22

Personal Safety

TEST YOUR KNOWLEDGE

1. **More people are killed each year through intentional acts of violence than through unintentional injuries (accidents).**
   True or False?

2. **You should not wear a seat belt because, in a collision, your car might catch on fire or become submerged in water.**
   True or False?

3. **Your odds are greatest for being killed in which of the following incidents?**
   a. A plane crash
   b. A car crash
   c. An unintentional poisoning

4. **Talking on a cell phone while driving increases the chances of severe injuries, especially for younger and older drivers.**
   True or False?

5. **Strangers commit about what percentage of sexual assaults against women?**
   a. 20%
   b. 40%
   c. 80%

ANSWERS

1. **FALSE.** The death rate for unintentional injuries is 48 (deaths per 100,000), whereas the rate for murder is 5.

2. **FALSE.** These kinds of crashes are rare, and the greatest danger is the impact that precedes them.

3. **C.** The odds of dying by unintentional poisoning—most commonly through prescription drug overdoses, such as with painkillers—are estimated at 1 in 96. The odds of being killed in a car crash are similar, 1 in 114, and the odds of a fatal plane crash, 1 in 9821.

4. **TRUE.** For drivers under age 25 or over age 64, talking on cell phones has been found to increase the odds for severe injuries.

5. **A.** The vast majority of sexual assaults against women are committed by friends, acquaintances, or intimate partners.

According to the latest data from the National Center for Health Statistics, more than 169,000 Americans die each year from injuries, and many more are temporarily or permanently disabled. The economic cost of injuries is high, with almost $1.06 trillion spent each year for medical care and rehabilitation of injured people. Injuries also cause emotional suffering for injured people and their families, friends, and colleagues.

You can take many steps to reduce the risk of injuries. Public health measures also attempt to reduce injury. Engineering strategies such as seat belts can help lower injury rates, as can the passage and enforcement of safety-related laws, such as those requiring tamper-proof containers for over-the-counter medications. Public education can also help prevent injuries.

Ultimately, though, it is up to each person to take responsibility for his or her actions and make wise choices, such as buckling a seat belt. Many of the same sensible attitudes, responsible behaviors, and informed decisions that optimize your wellness can improve your chances of avoiding injuries. This chapter explains how you can protect yourself and those around you from becoming victims of unintentional and intentional injuries.

If an injury occurs when no harm is intended, it is considered an **unintentional injury.** Motor vehicle crashes, falls, and fires often result in unintentional injuries. Public health officials prefer not to use the word *accidents* to describe unintentional injuries because it suggests events beyond human control. *Injuries* are predictable outcomes that can be controlled or prevented. In contrast, an **intentional injury** is one that is purposely inflicted by you or by another person.

Although Americans tend to express more concern about intentional injuries, unintentional injuries are far more common. Unintentional injuries are the leading cause of death for Americans aged 1 to 45 and the third leading cause of death for all age groups.

Because unintentional injuries are so common, they account for more **years of potential life lost** than any other cause of death. Let's look closely at the most common types of unintentional injuries.

TERMS

unintentional injury An injury that occurs when no harm was intended.

intentional injury An injury that is purposely inflicted by you or by another person.

years of potential life lost The difference between an individual's life expectancy and his or her age at death.

home injuries Unintentional injuries and deaths that occur in the home and on home premises to occupants, guests, domestic servants, and trespassers; falls, burns, poisonings, suffocations, unintentional shootings, drownings, and electrical shocks are examples.

UNINTENTIONAL INJURIES

Unintentional injuries are the leading cause of death in the United States for people aged 1 to 45. Injury situations are generally categorized into four general classes, based on where they occur: home injuries, motor vehicle injuries, leisure injuries, and work injuries. The greatest number of disabling injuries occur in the home; falls are the leading cause of nonfatal, unintentional injuries that are treated in hospital emergency departments. Wherever an injury occurs, however, your response can have a dramatic influence on the outcome.

What Causes an Injury?

Most injuries are caused by a combination of human and environmental factors. Human factors are inner conditions or attitudes that lead to an unsafe state, whether physical, emotional, or psychological. A common human factor that leads to injuries is risk-taking behavior. People vary in the amount of risk they tend to take in life, but young men are especially prone to taking risks (see the box "Injuries among Young Men"). Some people take risks to win the admiration of their peers. Other people simply overestimate their physical abilities or enjoy defying the laws of nature. Alcohol and drug use is another common risk factor that leads to many injuries and deaths.

Psychological and emotional factors can also play a role in injuries. People sometimes act on the basis of inadequate or inaccurate beliefs about what is safe or unsafe. For example, a person who believes that seat belts trap people in cars when a crash occurs and decides not to wear a seat belt is acting on inaccurate information. However, many people who have accurate information still decide to engage in risky behavior. Young people often have unsafe attitudes, such as "I won't get hurt" or "It won't happen to me." Such attitudes can lead to risk taking and ultimately to injuries.

Environmental factors leading to injury are external conditions and circumstances. They may be natural (weather conditions, the undertow of the ocean at the beach), social (a drunk driver), work-related (defective equipment, a slippery surface), or home-related (faulty wiring). Making the environment safer is an important aspect of safety. Laws are often passed to try to make our environment safer. Examples include speed limits on highways and workplace safety requirements.

Home Injuries

People spend a great deal of time at home and feel that they are safe and secure there. However, home can be a dangerous place. The most common fatal **home injuries** are the result of poisonings and falls (Table 22.1). The number of fatal injuries from firearms—in homicidal and suicidal shootings—has greatly increased.

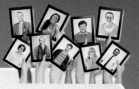

DIVERSITY MATTERS
Injuries among Young Men

Males significantly outnumber females in early deaths, whether unintentional or intentional. Except among adults aged 70 and over, the nonfatal injury rate is substantially higher in males than in females—and it peaks among young adult males (see the figure). Women are more likely to *attempt* suicide, but men are more likely to actually kill themselves. Deaths due to drug poisoning have occurred in men 1.8 times more frequently than in women. And four out of five DUI (driving under the influence) incidents involved a male driver, according to recent Centers for Disease Control and Prevention (CDC) statistics. Gender stereotypes about men and injuries do not apply in every case. For example, in 2009 and 2010, female soldiers deployed to Afghanistan had more injuries and more severe ones than male soldiers. But speaking generally, why do men, especially young men, have such high rates of injury?

Some researchers suggest that the male hormone testosterone plays a role in risky and aggressive behavior. Differences in brain structure and brain activity may also influence how men and women respond to stressors and how quickly and to what degree they become verbally or physically aggressive in response to anger. Moreover, cultural ideologies that men should inhabit rigid social roles—for example, as the breadwinner, protector, or stoic warrior—can lead to emotional stress when men are faced with a reality that requires more

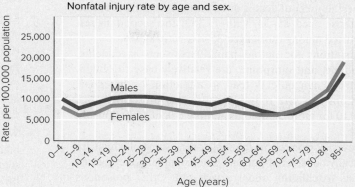

Nonfatal injury rate by age and sex.

flexibility. Ideologies that men are self-sufficient may conflict with notions about love and affection; thus, if a man cannot meet a partner's expectations for intimacy and a relationship fails, he may feel unable to ask for help and respond with a self-destructive reaction.

As gender dynamics change, the breadwinner role associated with men is now often shared with women. Both men and women work, and in some cases women are the sole breadwinners. Even as ideas about men as providers still prevail, fathers are expected to participate more fully in raising their children. In divorce cases, men are more likely to lose their home, children, and family, losses cited as factors in suicide.

Men may also have greater exposure to injury. Compared with women, men drive more miles, have greater access to firearms, and are more likely to ride

motorcycles, operate machinery, and have jobs associated with high rates of workplace injuries. They are also more likely to engage in sports and other recreational activities that are associated with high rates of injuries. Greater access to and use of firearms plays a role in higher rates of deaths among men from assault and suicide.

SOURCES: Centers for Disease Control and Prevention: Data and Statistics (WISQARS). 2019. *Leading Causes of Nonfatal Injuries 2000–2017, United States, All Races, Both Sexes, All Ages* (http://www.cdc.gov/injury/wisqars/nonfatal.html); Scourfield, J., and R. Evans. 2015. Why might men be more at risk of suicide after a relationship breakdown? Sociological insights. *American Journal of Men's Health* 9(5): 380–384; Stergiou-Kita, M., et al. 2016. Gender influences on return to work after mild traumatic brain injury. *Archives of Physical Medicine and Rehabilitation*. 97(2): S40–S45.

Table 22.1	Leading Causes of Deaths from Unintentional Injury, 2018

RANK	ALL AGE GROUPS TOTAL	15–24 YEARS OLD	25–34 YEARS OLD	35–44 YEARS OLD
1	Poisoning (62,399)	Motor vehicle traffic (6,308)	Poisoning (15,353)	Poisoning (14,978)
2	Motor vehicle traffic (37,991)	Poisoning (4,245)	Motor vehicle traffic (6,886)	Motor vehicle traffic (5,068)
3	Fall (37,455)	Drowning (431)	Drowning (482)	Fall (502)
4	Suffocation (6,701)	Fall (199)*	Fall (345)	Drowning (414)

SOURCE: Centers for Disease Control and Prevention. 2020. *10 Leading Causes of Injury Deaths by Age Group Highlighting Unintentional Injury Deaths, United States—2018* (http://www.cdc.gov/injury/wisqars/leadingcauses.html).

* 2017 *data*

Poisoning   More than 1 million nonfatal poisonings and 62,399 fatal poison-related incidents occur every year in the United States; 81% of poison exposures are unintentional, mainly due to prescription drug overdose. In the latest data, the highest number of deaths due to drug poisoning occurred among those aged 25–34, with 15,353; the second-highest rate occurred among those aged 35–44, with 14,978.

Prescriptions for opioid painkillers, such as codeine, hydrocodone, and morphine, are relatively easy to obtain. These drugs can quickly lead to addiction or overdose. Medications are safe only when used as prescribed. See Chapter 10 for more on opioids and the risk of addiction and overdose.

However, poisons come in many forms, some of which are not typically considered poisons. For example, honey can be poisonous to children under a year old. Other poisonous substances include cleaning agents, petroleum-based products, insecticides and herbicides, cosmetics, nail polish and remover, and many houseplants. All potentially poisonous substances should be used only as directed and stored out of the reach of children.

The most common type of gas poisoning is by carbon monoxide. Carbon monoxide gas is emitted by motor vehicle exhaust and heating equipment that runs on a fuel (e.g., gas, oil, kerosene, wood, charcoal). To prevent poisoning by gases, never operate or idle a vehicle in an enclosed space, like a garage, have your furnace inspected yearly, and use caution with any substance or device that produces potentially toxic fumes.

To be prepared for an unintentional poisoning, keep the national poison control hotline number (800-222-1222) in a convenient location. A call to the hotline will be routed to a local poison control center, which provides expert emergency advice 24 hours a day. If a poisoning occurs, act quickly. Remove the poison from contact with the victim's eyes, skin, or mouth, or move the victim away from contact with poisonous gases. Call the poison control center immediately. Do not follow the emergency instructions on product labels because they may be incorrect. Depending on the situation, you may be instructed to give the victim water to drink, or to flush affected parts of the skin or eyes with water. Do not induce vomiting. If you are advised to go to a hospital emergency department, take the poisonous substance or container with you.

Falls   Falls are the leading cause of death among people aged 65 and over. For people under age 44, falls are also a significant cause of unintentional death and injury. Most deaths from falls occur on stairs. Alcohol is a contributing factor in many falls. Strategies for preventing falls include the following:

- Install handrails and nonslip surfaces in the shower and bathtub.
- Keep floors, stairs, and outside areas clear of objects or conditions that could cause slipping or tripping, such as ice, snow, electrical cords, and toys.
- Put a light switch by the door of every room so that no one has to walk across a room to turn on a light. Use night lights in bedrooms (placed so as not to disrupt sleep), halls, stairs, and bathrooms.
- When climbing a ladder, use both hands. Never stand higher than the third step from the top. When using a stepladder, make sure the spreader brace is in the locked position. With straight ladders, set the base out one foot for every four feet of height.
- Don't stand on chairs to reach things.
- If there are small children in the home, place gates at the top and bottom of stairs. Never leave a baby unattended on a bed or table.

> **QUICK STATS**
> Since 1999, the age-adjusted drug-poisoning death rate has more than tripled, from 6.1 per 100,000 in 1999 to 20.7 per 100,000 in 2018.
> —National Center for Health Statistics, 2020

Fires   The National Fire Protection Association reported 363,000 home fires in 2018. Most fires begin in the kitchen, living room, or bedroom. Cooking is now the leading cause of home fire injuries; careless smoking is the leading cause of fire deaths, followed by problems with heating equipment and arson. A study of campus fire fatalities found that smoking materials left to smolder over time in a couch accounted for half of those fatalities in which smoking was involved.

To prevent fires, dispose of all cigarettes in ashtrays and never smoke in bed. Other strategies include proper maintenance of fireplaces, furnaces, heaters, chimneys, and electrical outlets, cords, and appliances. If you use a portable heater, keep it at least three feet away from curtains, bedding, and anything else that might catch fire. Never plug heaters into a surge protector or power strip, and never leave heaters on unattended.

Also, be prepared to handle fire-related situations. Plan at least two escape routes out of each room, and designate a location outside the home as a meeting place. For practice, stage a home fire drill; do this at night because that's when most deadly fires occur.

Data show that about three in five home fire deaths occur in homes with no working smoke alarms. Install smoke detectors on every level of your home. Your risk of dying in a fire is almost twice as high if you do not use them. Clean the detectors and check the batteries once a month, and replace the batteries at least once a year. Be sure that all

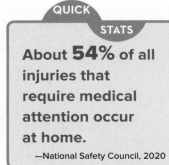

> **QUICK STATS**
> About **54%** of all injuries that require medical attention occur at home.
> —National Safety Council, 2020

residents are familiar with the sound of the alarm; when it goes off, take it seriously.

These strategies can help prevent injuries in a fire:

- Get out as quickly as possible, and go to the designated meeting place. Don't stop for a keepsake or pet. Never hide in a closet or under a bed. Once outside, count heads to see if everyone is out. If you think someone is still inside the burning building, tell the firefighters. Never go back inside a burning building.

- If you're trapped in a room, feel the door. If it is hot or if smoke is coming in through the cracks, don't open it; use the alternative escape route. If you can't get out, go to the window and shout for help.

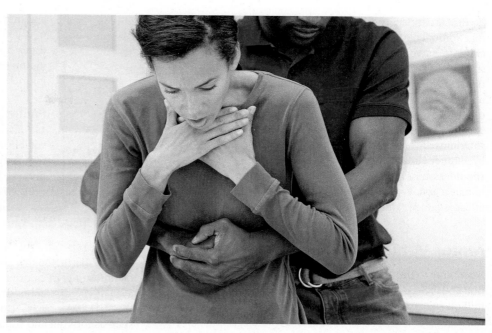

The Heimlich maneuver can save someone who is choking. Reach around the victim, making a fist and placing the thumb side of the fist just above the navel. Grasp your fist with the other hand and thrust upward and inward into the victim's abdomen. Continue with quick jerks until the object is expelled. Science Photo Library/Getty Images

- Smoke inhalation is the greatest cause of death and injury in fires. To avoid inhaling smoke, crawl along the floor away from the heat and smoke. Cover your mouth and nose, ideally with a wet cloth, and take short, shallow breaths.

- If your clothes catch fire, don't run. Drop to the ground, cover your face, and roll back and forth to smother the flames. Remember: stop–drop–roll.

Although house fires cause the most deaths, hot water causes the most nonfatal burns. Set your water heater no higher than 120°F. Young children are particularly at risk of being burned. Place barriers around stoves and radiators, and keep young children out of the kitchen, where they might be burned by spills. Put pans on rear burners, and turn pot handles toward the back of the stove. Keep hot foods away from the edge of counters and tables, and don't put them on a tablecloth that a small child can pull. Always test the contents of a baby bottle; when bottles are heated in microwave ovens, the liquid can become scalding before the outside of the bottle gets hot.

Suffocation and Choking
Suffocation and choking represented the fourth most common cause of death in the home. Elderly people and children are especially vulnerable. Children can suffocate if they put small items in their mouths, get tangled in their crib bedding, or get trapped in airtight appliances like old refrigerators. Keep small objects out of reach of children under age 3, and don't give them raw carrots, hot dogs, popcorn, gum, or hard candy. Examine toys carefully for small parts that could come loose. Don't give plastic bags or balloons to small children.

Adults can also become choking victims, especially if they fail to adequately chew food, or eat hurriedly or try to talk and eat at the same time. Many choking victims can be saved with the **Heimlich maneuver.** The American Red Cross recommends abdominal thrusts as the easiest and safest thing to do when an adult is choking. Back blows in conjunction with two-finger abdominal thrusts are an acceptable procedure for dislodging an object from the throat of an infant.

Firearms
When researchers compared rates of firearm deaths in high-income countries, they found that although the rates in most countries had declined since 2003, those in the United States, already the highest, remained unchanged. Over one-third of all unintended U.S. firearm deaths and nonfatal injuries involve children and young adults under 25 years of age. People who use firearms should remember the following:

- Always treat a gun as though it is loaded, even if you know it isn't.

- Never point a gun—loaded or unloaded—at anything you do not intend to shoot.

- Always unload a gun before storing it. Store unloaded firearms under lock and key, separate from ammunition.

- Always inspect firearms carefully before handling.

- If you ever plan to handle a gun, take a firearms safety course first.

- If you own a gun, use a gun lock designed specifically for that weapon.

Heimlich maneuver   A maneuver developed by Henry J. Heimlich, MD, to help force an obstruction from a person's windpipe or throat.   **TERMS**

Proper storage is critical. Do not assume that young children cannot fire a gun. Even children as young as 3 have enough finger strength to pull a trigger. One study estimated that 110 children aged 0–14 die each year as a result of unintentional firearm injuries. In the overwhelming majority of cases, victims and shooters are male, and the victim has either shot himself (one-third of cases) or been shot by another child. Anyone who picks up a gun should assume it is loaded. If you plan to handle a gun, avoid alcohol and drugs, which affect judgment and coordination.

Motor Vehicle Injuries

According to the National Highway Traffic Safety Administration (NHTSA), 38,800 Americans were killed and almost 4.5 million injured in motor vehicle crashes in 2019. The good news is that motor vehicle deaths in this country have decreased 25% in the past decade. Worldwide, motor vehicle crashes kill 1.25 million and injure up to 50 million people each year, placing motor vehicle injuries within the top 10 leading causes of death overall. Motor vehicle injuries also result in the majority of cases of paralysis due to spinal injuries,

and they are the leading cause of severe brain injury in the United States. Table 22.2 illustrates how likely Americans are to die from motor vehicle crashes versus other types of injuries.

Factors Contributing to Motor Vehicle Injuries Common causes of motor vehicle injuries are speeding; aggressive driving; fatigue; inexperience; the use of cell phones, handheld devices, and other distractions; the use of alcohol and other drugs; and the incorrect use of seat belts and other safety devices.

DISTRACTED DRIVING In 2018, motor vehicle crashes involving distracted drivers caused 2841 deaths and hundreds of thousands of injuries. Drivers in their twenties make up 27% of the distracted drivers in fatal crashes, according to the NHTSA. Distractions include visual-manual activity such as looking and using hands to type a text message (see the box "Cell Phones and Distracted Driving"), and cognitive tasks such as calculating numbers or formulating a sentence. Distractions can also intrude from outside the car—for example, billboards and roadside accidents—and from inside the car, as in the case of a conversation with a passenger, or eating, smoking, reaching for controls, preoccupation, and daydreaming.

SPEEDING After distracted and drunk driving, the next most common cause for car crashes is speeding and other errors in decision making (e.g., false assumption of others' actions, misjudgment of a gap or others' speed). As speed increases, momentum and the force of impact increase, and the time allowed for the driver to react (reaction time) decreases. Speed limits are posted to establish the safest maximum speed limit for a given area under ideal conditions; if visibility is limited or the road is wet, the safe maximum speed may be considerably lower. Many states have raised their highway speed limits since the 1995 repeal of the National Maximum Speed Limit of 55 miles per hour, and overall motor vehicle fatalities have since increased. Raising speed limits on rural interstates contributed to a 35% increase in crash death rates.

AGGRESSIVE DRIVING Speeding is also a hallmark of aggressive drivers—those who operate motor vehicles in an unsafe and hostile manner. Aggressive driving has increased more than 50% since 1990, and one in four U.S. drivers admits to driving aggressively at least some of the time. Other characteristics of aggressive driving include frequent, erratic, and abrupt lane changes; tailgating; running red lights or stop signs; passing on the shoulder; and blocking other cars trying to change lanes or pass. Extreme aggression can result from road rage and includes making obscene gestures, throwing objects, and ramming or sideswiping other vehicles. Aggressive driving is a traffic violation; road rage can be a criminal offense. For more about aggressive driving, take the quiz and review the strategies in the box "Are You an Aggressive Driver?"

VITAL STATISTICS

TABLE 22.2 Lifetime Odds of Death Due to Selected Types of Injury

INJURY TYPE	LIFETIME ODDS
Suicide	1 in 86
Opioid overdose	1 in 98
Motor vehicle crash	1 in 106
Fall	1 in 111
Homicide (assault by firearm)	1 in 298
Pedestrian incident	1 in 541
Motorcycle rider incident	1 in 890
Drowning	1 in 1121
Exposure to fire, flames, or smoke	1 in 1399
Choking from inhalation and ingestion of food	1 in 2618
Exposure to excessive natural heat	1 in 7770
Accidental gun discharge	1 in 9077
Electrocution, radiation, extreme temperatures, and pressure	1 in 12,484
Contact with sharp objects	1 in 29,483
Hornet/bee/wasp sting	1 in 53,989
Cataclysmic storm	1 in 54,699
Being bitten or attacked by a dog	1 in 118,776
Lightning strike	1 in 180,746
Airplane incident	Too few deaths in 2018 to calculate odds

SOURCE: National Safety Council. 2020. *Lifetime Odds of Deaths for Selected Causes, U.S.* Itasca, IL: National Safety Council.

WELLNESS ON CAMPUS
Cell Phones and Distracted Driving

A survey of nearly 5000 students from 12 colleges found that 91% reported phoning and/or texting while driving. This included 87% who text at traffic lights, 60% who text on city streets or in stop-and-go traffic, and 50% who send texts while driving on the freeway. Nearly half of the respondents said they were capable or very capable of safely talking on a cell phone while driving, but only 8.5% felt that other drivers were capable of doing so. These students overestimate their ability to multitask while driving.

The visual-manual distraction of locating, dialing, text messaging, browsing, and ending a call on handheld phones increases the risk of a crash by three times. Tasks that keep your hands and eyes from being engaged in driving the car have been shown to have a greater impact than cognitive distractions such as calculating numbers, formulating a sentence, listening to the radio, or talking with passengers. Many drivers assume that hands-free devices (like headsets, Bluetooth, and voice-control features on a phone or built into an automobile) are safer. However, research conducted by the National Safety Council has found that the cognitive distractions of using hands-free devices are just as unsafe.

Drivers using any phone—hands-free or handheld—have a tendency to "look at" objects without "seeing" them. Estimates indicate that drivers using cell phones fail to see up to 50% of the information in their driving environment. Distracted drivers experience what researchers call *inattention blindness*, similar to that of tunnel vision. Drivers look out the windshield, but they do not process everything that they need to know to effectively monitor their surroundings, seek and identify potential hazards, and respond to unexpected situations.

Drivers under age 25, who are the heaviest users of social media and cell phone technology, also generally have less skill in controlling vehicles and less efficiency in visual scanning, and they generally take more risks. Their lack of experience includes less ability to handle the effects of distraction, compared to the abilities of drivers aged 25 to 64.

Phone applications designed to prevent distracted driving have had some success. However, they have not solved all the problems of breaking the driver's focus on the road. The technology still needs to find a balance between allowing specific contacts and phone functions to work and blocking those that have proven dangerous. Developers are still working to resolve these problems: (1) poor integration with other phone functions, (2) battery drainage, (3) integrating languages other than English, and (4) managing pop-up messages outside of texts, for example, Facebook Messenger and WhatsApp messages.

For people who live where cell phone use is legal while driving and who choose to use a phone regardless of the risk, the following strategies may increase safety:

- Minimize phone use while driving.

- Use a hands-free device so that you can keep both hands on the steering wheel.

- Be familiar with your phone and its functions, especially speed dial and redial.

- Store frequently called numbers on speed dial so that you can place calls without looking at the phone.

- If your phone has voice-activated dialing, use it.

- Let the person you are speaking with know you are driving, and be prepared to end the call at any time.

- Don't place or answer calls in heavy traffic or hazardous weather conditions.

- Don't take notes or look up phone numbers while driving.

- Time calls so that you can place them when you are at a stop.

Any kind of distraction—visual, manual, or cognitive—can contribute to an unsafe driving situation.

SOURCES: Hill, L., et al. 2015. Prevalence of and attitudes about distracted driving in college students. *Traffic Injury Prevention* 16(4): 362–367; National Highway Traffic Safety Administration. *Facts and Statistics: What Is Distracted Driving?* (https://www.nhtsa.gov/campaign/distracted-driving); National Safety Council. 2018. *Technologies Can Reduce Cell Phone Distracted Driving* (https://www.nsc.org/road-safety/safety-topics/distracted-driving/technology-solutions); Oviedo-Trespalacios, O., V. Truelove, and M. King. 2020. "It is frustrating to not have control even though I know it's not legal!": A mixed-methods investigation on applications to prevent mobile phone use while driving. *Accident Analysis & Prevention* 137 (https://doi.org/10.1016/j.aap.2019.105412).

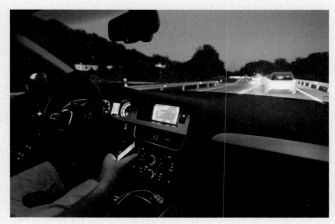

Ben Welsh/Design Pics/Getty Images

ASSESS YOURSELF
Are You an Aggressive Driver?

To find out if you are an aggressive driver, check any of the following statements that are true for you:

_____ I'm often unaware of both my speed and the speed limit.

_____ I often follow closely behind the car in front of me.

_____ If I feel the car in front of me is going too slowly, I tailgate.

_____ I change lanes frequently to pass people.

_____ I seldom use turn signals when changing lanes or turning.

_____ I often run red lights or roll through stop signs.

_____ I react to what I feel is another driver's mistake by cursing, shouting, or making rude gestures; by blocking a car from passing or changing lanes; by using high beams; or by braking suddenly in front of a tailgater.

_____ I become more competitive when I get behind the wheel.

_____ I often get angry or impatient with other drivers and with pedestrians.

_____ I would consider pulling over for a personal encounter with a bad driver.

Each of these statements is characteristic of aggressive drivers; the more items you checked, the greater your proclivity to drive aggressively and submit to road rage. If you checked even one statement, consider taking some of the following steps to reduce your hostility behind the wheel:

• Allow enough time to reach your destination without speeding.

• Avoid driving during periods of heavy traffic.

• Don't drive when you are angry, tired, or intoxicated.

• Imagine that the other drivers are all people you know and like. Be courteous and forgiving.

• Listen to soothing music or a book on tape, or practice a relaxation technique such as deep breathing (see Chapter 2).

• Take a course in anger management.

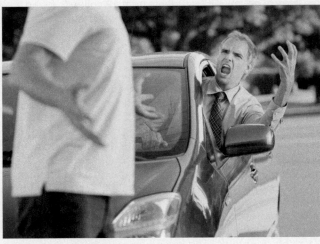

Chris Ryan/OJO Images/age fotostock

Even if you control your own aggressive impulses, you may still encounter an aggressive driver on the road. The AAA Foundation for Traffic Safety recommends these strategies:

• Avoid behaviors that may enrage an aggressive driver; these include cutting off cars when merging, driving slowly in the left lane, tailgating, and making rude gestures.

• If you make a mistake while driving, apologize. In surveys, the most popular and widely understood gestures for apologies include raising or waving a hand and touching or knocking the head with the palm of your hand (to indicate "What was I thinking?").

• Refuse to join in a fight. Avoid eye contact with an angry driver, and put distance between your car and his or her vehicle. If you think another driver is following you, call the police on a cell phone or drive to a public place.

SOURCES: New York State Department of Motor Vehicles. 2020. *Chapter 8: Defensive Driving* (https://dmv.ny.gov/about-dmv/chapter-8-defensive-driving#agg-drv); AAA Foundation for Traffic Safety. 2016. *Are You an Aggressive Driver?* (https://www.aaafoundation.org/are-you-aggressive-driver).

FATIGUE AND SLEEPINESS Driving requires mental alertness and attentiveness. Studies have shown that sleepiness causes slower reaction times, reduced coordination and vigilance, and delayed information processing. Drowsiness can be caused by not getting enough hours of sleep, by sleep disorders that prevent deep, necessary REM sleep, or by disruptions from shift work that force people to sleep at irregular hours. Research shows that even mild sleep deprivation causes deterioration in driving ability comparable to that caused by a 0.05% blood alcohol concentration—a level considered hazardous while driving. Being awake for 18 hours can impair driving ability as much as drinking two alcoholic beverages. Insufficient sleep can also cause

microsleeps—brief moments of sleep while driving that can have deadly results. (See Chapter 4 for more on drowsy driving.)

ALCOHOL AND OTHER DRUGS Alcohol is involved in about one-third of fatal crashes. Alcohol-impaired driving is illegal in all states and the District of Columbia. The legal limit for blood alcohol concentration (BAC) is 0.08%, but people can be impaired at much lower BACs. A driver with a BAC between 0.05% and 0.09% is nine times more likely to be involved in a crash than a person who has not been drinking. The combination of fatigue and alcohol use increases the risk even further. Because alcohol affects reason and judgment as well as the ability to make fast, accurate, and coordinated movements, a person who has been drinking will be less likely to recognize that he or she is impaired.

Other substances also affect judgment and driving ability. A recent study found that hay fever sufferers who had taken diphenhydramine (an antihistamine found in over-the-counter allergy medications such as Benadryl) were as impaired as if they were legally drunk. The effects of medicines that impair driving include blurred vision, confusion, dizziness, and drowsiness. The use of many over-the-counter drugs is potentially dangerous if you plan to drive (see Chapters 10 and 11). In most states, driving under the influence of specified medication carries the same penalty as a DUI. The use of prescription narcotics and depressants can also impair driving, as can marijuana. One year after legalizing recreational marijuana, Washington State's fatal crashes involving cannabis use rose from 8% to 17%. Use of many over-the-counter and all psychoactive drugs is potentially dangerous if you plan to drive (see Chapters 10 and 11).

SEAT BELTS, AIRBAGS, AND CHILD SAFETY SEATS The improper use of seat belts, airbags, and child safety seats contributes to injuries and deaths in motor vehicle crashes. Although mandatory seat belt laws for adults are in effect in 49 states (excluding New Hampshire) and the District of Columbia, only 90% of motor vehicle occupants used seat belts in 2018, even though they are the single most effective way to reduce the risk of crash-related death. The good news is that seat belt usage was at its highest level ever. Of drivers not wearing seat belts who have been killed in automobile crashes, an estimated 60–70% would have survived if they had been wearing one. Some people think that if they are involved in a crash they are better off being thrown free of their vehicle. In fact, the chances of being killed are 25 times greater if you are thrown from a vehicle, whether it is due to injuries caused by hitting a tree or the pavement or by being hit by another vehicle. Seat belts not only prevent you from being thrown from the car at the time of the crash but also provide protection from second collisions: If a car is traveling at 65 miles per hour (mph) and hits another vehicle, the car stops first; then the occupants stop because they, too, are traveling at 65 mph. Second collisions occur when occupants hit something inside the car, such as the dashboard or windshield. Seat belts prevent these second collisions and spread the force of the first collision over the occupants' bodies.

Since 1998, all new cars and light trucks have been equipped with dual airbags—one for the driver and one for the front passenger. Many vehicles also offer side airbags, which further reduce the risk of injury. Advanced airbag systems include risk reduction technologies such as sensors to detect crash severity, seat position, passenger size, and whether a passenger is wearing a seat belt. Although airbags provide supplementary protection in the event of a collision, most are useful only in head-on collisions. They also deflate immediately after inflating and therefore do not provide protection in collisions involving multiple impacts. Airbags are not a replacement for seat belts; everyone in a vehicle should buckle up.

Airbags deploy forcefully and can injure a child or short adult who is improperly restrained or sitting too close to the dashboard, although second-generation airbags are somewhat safer for children than older devices. To ensure that airbags work safely, always follow these basic guidelines: Place infants in rear-facing infant seats in the back seat, transport children aged 12 and under in the back seat, always use seat belts and appropriate safety seats, and keep 10 inches between the airbag cover and the breastbone of the driver or passenger. If necessary, adjust the steering wheel or use seat cushions to ensure that an inflating airbag would hit you in the chest and not in the face.

Another adjustment should be made for children who have outgrown child safety seats but are still too small for adult seat belts alone (usually aged 4–8). These children should be secured using booster seats that ensure that the seat belt is positioned low across the hips and thighs. About 70% of injured children are not properly restrained in the vehicle. All 50 states and the District of Columbia have child restraint laws, with 48 states mandating the use of booster seats for children who are too big for child safety seats. Before driving with a child, make sure that you know your state's laws, that you have an appropriate safety seat for the child, that the seat is installed correctly, and that the child is properly secured in the seat. Go to SeatCheck.org for resources on installing child seats.

Preventing Motor Vehicle Injuries Defensive driving can also help you avoid a motor vehicle collision. It entails the following:

- Be aware of traffic conditions around you by checking your rearview and side mirrors frequently.

- Be aware of the driving behaviors of other drivers, especially those who may be following too closely, driving erratically, speeding, or frequently shifting lanes. Anticipate the actions—and the possible errors—of other drivers.

- Don't follow other cars closely, and choose outside lanes to avoid getting boxed in by other vehicles.

- Never assume other drivers see you or that they anticipate an action you intend to make. Use your turn signals (even if you see no vehicles or pedestrians), make eye contact if possible, and allow enough road space and time for other drivers to prepare for and adjust to any action you take in traffic. Avoid driving in another driver's blind spot. Brake early, especially in poor weather conditions, allowing drivers behind you extra time for braking.

- Take special care at intersections. Make sure you have time to complete your maneuver in the intersection.

- Always allow enough following distance. Use the three-second rule: When the vehicle ahead passes a reference point, count out three seconds. If you pass the reference point before you finish counting, drop back and allow more following distance. This rule works well at slower speeds when roads are dry and weather conditions are good. When traveling on highways or the interstate, use the four-second rule.

- Slow down if weather or road conditions are poor. In those kinds of situations, the minimum recommendation is to follow four seconds behind the car in front of you.

Motorcycles and Motor Scooters   About one in seven traffic fatalities involves someone riding a motorcycle. In recent years, riders aged 50 years and over have represented one-third of these fatalities. The data also reveal that, per mile traveled, motorcycle riders are 28 times more likely to die in a crash than occupants of a car or other motor vehicle. Injuries from motorcycle collisions are generally more severe than those involving automobiles because motorcycles provide little, if any, protection. Because head injuries are the major cause of death, the use of a helmet is critical for rider safety. Thus, the District of Columbia and nearly all states (except Illinois, Iowa, and New Hampshire) have helmet laws, although only 19 of those states require the use of helmets by all riders. Still, only 59% of motorcyclists killed were wearing helmets. Riders also need to know how to operate a motorcycle safely. Operator error is a factor in approximately 75% of fatal motorcycle crashes.

People riding motor scooters face additional challenges. Such vehicles usually have a maximum speed of 35–40 mph and have less power for maneuverability, especially in an emergency. Drivers should use caution and learn how to handle these vehicles in traffic.

Additional strategies for preventing motorcycle and motor scooter injuries include the following:

- For maximum visibility, wear light-colored clothing, drive with your headlights on, and correctly position yourself in traffic.

- Develop the necessary skills. Lack of skill is a major factor in motorcycle and motor scooter injuries. Skidding from improper braking is the most common cause of loss of control.

- Wear a helmet. Helmets should be marked with the DOT symbol, certifying that they conform to federal safety standards established by the U.S. Department of Transportation. Helmet use is required by law in most states.

- Protect your eyes with goggles, a face shield, or a windshield. Wear protective clothing.

- Drive defensively, particularly when changing lanes and at intersections, and never assume that other drivers can see you.

Bicycles   Bicycle injuries result primarily from riders not knowing or understanding the rules of the road, failing to follow traffic laws, not having sufficient skill or experience to handle traffic conditions, or being intoxicated. Bicycles are considered vehicles; bicyclists must obey all traffic laws that apply to automobile drivers, including stopping at traffic lights and stop signs.

Head injuries are involved in about three out of four bicycle-related deaths. Currently, no state mandates that adult bicyclists wear helmets, but 21 states, the District of Columbia, and many counties and cities have laws requiring youth and adult cyclists to wear helmets. Research shows that wearing a helmet reduces the risk of head injury by 66–88%. Safe cycling strategies include the following:

- Wear safety equipment, including a helmet, eye protection, gloves, and proper footwear. To prevent clothes from tangling in the bike chain, secure the bottom of your pant legs with clips, and secure your shoelaces.

- Wear light-colored, reflective clothing. Equip your bike with reflectors, and use lights, especially at night or when riding in wooded or other dark areas.

- Ride with the flow of traffic, not against it, and follow all traffic laws. Use bike paths when they are available.

- Ride defensively; never assume that drivers have seen you. Be especially careful when turning or crossing at corners and intersections. Watch for cars turning right.

- Stop at all traffic lights and stop signs. Know and use hand signals.

Pedestrians   About one in seven motor vehicle deaths involves pedestrians, and more than 66,000 pedestrians are injured each year. Pedestrian deaths make up a larger proportion of traffic fatalities than they have in the past 33 years. The highest rates of death and injury occur among the very young and the elderly. Pedestrians are more likely to be hit head-on by the front of a vehicle than by the rear or sides. Pedestrian alcohol intoxication plays a significant role in up to half of all adult pedestrian fatalities, and researchers are also exploring the role of marijuana. The seven states that legalized recreational marijuana before 2016 saw a 16.4% increase in pedestrian deaths in early 2017, while all other states reported a 5.9% decrease. Walking while distracted with a cell phone may also account for more injuries and deaths. In hopes of cutting down injuries and deaths, cities in China have gone so far as to introduce special lanes on sidewalks for people looking down at electronic devices, and a city in Germany installed traffic signals on street surfaces.

The following strategies can help prevent injuries when you're walking or jogging:

- Walk or jog in daylight.
- Wear light-colored, reflective clothing.
- Face traffic when walking or jogging along a road, and follow traffic laws.
- Avoid busy roads or roads with poor visibility.
- Cross only at marked crosswalks and intersections.
- Don't use headphones.
- Don't hitchhike—it places you in a potentially dangerous situation.

Leisure Injuries

Most people enjoy some form of leisure activities, so it is not surprising that **leisure injuries** are a significant health-related problem in the United States. Key factors in leisure injuries include misuse of equipment, lack of experience and skill, use of alcohol or other drugs, and failure to use appropriate safety equipment. Specific safety strategies for activities associated with leisure injuries include the following:

- Don't swim alone, in unsupervised places, under the influence of alcohol, or for an unusual length of time. Use caution when swimming in unfamiliar surroundings or in water colder than 70°F. Check the depth of water before diving. Make sure that residential pools are fenced, and never allow children to swim unsupervised.

- Always use a **personal flotation device** (also known as a life jacket) when on a boat.

- For all sports and recreational activities, make sure facilities are safe, follow the rules, and practice good sportsmanship. Develop adequate skill in the activity, and use proper safety equipment, including, where appropriate, a helmet, eye protection, correct footwear, and knee, elbow, and wrist pads (see the box "Head Injuries in Contact Sports").

- If using equipment such as skateboards, snowboards, mountain bikes, or all-terrain vehicles, wear a helmet and other safety equipment, and avoid excessive speeds and unsafe stunts. Use playground equipment only for those activities for which it is designed.

- If you are active in excessively hot and humid weather, drink plenty of fluids, rest frequently in the shade, and slow down or stop if you feel uncomfortable. Danger signals of heat stress include excessive perspiration, dizziness, headache, muscle cramps, nausea, weakness, rapid pulse, and disorientation.

- Do not use alcohol or other drugs during recreational activities—such activities require coordination and sound judgment.

For more about exercise safety, see Chapter 14.

In-Line Skating and Skateboarding Injuries

Although in-line skating and skateboarding are not as popular as in the past, many American skaters are still injured badly enough each year to end up in a hospital emergency department. Injuries to the wrist and head are most common; many injuries occur because users do not wear appropriate safety gear. If you skate, wear a helmet, elbow and knee pads, wrist guards, a long-sleeved shirt, and long pants. Alcohol use appears to be a significant factor in in-line skating injuries that occur on college campuses. Because skating involves skill, judgment, and coordination, it makes sense not to mix skating and drinking.

Kick Scooter Injuries

Scooters are lightweight and have low-friction wheels for quickness and maneuverability. The most common injuries are arm or hand fractures and dislocations, cuts and bruises, and sprains; 85% of injuries involve children under age 15 years. Viewing scooters as toys more than transportation may lead riders to ignore these important safety precautions:

- Wear a helmet that meets bicycle helmet standards, along with knee and elbow pads.

- Be sure that handlebars, the steering column, and all nuts and bolts are securely fastened.

- Ride on smooth, paved surfaces away from motor vehicle traffic. Avoid streets and surfaces with water, sand, gravel, or dirt.

- Don't ride after dark.

- Closely supervise young children.

Weather-Related Injuries

Although you can't control the weather, the best approach is to be prepared for inclement weather that may occur in your area. Even though conditions may seem harmless at times, they can become dangerous quickly.

- *Heat.* Extreme heat is the leading weather-related killer in the United States, according to the National Weather Service. Heat-related illness such as heat stroke and heat exhaustion can be fatal, especially for children, older adults, and people who are dehydrated. The best way to deal with excessive heat is to stay indoors as much as possible, with a fan or air conditioner on. Wear lightweight, light-colored clothing; drink plenty of water to stay hydrated; and avoid heavy meals. If you must go out, move slowly and rest frequently in the shade. See Chapter 14 for advice on exercising in hot weather.

- *Cold.* Each year dozens of Americans die from exposure to cold temperatures. Conditions such as hypothermia (low body temperature) and frostbite (frozen skin or flesh) can be deadly. Most injuries and deaths in cold weather are due to a lack of preparedness or understanding of the dangers of low temperatures and wind chill. If you must go outdoors in very cold weather, dress in layers and cover your face, fingers, and ears to protect them from frostbite. Make sure your home and car are prepared with plenty of fuel, drinking water, warm clothes and blankets, batteries, and other emergency supplies. See Chapter 14 for advice on exercising in cold weather.

TERMS

leisure injuries Unintentional injuries and deaths that occur in public places, or places used in a public way, not involving motor vehicles; include most sports and recreation deaths and injuries; examples are falls, drownings, burns, and heat and cold stress.

personal flotation device A device designed to save a person from drowning by buoying up the body while in the water.

TAKE CHARGE
Head Injuries in Contact Sports

Reports of bizarre behavior, suicides, and middle-aged dementia among former professional football players, boxers, and soccer players have focused worldwide media attention on sports concussions. Death from chronic traumatic encephalopathy (CTE), a disease caused by repetitive brain trauma, was the diagnosis for 87% of over 200 football players whose brains were donated for a 2017 study. (CTE can be diagnosed only by autopsy.) Of 111 brains donated by National Football League players, 110 were diagnosed with CTE.

CTE has been found in younger athletes as well. An amateur football player in his early twenties suffered a variety of symptoms before dying at age 25. He had received repeated concussions since starting to play football at age six and continuing through college. He was an above-average student, but because of his symptoms—first, ongoing headaches, insomnia, anxiety, and difficulty with memory and concentration; and later, apathy, feelings of worthlessness, and suicidal thoughts—he had to stop both playing football and attending college. The diagnosis at his autopsy was CTE.

Concussions, or mild traumatic brain injuries (MTBIs), can be diagnosed immediately or after some cognitive and neurological testing. An MTBI is a traumatic injury to the brain or spinal cord resulting from a direct blow to the head or indirect blows elsewhere that can cause violent brain movement in the skull. A concussion, for example, can result from a blow to the chest that makes the head snap forward. Symptoms include headache, nausea, vomiting, sleep disturbances, depression, and loss of concentration. Unconsciousness occurs in only 10% of concussions.

Forty million people worldwide suffer concussions every year. Concussions account for 5% of the nearly 225,000 sports injuries occurring in the United States each year. They are most common in football, hockey, skiing, wrestling, rugby, basketball, and soccer. The incidence is higher in men than in women, but women are at greater risk when playing the same sport—for example, soccer. Concussions and their neurodegenerative fallouts also occur in soldiers and, generally, in people of all ages and careers if they have a fall or sustain an injury in a motor vehicle crash.

Although the National Football League continues to downplay the risk of injury in football, researchers and journalists have documented that repeated concussions in childhood sports can cause progressive damage to the brain.

Can we predict brain injuries before they become fatal? Researchers are working to predict injury risk—both of MTBI in the moment it happens and of CTE as it develops. For example, bioengineers at Stanford University outfitted athletes with mouth guards that monitored symptoms of MTBI and recorded more than 500 moments of impact during regular sporting events. This is especially significant because athletes often fail to recognize—let alone report—that they have suffered an injury. Because sustaining a second injury shortly after the first can result in much greater damage, an instantaneous indication of concussion should require medical professionals to pull a player to the sidelines.

What can individuals do to reduce their risk of concussion? Always wear a helmet when cycling, skiing, snowboarding, rock climbing, or skateboarding. Wearing seat belts and ensuring that car airbags are functioning properly can also help. Older adults can reduce their risk of concussions by keeping living spaces free of clutter, wearing stable footwear, and maintaining strength and balance through regular exercise.

Preventing concussions in contact sports is more challenging. The pre-participation physical examination can identify athletes with a history of concussion and assess their readiness to compete. Helmets in sports like football and hockey protect the skull from impact injuries (fractures and lacerations) but have little effect on the incidence or severity of concussions. Coaching fundamentals can teach athletes to avoid dangerous techniques such as spear blocking and tackling but do little to change the nature of high-impact collision sports. Professional officiating can cut down on dangerous play. Rule changes such as eliminating zone coverage in football or heading in soccer might reduce the concussion rate. Recognizing concussion injuries is important for preventing long-term disability. Finally, education can teach athletes about the symptoms and seriousness of concussions.

SOURCES: Daneshvar, D. H., et al. 2013. *Clinics in Sports Medicine*. 30(1): 1–17; Gregory, S. 2016. The NFL still won't tackle brain trauma at the Super Bowl. *Time*, February 6 (http://time.com/4210564/nfl-super-bowl-brain-trauma-cte/); Harmon, K. G., et al. 2013. American Medical Society for Sports Medicine Position Statement: Concussion in sport. *British Journal of Sports Medicine* 47(1): 15–26; Hernandez, F., et al. 2015. Six degree-of-freedom measurements of human mild traumatic brain injury. *Annals of Biomedical Engineering* 43(8): 1918–1934; McCarthy, M. 2016. Chronic traumatic encephalopathy is reported in 25 year old former American football player. *British Medical Journal* 352: 7027; Misra, A. 2014. Common sports injuries: Incidence and average charges. *ASPE Issue Brief*, March 17 (https://aspe.hhs.gov/pdf-report/common-sports-injuries-incidence-and-average-charges).

- *Wind.* Sustained winds as slow as 30 mph can make it difficult or impossible to walk or stand. In severe hurricanes and tornadoes, sustained winds near the storm's center can blow at speeds faster than 200 mph—strong enough to sweep a house off its foundation. In extremely windy conditions, take cover in a sturdy shelter, preferably a permanent structure with a foundation. In a severe storm such as a tornado, move to the lowest portion of the building or to a small interior room away from windows. If you're outdoors when a severe storm or tornado strikes, lie flat in a low spot or ditch. Don't stay inside a car or hide under an open-sided structure such as a bridge; such structures can act as a funnel and intensify the wind.

- *Lightning.* About 400 Americans are struck by lightning every year, and about 10% of them die. Lightning can strike even when it's not raining, and it often strikes with no warning. If you hear thunder, you are close enough to the lightning's source to be struck. The National Weather Service recommends that you go indoors when conditions are right for lightning. You are safer in a house, as long as you avoid anything that conducts electricity, including corded telephones, electrical appliances, computers, plumbing, and metal doors and windows. If you are not near a building, the next best option is a car. If there is no shelter, stay low, such as in a ditch, and avoid bodies of water. Tents or pavilions should be avoided.

- *Flooding.* Stay away from rapidly rising or moving water; it can carry you away in an instant. Even fairly shallow water can sweep away a car if the current is fast enough. If you're near rapidly rising water, move to higher ground and call for help. Don't attempt to drive or walk through flooded streets, and don't traverse a bridge if it is being pounded by high, fast-moving water. During heavy rain, stay alert for flash flood warnings and be ready to evacuate if necessary.

Work Injuries

Since 1912, when industrial records were first kept in the United States, the worksite has become a much safer place, as evidenced by a nearly 90% reduction in the unintentional death rate there. That figure becomes even more impressive when you realize that the size of the labor force has more than doubled and production has increased more than 10-fold in the same time period. A significant factor that accounts for the marked decline in **work injuries** has been the Occupational Safety and Health Act of 1970. As a result of that act, the Occupational Safety and Health Administration (OSHA) was created within the U.S. Department of Labor to ensure a safer and healthier environment for workers.

The Bureau of Labor Statistics estimates that in 2018 there were over 2.8 million nonfatal workplace injuries and illnesses; of these, 1.6 million cases resulted in days away from work, job transfer, or a job restriction. Although people who do extensive manual labor and lifting on the job make up less than half the workforce, they account for more than 75% of all work-related injuries and illnesses. Skin disorders are the most commonly reported occupational illnesses; the introduction of more hazardous chemicals at the worksite means that these disorders are of increasing concern.

Nonfatal injuries and illnesses in the workplace remained the same from 2017, although the number of fatalities rose. Transportation incidents accounted for the largest number of deaths, followed by slips and falls. Opioid fatalities also increased in 2017 and have increased by at least 25% annually since 2013. Other fatalities on the job involve crushing injuries, severe lacerations, burns, and electrocutions.

Back Injuries   Back problems account for hundreds of thousands of work injuries each year, although it is estimated

that twice as many workers experience some kind of minor back injury each year. According to the Bureau of Labor Statistics, back injuries account for almost one of five workplace injuries or illnesses. Many back injuries that occur on the job could be prevented through the use of proper lifting techniques:

- Bend at the knees and hips, not at the waist. Remain in an upright position and crouch down if you need to lower yourself to grasp the object.

- Place feet securely about shoulder-width apart; grip the object firmly.

- Lift gradually, with straight arms. Avoid quick, jerky motions. Lift by standing up or pushing with your leg muscles. Keep the object close to your body.

- If you have to turn, change the position of your feet. Twisting is a common and dangerous cause of injury. Plan ahead so that your pathway is clear and turning can be minimized.

Put the object down gently, reversing the steps for lifting.

Repetitive Strain Injuries   Musculoskeletal injuries and disorders in the workplace include **repetitive strain injuries (RSIs).** RSIs are caused by repeated strain on a particular part of the body. Twisting, vibrations, awkward postures, and other stressors may contribute to RSIs. **Carpal tunnel syndrome** is one type of RSI that has increased in recent years due to increased use of computers, both at work and in the home (see the box "Repetitive Strain Injury" for more information).

TERMS

work injuries   Unintentional injuries and deaths that arise out of and in the course of gainful work, such as falls, electrical shocks, exposure to radiation and toxic chemicals, burns, cuts, back sprains, and loss of fingers or other body parts in machines.

repetitive strain injury (RSI)   A musculoskeletal injury or disorder caused by repeated strain on the hand, arm, wrist, or other part of the body; also called *cumulative trauma disorder (CTD).*

carpal tunnel syndrome   Compression of the median nerve in the wrist, often caused by repetitive use of the hands, such as in computer use; characterized by numbness, tingling, and pain in the hands and fingers; can cause nerve damage.

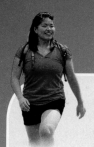

TAKE CHARGE
Repetitive Strain Injury

Repetitive strain injuries (RSIs) impact the musculoskeletal and nervous systems of the body and affect many people around the world. Other terms to describe this condition include *repetitive motion disorder (RMD), cumulative trauma disorder (CTD),* and *occupational overuse syndrome (OOS).*

An RSI can be caused by a combination of physical and psychosocial stressors, but the injury typically involves some kind of repetitive action or forceful exertion on the body over time. Pain in the extremities as well as the back and shoulders is commonly cited and tends to worsen with extended activity.

The task associated with an RSI may be something relatively simple and nonexertive like typing, writing, or clicking a computer mouse. One of the most common work-related injuries is *carpal tunnel syndrome (CTS),* which is characterized by pressure on the median nerve in the wrist that also affects tendons and ligaments in the forearm. Symptoms of CTS include numbness, tingling, burning, and/or aching in the hand, particularly in the thumb and the first three fingers. The pain may worsen at night and may shoot up from the hand as far as the shoulder. If it does not clear up on its own, immobilization of the joint at night can be helpful; other options may involve anti-inflammatory drugs or even surgery in extreme cases.

Examples of RSIs from physical activity by athletes include conditions commonly referred to as "golfer's elbow" or "tennis elbow," in which the joints are continually exposed to extreme stress in order to complete an action accurately with speed and force.

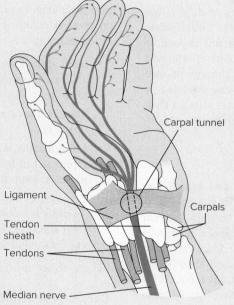

Carpal tunnel

Ligament

Tendon sheath

Carpals

Tendons

Median nerve

With new technologies being introduced every day, another type of RSI is now being recognized. Many people who use their thumbs to text suffer from a condition referred to as "texting thumb." Similarly, people who spend countless hours using handheld controls to play video games are experiencing "gamer's thumb."

In all cases, research indicates the primary risk factors are usually associated with poor posture, improper techniques for completing an activity, and overuse of a certain part of the body. The good news is that a person can make adjustments to reduce the risk of an RSI, either in what is being done or through modification of the environment. Warm up your wrists before you begin any repetitive motion activity, and take frequent breaks to stretch and flex your wrists and hands:

• Extend your arms out in front of you and stretch your wrists by pointing your fingers to the ceiling; hold for a count of five. Then straighten your wrists and relax your fingers for a count of five.

• With arms extended, make a tight fist with both hands and then bend your wrists so that your knuckles are pointed toward the floor; hold for a count of five. Then straighten your wrists and relax your fingers for a count of five.

Repeat these stretches several times, and finish by letting your arms hang loosely at your sides and shaking them gently for several seconds. It's also important to maintain a physically active lifestyle, take plenty of breaks to avoid hours of sedentary activity, stretch, apply proper ergonomic principles, and minimize other stress factors.

VIOLENCE AND INTENTIONAL INJURIES

Violence—the use of physical force with the intent to inflict harm, injury, or death upon yourself or another—is a major public health concern in the United States. According to the Federal Bureau of Investigation (FBI), 1.2 million violent crimes occurred in the United States in 2018. Examples of violence are assault, homicide, sexual assault, domestic violence, suicide, and child abuse.

Research comparing the rates of violence in countries belonging to the Organisation for Economic Co-operation and Development (OECD) shows that the United States has much higher rates of violence than other countries (as do Mexico and Estonia), with 4–10 times the homicide death rates found in economically similar countries.

Factors Contributing to Violence

Most intentional injuries and deaths are associated with an argument or a crime. However, there are many forms of violence, and no single factor can explain all of them.

Social Factors Rates of violence are not the same throughout society; they vary by geographic region, neighborhood, socioeconomic level, and many other factors. According to the FBI, violence rates were highest in the

South in 2018, followed by the West, Midwest, and Northeast regions of the country. Neighborhoods that are disadvantaged in status, power, and economic resources typically experience the most violence. In 2018, 30% of violent crimes were committed by people under 25 years old.

People who feel they are a part of society (with strong family and social ties), who are economically integrated (having a reasonable chance at getting a decent job), and who grow up in areas with a feeling of community (with good schools, parks, and neighborhoods) are significantly less likely to engage in violence. U.S. society, where more than one out of five children lives in poverty and where the gap between rich and poor keeps growing, should be expected to breed violence. In the view of many criminologists, the United States has a growing underclass of people who cannot expect to have even the worst permanent jobs. The absence of hopes and dreams, combined with family devastation and poverty, certainly contribute to violent behavior.

College campus environments can also contribute to violence. Because college campuses are transitory communities, some people may have less incentive to cooperate and coexist amicably. Some campus groups are known to promote bias toward others. For example, fraternities have been strongly associated with *pro-abuse peer support*—advice and materials that are hostile to women and espouse violence toward intimate partners. In a recent study, sorority members, who frequently associate with fraternity members, were found to be one group of women likely to experience negative peer support, as well as to associate with patriarchal and sexually abusive peers (see Table 22.3).

Violence in the Media   The mass media play a major role in exposing audiences of all ages to violence as an acceptable and effective means of solving problems. On average, children in the United States watch about four hours of television daily and may view as many as 10,000 violent acts on television and in movies each year. Computer and video games also include many violent acts, leading to concern that children's exposure to violence will make them more accepting or tolerant of it. The consequences of violence are depicted in the media much less frequently.

Researchers studying the links between TV viewing and bullying among children have found that the more hours per day a 4-year-old spent watching TV, the more likely the child was to engage in bullying behavior in later years. Factors that reduced the rate of bullying included cognitive stimulation, such as parents reading to a child, and emotional support and attention. Emotional support from parents may help children develop empathy, social competence, and self-regulation—skills that enable them to deal with peers without resorting to aggressive or bullying behavior.

Researchers have found that exposure to media violence at least temporarily increases aggressive feelings in children, making them more likely to engage in violent or fearful behavior; the direct, short-term effects on teens and adults are less clear. It makes sense for parents to be aware of the potential influence of the media on their children. A child may not clearly understand the distinctions between the fantasy world portrayed in the media and the complexities of the real world. Parents should monitor the TV shows, movies, video games, music, and other forms of media to which their children are exposed. Watching programs with children gives parents the opportunity to talk to them about violence and its consequences, to explain that violence is not the best way to resolve conflicts or solve problems, and to point out examples of positive behaviors such as kindness and cooperation.

Gender   In most cases, violence is committed by men. Males are nine times more likely than females to commit murder, and three times more likely than females to be murdered. Male college students are twice as likely as female students to be the victims of violence. As noted, some researchers have suggested that the male hormone testosterone is linked to aggressive behavior. Others point to prevailing cultural attitudes about male roles (i.e., men as dominant and controlling) as an explanation for the high rate of violence among men. However, these theories do not explain why violent men are more likely to live in the South, belong to minorities, be poor, and be young.

Women do commit acts of violence, including a small but substantial proportion of murders of spouses. This fact has been used to argue that women have the same capacity to commit violence as men, but most researchers note substantial differences. Men often kill their wives as the culmination of years of violence or after stalking them; they may kill their entire families and themselves at the same time. Women virtually never kill in such circumstances; rather, they kill their husbands after repeated victimization or while being beaten.

Table 22.3	Women at a Southern Atlantic College Most Likely to Experience Peers Who Generally Espouse Misogyny and Who Are Sexually Abusive Themselves	
ASSOCIATE WITH SEXUALLY ABUSIVE PEERS		**EXPERIENCE PRO-ABUSE PEER SUPPORT**
International students		Intercollegiate athletes
Sorority members		Sorority members
Members of social and political action coalitions		Members of social and political action coalitions

SOURCE: DeKeseredy, W. S., A. Hall-Sanchez, and J. Nolan. College campus sexual assault: The contribution of peers' proabuse informational support and attachments to abusive peers. *Violence Against Women* 24(8): 922–935.

Interpersonal Factors Although most people fear attack from strangers, the majority of victims are acquainted with their attackers. More than half of murders of women and three-fourths of sexual assaults are committed by someone the woman knows. Crime victims and violent criminals tend to share many characteristics—that is, they are likely to be young, male, from a minority group, and poor. Being a victim of teasing, bullying, or social exclusion may lead to aggressive behavior or violence.

Alcohol and Other Drugs Substance misuse and dependence are consistently associated with interpersonal violence and suicide. Intoxication affects judgment and increases aggression in some people, causing a small argument to escalate into a serious physical confrontation. On college campuses, alcohol is involved in about 95% of all violent crimes.

Firearms Many criminologists argue that the high rate of homicide in the United States is directly related to the very widespread handgun ownership and the relative ease of obtaining firearms, considering that the United States is the only industrialized country so unregulated. Whereas most victims of assaults with other weapons don't die, the death rate from assault by handgun is extremely high. The use of a handgun can change a suicide attempt to a completed suicide and a violent assault to a murder.

Assault

Assault is the use of physical force by a person or people to inflict injury or death on another. Homicide, aggravated assault, and robbery are examples of assault. Research indicates that the victims of assaultive injuries and their perpetrators tend to resemble one another in terms of ethnicity, educational background, psychological profile, and reliance on weapons.

Homicide

According to the FBI, 16,214 Americans were murdered in 2018. Men, teenagers, young adults, and members of minority groups, particularly African Americans and Latinos, are most likely to be murder victims. Although homicide rates for African Americans have declined dramatically in the past 25 years, the death rate from homicide for black males is much higher than the rate for the U.S. population as a whole (32.3 per 100,000 population for black males compared with 5.1 for the United States as a whole and 8.0 for all males). Poverty and unemployment have been identified as key factors in homicide, and these factors may account for the high rates of homicide among blacks and other minority groups.

> **QUICK STATS**
>
> **393 million guns are owned by U.S. civilians, ranking the United States first out of 178 countries in the number of privately owned guns.**
>
> —*Small Arms Survey*, 2018

Most homicides are committed with a firearm, occur during an argument, and occur among people who know one another. Intrafamilial homicide, in which the perpetrator and the victim are related, accounts for about one out of every eight homicides. About 40% of family homicides are committed by male spouses, usually following a history of physical and emotional abuse directed at the woman. Wives are more likely to be murdered than husbands, and when a wife kills her husband, it is usually in self-defense. Mass shootings receive a great deal of media coverage but represent a relatively small fraction of firearm-related deaths; 90% of homicides are single-victim incidents.

Deaths due to "legal interventions"—killings by police or other peace officers—are not technically classified as homicides. Newer methods that include such killings calculate that since 2015, about 1000 people per year lose their lives in law enforcement–related incidents. While more whites are killed by police than blacks and Hispanics, studies show that black men aged 15 to 34 are significantly more likely to be killed by police than are other people.

Gang-Related Violence

Violence results not only from acts of single individuals, as evidenced by the number of injuries and deaths resulting from gang activities. Gangs are most frequently associated with large cities, but gang activity also extends to the suburbs and even to rural areas. It is estimated that about 1.4 million Americans belong to gangs. The average age for joining a gang is 14, so 40% of gang members are younger than 18 years of age. Most gangs control a particular territory and oppose other gangs, as well as police and community efforts to eliminate them. Gangs may be involved in illegal drug trade, extortion, and protection schemes. Gang members are more likely than non–gang members to possess weapons, and violence may result from conflicts over territory or illegal activities.

Gangs are most common in areas where residents are poor and unemployment rates, population density, and crime rates are high. In these areas, young people may feel that legitimate success in life is out of reach and know that involvement in the drug market makes some gang members rich. Often gangs serve as a mechanism for companionship, self-esteem, support, and security. Indeed, gang membership may be viewed as the only possible means of survival in some areas.

Hate Crimes

When criminal acts are motivated by bias against another person's race or ethnicity, national origin, religion, sexual orientation, or disability, the offense is classified as a hate crime. Hate crimes may be committed against people or property. Those committed against people may include intimidation, assault, and even rape or murder. Crimes against property most frequently involve graffiti, the desecration of synagogues, cross burnings, and other acts of vandalism or property damage.

Over 7100 hate crimes were reported in 2018, but many go unreported. Crimes against people made up about two-thirds of all incidents, with intimidation and assault as the most common offenses. Hate crimes in 2016 and 2017 increased, and 6 in 10 victims were targeted because of their race or ethnicity. Hate crimes based on religion and ethnicity also rose, particularly against Jews and Muslims, as did hate crimes based on sexual orientation.

Hate crimes may be extremely brutal acts perpetrated at random on total strangers by multiple offenders. Suspects frequently are not identified, but research indicates that a substantial number of hate crimes are committed by males under age 20. Hate crimes are frequently associated with fringe groups that have extremist ideologies, such as the Ku Klux Klan and neo-Nazi groups. The Southern Poverty Law Center tracks hundreds of hate groups currently active in the United States; the rapid growth of hate sites on the internet is another area of concern.

A variety of factors lead to the prejudice and intolerance that are a major force behind hate crimes. The FBI has reported a substantial increase in hate-motivated crimes in the past several years, especially since the terrorist attacks of September 11, 2001. Hate crimes against lesbian, gay, bisexual, and transgender (LGBT) people have more than tripled in recent years. A social context of unemployment and hard economic times, an influx of immigrants, and the growth of visible minority rights movements have been associated with the recent increases in hate crimes in the United States.

School Violence

According to the National School Safety Center, over 450 school-associated violent deaths of students, faculty, and administrators occurred in the past decade. This figure includes homicides, suicides, and legal interventions. Most of these deaths occurred in urban areas or at high schools and involved the use of a firearm. As with other types of violence, both victims and offenders were predominantly young men. Homicide and suicide are the most serious but least common types of violence in schools; an estimated 836,000 nonfatal victimizations occurred at schools in 2018, including theft, vandalism, and assault.

How risky is the school environment? Since 2001, the rate of serious and less violent crimes at school has been higher than or about the same as away from school. Since 2009, the rates of serious violent incidents at and away from school (rape, other sexual assaults, physical attacks or fights with a weapon, threats of attack with a weapon, and robbery with or without a weapon) were not measurably different. Less than 3% of homicides of youths aged 5 to 19 occur at school. Total

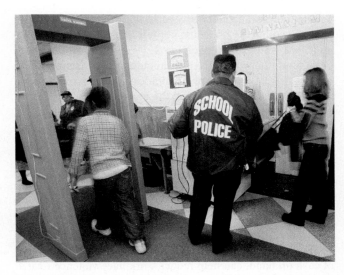

To increase safety, some high schools and middle schools (and even some elementary schools) have installed metal detectors. Dan Loh/Pool/AP Images

victimization rates for students aged 12 to 18 have declined both at school and away since 1992, and thefts and serious victimization declined both at and away from school.

Although schools are basically safe places, steps can be taken to identify at-risk youths and improve safety for all students. General characteristics of youths who have caused violent deaths in schools include the following:

- Uncontrollable angry outbursts
- Violent and abusive language and behavior
- Isolation from peers
- Depression and irritability
- Access to and preoccupation with weapons
- Lack of support and supervision from adults

Recommendations for reducing school violence include offering classroom training in anger management, social skills, and improved self-control; providing mental health and social services for students in need; developing after-school programs that help students build self-esteem and make friends; and keeping guns out of the hands of children and out of schools. Tragic school shootings over the past six years have also resulted in installation of security and surveillance systems throughout the country, as well as new protocols for entry into school buildings. But more needs to be done: in recent years, hundreds of students have been shot in more than 200 school incidents, and the numbers keep climbing.

Workplace Violence

Data show that workplace violence has decreased by 35% in the past decade. OSHA reports that nearly 2 million American workers are victims of workplace violence each year, including about 500 homicides. In about 60% of cases, workplace violence is committed by strangers;

acquaintances account for nearly 40% of cases; and intimates account for 1%. Most perpetrators of workplace violence are white males over age 21. Women's leading cause of death in the workplace is homicide. Firearms are used in nearly 80% of workplace homicides, and the majority of these homicides occur during the commission of a robbery or other crime.

Police and corrections officers have the most dangerous jobs, followed by taxi drivers, security guards, bartenders, mental health professionals, and workers at gas stations and convenience and liquor stores. According to the U.S. Department of Labor, state government workers experience more workplace violence of all types than do workers in local government or private industry.

General crime prevention strategies, including use of surveillance cameras and silent alarms and limits on the amount of cash on hand, can help reduce workplace violence related to robberies. A highly stressed workplace is a risk factor in cases of violence between acquaintances or coworkers; clear guidelines about acceptable behavior and prompt action after any threats or incidents of violence can help control this type of workplace violence.

Terrorism

In 2001, more Americans died as a result of terrorism than in any year before or since; the attacks on September 11 killed more than 3000 people, including citizens of 78 countries. But the chances of Americans dying from terrorist attacks are very, very low. The British Royal Statistical Society awarded its International Statistic of 2017 to the number 69 because it is the "annual number of Americans killed, on average, by lawnmowers—compared to two Americans killed annually, on average, by immigrant Jihadist terrorists." The FBI defines *terrorism* as the unlawful use of force or violence against people or property to intimidate or coerce a government, the civilian population, or any segment thereof in furtherance of political or social objectives. Terrorism can be domestic, carried out by groups based in the United States, or international. It comes in many forms, including biological, chemical, nuclear, and cyber. Its intent is to promote helplessness by instilling fear of harm or destruction.

Terrorism-prevention activities occur at all levels of government. U.S. government efforts include close work with the diplomatic, law enforcement, intelligence, economic, and military communities. The mission of the U.S. Department of Homeland Security is to help prevent, protect against, and respond to acts of terrorism on U.S. territory. It coordinates efforts to protect electric and water supply systems, transportation, gas and oil supplies, emergency services, computer infrastructure, and other systems.

> **intimate-partner violence (IPV)** Physical, sexual, or psychological harm by a current or former partner or spouse.
>
> **TERMS**

Do you have a role in preventing terrorism? You can be proactive by reporting anything you see or hear that is suspicious or threatening. You can also take personal responsibility and not let fear of terrorism immobilize or impede your ability to act.

Family and Intimate-Partner Violence

Violence in families challenges some of our most basic assumptions. *Family violence* generally refers to any illegitimate use of physical force, aggression, or verbal abuse by one family member toward another. Once referred to as domestic violence, the term **intimate-partner violence (IPV)** is now used to describe physical, sexual, or psychological harm imposed by a current or former partner or spouse. IPV consists of physical and sexual violence, stalking, and psychological aggression (like verbal abuse). IPV is widespread. An estimated 8.5 million women and 4 million men are victimized by an intimate partner in their lifetime. Child abuse consists of physical, sexual, or emotional abuse or neglect; an estimated one in four children experience some form of abuse or neglect in their lifetime. Nearly five children die every day as a result of abuse and neglect.

Battering Battery refers to harmful contact made without consent against another person. Studies reveal that over 85% of intimate-partner violence victims are women; 20–35% of women who visit emergency departments are there for injuries related to ongoing abuse. Of all women murdered in the United States each year, about one-third are killed by an intimate partner. Violence against wives or intimate partners as a result of battering occurs at every level of society, although it is more common at lower socioeconomic levels. It occurs more frequently in relationships with a high degree of conflict—an apparent inability to resolve arguments through negotiation and compromise. Almost 30% of women report having been physically assaulted or raped by an intimate partner, and more than 50% report having experienced some type of abuse—physical or psychological—in a relationship. In more than 10% of cases, the violence continues for 20 years or longer. The problem of intimate violence is apparent even among high school students. Among the students who had begun dating, 8% reported having been physically abused or hurt on purpose.

The need to control another person is at the root of much of abusive behavior. Abusive partners (in most cases a man) are controlling partners. Abuse includes behavior that physically harms, arouses fear, prevents a person from doing what she wants, or compels her to behave in ways she does not freely choose. Controlling people can use a variety of psychological, emotional, and physical tactics to keep their partners tied to them. Early in a relationship, a person's tendency to be controlling may not be obvious (see the box "Recognizing the Potential for Abusiveness in a Partner (or Yourself)").

In abusive relationships, the abuser often has a history of violent behavior, traditional beliefs about gender roles, and problems with alcohol abuse. Having low self-esteem and taking credit for others' achievements are common. Studies have suggested a three-phase cycle of battering, consisting of a

Recognizing the Potential for Abusiveness in a Partner (or Yourself)

There are no sure ways to tell whether someone will become abusive or violent toward an intimate partner, but you can look for warning signs. Remember that, although most abusive relationships involve male violence directed at a woman, women can also be abusive, as can partners in a same-sex relationship. Because most abusers are male, the following material refers to the abuser as "he." If you are concerned that a person you are involved with has the potential for violence, observe his or her behavior, and ask yourself these questions:

• What is this person's attitude toward women? How does he treat his mother and his sister? How does he work with female students, female colleagues, or a female boss? How does he treat your women friends?

• What is his attitude toward your autonomy? Does he respect the work you do and the way you do it? Or does he mock it, tell you how to do it better, or encourage you to give it up? Does he tell you he'll take care of you?

• How self-centered is he? Does he want to spend leisure time on your interests or his? Does he listen to you? Does he remember what you say?

• Is he possessive or jealous? Does he want to spend every minute with you? Does he cross-examine you about things you do when you're not with him?

• What happens when things don't go the way he wants them to? Does he blow up? Does he always have to get his way?

• Is he moody, mocking, critical, or bossy? Do you feel as if you're walking on eggshells when you're with him?

• Do you feel you have to avoid arguing with him?

• Does he drink too much or use drugs?

• Does he refuse to use condoms or take other precautions for safer sex?

Listen to your own uneasiness, and stay away from any man who disrespects women, who wants or needs you intensely and exclusively, and who has a knack for getting his own way almost all the time.

If you are in a serious relationship with a controlling person, you may already have experienced abuse. (If you have put your partner in any of these situations, you are likely an abuser.) Consider the following questions:

• Does your partner constantly criticize you, blame you for things that are not your fault, or verbally degrade you?

• Does he humiliate you in front of others?

• Is he suspicious or jealous? Does he accuse you of being unfaithful or monitor your mail or phone calls?

• Does he track all your time? Does he discourage you from seeing friends and family?

• Does he prevent you from getting or keeping a job or attending school? Does he control your shared resources or restrict your access to money?

• Has he ever pushed, pulled, slapped, hit, kicked, bitten, or restrained you? Thrown an object at you? Used a weapon on you or pointed one at you?

• Has he ever destroyed or damaged your personal property or sentimental items, or threatened to do so?

• Has he ever forced you to have sex or to do something sexually you didn't want to do?

• Does he anger easily when drinking or taking drugs?

• Has he ever threatened to harm you or your children, friends, pets, or property?

• Has he ever threatened to blackmail you if you leave?

If you answered yes to one or more of these questions, you may be experiencing intimate-partner violence. (If you have seen any of these behaviors in yourself, seek immediate help to stop these behaviors.) If you believe you or your children are in imminent danger, look in your local telephone directory for a women's shelter, or call 911. If you want information, referrals to a program in your area, or assistance, contact one of the organizations listed in the For More Information section at the end of the chapter.

---

period of increasing tension, a violent explosion and loss of control, and a period of contrition and seeking forgiveness and promises that it will never happen again. The batterer is drawn back to this cycle over and over again but rarely achieves a change in behavior.

Battered women often stay in violent relationships for years. They may be economically dependent on their partners, feel trapped or fear retaliation if they leave, believe their children need a father, or suffer low self-esteem themselves. They may love or pity their partner, or they may believe they'll eventually be able to stop the violence. They often leave the relationship when they finally resolve their own ambiguous feelings.

Battered women's shelters offer physical protection, counseling, support, and other assistance.

Stalking and Cyberstalking   **Stalking** is a crime under laws of all 50 states, the District of Columbia, the U.S.

> **stalking**   Repeatedly harassing or threatening a person through behaviors such as following a person, appearing at a person's residence or workplace, leaving written messages or objects, making harassing phone calls, or vandalizing property; frequently directed at a former intimate partner.   **TERMS**

territories, and the federal government. Battering is closely associated with stalking, characterized by harassing behaviors such as following or spying on a person and making written, or implied threats.

In the United States, it is estimated that 1 in 6 women and 1 in 19 men are stalked each year; about two-thirds of stalkers are men. About three of four female victims are stalked by current or former intimate partners; of these, over two-thirds had been physically or sexually assaulted by that partner during the relationship. Weapons are used to threaten or harm victims in one out of five cases.

STALKING FEMALE COLLEGE STUDENTS Data indicate that the 18–24 age group experiences the highest rate of stalking and that stalking of female college students may be greater than that experienced by the general population. A stalker's goal may be to control or scare the victim or to keep her or him in a relationship. Most stalking episodes last a year or less.

The use of the internet, email, chat rooms, Facebook, Instagram, and other electronic means to stalk another person is known as **cyberstalking.** As with offline stalking, the majority of cyberstalkers are men, and the majority of victims are women, although there have been same-sex cyberstalking incidents. Although many cases are not reported, the U.S. Department of Justice estimates that about 900,000 people each year experience cyberstalking in which some kind of technology was used, like GPS or another form of electronic monitoring to track the victims. As the seriousness of the crime is being recognized, several states have passed cyberstalking or related laws, and a federal law is under consideration. The impersonal nature of electronic communication may lower the barriers to harassment and threats, making cyberstalking more common. The popularity of social networking and online dating sites may also increase cyberstalking, especially because new technologies can allow a stalker to be located anywhere in the world.

Cyberstalkers may send harassing or threatening messages to the victim, or they may encourage others to harass the victim—for example, by impersonating the victim and posting inflammatory messages and personal information on bulletin boards or in chat rooms. Guidelines for staying safe online include the following:

- Avoid using your real name on the internet. Select an age- and gender-neutral identity.

- Avoid filling out profiles for accounts with information that could be used to identify you.

- Do not share personal information in public spaces anywhere online or give it to strangers.

- Learn how to filter unwanted email messages.

- Always use unique passwords that contain many characters—preferably an alphanumeric combination to make it more difficult for someone to hack into your account.

- If you use a social networking site, set your profile to "private" if that is an option.

- If you experience harassment online, do not respond to the harasser. Log off or go to a different site. If harassment continues, contact the harasser's internet service provider (ISP) by identifying the domain of the stalker's account (after the "@" sign); most ISPs have an email address for complaints. Often an ISP can try to stop the conduct by direct contact with the harasser or by closing his or her account. Save all communications for evidence, and contact your ISP and your local police department. Many states have laws against cyberstalking.

Violence against Children Violence is also directed against children. In 2018, an estimated 678,000 children were abused or neglected in the United States. About 3.5 million children received preventive services from Child Protective Services.

Parents who abuse children tend to have low self-esteem, to believe in physical punishment, to have a poor marital relationship, and to have been abused themselves (although many people who were abused as children do not grow up to abuse their own children). Poverty, unemployment, and social isolation are characteristics of families in which children are abused. External stressors related to socioeconomic and environmental factors are most closely associated with neglect, whereas stressors related to interpersonal issues are more closely associated with physical abuse. Single parents, both men and women, are at especially high risk for abusing their children. Very often one child, whom the parents consider different in some way, is singled out for violent treatment.

When government agencies intervene in child abuse situations, their goals are to protect the victims and to assist and strengthen the families. Successful programs emphasize education and early intervention, such as home visits to high-risk first-time mothers. Educational efforts focus on stress management, money management, job-finding skills, and information

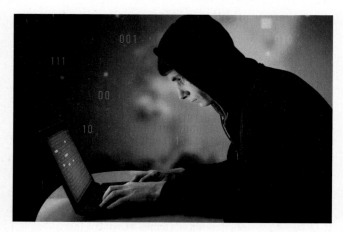

Set your social media profiles to "private." Artem Oleshko/Shutterstock

> **cyberstalking** The use of email, chat rooms, bulletin boards, or other electronic communication devices to stalk another person.

TERMS

about child behavior and development. Parents may receive counseling and be referred to substance abuse treatment programs. Support groups like Parents Anonymous are effective for parents committed to changing their behavior. Education, counseling, and support can help the victims of family violence.

Elder Abuse   Each year over 4 million older adults are abused, exploited, or mistreated by someone who is supposed to be giving them care and protection; only 1 in 24 incidents is reported. Most abusers are family members who are serving as caregivers.

Elder abuse can take different forms: physical, sexual, or emotional abuse; financial exploitation; neglect; or abandonment. Neglect accounts for about three out of five reported cases. Elders who have lost some mental or physical functions and must rely on others for care are most at risk and may suffer malnutrition, dehydration, mismanaged medication, or infection due to poor hygiene. Physical abuse accounts for about one out of six reported cases, and financial exploitation for about one out of eight reported cases. Experts also cite a growing concern about self-neglect among the elderly population. Self-neglect includes behavior that threatens a person's own health or safety and can include refusing to comply with doctors' orders or neglecting to eat a balanced diet.

Abuse often occurs when caring for a dependent adult becomes too stressful for the caregiver, especially if the elder is incontinent, shows mental deterioration, or is violent. Abuse may become an outlet for frustration. Many observers believe that the solution to elder abuse is support for both the elder and caregiver in the form of greater social and financial assistance, such as adult day care centers and education and public care programs.

Sexual Violence

The use of force and coercion in sexual interactions is one of the most serious problems in human relationships. The most extreme manifestation of sexual coercion—forcing a person to submit to another's sexual desires—is rape, but sexual coercion occurs in many subtler forms, including sexual harassment (see the box "The #MeToo Movement and Sexual Harassment").

Sexual Assault: Rape   **Sexual assault** is any unwanted sexual contact, including fondling and molestation. Rape is one type of sexual assault. Removing the term *forcible* from the offense name, the FBI redefined **rape** in 2013 as "penetration, no matter how slight, of the vagina or anus with any body part or object, or oral penetration by a sex organ of another person, without consent of the victim." When the victim is younger than the legally defined age of consent, the act constitutes **statutory rape,** whether or not coercion is involved. Coerced sexual activity in which the victim knows or is dating the rapist is often referred to as **date rape,** or *acquaintance rape.*

Most victims know their assailants, but fewer than 40% of all sexual crimes are reported.

Any woman—or man—can be a rape victim. Over 200,000 cases of rape are reported each year. An estimated 500,000 more women than men are raped each year, but those incidents are unreported. Research shows that 1 in 5 women and 1 in 71 men have experienced an attempted or completed rape. A study of college students also found that 1 in 5 college women experience a completed or attempted rape during their college years. Rape is the most underreported crime, and over 90% of sexual assault victims on college campuses do not report the crime. Most male-on-male rapes do not occur in prison.

WHO RAPES?   Men who commit rape may be any age and come from any socioeconomic group. Some rapists are exploiters in the sense that they rape on the spur of the moment and mainly want immediate gratification. Some attempt to compensate for feelings of sexual inadequacy and an inability to obtain satisfaction otherwise. Others are more hostile and sadistic and are primarily interested in hurting and humiliating a particular woman or women in general. Often the rapist is more interested in dominance, control, and power than in sexual satisfaction.

Most women are in much less danger of being raped by a stranger than of being sexually assaulted by a man they know or date. Surveys suggest that as many as 25% of women have had experiences in which the men they were dating persisted in trying to force sex despite the women's pleading, crying, screaming, or resisting. Surveys have also found that more than 60% of all rape victims were raped by a current or former spouse, boyfriend, or date.

Most cases of date rape are never reported to the police, partly because of the subtlety of the crime. Usually no weapons are involved, and direct verbal threats may not have been made. Rather than being terrorized, the victim usually is attracted to the man at first. Victims of date rape tend to shoulder much of the responsibility for the incident, questioning their own judgment and behavior rather than blaming the aggressor.

Strong evidence suggests that 15% of American women who have ever married have been raped by their husbands or ex-husbands; as many as 60% of battered women may have been raped by their husbands. A charge of spousal rape can now be taken to court in all states.

FACTORS CONTRIBUTING TO DATE RAPE   Although the general status of women in society has improved, the belief that

TERMS

sexual assault   Any unwanted sexual contact.

rape   Unwanted penetration—oral, anal, or vaginal.

statutory rape   Sexual interaction with someone under the legal age of consent.

date rape   Sexual assault by someone the victim knows or is dating; also called *acquaintance rape.*

The #MeToo movement against sexual harassment began in 2017 in the wake of sexual harassment, assault, and rape allegations against movie producer Harvey Weinstein. Using the hashtag #MeToo on social media websites, the campaign encourages people to share stories of sexual abuse and misconduct perpetrated against them in order to demonstrate the magnitude of the problem. Beginning with Hollywood celebrities, the movement's popularity has spread to the media, music, and technology industries, scientific fields, academia, politics, and some churches, resulting in the firing of numerous accused men in positions of power.

Although sexual harassment is forbidden by law, many cases go unreported. In a survey of 17,000 federal employees, 42% of women and 15% of men reported having been sexually harassed. If you are unsure what harassment is and whether you might be doing it, here are a few tips: Offer genuine compliments, but not about a person's body. Make conversation and jokes, but not those of a sexual nature. Greet others in a friendly way, not by whistling and leering. Be a kind, caring friend, coworker, or person; don't pat, rub, or touch someone without permission. Pursue friendships and romantic relationships, but not after the first one or two requests are turned down.

If you have been the victim of sexual harassment, you can take action to stop it. Be assertive with anyone who uses language or actions you find inappropriate. If possible, confront your harasser and tell him or her that the situation is unacceptable to you and you want the harassment to stop. Be clear. "Do not *ever* make sexual remarks to me" is an unequivocal statement. If assertive communication doesn't work, assemble a file or log documenting the harassment, noting the details of each incident and information about any witnesses who may be able to support your claims. You may discover others who have been harassed by the same person, which will strengthen your case. Then file a grievance with the harasser's supervisor or employer, such as someone in the dean's office if you are a student, or someone in the human resources office if you are an employee.

If your attempts to deal with the harassment internally are not successful, you can file an official complaint with your city or state Human Rights Commission or Fair Employment Practices Agency, or with the federal Equal Employment Opportunity Commission. You may also wish to pursue legal action under the Civil Rights Act or under local laws prohibiting employment discrimination. Often the threat of a lawsuit or other legal action is enough to stop the harasser.

nice women don't say yes to sex (even when they want to) and that real men don't take no for an answer is still prevalent among some groups.

Men and women also differ in their perception of romantic encounters and signals. In one study, researchers found that men interpreted women's actions on dates, such as smiling or talking in a low voice, as indicating an interest in having sex, whereas the women interpreted the same actions as being friendly.

Men who rape their dates tend to have certain attributes, including hostility toward women, a belief that dominance alone is a valid motive for sex, and an acceptance of sexual violence. They may feel that force is justified in certain circumstances, such as if they are sexually involved with a woman and she refuses to have sex, if the woman is known to have had sex with other men, or if the woman shows up at a party where people are drinking and taking drugs. The man often primes himself to force himself sexually on his date by drinking, which lowers his ordinary social inhibitions. Many college men who have committed date rape tried to seduce their dates by plying them with alcohol first.

DATE-RAPE DRUGS Studies have shown that drugs are a factor in more than 60% of sexual assaults. The most common form of drug-facilitated sexual assault (DFSA) is alcohol, where the victim consumes alcohol voluntarily and reaches a state of intoxication. An estimated 85% of sexual assaults among college students involve alcohol or other drugs.

About 5% of DFSA victims are given date-rape drugs. Also called predator drugs, the drugs include flunitrazepam (Rohypnol), gamma hydroxybutyrate (GHB), and ketamine ("Special K"). Rohypnol is not legal in the United States, but ketamine and GHB can be obtained legally because they are used for legitimate medical purposes.

These drugs have a variety of effects, including sedation; if slipped surreptitiously into a drink, they can incapacitate a person within about 20 minutes and make her or him more vulnerable to assault. Rohypnol, GHB, and other drugs also often cause anterograde amnesia, meaning victims have little memory of what happened while they were under the influence of the drug. (See Chapter 10 for more about the effects of these and other psychoactive drugs.)

The Drug-Induced Rape Prevention and Punishment Act of 1996 adds up to 20 years to the prison sentence of any rapist who uses a drug to incapacitate a victim. Supporters of the law likened dropping a drug in a victim's drink to putting a knife to her throat. The makers of Rohypnol are modifying the pills so that they will be a more noticeable color and will dissolve more slowly, thereby reducing the likelihood that Rohypnol can be used as a date-rape drug; however, other drugs in powdered or liquid form can be slipped into drinks unnoticed. Strategies such as the following can help ensure that your drink is not tampered with at a bar or party:

- Check with campus or local police to find out if drug-facilitated sexual assault has occurred in your area and, if so, where.

- Drink moderately and responsibly. Avoid group drinking and drinking games.

- Be wary of opened beverages—alcoholic or nonalcoholic—offered by strangers. When at an unfamiliar bar, watch the bartender pour your drink.

- Let your date be the first to drink from the punch bowl at a bar, club, or rave.

- If an opened beverage tastes, looks, or smells strange, do not drink it. If you leave your drink unattended, such as when you dance or use the restroom, get a fresh drink when you return to your table. Also, finish your food before leaving it unattended at the table.

- If you go to a party, club, or bar, go with friends. Arrange to arrive and leave together. Have a prearranged plan for checking on each other visually and verbally. If you feel giddy or lightheaded, get assistance.

Both males and females can take actions that will reduce the incidence of acquaintance rape.

DEALING WITH A SEXUAL ASSAULT Experts disagree about whether a woman who is faced with a rapist should fight back or give in quietly to avoid being injured or to gain time in the hope of escaping. Some rapists say that if a woman had screamed or resisted loudly, they would have run; others report they would have injured or killed her. (If a rapist is carrying a weapon, most experts advise against fighting unless absolutely necessary.) A woman who is raped by a stranger is more likely to be physically injured than a woman raped by someone she knows. Each situation is unique, and a woman should respond in whatever way she thinks best.

If you are threatened by a rapist and decide to fight back, here is what Women Organized Against Rape (WOAR) recommends:

- Trust your gut feeling. If you feel you are in danger, don't hesitate to run and scream. It is better to feel foolish than to be raped.

- Yell—and keep yelling. It will clear your head and start your adrenaline going; it may scare your attacker and also bring help. Don't forget that a rapist is also afraid of pain and afraid of getting caught.

- If an attacker grabs you from behind, use your elbows for striking his neck, his sides, or his stomach.

- Try kicking. Your legs are the strongest part of your body, and your kick is longer than his reach. Kick with the foot that is farther back and with the toe of your shoe. Aim low to avoid losing your balance.

- His most vulnerable spot is his knee; it's low, difficult to protect, and easily knocked out of place. Don't try to kick a rapist in the crotch; he has been protecting this area all his life and will have better protective reflexes there than at his knees.

- Once you start fighting, keep it up. Your objective is to get away as soon as you can.

- Remember that ordinary rules of behavior don't apply. It's OK to vomit, act crazy, or claim to have a sexually transmitted infection.

If you are raped, tell the first friendly person you meet what happened. Call the police, tell them you were raped, and give your location. Try to remember as many facts as you can about your attacker; write down a description as soon as possible. Don't wash or change your clothes, or you may destroy important evidence. The police will take you to a hospital for a complete exam; show the physician any injuries. Tell the police simply, but exactly, what happened. Be honest, and stick to your story.

If you decide that you don't want to report the rape to the police, be sure to see a physician as soon as possible. You need to be checked for pregnancy and sexually transmitted infections.

THE EFFECTS OF RAPE Rape victims suffer both physical and psychological injury. For most, physical wounds heal within a few weeks. Psychological pain may endure and be substantial. Even the most physically and mentally strong are likely to experience shock, anxiety, depression, shame, and a host of psychosomatic symptoms after being victimized. These psychological reactions following rape constitute rape trauma syndrome, which is characterized by fear, nightmares, fatigue, crying spells, and digestive upset. (Rape trauma syndrome is a form of posttraumatic stress disorder; see Chapter 3.) Self-blame is very likely; society has contributed to this tendency by perpetuating the myths that women can actually defend themselves and that no one can be raped if she doesn't want to be. Fortunately these false beliefs are dissolving in the face of evidence to the contrary.

Many organizations offer counseling and support to rape victims. Look in the telephone directory under Rape or Rape Crisis Center for a hotline number to call. Your campus may have counseling services or a support group.

Child Sexual Abuse Child sexual abuse is any sexual contact between an adult and a child who is below the legal age of consent. Adults and older adolescents are able to coerce children into sexual activity because of their authority and power over them. Threats, force, or the promise of friendship or material rewards may be used to manipulate a child. Sexual contacts are typically brief and consist of genital manipulation; genital intercourse is much less common.

Sexual abusers are usually male, heterosexual, and known to the victim. The abuser may be a relative, a friend, a neighbor, or another trusted adult acquaintance. Child abusers are often pedophiles, people who are sexually attracted to children. They may have poor interpersonal and sexual relationships with other adults and feel socially inadequate and inferior.

One highly traumatic form of sexual abuse is **incest**: sexual activity between people too closely related to legally marry. The most common forms of incest are father-daughter (which includes stepfather-stepdaughter) abuse, brother-sister abuse (usually an adolescent boy abusing a preadolescent girl), and uncle-niece abuse; mother-son sexual activity is rare. Adults who commit incest may be pedophiles, but

incest Sexual activity between close relatives, such as siblings or parents and their children. TERMS

often they are simply sexual opportunists or people with poor impulse control and emotional problems.

Most sexually abused children are between ages 8 and 12 when the abuse first occurs. More girls are sexually abused than boys. The degree of trauma for the child can be very serious, but it varies with the type of encounters, their frequency, the child's age and relationship to the abuser, and the parents' response. Father–daughter abuse may be the most traumatic form, in part because it is a violation of the basic parent–child relationship and because the abuse tends to be more frequent. Abused children may be depressed or moody, exhibit hyperactivity, play violently with others or with inanimate objects, talk nonsense, or intentionally injure themselves.

Child sexual abuse is often unreported. Surveys suggest that as many as 27% of women and 16% of men were sexually abused as children. An estimated 150,000–200,000 new cases of child sexual abuse occur each year. It can leave lasting scars; victims are more likely to suffer as adults from low self-esteem, depression, anxiety, eating disorders, self-destructive tendencies, sexual problems, and difficulties in intimate relationships.

If you were a victim of sexual abuse as a child and feel it may be interfering with your functioning today, you may want to address the problem. A variety of approaches can help, such as joining a support group of people who have had similar experiences, confiding in a partner or friend, or seeking professional help.

Sexual Harassment Unwelcome sexual advances, requests for sexual favors, and other verbal, visual, or physical conduct of a sexual nature constitute **sexual harassment** if such conduct explicitly or implicitly does any of the following:

- Affects academic or employment decisions or evaluations
- Interferes with an individual's academic or work performance
- Creates an intimidating, hostile, or offensive academic, work, or student living environment

Extreme cases of sexual harassment occur when a manager, a professor, or another person in authority uses his or her ability to control or influence jobs or grades to coerce people into having sex or to punish them if they refuse. A hostile environment can be created by conduct such as sexual gestures, display of sexually suggestive objects or pictures, derogatory comments and jokes, sexual remarks about clothing or appearance, obscene letters, and unnecessary touching or pinching. Sexual harassment can occur between people of the same or opposite sex.

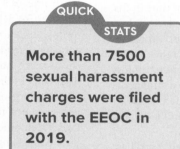

QUICK STATS

More than 7500 sexual harassment charges were filed with the EEOC in 2019.

—U.S. Equal Employment Opportunity Commission, 2019

> **sexual harassment** Unwelcome sexual advances, requests for sexual favors, and other conduct of a sexual nature that affects academic or employment decisions or evaluations; interferes with an individual's academic or work performance; or creates an intimidating, hostile, or offensive academic, work, or student living environment.
>
> **TERMS**

What You Can Do about Violence

Violence in our society is a serious threat to our collective health and well-being. This is especially true on college campuses, which in a sense are communities in themselves but sometimes lack the authority or guidance to tackle the issue of violence directly (see the box "Gun Violence"). Schools are now providing training for conflict resolution and are educating people about the diverse nature of our society, thereby encouraging tolerance and understanding. New programs are being developed at the grassroots level to deal with problems of violence directly.

As with any public health problem, one potential approach is to identify and target high-risk groups for intervention. Violence prevention programs currently focus on conflict resolution training and the development of social skills. These measures have proven effective; but for behavior change to be lasting, the focus of such programs must expand beyond individual intervention to include social and environmental factors.

Reducing gun-related injuries may require changes in the availability, possession, and lethality of the 10–14 million firearms sold legally in the United States each year with the appropriate supporting documentation. As part of the Brady gun control law, computerized instant background checks are performed for about 60% of gun sales (those by federally licensed dealers) to prevent purchases by convicted felons, people with a history of mental instability, and certain other groups. In some states, waiting periods are required in addition to the background checks. Some

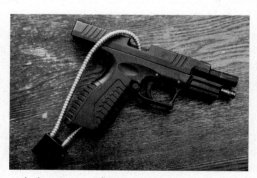

Using a gun lock can prevent firearm accidents. Tippman98x/Shutterstock

Ask Yourself

QUESTIONS FOR CRITICAL THINKING AND REFLECTION

Are you or is anyone you know a survivor of a violent act? If so, what were the circumstances surrounding the event? What was the outcome? How did the event affect your life or the life of the person you know?

When Americans face health threats like a virus or disease, our health care providers take immediate action to control the epidemic. Should we take a similar approach to gun violence?

Statistics on gun violence are grim. Each year in the United States, the use of firearms takes the lives of over 36,000 people (including suicides) and injures almost 28,000 more. It disproportionately affects young people, particularly males, and socially disadvantaged groups. Gun violence is a uniquely American problem. Making up only 5% of the world population, Americans nevertheless own 42% of privately held guns. In the United States there are more guns than people.

Should gun violence be viewed as any other contagion that can spread and endanger life? Special interest groups like the National Rifle Association have lobbied hard to prevent a public health approach. In 1997 Congress passed the Dickey Amendment, which prohibits government-sponsored health institutions from using funds to "advocate or promote gun control." Gun violence has not been seriously funded or studied as a public health threat for over 20 years. In 2016, over 140 medical institutions signed a letter to Congress urging it to lift restrictions on funding for gun violence research.

The American Public Health Association (APHA) suggests we need better surveillance and data reporting. Currently, the best database tracking system for gun-related deaths is the CDC's National Violent Death Reporting System. Because the process is voluntary and expensive, only 32 states currently report data.

One consistent theme that emerges from the limited research in this country and from research abroad is that more firearms and more permissive laws are associated with more gun-related deaths, whereas fewer guns and more restrictive laws are associated with fewer gun fatalities. In states such as New York, New Jersey, and Rhode Island, where gun ownership was 5–10% in 2013, there were roughly 5 gun deaths per 100,000 residents. By contrast, states such as Idaho, Arkansas, and West Virginia had a gun ownership rate of 55–60% and a gun death rate of around 15 per 100,000 residents.

The AHPA calls for "common sense" gun laws:

- Universal background checks for all, including purchasers online or at gun shows

- The reinstatement of the federal ban on high-powered assault rifles, which expired in 2004

- Expanded access to mental health services. It's important to note, however, that people with mental illnesses are more likely to be victims of gun violence, not perpetrators

- Expanded resources for school and community prevention strategies

- Greater investment in gun safety technologies

Since the 2012 shootings at Sandy Hook Elementary School in Connecticut, when 6 adults and 20 young children were killed by a 20-year-old gunman, a movement of young activists started to take shape. The #neveragain movement has blossomed as mass shootings continue to take out high school and college students, and politicians continue to listen to gun lobbyists. A poll by Harvard University's Institute of Politics shows that two-thirds of American voters under age 30 support stricter gun-control laws. They are marching, protesting, speaking up, and may be shifting the debate.

SOURCES: Alter, C. 2018. 'We just had a gun to our heads.' The Florida shooting survivors are transforming America's gun debate. *Time*, February 21 (http://time.com/5169436/florida-shooting-kids-gun-control-debate/); American Public Health Association. 2018. *Preventing Gun Violence* (https://www.apha.org/-/media/files/pdf/factsheets/160317_gunviolencefs.ashx?la=en&hash=AB71DE1BEDEBB2A797F8EC378E672791904FCF87); Gun Violence Archive. 2018. Past Summary Ledgers (http://www.gunviolencearchive.org/past-tolls); Lopez, G. 2018. America's gun problem, explained. *Vox* (https://www.vox.com/2015/10/3/9444417/gun-violence-united-states-america); Pew Research Center. 2013. *Section 3: Gun Ownership Trends and Demographics* (http://www.people-press.org/2013/03/12/section-3-gun-ownership-trends-and-demographics/#who-owns); Wagner, J. 2018. Poll shows growing support for stricter gun control among younger Americans. *The Washington Post*, April 18 (https://www.washingtonpost.com/news/post-politics/wp/2018/04/18/new-poll-shows-growing-support-for-stricter-gun-control-among-younger-americans/?noredirect=on&utm_term=.2b1cc431bd98); Zhang, S. 2018. Why can't the U.S. treat gun violence as a public-health problem? *The Atlantic* (https://www.theatlantic.com/health/archive/2018/02/gun-violence-public-health/553430/).

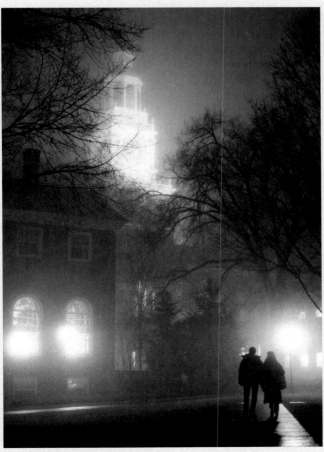

George Robinson/Alamy Stock Photo

groups advocate a complete and universal federal ban on the sale of all firearms.

Safety experts also advocate the adoption of consumer safety standards for guns, including features such as childproofing and indicators to show whether a gun is loaded. Technologies are now available to personalize handguns to help prevent unauthorized use. Owner identification through magnetic encoding, touch memory, radio frequency, or fingerprint reading can prevent others from using a personalized handgun. Education about proper storage is also important. Surveys indicate that more than 34% of homes with children contain guns. Data also show that in only 39% of those homes are firearms stored properly: locked, unloaded, and separate from ammunition. Unfortunately, over 7000 children are admitted to U.S. hospitals with gunshot wounds each year. To be effective, any approach to firearm injury prevention must have the support of law enforcement and the community as a whole.

PROVIDING EMERGENCY CARE

No matter how hard you try to avoid them, some injuries will inevitably occur. Therefore, it is important to prepare for situations in which you may need to provide emergency care for yourself or others. If you are prepared to help, you can improve someone else's chances of surviving or avoiding permanent disability.

A course in **first aid** can help you respond appropriately when someone is injured. One important benefit of first aid training is learning what *not* to do in certain situations. For example, a person with a suspected neck or back injury should not be moved unless there are other life-threatening conditions. A trained person can assess emergency situations accurately before acting.

Emergency rescue techniques can save the lives of people who are choking, who have stopped breathing, or whose hearts have stopped beating. As described earlier, the Heimlich maneuver is used when a victim is choking. Pulmonary resuscitation (also known as rescue breathing, artificial respiration, or mouth-to-mouth resuscitation) is used when a person is not breathing. Cardiopulmonary resuscitation (CPR) is used when a pulse cannot be found. In 2010, the American Heart Association made significant changes in its CPR guidelines for laypersons. Previous guidelines were to clear the airway, check for breathing, and begin chest compressions (ABC). The current guidelines are to begin chest compressions, clear the airway, and check for breathing (CAB). Starting with compressions gets the blood circulating, which is critical to keeping the person alive until help arrives. Compressions should be delivered fast, about 100 times a minute. The American Heart Association also authorizes use of a hands-only CPR technique on a teen or adult who suddenly collapses due to cardiac arrest;

first aid Emergency care given to an ill or injured person until medical care can be obtained.

emergency medical services (EMS) system
A system designed to network community resources for providing emergency care.

TERMS

Ask Yourself

QUESTIONS FOR CRITICAL THINKING AND REFLECTION

What kinds of emergency training have you had? What kinds of skills do you have that would enable you to help someone who was hurt, was trapped, or needed some other kind of assistance?

learn more and watch training videos at the association's website (heart.org/handsonlycpr). Courses in first aid and CPR are offered by the American Heart Association and the American Red Cross.

A new feature of some of these courses is training in the use of automated external defibrillators (AEDs), which monitor the heart's rhythm and, if appropriate, deliver an electrical shock to restart the heart. Because of the importance of early use of defibrillators in saving heart attack victims, these devices are being installed in public places, including casinos, airports, and many office buildings.

No matter how much training you get and how much experience you have, you will never be completely prepared for an emergency because it usually happens unexpectedly. Each emergency situation has unique variables that require you to use your knowledge and skills to help someone in need. And, as a person providing assistance, you are the first link in the **emergency medical services (EMS) system,** a system designed to network community resources for providing emergency care.

TIPS FOR TODAY AND THE FUTURE

Protecting yourself from injuries means taking sensible safety precautions every day, and preparing yourself to deal with an emergency.

RIGHT NOW YOU CAN:
- Check your home for any object or situation that could cause an injury, such as a tripping hazard, top-heavy shelves, and so on.
- Test the batteries in your home's smoke detectors, and change them if necessary. Test the detectors to make sure they work properly.
- If you ride a bike, check your helmet to ensure that it fits properly and will protect you in a crash. If you have any doubts, throw it away and buy a new one.

IN THE FUTURE YOU CAN:
- Get trained in CPR, rescue breathing, and the use of an automated external defibrillator. If you have already had such training, take a refresher course.
- Be watchful for hazardous situations at your school or workplace. If you notice anything suspicious, report it to an appropriate person right away.
- Prepare for a poisoning emergency by putting the number of your local poison control hotline in a conspicuous place.

SUMMARY

• Injuries are caused by a dynamic interaction of human and environmental factors. Risk-taking behavior is associated with a high rate of injury.

• The home can contain many poisonous substances, including medications, cleaning agents, plants, and fumes from cars and appliances.

• Most fall-related injuries occur on stairs or steps. Alcohol, chairs, and ladders are also involved in a significant number of falls.

• Careless smoking and problems with cooking or heating equipment are common causes of home fires. Being prepared for fire emergencies means planning escape routes and installing smoke detectors.

• Performing the Heimlich maneuver can prevent someone from choking to death.

• The proper storage and handling of firearms can help prevent injuries; assume that any gun is loaded.

• Key factors in motor vehicle injuries include aggressive driving, speeding, a failure to wear seat belts, alcohol and drug intoxication, fatigue, and distraction.

• Motorcycle, motor scooter, and bicycle injuries can be prevented by developing appropriate skills, driving or riding defensively, and wearing proper safety equipment, especially a helmet.

• Many injuries during leisure activities result from the misuse of equipment, lack of experience, use of alcohol, and a failure to wear proper safety equipment.

• Most work-related injuries involve extensive manual labor; back problems and repetitive strain injuries are most common.

• Factors contributing to violence include poverty, the absence of strong social ties, the influence of the mass media, cultural attitudes about gender roles, problems in interpersonal relationships, alcohol and drug abuse, and the availability of firearms.

• Types of violence include assault, homicide, gang-related violence, hate crimes, school violence, workplace violence, terrorism, family and intimate-partner violence, and sexual violence.

• Battering occurs at every socioeconomic level. The core issue is the abuser's need to control other people.

• Most rape victims are women, and most know their attackers. Factors in date rape include different standards of appropriate sexual behavior for men and women and different perceptions of actions.

• Child sexual abuse often results in serious trauma; usually the abuser is a trusted adult.

• Sexual harassment is unwelcome sexual advances or other conduct of a sexual nature that affects academic or employment performance or evaluations or that creates an intimidating, hostile, or offensive academic, work, or student living environment.

• Strategies for reducing violence include conflict resolution training, social skills development, and education programs that foster tolerance and understanding among diverse groups.

• Steps in giving emergency care include making sure the scene is safe for you and the injured person, conducting a quick examination of the victim, calling for help, and providing emergency first aid.

FOR MORE INFORMATION

American Association of Poison Control Centers. Provides free, confidential, and expert advice related to poisoning.

800-222-1222

http://www.aapcc.org

American Automobile Association Foundation for Traffic Safety. Provides consumer information about all aspects of traffic safety; the website has online quizzes and extensive links.

http://www.aaafoundation.org/home

American Bar Association: Domestic Violence. Provides information about statistics, research, and laws relating to domestic violence.

https://www.americanbar.org/groups/domestic_violence/

Consumer Product Safety Commission. Provides information and advice about safety issues relating to consumer products.

http://www.cpsc.gov

Governor's Highway Safety Association. Provides up-to-date information about cell phone and texting laws, as well as general information and publications related to traffic safety.

http://www.ghsa.org/html/stateinfo/laws/cellphone_laws.html

Insurance Institute for Highway Safety. Provides information about crashes on the nation's highways, as well as reports on topics such as speeding and crashworthiness of vehicles.

http://www.iihs.org

National Center for Health Statistics (Centers for Disease Control and Prevention). Monitors the health of the United States and provides up-to-date information and statistical data to the public and professionals.

http://www.cdc.gov/nchs

National Center for Injury Prevention and Control. Provides consumer-oriented information about unintentional injuries and violence.

http://www.cdc.gov/injury

National Center for Victims of Crime. An advocacy group for crime victims; provides statistics, news, safety strategies, tips on finding local assistance, and links to related sites.

http://www.victimsofcrime.org

National Children's Alliance. Helps local communities respond to allegations of child abuse.

http://nationalchildrensalliance.org

National Fire Protection Agency. Gives information about fire, electrical, and related hazards.

www.nfpa.org

National Highway Traffic Safety Administration. Supplies materials about reducing deaths, injuries, and economic losses from motor vehicle crashes.

http://www.nhtsa.gov

National Safety Council. Provides information and statistics about preventing unintentional injuries.

http://www.nsc.org

National Violence Hotlines. Provide information, referral services, and crisis intervention.

800-799-SAFE (7233) (domestic violence), http://www .thehotline.org

800-422-4453 (child abuse), http://www.childhelp.org

800-656-HOPE (4673) (sexual assault), http://www.rainn.org

Occupational Safety and Health Administration. Provides information about topics related to health and safety issues in the workplace.

http://www.osha.gov

Prevent Child Abuse America. Provides statistics, information, and publications relating to child abuse, including parenting tips.

http://www.preventchildabuse.org

Rape, Abuse, and Incest National Network (RAINN). Provides guidelines for preventing and dealing with sexual assault and abuse.

http://www.rainn.org

Tolerance.Org. Offers suggestions for fighting hate and promoting tolerance; sponsored by the Southern Poverty Law Center.

http://www.tolerance.org

World Health Organization: Violence and Injury Prevention and Disability. Provides statistics and information about the consequences of intentional and unintentional injuries worldwide.

http://www.who.int/violence_injury_prevention

The following sites provide statistics and background information about violence and crime in the United States:

Bureau of Justice Statistics: http://www.bjs.gov

Federal Bureau of Investigation: http://www.fbi.gov

National Criminal Justice Reference Service: http://www.ncjrs.gov

SELECTED BIBLIOGRAPHY

Administration for Children & Families. 2019. Child abuse, neglect data released. *28th edition of the Child Maltreatment Report.* Washington, DC: U.S. Department of Health & Human Services (https://www.acf.hhs .gov/media/press/2019/child-abuse-neglect-data-released)

Aizenman, N. 2017. Gun violence: How the U.S. compares with other countries. *National Public Radio,* October 6 (https://www.npr.org/sections/goatsandsoda /2017/10/06/555861898/gun-violence-how-the-u-s-compares-to-other -countries).

American College Health Association. 2008. *Shifting the Paradigm: Primary Prevention of Sexual Violence.* Linthicum, MD: American College Health Association.

Anderson, C. A., et al. 2010. Violent video game effects on aggression, empathy, and prosocial behavior in eastern and western countries: A meta-analytic review. *Psychological Bulletin* 136(2): 151–173.

Bureau of Aircraft Accidents Archives. 2000–2017. *Death Rate per Year* (http://www.baaa-acro.com/statistics/death-rate-per-year).

Bureau of Labor Statistics. 2019. Employer-related workplace injuries and illnesses—2018. *News Release.* Washington, DC: U.S. Department of Labor (https://www.bls.gov/news.release/pdf/osh.pdf).

Burgess, M., and S. Burpo. 2012. The effect of music videos on college students' perceptions of rape. *College Student Journal* 46(4): 748–763.

Centers for Disease Control and Prevention. 2016. *Impaired Driving: Get the Facts. Injury Prevention and Control: Motor Vehicle Safety.* Atlanta, GA: Centers for Disease Control and Prevention (https://www.cdc.gov /motorvehiclesafety/impaired_driving/impaired-drv_factsheet.html).

Centers for Disease Control and Prevention. 2017. *Nonfatal Injury Reports, 2001–2017.* Atlanta, GA: Centers for Disease Control and Prevention (https://webappa.cdc.gov/sasweb/ncipc/nfirates.html).

Centers for Disease Control and Prevention. 2017. *10 Leading Causes of Injury Deaths by Age Group Highlighting Unintentional Injury Deaths, United States–2017* (http://www.cdc.gov/injury/wisqars/leadingcauses.html).

Cramer, R., et al. 2013. An examination of sexual orientation and transgender-based hate crimes in the post–Matthew Shepard era. *Psychology, Public Policy, and Law* 19(3): 355–368.

Federal Bureau of Investigation. 2018. *Crime in the United States, 2018.* U.S. Department of Justice (https://ucr.fbi.gov/crime-in-the-u.s/2018/crime -in-the-u.s.-2018).

Federal Bureau of Investigation. 2019. *2018 Preliminary Semiannual Crime Statistics Released.* Washington, DC: U.S. Department of Justice.

Governors Highway Safety Association. 2020. *Child Passenger Safety Laws* (http://www.ghsa.org/html/stateinfo/laws/childsafety_laws.html).

Iqbal, S., et al. 2012. National carbon monoxide poisoning surveillance framework and recent estimates. *Public Health Reports* 127(5): 486–496.

Kann, L., et al. 2018. Youth Risk Behavior Surveillance—United States, 2017. *MMWR Surveillance Summaries* 67(8).

Kleisen, L. 2013. A positive view on road safety: Can 'car karma' contribute to safe driving styles? *Accident Analysis and Prevention* 50: 605–712.

Kochanek, K.D., et al. 2017. Deaths: Final data for 2017. *National Vital Statistics Reports* 68(9) (https://www.cdc.gov/nchs/data/nvsr/nvsr68 /nvsr68_09-508.pdf)

May, T. 2018. For Chinese pedestrians glued to their phones, a middle path emerges. *The New York Times,* June 8 (https://www.nytimes.com/2018 /06/08/world/asia/china-pedestrians-smartphones-path.html).

Levinson, A. A., B. Lannert, and M. Yalch. 2012. The effects of intimate partner violence on women and children survivors: An attachment perspective. *Psychodynamic Psychiatry* 40(3): 397–433.

Mendez, C., and B. Dillon. 2012. Workplace violence: Impact, causes, and prevention. *WORK* 42(1): 15–20.

Miller, M., et al. 2015. Firearms and suicide in U.S. cities. *Injury Prevention* 21(e1): e116–e119.

Monuteaux, M. C., et al. 2015. Firearm ownership and violent crime in the U.S.: An ecological study. *American Journal of Preventive Medicine* 49(2): 207–214.

Narang, P., et al. 2010. Do guns provide safety? At what cost? *Southern Medical Journal* 103(2): 151–153.

National Center for Education Statistics. 2020. Indicators of school crime and safety. Institute of Education Sciences (https://nces.ed.gov/programs /crimeindicators/ind_01.asp).

National Center for Health Statistics. 2015. *Deaths from Unintentional Injury among Adults Aged 65 and Over: United States, 2000–2013* (NCHS Data Brief No. 199). Atlanta, GA: National Center for Health Statistics (https://www.cdc.gov/nchs/products/databriefs/db199.htm).

National Center for Health Statistics. 2015. *National Estimates of the 10 Leading Causes of Nonfatal Injuries Treated in Hospital Emergency Departments, United States–2015* (https://www.cdc.gov/injury/wisqars/pdf /leading_causes_of_nonfatal_injury_2015-a.pdf).

National Center for Health Statistics. 2020. *Fact Sheet, NCHS Data on Drug Poisoning Deaths* (http://www.cdc.gov/nchs/data/factsheets/factsheet _drug_poisoning.pdf).

National Center for Statistics and Analysis. 2015. *2014 Crash Data Key Findings* (Report No. DOT HS 812 219). Washington, DC: National Highway Traffic Safety Administration.

National Health Care Provider Solutions. 2015. *AHA 2015 Guidelines Are Published: CPR Key Points* (https://nhcps.com/aha-2015-cpr-guidelines -published-key-points/).

National Highway Traffic Safety Administration. 2017. Traffic safety facts, 2015: Motorcycles. Report no. DOT HS-812-353. Washington, DC: US Department of Transportation.

National Highway Traffic Safety Administration. 2019. *2018 Fatal Motor Vehicle Crashes: Overview.* Report No. DOT HS-812-826. Washington, DC: U.S. Department of Transportation.

National Safety Council. 2020. *Injury Facts.* Itasca, IL: National Safety Council.

Pickrell, T. M., and E.-H. Choi. 2015. *Seat Belt Use in 2014—Overall Results* (Report No. DOT HS 812 113). Washington, DC: National Highway Traffic Safety Administration.

Reyns, B., B. Henson, and B. Fisher. 2012. Stalking in the twilight zone: Extent of cyberstalking victimization and offending among college students. *Deviant Behavior* 33(1): 1–25.

Ritchie, H. 2018. Is it fair to compare terrorism and disaster with other causes of death? *Our World in Data blog* (https://ourworldindata.org/is-it-fair-to-compare-terrorism-and-disaster-with-other-causes-of-death).

Ross, T., et al. 2010. The bicycle helmet attitudes scale: Using the Health Belief Model to predict helmet use among undergraduates. *Journal of American College Health* 59(1): 29–36.

Schmidt, M. 2018. How to not sexually harass someone: A simple guide to decency (https://inland360.com/more-news/2018/10/how-to-not-sexually-harass-someone-a-simple-guide-to-decency/).

Swogger, M. T., et al. 2012. Self-reported childhood physical abuse and perpetration of intimate partner violence: The moderating role of psychopathic traits. *Criminal Justice and Behavior* 39(7): 910–922.

U.S. Fire Administration. 2015. *Campus Fire Fatalities in Residential Buildings (2000-2015).* Washington, DC: U.S. Department of Homeland Security.

Victor, D. 2018. School shootings have already killed dozens in 2018. *The New York Times*, May 18 (https://www.nytimes.com/2018/05/18/us/school-shootings-2018.html).

Webster, D., Crifasi, C. K., and J. S. Vernick. 2014. Effects of the repeal of Missouri's handgun purchaser licensing law on homicides. *Journal of Urban Health* 91(2): 293–302.

Weinberger, S. E., et al. 2015. Firearm-related injury and death in the United States: A call to action from 8 health professional organizations and the American Bar Association. *Annals of Internal Medicine* 162(7): 513–517.

World Health Organization. 2020. *Road Traffic Injuries* (Fact Sheet No. 358) (http://www.who.int/mediacentre/factsheets/fs358/en/).

Xu, J. Q., et al. 2020. *Mortality in the United States, 2018.* NCHS Data Brief 355. Hyattsville, MD: National Center for Health Statistics (https://www.cdc.gov/nchs/data/databriefs/db355-h.pdf)

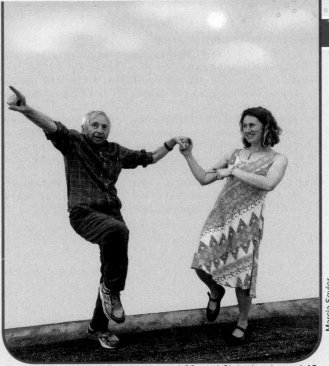

Authors Paul Insel, aged 82, and Claire Insel, aged 42.

Marcia Seyler

CHAPTER 23

CHAPTER OBJECTIVES

- List strategies for healthy aging
- Identify challenges that may accompany aging and explain how people can best confront them
- Explain the factors influencing life expectancy
- Understand the issues facing older adults in the United States

Aging: An Ongoing Process

TEST YOUR KNOWLEDGE

1. **Women should start taking preventive measures against osteoporosis after menopause.**
   True or False?

2. **What is the leading cause of physical disability in the United States?**
   a. Heart disease
   b. Arthritis
   c. Dementia

3. **On average, a woman will spend about the same amount of time during her life caring for an aging relative as she does raising children.**
   True or False?

4. **Exercise is beneficial for older people because it**
   a. Protects against osteoporosis
   b. Maintains alertness and intelligence
   c. Prevents falls

5. **When Social Security was initiated in 1935, the average life expectancy was _____ years lower than it is today.**
   a. 7
   b. 17
   c. 27

ANSWERS

1. **FALSE.** All people—but especially women—need to pay attention from their earliest years to diet and exercise in order to build bone mass.

2. **B.** According to the Centers for Disease Control and Prevention, arthritis is the leading cause of physical disability in the United States.

3. **TRUE.** On average, a woman will spend 17 years raising children and 18 years caring for an aging relative.

4. **ALL THREE.** Even for people over age 80, exercise can improve physical functioning and balance and reduce falls and injuries.

5. **B.** Life expectancy has increased by over 17 years since 1935 due to medical advances and improvements in diet and personal habits.

Nor, indeed, are we to give our attention solely to the body; much greater care is due to the mind and soul; for they, too, like lamps, grow dim with time, unless we keep them supplied with oil.

—On Old Age, Cicero (106–43 BCE)

Not long ago, it was rare to meet a centenarian. In 2019, the number of Americans aged 100 or older was about 80,000, compared with only about 4000 centenarians in 1950. And it's not only the extremely old who are increasing in number. The percentage of Americans aged 65 and up has nearly quadrupled since the beginning of the 20th century, from about 4% of the total population in 1900 to about 16% in 2020. In the United States, as in much of the world, people are living longer while birth rates are declining, resulting in a gradual but profound aging of our population.

Aging refers to the changes that occur in an organism over time. Aging is an inevitable process that begins at birth and ends when we die. Despite the inevitability of aging, there are many factors, some of which are in our control, that can modify the rate at which we age and the quality of our lives during our older years. There is no definitive age at which we become "old," but age 65 is commonly used in research and population statistics as the lower limit of old age. Throughout this text, the terms "older" and "elderly" refer to people aged 65 years and up.

PERSPECTIVES ON AGING

Most of us know someone who looks and acts years younger (or older) than what we might expect given their chronological age. How rapidly we age is the cumulative result of a host of genetic, social, and environmental factors. Our mindset also makes a difference in how we age. Aging may be described from different perspectives, including biological, psychological, and social aging.

In general, *biological aging* is associated with a reduction in the body's potential to repair and regenerate tissue. **Gerontology** is the scientific study of the physical changes that occur with aging. Despite an explosion of aging-related research, we have a long way to go before we fully understand the biological processes of aging. Current theories of aging fall into two main groups: programmed and damage related.

Programmed aging hypothesizes that our bodies age because of a hardwired pattern of shifts in gene expression that have been programmed through evolution. Advocates of this theory say that just as the growth of an embryo or a child occurs in a predetermined orderly manner, our genetic expression continues to change in a programmed manner throughout life, which ultimately results in the physical changes of aging and death. Damage-related aging theories postulate that environmental exposures such as disease, toxins, and natural radiation cause genetic and cellular damage that eventually exceeds the capacity of our bodies' repair systems. Regardless of why we age, getting older involves physical deterioration that can often be delayed or reduced by good diet, adequate exercise, sleep, and other wellness behaviors discussed in this chapter.

Psychological aging refers to the cognitive, emotional, and behavioral changes that naturally occur in humans over time. These include a gradual decline in cognitive processing speed, memory, and other mental functions, which occurs in most healthy older people. The normal cognitive changes associated with aging are relatively mild compared with the severe cognitive and behavioral deficits that occur in neurodegenerative diseases such as Alzheimer's disease. There are some "super-agers" who seem to have little or no loss in cognitive function even in very old age. In general, these people tend to be well educated, intelligent, and mentally active. Experts believe that this phenomenon may be partially genetic, but also, to some extent, due to "cognitive reserve," so that even if some brain tissue is damaged by the aging process, other parts of the brain can compensate.

Finally, *social aging* refers to the shifts in our relationships and societal roles as we age. These changes are often the result of major life events such as retirement, changes in income, deaths of family members and friends, or moving to a new location. These changes may occur abruptly and can sometimes result in rapid deterioration in self-identity and social functioning. Social aging also encompasses many positive aspects of aging. Many older people enjoy a degree of freedom that they have never previously experienced. Elders often report that they finally have time to pursue their natural interests and to truly savor their lives. Many seniors also say that now that they are older, they feel freer to "just be themselves," rather than worrying so much about what other people think of them.

Old age can be a wonderful part of life's journey. Many people live out their later years in loving and stable relationships and are in good psychological and physical health until they reach very old age. Others experience great challenges during the aging process. These can include severe decline in physical abilities, lack of social support, financial adversity, loneliness, and loss of self-esteem. The "age-old" question has been, what can we do to slow the physical aging process and lengthen our healthy, happy life span? Research shows that if we optimize wellness starting from our early years, we have a much greater chance of thriving during old age. Our perception of old age also makes a difference. Studies reveal that people who view aging in a more positive light are much more likely to thrive than those who have a generally negative attitude toward aging.

TERMS

aging A normal process of getting older, which includes physical, mental, and social changes.

gerontology The scientific study of the physical changes that occur with aging.

Many diseases, such as cancer, cardiovascular disease, arthritis, diabetes, and progressive neurological disorders such as dementia, become increasingly common with advancing age. But none of these diseases is inevitable, and your odds of acquiring these diseases is less if you follow lifelong healthy habits. Not smoking, eating well, exercising regularly throughout life, maintaining strong social bonds, and avoiding chronic stress all reduce the risk of acquiring these and many other diseases.

Of course, even with the healthiest behavior and environment, biological aging inevitably occurs. It results from genetic and biochemical processes we don't yet fully understand, but which include accumulated DNA damage, genetically programmed aging, impaired protein metabolism, changes in energy metabolism, and likely many other processes. These biological changes increase the risk for many diseases. Together, gradual aging and impairment from disease cause physiological changes throughout the body. Because of redundancy in most organ systems, the body's ability to function is not affected until damage is fairly extensive. Further research may help pinpoint the causes of aging and develop therapies to repair and even prevent damage to aging organs.

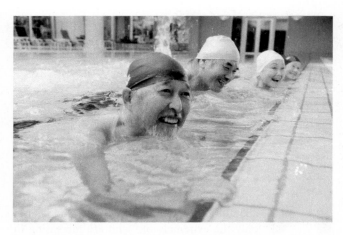

Regular exercise is a key to successful, healthy aging. Indeed/Taxi Japan/Getty Images

This may delay the onset of symptoms caused by a dementing disease, without actually changing the disease's underlying biological course.

Life-Enhancing Measures

Through good habits you can prevent, delay, lessen, or even reverse some of the negative changes associated with aging. Simple, daily practices can make a great difference to your level of energy and vitality now and throughout life. The following suggestions are mentioned throughout this text, but because they are profoundly related to health in later life, we highlight them here.

Don't Smoke The average pack-a-day smoker can expect to live about 13 to 14 fewer years than a nonsmoker. Furthermore, smokers suffer more illnesses and recover from illnesses more slowly than nonsmokers (see Chapter 12). About 10% of people age 65 and up are current smokers. It is never too late to quit smoking, and although all the damage from a lifetime of smoking can't be undone, quitting has important and immediate health benefits.

Challenge Your Mind Your level of education and mental activity throughout life seems to reduce your risk for developing dementia in old age. Reading, writing, doing puzzles, learning a language, and studying music are good ways to stimulate the brain. The more complex the activity, the more protective it may be. However, the causal relationship between such activities and cognitive diseases is not fully understood. For example, some effects of mental exercise may be related to a buildup of cognitive reserve, your brain's ability to find alternative routes to get the job done.

> **QUICK STATS**
>
> **The world's older population continues to grow at an unprecedented rate. Today, 9% of people worldwide (703 million) are aged 65 and over.**
> —United Nations, World Population Aging, 2019

Develop Physical Fitness Exercise significantly enhances psychological, cognitive, and physical health. A review of more than 70 scientific studies cited in the 2018 *Physical Activity Guidelines Advisory Committee Report* found that physically active people have a significantly lower risk of dying prematurely compared with inactive people. Poor fitness and low physical activity levels were found to be better predictors of premature death than smoking, diabetes, or obesity. The committee found that about 150 minutes (2.5 hours) of physical activity per week is sufficient to decrease risk of death.

Exercise produces many positive effects, including

- Lower blood pressure and healthier cholesterol levels
- Better protection against heart attacks and an increased chance of survival if one occurs
- Sustained or increased lung capacity
- Increased muscle mass and less accumulation of fat
- Maintenance of strength, flexibility, and balance
- Decreased risk of falls
- Improved sleep
- Longer life expectancy
- Protection against osteoporosis and type 2 diabetes
- Increased effectiveness of the immune system
- Maintenance of mental agility and flexibility, response time, memory, and hand–eye coordination

The stimulus that exercise provides also seems to protect against the loss of **fluid intelligence,** which is the ability to find solutions to new problems. Fluid intelligence depends on rapidity of responsiveness, memory, and alertness. Individuals who exercise regularly are also less susceptible to depression and dementia.

Regular physical activity also fends off age-related *sarcopenia*, which is the loss of muscle mass (see Chapter 14). Gradual loss of skeletal muscle mass occurs in nearly all people over age 30, with a typical decline of about 3% of skeletal muscle mass per year. Besides resulting in loss of strength and function, decreased skeletal muscle mass affects numerous metabolic pathways and is associated with many chronic diseases. Recent studies have shown that physical activity can reduce and even reverse the rate of loss of skeletal muscle mass that typically occurs with aging, which in turn decreases the risk for cardiovascular and many other chronic diseases.

Regular physical activity is essential for healthy aging, as well as for vitality throughout life. The National Institute on Aging has developed the exercise program Go4Life (https://go4life.nia.nih.gov) to help adults 50 and older incorporate more physical activity into their lives. The program offers four key types of exercises—with the goals of improving endurance, strength, balance, and flexibility. Elderly people should try to do strength exercises for all major muscle groups on two or more days a week, and they should also strive for at least 30 minutes of moderate-to-intense endurance activity on most or all days of the week. The principal recommendation is to avoid inactivity: Any amount or type of physical activity is better than none. Older adults with chronic conditions should seek guidance from their health care provider to find out what physical activities are effective, enjoyable, and safe given their particular strengths and challenges. For more about the beneficial effects of exercise for older adults, see the box "Can Exercise Delay the Effects of Aging?"

Eat Wisely   Good health at any age is enhanced by eating a varied, nutrient-dense diet (see Chapter 13). For many adults, that means eating more fruits, vegetables, and whole grains while eating fewer foods high in saturated and trans fats and added sugars. Special guidelines for older adults include the following:

- Get enough vitamin B-12 (eggs, dairy products, meat) and extra vitamin D from fortified foods or supplements.

- Limit sodium intake to 1500 mg per day (3/4 teaspoon salt), and get enough potassium (4700 mg per day) from foods. Many vegetables, legumes, fruits, and fish (such as salmon) are good dietary sources of potassium. In particular, yams, winter squash, potatoes, avocados, white beans, and bananas are high in potassium. High blood pressure becomes more common as we age, and studies show that older adults are particularly sensitive to the blood pressure–raising effects of excessive sodium intake.

- Eat foods rich in dietary fiber and drink plenty of water to help prevent constipation.

- Pay special attention to food safety. Older adults are often more susceptible to foodborne illness.

- Eat foods that are nutrient dense, including fruits and vegetables, and foods that contain healthy fats such as avocados, olive oil, and salmon.

Maintain a Healthy Weight   About 35% of older people are obese, which increases their risk for many chronic diseases, including cardiovascular disease, diabetes, and many cancers (see Chapter 15). On the other hand, being underweight has also been linked to increased risk of death in the elderly. Mortality rates in those over 65 years were lowest in people whose weight fell in the normal to slightly overweight range.

QUICK STATS

Among people ages 65 and older in 1965 only 5% had completed a bachelor's degree or more. By 2018, this share had risen to 29%.

US Census Bureau, Current Population Survey Annual Social and Economic Supplement, 2019

Control Drinking and Overdependence on Medications   Alcohol abuse ranks with depression as a common hidden mental health problem, affecting about 10% of older adults. Elders are especially vulnerable to the toxic effects of alcohol, in part because the ability to metabolize alcohol decreases with age. The same amount of alcohol will produce a higher blood alcohol level and more impairment in an elder compared with a young person. Alcohol overuse is often not identified in the elderly because the effects of alcohol or drug dependence can mimic disease, such as Alzheimer's disease.

Many people, including health professionals, don't realize that alcohol abuse is a common problem in the elderly. But in fact, widowers over age 75 have the highest rate of alcoholism of any group in the United States.

Opioid and benzodiazepine overuse is becoming increasingly common in the elderly. Misuse of these medications is especially dangerous for older people. Their use is associated with increased risk for falls and serious cognitive impairment. Older people are more likely to have reduced kidney or liver function, so they are less able to break down medication and more likely to overdose than younger people with normal drug metabolism.

fluid intelligence   The capacity to analyze new problems, reason, and identify patterns and relationships, independent of past knowledge.   **TERMS**

Can physical activity and exercise combat the degenerative effects of aging in middle-aged and older adults? The evidence indicates that they can. In reviewing the research, the U.S. government's Physical Activity Guidelines Advisory Committee concluded that physical activity can prevent or delay the onset of limitations and declines in functional health in older adults, can maintain or improve functional health in those who already have limitations, and can reduce the incidence of falls and fall-related injuries.

One mechanism by which physical activity prevents decline in functional health is through maintenance or improvement of the physiological capacities of the body, such as aerobic power, muscular strength, and balance—in other words, through improvements in physical fitness. Declines in these physiological capacities occur with biological aging and are often compounded by disease-related disability. But evidence shows that older adults who participate in regular aerobic exercise are 30% less likely than inactive individuals to develop functional limitations (such as a limited ability to walk or climb stairs) or role limitations (such as a limited ability to be the family grocery shopper). Although studies found that both physical activity and aerobic fitness were associated with reduced risk of functional limitations, aerobic fitness was associated with a greater reduction of risk. Evidence also suggests that regular physical activity is safe and beneficial for older adults who already have functional limitations.

Numerous studies have shown that regular exercise—particularly strength training, balance training, and flexibility exercises—can improve muscular strength, muscular endurance, and stability and provide some protection against falls. Aerobic activity, especially walking, also helps reduce the risk of falls, and some evidence indicates that tai chi exercise programs are beneficial as well. Regular exercise not only reduces the incidence of falls but also greatly enhances mobility, allowing older people to live more independently and with greater confidence. Research also shows that regular physical activity can reduce anxiety and depression in older adults. Exercise stimulates blood flow to the brain and may help the brain to function more efficiently and improve memory. There is some evidence that exercise may stave off mental decline and the occurrence of age-related dementia.

Current physical activity recommendations for older adults from the American Heart Association and the American College of Sports Medicine include moderate- to vigorous-intensity aerobic activity, strength training, and flexibility exercises, as well as balance exercises for older adults at risk for falls. Unfortunately, only about 12% of people aged 65 and over get the recommended amounts of physical activity, and many get no exercise at all beyond the activities of daily living. Older adults are the least active group of Americans. Although it is important to exercise throughout life, the evidence indicates that older adults who become more active even late in life can experience improvements in physical fitness and functional health.

SOURCES: Physical Activity Guidelines Advisory Committee. 2018 *Physical Activity Guidelines Advisory Committee Report, 2018.* Washington, DC: U.S. Department of Health and Human Services; Simonsick, E. M., et al. 2005. Just get out the door! Importance of walking outside the home for maintaining mobility: Findings from the Women's Health and Aging Study. *Journal of the American Geriatrics Society* 53(2): 198–203; Federal Interagency Forum on Aging-Related Statistics. 2018. *Older Americans 2016: Key Indicators of Well-Being.* Washington, DC: U.S. Government Printing Office; Rebelo-Marques, A., et al. 2018. Aging hallmarks: The benefits of physical exercise. *Frontiers in Endocrinology* (https://www.ncbi.nlm.nih.gov/pmc/articles/PMC5980968/).

Signs of potential alcohol or drug misuse include unexplained falls or frequent injuries, forgetfulness, depression, and malnutrition. Family, friends, and health care providers should be alert to changes in an older person's behavior that might be related to drug or alcohol misuse.

Schedule Physical Examinations to Detect Treatable Diseases   When detected early, many diseases, including hypertension, diabetes, glaucoma, and many types of cancer, can be successfully controlled by medication and lifestyle changes. Recommended screenings and immunizations can protect against preventable chronic and infectious diseases (see Chapters 16–18).

Recognize and Reduce Stress   Stress-induced physiological changes increase wear and tear on the body, and worsen cognitive decline in the elderly. Like people of all ages, elders benefit from reducing stress, getting enough sleep, not overworking, and avoiding substance misuse. The relaxation techniques described in Chapter 2 can help people of any age deal with stress.

Nurture Social Connections   Research shows that social connectedness is strongly associated with a longer, healthier, and happier life. Indeed, studies have shown that loneliness and social isolation are major risk factors for mortality, ranking similarly to other well-known risk factors such as smoking and physical inactivity. Strong relationships with friends and family are life enhancing in a multitude of ways.

DEALING WITH THE CHANGES OF AGING

Just as you can act to limit or delay some of the physical changes of aging, you can also prepare psychologically, socially, and financially for changes that may occur later in life.

If you have aging parents, grandparents, and friends, the following information may give you insight into their lives and encourage you to begin cultivating appropriate and useful behaviors that will benefit you now and throughout your life.

Changing Roles and Relationships

Changes in social roles are a major feature of life as we age. Retirement marks a major life change for many. Compared to 50 years ago, people spend a larger proportion of their lives (18 years or more on average) in retirement. This is mostly because people are living longer. Retirement has become more difficult to define as many people's working lives have become more flexible. Many people "retire" from their full-time job, but then continue to work part time. Others may retire, then start a new career. For independent workers, such as those who work in the "gig economy," pensions are rare, and saving for retirement may be especially challenging. For those who go abruptly from full-time employment to total retirement, the adjustment can be particularly difficult. People who have well-developed leisure pursuits and meaningful relationships adjust better to retirement than those with few interests outside work. Although retirement may be a desirable milestone for most people, it may also be viewed as a threat to prestige, purpose, and self-respect. Retired people may suffer as a result of the loss of their former roles in life.

Retirement and the end of child rearing also bring about changes in the relationship between marriage partners. The amount of time a couple spends together will likely increase, and activities will change. Couples may need a period of adjustment in which they get to know each other as individuals again. Discussing what types of activities each partner enjoys can help couples set up a mutually satisfying routine of shared and independent activities. But not all elderly people live as couples. Death of a spouse, divorce, and separation are all common reasons that older people become single. Older couples are much more likely to divorce or separate today than in the past. The loss of a spouse, whether through separation, divorce, or death, is one of the most serious stressors anyone can face. In particular, during the first three months after the death of a spouse, the risk of death for the surviving spouse increases by 66%. Loving social support from family, friends, and community support groups is critical for helping elders cope with major losses.

Increased Leisure Time Although retirement and freedom from child care responsibilities may confer the advantages of leisure time and freedom from work-related stress, many people who have spent most of their lives focused primarily on their careers may not know how to enjoy their free time. If you have developed diverse interests throughout life, retirement can be a joyful and fulfilling period of your life. It can provide opportunities for you to expand your horizons, try new activities, take classes, and meet new people. Volunteering in your community can enhance self-esteem through opportunities to contribute to society.

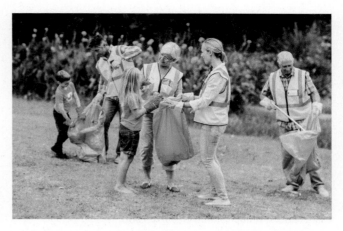

The retirement years can be the best part of your life socially, with increased opportunities to meet and interact with new and different people through volunteer work.
wavebreakmedia/Shutterstock

The Economics of Retirement Retirement may mean a severely restricted budget or possibly even financial disaster if you have failed to put aside adequate savings. Financial planning for retirement should begin early in life. People in their twenties and thirties should estimate how much money they need to support themselves comfortably, calculate their projected income, and begin a savings program. The earlier people begin such a program, the more money they will have at retirement.

Financial planning for retirement is especially critical for women. American women are much less likely than men to be covered by pension plans, 401(k) plans, and other retirement programs, reflecting the fact that women tend to have lower-paying jobs, work part time, or not work at all because of caregiving for children or elderly family members. Although the gap is narrowing, women currently outlive men by about five to six years, and they are more likely to develop chronic conditions that impair their daily activities later in life. The net result of these factors is that nearly twice as many older women than older men live in poverty.

Vulnerability to Crime Elderly people are especially vulnerable to crime, including physical, sexual, and emotional abuse, neglect, and financial victimization. Studies show that elder abuse, especially by family members, is grossly underreported. The consequences of crime against vulnerable elders are particularly severe; elder abuse triples the risk of premature death. Financial scams that target seniors have become increasingly common because scammers may believe that seniors are more likely to have access to money and may be easier to fool than younger people. Education about scams and abuse can help elders and those who care for them be alert for potential problems.

Adapting to Physical Changes

A person can do many things to minimize the effects of the physical changes associated with aging. However, some changes in physical functioning are inevitable, and successful aging involves anticipating and accommodating these changes. Adapting rather than giving up favorite activities may be the best strategy for dealing with physical limitations. Older people with limited strength may have to develop priorities for how to best use their energy. Paying close attention to the need for rest and sleep is crucial for enjoying life at all ages, but especially for elders. Coping with chronic health issues is, unfortunately, part of life for most elderly people. According to the National Council on Aging, approximately 80% of older adults have at least one chronic disease, and nearly as many have at least two. The most frequently occurring conditions in older people include arthritis, heart disease, cancer, diabetes, and hypertension.

Hearing Loss   The loss of hearing is a common physical change that can profoundly affect the lives of older adults. Loss of hearing occurs in virtually everyone as they age—a condition known as *presbycusis*, which can range from mild to severe. Hearing loss due to aging is often compounded by factors such as exposure to loud noise, certain medications that can damage hearing, trauma, and some diseases. Exposure to loud noise is the most important preventable cause of hearing loss.

Damage accumulates over the years, and it often results in significant hearing loss by middle and older age. Exposure to loud noises such as those made by lawnmowers, motorcycles, gunshots, loud music, and the use of headphones at excessive volume can significantly damage your hearing. Chronic exposure to even lower levels of noise, such as constant sound from a nearby freeway, can also result in permanent hearing loss (see Chapter 20). You can reduce the damaging impact of noise by keeping the volume down on your headphones, being alert to hazardous noise in the environment, wearing earplugs when you know you will be exposed to loud sounds, and staying as far as possible from the sound's source.

About one-third of people aged 65 and older and over half of people over 80 have significant hearing loss. Difficulty hearing affects a person's ability to interact with others and can lead to isolation and depression. Recent studies show that the risk of developing dementia doubles for older people with mild hearing loss and is five times greater for people with severe hearing loss compared with elderly people who do not have hearing loss.

Hearing loss should be assessed and treated by a health care professional. Hearing aids are often effective in improving quality of life, and they may even help to decrease the risk for developing dementia. Some people resist wearing hearing aids because of cost or fear of social stigma, but the benefits of using hearing aids—or personal amplification devices (which are much less expensive and available without a prescription)—can make the adjustment to these devices well worth the effort.

Vision Changes   Vision usually declines with age, making it difficult to perform far-away activities like driving and up-close activities like reading. By the time we reach our forties, nearly all of us will have developed *presbyopia*—a gradual decline in the ability to focus on close objects. This decline occurs because the lens of the eye becomes stiffer as we age, making it difficult or impossible to focus on nearby objects. Vision loss is also caused by other common eye diseases, such as **glaucoma**, **age-related macular degeneration (AMD)**, **cataracts**, and **diabetic retinopathy,** all of which can be detected with regular screening and treated with medication, laser treatment, or surgery.

Glaucoma is caused by increased pressure within the eye. The optic nerve can be permanently damaged by this increased pressure, resulting in a loss of side vision and, if untreated, blindness. Medication can relieve the pressure by decreasing the amount of fluid produced or by helping it drain more efficiently. Laser and conventional surgery are other options. Of the more than 3 million Americans with glaucoma, only half know that they have it; those who have not been diagnosed lose the opportunity to control it and preserve their sight. People over age 60, African Americans over age 40, and anyone with a family history of glaucoma are at a higher risk.

AMD is a slow disintegration of the *macula*—the tissue at the center of the retina where fine, straight-ahead detail is distinguished. AMD usually occurs after age 50 and is the leading cause of vision loss in Americans age 60 and up. Risk factors for AMD are age, family history, excessive unprotected sun exposure, and poor diet. Some cases of AMD can be treated with injections or laser surgery.

Cataracts are a clouding of the lenses of the eyes. Most cataracts develop as a result of aging, disease (such as diabetes), injury to the lens, or previous eye surgery. Smoking, excessive ultraviolet radiation exposure, and high blood pressure are also associated with increased risk for cataracts. Surgery is usually very effective.

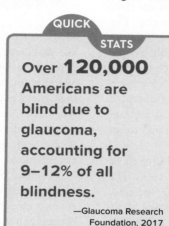

QUICK STATS

Over **120,000** Americans are blind due to glaucoma, accounting for 9–12% of all blindness.

—Glaucoma Research Foundation, 2017

TERMS

glaucoma   An increase in pressure in the eye due to fluid buildup that can result in loss of side vision and, if left untreated, blindness.

age-related macular degeneration (AMD)   A deterioration of the macula (the central area of the retina) leading to loss of vision in the center of the visual field, making it hard to read, drive, or recognize faces.

cataracts   Opacity of the lens of the eye that impairs vision and can cause blindness.

diabetic retinopathy   Damage to the blood vessels of the light-sensitive tissue at the back of the eye (retina) in people who have diabetes.

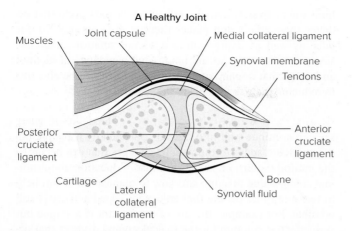

A Healthy Joint

- Muscles
- Joint capsule
- Medial collateral ligament
- Synovial membrane
- Tendons
- Posterior cruciate ligament
- Anterior cruciate ligament
- Cartilage
- Lateral collateral ligament
- Synovial fluid
- Bone

A Joint with Severe Osteoarthritis

- Muscles
- Bone spurs
- Medial collateral ligament
- Synovial membrane
- Tendons
- Posterior cruciate ligament
- Anterior cruciate ligament
- Worn-away cartilage
- Lateral collateral ligament
- Cartilage fragments in fluid
- Synovial fluid
- Bone

FIGURE 23.1 Osteoarthritis. When cartilage wears away within a joint, sharp spurs form and the amount of fluid increases, causing pain and swelling.

SOURCE: *Handout on Health: Osteoarthritis.* National Institute of Arthritis and Musculoskeletal and Skin Diseases. National Institutes of Health, April 2015.

Diabetic eye disease occurs in most people who have had diabetes for over two decades. Early diabetic retinopathy, which is treatable, often has no symptoms. It is crucial that people with diabetes have frequent eye examinations so that retinopathy and other eye diseases can be identified and treated before they result in permanent vision loss and blindness.

Arthritis About half of older people report having doctor-diagnosed **arthritis**, and many more elders have undiagnosed arthritis. The term *arthritis* simply means inflammation involving a joint. Of the more than 100 types of arthritis, osteoarthritis is by far the most common. Rheumatoid arthritis, an autoimmune disorder, is the second most common and is discussed in Chapter 18.

Osteoarthritis is a wear-and-tear disease that first affects the joint cartilage (the covering over the ends of bones that allows smooth movement at the joint). As the cartilage wears away, bone rubs directly against bone, causing damage to the joint. The involved bone often forms sharp spurs that can increase pain and further impair joint movement (Figure 23.1). Osteoarthritis most often affects the hands and the weight-bearing joints of the body—the knees, ankles, hips, and spine. Risk factors for osteoarthritis include aging, previous trauma, chronic overuse of the joints, being overweight, and genetic factors.

The prevention and treatment of osteoarthritis are similar. These strategies include exercise (which can protect the joint by lubricating it and strengthening the muscles that surround it), weight management (which lightens the load on weight-bearing joints), and avoidance of heavy or repetitive use of the joint. Swimming, walking, cross-country skiing, cycling, and tai chi are good low-impact exercises that can be helpful for people with osteoarthritis. Rotating between several types of exercise is helpful in order to avoid overstressing a particular set of joints. Assistive devices such as kitchen utensils and repair tools with large handles and devices that help open jars can help prevent further damage to the joints of the hands.

It is important to visit a physician as soon as arthritis symptoms occur so that the type of arthritis can be determined and appropriate treatment can be started. Exercise, physical therapy, and medications are usually the first treatments used to relieve inflammation and reduce pain, but if a joint is severely damaged and activity is limited, surgery to repair or replace the joint may be considered.

Osteoporosis As described in Chapter 13, **osteoporosis** is a condition in which bones become dangerously thin and fragile, making them very easy to break, even with relatively minor injury. Older women are at higher risk for osteoporosis than men, due in part to bone loss associated with postmenopausal decrease in estrogen. Fractures are the most serious consequence of osteoporosis. In particular, hip fractures take a high toll on the elderly, with up to a 20% incidence of death within a year of the injury. Vertebral compression fractures are also common in people with osteoporosis and a source of significant disability. The collapse of one or more vertebrae can cause loss of height, stooped posture, severe back pain, and breathing problems resulting from changes in the shape of the skeleton.

More than 50 million people in the United States either already have osteoporosis or are at high risk due to low bone mass that is not yet severe enough to meet criteria for osteoporosis. Women are at greater risk for osteoporosis than men because adult women typically have less overall bone mass than men. Bone loss accelerates in women during the first 5 to 10 years after the onset of menopause because of the

arthritis Inflammation and swelling of a joint or joints, usually causing pain and stiffness.

TERMS

osteoporosis The loss of bone density, causing bones to become weak, porous, and more prone to fractures, usually at the hip, spine, or wrist.

drop in estrogen, a hormone that, among many other things, helps to maintain bone mass. That, combined with the fact that women tend to live longer than men, makes osteoporosis much more common in women, although men who live into their eighties and nineties often develop osteoporosis.

Risk factors for osteoporosis include gender, older age, and race (black and Latino women have lower rates of osteoporosis than white and Asian women). Other risk factors include tobacco use, excessive use of alcohol (more than two drinks per day), poor diet (especially long-term low calcium intake), thyroid disease, a family history of osteoporosis, early menopause (before age 45), abnormal or irregular menstruation, a history of anorexia, and a thin, small frame. Thyroid medication, corticosteroid drugs (which are often used to treat conditions such as arthritis or asthma), and certain antiseizure drugs are among the many medications that can increase the risk of osteoporosis.

Preventing osteoporosis requires building as much bone as possible during your young years and then maintaining it as you age. Girls aged 9–18 are in their critical bone-building years, and they should eat foods rich in calcium and vitamin D and get adequate exercise. Weight-bearing activities must be performed regularly throughout life to have lasting effects. Strength training improves bone density, muscle mass, strength, and balance, protecting against both bone loss and falls, a major cause of fractures. Even the very elderly benefit from low-intensity strength training and weight-bearing exercises. These activities can improve bone density and can also improve balance, reducing the risk for falls.

Bone mineral density scans use X-rays to gauge an individual's risk of fracture and help determine if any medical treatment is needed. Screening tests are recommended for all women over 65, all men over 70, and postmenopausal women and men over 50 who have had a fracture or other risk factors. Below-normal bone density that is not severe enough to meet criteria for full-blown osteoporosis may be classified as *osteopenia*, which is usually treated with exercise, nutrition, and sometimes medication. Osteoporosis is treated with lifestyle modifications and medications.

Increased Risk for Falls Weakness, poor vision, impaired balance, cognitive deficits, and environmental hazards all contribute to the risk for falls in the elderly. Older people fall more often than younger adults, and the consequences of their falls tend to be much more severe. About one-third of all people age 65 and older have a significant fall each year. Even relatively minor falls can result in devastating, even lethal, injuries in the elderly. Brittle bones (see "Osteoporosis" above), increased tendency to develop brain bleeds, and general frailty make falls especially dangerous for older people. Older people often have a profound fear of falling that can

> **dementia** A loss of cognitive functioning that can interfere with daily life and cause a loss of the ability to function independently.   **TERMS**

limit their physical activity, creating a vicious cycle that reduces their fitness and makes them at even greater risk for falls, as well as depression and social isolation. Exercise, safety modifications to the home, and avoidance of alcohol and drugs that impair balance and judgment can be effective in reducing the risk for falls in the elderly.

Changes in Sexual Functioning The ability to enjoy sex can continue well into old age, particularly if people understand and adapt to the various changes that age brings to the natural pattern of sexual response. Education about normal changes due to aging and how to manage them can help to reassure older people that enjoyable sexual activity is still possible. For example, the use of a lubricant is a simple but very effective solution for the typical vaginal dryness that occurs after menopause and contributes to difficulties with intercourse. Erectile dysfunction becomes more common as men age but is often treatable with a combination of counseling and medications. In addition, couples can explore enjoyable sexual activities that do not involve intercourse. The mechanics of sexual activity may change as people age, but sexuality can remain a source of pleasure throughout life.

Sexually transmitted infections are on the rise in all age groups, including people over 50. Practicing safe sex, including using condoms, remains important at all ages.

Psychological and Cognitive Changes

Normal aging is associated with many structural, chemical, and functional changes in the brain. The brain as a whole, and certain areas in particular, shrink with aging. Older adults typically experience mild reduction in speed of thinking, memory function, ability to pay attention, and certain aspects of language function (especially the ability to retrieve words). Normally aging adults may experience temporary worsening of cognitive function when they are under extra stress due to information overload, fatigue, illness, or reaction to medications. Beyond brain changes associated with normal aging, older people are also at increased risk for many types of degenerative neurological diseases.

Cognitive Impairment **Dementia** refers to a set of symptoms associated with cognitive decline, such as problems with memory, language, attention, problem solving, and decision making. Diseases that lead to progressive cognitive impairment include, among others, Alzheimer's disease (AD), vascular dementia, cerebrovascular disease, Lewybody dementia (LBD), and frontotemporal lobe dementia. Symptoms of these diseases can include changes in memory, thinking, language, visuospatial function, judgment, and behavior. Early disease stages can sometimes be difficult to differentiate from normal aging, but eventually problems become more apparent, and the person may lose the ability to function independently. Some patients with relatively mild symptoms may fulfill criteria for a diagnosis of *mild cognitive impairment*, which is defined as objective cognitive impairment that can be detected with psychological testing, but the person is still able to function in most activities of daily life. For example, a patient may not recall as many details of a story as others, but she can still live alone, cook for herself, and enjoy a satisfying social life. It is important that people with changes in behavior or cognition be evaluated by a health care professional because some of the over 50 known causes of dementia-like symptoms are treatable (e.g., depression, hypothyroidism, normal pressure hydrocephalus, vitamin B-12 deficiency, overuse of alcohol, and misuse of medications). Even for conditions that cannot be cured, such as AD, different therapies can be tried to ease some symptoms.

The overall prevalence of dementia in the United States is about 10% in people over age 65. The prevalence roughly doubles with every five years of age; about one-third of people age 85 and older have some form of dementia. Globally, approximately 50 million people have dementia. This number is expected to rise over the next several decades due to increased life expectancy. However, some studies suggest that the age-adjusted prevalence of dementia in many developed countries may be decreasing, perhaps due to increased educational attainment and improvements in health (for example, reduced smoking and better control of cardiovascular risk factors).

Alzheimer's disease (AD) is the most common disease leading to dementia and is the cause for an estimated 60–80% of all cases of dementia. AD is a progressive brain disorder that is characterized by a gradual accumulation of the proteins beta-amyloid and tau in the brain. These proteins, in combination with inflammation and other incompletely understood processes, eventually destroy brain cells, leading to impairment of memory, cognition, and other brain functions. AD probably begins 20 years or more before symptoms are first noticed. Once symptoms occur, the disease gradually progresses until the person loses the ability to walk, speak, or even swallow. AD is irreversible and eventually fatal. The diagnosis of early AD can be challenging, and doctors may use biomarkers in cerebrospinal fluid or neuroimaging to confirm that AD is the cause of the symptoms. Research is ongoing to develop a simple and accurate blood test to diagnose AD, but no such test is currently available. On average, people with AD live about eight years after their symptoms become clearly identified. There are several medications that may slightly improve symptoms in some patients, but none of the currently available medications slows or stops the progression of the disease.

In 2019, an estimated 5.8 million Americans of all ages had AD, which usually occurs in people over age 65 but can occur in people as young as age 40. Besides age, the strongest risk factor for late onset AD is the gene variant *APOE ε*4. Other major risk factors include type 2 diabetes, high blood pressure, high total cholesterol, and obesity. Many other genetic and environmental factors may also contribute to the

Ask Yourself

QUESTIONS FOR CRITICAL THINKING AND REFLECTION

Scientists have identified genes that strongly increase the risk for Alzheimer's disease. Would you want to know whether you carried these genes?

risk for AD. Factors that seem to decrease the risk for AD include higher educational attainment and lifestyle factors such as regular physical activity, not smoking, healthy diet, avoiding excess alcohol use, and maintaining a healthy weight. Notice that these are the same lifestyle factors that seem to reduce the risk for heart disease, some cancers, stroke, and other serious diseases associated with aging.

Worrying about developing dementia is very common among middle-aged and older adults. Nearly three out of four adults aged 54 to 60 report using strategies such as playing brain games or taking vitamins or other supplements in the hope of preventing dementia. Unfortunately, many of these strategies are unproven. Supplements for brain health have become a huge business despite the fact that none of these supplements has been proven to be effective in preventing or reducing the risk of dementia. The U.S. Food and Drug Administration strictly regulates prescription drugs but does not regulate supplements. Sellers of supplements can claim that a product helps improve symptoms such as mental alertness or memory, as long as they do not advertise that their product helps prevent or improve a specific disease.

Vascular dementia, or **vascular cognitive impairment,** is a broad term describing cognitive changes that occur due to cerebrovascular disease, which can impair blood flow to the brain, resulting in damage or death of brain tissue. Vascular dementia accounts for about 10% of all dementia, although many experts believe that vascular issues often coexist with and contribute to the brain damage seen in other types of dementia such as AD. The symptoms of vascular dementia vary widely, depending on the type of vascular insult and its location in the brain. Sometimes symptoms start or worsen

TERMS

Alzheimer's disease (AD)   A disease characterized by the accumulation of beta-amyloid and tau in the brain, causing a progressive loss of memory and other brain functions, leading to dementia.

vascular dementia   Cognitive changes that occur due to cerebrovascular disease, when brain cells die due to inadequate blood flow.

cognitive impairment   Reduced mental functioning that may include memory, concentration, and judgment.

after a major stroke, and in other cases symptoms develop gradually due to progressive occlusion of small vessels deep in the brain. High blood pressure, cigarette smoking, diabetes, and hyperlipidemia are some risk factors that may be treated to reduce the risk of vascular cognitive impairment.

Lewy-body dementia (LBD) is a progressive brain disorder in which Lewy bodies (abnormal protein deposits) build up in areas of the brain, causing changes in behavior, cognition, and movement. It is similar to AD in many ways but is more likely than AD to cause fluctuations in cognitive ability, attention, or alertness. People with LBD are also much more likely to have visual hallucinations than people with AD. Additionally, LBD is associated with Parkinson-like changes in walking and movement, sleep disorders, and autonomic problems, such as loss of blood pressure control and disturbed bladder and bowel function. Treatment of symptoms may provide some benefit for patients with LBD, but the disease is not curable.

Mixed dementia is the condition describing what most older people with significant cognitive impairment often have—several brain pathologies simultaneously, which may all contribute to the impairment. The most common scenario is a combination of AD and vascular brain changes.

Grief A common psychological and emotional challenge of aging is dealing with grief. Aging is usually associated with multiple significant losses: deaths of friends and family members, loss of physical strength and appearance, loss of health, and often material losses. Grief is an emotional response to loss. Grief is a natural part of human experience but can be extremely painful and sometimes debilitating and slow to resolve. People of all ages often find help through in-person or online support groups with others who have experienced similar losses. (See Chapter 24 for more information about responses to loss and how to support a grieving person.)

Depression Unresolved grief and chronic health conditions, as well as many other issues, can lead to depression (see Chapter 3). Depression is not a part of normal aging and is important to diagnose and treat. A loss of interest in usually pleasurable activities, decreased appetite, insomnia or increased sleep, fatigue, and feelings of worthlessness are signs of depression.

Many people are surprised to learn that suicide is relatively common among the elderly; in particular, white men aged 65 and over commit suicide nearly six times as often as the general population.

Factors that increase the risk of suicide in the elderly include the recent death of a loved one, physical illness, uncontrolled pain, perceived poor health, social isolation and loneliness, and major changes in social roles (such as retirement). Depression is usually the single most significant factor associated with suicidal behavior in older adults.

LIFE EXPECTANCY

Life expectancy is a statistical average of the ages at death of a group of people over a certain period. In 2018, the overall life expectancy for the total U.S. population was 78.7 years, but those who survive to age 65 can expect to live even longer. A man reaching age 65 today can expect to live, on average, until age 83. A woman turning age 65 today can expect to live, on average, until age 86. In general, women have a longer life expectancy than men (see the box "Why Do Women Live Longer?").

Life expectancy varies among groups due to differences that include socioeconomic, genetic, and lifestyle factors. In the United States and several other countries, life expectancy increased dramatically in the 20th century due to medical and technological advances (see Chapter 1). But these improvements are not evenly distributed throughout society. Between 2001 and 2014, life expectancy didn't change for people in the lowest 5% of income, but it increased by about 3 years for men and women in the top 5%.

The number of very old people is increasing. It has been suggested that the biological **maximum life span** of humans is about 120 years, but recently there has been increasing interest from industry in developing drugs and other treatments that not only extend life but also target the aging process itself.

Although research is making some progress in that area, no magic bullet exists to prevent aging. So far, the only known way to potentially increase your healthy life span is through good diet, exercise, lowered stress, and all the usual measures that reduce risk for heart disease, cancer, stroke, and other common diseases of old age. Despite this, many businesses peddle unproven, often expensive, and sometimes harmful treatments, supplements, and other products that claim to slow down the aging process. These products can be sold as long as they are referred to as a "dietary supplement" and do not claim to treat or prevent any specific disease.

> **QUICK STATS**
>
> Men with the top 1% in income lived **15** years longer than men with the lowest 1% in income; for women, that gap was **10** years.
> —Chetty et al., 2016

> **TERMS**
>
> **Lewy-Body dementia** A progressive brain disorder in which Lewy bodies (abnormal protein deposits) build up in areas of the brain, causing changes in behavior, cognition, and movement.
>
> **life expectancy** The average length of time a person is expected to live.
>
> **maximum life span** A theoretically projected length of life based on the maximum potential of the human body in the best environment.

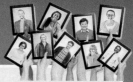
Women live longer than men in nearly every country around the world, even in places where maternal mortality rates are high. In the United States women on average can expect to live about five years longer than men (see the table in this box). As a consequence, the majority of people age 65 and older are women, with over 27 million older women versus about 22 million older men in the United States. Worldwide, women comprise more than 85% of the population that is more than 100 years old. From before birth through old age, human males have higher mortality rates than females. The female advantage in longevity is also seen in many other mammalian species, including great apes and most monkeys.

The reason for the gender gap in life expectancy is not entirely understood but is likely influenced by many biological, social, and lifestyle factors. The fact that females have two X chromosomes while males have only one, as well as differences in mitochondrial inheritance, may provide a genetic advantage that protects females from many diseases. In addition, the female hormone estrogen is also believed to be protective against many health conditions, especially cardiovascular disease. Conversely, the male hormone testosterone may have some negative effects on longevity. Interestingly, males who were castrated before puberty (who have very low levels of testosterone) seem to live much longer on average than men with normal testosterone levels. Hormonal levels may also help explain why men tend to have more visceral fat (fat surrounding the vital organs, such as the heart, that increases the risk for cardiac disease) than women do. Some experts believe that testosterone may also have a negative effect on the immune system.

In general, males are more likely to behave in ways that put them at higher risk for early death. Men are more likely to take more life-threatening risks than women, so they have higher rates of death due to trauma. Suicide rates are considerably higher in males than in females. Men are more likely to smoke and drink excessively than are women. Some experts hypothesize that women cope better with stress than men do.

The news for women is not all good, however, because not all their extra years are likely to be healthy years. They are more likely than men to suffer from chronic, but generally nonlethal, conditions like arthritis and osteoporosis. Women's longer life spans, combined with the fact that men tend to marry younger women and that widowed men remarry more often than widowed women do, mean there are many more single older women than men. Older men are more likely to live in family settings, whereas older women are more likely to live

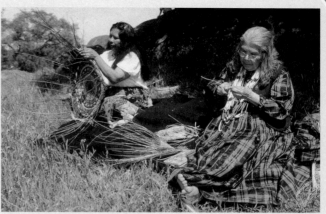

These Kashia Pomo women weave baskets together, which helps them stay active and maintain social and community ties, enhancing wellness as they age. inga spence/Alamy Stock Photo

alone. For many reasons, older women are much more likely than older men to be poor.

Life Expectancy

Year of Birth	Men	Women
Life expectancy at birth		
1900	46.3	48.3
1950	65.6	71.1
2000	74.1	79.3
2010	76.2	81.1
2019	75.4	81.6
Added expected years from age 65		
1900	11.5	12.2
1950	12.8	15.0
2000	16.0	19.0
2010	17.7	20.3
2019	17.4	20.5

SOURCES: National Center for Health Statistics. 2016. *Health, United States, 2015*. Hyattsville, MD: National Center for Health Statistics; World Health Organization. 2019. *World Population Aging 2019*. Geneva: World Health Organization; World Health Organization 2019. *Female life expectancy*.

LIFE IN AN AGING SOCIETY

As life expectancy increases and the birth rate drops, a larger proportion of people will be elderly. Society will need to adapt to a population that is increasingly skewed toward older people. This will necessitate changes in every aspect of our culture, including economics, governmental policies, and changes in our general attitudes toward older adults.

The Aging Minority

People age 65 and over are a large minority in the U.S. population. The number of U.S. elders exceeded 52 million and comprised about 16% of the total U.S. population in 2019. That number is expected to more than double by the year 2060 (Figure 23.2). In that same year, 4.3% of the U.S. population will be older than 85 years. Globally, the population

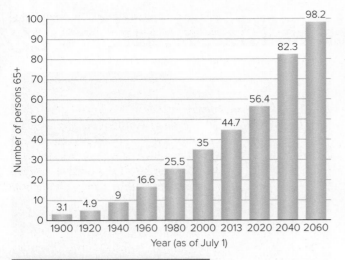

VITAL STATISTICS

FIGURE 23.2   Number of persons aged 65+, 1900–2060 (in millions).

SOURCES: Administration on Aging. 2018. *A Profile of Older Americans: 2017* (https://www.acl.gov/sites/default/files/Aging%20and%20Disability%20in%20America/2017OlderAmericansProfile.pdf); U.S. Census Bureau. 2017. *An Aging Nation* (https://www.census.gov/library/visualizations/2017/comm/cb17-ff08_older_americans.html).

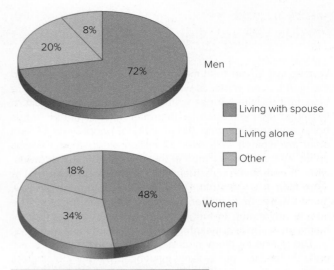

VITAL STATISTICS

FIGURE 23.3   Living arrangements of persons aged 65+, 2017. The majority of older noninstitutionalized Americans live with their spouses, although the rate is significantly higher for men than women. The gender gap is due in part to women's longer life expectancy; in addition, men are less likely than women to be widowed and more likely than women to remarry if their spouse dies.

SOURCE: Administration on Aging. 2018. *A Profile of Older Americans: 2017* (https://www.acl.gov/sites/default/files/Aging%20and%20Disability%20in%20America/2017OlderAmericansProfile.pdf).

over age 60 is expected to reach 2 billion by 2050. The enormous increase in the population of older people is likely to change many of our ideas about what it means to grow old. The depressing stereotype of old people as grumpy, ill, and useless burdens on their families and society will hopefully shift to a more positive picture that reflects the fact that most older people are happy, healthy, and self-sufficient.

Elderly people are often the glue that holds families and communities together. When parents are unable to care for their own children, grandparents often step in and take over the job of parenting. Older people provide untold years of caregiving to their ailing spouses, friends, and others who need their assistance. Just as our society is evolving toward a less prejudiced view of racial and sexual minorities, we need to drop our ingrained stereotypes regarding elders and treat them as individuals, each with unique capacities that add to the richness of our society.

What are the financial and social conditions of elderly people? Many fare quite well. The homeownership rate exceeds 80% for those aged 65–84, which is much higher than the homeownership rate for those under age 65 (about 65%). Older people's living expenses are often lower after retirement, which can help compensate for the decreased income that usually occurs with retirement. Some elders continue working part time, or even full-time, for years after retirement from their previous primary job. Many "retired" people continue to do paid work well into their seventies and beyond.

Unfortunately, the financial status of a substantial proportion of elders in the United States is precarious. Most older Americans rely on fixed sources of income, such as **Social Security** and pensions, that are eroded by inflation and are often not enough to live on comfortably.

Health care is the largest expense for older adults. On average, they visit a physician 10–12 times a year, are hospitalized more frequently, and require twice as many prescription drugs as the general population. Many elderly people with low incomes must choose between paying for medications and buying food. Health care costs are the most common reason for bankruptcy among Americans of all ages, including the elderly.

About 9% of elderly people lived below the official poverty level in 2017. Older women are more likely to be poor than are older men. Older people who live alone are also more likely to be poor than are those who live with families. Elderly whites who live alone are less likely to be poor than Hispanic and African American seniors. The highest poverty rates occur in older Hispanic women who live alone.

Family and Community Resources for Older Adults

With help from friends, family members, and community services, people in their later years can often remain active and independent. Over half of noninstitutionalized older Americans live with a spouse (Figure 23.3); some live with a family

Social Security   A government program that provides financial assistance to retirees, disabled persons, and families of retired, disabled, or deceased workers, financed through taxes on business and workers.   **TERMS**

member other than a spouse, and about 29% live alone. Only about 3% of people age 65 and over live in institutional settings, but among those over age 85, about 9% live in a nursing home.

Family Involvement in Caregiving

Surveys show that three out of four adults age 50 and over say they want to stay in their own home and community as they age. When elderly people are no longer able to live independently, the care they need is usually provided by family members and friends. Two-thirds of older people with long-term care needs receive all their care from unpaid relatives and friends in the family home. Most often, the bulk of the caregiving is provided by the elderly person's spouse, grown daughter, or daughter-in-law. With more people living into their eighties and beyond, and with fewer children per family, many people will face the dilemma of how best to care for an aging relative. Many caregivers are elderly themselves; over a third of caregivers are over age 65. Women provide the bulk of caregiving; surveys indicate that the average woman will spend about 17 years raising children and 18 years caring for an aging relative.

Caregiving can be rewarding, but it is also hard work. When the experience is stressful and long term, family members may become emotionally and physically exhausted. Caregivers are often juggling work, child care, and other home responsibilities in addition to caring for their elderly loved one. Caregivers often need to cut back on work or even quit when caregiving demands increase, which can place them and their families in financial peril. There are a few forward-thinking corporations that respond to the needs of their employees who are family caregivers by providing services such as flexible schedules, leaves, and even on-site adult care. Unfortunately, the majority of family caregivers experience considerable personal and financial strain.

Many caregivers can get some help through free community resources such as adult day care centers. Federal, state, and local governments fund a program called "In Home Supportive Services" that can sometimes help eligible low-income families. For those with the financial means, hiring a professional in-home caregiver for at least a few hours a day can make a huge difference for families that are caring for elderly relatives, especially when the physical demands of care are high, or if round-the-clock care is needed.

Other Living and Care Options

A wide variety of living and care options are available to older people. Retirement communities can be a good choice for people in reasonably good health and with a good income who want to maintain homeownership. Other types of facilities are available for people who need more assistance with daily living (see the box "Choosing a Place to Live").

QUICK STATS

Approximately **42 million** Americans have provided care to an adult aged 50 or over—without pay—in the prior 12 months.

—AARP, 2020

Many agencies also recruit and match people for shared living situations. Home-sharing arrangements can make housing more affordable and offer older adults the opportunity for new relationships, either with peers or with a younger person or family. Intergenerational homesharing may have the advantage of providing elders with the help of younger roommates for things such as demanding physical tasks, while elders in good health can help busy working families with tasks such as child care or household chores.

Long-term care insurance is a way to help meet the financial challenge of senior housing and caregiving needs. Unfortunately, long-term care insurance is very expensive, and often beyond the reach of those who need it the most.

Community Resources

Many communities provide numerous resources to help older adults remain active and in their own homes. Typical services, especially in urban areas, include the following:

- *Senior citizen centers or adult day care centers* provide meals, social activities, and sometimes health care services for those unable to be alone during the day. Many of these centers are operated by state or local governments and are free of charge.
- *Homemaker services* offer housekeeping, cooking, errand running, and escort services, usually for a fee.
- *Visiting nurses* provide basic health care and may be covered by health insurance.
- *Friendly visitor or daily telephone reassurance services* provide social contact for older people who live alone.
- *Home food delivery services* such as "Meals on Wheels" provide meals to homebound people at low cost or for free.
- *Low-cost senior legal aid* helps people manage their finances and legal needs.
- *Transportation services* offer rides for free or at low rates.
- *Geriatric care managers* can help seniors and their families with planning and decision making regarding all aspects of elder care. Geriatric care managers can be especially helpful if family members live far from the elderly person. Insurance doesn't usually cover the cost of a geriatric care manager.

Driving Challenges

Because they tend to be more cautious, older drivers usually have safer driving records than young adults. However, crashes in the older age group are more likely to be fatal. Many states require special driver testing for people over age 70 and may restrict some drivers as to the time, distance, or areas in which they may drive. Because of vision changes, cognitive problems, or other health issues, some older drivers may be required to give up their licenses

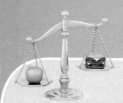

CRITICAL CONSUMER
Choosing a Place to Live

Polls show that a large majority of U.S. adults would like to stay in their homes and communities throughout their elder years. "Aging in place" can be a good option for elders who are functioning well and have the resources to obtain help when their needs increase. Over time, most of us will need help with everyday activities like shopping and cooking, and eventually with walking, dressing, or bathing.

Indeed, about two-thirds of American elders spend their older years in their own home or in the home of relatives or friends who provide their caregiving needs. This arrangement may become unworkable if the person needs round-the-clock attention or has physically demanding care needs. Paid in-home caregivers can be a huge help but are potentially very expensive.

Twenty-four-hour, in-home caregiving costs $250 per day or more in most parts of the United States. For elders with extensive caregiving needs, or who do not have friends or relatives who can care for them, moving to a facility that offers more services often makes the most sense. In addition, aging at home can be isolating for many seniors, who may prefer living in a place with more options for socialization and planned activities. Options besides the family home for elder living include the following:

- *Retirement communities* allow maximum independence with very little supervision. They often provide transportation, activities, and other services but do not routinely offer assistance with basic needs.

- *Residential care homes* (or *adult foster care homes)* are licensed to provide services to three or more residents in a smaller environment, typically in a private home. They usually provide assistance with medications, bathing, dressing, transportation, daily laundry, daily housekeeping, and meals.

- *Assisted living facilities* tend to be larger than residential care homes. They usually provide meals, housekeeping and laundry, transportation, medication management, security, activities, and care management and monitoring. They are not considered medical facilities, and often they are unable to meet the needs of residents who develop conditions that require nursing care. Fees are usually based on the needs of the resident, with higher costs for residents who need more extensive care.

- *Memory care facilities* provide residential care for people with memory loss, usually due to dementia, who are no longer able to safely care for themselves. Ideally, their staff receives specialized training that helps them manage the challenging needs of people with dementia. These facilities can be free-standing or a separate section of an assisted living facility.

- *Nursing homes* (also called skilled nursing facilities) provide 24-hour supervision, nursing care, and rehabilitation services for residents, who usually have significant medical needs. Some nursing home residents stay for short periods of rehabilitation, usually following a hospitalization. However, many nursing home patients are long-term residents who spend months or years receiving care for conditions such as advanced dementia or other severely debilitating conditions.

- Some providers offer all levels of care at one site. These *continuing care communities* allow people to move from one level to another as their needs change.

Finding the right place to live takes considerable investigation and thoughtful planning. It is important to be realistic about not only the person's current needs, but also about anticipating future ones. Consulting with a doctor or other geriatric health professional can be helpful in guiding your choices.

Cost is a major factor for most people. Retirement communities range from modest senior mobile home communities to luxurious accommodations with gourmet meals, extensive recreational facilities, and lavish grounds. Assisted living facilities have variable costs, often depending on the care needs of the resident. The median cost for assisted living in the United States is about $4000 per month. Residential care homes may be somewhat less expensive than assisted living facilities. Many people are surprised to learn that, most of the time, private health insurance and government programs (such as Medicare and Medicaid) do not pay for housing in retirement communities, residential care homes, or assisted living facilities.

Most nursing homes are very expensive; in the United States, the average cost for a nursing home is $245 per day (over $7000 per month). Private long-term care insurance can help pay for some types of long-term care (including in-home caregiving), but fewer than 10% of adults have this type of insurance, mostly due to its limited availability and high cost. A part of the cost of nursing home care may be covered by Medicare in some situations; Medicaid covers nursing home care if the applicant's income and financial assets are low enough.

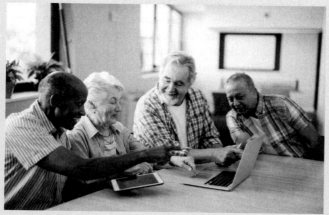

wavebreakmedia/Shutterstock

SOURCES: AARP. 2019. *2018 Home and Community Preferences: A National Survey of Adults Age 18-Plus* (https://www.aarp.org/research /topics/community/info-2018/2018-home-community-preference.html); Senior Living. 2019. *Senior Housing Options and Retirement Guide* (https://www.seniorliving.org/housing/); National Institute on Aging. 2019. *Aging in Place: Growing Older at Home* (https://www.nia.nih.gov/health /aging-place-growing-older-home#place).

before they feel ready. Elderly people report that the loss of a driver's license, and the loss of the independence it brings, is one of the most severe hardships they face. Community senior transportation services and ridesharing are helpful for nondrivers. In the future, self-driving cars are likely to be a boon to seniors who want to remain independent but are no longer able to drive.

Government Aid and Policies

The federal government helps older Americans through several programs, such as food assistance, housing subsidies, Social Security, Medicare, and Medicaid. Social Security, the life insurance and old-age pension plan, has saved many people from destitution, although it is intended as a supplement to other income rather than a sole source. Funding for Social Security comes primarily from American workers who pay into the system, and it depends on a sufficient number of current workers to support the number of retired people who are receiving benefits. As longevity increases and the birth rates decline in the United States, fewer workers will be supporting growing numbers of elderly beneficiaries.

Currently, there are about four working-age adults for every senior citizen in the United States, but this ratio will fall to about 2.6 to 1 by 2050, according to the Social Security Administration. For comparison, there were eight working-age adults for every senior citizen in 1945. Adjustments to the retirement age are being made to ease the strain on the Social Security system. Over a period of years, the age requirement for full Social Security benefits will be gradually increased from age 65 to 67. This and other financial remedies are important to keeping the Social Security system solvent.

Medicare is a major federal health insurance program for older adults and disabled persons. Medicare Part A is financed by part of the payroll (FICA) tax that also pays for Social Security. Medicare Part B is financed by premiums paid by people who choose to enroll. Part A helps pay for inpatient hospital care, some inpatient care in a skilled nursing facility, and some types of home and hospice care. Medicare Part B helps pay for physicians' services and other services not covered by Part A. Medicare parts C and D are optional private plans that help cover health care and prescription costs.

Overall, Medicare pays about half of all health care costs for older Americans as a group. It provides basic health care coverage for acute episodes of illness that require skilled professional care. It pays for some preventive services, including an initial physical exam, vaccinations, and screenings for cardiovascular disease, certain cancers, and many other conditions. It does not pay for many office visits, dental care, or dentures. The vast majority of nursing home care, especially long-term care, is not covered by Medicare. About 1.3 million older people currently live in nursing homes, but Medicare pays less than 2% of nursing home costs, and private insurers pay less than 1%, creating a tremendous financial burden for nursing home residents and their families.

When their financial resources are exhausted, people may apply for Medicaid. Created by a 1965 amendment to the Social Security Act, Medicaid provides medical insurance to low-income people of any age. Funded by state and federal contributions, the services vary from state to state but typically include hospital, nursing home, and home health care; physician services; and some medical supplies and services.

A crucial question regarding aid for elderly people is who will pay for it as our aging population expands. Currently, the government picks up many of these health care expenses, primarily through Medicare and Medicaid. Total health care expenditures are about 18% of the U.S. gross domestic product; people aged 55 and older account for more than half of total health care spending. Most countries throughout the world have some form of universal health care coverage for people of all ages. The United States is unique among developed nations in not having a health care system that provides care for all people.

Reimagining Aging

All too often, we have a negative view of aging. There are many benefits of older age. As we age, we acquire skills, wisdom, and a sense of history and perspective that can come only with spending lots of time on this earth. Although seniors generally score lower on tests of cognitive processing speed than younger people, in "real life" many of the most successful and respected leaders in our society are senior citizens who provide knowledge and wisdom that more than make up for a slight decrease in cognitive speed.

Contrary to the stereotype of the grumpy old man, studies show that our older years, along with childhood, are often the most contented times of our lives. According to researchers, our happiness tends to follow a U-shaped curve

QUICK STATS

For about half of seniors, Social Security provides at least **50**% of their income; for about **1 in 4** seniors, it provides at least **90**%.

—Center on Budget and Policy Priorities, 2019

Ask Yourself

QUESTIONS FOR CRITICAL THINKING AND REFLECTION

What do you want your life to be like when you are older? Do you hope to retire, or keep working indefinitely? Where would you like to live? How much time do you spend thinking about these questions? What have you planned for your later years?

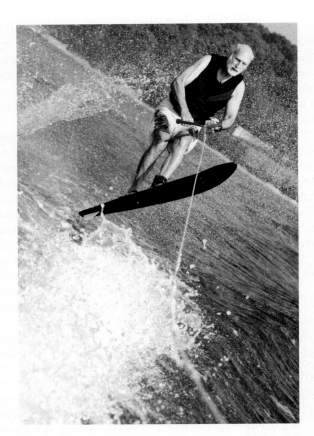

Some individuals defy all preconceived ideas about age and continue to live vigorous lives into their seventies, eighties, and beyond. durdenimages/123RF

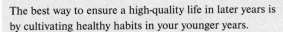
throughout our life span, with the least happy years being middle age, and the happiest times being when we are youngest and oldest.

Age is no guarantee of either wisdom or happiness. But why might a 70-year-old be more content or even happier than a 40-year-old? One reason could be that by old age, many of us will have developed a more peaceful acceptance of life that replaces the constant stress and striving of our middle years. Older people have often weathered devastating experiences such as the loss of loved ones, divorce, lost jobs, and other disappointments and personal tragedies. Many older people have finally figured out, often by adjusting expectations, what is most important to them and have stopped worrying so much about all the rest.

Younger people often find it very hard to imagine that they will one day be old, but being realistic about the opportunities and challenges of aging can help us best prepare for our older years. Whether you realize it or not, right now you are setting the stage for your aging experience. If you value wellness throughout life by being physically active, eating well, and cherishing close relationships, you greatly increase your chances of being healthy and happy in old age. If you treat old age as something to embrace, it should ease the adjustment to inevitable changes when you reach that stage of life.

SUMMARY

- People who take charge of their health during their youth have greater control over the physical and mental aspects of aging.

- Biological aging takes place over a lifetime, but some other changes associated with aging are more abrupt.

- A lifetime of interests and hobbies helps maintain creativity and intelligence.

- Exercise and a healthful diet throughout life enhance physical and psychological health.

- Alcohol and drug misuse is a common but often hidden problem among older adults.

- Tobacco use shortens life and may cause severe health impairment for many years.

- Keeping up with immunizations and participating in recommended health screening can help us live a longer, healthier life.

- Stress translates to wear and tear on the body; getting enough sleep, nurturing social connections, and practicing relaxation can be effective in reducing stress and increasing vitality and happiness.

- Retirement can be one of the most fulfilling and enjoyable times of life. Adjusting to new roles, participating in a variety of activities, having enough money to live comfortably, and having a sense of purpose in life are all important factors in successful retirement.

• Successful aging also involves anticipating and accommodating physical changes and limitations.

• Occasional slight confusion and forgetfulness are a part of normal aging, but more severe symptoms could be signs of a neurodegenerative disease, such as Alzheimer's disease, and should prompt a medical evaluation.

• Learning to cope with loss is an important part of the aging journey.

• Older adults can be role models for the successful integration of life's experiences and the ability to adapt to challenges.

• People over age 65 form a large and growing minority in the United States and throughout the world.

• Family and community resources can help older adults stay active and independent.

• Government aid to older adults includes food assistance, housing subsidies, Social Security, Medicare, and Medicaid.

FOR MORE INFORMATION

AARP. Provides information about all aspects of aging, including health promotion, health care, and retirement planning.

http://www.aarp.org

Administration on Aging. Provides fact sheets, statistical information, and internet links to other resources on aging.

http://www.acl.gov

Alliance for Aging Research. A nonprofit organization that supports medical and psychological research on aging.

http://www.agingresearch.org

Alzheimer's Association. Offers tips for caregivers and patients and information on the causes and treatment of Alzheimer's disease.

http://www.alz.org

American Diabetes Association. Provides information about treatment and management of the disease.

http://www.diabetes.org

Arthritis Foundation. Provides information about arthritis, including free brochures, referrals to local services, and research updates.

http://www.arthritis.org

Family Caregiver Alliance. Provides extensive educational material for caregivers, including written material in many languages, videos, and classes; provides support such as respite care; advocates for caregivers through public policy.

http://www.caregiver.org

Healthy Aging: U.S. Department of Health and Human Services. Lists numerous significant resources for all aspects of aging healthfully: brain and mental health, nutrition, exercise training, networking, how to locate benefits and find care, retirement planning, and many other aspects.

http://www.hhs.gov/aging/healthy-aging/index.html#

Medicare. Provides signup information; listings to compare doctors, providers, hospitals, plans, and suppliers available through the program; and details on costs and coverage.

http://www.medicare.gov

National Council on Aging. Provides helpful information about retirement planning, health promotion, and lifelong learning.

http://www.ncoa.org

National Institute on Aging. Provides fact sheets and brochures about aging-related topics.

http://www.nia.nih.gov

https://www.nia.nih.gov/health/exercise-physical-activity

National Osteoporosis Foundation. Provides information about the causes, prevention, detection, and treatment of osteoporosis.

http://www.nof.org

World Health Organization. Information about the global impact of dementia and several other age-related diseases.

http://www.who.int/mental_health/neurology/dementia/en/

SELECTED BIBLIOGRAPHY

AARP Public Policy Institute and National Alliance for Caregiving. 2020. *Caregiving in the United States 2020* (http://www.aarp.org/ppi/info-2020/caregiving-in-the-united-states.html).

Administration on Aging. 2018. *A Profile of Older Americans: 2017* (https://www.acl.gov/sites/default/files/Aging%20and%20Disability%20in%20America/2017OlderAmericansProfile.pdf).

Agency for Healthcare Research and Quality. 2016. *Statistical Brief #491: National Health Care Expenses in the U.S. Civilian Noninstitutionalized Population, Distributions by Type of Service and Source of Payment, 2013* (https://meps.ahrq.gov/data_files/publications/st491/stat491.shtml).

Agronin, M. 2019. Sexual dysfunction in older adults. *Up To Date* (https://www.uptodate.com/contents/sexual-dysfunction-in-older-adults).

Alzheimer's Association. 2019. *2019 Alzheimer's Disease Facts and Figures* (https://www.alz.org/media/documents/alzheimers-facts-and-figures-2019-r.pdf).

Alcohol Addiction Center. 2020. *Six Facts About Elderly Alcohol Abuse.* (https://alcoholaddictioncenter.org/elder-alcohol-abuse/).

America's Health Ratings. 2020. *Poverty in United States Summary 2020* (https://www.americashealthrankings.org/explore/senior/measure/poverty_sr/state/ALL).

Arias, E., and J. Xu. 2019. *United States Life Tables, 2017.* National Vital Statistics Reports. (https://www.cdc.gov/nchs/data/nvsr/nvsr68/nvsr68_07-508.pdf).

Armstrong, S. 2019. *Borrowed Time: The Science of How and Why We Age.* London: Bloomsbury Sigma.

Axelrod, J. et al. 2019. Isolated and struggling, many seniors are turning to suicide. *National Public Radio* (https://www.npr.org/2019/07/27/745017374/isolated-and-struggling-many-seniors-are-turning-to-suicide).

Binette, J., and K. Vasold. 2018. *2018 Home and Community Preferences: A National Survey of Adults Age 18-Plus.* Washington, DC: AARP Research, August (https://www.aarp.org/research/topics/community/info-2018/2018-home-community-preference.html?CMP=RDRCT-PRI-OTHER-LIVABLECOMMUNITIES-032218).

Bleiberg, L. 2019. Congress approves over-the-counter hearing aids. AARP (https://www.aarp.org/health/conditions-treatments/info-2019/otc-hearing-aids.html).

Castel, A. 2018. *Better with Age: The Psychology of Successful Aging.* Oxford: Oxford University Press.

Centers for Disease Control and Prevention. 2012. Prevalence of doctor-diagnosed arthritis and arthritis-attributable activity limitation—United States, 2010–2012. *Morbidity and Mortality Weekly Report* 55(40): 1089–1092.

Centers for Disease Control and Prevention. 2020. *Alzheimer's Disease and Healthy Aging* (https://www.cdc.gov/aging/publications/features/dementia-not-normal-aging.html).

Cheng, F., et al. 2016. Body mass index and all-cause mortality among older adults. *Obesity* (https://www.ncbi.nlm.nih.gov/pubmed/27570944).

Chetty, R., et al. 2016. The association between income and life expectancy in the United States, 2001–2014. *Journal of the American Medical Association* 315(16): 1750–1766.

Chin-Mei, L., and C. Lee. 2019. Association of hearing loss with dementia. *JAMA Network Open* (https://jamanetwork.com/journals/jamanetworkopen/fullarticle/2740068).

Cicero. 1923. *On Old Age. On Friendship. On Divination.* Translated by W. A. Falconer. Loeb Classical Library 154. Cambridge, MA: Harvard University Press.

Cubanski, J., et al. 2018. *How Many Seniors Live in Poverty?* Kaiser Family Foundation (https://www.kff.org/medicare/issue-brief/how-many-seniors-live-in-poverty/).

Devitt, M. 2018. *CDC Data Show U.S. Life Expectancy Continues to Decline: Suicides, Drug Overdose Deaths Named as Key Contributors.* American Academy of Family Practice (https://www.aafp.org/news/health-of-the-public/20181210lifeexpectdrop.html)

Family Caregiver Alliance. 2019. *Caregiver Statistics: Demographics* (https://www.caregiver.org/caregiver-statistics-demographics).

Fulmer, T., and D. Volmert. 2018. Reframing aging: Growing "old at heart." *Stanford Social Innovation Review* (https://ssir.org/articles/entry/reframing_aging_growing_old_at_heart#).

Gawande, A. 2014. *Being Mortal: Medicine and What Matters in the End.* New York: Metropolitan Books/Henry Holt & Company.

Gollub, J., et al. 2019. Association of subclinical hearing loss with cognitive performance. *JAMA Otolaryngology Head Neck Surgery* (https://jamanetwork.com/journals/jamaotolaryngology/fullarticle/2755646?guestAccessKey=9854eff1-fb55-4f64-88a0-4fc1466f9475&utm_content=weekly_highlights&utm_term=112319&utm_source=silverchair&utm_campaign=jama_network&cmp=1&utm_medium=email).

Hellmuth, J., G. D. Rabinovici, and B. L. Miller. 2019. The rise of pseudo-medicine for dementia and brain health. *Journal of the American Medical Association* 321(6): 543–544.

Hall, K. S., et al. 2017. Physical performance across the adult life span: Correlates with age and physical activity. *The Journals of Gerontology. Series A, Biological Sciences and Medical Sciences* 72(4): 572–578.

Harvard Men's Health Watch. 2019. *Don't Buy Into Brain Health Supplements.* Harvard Health Publishing (https://www.health.harvard.edu/mind-and-mood/dont-buy-into-brain-health-supplements).

House Committee on the Budget. 2018. *Retirement Security for an Aging Population Requires Higher Federal Spending* (https://budget.house.gov/publications/report/retirement-security-aging-population-requires-higher-federal-spending).

Hyams, J. 2011. *Time to Help Your Parents.* London: Piatkus.

Jellmuth, J., et al. 2019. The rise of pseudomedicine for dementia and brain health. *Journal of the American Medical Association* 321(6): 543–544.

Joshi, P. K., et al. 2017. Genome-wide meta-analysis associates *HLA-DQA1/DRB1* and *LPA* and lifestyle factors with human longevity. *Nature Communications* 8: 910.

Kaiser Family Foundation. 2019. *An Overview of Medicare* (https://www.kff.org/medicare/issue-brief/an-overview-of-medicare/).

Khan, S. S., et al. 2017. Molecular and physiological manifestations and measurement of aging in humans. *Aging Cell* 16(4): 624–633.

Langa, K. M., et al. 2017. A comparison of the prevalence of dementia in the United States in 2000 and 2012. *JAMA Internal Medicine* 177(1): 51–58.

Kirkwood, T. 2010. Why women live longer: Stress alone does not explain the longevity gap. *Scientific American*, October, 21.

Lewy Body Dementia Association. 2019. *What Is LBD?* (https://www.lbda.org/go/what-lbd-0).

Meyer, J. 2012. Centenarians: 2010. 2010 Census Special Reports (https://www.census.gov/prod/cen2010/reports/c2010sr-03.pdf).

National Council on Aging. 2015. *Falls Free: 2015 National Falls Prevention Action Plan* (www.ncoa.org/wp-content/uploads/FallsActionPlan_2015-FINAL.pdf).

National Center for Victims of Crimes. 2018. *Crimes Against Older Adults* (https://ovc.ncjrs.gov/ncvrw2018/info_flyers/fact_sheets/2018NCVRW_OlderAdults_508_QC.pdf).

National Council on Aging. 2019. Healthy Aging—Fact Sheet (https://d2mkcg26uvg1cz.cloudfront.net/wp-content/uploads/2018-Healthy-Aging-Fact-Sheet-7.10.18-1.pdf).

National Council on Aging. 2019. *Top 10 Financial Scams Targeting Seniors* (https://www.ncoa.org/economic-security/money-management/scams-security/top-10-scams-targeting-seniors/).

National Eye Institute. 2020. *Age-Related Macular Degeneration* (https://www.nei.nih.gov/learn-about-eye-health/eye-conditions-and-diseases/age-related-macular-degeneration).

National Eye Institute. 2019. *Diabetic Retinopathy* (https://www.nei.nih.gov/learn-about-eye-health/eye-conditions-and-diseases/diabetic-retinopathy).

National Institute on Aging. 2020. *Exercise & Physical Activity:* Getting Fit for Life (https://www.nia.nih.gov/health/exercise-and-physical-activity-getting-fit-life).

National Institute on Aging. 2019. *Long Term Care: Residential Facilities, Assisted Living, and Nursing Homes* (https://www.nia.nih.gov/health/residential-facilities-assisted-living-and-nursing-homes).

National Poll on Healthy Aging. 2019. *Thinking About Brain Health.* University of Michigan. (https://www.healthyagingpoll.org/report/thinking-about-brain-health).

NIH Osteoporosis and Related Bone Diseases National Resource Center. 2019. *Osteoporosis Overview* (https://www.bones.nih.gov/health-info/bone/osteoporosis/overview).

Ortman, J. M., V. A. Velkoff, and H. Hogan. 2014. *Aging Nation: The Older Population in the U.S.* (http://www.census.gov/prod/2014pubs/p25-1140.pdf).

Partnership to Fight Chronic Disease. 2019. *What Is the Impact of Chronic Disease on America?* (http://www.fightchronicdisease.org/sites/default/files/pfcd_blocks/PFCD_US.FactSheet_FINAL1%20(2).pdf).

Population Reference Bureau. 2019. Fact Sheet: Aging in the United States (https://www.prb.org/aging-unitedstates-fact-sheet/).

Rauch, J. 2019. *The Happiness Curve: Why Life Gets Better After 50.* London: Picador Publishing/Macmillan Publishers.

Rico-Uribe, L. et al. 2018. Association of loneliness with all-cause mortality: A meta-analysis. *PLoS One* (https://www.ncbi.nlm.nih.gov/pmc/articles/PMC5754055/).

Sacks, O. 2015. *Gratitude.* Canada: Knopf.

Sawyer, B., and G. Claxton. 2019. *How Do Health Expenditures Vary Across the Population?* Peterson-Kaiser Family Foundation (https://www.healthsystemtracker.org/chart-collection/health-expenditures-vary-across-population/#item-start).

Simon, S. 2015. *Unforgettable: A Son, a Mother, and the Lessons of a Lifetime.* New York: Flatiron Books, Macmillan.

Social Security Administration. 2015. *Fast Facts & Figures About Social Security, 2015* (SSA Publication No. 13-11785). Washington, DC: Social Security Administration.

Stern, C., and Z. Munn. 2010. Cognitive leisure activities and their role in preventing dementia: A systematic review. *International Journal of Evidence-Based Healthcare* 8(1): 2–17.

Tavernise, S. 2016. Centenarians proliferate, and live longer. *The New York Times,* 21 January.

Tyrovolas, S, et al. 2019. Skeletal muscle mass in relation to 10 year cardiovascular disease incidence among middle aged and older adults: The ATTICA study. *Journal of Epidemiology and Community Health.* Published online 11 November (https://jech.bmj.com/content/early/2019/10/16/jech-2019-212268.full).

United States Census Bureau. 2017, June 22. The nation's older population is still growing, Census Bureau reports. Release number CB17-100 (https://www.census.gov/newsroom/press-releases/2017/cb17-100.html).

United States Census Bureau. 2018, March 13. Older people expected to outnumber children for first time in U.S. history. Release number CB18-41 (https://www.census.gov/newsroom/press-releases/2018/cb18-41-population-projections.html)

University of Pennsylvania. 2013. Balancing act: Cell senescence, aging related to epigenetic changes. Perelman School of Medicine news release, August 30.

U.S. Department of Health and Human Services. 2018. *Physical Activity Guidelines for Americans,* 2nd ed. (https://health.gov/paguidelines/second-edition/pdf/Physical_Activity_Guidelines_2nd_edition.pdf).

Design Elements: Take Charge icon: VisualCommunications/Getty Images; Diversity Matters icon: Rawpixel Ltd/Getty Images; Critical Consumer icon: pagadesign/Getty Images.

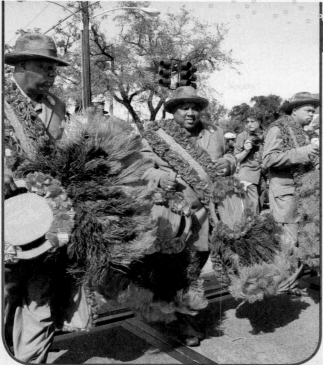

Ninette Maumus/Alamy Stock Photo

CHAPTER 24

Dying and Death

TEST YOUR KNOWLEDGE

ANSWERS

1. **What are the top three leading causes of death, in order, for Americans aged 15–34?**
   a. Cancer, unintentional injury, homicide
   b. Homicide, suicide, cancer
   c. Unintentional injury, suicide, homicide

2. **If you die in a car crash, your organs will automatically be donated to people waiting for transplants.**
   True or False?

3. **How many Americans die each day while waiting for an organ transplant?**
   a. 3
   b. 9
   c. 20

4. **Physician-assisted death is considered murder and is illegal in all 50 states.**
   True or False?

5. **The best way to help a friend who is grieving is to distract her or him from the loss by talking about sports, gossip, or other lighthearted topics.**
   True or False?

1. **C.** Unintentional injury is the number-one cause of death in young adults in the United States. This includes everything from car crashes to unintentional drug overdoses. Suicide is next, followed by homicide. Cancer and heart disease deaths rank fourth and fifth.

2. **FALSE.** For your organs to be donated, you must have authorized it prior to your death, or the donation must be authorized by relatives at the time of your death.

3. **C.** Every day in the United States, about 80 people receive an organ transplant, but another 20 people die while waiting for a needed organ.

4. **FALSE.** As of January 1, 2020, physician-assisted death (PAD) is legal in Oregon, Washington, Vermont, California, New Jersey, Colorado, Hawaii, Maine, and Washington, DC.

5. **FALSE.** Many people who are grieving want to talk about their loss, and a friend who will let them talk freely is valuable. The best strategy is simply to be a good listener and follow your grieving friend's lead.

Whether it is victims of a terrorist attack, an earthquake or a car crash, or a woman in her nineties dying peacefully with her family close by, images of death are all around us. Nevertheless, we rarely think about the inevitability of death in our own lives. Most of us live as if we are immortal. Accepting and dealing with death presents unique challenges to our sense of self, our relationships with others, and our understanding of the meaning of life itself.

Although pain and distress may accompany the dying process, facing death also presents an opportunity for growth as well as affirmation of the preciousness of our daily lives. Dealing with the death of a loved one can tear families apart, but it can also bring them together. The way we choose to confront death can greatly influence how we live.

This chapter discusses some of the many questions surrounding the end of life, including its meaning and function, steps individuals can take to make their death a bit easier for their loved ones, and tasks you may need to consider in preparing for your own death. This chapter also examines the process of grieving and provides advice that can help in dealing with the death of a loved one.

UNDERSTANDING AND ACCEPTING DEATH AND DYING

From a personal point of view, death challenges our emotional and intellectual security. We may acknowledge the fact that all living things die eventually and that this is nature's way of renewal, but this recognition offers little comfort when death touches our own lives. Questions about the meaning of death and what happens when we die are central to the great religions and philosophies of the world. Some promise a better life after death. Others teach that everyone is evolving toward perfection or divinity, a goal reached after successive rounds of life, death and rebirth. Still others suggest that it is not possible to know what—if anything—happens after death and that any judgment about life's worth and meaning must be made on the basis of satisfactions or rewards we create for ourselves and those around us in our lifetimes.

Even for the most secular individuals, spiritual beliefs and traditions can shape attitudes and behaviors surrounding death. Spirituality and religion offer solace to the extent that they may provide some meaning in dying. Mourning rituals and ceremonies associated with various religions ease the pangs of grief for many people. Dying and death are more than biological events; they have social and spiritual dimensions. Our beliefs—religious or philosophical—can be a key to how we relate to the prospect of our own death as well as the deaths of others.

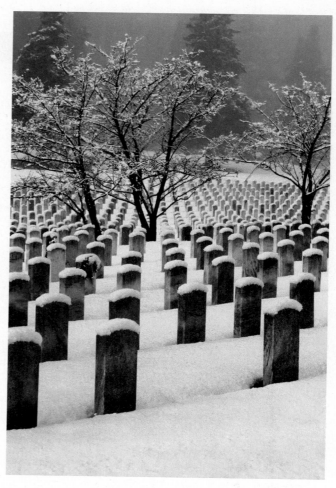

Death awaits all of us, and accepting and dealing with it are difficult but important tasks. Tom Mareschal/Photographer's Choice/Getty Images

Ultimately, we have no fully satisfying answer to the question of why death exists. When we look at the big picture, we see that death promotes variety through the evolution of species. The average human life is long enough to allow a person to reproduce and ensure that the species continues. Yet it is brief enough to allow for new genetic combinations, thereby providing a means of adaptation to changing conditions in the environment. From the perspective of species survival, the cycle of life and death makes sense.

Senescence, the biological process of aging, is complex, rooted in genetics, and universal in all mammals, including humans. Organisms age on both a cellular and a whole-organism level, ultimately resulting in death. Although scientific understanding of senescence is progressing, and average life spans are increasing, death remains an inevitable event for humans and nearly all other living beings.

Defining Death

Paradoxically, as our scientific understanding of death increases, defining death has become increasingly difficult.

senescence The biological process of aging. **TERMS**

Traditionally death has been defined as cessation of the flow of vital body fluids. This cessation occurs when the heart stops beating and breathing ceases, referred to as **clinical death.** These traditional signs are adequate for determining death in most cases. However, over the past several decades, the use of cardiopulmonary resuscitation (CPR) and other medical techniques have brought many "dead" people (by the traditional definition) back to life. The use of ventilators, artificial heart pumps, and other **life support systems** allow many body functions to be sustained artificially. In such cases, making a determination of death can be difficult and often controversial. The concept of **brain death** was developed to determine whether a person is alive or dead when traditional signs are inadequate because of supportive medical technology. The way death is defined has significant legal, ethical, and social consequences, including potential effects on criminal prosecution, inheritance, treatment of the corpse, and even mourning.

The Uniform Determination of Death Act, developed in 1981, provides criteria for determining brain death, which is defined as the complete and irreversible loss of function of the entire brain. The concept of brain death is particularly crucial for organ donation and transplantation. Medical technologies such as ventilators are used so that organs will remain viable over the hours or days that are needed to arrange for transplantation. Some organs—hearts, most obviously—must be harvested from a human being who is declared legally dead. Timing is critical in removing a heart from someone who has been declared dead and transplanting it into a person whose life can thereby be saved.

Safeguards are necessary to ensure that the determination of death occurs without regard to any plans for subsequent transplantation of the deceased's organs. Several thorough examinations need to be performed over a period of time in order to determine that both higher brain and brain-stem functions (which regulate heartbeat and breathing) have ceased irreversibly. The American Academy of Neurology published guidelines in 2010 for determination of brain death, but state laws are often nonspecific, and individual medical facilities have varying policies for determining brain death. The Academy has called for uniform legal standards for brain death in all states, as well as standard policies and practices regarding determination of brain death for all medical facilities throughout the United States.

As medical and technological advances occur, it has become increasingly clear that biological death consists of a series of events that occur over a period of time. In contrast to clinical death (irreversible cessation of heartbeat and breathing) or brain death, **cellular death** refers to a gradual process that occurs when heartbeat, respiration, and brain activity have stopped. Many cells throughout the body continue to survive for seconds, minutes, or hours after clinical and brain death, but gradually die as they utilize remaining oxygen and glucose. Cellular death encompasses the breakdown of metabolic processes and results in complete nonfunctionality at the cellular level. In a biological sense,

therefore, death can be defined as the cessation of life due to irreversible changes in cell metabolism.

Learning about Death

Our understanding of death changes as we grow and mature, as do our attitudes toward it. Very young children view death as an interruption and an absence, but their lack of a mature time perspective means that they do not understand death as final and irreversible. A child's understanding of death evolves greatly from about age 6 to age 9. During this period, most children begin to understand that death is final, universal, and inevitable. A person who consciously recognizes these facts is said to possess a **mature understanding of death.** Based on work done by Mark Speece and Sandor Brent, a formal understanding of the empirical, or observable, facts about death includes four components:

1. *Universality.* All living things die eventually. Death is all-inclusive, inevitable, and unavoidable (although unpredictable with respect to its exact timing). The bottom line is that we know we will die, but we don't know when.

2. *Irreversibility.* Organisms that die cannot be made alive again.

3. *Nonfunctionality.* Death involves the cessation of all physiological functioning, or signs of life.

4. *Causality.* There are biological reasons for the occurrence of death.

However, even individuals who possess a mature understanding of death commonly also hold nonempirical ideas about it. Such nonempirical ideas—that is, ideas not subject to scientific proof—deal mainly with the notion that human beings survive in some form beyond the death of the physical body. What happens to an individual's personality after he or she dies? Does the self or soul continue to exist after the death of the physical body? If so, what is the nature of this afterlife?

clinical death   The medical term applied to the TERMS point at which there is no longer blood flow in the body (the heart has stopped beating) and breathing has ceased.

life support systems   Medical technologies, such as a ventilator, that allow vital body functions to be sustained artificially.

brain death   A complete and irreversible cessation of brain activity indicated by various diagnostic criteria; this medical determination may be necessary when intensive hospital-based life support systems have been used to artificially sustain organ systems in the body.

cellular death   The breakdown of metabolic processes at the level of the body's cells.

mature understanding of death   The recognition that death is universal and irreversible, that it involves the cessation of all physiological functioning, and that there are biological reasons for its occurrence.

Developing personally satisfying answers to such questions, which involve what Speece and Brent term **noncorporeal continuity,** is also part of the process of acquiring a mature understanding of death.

In the United States, with its relative affluence and orderliness, death is not a part of the day-to-day existence of most young people. The death of a beloved pet is often a child's first experience of the reality and permanence of death. Even by college age, most Americans have experienced few, if any, deaths among their loved ones. There are exceptions, however, especially among those who have grown up in relatively dangerous environments, such as neighborhoods with high rates of violence or in places where deaths due to drug overdose are particularly frequent. However, even when death strikes those around us, many of us continue to feel a sense of invulnerability—that is, "It won't happen to me." By the time we reach old age, reminders of aging and death are frequent, especially as we experience the loss of many of our peers. The very old have often lost nearly everyone of significance in their lives. Coping with the death of loved ones and the loneliness that often follows, and preparing for our own impending death are central developmental tasks for the very elderly.

Denying versus Acknowledging Death

Understanding death in a mature fashion does not imply that we never experience anxiety about the deaths of those we love or about the prospect of our own deaths. The news of a friend's or loved one's serious illness can shock us into an encounter with mortality—not only that of our friend or loved one, but also of our own. The ability to find meaning and comfort in the face of mortality depends not only on having an understanding of the facts of death but also on our attitudes toward it.

Many people avoid any thought or mention of death. The sick and old are often isolated in hospitals and nursing homes. Relatively few Americans have been present at the death of a loved one. Where the reality of death is concerned, "out of sight, out of mind" is often the rule of the day. Instead of facing death rationally, our cultures are filled with unrealistic portrayals of death in movies, television, and video games. Children and many adults consume a daily fare of fake death. Cartoons and video games present death in a two-dimensional world where you can die and then be reborn to play again only seconds later.

Although many commentators characterize the predominant attitude toward death in the United States as "death denying," others are reluctant to generalize so broadly. People often maintain conflicting or ambivalent attitudes

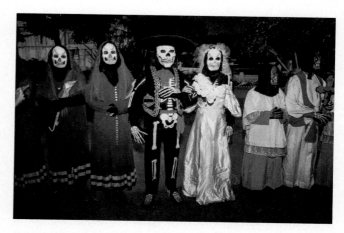

In Mexico, individuals publicly celebrate departed loved ones on the annual holiday *Día de los Muertos* (Day of the Dead). fitopardo.com/Getty Images

toward death. Those who view death as a relief or release from insufferable pain may have at least a sense that death is sometimes welcomed, but few people wholly avoid or wholly welcome death. In the past several decades, attitudes toward death in our culture have begun to change slowly. The hospice movement (discussed later in this chapter) has provided support and guidance for many families who choose to be present during the dying process of their loved ones, often in their own homes. Dying in a home setting fulfills the wishes of many patients and can also be a great comfort to friends and family.

Some cultures not only acknowledge the reality of death, but actually embrace it, even at times in a joyous way. For example, traditional Mexican culture honors the dead by remembering them often, especially during the annual holiday *Día de los Muertos* (Day of the Dead), in which families include their departed loved ones in their celebrations. This holiday is festive, tinged with some sadness, but mostly full of love, fun, and good humor. Similar celebrations that honor the dead in a festive manner are common in many cultures throughout the world. In the United States, Halloween—originally celebrated in church liturgy to remember their faithful dead—is now just a "spooky" holiday; witches, ghosts, and scary entities of all types abound, but our own departed loved ones are not invited to the party. Although specific religions have their own ways of honoring the dead, the general American culture lacks outlets for remembering departed loved ones and honoring their place in our hearts.

noncorporeal continuity   The notion that human beings survive in some form after the death of the physical body.

TERMS

Ask Yourself

QUESTIONS FOR CRITICAL THINKING AND REFLECTION
What situations or events make you think seriously about your own mortality? Is this something you consider now and then, or do you avoid thinking about death? What has influenced your willingness or reluctance to think about death?

PLANNING FOR DEATH

Acknowledging the inevitability of death allows us to plan for it. Adequate planning can help ensure that a sudden, unexpected death is not made even more difficult for survivors. Even when death is not sudden, individuals with a debilitating illness may become unable to make decisions for themselves. Many decisions can be anticipated, considered, and discussed with close relatives and friends long before death occurs.

Basic tasks in planning for death include making a will, appointing a health care power of attorney, setting up an advance health care directive, anticipating medical care needs, expressing preferences for end-of-life care, considering whether to become an organ donor, and helping survivors manage responsibilities. It is reasonable to begin some of these plans even during your college years, particularly with regard to issues such as organ donation, advance directives, and power of attorney for health care, and to review and revise these decisions periodically throughout life. Young people can also help their older relatives by urging them to complete these important tasks.

Making a Will

Surveys indicate that nearly 6 in 10 adult Americans do not have a will. Common reasons for not making a will include not wanting to deal with a "depressing subject," wanting to avoid the expense of legal services, the idea that "I don't need a will because I don't have much money," and "I just haven't gotten around to it." Whatever the reason, dying without a will can lead to unnecessary hardships for survivors, even when an estate is modest in size.

A **will** is a legal instrument expressing a person's intentions and wishes for the disposition of his or her property after death. It is a declaration of how your **estate**—that is, money, property, and other possessions—will be distributed after your death. During the life of the **testator** (the person making the will), a will can be changed, replaced, or revoked. When the testator dies, it becomes a legal instrument governing the distribution of the estate.

When a person dies **intestate**—that is, without having left a valid will—property is distributed according to rules set up by the state. The failure to execute a will may result in a distribution of property that is not compatible with a person's wishes or best suited to the interests and needs of heirs. In making a will, involving close family members may prevent the kinds of problems that can arise when actions are taken without the knowledge of those who will be affected. You don't necessarily need an attorney to make a will. If your needs are simple, online wills or legal forms sold in stores can be adequate if you follow instructions carefully.

You can also help your family members by writing down information that would be crucial to them should you die or become incapacitated. This document should include information such as bank accounts, credit cards, insurance policies, the location of documents and keys, the names of professional advisers, passwords for online accounts, the names of people who should be notified of your death, and so on.

You may feel that you are too young to be thinking about your own will, and if you are a young student, that may be reasonable. But this is a good time to be courageous and broach the subject with family members. Do your parents have a will? Do you know where they keep their important information should something happen to them? Let your family members know that you will greatly appreciate their efforts to plan ahead and keep you informed.

Completing an Advance Directive

An **advance directive** is a legal document that states your preferences about medical treatment. Having an advance directive is worthwhile for adults of any age, not just for the elderly. In a general sense, an advance directive is any statement made by a competent person about choices for medical treatment should he or she become unable to make such decisions or communicate them at some time in the future. Although specific requirements vary, all states authorize some type of advance directive.

Two forms of advance directives are legally important. First is the **living will,** which enables individuals to provide instructions about the kind of medical care they wish to receive or prohibit if they become incapacitated or otherwise unable to participate in treatment decisions (Figure 24.1). Many people believe that living wills are appropriate only for stating a desire to forgo life-sustaining procedures or to avoid medical heroics when death is imminent; indeed, most standard forms for completing a living will reflect this purpose. In fact, however, a living will can be drafted to express a range of ideas about the kinds of treatment a person would or would not want, and they can be written to cover various contingencies. Most living wills also include your preferences regarding organ donation (see below).

TERMS

will A legal instrument expressing a person's intentions and wishes for the disposition of his or her property after death.

estate The money, property, and other possessions belonging to a person.

testator The person who makes a will.

intestate Not having made a legal will.

advance directive Any legally recognized statement made by a competent person about his or her choices for medical treatment should he or she become unable to make such decisions or communicate them in the future.

living will A type of advance directive that allows individuals to provide instructions about the kind of medical care they wish to receive, or not receive, if they become unable to participate in treatment decisions.

	NEW YORK LIVING WILL – PAGE 1 OF 2
INSTRUCTIONS	*This Living Will has been prepared to conform to the law in the State of New York, as set forth in the case In re Westchester County Medical Center, 72 N.Y.2d 517 (1988). In that case the Court established the need for "clear and convincing" evidence of a patient's wishes and stated that the "ideal situation is one in which the patient's wishes were expressed in some form of writing, perhaps a 'living will.'"*
PRINT YOUR NAME	I, _____, being of sound mind, make this statement as a directive to be followed if I become permanently unable to participate in decisions regarding my medical care. These instructions reflect my firm and settled commitment to decline medical treatment under the circumstances indicated below:
	I direct my attending physician to withhold or withdraw treatment that merely prolongs my dying, if I should be in an **incurable or irreversible mental or physical condition with no reasonable expectation of recovery,** including but not limited to: (a) **a terminal condition**; (b) **a permanently unconscious condition**; or (c) **a minimally conscious condition in which I am permanently unable to make decisions or express my wishes.**
	I direct that my treatment be limited to measures to keep me comfortable and to relieve pain, including any pain that might occur by withholding or withdrawing treatment.
	While I understand that I am not legally required to be specific about future treatments **if I am in the condition(s) described above I feel especially strongly about the following forms of treatment:**
CROSS OUT ANY STATEMENTS THAT DO NOT REFLECT YOUR WISHES	I do not want cardiac resuscitation. I do not want mechanical respiration. I do not want artificial nutrition and hydration. I do not want antibiotics. However, I **do want** maximum pain relief, even if it may hasten my death.
© 2005 National Hospice and Palliative Care Organization	

	NEW YORK LIVING WILL – PAGE 2 OF 2
ADD PERSONAL INSTRUCTIONS (IF ANY)	Other directions: These directions express my legal right to refuse treatment, under the law of New York. I intend my instructions to be carried out, unless I have rescinded them in a new writing or by clearly indicating that I have changed my mind.
SIGN AND DATE THE DOCUMENT AND PRINT YOUR ADDRESS	Signed _____ Date _____ Address _____
WITNESSING PROCEDURE	I declare that the person who signed this document appeared to execute the living will willingly and free from duress. He or she signed (or asked another to sign for him or her) this document in my presence.
YOUR WITNESSES MUST SIGN AND PRINT THEIR ADDRESSES	Witness 1 _____ Address _____ Witness 2 _____ Address _____
© 2005 National Hospice and Palliative Care Organization	*Courtesy of Caring Connections 1700 Diagonal Road, Suite 625, Alexandria, VA 22314 www.caringinfo.org, 800/658-8898*

FIGURE 24.1 **A sample living will.** Because of differences in state law, each state has its own format for advance directives.

SOURCE: Valid copies of this and other state-specific advance directives can be found at www.caringinfo.org. Reprinted with permission of the National Hospice and Palliative Care Organization. Copyright © 2005 National Hospice and Palliative Care Organization. All rights reserved. Reproduction and distribution by an organization or organized group without the written permission of the National Hospice and Palliative Care Organization is expressly forbidden.

The second important form of an advance directive is the **health care proxy,** which is also known as a *durable power of attorney for health care.* This document allows you to appoint another person to make decisions about medical treatment if you become unable to do so. This decision maker may be a family member, a close friend, or an attorney with whom you have discussed your treatment preferences. The proxy is expected to act in accordance with your wishes as stated in an advance directive or as otherwise made known. If no proxy is chosen, most states assign the task to the patient's spouse, parents, or closest relative.

For advance directives to be of value, you must do more than merely complete the paperwork. Discuss your wishes ahead of time with caregivers and family members as well as with your physician. Advance directive forms vary somewhat from state to state, so it is important to use forms that are accepted in your state. You can download free forms, often from your state public health department, along with instructions and useful additions to the form. The popular *Five Wishes* form is another advance directive tool designed to promote family dialogue about how a person wishes to be treated when they cannot speak for themselves. The form specifies who you want to make care decisions for you; it also addresses your wishes about medical treatments, the level of comfort you would desire, and what you want your loved ones to know, including issues of forgiveness and preferences regarding memorial services. It is important to read and understand the entire document because *Five Wishes* can include conflicting directives (i.e., I do not want anything done or omitted by my doctors or nurses with the intention of taking my life) that have defeated end-of-life wishes when signers did not realize the meaning. Six states require the use of their own documents for advance directives.

Even with an advance directive, a patient's wishes to avoid aggressive medical interventions are often not followed. One reason is that, when every minute counts, emergency responders do not waste time looking for paperwork. Even if the advance directive is readily available, it does not constitute medical orders. For this reason, a separate document, called the *Physician Orders for Life-Sustaining Treatment* (POLST), has been developed and is available in most states. This document constitutes actual medical orders signed by

health care proxy A type of advance directive **TERMS** that allows an individual to appoint another person as an agent in making health care decisions in the event he or she becomes unable to participate in treatment decisions; also known as a *durable power of attorney for health care.*

your physician and is more likely to be followed, even in the event of an emergency situation. The POLST is intended primarily for people who are relatively near the end of life. In addition, people who are near the end of life and wish to avoid resuscitation and other forms of aggressive treatment often keep a signed document stating in bold letters "Do Not Resuscitate" or "Allow Natural Death" displayed in their home or hospital room.

Planning ahead entails different actions at different stages of life. For elderly people, or those with a potentially terminal illness, making specific plans for what lies ahead becomes an urgent matter. For most young adult students reading this book, extensive planning for your eventual death is probably not necessary or even desirable at this time. But thinking about some of these issues now will help you down the road, both in dealing with your own life and in helping your loved ones as they near the end of their lives. Completing an advance directive that includes your wishes regarding organ donation is appropriate at any age. If you fill out an advance directive and share it with your parents (or grandparents), they may be encouraged to follow your example.

Giving the Gift of Life

People at all stages of life should consider the pros and cons of becoming an organ donor. Of all the advances in medical techniques for helping patients who were formerly beyond recovery, perhaps the best known, and most effective, is the transplantation of human organs. Yet the demand for organs continues to dramatically outpace the number of organ donations. Each day about 80 people receive an organ transplant, but another 20 people on transplant waiting lists die because not enough organs are available. As of March 2020, more than 112,000 Americans were waiting for organ transplants. Many of these people will wait months or even years for a transplant, and many will die while they wait.

Organs and tissues that are used for transplant come from several sources. *Deceased donors* are the only source of hearts, whole lungs, or other body parts that can't be removed safely from living donors. Currently, about 80% of organs come from deceased donors. Eyes, bone, tendons, skin, and heart valves are some other tissues that are often donated by deceased donors. *Living donors* account for a little less than 20% of organ donations. Living donors can donate a single kidney, and parts of organs such as the liver, lungs, intestine, and pancreas. Living organ donors must be between the ages of 18 and 60 and in good health.

The benefits of being a living donor must be weighed against the risk of major surgery and many other factors that might impact the life of the donor. Living donors can also donate blood and bone marrow, skin (obtained after certain surgeries such as abdominoplasty), bone (obtained after knee

and hip replacements), and tissues that can be obtained after normal childbirth.

Organ and tissue donors are matched with potential recipients based on many factors including blood and tissue types. Generally, the most successful transplants occur when the donor and recipient are as genetically similar as possible. To help prevent rejection, transplant recipients nearly always need to take medications to suppress their immune systems.

There are many reasons for the shortage of donor organs. The number of people in need of transplants is growing because modern medical care tends to keep people with serious health problems alive longer. In addition, as transplant technology improves, more medical conditions can be treated effectively with transplantation. Although the need for transplantation grows, the organ supply has not kept pace. Not enough people register as donors and inform their families of their desire to be an organ donor. Although the recent spike in drug overdose deaths has resulted in a modest increase in deceased organ donation, the need for donor organs continues to far exceed supply.

The shortage of organs is particularly acute among some racial and ethnic groups, including African Americans, Asians and Pacific Islanders, and Hispanics/Latinos. This is mostly because the incidence of conditions such as high blood pressure and diabetes is disproportionately high in these groups, leading to an increased incidence of organ failure. For example, the incidence of kidney failure is three times higher in these groups than in non-Hispanic whites. Although organs are not matched by race, the chances for compatible blood type and tissue markers are more likely to be found among members of the same racial/ethnic group. This need for compatibility makes it crucial that people of all ethnicities contribute to the pool of organ donors.

People of any age or health status can register as donors. Even an elderly person or someone with cancer may be able to donate some types of tissue. It is crucial that people of all ages who are willing to donate organs and tissue let their families know and register as donors. In particular, it is important that young people consider becoming donors. The sudden unexpected death of a young person is a horrendous tragedy, but some good can come from such a loss through donating organs. Knowing that their loved one saved or improved the life of one or many people can be a lasting comfort to grieving family and friends.

There are several long-standing myths and fears about organ donation. A common unfounded fear is that if you are seriously injured or ill, physicians won't work as hard to save your life if they know you are a donor. Not true! Saving your life is always the first priority. Another common myth is that organ donation disfigures the body and makes an

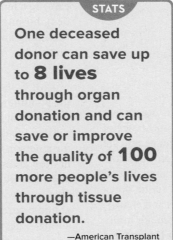

QUICK STATS

One deceased donor can save up to **8 lives** through organ donation and can save or improve the quality of **100** more people's lives through tissue donation.

—American Transplant Foundation, 2019

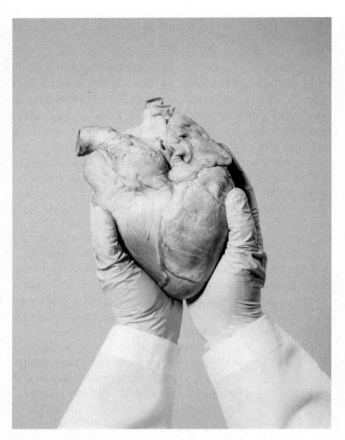

PM Images/Getty Images

open-casket funeral impossible. In fact, donated organs are removed surgically, which does not change the appearance of the body for the funeral service. In addition, some people are concerned that their religion may prohibit organ donation. When in doubt, you can discuss this with your clergy. But all major organized religions approve of organ and tissue donation, and most consider it an act of great kindness and charity.

If you decide to become an organ donor, there are multiple ways to register. You can complete a **Uniform Donor Card** either physically or online (go to organdonor.gov). Alternatively, in many states you can indicate your wish on your driver's license. You can also register online through the nonprofit website Donate Life America (donatelife.net), which manages a national registry for organ donors. Regardless of how you register, you are free to revoke your decision to be a donor at any time while you are alive.

Once you are dead, your family technically cannot overrule your decision to be an organ donor, though in practice, many hospitals ask family for permission even if you may have previously registered as a donor. For that reason, it is crucial that you discuss your decision with your family. If you die and are not a registered donor, your next of kin or power of attorney may be asked permission to donate your organs, and they are legally responsible for making that decision. Surveys show that most Americans would donate a family member's organs if they knew that was what their loved one wanted.

Considering Options for End-of-Life Care

The timeline of dying has changed radically over the past several generations. Not only do we, on average, tend to live longer, but we also are much more likely to live with chronic disease and disability for months or years before we die, compared to past generations who tended to be relatively healthy to nearly the end of life, and die after a brief, acute illness. Currently, the reality is that most of us will need caregiving help for days, weeks, months, or even years as we near the end of our lives.

The help needed can involve any combination of home care, residential facility care (such as assisted-living facilities), hospital stays, nursing home care, and hospice care. By becoming aware of the options, we and our families are empowered to make more informed and appropriate choices.

Home Care   The majority of people express a preference for at-home care during the end of life. An obvious advantage of home care is the fact that the person is in a familiar setting, ideally in the company of family and friends. Care for a person in the very last stage of life is often a 24-hour-a-day job and requires varying degrees of skill, medical knowledge, and physical strength. Family members are not always able to provide the level of care that is needed. Professional at-home caregivers can often make a huge difference in enabling a person to continue to live at home. This type of home care can be quite expensive, especially if it is needed on a 24-hour-per-day basis and is usually not covered by private or government health insurance plans. Although private long-term care insurance is available and can help pay for home and residential care, fewer than 1 in 10 Americans over age 50 have this type of insurance, in part because it is very costly.

When a patient has more extensive medical needs or does not have access to qualified in-home caregivers, institutional care may be necessary. When possible, however, home care is generally the most satisfying option for care as a person's life is reaching its end. In 2017, for the first time since the early part of the 1900s, more people who died a natural death were at home than in a hospital. Terminally ill people who wish to die at home, in their residential care facility, or in a more peaceful hospital environment are often aided by **hospice** programs, which are widely available throughout the United States and are providing a growing number of terminally ill patients much-needed assistance.

Uniform Donor Card   A consent form authorizing the use of the signer's body parts for transplantation or medical research upon his or her death.

hospice   A system of palliative care specifically for patients who are likely to die within six months, often at home, to optimize the quality of life for dying patients and their families.

TERMS

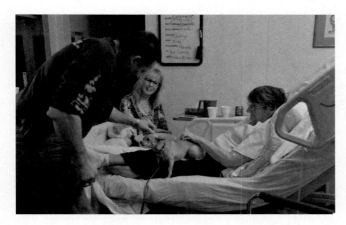

Hospice care focuses on relieving pain and other distressing symptoms in dying people and on providing support for family members. Jahi Chikwendiu/The Washington Post/Getty Images

Hospice is a system of **palliative care,** a collaborative, team-based approach to treatment that aims to prevent and relieve suffering in patients with serious or life-threatening illness. The overarching goal of palliative care is to improve the quality of life for the patient and his or her family during this period in their lives. The care team generally includes physicians, nurses, pharmacists, chaplains, social workers, home-health aides, and trained volunteers.

Hospice Programs   Hospice is a special kind of compassionate care for people in the final phase of a terminal illness, specifically for patients who are likely to die within six months or less. Hospice focuses on providing comfort care to patients at the end of life. Most hospice patients have previously undergone extensive medical efforts at curing their illnesses. The decision to switch from curative efforts to hospice care usually comes when cure is no longer a likely possibility, and the downsides of aggressive medical intervention outweigh the benefits of comfort care in a homelike setting. Generally, hospice patients and their families do not receive any bills for hospice care. Government programs, especially Medicare, pay the vast majority of hospice costs.

About two-thirds of hospice patients receive care in the place they call "home," which is most frequently their private residence, but also can be a nursing home or a residential care facility. It is also offered in hospitals and freestanding hospice facilities. Hospice care is available to people of all ages who are judged to be in their last six months of life. Typically, a patient who lives at home is cared for primarily by family members, with support from hospice workers who make regular visits to the home. Hospice does not routinely provide round-the-clock physical care, but hospice services often make it possible for family, friends, and paid caregivers to care for patients in

their own homes until death. Hospice staff members are available on call 24 hours per day, seven days a week. If there are concerns about the patient, the family or other caregivers can call at any time of day or night. A hospice nurse will evaluate the patient and provide treatment as needed. This service generally makes it possible for the patient to avoid going to the emergency room or being admitted to the hospital.

The availability of hospice care has grown at a remarkable rate since the first hospice program in the United States was established in 1974. Today there are well over 4000 Medicare-certified hospice programs in the United States. Approximately 48% of Medicare beneficiaries who died in the United States in 2017 were under the care of a hospice program. Referrals to hospice can be made by physicians, family members, friends, clergy, other health professionals, or the patients themselves. Qualifying for hospice care usually requires that two physicians certify that a patient's life expectancy is six months or less. Patients who enroll in hospice state that they choose to receive hospice care rather than curative treatment for their terminal illness. Should the patient decide that he or she wishes to resume curative treatment, hospice care can be revoked, and regular Medicare or other insurance coverage can be reinstated immediately.

When hospice care first became available in the United States, most hospice patients had cancer. Today cancer accounts for less than a third of hospice diagnoses. Other common diagnoses include heart disease, dementia (such as Alzheimer's disease), stroke, and lung disease. Any patient who is likely to die within six months is eligible for hospice care, regardless of the specific diagnosis. Over 75% of hospice patients are over 75 years old, although hospice programs take care of patients of all ages, including children.

In addition to nursing and medical care, hospices also provide social work services and spiritual support. The emphasis is on enhancing the quality of life rather than extending its length. Hospice patients often live longer than expected, at least in part due to the extra care and support they receive. In addition to helping patients achieve a good and peaceful death, an important goal of hospice care is to help patients and families discover how much can be shared at the end of life through personal and spiritual connections. Hospices continue to serve families after their loved one dies by providing bereavement care, which can include personal counseling and group support programs.

QUICK STATS

In 2018, **249** people received prescriptions under Oregon's Death with Dignity Act; **168** of those patients actually took the drugs and died as a result.

—Oregon Public Health Division, 2019

palliative care   A collaborative, team-based approach to treatment that aims to prevent and relieve suffering in patients with serious or life-threatening illness.

TERMS

Difficult Decisions at the End of Life

When death is approaching, medical interventions may increase suffering without improving the quality, or even quantity, of life. The decision to stop doing tests and treatments is often a difficult one for patients and their families, especially if their loved one is not receiving hospice care. Out of a desire to do "everything possible," families may unintentionally subject their loved one to unnecessary suffering. A medical philosophy that strives to keep people alive by all means and at any cost is increasingly being questioned.

Modern medicine can sometimes keep the human organism alive despite the cessation of normal heart, brain, respiratory, or kidney function. But should a patient without any hope of recovery be kept alive by means of artificial support? At what point does such treatment become futile, or even cruel? What if a patient has fallen into a **persistent vegetative state,** a condition of extensive and irreversible brain damage with absence of higher brain function, for an extended period, with no reasonable hope of improvement?

Ethical questions about a person's right to die have become prominent since the landmark case of Karen Ann Quinlan in 1975. At age 22 she was admitted in a comatose state to an intensive care unit, where her breathing was sustained by a mechanical ventilator. When she remained unresponsive, in a persistent vegetative state, her parents asked that the respirator be disconnected, but the medical staff responsible for Karen's care denied their request. The request to withdraw treatment eventually reached the New Jersey Supreme Court, which ruled that artificial respiration could be discontinued.

Since then, courts have ruled on removing other types of life-sustaining treatment, in certain circumstances. Notable was the case of Terri Schiavo, a married 26-year-old woman, who sustained a cardiac arrest that caused extensive brain damage. As a result, she entered a persistent vegetative state; she could breathe on her own but required a feeding tube for nutrition. She lacked awareness, showed no sign of voluntary movement, and her condition was irreversible. Contending that she would not want to continue living on life support, Terri's husband requested that her feeding tube be removed. Terri's parents contested the request, and a series of legal and political actions ensued, eventually involving the U.S. president and Congress.

Finally, after she had continued for 15 years in a persistent vegetative state, the U.S. Supreme Court intervened, allowing physicians to remove the tube. Schiavo died two weeks later. Autopsy showed profound, irreversible brain damage. Cases like this highlight the importance of expressing your wishes about life-sustaining treatment, in an advance directive or other document, before the need arises.

Withholding or Withdrawing Treatment The right of a competent patient to refuse unwanted treatment is now generally established in both law and medical practice. The consensus is that there is no medical or ethical distinction between withholding (not starting) a treatment and withdrawing (stopping) a treatment once it has been started. The right to refuse treatment remains constitutionally protected even when a patient is unable to communicate. In this situation, decisions are made by the patient's designated power of attorney for health care, or closest family member, who must do their best to determine what the patient would have wanted under the current circumstances. Having a clear advance directive, written when the patient was competent to make health care decisions, is extremely helpful for families who are faced with these difficult decisions.

Physician-Assisted Death and Voluntary Active Euthanasia *Physician-assisted death* and *voluntary active euthanasia* refer to practices that intentionally hasten the death of a person; both require the full informed consent of the patient.

Physician-assisted death (PAD) occurs when a doctor provides a prescription for a lethal dose of medication (usually a sedative, sometimes in combination with other medications)—at the patient's request—with the understanding that the patient plans to use the medication to end his or her life. The patient chooses if and when he or she wishes to take the fatal dose, usually in a home setting without the physician present. As of 2020, physician-assisted death is legal in California, Colorado, the District of Columbia, Hawaii, Maine, Montana, New Jersey, Oregon, Vermont, and Washington.

Oregon was the first state to legalize PAD following a citizens' initiative called the Death with Dignity Act. Even though PAD has been legally available in Oregon since 1994, the practice remains rare; in 2018 there were 36,191 total deaths in the state of Oregon, and only 168 (.46%) were physician-assisted deaths. The majority of patients who have chosen to use PAD to end their lives have been in the late phases of terminal cancer.

Oregon's Death with Dignity Act has been the model for other states who have legalized physician-assisted death, and all these states have similar regulations and safeguards. In Oregon, a patient who wishes to pursue an assisted death must orally request PAD from the attending physician on two occasions at least 15 days apart. The request must also be submitted in writing to the attending physician and signed in the presence of two witnesses. There is a 48-hour waiting period between the patient's written request and the writing of

---

persistent vegetative state A condition of **TERMS** extensive and irreversible brain damage with absence of higher brain function for an extended period. The person may have sleep-wake cycles, and occasional eyelid opening and movement, but lacks awareness or any cognitive function.

physician-assisted death (PAD) The practice of a physician intentionally providing, at the patient's request, a lethal overdose of drugs or other means for a patient to hasten death with the understanding that the patient plans to use them to end his or her life. The patient administers the drugs to himself or herself.

the prescription (starting in 2020, Oregon law allows patients who have less than 15 days to live to be exempt from some of the waiting periods). Additionally, the attending physician plus a consulting physician must confirm that the patient has a terminal illness that will likely lead to death within six months, whether the person is capable of making such a decision, and whether the patient may have any psychological disorder (such as depression). If either physician suspects any psychological disorder, the patient must be referred for a psychological evaluation. The patient must also be informed of alternatives to PAD, such as pain control and comfort and hospice care. In practice, the majority of patients who request PAD are already receiving hospice care.

A patient can rescind a PAD request at any time. Experience has shown that about one-third of patients who have received a prescription for lethal medication from their physician have chosen not to use it. Some patients who ultimately did not use the medication have said that merely having the means to end their own suffering gave them great comfort and enabled them to let nature take its course.

Patients who choose PAD generally have strong beliefs in personal autonomy and a determination to control the end of their lives. They do not wish to experience extreme suffering for themselves and their families and choose PAD as a more gentle, peaceful death. Patients must be able to ingest the oral medications used for PAD on their own.

Physicians and organizations can choose whether they wish to participate in the Death with Dignity Act. So far, only a very small percentage of physicians have opted to actively participate in the Death with Dignity Act. Because of this, many terminally ill people who are considering PAD have had difficulty finding doctors who are willing to help them.

In 1997 and again in 2006, the U.S. Supreme Court affirmed that individual states have the right to craft policy concerning PAD. The Supreme Court has also ruled on a related topic: the doctrine of **double effect** in the medical management of pain. The doctrine says that a harmful effect of treatment, even if it results in death, is permissible if the harm is not intended and occurs as a side effect of a beneficial action. The significance of this ruling as it relates to end-of-life care is that if the doctor's intent is to relieve a patient's severe pain, it is permissible to give the dose of medication needed to relieve the pain even if that dose, as a side effect, could cause respiratory depression, which could possibly hasten the patient's death. The doctrine of double effect allows physicians throughout the United States to do what is necessary to relieve a patient's pain, even if there is a chance that the medication may hasten death.

Active euthanasia is different from PAD, and it is illegal in the United States. Active euthanasia is defined as the intentional act of killing someone who would otherwise suffer from an incurable and painful disease. Active euthanasia can be involuntary, nonvoluntary, or voluntary. *Involuntary active euthanasia* refers to the ending of a patient's life by a medical practitioner without the patient's consent. This is considered highly unethical and is illegal throughout the world. The most notorious example of involuntary euthanasia was the medical killing programs of the Nazi regime. *Nonvoluntary euthanasia* occurs when a surrogate decision maker (not the patient) asks a physician for assistance to end another person's life.

Voluntary euthanasia (also known as voluntary active euthanasia, or VAE) is the intentional termination of life at the patient's request by someone other than the patient, usually a doctor or nurse. This means that a mentally competent patient requests direct assistance to die, and he or she receives active assistance from a qualified medical practitioner.

The difference between PAD and VAE is that PAD requires that patients must ingest the medication themselves, whereas with VAE, the health professional can administer the medication to the patient. In practice, PAD medications are typically swallowed by the patient, whereas VAE medications are usually given to the patient intravenously. The distinction is important because many patients at end of life are unable to swallow or to absorb oral medication, making them unable to use PAD. For example, people with amyotrophic lateral sclerosis (ALS, also called Lou Gehrig's disease) often lose the ability to lift a cup, or to swallow, even though they are usually mentally alert and capable of making their own medical decisions. Under these circumstances they would not be eligible for PAD.

Voluntary active euthanasia is legal under very strict guidelines in Belgium, Luxembourg, the Netherlands, Colombia, and Canada but is currently unlawful in the United States and the rest of the world. In the United States, taking active steps to end someone's life is a crime—even if the motive is mercy.

Many people believe that the demand by some patients for PAD or euthanasia results, at least in part, from the health care system's inattention to the needs of the dying. Advocates of hospice and palliative care have highlighted the need for adequate pain management, not only for patients with terminal illness, but for all patients with untreated or undertreated pain and suffering.

Health care providers vary tremendously with respect to how they assess and manage pain. Many physicians are uncomfortable prescribing or administering strong pain medications because they lack experience and may fear scrutiny by authorities such as the U.S. Drug Enforcement Agency. Physicians also worry about contributing to the current epidemic of opioid addiction and overdose death.

TERMS

double effect   A situation in which a harmful effect occurs as an unintended side effect of a beneficial action, such as when medication intended to control a patient's pain has the unintended result of causing the patient's death.

active euthanasia   A deliberate act intended to end another person's life; voluntary active euthanasia involves the practice of a physician's administering—at the request of a patient—medication or some other intervention that causes death.

When a person is near death and still having severe suffering despite optimal treatment, sometimes **palliative sedation** will be used. Palliative sedation involves giving a sedative medication that keeps the patient in an unconscious or semiconscious state until pain is brought under control or the patient dies as a result of his or her underlying disease. Palliative sedation is not meant to hasten death; rather it is used as a last resort when physician, patient, and family agree that this is the best way to relieve otherwise intractable suffering. Palliative sedation is legal in the United States and is accepted by the American Medical Association and many other medical organizations when used as a last resort in appropriately selected cases.

Planning a Funeral or Memorial Service

Funerals, memorial services, and celebrations of life are rites of passage that commemorate a person's life and acknowledge his or her passing from the community. Funerals and memorials allow survivors to support one another as they cope with their loss and express their grief. The presence of death rites in nearly every human culture suggests that these ceremonies serve deep-seated human needs.

Disposition of the Body   When a death occurs, one immediate concern of survivors is how to care for the body of their loved one. The care of the body after death varies greatly in different cultures. In the United States, the body is usually taken away from the home, hospital, or other site of death within a matter of minutes or hours. Contrary to popular myth, having a dead body in a home for a few hours, or even a few days, does not normally constitute a health risk. Keeping a loved one's body at home, at least for a few hours, can give the family a final chance to be with and care for the deceased. When the family is ready, the body can be transported for cremation or burial.

In some cases, an *autopsy* (a medical procedure performed after death to determine the cause of death or the extent of disease) may be performed. Families may request an autopsy in order to learn more about the cause of a loved one's death. An autopsy may be required by law if the death was sudden or unexpected, or if the death was due to injury, drug overdose, poisoning, or suspicious circumstances, such as possible homicide or suicide.

palliative sedation   The practice of using a sedative medication to keep a patient in an unconscious or semiconscious state until pain is brought under control or the patient dies as a result of the underlying disease.

embalming   The process of removing blood and other fluids and replacing them with chemicals to disinfect and temporarily retard deterioration of a corpse; some of the chemicals used, such as formaldehyde, are toxic and carcinogenic.

TERMS

People generally have a preference about the final disposition of their own body. For most Americans, the choice is either burial or cremation, and often depends on cultural and religious norms. *Burial* involves a grave dug into the earth (often with a cement liner) or entombment in a mausoleum (a building that houses dead bodies or remains). If a body is to be buried and the family wishes that the body be viewed during a wake or in an open-casket funeral, **embalming** is generally done. Embalming involves replacing body fluids with chemicals that delay, but do not prevent, decomposition. Many of these fluids are toxic and may pose environmental hazards as the body eventually decomposes and the chemicals slowly leach into the soil and water. Embalming is neither necessary nor legally required. Embalming was very common in 20th-century North America but is now declining in popularity for many reasons, including expense, environmental concerns, and cultural shifts. Embalming is rare throughout most of the world and is prohibited by many religions, such as Judaism and Islam, and it is not required or encouraged by any religion.

Bodies that are to be buried are generally placed in a casket, which can be made of almost anything from cardboard to steel. Caskets can cost thousands of dollars, and bereaved family members are sometimes convinced by unscrupulous funeral homes to buy very expensive caskets that they cannot afford. No casket can prevent a body from decomposing. A less expensive and more environmentally friendly option is an inexpensive wooden or cardboard casket that can be draped with cloth or a flag if desired. Some religions, such as Judaism and Islam, mandate very simple burials, with plain wooden coffins (or no coffin at all) and no embalming. Green, or natural, burial is an increasingly common option in some parts of the United States. The intent is to allow the body to recycle naturally and to protect the surrounding environment. Bodies are placed in the ground wrapped in cloth or rapidly degrading wooden or cardboard coffins, with no cement vault. Some green cemeteries are located in a park or nature preserve; others can be a special section of a larger conventional cemetery.

Cremation involves subjecting a body to intense heat, thereby reducing its organic components to a mineralized skeleton. The remaining bone fragments are then usually put through a cremulator, which reduces them to a granular state, often referred to as ashes (which actually resemble coarse sand). Only a decade ago, burial was more common than cremation in the United States, but now cremation is the more popular choice. Cremation is acceptable to many Christian sects and is the norm for most Hindus, Sikhs, Jains, and many Buddhists. In contrast, cremation is forbidden for Muslims, many Jewish sects, and the Eastern Orthodox Church (for more on cremation, see the box "A Consumer Guide to Funerals").

Arranging a Service   Commemorating a person's life and death may involve a traditional funeral ceremony, a simple memorial service, or other celebration of life. Whereas the casketed body is typically present at a funeral, the body is not at a memorial service. In some cases, both a funeral and

A traditional funeral with a casket costs about $7000, and many funerals cost $10,000 or more. When no preplanning has been done, as often occurs, family members have to make decisions under time pressure and in the grip of strong feelings. As a result, they may make poor decisions and spend more than they need to. To avoid these problems, millions of consumers are now making funeral arrangements in advance, comparing prices and services so that they can make well-informed purchasing decisions. Many people see funeral planning as an extension of will and estate planning.

Alternatives to traditional funerals exist. Cremation is now used in over 50% of deaths in the United States, with the rate of cremation increasing rapidly in recent years. According to the National Funeral Directors Association, by 2040 the U.S. cremation rate is projected to be over 78%. Cremation is a much less expensive alternative to a traditional burial. A direct cremation (no service or visitation at the funeral home) can cost as little as $600 in some cities and has a lower environmental impact than traditional burial. Cremated remains can be buried, placed in a columbarium niche, put into an urn kept by the family, interred in an urn garden, or scattered at sea or on land. Scattering ashes is regulated by a variety of federal, state, and local laws, so check these first. Whole-body donation (usually to a medical school) is another option chosen by many people for altruistic reasons, as well as for the fact that there is usually no cost.

Another alternative to an expensive traditional funeral is a more personalized, "do-it-yourself" family-centered funeral, with minimal costs because most of the tasks needed to care for the deceased person are provided by family and friends.

To ensure that you make the best possible decisions when planning a funeral, consider these options:

• Plan ahead. Think about what type of funeral you want and ask your loved ones about their preferences.

• Shop around. If you are going to use a funeral home, look for a few that belong to the National Funeral Directors Association (NFDA), and compare prices.

• Ask for a price list. The Funeral Rule requires funeral directors to give you an itemized price list when you ask either in person or over the telephone. Many funeral homes offer package funerals that cost less than individual items, but you may not need or want everything included in the package.

• Decide on the goods and services you want. Basic services include planning the funeral and coordinating arrangements with the cemetery or crematory. The casket is usually the single most expensive item; an average casket costs slightly more than $2000, but some caskets sell for as much as $10,000. You do not have to buy the casket from the funeral home you use. Many "big box" stores now sell caskets at much lower cost than funeral homes. Special body bags or very simple wood or cardboard caskets are also used and generally cost well under $1000.

• Resist pressure to buy goods and services you don't really want or need. Funeral directors are required to inform you that you need buy only those goods and services you want. If you feel you are being pressured, go elsewhere.

• In choosing a cemetery, consider its location, religious affiliation, the types of monuments allowed, and cost. Visit ahead of time to make sure it's suitable. Consider green burial if this option would have pleased your loved one. Use of a cemetery is optional for cremation.

• Once decisions have been made, put them in writing, give copies to family members, and keep a copy accessible. Review these decisions every few years and revise them if necessary.

SOURCE: National Funeral Directors Association. 2020. *Statistics* (https://www.nfda.org/news/statistics)

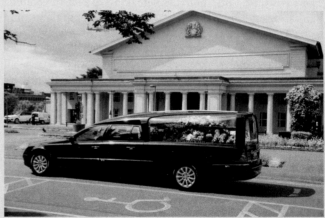

David Warren/Alamy Stock Photo

a memorial service are held, the former occurring within a few days after death and the latter being held sometime later. Some individuals express a preference for not having any sort of service, but in general, bereaved relatives and friends derive important benefits from having an opportunity to honor the deceased and express their grief through ceremony.

A funeral or memorial service can be a healing experience that allows loved ones to share memories and support one another. Memorial services can be held almost anywhere, including outdoors, in a home, or in a chapel. The service is often led by clergy, but many nontraditional services are led by a family member or close friend. The more the service fits the personality of the deceased person and meets the practical and emotional needs of the family, the better. A memory book or other photo display is common, and such items help bring back cherished memories of the person at different

Ask Yourself ?

QUESTIONS FOR CRITICAL THINKING AND REFLECTION

Have you ever been involved in a funeral? What role did you play? Did you feel that the service reflected the values and beliefs of the deceased person? Did the service provide healing and comfort to family and friends? Did the experience cause you to think about your own funeral and what it should be like?

stages in his or her life. A home-based or outdoor service with a potluck meal or snacks afterward can be meaningful and healing while not placing a great financial burden on the grieving family.

People who have a terminal illness sometimes find comfort and satisfaction in helping to plan for their own memorial services. A memorial service can be the joint creation of the dying person and family members who wish to be part of the project. Making at least some plans ahead of time can help ease the burden on survivors, who will undoubtedly face a great number of tasks and decisions when the death occurs. If your loved one has hospice care, the social worker and chaplain can often help guide you through the process of planning a memorial service.

COPING WITH IMMINENT DEATH

There is no one right way to live with or die of a life-threatening illness. Every disease has its own set of problems and challenges, and each person copes in his or her own way. Much of the suffering experienced by people with a life-threatening illness comes from overwhelming feelings of loss on all levels. Besides the many physical and emotional losses, there are often fears about loss of independence, physical pain, and concerns about costly medical care, and becoming a burden for family. How a person copes with such an experience is likely to reflect his or her personality and life history, as well as the nature of family relationships and patterns of interaction in the person's wider social environment. Spiritual strength can be a major factor in how we deal with these losses. The support of loving family, friends, clergy or other spiritual guides, and health care professionals, including a hospice team, can make the journey easier to bear.

The Tasks of Coping

In her groundbreaking 1969 book *On Death and Dying,* Elisabeth Kübler-Ross, a Swiss American psychiatrist and one of the first medical experts to focus on the topic of end of life, suggested that the response to an awareness of imminent death involves five psychological stages: denial, anger, bargaining, depression, and acceptance. The notion that these five stages occur in a linear progression has since become a kind of modern myth of how people *ought* to cope with dying.

Unfortunately, such thinking can lead to the idea that a person's task is to move sequentially through these stages, one after another, and that if this is not accomplished, the person has somehow failed. In fact, however, Kübler-Ross said that individuals go back and forth among the stages during the course of an illness, and stages can occur simultaneously.

The stage-based model devised by Kübler-Ross almost 50 years ago has been a stimulus toward a better understanding of how people cope with dying. Today the notion of stages has been deemphasized in favor of highlighting the tasks that require attention in order to cope well with a life-threatening illness. Psychologist and author Charles Corr, for example, distinguishes four primary dimensions in coping with dying:

1. *Physical.* Satisfying bodily needs and minimizing physical distress
2. *Psychological.* Maximizing a sense of security, self-worth, autonomy, and richness in living
3. *Social.* Sustaining significant relationships and addressing the social implications of dying
4. *Spiritual.* Identifying, developing, or reaffirming sources of meaning and fostering hope

Helping a dying person, and her or his loved ones, requires attention and support to all four dimensions.

In addition, though, we must remember that a person's death is as unique as his or her life. Thus, although models can help us gain understanding, they need to be balanced by paying attention to the dying person's own unfolding life story. Each person's pathway through life-threatening illness is determined by factors such as the specific disease and its course, his or her personality, and the available supportive resources.

Some people with life-threatening illness respond with a fighting spirit that views the illness not only as a threat but also as a challenge. These people strive to inform themselves about their illness and take an active part in treatment decisions, as much as they are able. They attempt to continue to set and accomplish goals, maintain relationships, and sustain a sense of personal vitality, competence, and power despite life-threatening illness. Other people with terminal disease, particularly in the later stages, tend to withdraw, and they sometimes find their peace in quietly letting go of striving. For many dying people, the world around them becomes smaller and more intimate. They may find it most helpful to ease into a peaceful place, in the presence of calm and loving people who respect their need for quiet companionship.

Supporting a Person in the Last Phase of Life

People often feel uncomfortable in the presence of a person who is in the final stage of life. How should we act? What can we say? Perhaps the most important and comforting thing we can do for a dying person is to simply be present. Sitting quietly and listening carefully, we can take our cues from the person who is dying. If the person is capable of speaking, and wishes to talk, attentive listening is an act of great kindness. If the person doesn't wish to talk, or is not able to, physical touch such as holding hands or putting a hand on the person's shoulder can be the most effective way to express your love and concern.

Attempting to cheer up a dying person by saying something like "you are going to be just fine" or "you can fight this and be well again" can be frustrating for a patient at the end of life, who knows that your words are simply not true. You cannot fix all the difficulties your dying loved one is facing, but you can listen, and show by your loving presence that you care. Simple words that come from the heart can be healing for the speaker and for the loved one whose time is short.

The level of alertness of a dying person often fluctuates. A patient who has been nonverbal may have moments of clear speech in the days or hours before death. People with dementia may have lucid periods. Even those who appear to be in a coma or deep sleep may be able to hear what is going on around them. Most experts think that hearing and touch are the last senses to go. Always assume that a dying person can hear what you say; be sure to keep that in mind when you speak to others in the room. Don't hesitate to speak lovingly to a dying person whether or not she or he shows outward signs of hearing you.

Besides having the loving presence of friends and family, the dying person may need other supportive resources. In the last hours and days before death it is very common for people to experience agitation or delirium, as brain function becomes increasingly impaired. Dealing with agitation, or the paranoid aspects of delirium, can be very hard on loved ones as well as on the person who is dying. A calm presence, and the support of hospice or other people who are experienced in caring for the dying, can be very helpful in coping with these difficult symptoms.

The Trajectory of Dying

Your ideas about dying may be quite different from what most people actually experience. The concept of a **trajectory of dying** is useful for understanding people's experiences as they near death. Although sudden death from an unexpected cause—a massive heart attack or an unintentional injury, for example—is one type of dying trajectory, our focus here is on deaths that occur with forewarning. Among these, some trajectories involve a steady and fairly predictable decline. This is the case with many cancers, which tend to follow the course of a progressive disease with a rapid terminal phase. Other kinds of advanced, chronic illness involve a long period of slow decline marked by episodes of crisis, the last of which proves to be fatal.

We can also distinguish between stages in a dying trajectory—namely, a period when a person is known to be terminally ill but is living with a life expectancy of perhaps weeks or months, possibly years, and a later period when dying is imminent and the person is described as *actively dying*. The way in which such trajectories are estimated—their duration and expected course—can affect both patients and caregivers and influence their actions. Deaths that happen

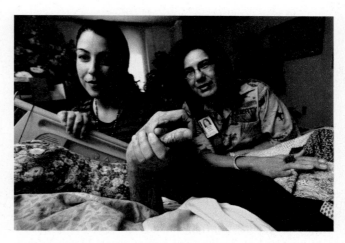

The simple acts of listening and loving touch can be extremely supportive to someone who is facing death. John Walker/The Fresno Bee/ZumaPress/Newscom

much sooner or much later than the patient and family expected may pose special difficulties. A family may experience more shock and guilt if the death occurs before they have had time to say their good-byes and emotionally prepare. When death is slow in coming, and the dying process lingers for days, weeks, or months longer than anticipated, families and the dying person may become physically, emotionally, and spiritually exhausted. The support of extended family, friends, hospice, and clergy can make the difference between an unbearable situation and one that is tolerable. In the best scenarios, the dying process can be a time when bonds of family and friendship are strengthened, and personal growth occurs for the dying person and his or her loved ones.

When a person is actively dying, his or her death is expected to occur within hours or, at most, a few days. During the last phase of a fatal illness, a dying person may exhibit any or all of these symptoms: irregular breathing or shortness of breath, decreased appetite and thirst, nausea and vomiting, incontinence, restlessness and agitation, disorientation and confusion, and diminished consciousness. These symptoms usually can be managed by skilled palliative care. Pain, if it is present, should be treated aggressively as part of a comprehensive approach to comfort care. Narcotic pain medications are generally the most effective and are routinely used at the end of life at whatever dose is needed to provide the pain control the patient desires. The stopping of eating and drinking is a normal part of the last phase of a terminal condition. As the body shuts down, food cannot be assimilated and may only contribute to a patient's discomfort. Forcing food or liquids often results in choking or nausea. If a person's mouth is dry, giving ice chips, dropping small amounts of water into the mouth from a straw or syringe, or using a moistened swab can help.

trajectory of dying The duration and nature of a person's experience of approaching death as influenced by the underlying cause of dying. TERMS

As death is drawing near, the patient's extremities may feel cold to the touch; lips, fingers, and toes may appear bluish; urination becomes less frequent; and the ability to communicate may be lost. In the final hours, purple blotches (mottling) may appear on the legs or arms. Simple steps—such as repositioning the patient, covering him or her with a light blanket, dimming the room's lighting, playing soft favorite music, or holding hands—can provide great relief and reassurance in the last moments. Just before death, the person may take a deep breath and sigh or shudder.

It is not unusual for a dying person to seem to wait until loved ones have left the room before taking her or his last breath. You should not feel guilty or rejected if you are not present at the moment of death. Some dying people seem to need to be alone in the moment of passing. The Hollywood version of death, where the dying person speaks meaningful last words to loved ones, then dies immediately, is much less common than a period of hours or days of apparent unresponsiveness before death finally comes.

COPING WITH LOSS

Even if you have not experienced the death of someone close, you have likely experienced many losses related to life changes. The loss of a job, the ending of a relationship, transitions from one school or neighborhood to another—these are the kinds of losses that occur in all our lives. Such losses are sometimes called little deaths, and in varying degrees they all involve grief.

As noted earlier in the chapter, for many people, the first really significant loss is the death of a special pet. The intensity of grief after losing a beloved companion animal is often comparable to the grief experienced following the loss of a human loved one. Never assume that the loss of a pet is "no big deal." The pain following the loss of a pet is even harder

grief A person's reaction to loss as manifested physically, emotionally, mentally, and behaviorally.

bereavement The period of sorrow that follows the death of a loved one.

mourning The process whereby a person actively copes with grief in adjusting to a loss and integrating it into his or her life.

to bear if the experience of the grieving person is belittled. The comments here about grief are relevant to many types of loss, not just the loss of a human friend or relative.

Experiencing Grief

Grief is the reaction to loss. It encompasses thoughts and feelings as well as physical and behavioral responses. Mental distress may involve disbelief, confusion, anxiety, disorganization, and depression. The emotions that can be present in normal grief include not only sorrow and sadness, but also relief, anger, guilt, and self-pity, among others. Bereaved people experience a range of feelings, including conflicting ones. Observing the faces of families at the funeral of a beloved relative often reveals smiles and moments of laughter in addition to solemn expressions and tears. Recognizing that grief can involve many feelings—not just sadness—makes us more able to cope with it. Common behaviors associated with grief include crying and talking repetitively about the deceased and the circumstances of the death. Bereaved people may be restless, as if not knowing what to do with themselves. Outward signs of grief may involve frequent sighing, crying, inappropriate laughter, insomnia, loss of appetite, and marked fatigue. Grief may also evoke a reexamination of religious or spiritual beliefs as a person struggles to make meaning of the loss. Guilt is a common emotion after the death of a loved one. People may blame themselves in some way for the death, or for not doing enough for the deceased, or for feeling a sense of relief that their loved one is gone. All such manifestations of grief can be present as part of our total response to **bereavement**—that is, the event of loss.

Mourning is closely related to grief and is often used as a synonym for it. However, mourning refers not so much to the *reaction* to loss but to the *process* by which a bereaved person adjusts to loss and incorporates it into his or her life. How this process is managed is determined, at least partly, by cultural and gender norms for the expression of grief.

The Course of Grief Grieving, like dying, is highly individual. In the first hours or days following a death, a bereaved person is likely to experience shock and numbness, as well as a sense of disbelief, especially if the death was unexpected. Consider the ways in which people die: a young child pronounced dead on arrival after a bicycle crash, an aged grandmother dying quietly in her sleep, a despondent executive who commits suicide, a young soldier killed in battle, a chronically ill person who dies a lingering death. The cause or mode of death—natural, accidental, homicide, or suicide—influences how grief is experienced. Even when a death is anticipated, grief is not necessarily diminished when the loss becomes real.

The death of a loved one is frequently a severe physical as well as emotional stressor. For example, in the first day after the death of a loved one, the rate of heart attack in the survivor increases by as much as 21 times. The risk of death decreases gradually over time but still remains above normal for several months after a loved one dies. After a death, grieving people often have difficulty sleeping, may neglect

- Recognize and acknowledge your loss.

- React to grief in the way that feels most natural to you. There is no "right" way to grieve.

- Take time for nature's process of healing. The odds are good that you will be functioning well again before long. Be patient with yourself.

- Know that powerful, overwhelming feelings will change with time. Grief is often experienced as a long series of ups and downs, with the intensity of feelings decreasing gradually over time.

- Beware of the lure of drugs and alcohol to reduce the pain of your grief, especially if you have had substance abuse issues in the past. Using alcohol or drugs to numb yourself will ultimately backfire and make your healing more difficult.

- Honor your loved one in a way that is meaningful to you. Consider creating a small memorial with a photo and flowers, start a scholarship in your loved one's name, plant a memorial tree, or write a song or poem in his or her honor.

- Consider joining a bereavement support group (in person or online) to connect with others who have had recent losses.

- Surround yourself with life: go out in nature, enjoy the healing companionship of a pet, connect with friends and family.

- If you are having difficulty functioning at school, work, or home after a few weeks, consider counseling or a support group.

- People who have had a recent loss are at higher risk for suicide. If you are having thoughts of suicide, or feeling hopeless, seek help right away.

- Care for yourself by finding time to eat, sleep, and move your body.

- Don't be afraid to let laughter and joy remain in your life. Experiencing positive feelings during mourning does not indicate a lack of respect or love for the deceased.

to eat nourishing food, and may forget to take their usual medications. These factors add to the health risks associated with recent loss. Recent loss also has a cognitive impact on many grievers. People often report that they feel confused and have difficulty concentrating following a significant loss.

After the initial shock begins to fade, the course of grief is characterized by anxiety, apathy, and pining for the deceased. The pangs of grief are felt as the bereaved person deeply experiences the pain of separation. Mourners often experience despair as they repeatedly go over the events surrounding the loss, perhaps fantasizing that somehow everything could be undone and be as it was before. During this period, the bereaved person may also begin to look toward the future and take the first steps toward building a life without the deceased.

Psychiatrist Colin Murray Parkes points to three main influences on a person's course of grieving:

1. The urge to look back, cry, and search for what is lost

2. The urge to look ahead, explore the world that emerges out of the loss, and discover what can be carried forward from the past into the future

3. The social and cultural pressures that influence how the first two urges are inhibited or expressed

As these influences interact, at times the bereaved tries to avoid the pain of grief and at other times confronts it. The goal is to achieve a balance between avoidance and confrontation that facilitates coming to terms with the loss. Attaining

this goal can be seen as an oscillation between what researchers Margaret Stroebe and Henk Schut call *loss-oriented* and *restoration-oriented* mourning. From this perspective, looking at old photographs and yearning for the deceased are examples of loss-oriented coping, whereas doing what is needed to reorganize life in the wake of the loss—for example, learning to do tasks that the deceased had always managed is part of restoration-oriented coping.

As time goes on, the acute pain and emotional turmoil of grief begin to subside. Physical and mental balance are gradually reestablished. The bereaved person becomes increasingly reintegrated into his or her social world. Sadness doesn't go away completely, but it recedes into the background much of the time. Although reminders of the loss stimulate waves of active grieving from time to time, the main focus is the present, not the past. Adjusting to loss may sometimes feel like a betrayal of the deceased loved one, but it is healthy to engage again in ongoing life and the future (see the box "Coping with Grief").

Social support for the bereaved is as critical during the later course of grief as it is during the first days after a loss. In offering support, we can reassure the grieving person that grief is normal, permissible, and appropriate. The anniversary of the loved one's death, birthdays, and major holidays following a significant loss can renew grieving, and the support of others is especially important and appreciated during those times. Connecting with friends and family to acknowledge the loss and reaffirm your ongoing relationship can be extremely comforting throughout the grieving experience.

Bereaved people may find it helpful to share their stories and concerns through organized support groups. Hospices provide bereavement support groups and counseling free of charge, usually for 13 months after the death. Many online and in-person support groups are organized around specific types of bereavement. The Compassionate Friends, for example, is a nationwide organization composed of parents who have experienced a child's death. This organization provides both local and online support groups. Losing a loved one to suicide is an especially traumatic loss that is often best understood by others who have had a similar loss. Suicide support groups are available in most communities. The American Foundation for Suicide Prevention has an online directory of suicide survivor support groups, as well as a program called "Healing Conversations," where people who have lost someone to suicide can talk by phone, video chat, or in person with trained volunteers who have also experienced the loss of a loved one to suicide. If you have lost a loved one to drugs or alcohol, GRASP (Grief Recovery After Substance Passing) has support groups in many communities as well as online support. (See For More Information at the end of this chapter for web addresses for these groups.)

There is no hard and fast "normal" amount of time that grief should last, but when the duration and intensity far exceed what is usually expected, it is often referred to as **complicated grief.** If the griever remains seriously impacted by disabling grief many months or years after a death, she or he may be experiencing complicated grief. Rates of complicated grief in Western countries tend to be highest when a child is lost, or when the death was violent and unexpected (see the box "Surviving the Sudden or Violent Death of a Loved One"). A history of mood disorder such as depression, as well as previous or ongoing substance abuse, increases the risk for complicated grief. Psychotherapy, with or without medication, can be critical for someone who is suffering from prolonged and debilitating grief.

Supporting a Grieving Person

When a person finds out that a loved one has died, the initial reaction may be profound shock and overwhelming distress. Such a person may initially respond best to the physical comfort of hugging and holding. Later, simply listening may be the most effective way to help someone who is grieving. Talking about the loss is an important way that many survivors cope with the changed reality, and they may need to tell their story over and over. The key to being a good listener is to avoid speaking too much, and to refrain from making judgments about whether the thoughts and feelings expressed by a survivor are right or wrong, good or bad. The emotions, thoughts, and behaviors evoked by loss may not be the ones we expect, but they can nonetheless be valid and appropriate within a survivor's experience of loss.

> **complicated grief** Grief that is unusually intense, prolonged, and debilitating.   **TERMS**

If a grieving friend or relative talks about suicide or seems in danger of causing harm to himself or herself or others, seek professional help right away. Most people are resilient and cope well with loss, but the recent loss of a loved one is a major risk factor for suicide and self-harm. Be alert to signs that a grieving person is in serious danger.

Although some people respond to loss with a feeling of helplessness, other people may react by taking charge. Making arrangements, taking care of tasks, and generally keeping busy may help them cope. Be aware that some people do not find it helpful to dwell on their feelings or talk a lot about their loss. Find out what *they* want to do—when the time is right, take a walk, go shopping together, go to a ball game, or see a movie. Your companionship while doing everyday activities may be the best gift you can give. Remember also that some grieving people may not appear sad or distressed. This lack of outward grieving does not mean that they didn't care about the deceased, are "in denial," or have a cold personality. Accept that this response is their way of coping with loss and show your support with your loving presence.

When a Young Adult Loses a Friend

Among young people aged 18–24 in the United States, the leading causes of death tend to be sudden and unexpected: unintentional injuries, overdose, homicide, and suicide. Losing a close friend to an unexpected death can be particularly traumatic. As a friend, you may feel unsupported and left out of the family's grieving. Also, you may blame yourself in some way for your friend's death or feel you should have somehow prevented the tragedy. If you lose a friend, be sure to look for support from friends, family, clergy, or health professionals, especially if the intense sadness or guilt feelings last for more than a few days or weeks. Friends can often help each other by working together to create their own way of celebrating the life of their lost friend. Many hospices have support groups specifically for young adults who have lost loved ones. These organizations welcome anyone, regardless of whether the deceased person used the services of hospice. Online support groups can also be extremely helpful.

Helping Children Cope with Loss

Children tend to cope with loss in a healthier fashion when they are included as part of their family's experience of grief and mourning. Although adults may be uncomfortable about sharing potentially disturbing or painful news with children, a

Ask Yourself

QUESTIONS FOR CRITICAL THINKING AND REFLECTION

Have you ever been in a close relationship with a bereaved person? What kind of support did he or she seem to appreciate most? Why do you think that was the case? How did the experience affect you?

Coping with the death of a loved one is among the greatest challenges a person faces in a lifetime. When the death is due to sudden or violent causes, such as injury, homicide, suicide, or unintentional drug overdose, the challenges of grieving are multiplied many fold. Experts estimate that one out of three of us will experience the traumatic loss of a close friend or relative to sudden violent death. Motor vehicle crashes, by their nature sudden and unpredictable, are one of the most common causes of traumatic death in young people. Hardly anyone makes it through high school without losing at least one classmate in an automotive crash. A fatal car crash leaves behind many victims besides those who died. Friends and relatives are devastated by the loss of a beloved young person. Any occupants of the vehicle who survive the crash typically suffer from injuries and psychological trauma, in addition to their grief for the ones who died. Posttraumatic stress is a common outcome for survivors. If the driver was intoxicated, or otherwise at fault for the crash survivors must also cope with that difficult knowledge. Feelings of anger and guilt are often mixed in with the sadness and loss.

Although homicide is far less common in the United States than motor vehicle crashes, young people who grow up in high-crime neighborhoods all too often experience the loss of relatives, friends, or acquaintances due to killings. When a loved one is murdered, grievers may agonize over the circumstances of the crime and imagine the horrible suffering their loved one might have endured. Survivors may be haunted by memories of the person's mangled body or may obsess over missing details of the crime. Survivors may also fear for their own safety. The police and legal system may add to the trauma through insensitivity at best, and offensive behavior toward survivors at worst.

People who survive a loved one's suicide or unintentional drug overdose also experience great suffering as a result of the stigma attached to these types of death. They often feel terrible guilt, wondering if they were in part responsible for their loved one's distress, or whether they could have done something to prevent the death. Perhaps the most difficult aspect of coping with sudden or violent death, and suicide in particular, is the societal stigma frequently directed at the survivors. The spouse or parent of someone who has committed suicide is often suspected of having been a source of the victim's unhappiness, or at least guilty for not sensing the trouble and doing something about it.

Thus, beyond the challenges of coping with a "natural" death, those who lose a loved one to a sudden or violent death face many additional sources of anguish. The sense of the world as a benevolent, safe, and predictable place is often lost when loved ones die in traumatic circumstances. Survivors often face questions of blame, legal issues, financial distress, and lack of social support. A grieving survivor may be called upon to relive the trauma and its horrifying memories over and over again during encounters with police and in legal proceedings. Moreover, friends and community members often avoid survivors, or respond with morbid curiosity or judgmental comments, rather than providing the loving support that is so desperately needed. Or they may back away from someone whose loss is too frightening to contemplate. The instinct to blame the deceased and the survivors for some aspect of a violent death is also common and often represents our attempt to reassure ourselves that if only we are vigilant, and do the right thing, this kind of tragedy won't happen to us or our loved ones.

Some experts refer to the grief experience related to violent loss as "traumatic grief," a term used by Marilyn Armour, a prominent researcher in the field. Traumatic grief involves symptoms of separation-related distress, resulting from the loss of a loved one, as well as symptoms of traumatic distress related to the horrible ordeal the mourner has experienced. Posttraumatic stress often complicates a survivor's ability to recover, and severe, prolonged grief may result. Finding meaning in a sudden and violent death is often much more challenging than in a death from old age or a lengthy illness. When someone dies of natural causes, the survivors are often comforted by the belief that at least their loved one is no longer suffering or that the person "died peacefully." In the case of violent death, there are no similar thoughts to soften the blow.

Despite the great challenges, most people who lose someone to a violent death do eventually recapture a sense of normalcy. Helping survivors starts with all of us reaching out with nonjudgmental love and kindness. For all survivors, the support of friends and community is crucial for regaining a sense of peace. A number of excellent organizations support survivors of loved ones whose deaths were through accidents, overdose, suicide, homicide, and other types of violence (see For More Information at the end of this chapter). Most of these organizations provide information about joining online and in-person support groups, as well as finding professional help for those who are having difficulty coping with traumatic loss.

child's natural curiosity usually negates the option of completely withholding information. Mounting evidence shows that it is best to include children from the beginning—as soon as a terminal prognosis is made, for example—to help them understand what is happening. Children should spend time with the dying person, if possible, to learn, share, offer, and receive comfort.

In talking about death with children, the most important guideline is to be honest. Offer an explanation at the child's level of understanding. Find out what the child wants to know. Keep the explanation simple, stick to basics, and verify what the child has understood from your explanation. A child's readiness for more details can usually be assessed by paying attention to his or her questions. Many hospices and other organizations, such as the Dougy Center in Portland, Oregon, provide bereavement help for children, utilizing art, games, music, and other activities appropriate to a child's developmental stage.

COMING TO TERMS WITH DEATH

We may wish we could keep death out of view and protect ourselves and others from the pain associated with it. But this wish cannot be fulfilled. With the death of a beloved friend or relative, we are confronted with emotions and thoughts that relate not only to the immediate loss but also to our own mortality. Our exposure to death can offer opportunities for extraordinary growth in the midst of loss. Encounters with dying and death, painful as they may be, can help us more fully appreciate the infinite preciousness of life and love.

TIPS FOR TODAY AND THE FUTURE

RIGHT NOW YOU CAN:

- Think about life's impermanence and appreciate the now.
- Don't miss out on opportunities to let your friends and loved ones know that you care for them. Let your awareness of death guide you into leading a loving and purposeful life.
- Consider organ donation as a lasting gift of life to others. If you want to be an organ donor, make the appropriate arrangements now, as described in this chapter.

IN THE FUTURE YOU CAN:

- Talk to your parents or grandparents about their wishes for the end of life. Let them know you care for them and want to be involved. Suggest that you look together at an advance directive form.
- Make a difference for a grieving friend or relative. Show that you care by your loving presence and your willingness to listen quietly.

SUMMARY

- The existence of death makes rational sense in terms of species survival and evolution; grappling with the philosophical and spiritual aspects of our own death is a major part of life's journey.

- Dying and death are more than biological events; they have social and spiritual dimensions.

- The traditional criteria for clinical death are the cessation of breathing and heartbeat. Brain death is an irreversible cessation of brain activity indicated by various diagnostic criteria.

- Between ages 6 and 9, most children begin to develop an understanding that death is final, universal, and inevitable.

- A mature understanding of death can include ideas about the survival of the human personality or soul after death. Problems arise when avoidance or denial of death fosters the notion that it happens only to others.

- A will is a legal instrument that governs the distribution of a person's estate after death.

- Advance directives, such as living wills, are used to express your wishes about the use of life-sustaining treatment and how you would wish to be treated if you could not speak for yourself. The health care proxy (also called durable power of attorney) specifies who will make medical decisions for you if you are unable.

- Palliative care is a team-based approach to improving the quality of life for seriously ill patients by controlling pain and relieving physical and psychological suffering.

- Hospice programs are a type of palliative care specifically for patients who are likely to die within six months, often at home, to optimize the quality of life of dying patients and their families.

- Choices about end-of-life care include making decisions about attempting to prolong life through artificial means or allowing natural death to occur if you have a terminal condition with no reasonable chance of recovery.

- The right of a competent patient to refuse unwanted treatment, or to terminate an undesired treatment, is now generally established in both law and medical practice.

- Physician-assisted death occurs when a physician prescribes medication at a patient's request, with the understanding that the patient plans to take the medicine to end his or her life. PAD is legal, with strict regulations, in some states in the United States. Voluntary active euthanasia refers to the intentional ending of a patient's life, at his or her request, by someone other than the patient, such as a doctor or nurse.

- People can donate their bodies or specific organs for transplantation and other medical uses after death. People of all ages can make their wishes to donate their organs known on their driver's license or other state forms, or through the National Donate Life Registry. They also need to let their families know that they wish to be organ donors.

- Living donors can donate a single kidney or parts of other organs. Living donations account for nearly 20% of organ transplantation.

- Bereaved people usually benefit from participating in a funeral or other type of memorial service to commemorate a loved one's life and death.

- For Americans, the decision about what to do with the body after death usually involves choosing between burial or cremation.

- Coping with dying involves physical, psychological, social, and spiritual dimensions.

- The gift of listening and loving touch can be especially important to someone who is dying.

- It is useful for patients and caregivers to understand the trajectory, or course, of dying.

- Grief encompasses thoughts and feelings as well as physical and behavioral responses. Complicated grief occurs when someone is debilitated by severe grief over a lengthy period of time.

- Mourning, the process by which a person integrates a loss into his or her life, is determined partly by social and cultural norms for expressing grief.

- Children tend to cope with death in a healthier fashion when they are included in their family's experience of grief and mourning.

- Dying and death offer opportunities for growth in the midst of loss.

FOR MORE INFORMATION

Aging with Dignity: Five Wishes. Source for an advance directive that includes designation of a health care proxy (durable power of attorney), and the kind of medical treatment you want or want to avoid. In addition, it has sections regarding your wishes about pain control, how you want people to treat you, and what you want your loved ones to know when you are dying. Cost is $5 for an online copy; also available are conversation guides for speaking with family and friends about advance directives, as well as instructional videos.

http://fivewishes.org

American Foundation for Suicide Prevention. The "Find Support" section of this website has information for people whose lives have been touched by suicide, including support groups, individual help, and crisis care for those who are considering suicide, have attempted suicide, have lost someone to suicide, or have a loved one who has attempted suicide.

https://afsp.org/find-support/

Caring Connections (a program of the National Hospice and Palliative Care Organization). Provides resources for end-of-life decision making with the goal of planning before a crisis occurs, including information about state-specific advance directives. Extensive information about end-of-life-caregiving, hospice, and palliative care.

http://www.caringinfo.org

The Compassionate Friends. Provides grief support after the death of a child, including local chapters and online support groups.

http://www.compassionatefriends.org

Donate Life America. Extensive information about organ donation and transplantation. This website allows you to add your information to be on the national registry of organ donors.

http://www.donatelife.net

The Dougy Center. Offers education about childhood bereavement and support groups for bereaved children, teens, young adults, and parents.

http://www.dougy.org

Funeral Consumers Alliance. A site with extensive information about how to plan a dignified family-centered funeral, details of cremation and burial, and dealing with death and grief.

http://www.funerals.org

GRASP: Grief Recovery After a Substance Passing. Website for friends and family of people who have died as a result of substance use. Local and online support groups are available.

http://grasphelp.org

GriefNet. A site where you can communicate with others via email support groups in the areas of death, grief, and major loss. You can create a memorial for your loved one on this website.

http://www.griefnet.org

Hospice Foundation of America. Provides extensive information about hospice care, end-of-life care, grief, and grief support groups.

http://www.hospicefoundation.org

National Cancer Institute: Grief, Bereavement and Coping with Loss. Provides information about types of grief reactions, complicated grief, treatment for complicated grief, children and loss, and cultural aspects of grief.

http://www.cancer.gov/about-cancer/advanced-cancer/caregivers /planning/bereavement-pdq

National Hospice and Palliative Care Organization (NHPCO). Provides information about hospice care and advance directives, including an online national directory of hospices listed by state and city.

http://www.nhpco.org

The following organizations provide information about organ donation and donor cards:

Coalition on Donation: http://www.donatelife.net

Organ Procurement and Transplantation Network:

http://www.organdonor.gov

Transplant Living: http://www.transplantliving.org

SELECTED BIBLIOGRAPHY

American Academy of Hospice and Palliative Medicine. 2014. *Palliative Sedation Position Statement* (http://aahpm.org/positions/palliative -sedation).

American Transplant Foundation. 2019. *Facts and Myths* (http://www .americantransplantfoundation.org/about-transplant/facts-and-myths/).

Burkle, C. M., et al. 2014. Why brain death is considered death and why there should be no confusion. *Neurology,* September 12 (epub).

Bonanno, G. A. 2009. *The Other Side of Sadness: What the New Science of Bereavement Tells Us about Life after Loss.* New York: Basic Books.

Bratton, C., et al. 2011. Racial disparities in organ donation and why. *Current Opinion in Organ Transplantation* 16(2): 243-249.

Callanan, M., and P. Kelley. 1992. *Final Gifts: Understanding the Special Awareness, Needs, and Communications of the Dying.* New York: Bantam Books.

Carey, I. M., et al. 2014. Increased risk of acute cardiovascular events after partner bereavement: A matched cohort study. *JAMA Internal Medicine* 174(4): 598–605.

Centers for Disease Control and Prevention. 2018. 10 *Leading Causes of Death by Age Group, U.S.-2018* (https://www.cdc.gov/injury/wisqars /LeadingCauses.html).

Cherny, N. 2020. Palliative sedation. *Up to Date* (https://www.uptodate.com /contents/palliative-sedation#H21551864).

Corr, C. A., et al. 2008. *Death and Dying: Life and Living.* Florence, KY: Wadsworth Publishing.

Death with Dignity National Center. 2020. *Death with Dignity around the U.S.* (http://www.deathwithdignity.org/take-action).

Doka, K. J., and A. S. Tucci (Eds.). 2011. *Beyond Kübler-Ross: New Perspectives on Death, Dying and Grief.* Washington, DC: Hospice Foundation of America.

Donatelli, L. A., et al. 2006. Ethical issues in critical care and cardiac arrest: Clinical research, brain death, and organ donation. *Seminars in Neurology* 26(4): 452–459.

EthnoMed. 2018. Cultural relevance in end of life care. (https://ethnomed .org/clinical/end-of-life/cultural-relevance-in-end-of-life-care).

Gallup Poll. 2016. *Majority in U.S. Do Not Have a Will* (http://news.gallup .com/poll/191651/majority-not.aspx).

Gawande, A. 2014. *Being Mortal: Medicine and What Matters in the End.* New York: Metropolitan Books.

Glazier, A. 2018. Organ donation and the principles of gift law. *Clinical Journal of American Society of Nephrology* 13(8): 1283–1284.

Greer, D. M., et al. 2016. Variability of brain death policies in the United States. *JAMA Neurology* 73(2): 213–218.

Haberman, C. 2014. From private ordeal to national fight: The case of Terri Schiavo. *New York Times*, 20 April (https://www.nytimes.com/2014/04 /21/us/from-private-ordeal-to-national-fight-the-case-of-terri-schiavo.html).

Hahn, M. P. 2012. Review of palliative sedation and its distinction from euthanasia and lethal injection. *Journal of Pain and Palliative Care Pharmacotherapy* 26(1): 30.

Kolata, G. 2019. More Americans are dying at home than in hospitals. *New York Times*, 11 December (https://www.nytimes.com/2019/12/11/health /death-hospitals-home.html).

Konigsberg, R. D. 2011. *The Truth about Grief.* New York: Simon & Schuster.

Kristensen, P., Weisaeth, L., Heir, T. 2012. Bereavement and mental health after sudden and violent losses: A review. *Psychiatry* 75(1): 76–97.

Mayo Clinic. 2018. *Living Wills and Advance Directives for Medical Decisions* (http://www.mayoclinic.org/healthy-lifestyle/consumer-health/in-depth /living-wills/art-20046303?pg51).

Mostofsky, E., et al. 2012. Risk of acute myocardial infarction after the death of a significant person in one's life. *Circulation: Journal of the American Heart Association* 125: 491–496.

National Cancer Institute. 2020. *Grief, Bereavement, and Coping with Loss* (https://www.cancer.gov/about-cancer/advanced-cancer/caregivers /planning/bereavement-hp-pdq/#section/_149).

National Funeral Directors Association. 2020. *Statistics* (https://www.nfda .org/news/statistics).

National Hospice and Palliative Care Organization. 2019. *NHPCO Facts and Figures: 2018 Edition, revision 7-2-2019.* (https://39k5cm1a9u1968hg 74aj3x51-wpengine.netdna-ssl.com/wp-content/uploads/2019/07/2018 _NHPCO_Facts_Figures.pdf).

National Hospice and Palliative Care Organization. 2020. *History of Hospice Care* (https://www.nhpco.org/hospice-care-overview/history-of -hospice/).

Nuland, S. 1993. *How We Die: Reflections on Life's Final Chapter.* New York: Random House.

Oregon Death with Dignity Act. 2019. *Annual Reports: 2018* (https://www .deathwithdignity.org/oregon-death-with-dignity-act-annual-reports/).

Oregon Health Authority. 2020. *Frequently Asked Questions about the Death with Dignity Act* (https://www.oregon.gov/oha/PH/PROVIDERPARTNER RESOURCES/EVALUATIONRESEARCH/DEATHWITHDIGNITY ACT/Pages/faqs.aspx).

Parkes, C., P. Laungani, and W. Young (Eds.). 2015. *Death and Bereavement across Cultures,* 2nd ed. New York: Routledge.

Russell, J. A., et al. 2019. Brain death, the determination of brain death, and member guidance for brain death accommodation requests: AAN position statement. *Neurology* 92: 1–5.

Schulz, R., et al. 2006. Predictors of complicated grief among dementia caregivers: A prospective study of bereavement. *American Journal of Geriatric Psychiatry* 14(8): 650–658.

U.S. Department of Health and Human Services. 2020. *Organ Donation Statistics* (https://www.organdonor.gov/statistics-stories/statistics.html).

Design Elements: Critical Consumer icon: pagadesign/Getty Images; Take Charge icon: VisualCommunications/Getty Images.

NUTRITION RESOURCES

FIND OUT ABOUT NUTRITIONAL CONTENT OF COMMON FOODS

If you are developing a behavior change plan to improve your diet, or if you simply want to choose more healthful foods, you may want to know more about the nutritional content of common food items. You can look up the nutrient content of the foods you eat in the USDA Agricultural Research Service National Nutrient Database for Standard Reference (http://www.ars.usda.gov/Services/docs.htm?docid=17477), which lists foods both by description and by nutrient content. For example, under "protein," you can find out how much protein there is in a chicken pot pie or what foods have the most protein per serving. Although cumbersome, the database is comprehensive.

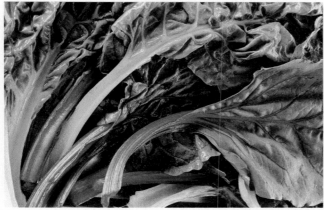

Andi Berger/Shutterstock

FIND OUT ABOUT NUTRITIONAL CONTENT OF FAST FOOD

Although most foods served at fast-food and casual restaurants are high in calories, fat, saturated fat, cholesterol, sodium, and sugar, some items are more healthful than others. If you eat at fast-food or casual restaurants, knowing the nutritional content of various items can help you make better choices. Chain restaurants provide nutritional information both online and in print brochures available at most restaurant locations. To learn more about the items you order, visit the restaurants' websites. A link to nutrition information is often found toward the bottom of the page or in a sidebar. It is usually placed under a heading with other links about the company.

Here are some helpful nutrition-oriented websites:

Self's NutritionData: nutritiondata.self.com
The Doc's Kitchen: thedocskitchen.com
American College Health Association: https://www.acha.org/
     ACHA/Resources/Topics/Nutrition.aspx
The World's Healthiest Foods: whfoods.org
NutritionFacts.org: nutritionfacts.org
Academy of Nutrition and Dietetics: https://www.eatright.org/

A SELF-CARE GUIDE FOR COMMON MEDICAL PROBLEMS

This self-care guide will help you manage some of the most common symptoms and medical problems, including the following:

- Fever
- Sore throat
- Cough
- Nasal congestion
- Ear problems
- Nausea, vomiting, or diarrhea
- Heartburn and indigestion
- Headache
- Low-back pain
- Strains and sprains
- Cuts and scrapes

The following sections describe symptoms in terms of what is going on in your body. Most symptoms are part of the body's natural healing response. Symptoms are usually self-limiting; that is, they resolve on their own with time and simple self-care.

This appendix also offers basic self-care advice, along with guidelines for getting professional help. No medical advice is perfect. You must decide whether to self-treat or get professional help. This guide is intended to give you information so that you can make better, more informed decisions. If the advice given here differs from that of your physician, follow your physician's instructions because they will be based on your condition, health status, medical history, and other factors that apply specifically to you.

The guidelines given here apply to *generally healthy adults*. If you are pregnant or nursing or if you have a chronic disease, particularly one that requires medication, check with your physician for appropriate self-care advice. Additionally, if you have an allergy or suspected allergy to any recommended medication—including over-the-counter (OTC) medicines—check with your physician before using it.

If you have several symptoms, read about your primary symptom first and then proceed to secondary symptoms. If you are particularly concerned about a symptom or confused about how to manage it, call your physician to get more information.

FEVER

A *fever* is an abnormally high body temperature, usually over 100°F (37.8°C). It is most commonly a sign that your body is fighting an infection. Fever may also be due to an inflammation, an injury, or a drug reaction. Chemicals released into your bloodstream during an infection reset the thermostat in your brain. The message goes out to your body to turn up the heat. The blood vessels in your skin constrict, and you curl up and throw on extra blankets to reduce heat loss. Meanwhile, your muscles may begin to shiver to generate additional body heat. The resulting rise in body temperature is a fever. Later, when your brain senses that the temperature is too high, you start sweating. As the sweat evaporates, it carries heat away from the body.

A fever may help you fight infections by making the body less hospitable to bacteria and viruses. A high body temperature appears to bolster the immune system and may inhibit the growth of infectious microorganisms.

Most generally healthy people can tolerate a fever as high as 103–104°F (39.4–40.0°C) without problems. If you are essentially healthy, there is little need to reduce a fever unless you are very uncomfortable. Older adults and people with chronic health problems such as heart disease may not tolerate a high fever, however, so fever reduction may be advised.

In small children (especially infants), even a low-grade fever can be a sign of a serious problem. Seek immediate medical help for any infant younger than 3 months whose temperature is 100.4°F (38.0°C) or higher, or for any child older than 3 months whose temperature is greater than 102°F (38.9°C). In small children, temperature should be checked with a digital rectal thermometer (and a temporal artery thermometer may also provide accurate readings). Do not attempt to take a baby's temperature orally; if you have trouble taking a child's temperature for any reason, contact a medical professional right away. Noncontact infrared thermometers, if used properly, present a fast and noninvasive way to get a temperature, whether from a healthy newborn infant or an adult during an infectious disease pandemic.

Most problems with fevers are due to loss of fluids from evaporation and sweating, which may cause dehydration.

Self-Assessment

1. If you are sick, take your temperature several times throughout the day. Oral temperatures should not be measured for at least 10 minutes after smoking, eating, or drinking a hot or cold liquid. Don't use a glass thermometer that contains mercury. Digital thermometers are accurate, easy to read, and inexpensive. Follow your thermometer's directions.

   "Normal" temperature varies from person to person, so it is important to know what is normal for you. Your normal temperature will also vary throughout the day, being lowest in the early evening. If you exercise or if it is a hot day, your temperature may normally rise. Women's body temperatures typically vary by a degree or more through the menstrual cycle, peaking around the time of ovulation. Rectal temperatures normally run about 0.5–1.0°F higher than oral temperatures.

   If your recorded temperature is more than 1.0–1.5°F above your normal baseline temperature, you have a fever.

2. If you have a fever, watch for signs of dehydration. They include excessive thirst; very dry mouth; infrequent urination with dark, concentrated urine; and light-headedness.

Self-Care

1. Drink plenty of fluids to prevent dehydration—at least eight ounces of water, juice, or broth every two hours.
2. Take a sponge bath using lukewarm water to increase evaporation and help reduce body temperature naturally. Don't use alcohol rubs, ice, or cold baths to reduce temperature.
3. Dress lightly. Bundling up interferes with the body's ability to shed excess heat.
4. Take an aspirin substitute (acetaminophen, ibuprofen, or naproxen sodium) to reduce the fever and the associated headache and achiness. Follow the product's dosage instructions carefully. Do not give aspirin to anyone younger than age 20 years because some younger people with chickenpox, influenza, or other viral infections can develop a life-threatening complication, called Reye's syndrome, after taking aspirin.

When to Call the Physician

- If the fever is higher than 103°F (39.4°C), or higher than 102°F (38.9°C) in a person over 60 years old.
- If a fever lasts more than three days.
- If you experience recurrent unexplained fevers.
- If a fever is accompanied by a rash, stiff neck, severe headache, difficulty breathing, discolored sputum, severe pain in the side or abdomen, painful urination, convulsions, or confusion.
- If you show signs of dehydration along with a fever.
- If a fever appears after starting a new medication.

SORE THROAT

A sore throat—called *pharyngitis*—is caused by inflammation of the throat lining resulting from an infection, allergy, or irritation (especially from cigarette smoke). If you have an infection, you may also notice some hoarseness from swelling of the vocal cords and "swollen glands," which are enlarged lymph nodes that produce white blood cells to help fight the infection. Lymph nodes may become tender and remain swollen for weeks after the infection subsides.

Viruses cause most throat infections, so antibiotics are not effective against them. Most viral sore throats clear up in about a week with no treatment. But if a sore throat is accompanied by other symptoms (like a high fever, fatigue, aches, rash, or localized swelling), a more serious viral illness is possible, such as the flu, mononucleosis, or measles. These conditions should be diagnosed and treated by a physician.

About 20–30% of throat infections are due to streptococcal bacteria ("strep throat"). This type of microbe can cause complications such as rheumatic fever and rheumatic heart disease and, therefore, should be diagnosed by a physician and treated with antibiotics. Strep throat is usually characterized by a very sore throat, a high fever, swollen lymph nodes, and a whitish discharge at the back of the throat.

Allergy-related sore throats may come with a runny nose, sneezing, and watery, itchy eyes.

Self-Assessment

1. Take your temperature.
2. Look at the back of your throat in a mirror. Is there a whitish discharge on the tonsils or in the back of the throat?
3. Feel the front and back of your neck. Do you feel enlarged, tender lymph nodes?

Self-Care

1. If you smoke, stop.
2. Drink plenty of liquids to soothe your inflamed throat.
3. Gargle with warm salt water (¼ tsp salt in four ounces of water) every hour or so to help reduce swelling and discomfort.
4. Suck on throat lozenges, cough drops, or hard candies to keep your throat moist.
5. Use throat lozenges, sprays, or gargles that contain an anesthetic to make swallowing less painful.
6. Try an aspirin substitute to ease throat pain.
7. For an allergy-related sore throat, try an antihistamine such as chlorpheniramine or loratadine.

When to Call the Physician

- If you have great difficulty swallowing saliva or breathing.
- If your sore throat is accompanied by a fever over 101°F (38.3°C), especially if you do not have other cold symptoms such as nasal congestion or a cough.
- If your sore throat is accompanied by a skin rash.
- If whitish pus appears on the tonsils.
- If you have a sore throat and recently had contact with a person who has had a positive throat culture for strep.
- If your lymph nodes have been enlarged for more than three weeks.
- If you have been hoarse for more than three weeks.

COUGH

A *cough* is a protective mechanism of the body to help keep the airways clear. There are two types of cough: a dry cough (without mucus) and a productive cough (with mucus). Common causes of cough include infection (viral or bacterial), allergies, and irritation from smoking and pollutants. If you have a cold, the cough may be the last symptom to improve because the airways may remain irritated for several weeks after the infection has resolved.

Your airways are lined with hairlike projections called *cilia,* which move back and forth to help clear the airways of mucus, germs, and dust. Infections and cigarette smoking paralyze and damage this vital defensive mechanism.

Self-Assessment

1. Take your temperature.
2. Observe your mucus. Thick brown or bloody mucus suggests a bacterial infection.

Self-Care

1. If you smoke, stop.
2. Drink plenty of liquids (at least six eight-ounce glasses a day) to help thin mucus and loosen chest congestion.
3. Use moist heat from a hot shower or vaporizer to help loosen chest congestion.
4. Suck on cough drops, throat lozenges, or hard candy to moisten your throat and relieve a dry, tickling cough.
5. If you have a dry, nonproductive cough or the cough keeps you from sleeping, you can use a cough syrup or lozenge that contains the nonprescription cough suppressant dextromethorphan. If your cough is productive, ask your physician before using a cough suppressant. Productive coughs are often protective.

When to Call the Physician

- If your cough is accompanied by thick brown or bloody sputum.
- If your cough is accompanied by a high fever—above 102°F (38.9°C)—and shaking chills.
- If you are experiencing severe chest pains, wheezing, or shortness of breath.
- If your cough lasts longer than three weeks (a chronic cough).

NASAL CONGESTION

Nasal congestion (a stuffy nose) is most commonly caused by infection or allergies. When infected, the nasal passages become congested because of increased blood flow and mucus production. This congestion is actually part of the body's defense to fight infection. The increased blood flow raises the temperature of the nasal passages, making them less hospitable to germs. The nasal secretions are rich in white blood cells and antibodies to help fight and neutralize the invading organisms and flush them away. Nasal congestion associated with sore throat, cough, and fever usually indicates a viral infection. Green nasal discharge is common with viral infections; it does not mean you need an antibiotic.

Nasal congestion caused by allergies is often accompanied by a thin, watery discharge, sneezing, and itchy eyes; it is sometimes associated with a seasonal pattern. In an allergic reaction, the offending allergen (such as pollen, dust, mold, or dander) triggers the release of histamine and other chemicals from the cells lining the nose, throat, and eyes. These chemicals cause swelling, discharge, and itching. Antihistamine drugs block the release of these irritating chemicals.

Self-Assessment

1. Take your temperature.
2. Observe your nasal secretions. Thick brown or bloody discharge suggests a bacterial infection.
3. Tap with your fingers over the sinus cavities above and below the eyes. If the tapping causes increased pain, you may have a bacterial sinus infection.

Self-Care

1. If you smoke, stop.
2. Use moist heat from a hot shower or vaporizer to help liquefy congested mucus.

3. Use a decongestant nasal spray or drops to temporarily relieve congestion. However, if these decongestants are used for more than three days, they can create more nasal congestion ("rebound congestion"). As an alternative, use salt water nose drops (¼ tsp salt in ½ cup boiled water, cooled before using) or a commercial saline spray several times a day.
4. Try an oral decongestant such as phenylephrine or pseudo-ephedrine to help shrink swollen mucous membranes and open nasal passages. In some people, these medications can cause nervousness, sleeplessness, or heart palpitations. If you have uncontrolled high blood pressure, heart disease, or diabetes, check with your physician before using decongestants.

When to Call the Physician

- If nasal congestion is accompanied by severe pain and tenderness in the forehead, cheeks, or upper teeth and a high fever (above 102°F or 38.9°C).
- If you have thick brown or bloody nasal discharge.
- If your nasal congestion and discharge are unresponsive to self-care and last longer than three weeks.

EAR PROBLEMS

Ear symptoms include earache, discharge, itching, stuffiness, and hearing loss. They may be caused by problems in the external ear canal, eardrum, middle ear, or eustachian tube (the passage that connects the middle ear space to the back of the throat). The ear canal can become blocked by excess wax, producing hearing loss and a sense that the ear is plugged. An infection of the external ear canal due to excessive moisture and trauma is often referred to as "swimmer's ear." It can cause pain, a sense of fullness, discharge, and itching. Congestion and blockage of the eustachian tube by a cold or allergy can result in pain, a sense of fullness, and hearing loss. A middle ear infection often produces severe pain, hearing loss, and fever.

Self-Assessment

1. Check for fever, which may be a sign of infection.
2. Have someone look into the ear canal with a flashlight. Look for wax blockage or a red, swollen canal indicating an external ear infection.
3. Wiggle the outer part of the ear. If this increases the pain, an infection or inflammation of the external ear canal is the likely cause.

Self-Care

1. If blockage of the ear canal with wax is the problem, first try a hot shower to liquefy the wax, and use a washcloth to wipe out the ear canal. You can also use a few drops of an over-the-counter wax softener and then flush the canal gently with warm water in a bulb syringe. Do not use sharp objects or cotton swabs; they can scratch the ear canal or push the wax in deeper.
2. To treat mild infections of the external ear canal, you must thoroughly dry the ear canal. A few drops of a drying solution (one part rubbing alcohol, one part white vinegar) on a piece of cotton gently inserted into the ear canal can act as a wick to dry the canal.

3. To relieve congestion and blockage of the eustachian tube, try a decongestant or a nasal spray (but for no longer than three days). Hot showers or a vaporizer may help loosen secretions, and yawning or swallowing may help open the eustachian tube. For a mild plugging sensation without fever or pain, pinch your nostrils and blow gently into your nose (not through your mouth) to force air up the eustachian tube and "pop" your ears.

When to Call the Physician

- If you have a severe earache accompanied by a fever.
- If puslike or bloody discharge comes from the ear.
- If you experience sudden hearing loss, especially if accompanied by ear pain or recent trauma to the ear.
- If you have ringing in the ears or dizziness.
- If you experience any ear symptom that lasts longer than two weeks.

NAUSEA, VOMITING, OR DIARRHEA

Nausea, vomiting, and diarrhea usually are defensive reactions of your body to rapidly clear your digestive tract of irritants. These symptoms may be caused by a viral infection, foodborne illness, medications, or other types of infection. Vomiting dramatically ejects irritants from your stomach, and nausea (feeling discomfort in the stomach or the sensation that you may vomit) discourages eating to allow the stomach to rest. With diarrhea, overstimulated intestines flush out the offending irritants.

The major complications of vomiting and diarrhea are dehydration from fluid loss and decreased fluid intake and a risk of bleeding from irritation of the digestive tract.

Self-Assessment

1. Take your temperature. A fever is often a clue that an infection is causing the symptoms.
2. Note the color and frequency of vomiting and diarrhea. This will help you estimate the severity of fluid losses and check for bleeding (red, black, or "coffee grounds" material in the stool or vomit; iron tablets and Pepto-Bismol can also cause black stools).
3. Watch for signs of dehydration. They include a very dry mouth; excessive thirst; infrequent urination with dark, concentrated urine; and light-headedness.
4. Look for signs of hepatitis, an infection of the liver. Symptoms include a yellow color in the skin and the white parts of the eyes.

Self-Care

1. To replace fluids, take frequent, small sips of clear liquids such as water, noncitrus juice, broths, flat ginger ale, or ice chips.
2. When the vomiting and diarrhea have subsided for at least six hours, try nonirritating, constipating foods like the BRAT diet: bananas, rice, applesauce, and toast.
3. For several days, avoid alcohol, milk products, fatty foods, aspirin, and other medications that might irritate the stomach.

Do not stop taking regularly prescribed medications without discussing this change with your physician.

4. Medications are not usually advised for vomiting. Loperamide, available without a prescription, can ease diarrhea.

When to Call the Physician

- If you cannot retain any fluids for 12 hours or show signs of dehydration.
- If you have severe abdominal pains that are not relieved by the vomiting or diarrhea.
- If you see blood in the vomit (red or "coffee grounds" material) or in the stool (red or black tarlike material).
- If the vomiting or diarrhea is accompanied by a high fever (above 102°F or 38.9°C).
- If you see a yellow coloring of the skin or the white parts of the eyes.
- If your vomiting is accompanied by a severe headache or if you have experienced a recent head injury.
- If vomiting or diarrhea lasts three days without improvement.
- If you are pregnant or have diabetes.
- If you experience recurrent vomiting and/or diarrhea.

HEARTBURN AND INDIGESTION

Indigestion and heartburn are usually a result of irritation of the stomach or the *esophagus* (the tube that connects the mouth to the stomach). The stomach lining is usually protected from stomach acids, but the esophagus is not. Therefore, if stomach acids "reflux," or back up into the esophagus, the result is usually a burning discomfort in the chest and throat. The esophagus is normally protected by a muscular valve—called a *sphincter*—that allows food to enter the stomach but prevents stomach contents from flowing upward into the esophagus. Certain foods (including chocolate, garlic, and onions), medications, and smoking can loosen and open this protective valve. Overeating, lying down, or bending over can also cause the stomach acids to gain access to the sensitive lining of the esophagus.

Self-Assessment

1. Look for a pattern in the symptoms. Do they occur after eating certain foods, taking certain medications, or when you bend over or lie down? Do certain foods or an antacid relieve the symptoms?
2. Observe your bowel movements. Black, tarlike stools may indicate bleeding in the stomach (iron tablets and Pepto-Bismol can also cause black stools).

Self-Care

1. Avoid irritants such as smoking, aspirin, ibuprofen, naproxen sodium, alcohol, caffeine (coffee, tea, cola), chocolate, onions, carbonated beverages, spicy or fatty foods, acidic foods (vinegar, citrus fruits, tomatoes), or any other foods that seem to make your symptoms worse.

2. Take nonabsorbable antacids such as Maalox, Mylanta, or Gelusil every hour or two and especially before bedtime, or try an acid reducer, now available without a prescription (Pepcid, Tagamet, Zantac, or Prilosec). These drugs work in different ways, so ask your physician to help you choose the right medication for you.
3. Avoid tight clothing.
4. Avoid overeating. Eat smaller, more frequent meals.
5. Don't lie down for one or two hours after a meal. Elevate the head of your bed with 4- to 6-inch blocks of wood or bricks. Adding extra pillows usually makes things worse by creating a posture that increases pressure on the stomach. Try sleeping on your left side, which may reduce reflux compared to sleeping on your back or right side.
6. If you are overweight in the abdominal area, weight loss may help. Abdominal obesity can increase pressure on the stomach when you are lying down.

When to Call the Physician

- If you produce stools that are black and tarlike or vomit that is bloody or contains material that looks like coffee grounds.
- If you suffer severe abdominal or chest pain.
- If you have pain that goes through to the back.
- If you get no relief from antacids.
- If you have trouble swallowing solid foods.
- If your symptoms last longer than three days.

Recurrent or persistent abdominal pain may be a symptom of an *ulcer*, a raw area in the lining of the stomach or *duodenum* (the first part of the small intestine). About 1 in 5 men and 1 in 10 women develop an ulcer at some time in their lives. Most ulcers are linked to infection with the bacterium *Helicobacter pylori*; people who regularly take nonsteroidal anti-inflammatory drugs like aspirin or ibuprofen are also at risk for ulcers because these drugs irritate the lining of the stomach. *H. pylori* infection is relatively easy to diagnose and treat, and other medications are available to treat ulcers linked to other causes. Many of the self-care measures described here are also frequently recommended for people with ulcers.

HEADACHE

Headache is one of the most common symptoms. There are four major types of headache: tension, migraine, cluster, and sinus. Tension headaches, migraines, and cluster headaches are described in Chapter 2. Sinus headaches are caused by blockage of the sinus cavities with resulting pressure and pain in the cheeks, forehead, and upper teeth. Headache caused by elevated blood pressure is uncommon and occurs only at very high pressure levels.

Self-Assessment

1. Take your temperature. The presence of fever may indicate a sinus infection. Fever, severe headache, and a very stiff neck suggest *meningitis*—a rare but extremely serious infection around the brain and spinal cord.

2. Tap with your fingers over the sinus cavities in your cheeks and forehead. If this causes increased pain, it may indicate a sinus infection.
3. For recurrent headaches, keep a headache journal. Record how often and when your headaches occur, associated symptoms, activities that precede the headache, and your food and beverage intake. Look for patterns that may provide clues to the cause(s) of your headaches.

Self-Care

1. Try applying ice packs or heat on your neck and head.
2. Gently massage the muscles of your neck and scalp.
3. Try deep relaxation or breathing exercises.
4. Take aspirin or an aspirin substitute for pain relief. Over-the-counter products containing a combination of aspirin, acetaminophen, and caffeine are approved by the FDA for treating migraines.
5. If the pain is associated with nasal congestion, try a decongestant medication.
6. Try to avoid emotional and physical stressors (such as poor posture and eyestrain).
7. Try avoiding foods that may trigger headaches, such as aged cheeses, chocolate, nuts, red wine, alcohol, avocados, figs, raisins, and fermented or pickled foods.

When to Call the Physician

- If you experience a headache that seems unusually severe or occurs suddenly.
- If your headache is accompanied by fever and a very stiff neck.
- If your headache occurs along with sinus pain, tenderness, and fever.
- If you get a severe headache following a recent head injury.
- If your headache is associated with slurred speech, visual disturbance, or numbness or weakness in the face, arms, or legs.
- If a headache persists longer than three days.
- If you get recurrent unexplained headaches.
- If your headaches increase in severity or frequency.
- If you experience severe migraine headaches.

LOW-BACK PAIN

Pain in the lower back is a very common condition; it is most often due to a strain of the muscles and ligaments along the spine, often triggered by bending, lifting, or other activity. Low-back pain can also result from bone growths (spurs) irritating the nerves along the spine or pressure from ruptured or protruding discs, which are the "shock absorbers" between the vertebrae. Sometimes back pain is caused by an infection or stone in the kidney. Fortunately, however, simple muscular strain is the most common cause of low-back pain and can usually be effectively self-treated.

Self-Assessment

1. Take your temperature. Back pain with high fever may indicate a kidney or other infection.
2. Check for blood in your urine or frequent, painful urination, which may also indicate a kidney problem.
3. Observe for tingling or pain traveling down one or both legs *below* the knee when you bend, cough, or sneeze. These symptoms suggest a disc problem.

Self-Care

1. Lie on your back or in any comfortable position on the floor or on a firm mattress, with knees slightly bent and supported by a pillow. Rest for a day if the pain persists.
2. Use ice packs on the painful area for the first three days, and then continue with cold or change to heat, whichever gives more relief.
3. Take aspirin or an aspirin substitute for pain relief.
4. After the acute pain has subsided, begin gentle back and stomach exercises. Practice good posture and lifting techniques to protect your back. Try to resume gentle, everyday activities like walking as soon as possible. Bed rest beyond one day is no longer advised and may make things worse; try gentle stretching, and resume activities that don't aggravate the problem. To learn more about proper back exercises and use of your back, consult a physical therapist or your physician.

When to Call the Physician

- When your back pain follows a severe injury such as a car crash or fall.
- If the pain radiates down the leg *below* the knee on one or both sides.
- If you experience persistent numbness, tingling, or weakness in the legs or feet.
- If you experience a loss of bladder or bowel control.
- If your back pain is associated with high fever (above 101°F or 38.3°C), frequent or painful urination, blood in the urine, or severe abdominal pain.
- If the pain does not improve after 72 hours of self-care.

STRAINS AND SPRAINS

Missteps, slips, falls, and athletic misadventures can result in a variety of strains, sprains, and fractures. A *strain* occurs when you overstretch a muscle or tendon (the connective tissue that attaches muscle to bone). *Sprains* are caused by overstretching or tearing ligaments (the tough fibrous bands that connect bone to bone). A *fracture* is a break in a bone, which may or may not go all the way through the bone. Depending on the severity and location, a sprain may actually be more serious than a fracture because bones generally heal very strongly, whereas ligaments may remain stretched and lax after healing. After a sprain, it may take six weeks for the ligament to heal.

After most injuries, you can expect pain and swelling. This is the body's way of immobilizing and protecting the injured part so that healing can take place. The goal of self-assessment is to determine whether you have a minor injury that you can safely self-treat or a more serious injury to an artery, nerve, or bone that should be treated by your physician.

Self-Assessment

1. Watch for coldness, blue color, or numbness in the limb beyond the injury. These may be signs of damage to an artery or a nerve.
2. Look for signs of a possible fracture, which include a misshapen limb, reduced length of the limb on the injured side compared to the uninjured side, an inability to move or bear weight, a grating sound with movement of the injured area, extreme tenderness at one point along the injured bone as you press with your fingers, or a sensation of snapping at the time of the injury.
3. Gently move the injured area through its full range of motion. Immobility or instability suggests a more serious injury.

Self-Care

1. Immediately immobilize, protect, and rest the injured area until you can bear weight on it or move it without pain. Remember: If it hurts, don't do it.
2. To decrease pain and swelling, immediately apply ice (a cold pack or ice wrapped in a cloth) for 15 minutes every hour for the first 24–48 hours. Then apply ice or heat as needed for comfort.
3. Immediately elevate the injured limb above the level of your heart for the first 24 hours to decrease swelling.
4. Immobilize and support the injured area with an elastic wrap or splint. Be careful not to wrap so tightly as to cause blueness, coldness, or numbness.
5. Take aspirin or an aspirin substitute for pain as needed.

When to Call the Physician

- If the injury occurred with great force, such as a high fall or a motor vehicle crash.
- If you hear or feel a snap at the time of the injury.
- If the injured limb is blue, cold, or numb.
- If the limb is bent, twisted, or crooked.
- If you feel tenderness at specific points along a bone.
- If you cannot move the injured area.
- If a joint becomes wobbly or unstable.
- If there is marked swelling of the injured area.
- If the injured area cannot bear weight after 24 hours.
- If you experience pain that increases or lasts longer than four days.

CUTS AND SCRAPES

Cuts and scrapes are common disruptions of the body's skin. Fortunately the vast majority of these wounds are minor and don't require stitches, antibiotics, or a physician's care. An *abrasion* involves a scraping away of the superficial layers of skin. Abrasions, though less serious than cuts, are often more painful because they disrupt more skin nerves. There are two types of cuts: *lacerations* (narrow slices of the skin) and *puncture wounds* (stabs into deeper tissues).

Normal healing of a cut or scrape is a remarkable process. After the bleeding stops, small amounts of serum, a clear yellowish fluid, may leak from the wound. This fluid is rich in antibodies to help prevent an infection. Redness and swelling normally occur as more blood is shunted to the area, bringing white blood cells and nutrients to speed healing. There may also be some swelling of nearby lymph nodes, which are another part of your body's defense against infection. Finally, a scab forms. This is "nature's bandage," which protects the area while it heals.

The main concerns about cuts are the possibility of damage to deeper tissues and the risk of infection. Damage to underlying blood vessels may lead to severe bleeding as well as blueness and coldness in areas beyond the wound. Injured nerves may produce numbness and a loss of the ability to move parts of the body beyond the injured area. Damaged muscles, tendons, and ligaments can also result in inability to move areas beyond the cut.

Wound infection usually does not take place until 24–48 hours after an injury. Signs of infection include increasing redness, swelling, pain, pus, and fever. One of the most serious, though fortunately uncommon, complications of puncture wounds is tetanus ("lockjaw"). This bacterial infection thrives in areas not exposed to oxygen, so it is more likely to develop in deep puncture wounds or dirty wounds. Tetanus is not likely to develop in minor cuts or wounds caused by clean objects like knives. You need a tetanus immunization shot following a cut under the following conditions:

- If you have never had the recommended tetanus immunization injections.
- If you have a dirty or contaminated wound and it has been longer than five years since your last tetanus immunization.
- If you have a clean, minor wound and it has been longer than 10 years since your last tetanus immunization.

Self-Assessment

1. Look for warning signs of complications: persistent bleeding, numbness, an inability to move the injured area, or the later development of pus, increasing redness, and fever.
2. Measure the cut. If your cut is shallow, less than ¼ inch deep, less than an inch long, and not in a high-stress area (such as a joint, which bends) and you can easily hold the edges of the wound closed, it probably won't need stitches.

Self-Care

1. Apply direct pressure over the wound until the bleeding stops. The only exception is puncture wounds, which should be encouraged to bleed freely (unless spurting a large amount of blood) for a few minutes to flush out bacteria and debris.
2. When bleeding stops, wash your hands thoroughly with soap and water, then carefully cleanse the wound with clean water. Avoid getting soap in the wound because it can irritate exposed tissues. Experts now advise against pouring hydrogen peroxide into a wound because it may damage sensitive tissue. Do not try to remove visible dirt, debris, or objects (such as splinters or shards) from the wound; such cleaning should be done by a medical professional. If you don't see anything in the wound but suspect something may be there, see a doctor immediately.
3. Pat the area dry with a clean towel, then apply an antiseptic ointment and a clean bandage.
4. If it is an abrasion, cover the area with a sterile adhesive bandage until a scab forms. For minor lacerations, close the cut with a butterfly bandage or a sterile adhesive tape, drawing the edges close together but not overlapping. If there is an extra flap of clean skin, leave it in place for extra protection. Do not attempt to close a puncture wound. Instead soak the wound in warm water for 15 minutes several times a day for several days. Soaking helps keep the wound open and thus prevents infection.

When to Call the Physician

- If you cannot control bleeding by applying direct pressure to the wound.
- If you develop numbness, weakness, or an inability to move the injured area.
- If the wound (any wound) is large or deep.
- If you get a cut in an area that bends and with edges that cannot easily be held together.
- If you are cut on the hands or face, unless the injury is clean and shallow.
- If the wound is contaminated and you cannot remove the foreign material.
- If the injury was caused by a human or animal bite.
- If you need a tetanus immunization (see the indications noted earlier).
- If the wound develops increasing redness, swelling, pain, or pus—or if you develop fever—24 hours or more after the injury.
- If the wound is not healing well after three weeks.

Note: Page references followed by b indicate boxes; f, figures; t, tables. Boldface numbers indicate pages on which key terms are defined.